Encyclopedia of Behavioral Medicine

Marc D. Gellman
Editor

Encyclopedia of Behavioral Medicine

Second Edition

Volume 3

P–Z

With 109 Figures and 54 Tables

Springer

Editor
Marc D. Gellman
Behavioral Medicine Research Center
Department of Psychology
University of Miami
Miami, FL, USA

ISBN 978-3-030-39901-6   ISBN 978-3-030-39903-0 (eBook)
ISBN 978-3-030-39902-3 (print and electronic bundle)
https://doi.org/10.1007/978-3-030-39903-0

1st edition: © Springer Science+Business Media New York 2013
2nd edition: © Springer Nature Switzerland AG 2020
This work is subject to copyright. All rights are reserved by the Publisher, whether the whole or part of the material is concerned, specifically the rights of translation, reprinting, reuse of illustrations, recitation, broadcasting, reproduction on microfilms or in any other physical way, and transmission or information storage and retrieval, electronic adaptation, computer software, or by similar or dissimilar methodology now known or hereafter developed.
The use of general descriptive names, registered names, trademarks, service marks, etc. in this publication does not imply, even in the absence of a specific statement, that such names are exempt from the relevant protective laws and regulations and therefore free for general use.
The publisher, the authors, and the editors are safe to assume that the advice and information in this book are believed to be true and accurate at the date of publication. Neither the publisher nor the authors or the editors give a warranty, expressed or implied, with respect to the material contained herein or for any errors or omissions that may have been made. The publisher remains neutral with regard to jurisdictional claims in published maps and institutional affiliations.

This Springer imprint is published by the registered company Springer Nature Switzerland AG.
The registered company address is: Gewerbestrasse 11, 6330 Cham, Switzerland

Opening Quotations to the First Edition

Some of the unhealthful behaviors that make the greatest contribution to the current burden of disease are cigarette smoking, the abuse of alcohol and drugs, the overeating and underexercise that produce obesity, and Type A behavior. Unfortunately, these behaviors are stubbornly resistant to change and discouragingly subject to relapse. Thus, for behavioral scientists to promise to achieve too much too soon is to court disastrous disillusionment. But any contributions that behavioral scientists can make to reduce any of them will have highly significant implications for health.

>   Miller, N. E. (1983). Behavioral medicine: Symbiosis between laboratory and clinic. *Annual Reviews of Psychology, 34*, 1–31.

As behavioral medicine researchers, we must become more directly involved in translating gains in the science of clinical and community (disease) prevention to gains in public policy. We have an unprecedented window of opportunity given the growing recognition at all levels of health care and government that clinical and community interventions that promote and support health behaviors will be essential for success in reducing the nation's most prevalent and costly health problems and untenable health-care costs and disparities. This is the kind of opportunity that propelled the founders of our field 25 years ago, and we are better prepared than ever in our history to seize it.

>   Ockene, J. K., & Orleans, C. T. (2010). Behavioral medicine, prevention, and health reform: Linking evidence-based clinical and public health strategies for population health behavior change. In A. Steptoe (Ed.), *Handbook of behavioral medicine: Methods and applications* (pp. 1021–1035). New York: Springer.

The extent to which behavioral medicine can become a successful part of health care delivery systems will in large part depend upon investigators in the field being able to master clinical translational research, moving from efficacy to effectiveness with a high ratio of benefit to cost. … Because Behavioral Medicine has been constructed based on the understanding of relationships among behavior, psychosocial processes and sociocultural contexts, the field is well-positioned to take a leadership role in informing future health care policies. The field of Behavioral Medicine appears to have a bright, important future.

>   Schneiderman, N. (2012). A personal view of behavioral medicine's future. This volume.

Foreword to the First Edition

Early Developments in the Field of Behavioral Medicine

At the editors' request, this Foreword provides a personal account of the early development of behavioral medicine. With many colleagues, I was fortunate to play a role in bringing together behavioral and biomedical sciences in such a way that the synergism resulting from this interaction resulted in ideas, conceptualizations, models, and ultimately interventions that were truly different from preexisting approaches to health and illness. As noted in the Preface, the contents of this encyclopedia bear witness to the manner in which behavioral medicine has matured during the past 30 years, illustrating current activities in the domains of basic research, clinical investigation and practice, and public health policy.

In 1963, I was a psychology intern in the Department of Medical Psychology at the University of Oregon Medical School (now called the Oregon Health Sciences Center). Under the guidance of Joseph Matarazzo, chair of the department, the relationship between medicine and psychology was undergoing an historic realignment. Joe had a fascinating and exciting perspective on the nature of such relationships and on psychology's potential to make those relationships mutually rewarding for both patients and practitioners. I consider myself fortunate to have been "in the right place at the right time" when a request came from the Division of Cardiothoracic Surgery for psychological and psychiatric consultation on a problem that was mystifying the surgeons.

Under the leadership of Albert Starr, surgeons were performing groundbreaking procedures known as "open heart surgery" on patients who had been incapacitated, typically for many years, by their heart conditions. These surgeries offered them the opportunity to reclaim their earlier lives as active members of society, and, in some cases, to take on roles that were denied to them since childhood. Paradoxically, following surgery, many patients, rather than expressing their gratitude for the opportunity to be "made whole again," become angry, depressed, and suicidal. With colleagues from the departments of psychology and psychiatry, we begin a search for the "underlying mental illness" that must have been uncovered by the stress of the surgery. However, rather than discovering the presence of psychiatric illness, it was found that the *absence of psychological strength* was a key factor associated with the behavioral anomalies. This finding led to the development of a program to psychologically evaluate a candidate's readiness to undergo surgery and to better prepare psychologically vulnerable candidates for the recovery experience.

My dissertation on psychological adjustment following open heart surgery led me to the Division of Psychosomatic Medicine in the Department of

Psychiatry at the Johns Hopkins University School of Medicine, and to the application of psychodynamic theory to problems as diverse as diabetes, cardiovascular disease, cancer, and transgender surgery. In 1974, I accepted a position at the National Heart, Lung, and Blood Institute (NHLBI) of the National Institutes of Health (NIH) as chief of a unit that would eventually become the Behavioral Medicine Branch. The first year was *very* difficult since I was essentially the only behavioral scientist at NHLBI, and no one understood exactly what I was supposed to do and why I was there. However, I considered this to be a singular opportunity to bring the behavioral and biological sciences together, if only we could come up with a model, a theoretical framework that made sense to both groups and was scientifically viable.

Good problem-solving strategies break the overall problem down into more manageable pieces. The first was to address the lack of fundable studies in the NHLBI portfolio, which comprised a total of four regular research grants (R01s). The institute director commented to me that behavioral scientists must not be very good scientists as their applications were routinely disapproved or failed to make the funding payline. However, investigation revealed that the 25 "behavioral" applications submitted for the current round were scattered among 14 different study sections. Two issues became evident: (1) many of the behavioral applications were biologically weak and (2) the multidisciplinary expertise necessary to properly review applications that had both behavioral and biological endpoints was missing from the various study sections to which the applications had been assigned.

It became clear that two efforts were needed. First, it was necessary to make both biomedical and behavioral scientists aware of the need for a collaborative "biobehavioral" approach involving top-tier expertise in both areas when submitting grant applications. Second, it was necessary to campaign within the NIH for a study section that could provide relevant peer review for these biobehavioral applications. NIH agreed to convene an "ad hoc" temporary review group (the Behavioral Medicine Study Section) to assess whether there really was a need for such a group. Clearly there was, since 3 years later the study section was formally chartered as a standing study section.

Meanwhile, it became obvious that to develop and sustain meaningful research programs within the NIH would require organized, active, outside constituencies of scientists and clinicians who could provide peer review to all aspects of NIH program development and scientific leadership, i.e., partnerships with academic and professional societies that could provide advice and guidance were needed. With specific regard to biobehavioral research, the need for credible representation led us to Neal Miller, a behavioral scientist who was well known to, and highly respected by, the biomedically oriented Institute staff. Neal had performed landmark studies of learning and biofeedback. He was persuaded to serve as keynote speaker for the 1975 NHLBI Working Conference on Health Behavior. The 3 days of intensive deliberations between senior behavioral and biomedical scientists were summarized and published as a proceedings to serve as the public blueprint for the Institute's future biobehavioral scientific agenda.

Along with the 1977 Yale Conference on Behavioral Medicine sponsored by NIH, this meeting set the stage for a 1978 organizational meeting hosted by

David Hamburg, President of the Institute of Medicine of the National Academy of Sciences. The deliberations of this two-day gathering of highly respected biomedical and behavioral scientists gave birth to two organizations, the Society of Behavioral Medicine (SBM) and the Academy of Behavioral Medicine Research (ABMR). The founding leaderships of these organizations agreed to be complementary rather than competitive in mission and purpose, with SBM serving both scientific and professional interests of all persons interested in the field and ABMR being a small invitation-only group of distinguished senior scientists dedicated to identifying and promoting "gold standard" science in behavioral medicine. SBM created a newsletter that became the high-quality scientific and professional journal *Annals of Behavioral Medicine*, and ABMR published an annual volume, *Perspectives on Behavioral Medicine*, summarizing scientific presentations at their annual retreat meeting.

During this early developmental period, a potentially divisive issue arose among the cadre of behavioral medicine pioneers: Exactly what is meant by the term "behavioral medicine?" Agreement on a common definition of the field was clearly necessary. One contingent defined behavioral medicine primarily as "behavior modification with medical patients," while another contingent took a broader view which included the aforementioned aspect, but challenged both the behavioral and biomedical communities to join forces as "the interdisciplinary field concerned with the development and integration of behavioral and biomedical science knowledge and techniques relevant to the understanding of health and illness, and the application of this knowledge and these techniques to prevention, diagnosis, treatment and rehabilitation." The latter became the agreed-upon definition by both behavioral medicine organizations and survived intact for a decade until the founders of the International Society of Behavioral Medicine proposed in 1990 that "psychosocial" be added to "behavioral and biomedical" to better align the definition with the charters of the emerging European national and regional behavioral medicine organizations.

The underlying concepts of behavioral medicine are perhaps thousands of years old. Prior to the emergence of behavioral medicine in the mid to late 1970s, the most recent effort to capture mind-body interactions can be attributed to those engaged in research and practice of psychosomatic medicine. Primarily psychodynamically oriented psychiatrists, they began to take note of behavioral medicine, initially identifying the fledgling organizations with the first definition mentioned previously (behavior modification with medical patients) whereas their interests were principally focused upon how the principles of psychoanalysis could be applied to the treatment of somatic disorders. However, as the second definition gained traction among the rank and file of the behavioral medicine community, psychosomatic medicine scientists and practitioners were challenged to either resist or join forces with the newcomers. Over the next decade, it became clear that, while psychoanalytic theory was intellectually provocative, it lacked the tools of modern day science to test its theories, and hence such theorizing remained in the realm of speculation. Behavioral medicine, on the other hand, took full advantage of the new monitoring instrumentation generated in large part by the U.S. space program's need for ambulatory monitoring of physiological processes via telemetry. Such instrumentation facilitated exploration in the laboratory and in real life of how variation in biological processes may be stimulated by behavioral inputs, as well as how biological processes may impact behavior. Over the next 20 years, the membership of the American Psychosomatic Society and the organization's flagship journal, *Psychosomatic Medicine*, shifted their emphasis to one indistinguishable from that of organized behavioral medicine.

During this time, biobehavioral scientific programs were beginning to develop within several institutes at NIH, and funding for biobehavioral research increased exponentially, albeit unevenly. An inter-institute Committee on Health and Behavior was formed, with Matilda White Riley from the National Institute on Aging as its first chair. This committee served in an advisory capacity to the individual institute directors as well as to the NIH director, becoming the precursor for the Office of Behavioral and Social Science Research, Office of the Director, NIH, which is now under the leadership of Robert Kaplan, past president of both SBM and ABMR.

Although research funding was increasing, another challenge became evident: Where were the *training* resources to support new entrants to the field? Typically, research training programs in the biological and biomedical sciences relied on NIH support; it became obvious that such resources needed to be developed to establish a pipeline for "biobehavioral" scientists-in-training to receive both individual and institutional support. Donald Cannon, chief of the training branch at NHLBI, the unit responsible for supporting both types of awards at NHLBI became interested in the issue, and met with senior behavioral medicine researchers who could apply for such awards based on their research programs and the resources of their institutions. Over the next 3 years, 12 institutional awards were made to support cardiovascular behavioral medicine training for both behavioral/social scientists and biomedical/biological scientists, further solidifying the scientific base for the field.

These developments within the United States were mirrored in other parts of the Western world, with emerging organizations in several European countries grappling with the relevance of the behavioral medicine concept to their perspectives on health and illness. In the mid-1980s, discussions at an SBM annual conference with international attendees resulted in an agreement to form an International Society of Behavioral Medicine (ISBM) dedicated to supporting the emergence of new as well as existing national and regional behavioral medicine organizations. Funds to support several planning meetings were provided by the Rockefeller family and the Duke University Behavioral Medicine Research Center, and the first International Congress of Behavioral Medicine took place in 1990 in Uppsala, Sweden. The International Society (members are national or regional societies rather than individuals) represented seven national and regional societies at this first meeting. *International Journal of Behavioral Medicine* became the scientific outlet for behavioral medicine studies of international relevance. By 2012, 26 (and counting...) national/regional societies from every continent formed the membership of ISBM.

Finally, one important element of the behavioral medicine paradigm deserves mention, as it is illustrative of the basic conceptual infrastructure of biomedical and behavioral *integration*. Often, biomedical and behavioral scientists pose the question of treatment efficacy in terms of which is more effective, pharmacologic or behavioral treatments. Rather than "either/or," the behavioral medicine position is to determine how both treatments, perhaps in combination or in sequence, may provide a more effective treatment than either alone. Several examples come to mind, for example, smoking cessation, hypertension treatment, and cardiovascular disease prevention. Using a drug to lower blood pressure or cholesterol can provide a window of opportunity to use non-pharmacologic strategies to maintain lowered blood pressure/cholesterol, thereby reducing/eliminating reliance on the medication. Smoking cessation programs typically are more effective when both behavioral and pharmacologic treatments are combined to sustain cessation. Pharmacologic agents are typically more efficient at creating the desired effect but may have long-term side effects; behavioral treatments may be less efficient at creating change but may be more effective at sustaining conditions that have been achieved pharmacologically. The bottom line is straightforward: Rather than asking which approach is superior, use the strengths of both areas of science creatively to achieve a sustainable treatment effect that minimizes unwanted side effects and could not be attained by using either approach by itself.

In summary, I have tried to provide a few personal insights into the events leading to the formalization of behavioral medicine as a viable, vibrant perspective on the promotion of health and the prevention and treatment of disease and as the multidisciplinary inquiry into the underlying mechanisms involving brain, genes, behavior, and physiology/biology. I hope that this provides a useful historical "snapshot" as you immerse yourself in the impressive array of accomplishments chronicled in this encyclopedia.

The following Foreword by Neil Schneiderman presents a personal view of behavioral medicine's future.

Stephen M. Weiss

Foreword to the First Edition

A Personal View of Behavioral Medicine's Future

The field of behavioral medicine appears to have a bright, important future. That is because contemporary scholarship in behavioral medicine has been constructed upon a solid foundation consisting of basic biological and behavioral science, population-based studies, and randomized clinical trials (RCT). The edifice that is emerging derives its strength and form from its interdisciplinary structure. It derives its reach and potential for future growth from its selection of key building materials and tools including the study of etiology, pathogenesis, diagnosis, treatment, rehabilitation, prevention, health promotion and community health. Because behavioral medicine approaches to prevention, treatment, and health promotion involve important relationships among behavior, psychosocial processes, and the sociocultural context, the roof of this structure will both consist of and benefit from the support of informed patients and populations, thoughtful educated health-care providers and involved communities.

Let us begin with population-based studies. During the second half of the twentieth century, epidemiological studies described important associations between traditional risk factors on the one hand and morbidity and mortality on the other, but elucidated relatively few of the variables mediating these associations. In my own area of cardiovascular disease (CVD) research, considerable attention has now focused upon obesity, inflammation, insulin resistance, oxidative stress, and hemostatic mechanisms as potential mediators. In this respect, traditional large-scale multicenter population-based studies have done a better job of describing the association between traditional risk factors (abnormal lipids, hypertension, smoking, diabetes, age) and CVD and their putative mediators than they have in describing the associations between biobehavioral, psychosocial, and sociocultural risk factors and CVD, and their mediators. However, this is now beginning to be addressed in such National Institute of Health (NIH) multicenter studies as the Hispanic Community Health Study/Study of Latinos (HCHS/SOL), Coronary Risk Development in Young Adults (CARDIA), and Multi-Ethnic Study of Atherosclerosis (MESA). Some of these studies are employing such preclinical measures of disease as carotid intimal-medial wall thickness and plaque by ultrasonography and coronary artery calcium by computed tomography to examine the progression of disease processes relating risk factors and CVD.

The examination of preclinical markers of disease as mediators between biobehavioral, psychosocial, and sociocultural risk factors on the one hand and chronic diseases on the other has been facilitated by the availability of commercial assays. These assays have permitted the study of biomarkers involved in preclinical disease processes including adhesion molecules, pro-inflammatory cytokines, and oxidative stress in both animal and human studies. We can expect that many further advances will be made in the development of commercially available research methods and that they will increase our understanding of relationships among biobehavioral, psychosocial, and sociocultural risk factors and the pathophysiology of CVD, cancer, and other chronic diseases.

Although a wide range of epidemiological studies have called attention to potentially modifiable risk factors, and most chronic disease risk factors are modifiable (Yusuf et al. 2004), it should be recognized that chronic disease outcomes are the result of the joint effects of risk genes, the environment, and behavior upon these risk factors. One can therefore expect that on the basis of genomic analyses, future studies will begin to identify the extent to which particular individuals are vulnerable to specific risk factors and diseases and may be candidates for targeted behavioral as well as pharmacological interventions. Thus, in the coming era of personalized or tailored medicine, we may expect that behavioral medicine research will play an important role both in understanding the antecedents of disease that interact with genomic predispositions and in selecting appropriate treatment interventions.

The future for behavioral medicine science playing an essential role in population-based observational studies appears to be inevitable. This will occur because both the fields of behavioral medicine and epidemiology have expanded their horizons based upon important scientific findings. Early epidemiological studies focused upon hygiene and infectious diseases. By the middle of the twentieth century, epidemiological studies were examining the prevalence of multiple risk factors (e.g., smoking, dyslipidemia, hypertension) and disease outcomes (e.g., coronary heart disease [CHD], stroke, cancers). However, more recent multicenter observational studies have increasingly identified behavioral, psychosocial, and sociocultural variables as potential risk factors for chronic diseases. Thus, future multicenter observational studies will likely include demographic (e.g., racial/ethnic background, sex, socioeconomic status, neighborhood environments), psychosocial (e.g., temperament and personality, marital and work stressors, social support), lifestyle (e.g., medication adherence, diet, sleep, physical activity, smoking), biomarkers (e.g., immune, inflammatory, hemostatic, imaging), and genomic factors that influence disease outcomes. An important trend that is likely to increase in the future is the development of consortia of population-based studies (e.g., Population of Architecture using Genomics and Epidemiology: PAGE) whose purpose is to investigate mature genetic variants associated with complex diseases in large diverse populations. Such consortium studies are each beginning to include well over 100,000 participants. Perhaps most importantly the constituent studies and the consortia will be able to follow participants over the course of many years, providing important incidence data that will allow us to examine the specific causal variables influencing the course of disease. This represents an important opportunity for behavioral medicine scientists.

Traditional observational studies have often reported findings using odds ratios, which provide estimates (with confidence interval) for the relationship between binary variables. Such studies have also permitted assessment of the effects of other variables on specific relationships using regression analyses. More recently, scientific interest in understanding the role of potential mediators of relationship between risk factors and disease outcomes has increasingly led to the use of analytic techniques such as structural equation modeling including path analysis, which until now have mostly been used in the social sciences. We can expect that a dramatic improvement in our understanding of the mediators between risk factors and disease outcomes will occur in the coming years.

The completion of the Human Genome Project in 2003 led to an increased interest in gene-environment interactions within the behavioral medicine research community. Such interactions occur when genetic factors affect measured phenotypes differentially, for example, when men with the E4 allele of the apolipoprotein E gene (APOE) were shown to have an increased smoking related risk for CHD events (Humphries et al. 2001). Other studies have shown that the interaction of the alpha 2ß-adrenergic receptor polymorphism with job strain is related to elevated blood pressure (Ohlin et al. 2007), and several other studies have related gene polymorphisms with cardiovascular reactivity to mental challenge. Most behavioral studies that have examined gene-environment interactions have been carried out on relatively small samples, but it appears inevitable that a large number of high-quality, well-powered, gene-environment studies of direct relevance to behavioral medicine will be initiated during the next few years.

In addition to the structural genomics exemplified in gene-environment interaction studies, functional genomic studies are also likely to become of increasing interest to behavioral medicine investigators. Briefly, functional genomics focuses on the basics of protein synthesis, which is how genes are "switched on" to provide messenger RNA (mRNA). Francis Crick, who along with James Watson discovered the structure of the DNA molecule, originally thought that each gene, consisting of a particular DNA sequence, codes for one specific mRNA molecule that in turn codes for a specific protein (Crick 1970). Subsequently, it became evident that after being transcribed, most mRNA molecules undergo an editing process with some segments being spliced out. In this way, a gene can lead to more than one type of mRNA molecule and consequently more than one type of protein. Thus human cells, which each contain about 25,000 genes, are able to synthesize more than 100,000 different proteins.

Epigenetics refers to the altering of gene function without changes in the DNA sequence. This can occur either by methylation of the DNA itself or by remodeling of the chromatin structure in which the DNA is packaged. Because of these processes, in utero exposure to nutrition or social factors can cause permanent modification of gene expression patterns that may lead to increased risk of mental disorders, diabetes, cancer, or cardiovascular diseases (Jirtle and Skinner 2007). As an example of how social exposure in early life can have long-duration epigenetic and phenotypic influences, Meaney and Szyf (2005) showed that neonatal rodents who received high levels of postpartum nurturing revealed diminished cortisol responses to stressful experiences when they reached adulthood. Such studies are providing a strong basis for future epigenetic behavioral medicine research.

The important advances made by observational and mechanistic studies relevant to behavioral medicine research are paralleled by a few RCT that have provided evidence that behavioral interventions aimed at modifying lifestyle or psychosocial variables can help prevent morbidity and/or mortality in high-risk populations. Thus, for example, the Diabetes Prevention Program trial (Knowler et al. 2002) in the United States and the Finnish Diabetes Prevention Trial (Tuomilehto et al. 2001) each observed that lifestyle interventions targeting weight loss and an increase in physical activity can reduce the incidence of diabetes in prediabetic patients. Based upon the success of these trials, the NIH has sponsored Look AHEAD (Action for Health in Diabetes), an RCT that is scheduled to last for 11.5 years. This trial is specifically examining whether an intensive lifestyle intervention similar to that used in the Diabetes Prevention Program can prevent major CVD events in obese participants with type 2 diabetes. Whereas the diabetes prevention projects and the Look AHEAD trial are essential for establishing that lifestyle interventions can prevent type 2 diabetes and reduce CVD risk in diabetic patients, subsequent investigation will be needed for us to learn how such interventions can be applied to clinical practice.

Although psychosocial-behavioral RCT conducted upon patients following major adverse coronary events (e.g., myocardial infarction) have yielded both positive and null results, the three major trials that have reported positive results share important similarities that differentiate them from the studies reporting null results (Friedman et al. 1986; Gulliksson et al. 2011; Orth-Gomér et al. 2009). Thus, the participants in the three major RCT reporting positive results all received group-based cognitive behavior therapy that included, in addition to cognitive behavior therapy, relaxation training and attention to lifestyle problems. The interventions all included up to 20 sessions over a year or more and used therapists specifically trained to use behavior change techniques in order to conduct behavioral interventions with cardiac patients. Treatment began at least several months after the CHD event and patients were followed up for an average of 4.5–7.8 years. Although the trials yielding positive results each studied between 237 and 862 participants, the size of each study was insufficient to permit assessment of the efficacy of specific intervention components, the role of potential biological mediators or the applicability of the intervention to populations differing in terms of important demographic characteristics. Thus there is still a need to replicate and amplify the results of the previously successful trials in rigorous, large-scale, multicenter RCT that can identify the demographic, psychosocial, and lifestyle variables that influence specific behavioral and biological determinants of risk.

In the future, evidence-based medicine will play an ever-increasing role in clinical health care. The extent to which behavioral medicine can become a successful part of health-care delivery systems will in large part depend upon investigators in the field being able to master clinical translational research, moving from efficacy to effectiveness with a high ratio of benefit to cost. Thus, for example, the Diabetes Prevention Program (Knowler et al. 2002) showed that in high-risk patients, a lifestyle intervention reduced the incidence of diabetes significantly better than a pharmacological intervention and that both interventions were superior to a placebo condition. However, the lifestyle intervention was labor intensive and required considerable effort to get participants to maintain improvement. In contrast, maintaining adherence to taking a pill once daily may pose a less daunting task. However, recent advances in web-based intervention research may level the playing field. Thus, automatic e-mail reminders, phone or e-mail based consultations with a health-care professional, interaction with web-based programs, and the instant availability of important specially tailored information on an interactive website can all help patient adherence. To the extent that weight loss programs that involve diet and exercise do more than only decrease the risk of type 2 diabetes but also improve other aspects of CVD risk, such programs are particularly valuable in terms of health promotion.

The RCT that decreased morbidity or mortality rate in CHD patients each required 20 or more group-based sessions (Friedman et al. 1986; Gulliksson et al. 2011; Orth-Gomér et al. 2009). When amortized over the length of the 4.5–7.8 year follow-up period, however, the cost compares favorably with that of most drugs also used in treatment. Participating in 20 or more sessions also poses a personal cost and some hardship for many people. However, the implementation of interactive web-based group sessions using both sound and video could obviate the need for most face-to-face meetings and allow interpersonal interactions to continue over long periods of time. It therefore seems apparent that the rapid advances taking place in science and practice during the internet era will prove helpful in making behavioral medicine an important ingredient of future health-care systems.

Future health-care systems could be strengthened by well-informed patients and by health-care providers who are grounded in behavioral medicine concepts as well as clinical medicine. Attention to the human and health-influencing aspects of neighborhoods (i.e., the built environment) are also important and dependent on informed public policy. Because Behavioral Medicine has been constructed based on the understanding of relationships among behavior, psychosocial processes, and sociocultural contexts, the field is well positioned to take a leadership role in informing future health-care policies. The field of behavioral medicine appears to have a bright, important future.

Neil Schneiderman

References

Crick, F. (1970). Central dogma of molecular biology. *Nature, 227*, 561–563. PMID: 4913914.

Friedman, M., Thoresen, C. E., Gill, J. J., Ulmer, D., Powell, L. H., & Price, V. A., et al. (1986). Alteration of type A behavior and its effect on cardiac recurrences in post myocardial infarction patients: Summary results of the recurrent coronary prevention project. *American Heart Journal, 112*, 653–655. PMID: 3766365.

Gulliksson, M., Burell, G., Vessby, B., Lundin, L., Toss, H., & Svärdsudd, K. (2011). Randomized controlled trial of cognitive behavioral therapy vs standard treatment to prevent recurrent cardiovascular events in patients with coronary heart disease: Secondary prevention in Uppsala primary health care project (SUPRIM). *Archives of Internal Medicine, 171,* 134–140. PMID: 21263103.

Humphries, S. E., Talmud, P. J., Hawe, E., Bolla, M., Day, I. N., Miller, G. J. (2001). Apolipoprotein E4 and coronary heart disease in middle-aged men who smoke: A prospective study. *Lancet, 385,* 115–119. PMID: 11463413.

Jirtle, R. L., & Skinner, M. K. (2007). Environmental epigenomics and disease susceptibility. *Nature Reviews Genetics, 8,* 253–262. PMID: 17363974.

Knowler, W. C., Barrett-Connor, E., Fowler, S. E., Hamman, R. F., Lachin, J. M., et al., & Diabetes Prevention Program Research Group. (2002). Reduction in the incidence of type 2 diabetes with lifestyle intervention or metformin. *The New England Journal of Medicine, 346,* 393–403. PMID: 11832527.

Meaney, M. J., &Szyf, M. (2005). Environmental programming of stress responses through DNA methylation life at the interface between a dynamic environment and a fixed genome. *Dialogues in Clinical Neuroscience, 7,* 103–123. PMID: 16262207.

Ohlin, S. E., Berglund, G., Nilsson, P., & Melander, O. (2007). Job strain, decision latitude and alpha 2ß-adrenergic receptor polymorphisms significantly interact and associate with high blood pressure in men. *Journal of Hypertension, 25,* 1613–1619. PMID: 18622236.

Orth-Gomér, K., Schneiderman, N., Wang, H., Walldin, C., Bloom, M., & Jernberg, T. (2009). Stress reduction prolongs life in women with coronary disease: The Stockholm Women's Intervention Trial for Coronary Heart Disease (SWITCHD). *Circulation: Cardiovascular Quality and Outcomes, 2,* 25–32. PMID: 20031809.

Tuomilehto, J., Lindström, J., Eriksson, J. G., Valle, T. T., Hämäläinen, H., et al., & Finnish Diabetes Prevention Study Group. (2001). Prevention of type 2 diabetes mellitus by changes in lifestyle among subjects with impaired glucose tolerance. *The New England Journal of Medicine, 344,* 1343–1350. PMID: 11333990.

Yusuf, S., Hawken, S., Ounpuu, S., Dans, T., Avezum, A., Lanas, F., & McQueen, M., et al. (2004). Effect of potentially modifiable risk factors associated with myocardial infarction in 52 countries: The INTERHEART study: case–control study. *Lancet, 364,* 937–952. PMID: 15364185.

Preface to the Second Edition

Since its initial publication in 2013, the Encyclopedia of Behavioral Medicine has been well utilized by professionals and students wishing to learn more about the interdisciplinary field of behavioral medicine. As noted in the Preface to that edition of the Encyclopedia, it provided a "snapshot in time" of its subject. It was also noted that the Editors hoped subsequent editions would provide additional snapshots in due course. Accordingly, I am very pleased that this second edition has now been published. As for the first edition, entries fall into three categories or domains that represent issues of interest: basic sciences, clinical investigation, and public health and public policy.

The continued growth of the field is witnessed by the increasing membership in, and attendance at the annual scientific meetings of, its primary professional organizations. A further example of its progression and evolution is the founding, in 2018, of the Behavioral Medicine Research Council, an autonomous joint committee of the Society for Health Psychology, the Academy of Behavioral Medicine Research, the American Psychosomatic Society, and the Society of Behavioral Medicine (Freedland 2019). With this rapid growth and expansion, many new terms have been established in the field, be they in public health, clinical medicine, or the physical and social sciences. Additionally, considerable progress has been made in existing areas within the field covered in the first edition of the Encyclopedia. This expansion brought about the need for this second edition of the Encyclopedia of Behavioral Medicine.

Many of the 1200 entries in the first edition have been updated considerably, and over 450 new entries have been added. These updated and new entries discuss new terms that are now part of the behavioral medicine lexicon. Several examples are highlighted here in bold font. In the area of digital health and mHealth/eHealth, new terms such as **behavioral informatics**, the collecting, analyzing, and interpreting heterogeneous data to model and shape human behavior (chapter "Behavioral Informatics" by Singh and Ghosh), and **digital health coaching**, using digital technologies to help patients identify and work toward behavior change, are now firmly established (chapter "Digital Health Coaching" by Sargent and Tomasino). In the basic sciences, researchers in behavioral medicine have begun examining brain–gut interactions and in particular the **gut microbiome** (chapter "Gut Microbiome" by Gellman). Within the domain of intervention research can be found the newly-emerging framework for developing efficient, cost-effective, and scalable behavioral interventions known as **multiphase optimization strategy** or MOST (chapter "Multiphase Optimization Strategy (MOST)" by Goldstein and Kugler). As for the first edition, it is hoped that this new edition will prove useful to students, teachers, researchers, clinicians, and individuals engaged in public health and public policy pursuits. In a world in which the pace of change seems always to be increasing, there is no doubt that the field of behavioral medicine will continue to evolve rapidly. In due course, therefore, another edition may be published. In the meantime, this edition provides a comprehensive current resource that encapsulates key aspects of our discipline and also generates an architectural framework for its further evolution. For readers who are students, it is also hoped that you will become motivated to contribute to behavioral medicine's future.

Miami, Florida   Marc D. Gellman
September 2020

References

Freedland, K. E. (2019). The Behavioral Medicine Research Council: Its origins, mission, and methods. *Health Psychology, 38*(4), 277–289. https://doi.org/10.1037/hea0000731.

Preface to the First Edition

The establishment, advancement, and maturation of the field of behavioral medicine bears witness to interest among research scientists, clinicians, and policy makers in psychological, behavioral, and social influences on health and disease from the perspective of both the individual patient and global public health. It has become increasingly clear that such influences may negatively impact health and well-being and, equally importantly, that behavioral interventions may be protective and curative.

Neal Miller (1909–2002), an American psychologist and recipient of the National Medal of Science in 1964, is often credited as being the founder of behavioral medicine. He made significant contributions to our understanding of the relationship between reinforcement mechanisms and the control of autonomic behavior, and in pioneering the field of biofeedback, which is used successfully today to treat a variety of medical conditions. The original definition of behavioral medicine was developed at the Yale Conference on Behavioral Medicine and later published by Gary Schwartz and Stephen Weiss (1977):

> "Behavioral medicine" is the field concerned with the development of behavioral science knowledge and techniques relevant to the understanding of physical health and illness, and the application of this knowledge and these techniques to diagnosis, prevention, treatment and rehabilitation.

While this definition remains the cornerstone of our interdisciplinary and integrative field, developments in many relevant subfields have advanced at rapid rates, and whole new specialties have arisen. This evolution was well exemplified by the publication in 2010 of the *Handbook of Behavioral Medicine* (Steptoe 2010). Relevant knowledge and understanding of issues of interest in behavioral medicine is now contributed by the disciplines of and expertise from anthropology, behavioral and molecular genetics, behavioral science, biostatistics, clinical medicine, cultural studies, epidemiology, health economics, general medicine, genomics, psychiatry, psychology, physiology, public health and public health policy, and sociology, to name but a few. It was therefore considered an opportune and appropriate time to create the *Encyclopedia of Behavioral Medicine*, whose publication coincides with the 12th International Congress of Behavioral Medicine, held on August 29th to September 1st, 2012, in Budapest, with attendees representing multiple disciplines and many countries around the globe. The theme of the meeting is "Behavioral Medicine: From Basic Science to Clinical Investigation and Public Health," the theme around which this *Encyclopedia* has been developed.

Accordingly, the *Encyclopedia* contains entries falling into three categories or domains that represent issues of interest: basic research, clinical investigation and practice, and public health and public health policy. The domain of basic research addresses the key questions of mechanisms of action, both in terms of how behavior can have a deleterious impact on health and how a change in behavior can be beneficial, either preventively or therapeutically. The domain of clinical investigation and practice translates this basic knowledge into clinical interventions on a patient-by-patient basis. Finally, the domain of public health and public health policy takes a broader view of how behavioral medicine research and interventions can impact the health of populations at the community, regional, national, and global levels. This includes addressing the system-wide/public education and advocacy/political activities that are needed to facilitate maximum benefits at the global level.

It can immediately be seen that behavioral medicine is indeed a multidisciplinary and interdisciplinary field. Researching mechanisms of action requires a detailed level of human biology, starting from the molecular genetic level and progressing from cellular to organ to whole-body study. A thorough understanding of environmental interactions with biological functioning is also necessary. The domains of basic research and clinical investigation and practice are linked by the increasingly important concept of translational medicine, that is, how to translate our mechanistic knowledge and understanding into successful clinical interventions most effectively and efficiently. The final challenge, likely the most challenging but ultimately providing the greatest benefit, is to address these interventions at the public health level.

Within these overarching categories, it is possible to group together various entries into categories of interest to individual readers or groups of readers pursuing their own research in cross-cutting areas. One example might be the impact of behavioral medicine research and interventions across the life span, that is, taking a life cycle approach. Entries in the *Encyclopedia* such as Children's Health Study, Elderly, End-of-Life Care, Geriatric Medicine, Life Span, Obesity in Children, and Successful Aging might be instructive in this case.

A second example might be looking at genetic predisposition to the deleterious impact of environmental factors and, equally of interest, to the therapeutic benefit of certain behavioral medicine interventions. Entries of interest here might be Family Studies (Genetics), Gene-Environment Interaction, Gene Expression, Genome-wide Association Study, and Twin Studies. While not always intuitively obvious, one of the most powerful ways to study the effects of environmental (behavioral) factors on a phenotype of interest (e.g., a given disease state or condition of clinical concern) is to study genetic influence on that phenotype (Plomin et al. 1997). Having done so, it is possible to remove from consideration the individual variation attributable to genetic influence and hence to focus on variation attributable to environmental and gene-environment interaction influences. We are certain that readers will find many such groupings of entries relevant to their own interests and research.

Additional evidence of the growth of the discipline of behavioral medicine is provided by the fact that training in the field can be found in universities around the world, ensuring that the next generation of researchers and practitioners will be trained by current experts. Before going on to specialize in behavioral medicine research or clinical practice, individuals often receive their terminal degrees in disciplines such as medicine, public health, nursing, and psychology. Such diversity is a tremendous strength in this interdisciplinary field.

Like all such printed endeavors, the *Encyclopedia* proves a "snapshot in time" of its subject. Research during the past 30 years has provided the solid foundation from which future advances will be made, and it will be of great interest to all of us in behavioral medicine to follow its further development. We are grateful to Stephen Weiss for providing a Foreword entitled "Early Developments in the Field of Behavioral Medicine," which reviews important events in the discipline's evolution, and to Neil Schneiderman for providing a Foreword entitled "A Personal View of Behavioral Medicine's Future," which provides an insightful view of likely trajectories and benefits of our discipline. We hope that subsequent editions will provide additional snapshots in due course.

Miami
July 2012

Marc D. Gellman
J. Rick Turner

References

Plomin, R., DeFries, J. C., McClearn, G. E., & Rutter, M. (1997). *Behavioral genetics* (3rd ed.). New York: WH Freeman & Company.

Schwartz, G., & Weiss, S. (1977). What is behavioral medicine. *Psychosomatic Medicine, 39*(6), 377–381.

Steptoe, A. (Ed.) (2010). *Handbook of behavioral medicine: Methods and applications*. New York: Springer.

List of Authors

David B. Abrams, P. 1, 2075
Howard Aizenstein, P. 1330
Tatsuo Akechi, P. 120, 633
Mustafa al'Absi, P. 143, 957, 1279, 1494, 1502, 1693
Jessica Alcorso, P. 1315
Melissa A. Alderfer, P. 1340, 1640
Sarah Aldred, P. 124, 1506, 1596, 2141
Katie E. Alegria, P. 496
Nida Ali, P. 87, 445
Julia Allan, P. 485, 2230
Peter Allebeck, P. 1000, 1024
Josh Allen, P. 161
Bruce S. Alpert, P. 267
Leila Anane, P. 1145
David E. Anderson, P. 1204
Giles M. Anderson, P. 972
Norman B. Anderson, P. 105
Gerhard Andersson, P. 2244
Tetusya Ando, P. 908, 1804
Mike Antoni, P. 1389
Hannah Appleseth, P. 1234
William Arguelles, P. 2183
Danielle Arigo, P. 1674
Wiebke Arlt, P. 1473
Arpo Aromaa, P. 1399
Elva Arredondo, P. 582
Lisa G. Aspinwall, P. 1713
Kristin J. August, P. 2095
Robin Austin, P. 538
Kieran Ayling, P. 215
Simon L. Bacon, P. 372, 409, 810, 882, 966
Rachel N. Baek, P. 15
Jonathan Z. Bakdash, P. 1107
Elizabeth Baker, P. 2069, 2071
Priya Balaji, P. 1094, 1100, 1101, 1104
Austin S. Baldwin, P. 179, 1170
Chad Barrett, P. 106, 233, 603, 1515, 1656, 1877, 2279

Jennifer A. Bartz, P. 1599
Abigail Batchelder, P. 979
Michele Crites Battié, P. 811
G. David Batty, P. 782, 1417, 2085, 2108
Carolyn Baum, P. 1546
Linda C. Baumann, P. 7, 55, 150, 260, 309, 544, 744, 755, 1010, 1175, 1738, 1977, 2242
Elliott A. Beaton, P. 293, 295, 1128, 1482
C. Andres Bedoya, P. 685
Catherine Benedict, P. 253, 356, 358, 786, 2147
M. Bernardine, P. 1665
Ryan M. Beveridge, P. 849, 861
Stephen Birch, P. 236, 567, 1007
Orit Birnbaum-Weitzman, P. 793, 1406, 2083, 2105, 2198, 2199
Kacie Allen Blackman, P. 1852
Twyla Blackmond Larnell, P. 1833, 1835
James A. Blumenthal, P. 2210
Guy Bodenmann, P. 851, 2234
Marie Boltz, P. 542, 1133
Susan J. Bondy, P. 1966
Stephan Bongard, P. 110
Brian Borsari, P. 248
Jos A. Bosch, P. 1141, 1145, 1149
Stephanie Bowlin, P. 2334
Sophia Brady, P. 1677
Nicole Brandt, P. 18, 123, 682, 701, 702, 1993
Lauren Brenner, P. 735
Dana Brimmer, P. 226
Carrie Brintz, P. 899, 1055
Caitlin A. Bronson, P. 383
J. F. Brosschot, P. 1245, 1650, 2359
Frankie F. Brown, P. 1319, 1323
Jennifer L. Brown, P. 2019
Bonnie Bruce, P. 997
Vaughn Bryant, P. 1462
Patrícia Cardoso Buchain, P. 26, 1794, 1799
Tony W. Buchanan, P. 1776
Ross Buck, P. 516
Romola S. Bucks, P. 2252
Donna C. Burdzy, P. 1729
Rachel J. Burns, P. 203
Michelle Nicole Burns, P. 729
Victoria E. Burns, P. 1145
David Busse, P. 1333
Natalie E. Bustillo, P. 1351, 1459
Colin D. Butler, P. 719
Jorie Butler, P. 727, 1983
Melissa M. A. Buttner, P. 2367

John T. Cacioppo, P. 1302
Demetria Cain, P. 1418
Matthew Calamia, P. 549
David Cameron, P. 1994, 2003, 2006
Linda D. Cameron, P. 496, 498
Nerissa Campbell, P. 1682
Tavis S. Campbell, P. 486, 868, 914, 926, 1348, 2289, 2323
Turhan Canli, P. 2016
Leeanne M. Carey, P. 1546
Rachel Carey, P. 206
Jordan Carlson, P. 807, 1283, 1291, 1293
Adriana Carrillo, P. 265, 865, 866, 1197, 1567, 1807
Douglas Carroll, P. 740, 1122, 1169, 1775, 1806, 2312
Judith Carroll, P. 2254
Linda Carroll, P. 25, 1631, 1737, 1747
Jennifer Carter, P. 168
Charles Carver, P. 550
Pedro C. Castellon, P. 1422
Fong Chan, P. 1780
Sherilynn F. Chan, P. 1646
Matthieu Chansard, P. 1627
Stephenie Chaudoir, P. 2142
Margaret A. Chesney, P. 425, 1204
Ornit Chiba-Falek, P. 924, 1481
Yoichi Chida, P. 1043
Olveen Carrasquillo Chief, P. 1001, 1020, 1078
Michael S. Chmielewski, P. 884
Julie Chronister, P. 1780
Linda Cillessen, P. 1396
Molly S. Clark, P. 130, 1123, 1709, 1987
Tyler Clark, P. 444, 1684
Benjamin L. Clarke, P. 58
Tainya C. Clarke, P. 333
Lindy Clemson, P. 835
Stephen Clift, P. 2041
Lorenzo Cohen, P. 29
Susan E. Collins, P. 8, 79
Persis Commissariat, P. 15
Félix R. Compen, P. 1396
Richard J. Contrada, P. 383
Michael James Coons, P. 959, 961, 963, 1117, 1603, 1608, 1611, 1617, 1620, 1623
Susannah D. Copland, P. 1166
Quirino Cordeiro, P. 26, 1794, 1799
Erin S. Costanzo, P. 1593, 2304
Simon J. Craddock Lee, P. 1447
Monique F. Crane, P. 1574
Jennifer Creek, P. 2240

Matthew Cribbet, P. 1651
Hugo Critchley, P. 741
Crista N. Crittenden, P. 503, 504, 505
Sierra Cronan, P. 1226
Andrea Croom, P. 763, 1087
Rick Crosby, P. 532
Jennifer Cumming, P. 972, 1800, 1801
Cassie Cunningham, P. 1638
Maurizio Cutolo, P. 790
Elizabeth da Silva Cardoso, P. 1780
Amber Daigre, P. 886
Catherine Darker, P. 1925
Karina Davidson, P. 469
Gary Davis, P. 825
Mary C. Davis, P. 153
Karen Dawe, P. 215
Marijke De Couck, P. 669, 1492
Stefanie De Jesus, P. 1682, 2078
Karla Espinosa de los Monteros, P. 872
Alexandra Martini de Oliveira, P. 26, 1794, 1799
Maartje de Wit, P. 645, 1024, 1818, 1820
Denise de Ybarra Rodríguez, P. 2073
Scott DeBerard, P. 159, 1039, 1068, 1282, 1284
Joost Dekker, P. 614
Alan M. Delamater, P. 1201, 1365, 1391, 1524, 2257, 2283
Kelly S. DeMartini, P. 78
Michael I. Demidenko, P. 1053, 1068
Johan Denollet, P. 1469, 2089, 2285
Ellen-ge Denton, P. 631
Stuart Derbyshire, P. 452
Martin Deschner, P. 103
Tamer F. Desouky, P. 995
Mary Amanda Dew, P. 1567
Sally Dickerson, P. 2098
Andrea F. DiMartini, P. 1567
Joel E. Dimsdale, P. 664
Ding Ding, P. 242, 312, 715
Genevieve A. Dingle, P. 2041
Beate Ditzen, P. 571, 769, 1338, 1660
Diane Dixon, P. 666
Kelly Doran, P. 870, 1941
Susan Dorsey, P. 1502
Monica Dowling, P. 635
Mark T. Drayson, P. 1177
Michelle Drerup, P. 229
Frank A. Drews, P. 1107
Suzana Drobnjak, P. 308, 1366
Joan L. Duda, P. 1677, 1971

Alejandra Duenas, P. 570
Joan Duer-Hefele, P. 469
Mariam Dum, P. 2198, 2199
Jennifer Duncan, P. 322
Christine Dunkel Schetter, P. 1732, 1899
Valerie Earnshaw, P. 2142
Lisa A. Eaton, P. 537
Moritz Thede Eckart, P. 410
Ulrike Ehlert, P. 945, 1886
Alexandre Elhalwi, P. 810, 966
Lorin Elias, P. 301
Helio Elkis, P. 1794, 1799
Lee Ellington, P. 408
Christopher G. Engeland, P. 2360
Elissa S. Epel, P. 2227
Jennifer Toller Erausquin, P. 919
Alexandra Erdmann, P. 2304
Sabrina Esbitt, P. 978
Shaniff Esmail, P. 1420, 1849
Paul Estabrooks, P. 1852
Susan A. Everson-Rose, P. 1094, 1100, 1101, 1104
Rachel Faller, P. 919
Anja C. Feneberg, P. 1439
Sally A. M. Fenton, P. 1509, 1677, 1958, 1971
Susan J. (Sue) Ferguson, P. 1082, 1711
Cristina A. Fernandez, P. 1452
Tania C. T. Ferraz Alves, P. 26
Angela Fidler Pfammatter, P. 798, 1895, 2259
Tiffany Field, P. 1338
Robyn Fielder, P. 2020, 2023
David J. Finitsis, P. 1265
Simona Fischbacher, P. 1886
Susanne Fischer, P. 1902, 2179
Skye Fitzpatrick, P. 251
Kelly Flannery, P. 1119
Magne Arve Flaten, P. 1508, 1693
Sara Fleszar, P. 498
Scrina Floyd, P. 844
Rachel Flurie, P. 18, 123, 682
Susan Folkman, P. 2177, 2327
Katherine T. Fortenberry, P. 130, 1123, 1709, 1987
Andrew Fox, P. 1370
Kristen R. Fox, P. 1567
Christopher France, P. 101, 261
Janis L. France, P. 261
Renée-Louise Franche, P. 1849
Anne Frankel, P. 1462
Elizabeth J. Franzmann, P. 53, 367, 369

Fred Friedberg, P. 874
Georita Marie Frierson, P. 1403, 1665
Shin Fukudo, P. 102, 912, 1190, 1247
Terry Fulmer, P. 10
Julianne Holt-Lunstad Fulton, P. 1335
Jens Gaab, P. 1080
Amiram Gafni, P. 236, 567, 1007
Elizabeth Galik, P. 911, 1196, 1514
Stephen Gallagher, P. 1871, 1881, 2123
Steven Gambert, P. 676, 677, 1517, 1521, 1742
Luis I. García, P. 918, 1113
M. Kay Garcia, P. 29
Ryan Garcia, P. 1563, 1564, 1656
Luz M. Garcini, P. 1403
Stephanie L. Garey, P. 350
Mariana Garza, P. 1063
Robert J. Gatchel, P. 1489
Klaus Gebel, P. 242
Pamela A. Geller, P. 1181
Marc D. Gellman, P. 35, 223, 267, 780, 974, 1810, 2015
Login S. George, P. 1349, 1876
William Gerin, P. 380
Denis Gerstorf, P. 1309, 2313
Isha Ghosh, P. 218
Yori Gidron, P. 34, 73, 85, 145, 158, 292, 472, 515, 672, 673, 724, 725, 815, 816, 878, 891, 913, 965, 971, 981, 1019, 1026, 1085, 1314, 1424, 1425, 1434, 1486, 1487, 1488, 1499, 1500, 1637, 1645, 1869, 1930, 1951, 1960, 1970, 2082, 2201, 2203, 2214, 2255, 2258
Supria K. Gill, P. 1053, 1068
Annie T. Ginty, P. 266, 275, 276, 466, 538, 655, 1047, 1770, 2220
Karen Glanz, P. 2044
Elizabeth Gleyzer, P. 523, 2290
Ronald Goldberg, P. 705
Carly M. Goldstein, P. 1429, 2092, 2138, 2308
Stephanie P. Goldstein, P. 2308
Peter M. Gollwitzer, P. 1159
Heather Honoré Goltz, P. 346, 354, 1752, 1753, 1837
Carley Gomez-Meade, P. 265, 865, 866, 1807
Jeffrey S. Gonzalez, P. 15, 978, 979, 1745
Patricia Gonzalez, P. 2105
Jeffrey L. Goodie, P. 472
Daniel Gorrin, P. 395, 611
John Grabowski, P. 624, 2188
Douglas A. Granger, P. 1933
Douglas P. Gross, P. 811, 900, 1420, 1537, 1849, 2318
Beth Grunfeld, P. 1912
Jessica Haberer, P. 1361
Tibor Hajos, P. 1024, 1818

Chanita H. Halbert, P. 584
Judith A. Hall, P. 693
Katherine S. Hall, P. 1282
Martica H. Hall, P. 1195, 1454, 2048, 2059, 2066
Peter A. Hall, P. 805, 1210, 1644, 1704, 1767, 2228
Heidi Hamann, P. 303
Mark Hamer, P. 1034, 1774, 1775, 2182, 2339
Fiona Louise Hamilton, P. 736
Kyra Hamilton, P. 2151
Margaret Hammersla, P. 1681
Reiner Hanewinkel, P. 2247
Nelli Hankonen, P. 1231
Kazuo Hara, P. 2325, 2326
Samantha M. Harden, P. 1852
Manjunath Harlapur, P. 43, 127, 867, 877, 1297, 1299, 1580, 1741, 2297
John Harlow, P. 66
Victoria Harms, P. 301
Lisa Harnack, P. 1519
Stacey L. Hart, P. 346, 354, 1752, 1753, 1837
Briain O. Hartaigh, P. 590, 2018
Alison Hartman, P. 1181
Steven Harulow, P. 2116
Toshihide Hashimoto, P. 1914
Masahiro Hashizume, P. 255
Brant P. Hasler, P. 683
Misty A. W. Hawkins, P. 1011
Louise C. Hawkley, P. 1303
Calvin Haws, P. 1537
Laura L. Hayman, P. 989
Jennifer Heaney, P. 20, 560, 778, 1127, 1693
Christine Heim, P. 1660, 2167
Eric B. Hekler, P. 66
Lois Jane Heller, P. 2221
Miranda Hellman, P. 573, 757, 1253, 1257, 1260, 1261, 1262, 1545, 1802, 2356
Whitney M. Herge, P. 407, 1720
Patricia Cristine Heyn, P. 1282
Emma Hiatt, P. 1780
Angela M. Hicks, P. 172
Benjamin Hidalgo, P. 246, 517
Catharina Hjortsberg, P. 1015
Clare Hocking, P. 1540
Richard Hoffman, P. 1496, 1961
Sara A. Hoffman, P. 798, 1895, 2259
Maxine Holmqvist, P. 1759, 1761, 1765
Emily D. Hooker, P. 982
Stephanie Ann Hooker, P. 244, 365, 377, 1930, 1975, 2009, 2035, 2105
Monica Webb Hooper, P. 325, 823, 2069, 2071, 2073

Christiane A. Hoppmann, P. 1309, 2313
M. Bryant Howren, P. 36, 1823
Brian M. Hughes, P. 270
Ryan Hulla, P. 1489
Mann Hyung Hur, P. 759
Seth Hurley, P. 114, 116
Mustafa M. Husain, P. 1627
John Hustad, P. 248
Shannon Idzik, P. 1740, 1742, 1743
Shuji Inada, P. 198, 2328
Salvatore Insana, P. 1513, 1827, 1882, 2056, 2068
Leah Irish, P. 1561
Daisuke Ito, P. 1768
Makiko Ito, P. 1803
Satoru Iwase, P. 1622
Karen Jacobs, P. 573, 757, 1253, 1257, 1260, 1261, 1262, 1545, 1802, 2213, 2356
Farrah Jacquez, P. 840
Denise Janicki-Deverts, P. 503, 504, 505
Kate L. Jansen, P. 130, 1123, 1709, 1987
Imke Janssen, P. 887
Lisa M. Jaremka, P. 849, 861
Elissa Jelalian, P. 1523, 1525, 1528
Chad D. Jensen, P. 1523, 1525, 1528
Jason Jent, P. 428, 435, 856
Rong Jiang, P. 925, 1642
Alvin Jin, P. 655
Debra Johnson, P. 57, 60, 92
Jillian A. Johnson, P. 486, 868, 914, 926, 1348, 2289, 2323
Sara B. Johnson, P. 1933
Derek Johnston, P. 94, 96
Marie Johnston, P. 206
Phil Jones, P. 940
Sarah Jones, P. 2138
Randall Steven Jorgensen, P. 1910
Melissa Julian, P. 1732, 1899
Kauhanen Jussi, P. 1271
Vanessa Juth, P. 2098
Yoshinobu Kanda, P. 1049
Maria Kangas, P. 12, 49
Afton N. Kapuscinski, P. 2120, 2127, 2218
Mardís Karlsdóttir, P. 1648
Yoko Katayori, P. 102
Erin E. Kauffman, P. 2099
Francine Kaufman, P. 640
Peter Kaufmann, P. 1266
Jacob J. Keech, P. 2151
Quinn D. Kellerman, P. 774

Alan Kessedjian, P. 1471, 2216
Riyad Khanfer, P. 1329, 1466
Falk Kiefer, P. 1279
Hiroe Kikuchi, P. 353, 991, 993, 1639, 1868
Kristin Kilbourn, P. 796
Christopher J. Kilby, P. 761, 1275
Tereza Killianova, P. 890, 1928
Jeong Han Kim, P. 2316
Youngmee Kim, P. 98, 2164
Pamela S. King, P. 670, 752, 753, 1357, 1410
Megan Kirouac, P. 79
Clemens Kirschbaum, P. 561, 2275
George D. Kitas, P. 1677, 1971
Mika Kivimaki, P. 2140
Predrag Klasnja, P. 66
Maria Kleinstäuber, P. 1413, 2373
Wendy Kliewer, P. 817
Christopher E. Kline, P. 20, 1700, 2061, 2064
Anna K. Koch, P. 575, 1203
Dorothea König, P. 746
Carolyn Korbel, P. 172, 609
Rachel Kornfield, P. 663
Emily Kothe, P. 1289, 2086
Michael Kotlyar, P. 316, 1973
Marc A. Kowalkouski, P. 346, 354, 1752, 1753, 1837
Tara Kraft, P. 2334
Jean L. Kristeller, P. 1392
Kurt Kroenke, P. 2110
Stefan Krumm, P. 1241
Ulrike Kübler, P. 2185
Laura D. Kubzansky, P. 1597
Brigitte M. Kudielka, P. 638
Kari C. Kugler, P. 1429
Masayoshi Kumagai, P. 200
Keiki Kumano, P. 2137
Yoshihiko Kunisato, P. 2284
Elyse Kupperman, P. 15
Annette M. La Greca, P. 407, 1646, 1720
Pearl La Marca-Ghaemmaghami, P. 945
Seppo Laaksonen, P. 2208
Lara LaCaille, P. 311, 711, 2231
Rick LaCaille, P. 1234, 1786, 2172
Laura H. Lacritz, P. 1435
Karl-Heinz Ladwig, P. 1359
Nathan Landers, P. 1489
Ryan R. Landoll, P. 407
Joshua Landvatter, P. 1226
Tanja Lange, P. 459

Brittney Lange-Maia, P. 887
Jost Langhorst, P. 575, 1203
David Latini, P. 346, 354, 1752, 1753, 1837
Emily Lattie, P. 735
Kim Lavoie, P. 125, 440
Lauren Law, P. 1980
Hannah G. Lawman, P. 1980
David J. Lee, P. 333, 1452
Emily E. Lenk, P. 769
Carter A. Lennon, P. 74
Wen B. Leong, P. 1377
Stephen J. Lepore, P. 817
Bonnie S. LeRoy, P. 931
Yvonne Leung, P. 1643
Bonnie Levin, P. 617
Helena Lewis-Smith, P. 283
Bingshuo Li, P. 143
Roselind Lieb, P. 1707
Jane Limmer, P. 844
Bernt Lindahl, P. 1920
Martin Lindström, P. 2079
Megan R. Lipe, P. 343
Steven E. Lipshultz, P. 1450
Cecilia W. P. Li-Tsang, P. 2240
Maria Magdalena Llabre, P. 2183
Judy D. Lobo, P. 1076
Valerie G. Loehr, P. 1170
Joanna Long, P. 1150, 1800, 1801
Kristin A. Long, P. 1340
Sana Loue, P. 577
William R. Lovallo, P. 1776
Travis I. Lovejoy, P. 321, 1053, 1068
Wei Lü, P. 270
Tana M. Luger, P. 999, 2215
Anna Luke, P. 2092
Mark A. Lumley, P. 107
M. Kathleen B. Lustyk, P. 1864
Faith S. Luyster, P. 703, 2052, 2055
Kristin L. MacGregor, P. 78
Anna MacKinnon, P. 1426
Shannon Madore, P. 796
Nicole E. Mahrer, P. 1732, 1899
Elizabeth A. Majka, P. 1302
Jamil A. Malik, P. 1273
Neena Malik, P. 855
Elizabeth M. Maloney, P. 1549
Tsipora Mankovsky, P. 453
Amy Jo Marcano-Reik, P. 31, 113, 122, 474

Judy A. Marciel, P. 588
Kristen K. Marciel, P. 588
Erin N. Marcus, P. 1020
Seth A. Margolis, P. 1745
Michela (Micky) Marinelli, P. 699
Jacqueline Markowitz, P. 573, 757, 1253, 1257, 1260, 1261, 1262, 1545, 1802, 2356
David G. Marrero, P. 644
Meghan L. Marsac, P. 1640
Elaine Marshall, P. 1786
Alexandra Martin, P. 26, 1794, 1799, 1917
Kevin S. Masters, P. 307, 679, 826, 1244, 2125
Della Matheson, P. 99, 1199
Yoshinobu Matsuda, P. 357
Hiromichi Matsuoka, P. 351
Yutaka Matsuyama, P. 1059
Sonia Matwin, P. 609
Alfred L. McAlister, P. 1003
Lisa M. McAndrew, P. 507, 995
Jeanette McCarthy, P. 933, 939, 1664
Shawn McClintock, P. 1627
Lance M. McCracken, P. 1609
James A. McCubbin, P. 766
Hayley McDonald, P. 148
Bonnie McGregor, P. 358
Brooke McInroy, P. 100
David McIntyre, P. 199
Tara McMullen, P. 1978, 1986, 1990
Marcia D. McNutt, P. 823
Tamar Mendelson, P. 2170
Luigi Meneghini, P. 246, 641, 642, 964, 991, 1202, 2282
Melissa Merrick, P. 428, 435
Shelby Messerschmitt-Coen, P. 851
Sarah Messiah, P. 276, 286, 288
Miriam A. Mestre, P. 1450
Elizabeth Mezick, P. 2058, 2063
Kathleen Michael, P. 643
Susan Michie, P. 206
Eleanor Miles, P. 63, 259
Donna Miller, P. 1452
Robert Miller, P. 2275
Tracie L. Miller, P. 1450
Rachel Millstein, P. 61, 137, 281
Faisal Mir, P. 2216
Karlie M. Mirabelli, P. 661
Akihisa Mitani, P. 162, 163, 166, 450, 1313, 1813
Jason W. Mitchell, P. 918, 1073, 2025
Laura A. Mitchell, P. 502

Koji Miyazaki, P. 476
Marilyn Moffat, P. 1685
David C. Mohr, P. 729
Kristine M. Molina, P. 793, 1005, 1833, 1835
Ivan Molton, P. 739, 941
Jane Monaco, P. 397, 500, 714, 1911, 2330
Enid Montague, P. 2294
Miranda Montrone, P. 2204
Pablo A. Mora, P. 507, 995, 1997
Theresa A. Morgan, P. 884, 1277
Matthis Morgenstern, P. 2247
Chica Mori, P. 1622
Yoshiya Moriguchi, P. 905
Alexandre Morizio, P. 882
Eleshia J. P. Morrison, P. 1403
Anett Mueller, P. 2016
Hanna M. Mües, P. 2028
Matthew Muldoon, P. 1552
Barbara Mullan, P. 1157
Tomohiko Muratsubaki, P. 1247
Elizabeth Murray, P. 736
Julie Murray, P. 159, 1039, 1284
Seema Mutti, P. 1332
Yoko Nagai, P. 741
Eun-Shim Nahm, P. 1586
Motohiro Nakajima, P. 1502
Misuzu Nakashima, P. 213, 231
Benjamin H. Natelson, P. 1360
Urs M. Nater, P. 87, 445, 788, 1368, 1439, 1660, 2028, 2179
Gabriana Navarrete, P. 1864
Astrid Nehlig, P. 477
Alexandra Nelson, P. 1181
Ashley M. Nelson, P. 1593
Kimberly Nelson, P. 628
Jonathan Newman, P. 1032, 1051, 1243, 1294, 1433, 1699, 1736, 2109, 2181, 2302, 2306, 2351
Sarah J. Newman, P. 859
Darren Nickel, P. 183
Nicole Nisly, P. 90
Karen Niven, P. 62, 63
Kyle R. Noll, P. 1435
Wynne E. Norton, P. 678
Kathryn Noth, P. 686
Ciara M. O'Brien, P. 1971
Eoin O'Brien, P. 1689
Julianne O'Daniel, P. 932
Michael O'Hara, P. 2347
Lindsay Oberleitner, P. 107

Gabriele Oettingen, P. 1159
Ken Ohashi, P. 2135
Keisuke Ohta, P. 44
Michele L. Okun, P. 293, 1505, 1724, 1735
Toru Okuyama, P. 141, 329, 1757
Ellinor K. Olander, P. 2357
Brian Oldenburg, P. 1550
Sheina Orbell, P. 977
Tracy Orlcans, P. 1578
Kristina Orth-Gomér, P. 1582
Patricia Osborne, P. 1745
Kenneth J. Ottenbacher, P. 1587
Margaret E. Ottenbacher, P. 1587
Nicole Overstreet, P. 1070
Jan R. Oyebode, P. 968, 969
Gozde Ozakinci, P. 1997
Debbie Palmer, P. 431
Steven C. Palmer, P. 340, 1093
Kenneth Pargament, P. 1729
Crystal L. Park, P. 1349, 1876
Joanne Park, P. 1420, 1537, 1849
Alyssa Parker, P. 392, 857, 1118, 1126
Kristen Pasko, P. 1674
Seema M. Patidar, P. 785
Anna Maria Patino-Fernandez, P. 118, 314, 712, 1376
David Pearson, P. 2354
Hollie Pellosmaa, P. 1090
Jennifer Pellowski, P. 917, 1457, 1461
Frank J. Penedo, P. 358
Watcharaporn Pengchit, P. 1713
Donald Penzien, P. 1383
Deidre Pereira, P. 343, 350, 785, 935
Edward L. Perkins, P. 690
Richard Peter, P. 1358
Anna C. Phillips, P. 1177, 1646
Alison Phillips, P. 507
Sarah Piper, P. 373, 1843, 1845
Alefiyah Z. Pishori, P. 622
Helene J. Polatajko, P. 1546
Lynda H. Powell, P. 887
Glenn Pransky, P. 1613, 1615
Harry Prapavessis, P. 674, 1682
Aric A. Prather, P. 2037
Courtney C. Prather, P. 2099
Sarah D. Pressman, P. 982, 2334
James O. Prochaska, P. 2266
Elizabeth R. Pulgaron, P. 147, 165, 1524, 1595, 2283
Naum Purits, P. 828

Pekka Puska, P. 2249
Conny W. E. M. Quaedflieg, P. 2161
Mashfiqui Rabbi, P. 1632
Whitney Raglin, P. 840
Jeanetta Rains, P. 1383
P. H. Amelie Ramirez, P. 1748
Isabel F. Ramos, P. 1732
Ashley K. Randall, P. 851, 2234
Sheah Rarback, P. 789, 1027, 1312, 1444
Holly Rau, P. 1136, 1138
Maija Reblin, P. 391
Jerrald Rector, P. 1145
Gabriela Reed, P. 842, 848
William Reeves, P. 1368
Emily W. Reid, P. 2270
Ulf-Dietrich Reips, P. 1216
Anthony Remaud, P. 1250
Kirsten Rene, P. 1773
Michiel F. Reneman, P. 900, 2318
Barbara Resnick, P. 71, 366, 943, 944, 1451, 1459, 2193
Spencer M. Richard, P. 1284
Michael Richter, P. 186, 188, 1626, 2211
Nina Rieckmann, P. 708
Winfried Rief, P. 2113, 2114
Kristen Riley, P. 240
Deborah Rinehart, P. 988
Lynnee Roane, P. 1115
Christopher Robert, P. 1489
Osvaldo Rodriguez, P. 1078
Laura Rodriguez-Murillo, P. 439, 555, 698, 922, 940, 1059, 1082, 1112, 1192, 1856
Kathryn A. Roecklein, P. 1964
Megan Roehrig, P. 322
Nicolas Rohleder, P. 1187, 1210, 2280
Chelsea Romney, P. 1899
Karen S. Rook, P. 2095
Jed E. Rose, P. 1504
Leah Rosenberg, P. 373, 375, 559, 881, 1123, 1295, 1649, 1843, 1845, 2257, 2305
Debra Roter, P. 693
Alexander J. Rothman, P. 203
Eric Roy, P. 299, 492, 493, 494
Rachel S. Rubinstein, P. 383
John Ruiz, P. 1063, 2099
John Ryan, P. 1330
Valerie Sabol, P. 707, 1046, 1815
Rany M. Salem, P. 439, 555, 698, 922, 940, 1059, 1082, 1112, 1192, 1856
Kristen Salomon, P. 655, 1373, 1648, 1688, 2146, 2158
Janine Sanchez, P. 543, 652, 760, 960, 1201

Lee Sanders, P. 521, 1017
Timothy S. Sannes, P. 935
Elizabeth Sargent, P. 658
Amy F. Sato, P. 1523, 1525, 1528
Eve Saucier, P. 1772
Shekhar Saxena, P. 2357
Wolff Schlotz, P. 2154
Havah Schneider, P. 978
Neil Schneiderman, P. 1062, 1212, 1955
Beth Schroeder, P. 151, 171, 612
James W. Schroeder, P. 782
Marie-Louise Schult, P. 1258
Brandon K. Schultz, P. 661
M. Di Katie Sebastiano, P. 278, 903
Sabrina Segal, P. 1515, 2212
Theresa Senn, P. 2026, 2032
Jonathan A. Shaffer, P. 422, 2129
Kelly M. Shaffer, P. 2164
Peter A. Shapiro, P. 1040
Leigh A. Sharma, P. 1501
Marianne Shaughnessy, P. 463, 533, 1755, 1893
Christopher Shaw, P. 2324
William S. Shaw, P. 1613, 1615
Tamara Goldman Sher, P. 686
Kerry Sherman, P. 283, 606, 761, 1275, 2204
Simon Sherry, P. 251, 1426
Vivek Shetty, P. 257
Akihito Shimazu, P. 1269
Daichi Shimbo, P. 43, 127, 376, 867, 877, 1297, 1299, 1580, 1741, 2297
Erica Shreck, P. 979
Koseki Shunsuke, P. 1985
Johannes Siegrist, P. 1534, 2038
Matthew A. Simonson, P. 936, 1830
Kit Sinclair, P. 2240
Abanish Singh, P. 54, 84, 529, 1706
Vivek K. Singh, P. 218
Bengt H. Sjölund, P. 1860
Celette Sugg Skinner, P. 2223
Michelle Skinner, P. 748, 750
Nadine Skoluda, P. 1906
Tom Smeets, P. 2161
Alicia K. Smith, P. 782
Barbara Smith, P. 438
Lauren Smith, P. 1063
Timothy W. Smith, P. 1035, 1223
Howard Sollins, P. 692, 1014, 2207
Colin L. Soskolne, P. 719
Ana Victoria Soto, P. 157, 370, 604
Anne E. M. Speckens, P. 1396

Mary Spiers, P. 291, 399, 2270
Kevin S. Spink, P. 183
Bonnie Spring, P. 798, 1895, 2259
Sara Mijares St. George, P. 2090
Tobias Stalder, P. 561
Annette L. Stanton, P. 304
Shannon L. Stark, P. 153
Adrienne Stauder, P. 2010
Michael E. Stefanek, P. 329
Jeremy Steglitz, P. 1603, 1617
Nikola Stenzel, P. 1241
Colleen Stiles-Shields, P. 1953, 2294
Anna M. Stone, P. 1377
Madison E. Stout, P. 1011
Mark Stoutenberg, P. 1670
Jana Strahler, P. 1381, 1929
Deborah M. Stringer, P. 1469
Victoria Anne Sublette, P. 1287
Madalina L. Sucala, P. 1556
Alyson Sularz, P. 322
Michael J. L. Sullivan, P. 197, 453
Hannah Süss, P. 1902
Shin-ichi Suzuki, P. 1760, 1768, 1797, 1985, 2284
Melanie Swan, P. 1824
C. Renn Upchurch Sweeney, P. 599, 654, 717
Sefik Tagay, P. 1943
Shahrad Taheri, P. 1377
Misato Takada, P. 1558
Yoshiyuki Takimoto, P. 791, 792, 957, 1191, 1196
Yukari Tanaka, P. 912, 1190
Molly L. Tanenbaum, P. 15
Asuka Tanoue, P. 1760
Marc Taylor, P. 2172
Robert N. Taylor, P. 769
Jacqueline A. ter Stege, P. 606
Julian F. Thayer, P. 187, 1048, 1650
Törös Theorell, P. 1254
G. Neil Thomas, P. 1377
Roland Thomeé, P. 1905
Dylan Thompson, P. 45
Rebecca C. Thurston, P. 1343
Warren Tierney, P. 1871, 1881, 2123
Jasmin Tiro, P. 1447
Emil C. Toescu, P. 402, 1477
Fumiharu Togo, P. 465
Akihiro Tokoro, P. 323, 324
Kathryn N. Tomasino, P. 658
A. Janet Tomiyama, P. 2227
Hansel Tookes, P. 1467

George J. Trachte, P. 400, 784, 1884, 2307
Lara Traeger, P. 400, 442, 487, 498, 681
Vincent Tran, P. 1022, 1708, 1727, 1769
William Trim, P. 45
Wendy Troxel, P. 229, 1193, 1335
Emiko Tsuchiya, P. 102
Viana Turcios-Cotto, P. 2174
Barbara Turner, P. 1748
J. Rick Turner, P. 6, 65, 83, 146, 201, 241, 247, 396, 398, 401, 416, 467, 468, 475, 521, 526, 535, 548, 576, 600, 601, 613, 622, 653, 677, 702, 726, 727, 812, 814, 839, 854, 879, 929, 930, 933, 939, 1061, 1129, 1192, 1215, 1246, 1301, 1335, 1349, 1354, 1374, 1388, 1409, 1410, 1439, 1473, 1512, 1531, 1532, 1625, 1658, 1691, 1700, 1744, 1745, 1756, 17771, 1817, 1841, 1857, 1859, 1866, 1892, 1945, 2043, 2132, 2133, 2136, 2186, 2217, 2294, 2301, 2302
James Edward Turner, P. 45, 367, 591, 1151, 1319, 1323, 1346
Bert N. Uchino, P. 1226
Jane Upton, P. 26, 202, 792, 1141, 1402, 1763, 1795, 2008
Antti Uutela, P. 2298
Julia R. Van Liew, P. 1302
Kavita Vedhara, P. 215
Jet J. C. S. Veldhuijzen van Zanten, P. 574, 771, 1677, 2158
Bart Verkuil, P. 1245, 1650, 2359
Andrea C. Villanti, P. 2075
Ana Vitlic, P. 1473
Adriana Dias Barbosa Vizzotto, P. 26, 1794, 1799
Catharina Vogt, P. 1906
John P. Vuchetich, P. 316, 1973
Katarzyna Wac, P. 1819
Amy Wachholtz, P. 523, 2290
Anton J. M. Wagenmakers, P. 1947
Melanie Wakefield, P. 1695
Andrea Wallace, P. 1992
Margaret Wallhagen, P. 1029, 1030
Melissa Walls, P. 2108
Kenneth A. Wallston, P. 1423
Jenny T. Wang, P. 650, 859, 864
Jennifer L. Warnick, P. 798, 1895, 2259
Andrew J. Wawrzyniak, P. 892, 896
Thomas L. Webb, P. 1994, 2003, 2006
Lisa Juliane Weckesser, P. 2275
Mark Vander Weg, P. 417
Stephen M. Weiss, P. 2331
Jennifer Wessel, P. 506, 531, 690, 1057, 1412, 1859, 2281
William Whang, P. 142, 157, 168, 370, 535, 557, 604, 1034, 1355, 1357, 1517, 2353
Anthony J. Wheeler, P. 159, 1282
Angela White, P. 2014
Anna C. Whittaker, P. 119, 121, 1281, 1925

Timothy Whittaker, P. 1056
Timothy H. Wideman, P. 197
Deborah J. Wiebe, P. 192, 985
Friedrich Wieser, P. 769
Diana Wile, P. 147
James D. Wilkinson, P. 1450
Paula Williams, P. 1136, 1138, 1651
Redford B. Williams, P. 2341, 2344
Virginia P. Williams, P. 2341
Dawn Wilson, P. 1980, 2090
Oliver J. Wilson, P. 1947
Kelly Winter, P. 1165
Katie Witkiewitz, P. 2376
Michael Witthöft, P. 795, 1634
Jutta M. Wolf, P. 1187, 1772, 1773
Oliver T. Wolf, P. 1086
Timothy Wolf, P. 1848
Patricia Woltz, P. 317
Cara Wong, P. 221
Patricia M. Wong, P. 1964
Jennifer Wortmann, P. 1873
Emily M. Wright, P. 442, 487
Rex A. Wright, P. 186, 188, 1626, 2211
Ellen Wuest, P. 573, 757, 1253, 1257, 1260, 1261, 1262, 1545, 1802, 2356
Alexandra Wuttke-Linnemann, P. 1439
Naoya Yahagi, P. 44, 200
Yu Yamada, P. 424, 1555
Yoshiharu Yamamoto, P. 86
Yuko Yanai, P. 1797
Betina R. Yanez, P. 304
Samantha Yard, P. 628
M. Taghi Yasamy, P. 2357
Siqin Ye, P. 31, 113, 371, 427, 530, 555, 557, 755, 1031, 1081, 1250
Jason S. Yeh, P. 650, 1166
Ilona S. Yim, P. 1333
Alyssa Ylinen, P. 7, 55, 150, 260, 309, 544, 744, 755, 1010, 1175, 1738, 1977, 2242
Deborah Lee Young-Hyman, P. 1455, 1456
Xiaohui Yu, P. 1094, 1100, 1101, 1104
Lauren Zagorski, P. 678
Ydwine Zanstra, P. 94
Alex Zautra, P. 153
Chris Zehr, P. 1354, 1644, 1704
Kristin A. Zernicke, P. 486, 868, 914, 926, 1348, 2289, 2323
Emily Zielinski-Gutierrez, P. 226
Cortney Taylor Zimmerman, P. 1720
Sheryl Zimmerman, P. 1630
Tanja Zimmermann, P. 571

Acknowledgments

For this second edition of the *Encyclopedia of Behavioral Medicine,* I must begin by acknowledging the original creator of the idea for this Encyclopedia, the now-retired former Senior Editor from Springer Nature, Janice Stern. Janice was the driving force for the first edition when she approached me at the International Congress of Behavioral Medicine held in Tokyo, August 2008, to discuss this project and subsequently assisted through the publication process with its release in the Summer of 2012, in conjunction the International Congress of Behavioral Medicine held in Budapest. It was a few short years after the publication of the first edition that Janice was busy convincing me that it was time to begin preparing the second edition that you are now reading. Janice stayed with the project until her retirement at the end of 2017. I am indebted to her for her friendship.

A heartfelt thanks to all authors of the entries in both editions of the Encyclopedia. You are experts in your respective fields, and you have done a great service to the discipline of behavioral medicine by contributing to this authoritative resource for researchers, practicing clinicians, and the students that are the future of our discipline.

While no longer serving as the co-editor for the *Encyclopedia of Behavioral Medicine,* J. Rick Turner has always been available as a consultant for this second edition. He has assisted on various projects and contributed with new entries. For this, I will always be grateful for his friendship, guidance, thoughtfulness, and writing skills.

Next I must acknowledge the Associate Editors. They come from multiple regions of the world and hence permit this work to be truly an international collaboration. Without their hard work and dedication to this project, we would not have the *Encyclopedia of Behavioral Medicine* in the form that you see it. They assisted in the selection of the terms that are included in the *Encyclopedia* and in the selection of the authors who developed each of the entries: sincere thanks to all of you.

I am beholden to the Springer Nature Major Reference Works team including Alexa Steele and Mary Baker. Mary was the editorial assistant that kept track of all of the new and updated entries, and in many ways was instrumental in bringing this second edition of the *Encyclopedia* to fruition.

Lastly, to my loving wife Jill. She has, and continues to be my co-pilot and life partner. Jill has been by my side throughout the development of both the first and second editions of the *Encyclopedia*. I could not have done this without your support.

Marc D. Gellman

About the Editor

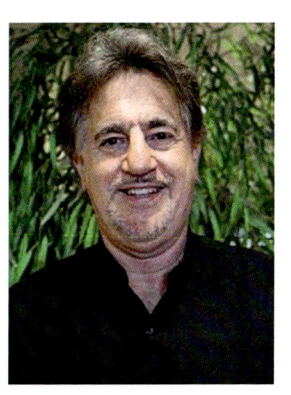

Marc D. Gellman Editor-in-Chief, Encyclopedia of Behavioral Medicine

Marc D. Gellman, Ph.D., is a Research Associate Professor of Psychology at the University of Miami. He is also the Associate Director of the Behavioral Medicine Research Center and Associate Director of the Training Program in Cardiovascular Behavioral Medicine, located at the Miller School of Medicine, University of Miami, where he holds a Secondary Appointment in the Department of Medicine. He has been a member of the faculty of the University of Miami since 1986, having previously received all of his formal training (B.S., M.S., and Ph.D. degrees) there.

Since 1986, Dr. Gellman has been continuously funded by the National Institutes of Health, primarily in the area of Cardiovascular Behavioral Medicine. He has published in a variety of journals including: *Journal of the American Medical Association*, *Psychosomatic Medicine; Health Psychology*, *Annals of Behavioral Medicine*, *Genome Biology*, *Addictive Behaviors*, *Psychophysiology*, and many others. Dr. Gellman currently serves on the Editorial Advisory Board for the McGraw Hill *Annual Editions: Drugs, Society and Behavior*. He previously served on the Editorial Board of the Sage Publications scientific book series Behavioral Medicine and Health Psychology from 1997 to 2004, edited by Dr. J. Rick Turner, his co-editor for the first edition of this Encyclopedia.

Dr. Gellman is a former Board Member of the International Society of Behavioral Medicine, serving as its Secretary from 2004 to 2008 and Chair of the Communications Committee from 2000 to 2004. From 2004 to 2006 he served as

Program Co-chair for the International Congress of Behavioral Medicine. He is a long-time Board Member of the Society of Behavioral Medicine, serving in various capacities from 1996 to 2007. He continues to serve as a member of the Wisdom Council for the Society of Behavioral Medicine.

Dr. Gellman is the recipient of the Distinguished Service Award from the Society of Behavioral Medicine (multiple times) and the Outstanding Service Award from the International Society of Behavioral Medicine. He is a Fellow of the Society of Behavioral Medicine, and also a member of American Psychological Association, Society for Health Psychology, American Psychosomatic Society, and the International Society of Behavioral Medicine. In 2016, he received the Distinguished Career Contribution Award from the International Society of Behavioral Medicine.

In his spare time, Dr. Gellman is an avid bicycle rider and enjoys "out of car experiences" with his wife Jill, touring numerous countries on their tandem bicycle. He is a wine aficionado, an enthusiast of rock, jazz, and reggae music, and occasionally lectures on the influence drugs have on culture, being inspired by his attendance at the historic Woodstock Music and Art Festival in 1969.

Associate Editors

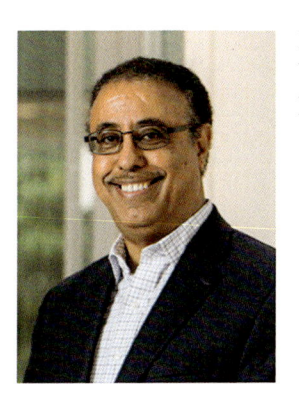

Mustafa al'Absi
University of Minnesota Medical School
Duluth, USA

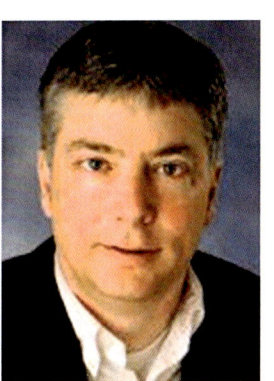

Alan J. Christensen
Department of Psychology
The University of Iowa Spence
Iowa City, USA

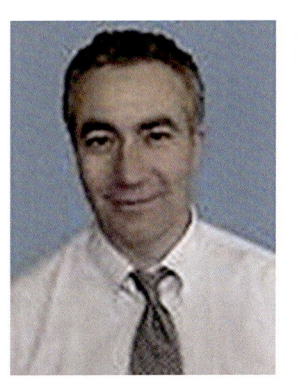

Alan M. Delamater
University of Miami Miller School of Medicine
Miami, USA

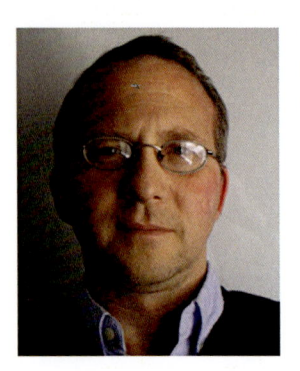

Yori Gidron
Lille 3 University and Siric Oncollile
Lille, France

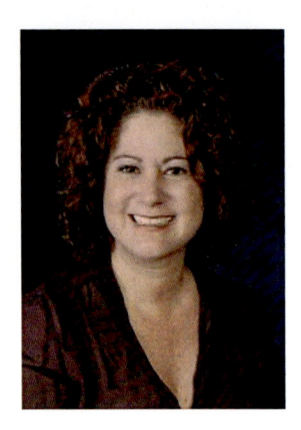

Michele L. Okun
University of Colorado Colorado Springs
Colorado Springs, USA

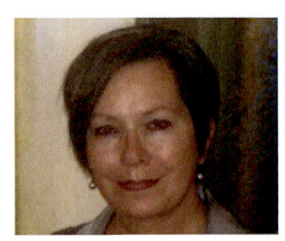

Martica H. Hall University of Pittsburgh
Pittsburgh, USA

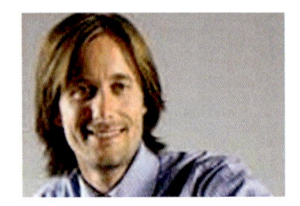

Tavis S. Campbell
University of Calgary
Calgary, Canada

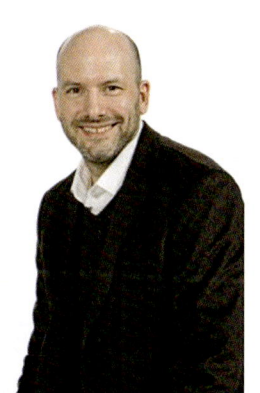

Simon L. Bacon
Concordia University and Montreal
Behavioural Medicine Centre
CIUSSS du Nord-de-l'île-de-Montréal
Montreal, Canada

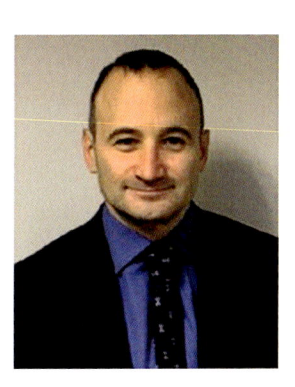

Steven A. Safren
University of Miami
Coral Gables, USA

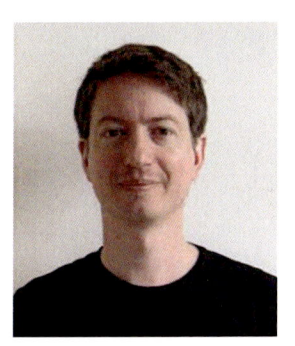

Urs M. Nater
University of Vienna
Vienna, Austria

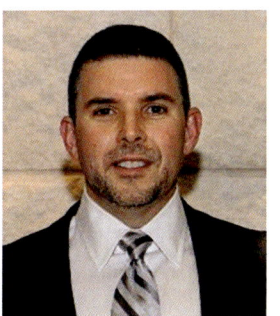

Frank J. Penedo
Northwestern University
Chicago, USA

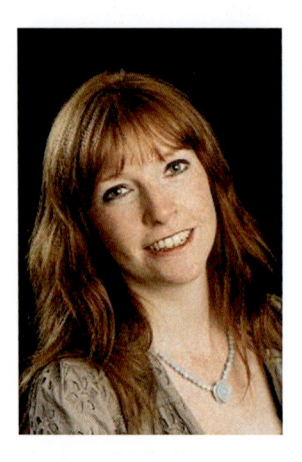

Anna C. Whittaker
University of Stirling
Stirling, UK

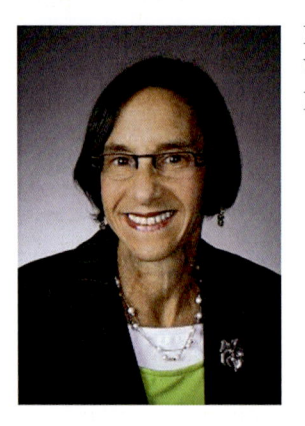

Barbara Resnick
University of Maryland
Baltimore, USA

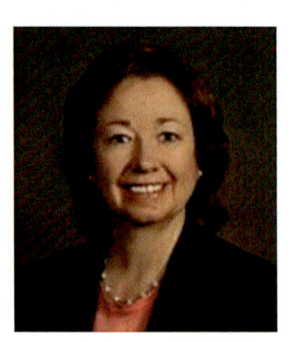

Marie Boltz
Pennsylvania State University
University Park, USA

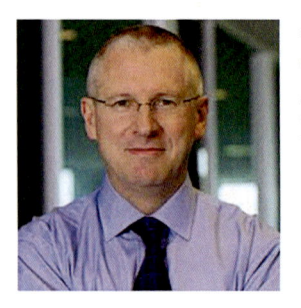

J. Rick Turner
Campbell University College of Pharmacy
and Health Sciences
Buies Creek, USA

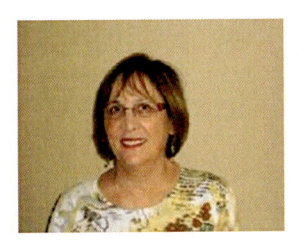

Linda C. Baumann
University of Wisconsin-Madison
Madison, USA

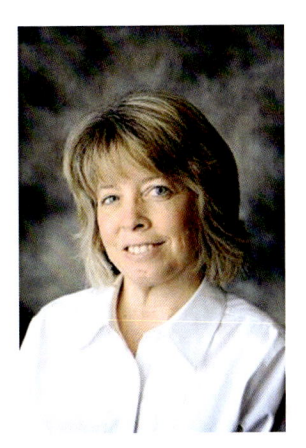

Deborah J. Wiebe
University of California, Merced
Merced, USA

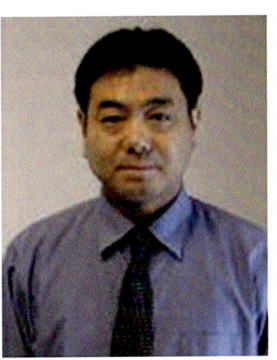

Kazuhiro Yoshiuchi
Department of Stress Sciences and
Psychosomatic Medicine
Graduate School of Medicine
Bunkyo-ku, Japan

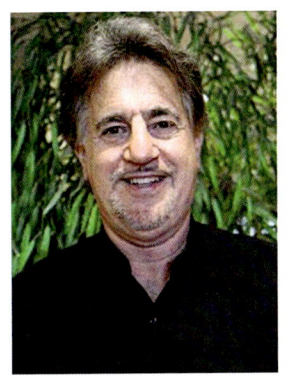

Marc D. Gellman
Behavioral Medicine Research Center
Department of Psychology
University of Miami
Miami, USA

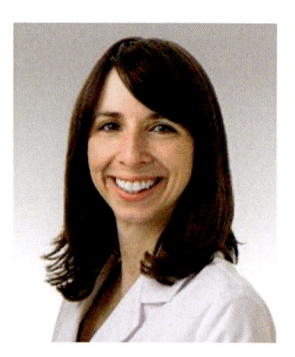

Emily Lattie
Northwestern University
Chicago, USA

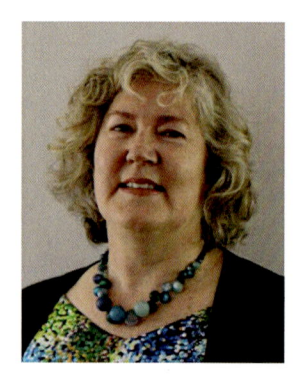

Kerry A. Sherman
Macquarie University
Sydney, Australia

Advisory Board

Linda D. Cameron The University of Auckland, Auckland, New Zealand

Margaret A. Chesney University of California, San Francisco, San Francisco, CA, USA

Joel E. Dimsdale University of California San Diego, La Jolla, CA, USA

Laura L. Hayman College of Nursing and Health Sciences, University of Massachusetts Boston, Director of Research, GoKids Boston, Boston, MA, USA

Norito Kawakami Graduate School of Medicine, University of Tokyo, Tokyo, Japan

Brian Oldenburg Department of Epidemiology and Preventive Medicine, Faculty of Medicine, Nursing and Health Sciences, Monash University, Victoria, Australia

Winfried Rief Philipps-Universität Marburg, Marburg, Germany

Neil Schneiderman Department of Psychology, University of Miami, Coral Gables, FL, USA

Andrew Steptoe Department of Epidemiology and Public Health, University College London, London, UK

Stephen M. Weiss Department of Psychiatry and Behavioral Sciences, University of Miami Miller School of Medicine, Miami, FL, USA

Redford B. Williams Division of Behavioral Medicine, Duke University, Durham, NC, USA

Contributors

David B. Abrams Johns Hopkins Bloomberg School of Public Health, The Schroeder Institute for Tobacco Research and Policy Studies at Legacy, Washington, DC, USA

Howard Aizenstein Geriatric Psychiatry Neuroimaging, Western Psychiatric Institute and Clinic, University of Pittsburgh Medical Center, Pittsburgh, PA, USA

Tatsuo Akechi Department of Psychiatry and Cognitive-Behavioral Medicine, Graduate School of Medical Sciences, Nagoya City University, Mizuho-cho, Mizuho-ku, Nagoya, Japan

Mustafa al'Absi University of Minnesota Medical School, School of Medicine, University of Minnesota, Duluth, MN, USA

Jessica Alcorso Macquarie University, Sydney, NSW, Australia

Melissa A. Alderfer Division of Oncology, The Children's Hospital of Philadelphia, Philadelphia, PA, USA

Sarah Aldred School of Sport and Exercise Sciences, The University of Birmingham, Edgbaston, Birmingham, UK

Katie E. Alegria Psychological Sciences, University of California, Merced, Merced, CA, USA

Nida Ali Department of Psychology, University of Vienna, Vienna, Austria

Julia Allan School of Medicine and Dentistry, University of Aberdeen, Aberdeen, Scotland, UK

Peter Allebeck Department of Public Health Sciences, Karolinska Institute, Stockholm, Sweden

Josh Allen Care and Compliance Group, Inc., American Assisted Living Nurses Association, Wildomar, CA, USA

Bruce S. Alpert Department of Pediatrics, University of Tennessee Health Science Center, Memphis, TN, USA

Leila Anane School of Sport and Exercise Sciences, The University of Birmingham, Edgbaston, Birmingham, UK

David E. Anderson Division of Nephrology, Department of Medicine, University of California, San Francisco, CA, USA

Giles M. Anderson Oxford Brookes University, Oxford, UK

Norman B. Anderson Faculty Leadership Development Program, Florida State University, Tallahassee, FL, USA

Gerhard Andersson Department of Behavioural Science and Learning, Linköping University, Linköping, Sweden

Tetusya Ando Department of Psychosomatic Research, National Institute of Mental Health, National Center of Neurology and Psychiatry, Kodaira-shi, Tokyo, Japan

Mike Antoni Department of Psychology, University of Miami, Sylvester Cancer Center, Miller School of Medicine, Miami, FL, USA

Hannah Appleseth University of Minnesota Duluth, Duluth, MN, USA

William Arguelles Department of Psychology, University of Miami, Coral Gables, FL, USA

Danielle Arigo Department of Psychology, Rowan University, Glassboro, NJ, USA

Wiebke Arlt Institute of Metabolism and Systems Research, The University of Birmingham, Birmingham, UK

Arpo Aromaa Health and Functional Capacity, National Institute for Health and Welfare, Helsinki, Finland

Elva Arredondo Division of Health Promotion and Behavioral Sciences, San Diego State University, San Diego, CA, USA

Lisa G. Aspinwall Department of Psychology, The University of Utah, Salt Lake City, UT, USA

Kristin J. August Department of Psychology, Rutgers University, Camden, NJ, USA

Robin Austin School of Nursing, University of Minnesota, Minneapolis, MN, USA

Kieran Ayling Division of Primary Care, School of Medicine, University of Nottingham, Nottingham, UK

Simon L. Bacon Department of Exercise Science, Concordia University and Montreal Behavioural Medicine Centre, CIUSSS-NIM: Hopital du Sacre-Coeur de Montreal, Montreal, QC, Canada

Department of Health, Kinesiology, and Applied Physiology, Concordia University and Montreal Behavioural Medicine Centre, CIUSSS du Nord-de-l'île-de-Montréal, Montreal, QC, Canada

Rachel N. Baek Clinical Psychology, Health Emphasis, Ferkauf Graduate School of Psychology, Yeshiva University, Bronx, NY, USA

Jonathan Z. Bakdash Department of Psychology and Special Education, Texas A&M–Commerce, Commerce, TX, USA

Elizabeth Baker Department of Psychology, University of Miami, Coral Gables, FL, USA

Priya Balaji Department of Medicine and Program in Health Disparities Research, University of Minnesota Medical School, Minneapolis, MN, USA

Austin S. Baldwin Department of Psychology, Southern Methodist University, Dallas, TX, USA

Chad Barrett Department of Psychology, University of Colorado, Denver, CO, USA

Jennifer A. Bartz Department of Psychology, McGill University, Montreal, QC, Canada

Abigail Batchelder Diabetes Research Center, Albert Einstein College of Medicine, Yeshiva University, Bronx, NY, USA

Michele Crites Battié Department of Physical Therapy, University of Alberta, Edmonton, AB, Canada

G. David Batty Department of Epidemiology and Public Health, University College London, London, UK

Carolyn Baum Program in Occupational Therapy, Washington University School of Medicine in St. Louis, St. Louis, MO, USA

Linda C. Baumann School of Nursing, University of Wisconsin-Madison, Madison, WI, USA

Elliott A. Beaton Department of Psychiatry and Behavioral Sciences and the M.I.N.D. Institute, University of California-Davis, Sacramento, CA, USA

C. Andres Bedoya Behavioral Medicine Service Department of Psychiatry, Massachusetts General Hospital, Harvard Medical School, Boston, MA, USA

Catherine Benedict Department of Psychology, University of Miami, Coral Gables, FL, USA

M. Bernardine Centers for Behavioral and Preventive Medicine, Brown University, Providence, RI, USA

Ryan M. Beveridge Department of Psychological and Brain Sciences, University of Delaware, Newark, DE, USA

Stephen Birch Clinical Epidemiology and Biostatistics (CHEPA), McMaster University, Hamilton, ON, Canada

Orit Birnbaum-Weitzman Department of Psychology, University of Miami, Miami, FL, USA

Kacie Allen Blackman Department of Human Nutrition, Foods, and Exercise, Virginia Tech, Blacksburg, VA, USA

Twyla Blackmond Larnell Loyola University Chicago, Chicago, IL, USA

James A. Blumenthal Department of Psychiatry and Behavioral Sciences, Duke University Medical Center, Durham, NC, USA

Guy Bodenmann Department of Psychology, University of Zurich, Zurich, Switzerland

Marie Boltz The Pennsylvania State University College of Nursing, State College, PA, USA

Susan J. Bondy Dalla Lana School of Public Health, University of Toronto, Toronto, ON, Canada

Stephan Bongard Department of Psychology, Goethe-University, Frankfurt am Main, Germany

Brian Borsari Department of Veterans Affairs Medical Center, Mental Health Service, San Francisco, CA, USA

Department of Behavioral and Social Sciences, Center for Alcohol and Addiction Studies, Brown University, Providence, RI, USA

Jos A. Bosch Department of Clinical Psychology, Faculty of Social and Behavioral Sciences, University of Amsterdam, Amsterdam, The Netherlands

Stephanie Bowlin Department of Psychology, University of Kansas, Lawrence, KS, USA

Sophia Brady School of Sport, Exercise and Rehabilitation Sciences, University of Birmingham, Birmingham, UK

Nicole Brandt School of Pharmacy, University of Maryland, Baltimore, MD, USA

Lauren Brenner Center for Behavioral Intervention Technologies, Northwestern University, Chicago, IL, USA

Dana Brimmer Division of High-Consequence Pathogens and Pathology, Centers for Disease Control and Prevention, McKing Consulting Corporation, Atlanta, GA, USA

Carrie Brintz Department of Psychology, University of Miami, Coral Gables, FL, USA

Caitlin A. Bronson Department of Psychology, Rutgers, The State University of New Jersey, Piscataway, NJ, USA

J. F. Brosschot Clinical, Health and Neuro Psychology, Leiden University, Leiden, The Netherlands

Frankie F. Brown Department for Health, University of Bath, Bath, UK

Jennifer L. Brown Department of Behavioral Sciences and Health Education, Emory University School of Public Health, Atlanta, GA, USA

Bonnie Bruce Division of Immunology and Rheumatology, Stanford University Department of Medicine, Palo Alto, CA, USA

Vaughn Bryant Behavioral and Social Sciences, Brown University, Providence, RI, USA

Patrícia Cardoso Buchain Occupational Therapist of the Occupational Therapy Service, Institute of Psychiatry – Hospital das Clínicas University of São Paulo Medical School, São Paulo, SP, Brazil

Tony W. Buchanan Department of Psychology, Saint Louis University, Saint Louis, MO, USA

Ross Buck Communication Sciences and Psychology, University of Connecticut, Storrs, CT, USA

Romola S. Bucks School of Psychological Science, The University of Western Australia (M304), Perth, WA, Australia

Donna C. Burdzy Department of Psychology, Bowling Green State University, Bowling Green, OH, USA

Rachel J. Burns Department of Psychiatry, McGill University, Montreal, QC, Canada

Michelle Nicole Burns Feinberg School of Medicine, Department of Preventive Medicine, Center for Behavioral Intervention Technologies, Northwestern University, Chicago, IL, USA

Victoria E. Burns School of Sport and Exercise Sciences, The University of Birmingham, Edgbaston, Birmingham, UK

David Busse Department of Psychology and Social Behaviour, University of California, Irvine, Irvine, CA, USA

Natalie E. Bustillo Department of Psychology, University of Miami, Coral Gables, FL, USA

Colin D. Butler National Centre for Epidemiology and Population Health, Australian National University, Canberra, ACT, Australia

College of Arts, Humanities and Social Sciences, Flinders University, Adelaide, Australia

Jorie Butler Department of Psychology, University of Utah, Salt Lake City, UT, USA

Melissa M. A. Buttner Department of Psychology, University of Iowa, Iowa City, IA, USA

John T. Cacioppo Department of Psychology, The University of Chicago, Chicago, IL, USA

Demetria Cain Center for Health Intervention and Prevention, University of Connecticut, Storrs, CT, USA

Matthew Calamia Department of Psychology, University of Iowa, Iowa City, IA, USA

David Cameron Information School, The University of Sheffield, Sheffield, UK

Linda D. Cameron Psychological Sciences, University of California, Merced, Merced, CA, USA

Nerissa Campbell Exercise and Health Psychology Laboratory, The University of Western Ontario, London, ON, Canada

Tavis S. Campbell Department of Psychology, University of Calgary, Calgary, AB, Canada

Turhan Canli Department of Psychology, Stony Brook University Psychology B-214, Stony Brook, NY, USA

Leeanne M. Carey Occupational Therapy, School of Allied Health, La Trobe University, Melbourne, VIC, Australia

Rachel Carey University College London, London, UK

Jordan Carlson Public Health, San Diego State University, University of California San Diego, San Diego, CA, USA

Adriana Carrillo Department of Pediatrics, Miller School of Medicine, University of Miami, Miami, FL, USA

Douglas Carroll School of Sport and Exercise Sciences, The University of Birmingham, Edgbaston, Birmingham, UK

Judith Carroll Cousins Center for Psychoneuroimmunology, University of California, Los Angeles, CA, USA

Linda Carroll Department of Public Health Sciences, University of Alberta, Edmonton, AB, Canada

Jennifer Carter The University of Iowa, Iowa City, IA, USA

Charles Carver Department of Psychology, University of Miami, Coral Gables, FL, USA

Pedro C. Castellon Epidemiology and Public Health, Miller School of Medicine, University of Miami, Miami, FL, USA

Fong Chan Department of Rehabilitation Psychology and Special Education, University of Wisconsin-Madison, Madison, WI, USA

Sherilynn F. Chan Cincinnati Children's Hospital Medical Center, University of Cincinnati College of Medicine, Cincinnati, OH, USA

Matthieu Chansard Department of Psychiatry, The University of Texas Southwestern Medical Center at Dallas Columbia University/New York State Psychiatric Institute, Dallas, TX, USA

Stephenie Chaudoir Department of Psychology, Bradley University, Peoria, IL, USA

Margaret A. Chesney Department of Medicine and Osher Center for Integrative Medicine, University of California, San Francisco, CA, USA

Ornit Chiba-Falek Duke University Medical Center, Durham, NC, USA

Yoichi Chida Faculty of Human Happiness Office 4, Happy Science University 4F, Chosei-mura, Chosei-gun, Japan
Department of Medical Science, Happy Science Clinic, Kawasaki City, Japan

Olveen Carrasquillo Chief Division of General Internal Medicine, Miller School of Medicine, University of Miami, Miami, FL, USA

Michael S. Chmielewski Department of Psychology, University of Toronto, Toronto, ON, Canada

Julie Chronister Department of Counseling, San Francisco State University, San Francisco, CA, USA

Linda Cillessen Center for Mindfulness, Department of Psychiatry, Radboud University Medical Center, Nijmegen, The Netherlands
Donders Institute for Brain, Cognition and Behaviour, Radboud University, Nijmegen, The Netherlands

Molly S. Clark Midwestern University College of Health Sciences, Clinical Psychology, Glendale, AZ, USA

Tyler Clark School of Psychology, The University of Sydney, Sydney, NSW, Australia

Benjamin L. Clarke Academic Health Center, School of Medicine-Duluth Campus, University of Minnesota, Duluth, MN, USA

Tainya C. Clarke Department of Epidemiology and Public Health, Miller School of Medicine, University of Miami, Miami, FL, USA

Lindy Clemson Ageing, Work and Health Research Unit, Faculty of Health Sciences, University of Sydney, Lidcombe, NSW, Australia

Stephen Clift Sidney de Haan Research Centre for Arts and Health, Canterbury Christ Church University, Canterbury, UK

Lorenzo Cohen Department of Palliative, Rehabilitation, and Interactive Medicine, Division of Cancer Medicine, The University of Texas MD Anderson Cancer Center, Houston, TX, USA

Susan E. Collins Department of Psychiatry and Behavioral Sciences, University of Washington, Harborview Medical Center, Seattle, WA, USA

Persis Commissariat Clinical Psychology, Health Emphasis, Ferkauf Graduate School of Psychology, Yeshiva University, Bronx, NY, USA

Félix R. Compen Center for Mindfulness, Department of Psychiatry, Radboud University Medical Center, Nijmegen, The Netherlands

Donders Institute for Brain, Cognition and Behaviour, Radboud University, Nijmegen, The Netherlands

Richard J. Contrada Department of Psychology, Rutgers, The State University of New Jersey, Piscataway, NJ, USA

Michael James Coons Department of Preventive Medicine, Feinberg School of Medicine, Northwestern University, Chicago, IL, USA

Susannah D. Copland Obstetrics and Gynecology, Division of Reproductive Endocrinology and Fertility, Duke Fertility Center, Durham, NC, USA

Quirino Cordeiro Department of Psychiatry and Psychological Medicine, Santa Casa Medical School, São Paulo, SP, Brazil

Erin S. Costanzo Department of Psychiatry, Carbone Cancer Center, University of Wisconsin-Madison, Madison, WI, USA

Simon J. Craddock Lee Department of Clinical Sciences, The University of Texas Southwestern Medical Center, Dallas, TX, USA

Monique F. Crane Macquarie University, North Ryde/Sydney, NSW, Australia

Jennifer Creek Occupational Therapist, Guisborough, North Yorkshire, UK

Matthew Cribbet Department of Psychology, University of Utah, Salt Lake City, UT, USA

Hugo Critchley Brighton and Sussex Medical School, University of Sussex, Brighton, East Sussex, UK

Crista N. Crittenden Department of Psychology, Carnegie Mellon University, Pittsburgh, PA, USA

Sierra Cronan Department of Psychology and Health Psychology Program, University of Utah, Salt Lake City, UT, USA

Andrea Croom Department of Psychology, University of Texas Southwestern Medical Center, Dallas, TX, USA

Rick Crosby University of Kentucky, Lexington, KY, USA

Jennifer Cumming School of Sport and Exercise Sciences, The University of Birmingham, Edgbaston, Birmingham, UK

Cassie Cunningham College of Public Health, University of Iowa, Liberty, IA, USA

Maurizio Cutolo Department of Internal Medicine, Research Laboratories and Academic Unit of Clinical Rheumatology, University of Genova, Genoa, Italy

Elizabeth da Silva Cardoso Department of Educational Foundations and Counseling Programs, The City University of New York-Hunter College, New York, NY, USA

Amber Daigre Department of Pediatrics, University of Miami Miller School of Medicine, Miami, FL, USA

Catherine Darker Public Health and Primary Care, Institute of Population Health, School of Medicine, Trinity College Dublin, The University of Dublin, Dublin, Ireland

Karina Davidson Department of Medicine, Columbia University Medical Center, New York, NY, USA

Gary Davis Medical School Duluth, University of Minnesota, Duluth, MN, USA

Mary C. Davis Department of Psychology, Arizona State University, Tempe, AZ, USA

Karen Dawe School of Social and Community Medicine, University of Bristol, Bristol, UK

Marijke De Couck Free University of Brussels (VUB), Jette, Belgium

Stefanie De Jesus Exercise and Health Psychology Laboratory, The University of Western Ontario, London, ON, Canada

Karla Espinosa de los Monteros Clinical Psychology, SDSU/UCSD Joint Doctoral Program in Clinical Psychology, San Diego, CA, USA

Alexandra Martini de Oliveira Occupational Therapy Service, Institute of Psychiatry – Hospital das Clínicas University of São Paulo Medical School, São Paulo, SP, Brazil

Maartje de Wit Medical Psychology, VU University Medical Center, Amsterdam, North Holland, The Netherlands

Denise de Ybarra Rodríguez Department of Psychology, University of Miami, Coral Gables, FL, USA

Scott DeBerard Department of Psychology, Utah State University, Logan, UT, USA

Joost Dekker Department of Psychiatry and Department of Rehabilitation Medicine, VU University Medical Centre, Amsterdam, The Netherlands

Alan M. Delamater Department of Pediatrics, University of Miami Miller School of Medicine, Miami, FL, USA

Kelly S. DeMartini Division of Substance Abuse, School of Medicine, Yale University, New Haven, CT, USA

Michael I. Demidenko VA Portland Health Care System, Portland, OR, USA

Oregon Health and Science University, Portland, OR, USA

Johan Denollet CoRPS – Center of Research on Psychology in Somatic diseases, Tilburg University, Tilburg, The Netherlands

Ellen-ge Denton Department of Medicine Center for Behavioral Cardiovascular Health, Columbia University Medical Center, New York, NY, USA

Stuart Derbyshire National University of Singapore, Singapore, Singapore

Martin Deschner Psychiatry, Division of Psychology, The University of Texas Southwestern Medical Center at Dallas, Dallas, TX, USA

Tamer F. Desouky Department of Psychology, The University of Texas at Arlington, Arlington, TX, USA

Mary Amanda Dew School of Medicine and Medical Center, University of Pittsburgh, Pittsburgh, PA, USA

Sally Dickerson Pace University, New York, NY, USA

Andrea F. DiMartini School of Medicine and Medical Center, University of Pittsburgh, Pittsburgh, PA, USA

Joel E. Dimsdale Department of Psychiatry, University of California San Diego, La Jolla, CA, USA

Ding Ding Graduate School of Public Health/Department of Family Preventive Medicine, San Diego State University/University of California San Diego, San Diego, CA, USA

Genevieve A. Dingle The University of Queensland, Brisbane, QLD, Australia

Beate Ditzen Department of Psychosocial Medicine, Heidelberg University, Heidelberg, Germany

Diane Dixon Department of Psychology, University of Strathclyde, Scotland, UK

Kelly Doran University of Maryland, Baltimore School of Nursing, Baltimore, MD, USA

Susan Dorsey School of Nursing, University of Maryland, Baltimore, MD, USA

Monica Dowling Miller School of Medicine, University of Miami, Miami, FL, USA

Mark T. Drayson College of Medical and Dental Sciences, University of Birmingham, Edgbaston, Birmingham, UK

Michelle Drerup Sleep Disorders Center Neurological Institute, Cleveland Clinic, Cleveland, OH, USA

Frank A. Drews Department of Psychology, University of Utah, Salt Lake City, UT, USA

Center for Human Factors in Patient Safety, VA Salt Lake City Health Care System, Salt Lake City, UT, USA

Suzana Drobnjak Department of Psychology, University of Zurich, Binzmuehlestrasse, Switzerland

Joan L. Duda School of Sport, Exercise and Rehabilitation Sciences, University of Birmingham, Birmingham, UK

Alejandra Duenas School of Management, IESEG, Paris, France

Joan Duer-Hefele Columbia University, New York, NY, USA

Mariam Dum Jackson Memorial Hospital, Miami, FL, USA

Jennifer Duncan Department of Preventive Medicine, Feinberg School of Medicine, Northwestern University, Chicago, IL, USA

Christine Dunkel Schetter Department of Psychology, University of California, Los Angeles (UCLA), Los Angeles, CA, USA

Valerie Earnshaw Department of Public Health, Yale University, New Haven, CT, USA

Lisa A. Eaton Center for Health, Intervention, and Prevention, University of Connecticut, New Haven, CT, USA

Moritz Thede Eckart General and Biological Psychology, Department of Psychology, University of Marburg, Marburg, Germany

Ulrike Ehlert Department of Psychology, University of Zurich, Zurich, Switzerland

Alexandre Elhalwi McGill University, Montreal, QC, Canada

Lorin Elias Department of Psychology, University of Saskatchewan, Saskatoon, SK, Canada

Helio Elkis Department and Institute of Psychiatry, University of São Paulo Medical School, São Paulo, SP, Brazil

Lee Ellington Department of Nursing, College of Nursing, University of Utah, Salt Lake City, UT, USA

Christopher G. Engeland Department of Biobehavioral Health, The Pennsylvania State University, University Park, PA, USA

Elissa S. Epel Department of Psychiatry, Weill Institute for Neurosciences, University of California, San Francisco, CA, USA

Jennifer Toller Erausquin Department of Public Health Education, University of North Carolina at Greensboro, Greensboro, NC, USA

Alexandra Erdmann Department of Psychiatry, Carbone Cancer Center, University of Wisconsin-Madison, Madison, WI, USA

Sabrina Esbitt Clinical Psychology, Health Emphasis, Ferkauf Graduate School of Psychology, Yeshiva University, Bronx, NY, USA

Shaniff Esmail Department of Occupational Therapy, University of Alberta, Edmonton, AB, Canada

Paul Estabrooks Department of Health Promotions, University of Nebraska Medical Center, Omaha, NE, USA

Susan A. Everson-Rose Department of Medicine and Program in Health Disparities Research, University of Minnesota Medical School, Minneapolis, MN, USA

Rachel Faller Department of Public Health Education, University of North Carolina at Greensboro, Greensboro, NC, USA

Anja C. Feneberg Department of Applied Psychology: Health, Development, Enhancement and Intervention, Faculty of Psychology, University of Vienna, Vienna, Austria

Sally A. M. Fenton School of Sport, Exercise and Rehabilitation Sciences, University of Birmingham, Birmingham, UK

Susan J. (Sue) Ferguson Department of Psychology, Macquarie University, Sydney, NSW, Australia

Cristina A. Fernandez Department of Epidemiology and Public Health, Miller School of Medicine, University of Miami, Miami, FL, USA

Tania C. T. Ferraz Alves Department and Institute of Psychiatry, University of São Paulo Medical School, São Paulo, SP, Brazil

Angela Fidler Pfammatter Feinberg School of Medicine, Northwestern University, Chicago, IL, USA

Tiffany Field Touch Research Institute, University of Miami, School of Medicine, Miami, FL, USA

Robyn Fielder Center for Health and Behavior, Syracuse University, Syracuse, NY, USA

David J. Finitsis Department of Psychology, University of Connecticut, Storrs, CT, USA

Simona Fischbacher Klinische Psychologie und Psychotherapie, Universität Zürich, Zürich, Switzerland

Susanne Fischer Clinical Psychology and Psychotherapy, Institute of Psychology, University of Zurich, Zurich, Switzerland

Skye Fitzpatrick Department of Psychology, Ryerson University, Toronto, ON, Canada

Kelly Flannery School of Nursing, University of Maryland Baltimore, Baltimore, MD, USA

Magne Arve Flaten Department of Psychology, University of Tromsø, Tromsø, Norway

Sara Fleszar University of California, Merced, Merced, CA, USA

Serina Floyd Obstetrics and Gynecology, Duke Hospital, Raleigh, NC, USA

Rachel Flurie University of Maryland, Baltimore, MD, USA

Susan Folkman Department of Medicine, School of Medicine, University of California San Francisco, San Mateo, CA, USA

Katherine T. Fortenberry Department of Family and Preventative Medicine, The University of Utah, Salt Lake City, UT, USA

Andrew Fox Recovery and Wellbeing Inpatient Services, Birmingham and Solihull Mental Health NHS Trust, Birmingham, West Midlands, UK

Kristen R. Fox Nationwide Childrens Hospital, Columbus, OH, USA

Christopher France Department of Psychology, Ohio University, Athens, OH, USA

Janis L. France Department of Psychology, Ohio University, Athens, OH, USA

Renée-Louise Franche School of Population and Public Health, University of British Columbia, Vancouver, BC, Canada

WorkSafe BC, Vancouver, BC, Canada

Institute for Work and Health, Toronto, ON, Canada

Anne Frankel Robert Stempel College of Public Health and Social Work, Florida International University, Miami, FL, USA

Elizabeth J. Franzmann Department of Otolaryngology, Division of Head and Neck Surgery, Miller School of Medicine, University of Miami, Miami, FL, USA

Fred Friedberg Psychiatry and Behavioral Sciences, Stony Brook University Medical Center, Stony Brook, NY, USA

Georita Marie Frierson Department of Psychology, Southern Methodist University, Dallas, TX, USA

Shin Fukudo Department of Behavioral Medicine, School of Medicine, Tohoku University Graduate, Seiryo-machi, Aoba-ku, Sendai, Japan

Terry Fulmer Bouvé College of Health Sciences, Northeastern University, Boston, MA, USA

Julianne Holt-Lunstad Fulton Department of Psychology, Brigham Young University, Provo, UT, USA

Jens Gaab Clinical Psychology and Psychotherapy, Department of Psychology, University of Basel, Basel, Switzerland

Amiram Gafni Department of Clinical Epidemiology and Biostatistics, Centre for Health Economics and Policy Analysis, McMaster University, Hamilton, ON, Canada

Elizabeth Galik School of Nursing, University of Maryland, Baltimore, MD, USA

Stephen Gallagher Department of Psychology, Faculty of Education and Health Sciences, University of Limerick, Castletroy, Limerick, Ireland

Steven Gambert Department of Medicine, School of Medicine, University of Maryland, Baltimore, MD, USA

Luis I. García Center for AIDS Intervention Research, Medical College of Wisconsin, Milwaukee, WI, USA

M. Kay Garcia Department of Palliative, Rehabilitation, and Interactive Medicine, Division of Cancer Medicine, The University of Texas MD Anderson Cancer Center, Houston, TX, USA

Ryan Garcia University of Texas Southwestern Medical Center at Dallas, Dallas, TX, USA

Luz M. Garcini Ethnic Minority and Multicultural Health SBM SIG Co-Chair, SDSU/UCSD Joint Doctoral Program in Clinical Psychology, San Diego, CA, USA

Stephanie L. Garey Department of Clinical and Health Psychology, College of Clinical Health and Health Professions, University of Florida, Gainesville, FL, USA

Mariana Garza Department of Psychology, University of North Texas, Denton, TX, USA

Robert J. Gatchel Department of Psychology, College of Science, University of Texas at Arlington, Arlington, TX, USA

Klaus Gebel School of Education, University of Newcastle, University Drive, Callaghan, NSW, Australia

City Futures Research Centre, University of New South Wales, Sydney, NSW, Australia

Pamela A. Geller Department of Psychology, Drexel University; Drexel University College of Medicine, Philadelphia, PA, USA

Marc D. Gellman Behavioral Medicine Research Center, Department of Psychology, University of Miami, Miami, FL, USA

Login S. George Department of Psychology, University of Connecticut, Storrs, CT, USA

William Gerin The College of Health and Human Development, University Park, PA, USA

Denis Gerstorf Institute of Psychology, Humboldt University, Berlin, Germany

Isha Ghosh School of Communication and Information, Rutgers University, New Brunswick, NJ, USA

Yori Gidron SCALab, Lille 3 University and Siric Oncollile, Lille, France

Supria K. Gill VA Portland Health Care System, Portland, OR, USA

Palo Alto University, Palo Alto, CA, USA

Annie T. Ginty School of Sport and Exercise Sciences, The University of Birmingham, Edgbaston, Birmingham, UK

Karen Glanz Schools of Medicine and Nursing, University of Pennsylvania, Philadelphia, PA, USA

Elizabeth Gleyzer Department of Psychology, William James College, Newton, MA, USA

Ronald Goldberg Diabetes Research Institute, University of Miami Miller School of Medicine, Miami, FL, USA

Carly M. Goldstein The Weight Control and Diabetes Research Center, The Miriam Hospital, Providence, RI, USA

Warren Alpert Medical School, Brown University, Providence, RI, USA

Stephanie P. Goldstein Warren Alpert Medical School, Brown University, Providence, RI, USA

Peter M. Gollwitzer Department of Psychology, New York University, New York, NY, USA

Heather Honoré Goltz HSR&D Center of Excellence, Michael E. DeBakey VA Medical Center (MEDVAMC 152), Houston, TX, USA

Department of Social Sciences, University of Houston-Downtown, Houston, TX, USA

Carley Gomez-Meade Department of Pediatrics, Miller School of Medicine, University of Miami, Miami, FL, USA

Jeffrey S. Gonzalez Departments of Medicine and Epidemiology & Public Health, Albert Einstein College of Medicine, Bronx, NY, USA

Patricia Gonzalez Institute for Behavioral and Community Health (IBACH), Graduate School of Public Health, San Diego State University, San Diego, CA, USA

Jeffrey L. Goodie Department of Medical and Clinical Psychology, Uniformed Services University of the Health Sciences, Bethesda, MD, USA

Daniel Gorrin Department of Physical Therapy, University of Delaware, Newark, DE, USA

John Grabowski Department of Psychiatry, Medical School, University of Minnesota, Minneapolis, MN, USA

Douglas A. Granger Center for Interdisciplinary Salivary Bioscience Research, School of Nursing, Bloomberg School of Public Health, and School of Medicine The Johns Hopkins University, Baltimore, MD, USA

Douglas P. Gross Department of Physical Therapy, University of Alberta, Edmonton, AB, Canada

Beth Grunfeld Department of Psychological Sciences, Birkbeck College, University of London, London, UK

Jessica Haberer Medicine and Center for Global Health, Massachusetts General Hospital, Harvard University, Boston, MA, USA

Tibor Hajos Medical Psychology, VU University Medical Center, Amsterdam, North Holland, The Netherlands

Chanita H. Halbert School of Medicine, University of Pennsylvania, Philadelphia, PA, USA

Judith A. Hall Department of Psychology, Northeastern University, Boston, MA, USA

Katherine S. Hall Durham VA Medical Center Geriatric Research, Education, and Clinical Center, Durham, NC, USA

Martica H. Hall Department of Psychiatry, University of Pittsburgh, Pittsburgh, PA, USA

Peter A. Hall Faculty of Applied Health Sciences, University of Waterloo, Waterloo, ON, Canada

Heidi Hamann Department of Psychiatry, UT Southwestern Medical Center, Dallas, TX, USA

Mark Hamer Epidemiology and Public Health, Division of Population Health, University College London, London, UK

Fiona Louise Hamilton University College London, London, UK

Kyra Hamilton School of Applied Psychology, Menzies Health Institute Queensland, Griffith University, Brisbane, QLD, Australia

Margaret Hammersla University of Maryland School of Nursing, Baltimore, MD, USA

Reiner Hanewinkel Institute for Therapy and Health Research, Kiel, Germany

Nelli Hankonen Department of Lifestyle and Participation, National Institute for Health and Welfare University of Helsinki, Helsinki, Finland

Kazuo Hara Department of Metabolic Diseases, Graduate School of Medicine, The University of Tokyo, Bunkyo-ku, Tokyo, Japan

Samantha M. Harden Department of Human Nutrition, Foods, and Exercise, Virginia Tech, Blacksburg, VA, USA

Manjunath Harlapur Center of Behavioral Cardiovascular Health, Division of General Medicine, Columbia University, New York, NY, USA

John Harlow School for the Future of Innovation in Society, Arizona State University, Tempe, AZ, USA

Victoria Harms Department of Psychology, University of Saskatchewan, Saskatoon, SK, Canada

Lisa Harnack Division of Epidemiology and Community Health, School of Public Health, University of Minnesota, Minneapolis, MN, USA

Stacey L. Hart Department of Psychology, Ryerson University, Toronto, ON, Canada

Briain O. Hartaigh School of Sport and Exercise Sciences, The University of Birmingham, Edgbaston, Birmingham, UK

Alison Hartman Department of Psychology, Drexel University, Philadelphia, PA, USA

Steven Harulow Royal College of Speech and Language Therapists, London, UK

Toshihide Hashimoto Division of Rehabilitation, Joumou Hospital, Maebashi, Japan

Masahiro Hashizume Department of Psychosomatic Medicine, Faculty of Medicine, Toho University, Ota-ku, Tokyo, Japan

Brant P. Hasler Western Psychiatric Institute and Clinic University of Pittsburgh School of Medicine, Pittsburgh, PA, USA

Misty A. W. Hawkins Department of Psychology, Oklahoma State University, Stillwater, OK, USA

Louise C. Hawkley Academic Research Centers, NORC at the University of Chicago, Chicago, IL, USA

Calvin Haws Workers' Compensation Board of Alberta Millard Health, Edmonton, AB, Canada

Laura L. Hayman College of Nursing and Health Sciences, University of Massachusetts Boston, Boston, MA, USA

Jennifer Heaney Clinical Immunology Service, The University of Birmingham, Birmingham, UK

Christine Heim Institute of Medical Psychology, Charité University Medicine Berlin, Berlin, Germany

Eric B. Hekler Nutrition Program, School of Nutrition and Health Promotion, Arizona State University, Phoenix, AZ, USA

Lois Jane Heller Department of Biomedical Sciences, University of Minnesota Medical School – Duluth, Duluth, MN, USA

Miranda Hellman Boston University, Boston, MA, USA

Whitney M. Herge Department of Psychology, Texas Scottish Rite Hospital for Children, Dallas, TX, USA

Patricia Cristine Heyn Department of Physical Medicine and Rehabilitation, University of Colorado Denver Anschutz Medical Campus School of Medicine, Aurora, CO, USA

Emma Hiatt Rehabilitaion Psychology and Special Education, University of Wisconsin-Madison, Madison, WI, USA

Angela M. Hicks Department of Psychology, Westminster College, Salt Lake City, UT, USA

Benjamin Hidalgo Department of Psychiatry, Medical College of Wisconsin, Milwaukee, WI, USA

Catharina Hjortsberg The Swedish Institute for Health Economics, Lund, Sweden

Clare Hocking Faculty of Health and Environmental Sciences, Auckland University of Technology, Auckland, New Zealand

Richard Hoffman Academic Health Center, School of Medicine-Duluth Campus University of Minnesota, Duluth, MN, USA

Sara A. Hoffman Feinberg School of Medicine, Northwestern University, Evanston, IL, USA

Maxine Holmqvist Clinical Health Psychology, University of Manitoba, Winnipeg, MB, Canada

Emily D. Hooker Psychology and Social Behaviour, University of California, Irvine, Irvine, CA, USA

Stephanie Ann Hooker Department of Psychology, University of Colorado Denver, Denver, CO, USA

Monica Webb Hooper Department of Psychology, University of Miami, Coral Gables, FL, USA

Christiane A. Hoppmann Department of Psychology, University of British Columbia, Vancouver, BC, Canada

M. Bryant Howren Department of Psychology, The University of Iowa and Iowa City VA Healthcare System, Iowa City, IA, USA

Brian M. Hughes School of Psychology, National University of Ireland, Galway, Galway, Ireland

Ryan Hulla Department of Psychology, College of Science, University of Texas at Arlington, Arlington, TX, USA

Mann Hyung Hur Public Administration, Chung-Ang University, Seoul, Korea

Seth Hurley Department of Psychology, University of Iowa, Iowa City, IA, USA

Mustafa M. Husain Department of Psychiatry, The University of Texas Southwestern Medical Center at Dallas Columbia University/New York State Psychiatric Institute, Dallas, TX, USA

John Hustad Department of Medicine and Public Health Sciences, Penn State College of Medicine, Hershey, PA, USA

Shannon Idzik University of Maryland School of Nursing, Baltimore, MD, USA

University of Maryland Upper Chesapeake Health Comprehensive CARE Center, Bel Air, MD, USA

Shuji Inada Department of Stress Science and Psychosomatic Medicine, Graduate School of Medicine, The University of Tokyo, Tokyo, Japan

Salvatore Insana Western Psychiatric Institute and Clinic, Pittsburgh, PA, USA

Leah Irish Department of Psychiatry, School of Medicine, Universitsy of Pittsburghe, Pittsburgh, PA, USA

Daisuke Ito Department Clinical Psychology, Graduate School of Education, Hyogo University to Teacher Education, Kato, Hyogo, Japan

Makiko Ito Department of Stress Science and Psychosomatic Medicine, Graduate School of Medicine, The University of Tokyo, Bunkyo-ku, Tokyo, Japan

Satoru Iwase Department Of Palliative Medicine, The University of Tokyo Hospital, Tokyo, Japan

Karen Jacobs Occupational Therapy, College of Health and Rehabilitation Science, Sargent College, Boston University, Boston, MA, USA

Farrah Jacquez Department of Psychology, University of Cincinnati, Cincinnati, OH, USA

Denise Janicki-Deverts Department of Psychology, Carnegie Mellon University, Pittsburgh, PA, USA

Kate L. Jansen Behavioral Health, Midwestern University, Glendale, AZ, USA

Department of Family Medicine, University of Mississippi Medical Center, Jackson, MS, USA

Imke Janssen Department of Preventive Medicine, Rush University Medical Center, Chicago, IL, USA

Lisa M. Jaremka Department of Psychological and Brain Sciences, University of Delaware, Newark, DE, USA

Elissa Jelalian Department of Psychiatry, Rhode Island Hospital, Brown Medical School, Providence, RI, USA

Chad D. Jensen Department of Psychology, Brigham Young University, Provo, UT, USA

Jason Jent Department of Pediatrics, Mailman Center for Child Development, University of Miami, Miami, FL, USA

Rong Jiang Department of Psychiatry and Behavioral Sciences, Duke University, Durham, NC, USA

Alvin Jin Department of Psychology, University of South Florida College of Arts and Sciences, Tampa, FL, USA

Debra Johnson Department of Psychology, University of Iowa, Iowa City, IA, USA

Jillian A. Johnson Department of Psychology, University of Calgary, Calgary, AB, Canada

Sara B. Johnson School of Medicine and Bloomberg School of Public Health, Johns Hopkins School of Medicine, Baltimore, MD, USA

Derek Johnston School of Psychology, University of Aberdeen, Aberdeen, UK

Marie Johnston School of Medicine and Dentistry, University of Aberdeen, Aberdeen, UK

Phil Jones School of Geography, Earth and Environmental Sciences, University of Birmingham, Edgbaston, Birmingham, UK

Sarah Jones Skidmore College, Saratoga Springs, NY, USA

Randall Steven Jorgensen Department of Psychology, Syracuse University, Syracuse, USA

Melissa Julian George Washington University, Washington, DC, USA

Kauhanen Jussi Institute of Public Health and Clinical Nutrition, University of Eastern Finland, Kuopio, Finland

Vanessa Juth Nursing Science, University of California Irvine, Irvine, CA, USA

Yoshinobu Kanda Division of Hematology, Jichi Medical University Saitama Medical Center, Omiya-ku, Saitama, Japan

Maria Kangas Department of Psychology, Centre for Emotional Health, Sydney, NSW, Australia

Afton N. Kapuscinski Psychology Department, Syracuse University, Syracuse, NY, USA

Mardís Karlsdóttir Department of Psychology, The University of Iceland School of Health Sciences, Reykjavík, Iceland

Yoko Katayori Department of Behavioral Medicine, School of Medicine, Tohoku University Graduate, Seiryo-machi, Aoba-ku, Sendai, Japan

Erin E. Kauffman Department of Psychology, University of North Texas, Denton, TX, USA

Francine Kaufman Medtronic, Northridge, CA, USA

Peter Kaufmann Division of Prevention and Population Sciences, National Heart, Lung, and Blood Institute Clinical Applications and Prevention Branch, Bethesda, MD, USA

Jacob J. Keech School of Applied Psychology, Menzies Health Institute Queensland, Griffith University, Brisbane, QLD, Australia

Quinn D. Kellerman Department of Psychology, University of Iowa, Iowa City, IA, USA

Alan Kessedjian Clinical Psychologist, Birmingham, UK

Riyad Khanfer School of Sport and Exercise Sciences, The University of Birmingham, Edgbaston, Birmingham, UK

Falk Kiefer Department of Addictive Behaviour and Addiction Medicine, Central Institute of Mental Health, Mannheim, Germany

Hiroe Kikuchi Department of Psychosomatic Medicine, Center Hospital, National Center for Global Health and Medicine, Tokyo, Japan

Kristin Kilbourn Department of Psychology, University of Colorado Denver, Denver, CO, USA

Christopher J. Kilby Centre for Emotional Health, Department of Psychology, Macquarie University, Sydney, NSW, Australia

Tereza Killianova Free University of Brussels (VUB), Jette, Belgium

Jeong Han Kim Department of Clinical Counseling and Mental Health, Texas Tech University Health Science Center, Lubbock, TX, USA

Youngmee Kim Department of Psychology, University of Miami, Coral Gables, FL, USA

Pamela S. King Pediatric Prevention Research Center, Department of Pediatrics, Wayne State University School of Medicine, Detroit, MI, USA

Megan Kirouac Department of Psychiatry and Behavioral Sciences, University of Washington, Harborview Medical Center, Seattle, WA, USA

Clemens Kirschbaum Department of Psychology, Faculty of Psychology, Technische Universität Dresden, Dresden, Germany

George D. Kitas Russells Hall Hospital, The Dudley Group NHS Foundation Trust, Dudley, UK

George D. Kitas Department of Rheumatology, Russells Hall Hospital, Dudley Group NHS Foundation Trust, Dudley, UK

Mika Kivimaki Epidemiology and Public Health, University College London, London, UK

Predrag Klasnja Group Health Research Institute, Seattle, WA, USA

School of Information, University of Michigan, Ann Arbor, MI, USA

Maria Kleinstäuber Department of Clinical Psychology and Psychotherapy, Philipps University, Marburg, Germany

Wendy Kliewer Department of Psychology, Virginia Commonwealth University, Richmond, VA, USA

Christopher E. Kline Department of Health and Physical Activity, University of Pittsburgh, Pittsburgh, PA, USA

Anna K. Koch University of Duisburg-Essen, Essen, Germany

Dorothea König Faculty of Psychology, University of Vienna, Vienna, Austria

Carolyn Korbel The Neurobehavioral Clinic and Counseling Center, Lake Forest, CA, USA

Rachel Kornfield Department of Communication Studies, Northwestern University, Evanston, IL, USA

Emily Kothe School of Psychology, University of Sydney, Sydney, NSW, Australia

Michael Kotlyar Department of Experimental and Clinical Pharmacology, College of Pharmacy, University of Minnesota, Minneapolis, MN, USA

Marc A. Kowalkouski HSR&D Center of Excellence, Michael E. DeBakey VA Medical Center (MEDVAMC 152), Houston, TX, USA

Department of Social Sciences, University of Houston-Downtown, Houston, TX, USA

Tara Kraft Department of Psychology, University of Kansas, Lawrence, KS, USA

Jean L. Kristeller Department of Psychology, Indiana State University, Terre Haute, IN, USA

Kurt Kroenke Department of Medicine, Indiana University, Indianapolis, IN, USA

Regenstrief Institute, Indianapolis, IN, USA

VA HSR&D Center for Implementing Evidence-Based Practice, Indianapolis, IN, USA

Stefan Krumm University of Muenster, Muenster, Germany

Ulrike Kübler Department of Psychology, University of Zurich, Binzmuehlestrasse, Zurich, Switzerland

Laura D. Kubzansky Department of Society, Human Development, and Health, Harvard School of Public Health, Boston, MA, USA

Brigitte M. Kudielka Department of Medical Psychology, Psychological Diagnostics and Research Methodology, University of Regensburg, Regensburg, Germany

Kari C. Kugler Department of Biobehavioral Health, The Pennsylvania State University, University Park, PA, USA

Masayoshi Kumagai Department of Metabolic Diseases, Graduate School of Medicine, The University of Tokyo, Tokyo, Japan

Keiki Kumano Department of Cell Therapy and Transplantation Medicine, The University of Tokyo, Bunkyo-ku, Tokyo, Japan

Yoshihiko Kunisato School of Human Sciences, Senshu University, Kawasaki, Kanagawa, Japan

Elyse Kupperman Clinical Psychology, Health Emphasis, Ferkauf Graduate School of Psychology, Yeshiva University, Bronx, NY, USA

Annette M. La Greca Department of Psychology, University of Miami, Miami, FL, USA

Pearl La Marca-Ghaemmaghami Department of Psychology, Clinical Psychology and Psychotherapy, University of Zurich, Zurich, Switzerland

Seppo Laaksonen University of Helsinki, Helsinki, Finland

Lara LaCaille Department of Psychology, University of Minnesota Duluth, Duluth, MN, USA

Rick LaCaille Psychology Department, University of Minnesota Duluth, Duluth, MN, USA

Laura H. Lacritz Department of Psychology, The University of Texas Southwestern Medical Center at Dallas, Dallas, TX, USA

Karl-Heinz Ladwig Institut für Epidemiologie, GmbH, Neuherberg, Germany

Nathan Landers Department of Psychology, College of Science, University of Texas at Arlington, Arlington, TX, USA

Ryan R. Landoll Uniformed Services University of the Health Sciences, F. Edward Hebert School of Medicine, Bethesda, MD, USA

Joshua Landvatter Department of Psychology and Health Psychology Program, University of Utah, Salt Lake City, UT, USA

Tanja Lange Department of Neuroendocrinology, University of Luebeck, Lübeck, Germany

Brittney Lange-Maia Department of Preventive Medicine, Rush University Medical Center, Chicago, IL, USA

Jost Langhorst Department for Internal and Integrative Medicine, Klinikum Bamberg, Bamberg, Germany

David Latini Scott Department of Urology, Baylor College of Medicine, Houston, TX, USA

Emily Lattie Center for Behavioral Intervention Technologies, Northwestern University, Chicago, IL, USA

Kim Lavoie Department of Psychology, Montreal Behavioural Medicine Centre, University of Québec at Montreal (UQAM), Montréal, QC, Canada

Lauren Law Department of Psychology, University of South Carolina, Columbia, SC, USA

Hannah G. Lawman Department of Psychology, University of South Carolina, Columbia, SC, USA

David J. Lee Department of Epidemiology and Public Health, Miller School of Medicine, University of Miami, Miami, FL, USA

Emily E. Lenk Wake Forest School of Medicine, Winston-Salem, NC, USA

Carter A. Lennon Department of Psychology, University of Connecticut, Center for Health, Intervention and Prevention, Storrs, CT, USA

Wen B. Leong Institute for Applied Health Research, The University of Birmingham, Birmingham, UK

Stephen J. Lepore Department of Public Health, Temple University, Philadelphia, PA, USA

Bonnie S. LeRoy Department of Genetics Cell Biology and Development, University of Minnesota, Minneapolis, MN, USA

Yvonne Leung Department of Psychosocial Oncology and Palliative Care, Princess Margaret Hospital, University Health Network/University of Toronto, Toronto, ON, Canada

Bonnie Levin Department of Neurology, Miller School of Medicine, University of Miami, Miami, FL, USA

Helena Lewis-Smith Centre for Appearance Research, University of the West of England, Bristol, UK

Bingshuo Li University of Minnesota Medical School, School of Medicine, University of Minnesota, Duluth, MN, USA

Roselind Lieb Department of Psychology, Division of Clinical Psychology and Epidemiology, Basel, Switzerland

Jane Limmer Obstetrics and Gynecology, Duke Hospital, Durham, NC, USA

Bernt Lindahl Occupational and Environmental Medicine, Department of Public Health and Clinical Medicine, Umeå University, Umeå, Sweden

Martin Lindström Department of Clinical Sciences, Malmö, Sweden

Megan R. Lipe Department of Clinical Health and Psychology, University of Florida, College of Public Health and Health Professions, Gainesville, FL, USA

Steven E. Lipshultz Wayne State University School of Medicine, Detroit, MI, USA

Cecilia W. P. Li-Tsang Department of Rehabilitation Sciences, The Hong Kong Polytechnic University, Kowloon, Hong Kong, China

Maria Magdalena Llabre Department of Psychology, University of Miami, Coral Gables, FL, USA

Judy D. Lobo Department of Psychology, University of Miami, Miami, FL, USA

Valerie G. Loehr Department of Psychology, Southern Methodist University, Dallas, TX, USA

Joanna Long School of Sport and Exercise Sciences, The University of Birmingham, Edgbaston, Birmingham, UK

Kristin A. Long Department of Psychology, University of Pittsburgh, Pittsburgh, PA, USA

Sana Loue Department of Epidemiology and Biostatistics, Case Western Reserve University, School of Medicine, Cleveland, OH, USA

William R. Lovallo Department of Psychiatry and Behavioral Sciences, University of Oklahoma Health Sciences Center and VA Medical Center, Oklahoma City, OK, USA

Travis I. Lovejoy Department of Psychiatry and School of Public Health, Oregon Health and Science University, Portland, OR, USA

Wei Lü Shaanxi Key Laboratory of Behavior and Cognitive Neuroscience, School of Psychology, Shaanxi Normal University, Xi'an, China

Tana M. Luger Department of Psychology, University of Iowa, Iowa City, IA, USA

Anna Luke Department of Psychology, Kent State University, Kent, OH, USA

Mark A. Lumley Department of Psychology, Wayne State University, Detroit, MI, USA

M. Kathleen B. Lustyk Department of Behavioral and Social Sciences, Embry–Riddle Aeronautical University, Prescott, AZ, USA

Faith S. Luyster School of Nursing, University of Pittsburgh, Pittsburgh, PA, USA

Kristin L. MacGregor Department of Psychology, Syracuse University, Syracuse, NY, USA

Anna MacKinnon Department of Psychology, McGill University, Montreal, QC, Canada

Shannon Madore Department of Psychology, University of Colorado Denver, Denver, CO, USA

Nicole E. Mahrer Department of Psychology, University of La Verne, La Verne, CA, USA

Elizabeth A. Majka Department of Psychology, The University of Chicago, Chicago, IL, USA

Jamil A. Malik National Institute of Psychology, Quaid-i-Azam University/VU University Amsterdam, Islamabad, Pakistan

Neena Malik Department of Pediatrics, Miller School of Medicine, University of Miami, Miami, FL, USA

Elizabeth M. Maloney Formerly of the Viral and Rickettsial Division, Centers for Disease Control and Prevention, Atlanta, GA, USA

Tsipora Mankovsky Department of Psychology, McGill University, Montreal, QC, Canada

Amy Jo Marcano-Reik Department of Bioethics, Cleveland Clinic, Cleveland, OH, USA

Center for Genetic Research Ethics and Law, Case Western Reserve University, Cleveland, OH, USA

Judy A. Marciel Perioperative Services, East Tennessee Children's Hospital, Knoxville, USA

Kristen K. Marciel Department of Psychology, University of Miami, Coral Gables, USA

Erin N. Marcus Division of General Internal Medicine, Miller School of Medicine, University of Miami, Miami, FL, USA

Seth A. Margolis Clinical Psychology, Health Emphasis, Ferkauf Graduate School of Psychology, Yeshiva University, Bronx, NY, USA

Michela (Micky) Marinelli Department of Cellular and Molecular Pharmacology, Rosalind Franklin University of Medicine and Science, North Chicago, IL, USA

Jacqueline Markowitz Occupational Therapy, College of Health and Rehabilitation Science, Sargent College, Boston University, Boston, MA, USA

David G. Marrero Diabetes Translational Research Center, Indiana University School of Medicine, Indianapolis, IN, USA

Meghan L. Marsac Department of Pediatrics, Kentucky Children's Hospital and College of Medicine, University of Kentucky, Lexington, PA, USA

Elaine Marshall University of Minnesota Duluth, Duluth, MN, USA

Alexandra Martin Friedrich-Alexander University Erlangen-Nürnberg, University Hospital, Erlangen, Erlangen, Germany

Kevin S. Masters Department of Psychology, University of Colorado Denver, Denver, CO, USA

Della Matheson Diabetes Research Institute, Miller School of Medicine, University of Miami, Miami, FL, USA

Yoshinobu Matsuda National Hospital Organization, Kinki-Chuo Chest Medical Center, Sakai shi, Osaka, Japan

Hiromichi Matsuoka Department of Psychosomatic Medicine, Kinki University Faculty of Medicine, Osakasayama, Osaka, Japan

Yutaka Matsuyama Department of Biostatistics, School of Public Health, The University of Tokyo, Bunkyo-ku, Tokyo, Japan

Sonia Matwin Department of Psychiatry, Harvard Medical School, Boston, MA, USA

Alfred L. McAlister Behavioral Sciences, University of Texas School of Public Health, Austin, TX, USA

Lisa M. McAndrew War Related Illness and Injury Study Center, Veterans Affairs NJ Healthcare System, East Orange, NJ, USA

Jeanette McCarthy Community and Family Medicine, Duke University Medical Center, Durham, NC, USA

Shawn McClintock Department of Psychiatry, The University of Texas Southwestern Medical Center at Dallas Columbia University/New York State Psychiatric Institute, Dallas, TX, USA

Lance M. McCracken Psychology Department, Institute of Psychiatry, King's College London, London, UK

James A. McCubbin Department of Psychology, Clemson University, Clemson, SC, USA

Hayley McDonald Centre for Emotional Health, Macquarie University, Macquarie Park, NSW, Australia

Bonnie McGregor Fred Hutchinson Cancer Research Center, Seattle, WA, USA

Brooke McInroy The University of Iowa, Iowa City, IA, USA

David McIntyre School of Sport and Exercise Sciences, The University of Birmingham, Edgbaston, Birmingham, UK

Tara McMullen Doctoral Program in Gerontology, University of Maryland Baltimore and Baltimore County, Baltimore, MD, USA

Marcia D. McNutt Department of Psychology, University of Miami, Coral Gables, FL, USA

Tamar Mendelson Mental Health, Johns Hopkins Bloomberg School of Public Health Johns Hopkins University, Baltimore, MD, USA

Luigi Meneghini Diabetes Research Institute, University of Miami, Miami, FL, USA

Melissa Merrick Division of Violence Prevention, Centers for Disease Control and Prevention, Atlanta, GA, USA

Shelby Messerschmitt-Coen Counselor Education and Supervision, The Ohio State University, Columbus, OH, USA

Sarah Messiah Department of Pediatrics, University of Miami, Miami, FL, USA

Miriam A. Mestre Department of Pediatrics, Wayne State University School of Medicine, Detroit, MI, USA

Elizabeth Mezick Department of Psychology, University of Pittsburgh, Pittsburgh, PA, USA

Kathleen Michael School of Nursing, University of Maryland, Baltimore, MD, USA

Susan Michie University College London, London, UK

Eleanor Miles Department of Psychology, The University of Sheffield, Sheffield, UK

Donna Miller Centers for Disease Control and Prevention, National Center for Health Statistics, Hyattsville, MD, USA

Robert Miller Faculty of Psychology, Technische Universität Dresden, Dresden, Germany

Tracie L. Miller Department of Pediatrics, Miller School of Medicine, University of Miami, Miami, FL, USA

Rachel Millstein Clinical Psychology, University of California, San Diego/San Diego State University, San Diego, CA, USA

Faisal Mir School of Sport and Exercise Sciences, University of Birmingham, Edgbaston, Birmingham, UK

Karlie M. Mirabelli East Carolina University, Greenville, NC, USA

Akihisa Mitani Department of Respiratory Medicine, The University of Tokyo Hospital, Tokyo, Japan

Department of Respiratory Medicine, Mitsui Memorial Hospital, Chiyoda-ku, Tokyo, Japan

Jason W. Mitchell Center for AIDS Intervention Research, Medical College of Wisconsin, Milwaukee, WI, USA

Laura A. Mitchell Department of Psychology, School of Life Sciences, Glasgow Caledonian University, Glasgow, Scotland, UK

Koji Miyazaki Department of Hematology, Kitasato University School of Medicine, Sagamihara, Kanagawa, Japan

Marilyn Moffat Department of Physical Therapy, New York University, New York, NY, USA

David C. Mohr Feinberg School of Medicine, Department of Preventive Medicine, Center for Behavioral Intervention Technologies, Northwestern University, Chicago, IL, USA

Kristine M. Molina Department of Psychological Sciences, University of California, Irvine, Irvine, CA, USA

Ivan Molton Department of Rehabilitation Medicine, University of Washington, Seattle, WA, USA

Jane Monaco Department of Biostatistics, The University of North Carolina at Chapel Hill, Chapel Hill, NC, USA

Enid Montague DePaul University, Northwestern University, Chicago, IL, USA

Miranda Montrone Counselling Place, Glebe, Sydney, NSW, Australia

Pablo A. Mora Department of Psychology, The University of Texas at Arlington, Arlington, TX, USA

Theresa A. Morgan Alpert Medical School of Brown University, Department of Psychiatry, Brown University, Providence, RI, USA

Matthis Morgenstern Institute for Therapy and Health Research, Kiel, Germany

Chica Mori Department of Palliative Medicine, The University of Tokyo Hospital, Tokyo, Japan

Yoshiya Moriguchi Department of Psychophysiology, National Institute of Mental Health, National Center of Neurology and Psychiatry, Kodaira, Tokyo, Japan

Alexandre Morizio Department of Exercise Science, Concordia University, Montreal Behavioral Medicine Centre, Montreal, QC, Canada

Eleshia J. P. Morrison Department of Psychology, Ethnic Minority and Multicultural Health SBM SIG Chair, The Ohio State University, Columbus, OH, USA

Anett Mueller Department of Psychology, State University of New York at Stony Brook, Stony Brook, NY, USA

Hanna M. Mües Department of Clinical and Health Psychology, Faculty of Psychology, University of Vienna, Vienna, Austria

Matthew Muldoon Department of Medicine, University of Pittsburgh, Pittsburgh, PA, USA

Barbara Mullan Centre for Medical Psychology and Evidence-based Decision-making, University of Sydney, Sydney, NSW, Australia

Tomohiko Muratsubaki Department of Behavioral Medicine, School of Medicine, Tohoku University, Sendai, Japan

Elizabeth Murray University College London, London, UK

Julie Murray Utah State University, Logan, UT, USA

Seema Mutti School of Public Health and Health Systems, University of Waterloo, Waterloo, ON, Canada

Yoko Nagai Brighton and Sussex Medical School, University of Sussex, Brighton, East Sussex, UK

Eun-Shim Nahm School of Nursing, University of Maryland, Baltimore, MD, USA

Motohiro Nakajima University of Minnesota Medical School, School of Medicine, University of Minnesota, Duluth, MN, USA

Misuzu Nakashima Hizen Psychiatric Center, Saga, Japan

Benjamin H. Natelson Department of Pain Medicine and Palliative Care, Beth Israel Medical Center and Albert Einstein College of Medicine, Bronx, NY, USA

Urs M. Nater Department of Psychology, University of Vienna, Vienna, Austria

Gabriana Navarrete Department of Behavioral and Social Sciences, Embry–Riddle Aeronautical University, Prescott, AZ, USA

Astrid Nehlig U666, INSERM, Faculty of Medicine, University of Strasbourg, Strasbourg, France

Alexandra Nelson Child and Family Psychological Services/Integrated Behavioral Associates, Weymouth, MA, USA

Ashley M. Nelson Massachusetts General Hospital, Boston, MA, USA

Kimberly Nelson Department of Psychology, University of Washington, Seattle, WA, USA

Jonathan Newman Columbia University, New York, NY, USA

Sarah J. Newman Duke University, Durham, NC, USA

Darren Nickel Department of Physical Medicine and Rehabilitation, University of Saskatchewan, Saskatoon, SK, Canada

Nicole Nisly Department of Internal Medicine, University of Iowa, Iowa City, IA, USA

Karen Niven Manchester Business School, The University of Manchester, Manchester, UK

Kyle R. Noll Department of Physical Medicine and Rehabilitation, Baylor College of Medicine, Houston, TX, USA

Wynne E. Norton Department of Health Behavior, School of Public Health, University of Alabama at Birmingham, Birmingham, AL, USA

Kathryn Noth Illinois Institute of Technology, College of Psychology, Chicago, IL, USA

Ciara M. O'Brien School of Sport, Exercise and Rehabilitation Sciences, University of Birmingham, Birmingham, UK

Eoin O'Brien The Conway Institute, University College Dublin, Belfield, Dublin, Ireland

Julianne O'Daniel Illumina Inc, San Diego, CA, USA

Michael O'Hara Department of Psychology, University of Iowa, Iowa City, IA, USA

Lindsay Oberleitner Department of Psychology, Wayne State University, Detroit, MI, USA

Gabriele Oettingen Department of Psychology, New York University, New York, NY, USA

Ken Ohashi Department of General Internal Medicine, National Cancer Center Hospital, Chuo-ku, Tokyo, Japan

Keisuke Ohta Department of Metabolic Diseases, Graduate School of Medicine, The University of Tokyo, Tokyo, Japan

Michele L. Okun Department of Psychology, University of Colorado Colorado Springs, Colorado Springs, CO, USA

Toru Okuyama Division of Psycho-oncology and Palliative Care, Nagoya City University Hospital, Nagoya, Aichi, Japan

Ellinor K. Olander City, University of London, London, UK

Brian Oldenburg School of Population and Global Health, The University of Melbourne, Melbourne, VIC, Australia

Sheina Orbell Department of Psychology, University of Essex, Essex, UK

Tracy Orleans Robert Wood Johnson Foundation, Princeton, NJ, USA

Kristina Orth-Gomér Department of Clinical Neuroscience, Karolinska Institute, Stockholm, Sweden

Patricia Osborne Clinical Psychology, Health Emphasis, Ferkauf Graduate School of Psychology, Yeshiva University, Bronx, NY, USA

Kenneth J. Ottenbacher Division of Rehabilitation Sciences, University of Texas Medical Branch, Galveston, TX, USA

Margaret E. Ottenbacher Institute for Translational Sciences, University of Texas Medical Branch, Galveston, TX, USA

Nicole Overstreet Social Psychology, University of Connecticut, Storrs, CT, USA

Jan R. Oyebode Dementia Care, University of Bradford, Bradford, UK

Gozde Ozakinci Health Psychology, School of Medicine, University of St Andrews, St Andrews, UK

Debbie Palmer Department of Psychology, University of Wisconsin-Stevens Point, Stevens Point, WI, USA

Steven C. Palmer Abramson Cancer Center, University of Pennsylvania, Philadelphia, PA, USA

Kenneth Pargament Department of Psychology, Bowling Green State University, Bowling Green, OH, USA

Crystal L. Park Department of Psychology, University of Connecticut, Storrs, CT, USA

Joanne Park Workers' Compensation Board of Alberta Millard Health, Edmonton, AB, Canada

Department of Occupational Therapy, University of Alberta, Edmonton, AB, Canada

Alyssa Parker UTSW Health Systems, South Western Medical Center, Dallas, TX, USA

Kristen Pasko Department of Psychology, Rowan University, Glassboro, NJ, USA

Seema M. Patidar Department of Clinical and Health Psychology, University of Florida, Gainesville, FL, USA

Anna Maria Patino-Fernandez Department of Pediatrics, University of Miami, Miami, FL, USA

David Pearson School of Psychology, University of Aberdeen, Aberdeen, UK

Hollie Pellosmaa Tusculum University, Greeneville, TN, USA

Jennifer Pellowski Department of Behavioral and Social Sciences, Brown University School of Public Health, Providence, RI, USA

Frank J. Penedo Department of Psychology, University of Miami and Cancer Survivorship Program, Sylvester Comprehensive Cancer Center, Miller School of Medicine, University of Miami, Miami, FL, USA

Watcharaporn Pengchit Faculty of Psychology, Chulalongkorn University, Bangkok, Thailand

Donald Penzien Wake Forest School of Medicine, Winston-Salem, NC, USA

Deidre Pereira Department of Clinical Health and Psychology, University of Florida, College of Public Health and Health Professions, Gainesville, FL, USA

Edward L. Perkins Biomedical Sciences, Mercer University School of Medicine, Savannah, GA, USA

Richard Peter Institute of Epidemiology and Medical Biometry, University of Ulm, Ulm, Germany

Anna C. Phillips School of Sport, Exercise and Rehabilitation Sciences, University of Birmingham, Edgbaston, Birmingham, UK

Alison Phillips Department of Psychology, Iowa State University, Ames, IA, USA

Sarah Piper Institute of Metabolic Science, Addenbrookes Hospital, Metabolic Research Laboratories, University of Cambridge, Cambridge, UK

Alefiyah Z. Pishori Department of Psychology, University of Connecticut, Storrs, CT, USA

Helene J. Polatajko Department of Occupational Therapy and Occupational Science, Faculty of Medicine, University of Toronto, Toronto, ON, Canada

Lynda H. Powell Department of Preventive Medicine, Rush University Medical Center, Chicago, IL, USA

Glenn Pransky Center for Disability Research, Liberty Mutual Research Institute for Safety, Hopkinton, MA, USA

University of Massachusetts Medical School, Worcester, MA, USA

Harry Prapavessis Faculty of Health Sciences, University of Western Ontario, London, ON, Canada

Aric A. Prather Center for Health and Community, University of California, San Francisco, CA, USA

Courtney C. Prather Department of Psychology, University of North Texas, Denton, TX, USA

Sarah D. Pressman Psychology and Social Behaviour, University of California, Irvine, CA, USA

James O. Prochaska Clinical and Health Psychology, University of Rhode Island, Kingston, RI, USA

Elizabeth R. Pulgaron Department of Pediatrics, University of Miami, Miami, FL, USA

Naum Purits Stockholm, Sweden

Pekka Puska National Institute for Health and Welfare (THL), Helsinki, Finland

Conny W. E. M. Quaedflieg Faculty of Psychology and Neuroscience, Maastricht University, Maastricht, MD, The Netherlands

Mashfiqui Rabbi Harvard University, Cambridge, MA, USA

Whitney Raglin Department of Psychology, University of Cincinnati, Cincinnati, OH, USA

Jeanetta Rains Center for Sleep Evaluation, Elliot Hospital, Manchester, NH, USA

P. H. Amelie Ramirez Department of Epidemiology and Biostatistics, The University of Texas Health Science Center at San Antonio, San Antonio, TX, USA

Isabel F. Ramos Department of Psychology, UCLA, Los Angeles, CA, USA

Ashley K. Randall College of Integrative Sciences and Arts, Arizona State University, Tempe, AZ, USA

Sheah Rarback Department of Pediatrics, University of Miami, Miami, FL, USA

Holly Rau Department of Psychology, University of Utah, Salt Lake City, UT, USA

Maija Reblin College of Nursing, University of Utah, Salt Lake City, UT, USA

Jerrald Rector Purdue University, West Lafayette, IN, USA

Gabriela Reed Psychiatry, Children's Medical Center, UT Southwestern Medical Center, Dallas, TX, USA

William Reeves Office of Surveillance, Epidemiology and Laboratory Services Centers for Disease Control and Prevention, Atlanta, GA, USA

Emily W. Reid Department of Psychology, Drexel University, Philadelphia, PA, USA

Ulf-Dietrich Reips Department of Psychology, Universität Konstanz, Konstanz, Germany

Anthony Remaud Elisabeth Bruyere Research Institute, University of Ottawa, Ottawa, ON, Canada

Kirsten Rene Department of Psychology, Brandeis University, Waltham, MA, USA

Michiel F. Reneman Department of Rehabilitation Medicine, University of Groningen, University Medical Center Groningen, Groningen, The Netherlands

Barbara Resnick School of Nursing, University of Maryland, Baltimore, MD, USA

E. W. Reid: deceased.

Spencer M. Richard Department of Psychology, Utah State University, Logan, UT, USA

Michael Richter Department of Psychology, University of Geneva, Geneva, Switzerland

Nina Rieckmann Berlin School of Public Health, Charité Universitätsmedizin, Berlin, Germany

Winfried Rief Department of Clinical Psychology and Psychotherapy, Philipps University of Marburg, Marburg, Germany

Kristen Riley Department of Psychology, University of Connecticut, Storrs, CT, USA

Deborah Rinehart Denver Health and Hospital Authority, Denver, CO, USA

Lynnee Roane School of Nursing, University of Maryland, Baltimore, MD, USA

Christopher Robert Department of Psychology, College of Science, University of Texas at Arlington, Arlington, TX, USA

University of Missouri, Columbia, MO, USA

Osvaldo Rodriguez Miami VA Healthcare System, Miami, FL, USA

Laura Rodriguez-Murillo Department of Psychiatry, Columbia University Medical Center, New York, NY, USA

Kathryn A. Roecklein Department of Psychology, University of Pittsburgh, Pittsburgh, PA, USA

Megan Roehrig Department of Preventive Medicine, Feinberg School of Medicine, Northwestern University, Chicago, IL, USA

Nicolas Rohleder Department of Psychology, Brandeis University, Waltham, MA, USA

Chelsea Romney University of California, Los Angeles (UCLA), Los Angeles, CA, USA

Karen S. Rook Department of Psychology and Social Behavior, University of California Irvine, Irvine, CA, USA

Jed E. Rose Department of Psychiatry, Duke Center for Nicotine and Smoking Cessation Research, Durham, NC, USA

Leah Rosenberg Department of Medicine, School of Medicine, Duke University, Durham, NC, USA

Debra Roter Johns Hopkins Bloomberg School of Public Health, Baltimore, MD, USA

Alexander J. Rothman Department of Psychology, University of Minnesota, Minneapolis, MN, USA

Eric Roy Department of Kinesiology, University of Waterloo, Waterloo, ON, Canada

Rachel S. Rubinstein Department of Psychology, Rutgers, The State University of New Jersey, Piscataway, NJ, USA

John Ruiz Department of Psychology, University of Arizona, Tuscon, AZ, USA

John Ryan Department of Psychiatry, Western Psychiatric Institute and Clinic, University of Pittsburgh, Pittsburgh, PA, USA

Valerie Sabol School of Nursing, Duke University, Durham, NC, USA

Rany M. Salem Broad Institute, Cambridge, MA, USA

Cambridge Center, Cambridge, MA, USA

Kristen Salomon Department of Psychology, University of South Florida College of Arts and Sciences, Tampa, FL, USA

Janine Sanchez Department of Pediatrics, University of Miami Miller School of Medicine, Miami, FL, USA

Lee Sanders Center for Health Policy and Primary Care Outcomes Research, Stanford University, Stanford, CA, USA

Timothy S. Sannes Department of Clinical and Health Psychology, College of Clinical Health and Health Professions, University of Florida, Gainesville, FL, USA

Elizabeth Sargent Northwestern University, Chicago, IL, USA

Amy F. Sato Department of Psychology, Kent State University, Kent, OH, USA

Eve Saucier Brandeis University, Waltham, MA, USA

Shekhar Saxena Department of Mental Health and Substance Abuse, World Health Organization, Geneva, Switzerland

Wolff Schlotz Institute of Experimental Psychology, University of Regensburg, Regensburg, Germany

Havah Schneider Ferkauf Graduate School of Psychology, Yeshiva University, Bronx, NY, USA

Neil Schneiderman Department of Psychology, Behavioral Medicine Research Center, University of Miami, Coral Gables, FL, USA

Beth Schroeder University of Delaware, Newark, DE, USA

James W. Schroeder Genetics and Molecular Biology Program, Emory University, Atlanta, GA, USA

Marie-Louise Schult Karolinska Institute, Department of Clinical Sciences, Department of Neurobiology, Care Sciences and Society, The Rehabilitation Medicine, University Clinic Danderyd Hospital, Stockholm, Sweden

Brandon K. Schultz East Carolina University, Greenville, NC, USA

M. Di Katie Sebastiano Kinesiology, University of Waterloo, Waterloo, ON, Canada

Sabrina Segal Department of Neurobiology and Behavior, University of California, Irvine, CA, USA

Theresa Senn Center for Health and Behavior, Syracuse University, Syracuse, NY, USA

Jonathan A. Shaffer Department of Medicine/Division of General Medicine, Columbia University Medical Center, New York, NY, USA

Kelly M. Shaffer University of Virginia School of Medicine, Charlottesville, VA, USA

Peter A. Shapiro Department of Psychiatry, Columbia University Medical Center, Columbia University, New York, NY, USA

Leigh A. Sharma Department of Psychology, University of Iowa, Kenosha, WI, USA

Marianne Shaughnessy School of Nursing, University of Maryland, Baltimore, MD, USA

Christopher Shaw Deakin University, Melbourne, VIC, Australia

William S. Shaw Center for Disability Research, Liberty Mutual Research Institute for Safety, Hopkinton, MA, USA
University of Massachusetts Medical School, Worcester, MA, USA

Tamara Goldman Sher The Family Institute at Northwestern University, Evanston, IL, USA

Kerry Sherman Department of Psychology, Centre for Emotional Health, Macquarie University, Sydney, NSW, Australia

Simon Sherry Department of Psychology, Dalhousie University, Halifax, NS, Canada

Vivek Shetty Oral and Maxillofacial Surgery, University of California, Los Angeles, CA, USA

Akihito Shimazu Department of Mental Health, Graduate School of Medicine, The University of Tokyo, Bunkyo-ku, Tokyo, Japan

Daichi Shimbo Center for Behavioral Cardiovascular Health, Columbia University, New York, NY, USA

Erica Shreck Yeshiva University, Bronx, NY, USA

Koseki Shunsuke Faculty of Psychology and Education, J. F. Oberlin University, Machida-shi, Tokyo, Japan

Johannes Siegrist Work Stress Research, Centre for Health and Society Faculty of Medicine, University of Düsseldorf, Life Science Center, Düsseldorf, Germany

Matthew A. Simonson Institute for Behavioural Genetics, Boulder, CO, USA

Kit Sinclair School of Medical and Health Sciences, Tung Wah College, Kowloon, Hong Kong, China

Abanish Singh Duke University Medical Center, Durham, NC, USA

Vivek K. Singh School of Communication and Information, Rutgers University, New Brunswick, NJ, USA

Bengt H. Sjölund University of Southern Denmark, Odense, DK, Denmark

Celette Sugg Skinner Clinical Sciences, The University of Texas Southwestern Medical Center at Dallas Harold C. Simmons Cancer Center, Dallas, TX, USA

Michelle Skinner Department of Psychology, University of Utah, Salt Lake City, UT, USA

Nadine Skoluda Faculty of Psychology, University of Vienna, Vienna, Austria

Tom Smeets Department of Medical and Clinical Psychology, Tilburg School of Social and Behavioral Sciences, Tilburg University, Tilburg, The Netherlands

Alicia K. Smith Psychiatry and Behavioral Sciences, Emory University SOM, Atlanta, GA, USA

Barbara Smith School of Nursing, University of Maryland, Baltimore, MD, USA

Lauren Smith Department of Psychology, University of North Texas, Denton, TX, USA

Timothy W. Smith Department of Psychology, University of Utah, Salt Lake City, UT, USA

Howard Sollins Attorneys at Law, Shareholder at Baker Donelson in the BakerOber Health Law Group, Baltimore, MD, USA

Colin L. Soskolne School of Public Health, University of Alberta, Edmonton, AB, Canada

Ana Victoria Soto Medicine – Residency Program, Columbia University Medical Center, New York, NY, USA

Anne E. M. Speckens Center for Mindfulness, Department of Psychiatry, Radboud University Medical Center, Nijmegen, The Netherlands

Mary Spiers Department of Psychology, Drexel University, Philadelphia, PA, USA

Kevin S. Spink College of Kinesiology, University of Saskatchewan, Saskatoon, SK, Canada

Bonnie Spring Department of Preventive Medicine, Feinberg School of Medicine, Northwestern University, Chicago, IL, USA

Sara Mijares St. George Department of Public Health Sciences, University of Miami Miller School of Medicine, Miami, FL, USA

Tobias Stalder University Siegen, Siegen, Germany

Annette L. Stanton Department of Psychology, University of California, Los Angeles, CA, USA

Shannon L. Stark Department of Psychology, Arizona State University, Tempe, AZ, USA

Adrienne Stauder Institute of Behavioural Sciences, Semmelweis University Budapest, Budapest, Hungary

Michael E. Stefanek Department of Psychological Sciences, Augusta University, Augusta, GA, USA

Jeremy Steglitz Department of Psychiatry and Behavioral Sciences, Clinical Psychology Division, Feinberg School of Medicine, Northwestern University, Chicago, IL, USA

Nikola Stenzel Department of Clinical Psychology and Psychotherapy, Philipps University of Marburg, Marburg, Germany

Colleen Stiles-Shields Loyola University, Chicago, IL, USA

Northwestern University, The University of Chicago, Chicago, IL, USA

Anna M. Stone Thornley Street Surgery, Wolverhampton, UK

Madison E. Stout Department of Psychology, Oklahoma State University, Stillwater, OK, USA

Mark Stoutenberg Department of Kinesiology, Temple University, Philadelphia, PA, USA

Jana Strahler Clinical Biopsychology, Department of Psychology, University of Marburg, Marburg, Germany

Deborah M. Stringer Department of Psychology, University of Iowa, Iowa City, IA, USA

Victoria Anne Sublette School of Public Health, University of Sydney, Sydney, NSW, Australia

Madalina L. Sucala Johnson & Johnson, Health and Wellness Solutions, New Brunswick, NJ, USA

Alyson Sularz Department of Preventive Medicine, Feinberg School of Medicine, Northwestern University, Chicago, IL, USA

Michael J. L. Sullivan Department of Psychology, McGill University, Montreal, QC, Canada

Hannah Süss Clinical Psychology and Psychotherapy, Institute of Psychology, University of Zurich, Zurich, Switzerland

Shin-ichi Suzuki Faculty of Human Sciences, Graduate School of Human Sciences, Waseda University, Tokorozawa-shi, Saitama, Japan

Melanie Swan Philosophy Department, Purdue University, West Lafayette, IN, USA

C. Renn Upchurch Sweeney Salt Lake City Healthcare System, Salt Lake City, UT, USA

Sefik Tagay Department of Psychosomatic Medicine and Psychotherapy, University of Duisburg-Essen, Essen, North Rhine-Westphalia, Germany

Shahrad Taheri Research Division, Weill Cornell Medicine, Doha, Qatar

Misato Takada Department of Socio-Economics, Faculty of Economics, Daito Bunka University, Higashimatsuyama-shi, Saitama, Japan

Yoshiyuki Takimoto Department of Stress Science and Psychosomatic Medicine, Graduate School of Medicine, The University of Tokyo, Bunkyo-ku, Tokyo, Japan

Yukari Tanaka Department of Behavioral Medicine, School of Medicine, Tohoku University Graduate, Seiryo-machi, Aoba-ku, Sendai, Japan

Molly L. Tanenbaum Clinical Psychology, Health Emphasis, Ferkauf Graduate School of Psychology, Yeshiva University, Bronx, NY, USA

Asuka Tanoue Advanced Research Center for Human Science, Waseda University, Tokorozawa, Saitama, Japan

Marc Taylor Behavioral Sciences and Epidemiology, Naval Health Research Center, San Diego, CA, USA

Robert N. Taylor Department of Obstetrics and Gynecology, Wake Forest School of Medicine, Winston-Salem, NC, USA

Jacqueline A. ter Stege Psychosocial Research and Epidemiology, Netherlands Cancer Institute, Amsterdam, The Netherlands

Julian F. Thayer Department of Psychology, The Ohio State University, Columbus, OH, USA

Töres Theorell Stress Research Institute, Stockholm University, Stockholm, Sweden

G. Neil Thomas Institute for Applied Health Research, The University of Birmingham, Birmingham, UK

Roland Thomeé Department of Rehabilitation Medicine, Sahlgrenska University Hospital, Göteborg, Sweden

Dylan Thompson Department for Health, University of Bath, Bath, UK

Rebecca C. Thurston Department of Psychiatry, School of Medicine, University of Pittsburgh, Pittsburgh, PA, USA

Warren Tierney Department of Psychology, Faculty of Education and Health Sciences, University of Limerick, Castletroy, Limerick, Ireland

Jasmin Tiro Department of Clinical Sciences, The University of Texas Southwestern Medical Center, Dallas, TX, USA

Emil C. Toescu Division of Medical Sciences, The University of Birmingham, Edgbaston, Birmingham, UK

Fumiharu Togo Graduate School of Education, The University of Tokyo, Bunkyo-ku, Tokyo, Japan

Akihiro Tokoro Department of Psychosomatic Medicine, National Hospital Organization, Kinki-Chuo Chest Medical Center, Sakai, Osaka, Japan

Kathryn N. Tomasino Northwestern University, Chicago, IL, USA

A. Janet Tomiyama Rutgers University, New Brunswick, NJ, USA

Hansel Tookes Department of Epidemiology and Public Health, Miller School of Medicine, University of Miami, Miami, FL, USA

George J. Trachte Academic Health Center, School of Medicine-Duluth Campus, University of Minnesota, Duluth, MN, USA

Lara Traeger Behavioral Medicine Service, Massachusetts General Hospital/Harvard Medical School, Boston, MA, USA

Vincent Tran Southwestern Medical Center, University of Texas, Dallas, TX, USA

William Trim Department for Health, University of Bath, Bath, UK

Wendy Troxel Psychiatry and Psychology, University of Pittsburgh, Pittsburgh, PA, USA

Emiko Tsuchiya Department of Behavioral Medicine, School of Medicine, Tohoku University Graduate, Seiryo-machi, Aoba-ku, Sendai, Japan

Viana Turcios-Cotto Department of Psychology, University of Connecticut, Storrs, CT, USA

Barbara Turner The University of Texas Health Science Center at San Antonio, San Antonio, TX, USA

J. Rick Turner Campbell University College of Pharmacy and Health Sciences, Buies Creek, NC, USA

James Edward Turner Department for Health, University of Bath, Bath, UK

Bert N. Uchino Department of Psychology and Health Psychology Program, University of Utah, Salt Lake City, UT, USA

Jane Upton Department of Psychology, William James College, Newton, MA, USA

Antti Uutela Department for Lifestyle and Health, National Institute for Health and Welfare, Helsinki, Province of Uusimaa, Finland

Julia R. Van Liew Department of Psychology, University of Iowa, Iowa City, IA, USA

Kavita Vedhara Division of Primary Care, School of Medicine, University of Nottingham, Nottingham, UK

Jet J. C. S. Veldhuijzen van Zanten School of Sport, Exercise and Rehabilitation Sciences, University of Birmingham, Birmingham, UK

Bart Verkuil Clinical, Health and Neuro Psychology, Leiden University, Leiden, The Netherlands

Andrea C. Villanti Johns Hopkins Bloomberg School of Public Health, The Schroeder Institute for Tobacco Research and Policy Studies at Legacy, Washington, DC, USA

Ana Vitlic University of Huddersfield, Huddersfield, UK

Adriana Dias Barbosa Vizzotto Occupational Therapist of the Occupational Therapy Service, Institute of Psychiatry – Hospital das Clínicas University of São Paulo Medical School, São Paulo, SP, Brazil

Catharina Vogt RespectResearchGroup, University of Hamburg, Hamburg, Germany

John P. Vuchetich Department of Psychiatry, University of Minnesota School of Medicine, Minneapolis, MN, USA

Katarzyna Wac University of Copenhagen, Copenhagen, Denmark

QoL Lab, University of Geneva, Geneva, Switzerland

Amy Wachholtz Department of Psychology, University of Colorado Denver, Denver, CO, USA

Anton J. M. Wagenmakers Research Institute for Sport and Exercise Sciences, Liverpool John Moores University, Liverpool, UK

Melanie Wakefield Centre for Behavioural Research in Cancer, Cancer Council Victoria, Melbourne, VIC, Australia

Andrea Wallace College of Nursing, University of Iowa, Iowa City, IA, USA

Margaret Wallhagen Department of Physiological Nursing, University of California San Francisco School of Nursing, San Francisco, CA, USA

Melissa Walls Biobehavioral Health and Population Sciences, University of Minnesota Medical School – Duluth, Duluth, MN, USA

Kenneth A. Wallston School of Nursing, Vanderbilt University, Nashville, TN, USA

Jenny T. Wang Department of Medical Psychology, Duke University, Durham, NC, USA

Jennifer L. Warnick University of Florida, Gainesville, FL, USA

Andrew J. Wawrzyniak Department of Psychiatry and Behavioral Sciences, University of Miami Miller School of Medicine, Miami, FL, USA

Thomas L. Webb Department of Psychology, The University of Sheffield, Sheffield, UK

Lisa Juliane Weckesser Faculty of Psychology, Technische Universität Dresden, Dresden, Germany

Mark Vander Weg Department of Internal Medicine, The University of Iowa and Iowa City VA Health Care System, Iowa City, IA, USA

Stephen M. Weiss Department of Psychiatry and Behavioral Sciences, Miller School of Medicine, University of Miami, Miami, FL, USA

Jennifer Wessel Public Health, School of Medicine, Indiana University, Indianapolis, IN, USA

William Whang Division of Cardiology, Columbia University Medical Center, New York, NY, USA

Anthony J. Wheeler Department of Psychology, Utah State University, Logan, UT, USA

Angela White Department of Psychology, University of Connecticut, Storrs, CT, USA

Anna C. Whittaker School of Sport, Faculty of Health Science and Sport, University of Stirling, Stirling, UK

Timothy Whittaker The International Register of Herbalists and Homeopaths, Cinderford, Glos, UK

Timothy H. Wideman Department of Psychology, McGill University, Montreal, QC, Canada

Deborah J. Wiebe Psychological Sciences, University of California, Merced, Merced, CA, USA

Friedrich Wieser Department of Gynecology and Obstetrics, Emory University School of Medicine, Atlanta, GA, USA

Diana Wile Department of Pediatrics, University of Miami, Miami, FL, USA

James D. Wilkinson Wayne State University School of Medicine, Detroit, MI, USA

Paula Williams Department of Psychology, University of Utah, Salt Lake City, UT, USA

Redford B. Williams Department of Psychiatry and Behavioral Sciences, Division of Behavioral Medicine, Duke University, Durham, NC, USA

Virginia P. Williams Williams LifeSkills, Inc., Durham, NC, USA

Dawn Wilson Department of Psychology, University of South Carolina, Columbia, SC, USA

Oliver J. Wilson Institute for Sport, Physical Activity and Leisure, Leeds Beckett University, Leeds, UK

Kelly Winter Epidemiology, Florida International University, Miami, FL, USA

Katie Witkiewitz University of New Mexico, Albuquerque, NM, USA

Michael Witthöft Psychologisches Institut Abteilung Klinische Psychologie und Psychotherapie, Johannes Gutenberg Universität Mainz, Mainz, Germany

Jutta M. Wolf Department of Psychology, Brandeis University, Waltham, MA, USA

Oliver T. Wolf Department of Cognitive Psychology, Ruhr-Universität Bochum, Bochum, Germany

Timothy Wolf Department of Occupational Therapy and Neurology, Program in Occupational Therapy, St. Louis, MO, USA

Patricia Woltz School of Nursing, University of Maryland, Baltimore, MD, USA

Cara Wong School of Psychology, University of Sydney, Sydney, NSW, Australia

Patricia M. Wong Department of Psychology, University of Pittsburgh, Pittsburgh, PA, USA

Jennifer Wortmann Mental Health and Chaplaincy, VA Mid-Atlantic MIRECC, Durham, NC, USA

Emily M. Wright Department of Psychiatry, Massachusetts General Hospital, Boston, MA, USA

Rex A. Wright Department of Psychology, College of Arts and Sciences, University of North Texas, Denton, TX, USA

Ellen Wuest Boston University, Boston, MA, USA

Alexandra Wuttke-Linnemann Center for Mental Health in Old Age, Landeskrankenhaus (AöR), Mainz, Germany

Department of Psychiatry and Psychotherapy, University Medical Center Mainz, Mainz, Germany

Naoya Yahagi Department of Metabolic Diseases, Graduate School of Medicine, The University of Tokyo, Tokyo, Japan

Yu Yamada Department of Psychosomatic Medicine, Kyushu University, Fukuoka, Japan

Yoshiharu Yamamoto Educational Physiology Laboratory, Graduate School of Education The University of Tokyo, Bunkyo-ku, Tokyo, Japan

Yuko Yanai Department of Psycho-Oncology, National Cancer Center Japan, Chuo-ku, Japan

Betina R. Yanez Department of Psychology, University of California, Los Angeles, CA, USA

Samantha Yard Department of Psychology, University of Washington, Seattle, WA, USA

M. Taghi Yasamy Department of Mental Health and Substance Abuse, World Health Organization, Geneva, Switzerland

Siqin Ye Division of Cardiology, Columbia University Medical Center, New York, NY, USA

Jason S. Yeh Obstetrics and Gynecology, Division of Reproductive Endocrinology and Fertility, Duke University Medical Center, Durham, NC, USA

Ilona S. Yim Department of Psychology and Social Behaviour, University of California, Irvine, Irvine, CA, USA

Alyssa Ylinen Allina Health System, St. Paul, MN, USA

Deborah Lee Young-Hyman Department of Pediatrics, Georgia Prevention Institute Georgia Health Sciences University, Augusta, GA, USA

Xiaohui Yu Department of Medicine and Program in Health Disparities Research, University of Minnesota Medical School, Minneapolis, MN, USA

Lauren Zagorski Department of Psychology, The University of Iowa, Iowa City, IA, USA

Ydwine Zanstra The Amsterdam University College, Amsterdam, The Netherlands

Alex Zautra Department of Psychology, Arizona State University, Tempe, AZ, USA

Chris Zehr Department of Health Studies and Gerontology, University of Waterloo, Waterloo, ON, Canada

Kristin A. Zernicke Department of Psychology, University of Calgary, Calgary, AB, Canada

Emily Zielinski-Gutierrez Division of Vector-Borne Diseases, Centers for Disease Control and Prevention, Ft. Collins, CO, USA

Cortney Taylor Zimmerman Department of Pediatrics, Baylor College of Medicine/Texas Children's Hospital, Houston, FL, USA

Sheryl Zimmerman School of Social Work, The University of North Carolina at Chapel Hill, Chapel Hill, NC, USA

Tanja Zimmermann Department of Clinical Psychology, Psychotherapy and Diagnostics, University of Braunschweig, Braunschweig, Germany

P

P-30 Antigen

▶ Prostate-Specific Antigen (PSA)

Pain

Michael James Coons[1] and Jeremy Steglitz[2]
[1]Department of Preventive Medicine, Feinberg School of Medicine, Northwestern University, Chicago, IL, USA
[2]Department of Psychiatry and Behavioral Sciences, Clinical Psychology Division, Feinberg School of Medicine, Northwestern University, Chicago, IL, USA

Synonyms

Pain management/control; Pain, psychosocial aspects; Pain threshold

Definition

Pain is a noxious sensory phenomenon that provides information to organisms about the occurrence or threat of injury. Pain is also a multidimensional experience that results from a complex interaction between biological and psychological components and is further influenced by behavioral and social factors. The temporal course of pain can range from acute, or time-limited states in response to injury, to chronic states in which pain persists beyond the point of tissue repair or healing. Although the Gate Control Theory (Melzack & Wall, 1967) provides a unified model of pain, a variety of pain subtypes exist that have different underlying mechanisms.

Description

Neurobiology of Pain

A primary function of the nervous system is to communicate information to alert organisms to the experience or threat of injury. Therefore, the noxious qualities of pain function to capture our attention and motivate action to minimize the risk of harm. Nociceptors are a specialized class of primary afferent nerves. Myelinated nociceptors signal sharp pain from heat and pressure stimuli on skin with hair. Unmyelinated nociceptors signal burning and pressure-induced pain on hairless skin. Both unmyleinated and myelinated nociceptors signal pain from chemical stimuli. Injury leads to increased pain sensitivity or hyperalgesia caused by inflammation.

CNS Mechanisms of Pain Modulation

At the level of the spinal cord, pain modulation occurs in the substantia gelatinosa (SG) of the dorsal horn. The SG serves an inhibitory or gating function that modulates pain signal transduction. Pain modulation also occurs in the periaqueductal

© Springer Nature Switzerland AG 2020
M. D. Gellman (ed.), *Encyclopedia of Behavioral Medicine*,
https://doi.org/10.1007/978-3-030-39903-0

gray (PAG) and rostral ventromedial medulla (RVM) of the midbrain, which function as a bidirectional relay station. The system is involved in the suppression of ascending responses to harmful stimuli and enhances nociceptive responses. The PAG-RVM system has connections to the hypothalamus and limbic forebrain structures including the amygdala, anterior cingulate cortex, and anterior insula. Consequently, fear, attention, and pain expectancies exert top-down processes that influence pain perception.

Clinical Classifications of Pain

Postoperative Pain and its Management

Acute postoperative pain is a product of a range of physiological mechanisms. It comprises a constellation of sensory, emotional, and psychological experiences that follow surgery and is associated with autonomic, endocrine-metabolic, physiological, and behavioral responses. Considerable progress has been made to understand the functions of the peripheral and central nervous systems, mechanisms of acute postoperative pain, side effects of analgesic drugs, and techniques and interventions in surgical patients. However, improvements in the management of acute postoperative pain are needed. Specifically, the use of acute pain management services may help to ensure that evidence-based analgesic techniques are implemented. Furthermore, improved collaboration would be useful between interdisciplinary care teams including anesthesiologists, surgeons, nurses, and mental health professionals to optimize postoperative pain management.

Deep Somatic Tissue Pain Deep tissue pain encompasses pain from the joints and muscles. The pain is often diffuse and characterized by dull and aching sensations. Major sources of deep somatic tissue pain are inflammatory diseases, trauma, overload, and degenerative diseases. Under normal conditions, these nociceptors are activated by stimuli that can lead to structural damage including overload, twisting, pressure, and ischemic contraction. Under conditions of inflammation or trauma, nociceptors of joint and muscle become increasingly sensitized, particularly to mechanical stimuli.

Two types of spinal cord neurons process nociceptive input from joint and muscle. These neurons show two distinct properties: (1) They converge inputs from the skin and deep tissue, and (2) they are activated by mechanical stimuli. Neurons in the thalamus and cortex process inputs from deep tissue.

Arthritis Osteoarthritis (OA) is a degenerative joint disease that results in pain localized to the joint cartilage and subchondral bone. It affects approximately 30% of adults 75 years and older. OA is classified by the location of the affected joints (e.g., hip or knee) and whether the pain is primary or secondary to other conditions or disease processes. OA pain may occur in response to mechanical stimuli but may be chemically mediated when joint tissues fail to adequately repair. Consequences of OA include loss of articular cartilage, new bone formation in the subchondral region, and formation of new cartilage and bone in the joints and are characterized by pain, stiffness, functional limitations, and impaired quality of life.

Rheumatoid arthritis (RA) is an autoimmune disease that results in significant joint inflammation and pain. It affects nearly 1% of the adult population. RA involves both the small and large joints and is distributed symmetrically. RA may eventually progress to joint failure, which can result in secondary OA. Age, sex, family history, and tobacco use are significant risk factors for RA.

Treatment for arthritis is multidimensional. Components may include education about the disease process, weight loss to minimize joint stress, increased physical activity and/or physical therapy, analgesics, anti-inflammatory drugs, and local steroid or hyaluronic acid injections. Specific to RA, antirheumatic drugs (DMARDs) may be used to reduce inflammation and slow the disease progression. In severe or advanced cases, surgical intervention including joint replacement may be indicated.

Fibromyalgia Syndrome Fibryomyalgia syndrome (FMS) is a persistent pain condition involving the soft tissues. It affects approximately 2% in the general population and is significantly more prevalent among women than men. Although its etiology is unknown, significant advances have been made in understanding its clinical presentation. Pain is believed to result from central sensitization of somatosensory pathways that induce enhanced pain perception. This includes persistent, diffuse pain to touch at localized areas in soft tissues. Other systemic symptoms include recurrent headaches, dizziness, fatigue, morning stiffness, irritable bowel syndrome, irritable bladder syndrome, insomnia, cognitive dysfunction, depression, and anxiety.

Treatment for FMS is similar to that of other persistent pain conditions and includes education, physical activity and/or physical therapy, cognitive-behavioral therapy, and pharmacological interventions that act on central neural pathways.

Low Back Pain Low back pain (LBP) is defined as pain, muscle tension, or stiffness that is localized between the costal margin and inferior gluteal folds. It also presents with or without radiating leg pain. It can also be classified as specific, or in response to a known pathology (e.g., hernia, fracture), or nonspecific or idiopathic. Nonspecific LBP accounts for 90% of all cases. Physical exercises are currently the only empirically supported intervention to prevent LBP. Many randomized controlled trials and systematic reviews have been published that examine its treatment. Physical activity, nonsteroidal anti-inflammatory drugs (NSAIDs), and muscle relaxants are effective treatments for acute LBP. Physical therapy and CB therapy in the context of interdisciplinary pain treatment programs are recommended for persistent LBP.

Visceral Pain Visceral pain is diffuse. It results in referred pain (pain perceived in sites other than the site of injury or pain stimuli). Unlike somatic nociceptors, the activation of visceral nociceptors does not require tissue damage. Rather, it can be caused by the distension of hollow organs, traction on the mesentery, ischemia, and endogenous chemicals associated with inflammatory processes.

Thorax Pain Angina pectoris is the most frequently occurring form of thorax pain. It is caused by myocardial ischemia but often produces chest pain that is distal to the ischemic event. Cardiac pain is mediated by interplay between autonomic reflexes and peripheral cardiac nerves. The thalamus and hypothalamus transmit cardiac pain to the prefrontal cortex. The occurrence of pain is slow and lacks spatial localization. The clinical presentation of myocardial ischemia can be different in men and women. Pharmacotherapy is the primary intervention for angina pectoris and acute myocardial infarction (MI) including beta-blockers, nitroglycerin, morphine, and anti-thrombotic agents. Percutaneous transluminal coronary intervention (PCI) and coronary artery bypass graft surgery (CAGB) are surgical interventions that improve coronary blood flow. Other forms of thorax pain include esophageal chest pain, aortic aneurysms, and pulmonary events including embolism.

Abdominal Pain Abdominal pain can be caused by chronic functional disorders or acute life-threatening conditions. Chronic disorders, such as irritable bowel syndrome, account for the majority of diagnoses that account for abdominal pain. Most chronic disorders result in enhanced pain perception in response to visceral stimuli, which results from central pain modulation mechanisms. In contrast, acute abdominal pain is caused by an identifiable stimulus or pathology (e.g., gastric ulcer). Although interventions for acute abdominal pain are highly effective, the development of efficacious treatments for chronic conditions is needed.

Orofacial Pain Orofacial pain is defined as pain experienced in the motor or sensory aspects of the trigeminal nerve system. Pain signals are transmitted to the nucleus caudalis in the medulla and project onward to the thalamus and cortex via the trigeminothalamic tract. Orofacial pain is exacerbated by central convergence, inflammation of the oral mucosa, and central sensitization to pain (increased spontaneous firing of nerves). Prevention strategies include preoperative administration of NSAIDs to block inflammatory processes and local anesthetics to reduce central sensitization. However, due to common adverse events when using systemic opioids, their outpatient use is limited. The etiology of persistent (unremitting or recurrent) orofacial pain is poorly understood. Consequently, pain management is imprecise, and the majority of therapies are not validated.

Neuropathic Pain Neuropathic pain occurs in response to injury (lesion or dysfunction) of the nervous system. Numerous animal models have been proposed to account for the underlying mechanisms. One of the earliest models originated from the observation that animals attack a limb in which the axons of neurons have been severed following injury. This model suggests that a central sensitization process occurs, such that severed nerves exhibit greater spontaneous firing frequencies than healthy intact nerves. Individuals experiencing neuropathic pain describe their pain as "electric shocks, burning, tingling, itching, and prickling." Examples of neuropathic pain conditions include neuropathies (e.g., peripheral, autonomic) and neuralgias (e.g., trigeminal). Pharmacological treatments may include topical analgesics, tricyclic antidepressants, anticonvulsants, and opioids.

Phantom Limb Pain This is a form of neuropathic pain and refers to perceived pain sensations in the anatomical space of a limb that has been amputated. Although the majority of individuals experience sensations related to the shape, posture, or movement of the missing limb, 60–80% of individuals experience intermittent or persistent pain. Although the specific mechanisms underlying phantom limb pain are not entirely understood, both the peripheral and central nervous systems are involved. Additional treatments may include sodium channel blockers, physical therapy, and transcutaneous electrical nerve stimulation.

Cancer Pain The neurobiology of cancer pain is poorly understood. However, new models have identified mechanisms that both produce and maintain cancer pain. Tumor cells and tumor-associated cells (macrophages, neutrophils, T-lymphocytes) are believed to sensitize primary afferent neurons in the periphery. Findings from these studies may lead to the development of novel therapies that act on these peripheral mechanisms and could improve the quality of life of individuals living with cancer.

Pain Assessment and Intervention Pain is a complex and subjective experience characterized by sensory-discriminative, motivational-affective, and cognitive-evaluative dimensions. Pain can be evaluated using a variety of tools including verbal and numerical self-report scales, visual analogue scales (VAS), self-report measures, behavioral observation, and physiological markers. A combination of these measures is recommended to yield the most valid information about this phenomenon.

Within clinical and research settings, the VAS, the McGill Pain Questionnaire (MPQ), and the Multidimensional Pain Inventory (MPI) are examples of commonly used instruments. Using a VAS, individuals are asked to rate their current pain intensity on a numeric scale that is anchored by 0 (no pain at all) and 10 (the most pain you could imagine experiencing). The McGill Pain Questionnaire was developed Melzack and Wall (Melzack 1975). It evaluates the specific location(s), intensity, and qualities of pain that individuals currently experience. It contains four domains including sensory, affective, evaluative, and miscellaneous. It can either be clinician-administered or completed independently by patients in a self-report manner. The McGill Pain Questionnaire is a reliable and valid tool to assess the multidimensional nature of pain experience. For research applications where time is limited to obtain information, a short-form McGill Pain Questionnaire (SF-MPQ) is also available. The MPI is a comprehensive self-report instrument designed to evaluate a full range of experiences with persistent pain conditions. It includes dimensions of pain intensity, emotional distress, cognitive and functional adaptation, and social support. It has also been shown to have solid psychometric properties.

Cognitive-Behavioral Approaches to Pain Management In the context of persistent pain conditions, cognitive-behavioral (CB) interventions focus on developing adaptive pain coping skills. These skills are intended to minimize the experience of pain, prevent or minimize pain exacerbations, and limit pain-related disability. A CB intervention addresses the subjective and contextual aspects of pain. First, patients receive education about theories of pain (e.g., Gate Control Theory) to foster an understanding of why pain persists beyond the point of tissue repair. Understanding this conceptual framework provides the foundation for deploying a series of related cognitive and behavioral interventions. Cognitive interventions may include cognitive restructuring to minimize pain catastrophizing, attention diversion and distraction techniques, and problem solving exercises. Behavioral interventions may include relaxation, paced diaphragmatic breathing, goal setting, behavioral activation, and graded exposure to feared physical activities. In the management of persistent pain, CB interventions are often most effective when implemented in the context of interdisciplinary care teams and can be used as an adjuvant to other physical, pharmacological, or surgical therapies.

Cross-References

▶ Gate Control Theory of Pain
▶ Pain Anxiety
▶ Pain Management/Control
▶ Pain Threshold
▶ Pain, Psychosocial Aspects
▶ Pain-Related Fear

References and Readings

Bielefeldt, K., & Gebhart, G. F. (2006). Visceral pain: Basic mechanisms. In S. B. McMahon & M. Koltzenburg (Eds.), *Wall and Melzack's textbook of pain* (pp. 721–736). Philadelphia: Elsevier.

Dahl, J. B., & Kehlet, H. (2006). Postoperative pain and its management. In S. B. McMahon & M. Koltzenburg (Eds.), *Wall and Melzack's textbook of pain* (5th ed., pp. 635–652). Philadelphia: Elsevier.

Dionne, R. A., Kim, H., & Gordon, S. M. (2006). Acute and chronic dental and orofacial pain. In S. B. McMahon & M. Koltzenburg (Eds.), *Wall and Melzack's textbook of pain* (5th ed., pp. 833–850). Philadelphia: Elsevier.

Mantyh, P. W. (2006). Cancer pain: Causes, consequences, and therapeutic opportunities. In S. B. McMahon & M. Koltzenburg (Eds.), *Wall and Melzack's textbook of pain* (5th ed., pp. 1087–1098). Philadelphia: Elsevier.

Melzack, R. (1975). The McGill Pain Questionnaire: Major properties and scoring methods. *Pain, 1*, 275–299.

Melzack, R., & Katz, J. (2006). Pain assessment in adult patients. In S. B. McMahon & M. Koltzenburg (Eds.), *Wall and Melzack's textbook of pain* (5th ed., pp. 291–304). Philadelphia: Elsevier.

Melzack, R., & Wall, P. D. (1967). Pain mechanisms: A new theory. *Science, 150*, 971–979.

Meyer, R. A., Ringkamp, M., Campbell, J. N., & Raja, S. N. (2006). Peripheral mechanisms of cutaneous nociception. In S. B. McMahon & M. Koltzenburg (Eds.), *Wall and Melzack's textbook of pain* (5th ed., pp. 3–34). Philadelphia: Elsevier.

Nikolasjsen, L., & Straehelin Jensen, T. (2006). Phantom limb. In S. B. McMahon & M. Koltzenburg (Eds.), *Wall and Melzack's textbook of pain* (5th ed., pp. 961–972). Philadelphia: Elsevier.

Ossipov, M. H., Lai, J., & Porreca, F. (2006). Mechanisms of experimental neuropathic pain: Integration from animal models. In S. B. McMahon & M. Koltzenburg (Eds.), *Wall and Melzack's textbook of pain* (5th ed., pp. 929–946). Philadelphia: Elsevier.

Russell, I. J., & Bieber, C. S. (2006). Myofascial pain and fibromyalgia syndrome. In S. B. McMahon & M. Koltzenburg (Eds.), *Wall and Melzack's textbook of pain* (pp. 669–682). Philadelphia: Elsevier.

Scadding, J. W., & Koltzenburg, M. (2006). Painful peripheral neuropathies. In S. B. McMahon & M. Koltzenburg (Eds.), *Wall and Melzack's textbook of pain* (5th ed., pp. 973–1000). Philadelphia: Elsevier.

Schaible, H. G. (2006). Basic mechanisms of deep somatic tissue. In S. B. McMahon & M. Koltzenburg (Eds.), *Wall and Melzack's textbook of pain* (5th ed., pp. 621–635). Philadelphia: Elsevier.

Scott, D. L. (2006). Osteoarthritis and rheumatoid arthritis. In S. B. McMahon & M. Koltzenburg (Eds.), *Wall and Melzack's textbook of pain* (pp. 653–668). Philadelphia: Elsevier.

Sylven, C., & Erikson, E. (2006). Thorax. In S. B. McMahon & M. Koltzenburg (Eds.), *Wall and Melzack's textbook of pain* (5th ed., pp. 737–752). Philadelphia: Elsevier.

Turk, D. C. (2002). A cognitive-behavioral perspective on treatment of chronic pain patients. In R. J. Gatchel & D. C. Turk (Eds.), *Psychological approaches to pain management: A practitioner's handbook* (pp. 138–158). New York: Guilford.

van Tulder, M. W., & Koes, B. (2006). Low back pain. In S. B. McMahon & M. Koltzenburg (Eds.), *Wall and Melzack's textbook of pain* (5th ed., pp. 699–708). Philadelphia: Elsevier.

Wong, H. Y., & Mayer, E. A. (2006). A clinical perspective on abdominal pain. In S. B. McMahon & M. Koltzenburg (Eds.), *Wall and Melzack's textbook of pain* (5th ed., pp. 753–776). Philadelphia: Elsevier.

Pain Anxiety

Michael James Coons
Department of Preventive Medicine, Feinberg School of Medicine, Northwestern University, Chicago, IL, USA

Synonyms

Pain-related fear

Definition

Pain anxiety is a future-oriented state of autonomic arousal that is triggered by the anticipation of pain. Similar to the tripartite model of anxiety, it is comprised of cognitive, physiological, and behavioral components. Pain anxiety is an affective manifestation of the autonomic nervous system that occurs in response to the anticipation of pain. Albeit to a lesser degree than that triggered by fear, the sympathetic nervous system becomes activated by the septo-hippocampal brain regions. Pain anxiety is characterized by cognitive, physiological, and behavioral symptoms. Cognitively, individuals become hypervigilant for pain-related cues by internally scanning their body (for internal signs and symptoms of pain) and the environment (for pain-inducing contexts or stimuli). They also anticipate experiencing pain in the future and may often expect their pain to be catastrophic (e.g., "Having to get my tooth fixed at the dentist will be excruciating"). In turn, individuals become motivated to engage in avoidance behaviors to minimize the likelihood of experiencing future pain. According to fear-avoidance models of pain, behavioral avoidance (typically of situations involving physical activity or movement) leads to physical deconditioning and muscle atrophy, which in turn, may result in greater pain intensity. Pain anxiety and related avoidance behavior greatly contributes to the progression of acute to persistent pain.

The most common mode of assessment of pain anxiety involves the administration of well-validated self-report instruments. Several published scales are available that assess the nature and extent of pain-related cognitions (e.g., "When I hurt, I think about pain constantly"), pain-related avoidance (e.g., "I try to avoid activities that cause pain"), and physiological symptoms (e.g., "When I sense pain, I feel dizzy or faint"). Examples of self-report instruments include the Pain Anxiety Symptom Scale (PASS) and the Burn-Specific Pain Anxiety Scale. Alternative modes of assessing pain-related fear include semi-structured clinical interviews and the direct observation of patient behavior.

Cognitive behavior therapy (CBT) is the most well-validated intervention for pain anxiety. Treatment components include psychoeducation and introduction, demonstration, and practice of a variety of adaptive coping skills (i.e., progressive muscle relaxation, diaphragmatic breathing, mental imagery, behavioral activation and pleasant activity scheduling, activity-rest cycling, physical therapy/exercise, problem-solving, cognitive restructuring, and calming self-statements). In treating pain-related fear, special emphasis is placed on graded in vivo exposure with behavioral experiments. These latter components allow individuals to identify situations through which they can gather information to test and challenge their distorted pain-related cognitions.

Cross-References

▶ Pain, Psychosocial Aspects
▶ Pain-Related Fear

References and Readings

Asmundson, G. J. G., Norton, P. J., & Vlaeyen, W. S. (2004). Fear-avoidance models of chronic pain: An overview. In G. J. G. Asmundson, J. W. S. Vlaeyen, & G. Crombez (Eds.), *Understanding and treating fear of pain* (pp. 3–24). New York: Oxford University Press.

de Williams, A. C., & McCracken, L. M. (2004). Cognitive behavioral therapy for chronic pain: An overview with specific reference to fear avoidance. In G. J. G. Asmundson, J. W. S. Vlaeyen, & G. Crobez (Eds.), *Understanding and treating fear of pain* (pp. 293–312). New York: Oxford University Press.

McNeil, D. W., & Vowles, K. E. (2004). Assessment of fear and anxiety associated with pain: Conceptualization, methods, and measures. In G. J. G. Asmundson, J. W. S. Vlaeyen, & G. Crombez (Eds.), *Understanding and treating fear of pain* (pp. 189–211). New York: Oxford University Press.

Pain Anxiety Symptoms Scale (PASS) and Short Version PASS-20

Lance M. McCracken
Psychology Department, Institute of Psychiatry, King's College London, London, UK

Definition

Short self-report questionnaires designed to measure aspects of pain-related anxiety and avoidance for use in clinical assessment and research.

Description

The 40-item Pain Anxiety Symptoms Scale (PASS) (McCracken et al. 1992) and a shorter 20-item version of the same assessment instrument (PASS-20) (McCracken and Dhingra 2002) measure pain-related anxiety, fear, and avoidance. They were designed for clinical and research purposes and mostly for use with adults with recurrent or chronic pain conditions. However, they have been validated and used in people without identified pain conditions, such as university students and people recruited from community settings (Abrams et al. 2007). The original PASS was developed at a time during the late 1980s and early 1990s when clinicians and researchers were beginning to focus greater attention on processes of fear and avoidance in relation to chronic pain. Since that time a model of chronic pain referred to as the "fear-avoidance" model has become a popular organizing framework guiding research and treatment development (Vlaeyen and Linton 2000). The PASS and PASS-20 have been used in research investigating models and mechanisms of pain-related disability, and in treatment process and outcome research (McCracken and Gross 1998; Vowles and McCracken 2008). They are also routinely used in clinical practice for analyzing and conceptualizing cases and in treatment-related decision making.

Both versions of the PASS include four subscales that reflect aspects of avoidance behavior (e.g., I will stop any activity as soon as I sense pain coming on), cognitive anxiety (e.g., During painful episodes it is difficult for me to think of anything else besides the pain), fear (e.g., When I feel pain I am afraid that something terrible will happen), and physiological anxiety (e.g., I find it hard to calm my body down after periods of pain). The four subscales are equal length in each version of the measure. All items are rated on a scale from 0 (never) to 5 (always). In the 40-item version five items are reverse-keyed and must be recoded before calculating summary scores. Summary scores for both versions are calculated by summing assigned items and then by summing the subscales to derive an overall score. There are no set cutoffs for interpreting scores from the instruments. One method to facilitate interpretation is to convert raw scores to standard scores or percentile ranks. As an example, a table of raw scores and percentile rank equivalents has been constructed from a large consecutive sample of patients seen at a tertiary care center in the UK (N = 339). From this raw scores of 15.0, 33.0, 60.0, and 78.0 from the PASS-20 correspond to the 5th, 25th, 75th, and 95th percentile, respectively.

The PASS and PASS-20 have been extensively validated. They both show very good internal consistency and temporal consistency (McCracken and Dhingra 2002; Roelofs et al. 2004) and a factor structure that generally matches the a priori subscale structure (Abrams et al. 2007; Larsen et al. 1997; Roelofs et al. 2004). Both versions of the instrument demonstrate adequate construct validity in relation to variables such as general anxiety and depression (e.g., Roelofs et al. 2004) and show mostly moderate to large correlations with important criterion variables, such as measures of physical and psychosocial disability (e.g., McCracken and Dhingra 2002). The original PASS (McCracken and Gross 1998) and the 20-item version (Vowles and McCracken 2008) both appear sensitive to the effects of multidisciplinary treatment for chronic pain.

For most uses currently the PASS-20 is preferred as it appears equivalent to the longer version in most important respects. The PASS-20 has been translated into Chinese, Dutch, French, Icelandic, Iranian, Polish, and Spanish, among other languages.

The fear-avoidance model of chronic pain has been a very useful model for understanding pain-related disability and for guiding the current generation of treatment developments for chronic pain. At the same there are other theoretical and treatment developments that appear wider in scope and possibly more progressive than the fear-avoidance model. These developments include contextual approaches within cognitive behavior therapy, approaches such as Acceptance and Commitment Therapy (ACT) (Hayes et al. 1999) and mindfulness-based approaches. In this work measures such as the PASS-20 remain useful. Other variables that are known to have strong relations with pain-related fear and avoidance are also now frequently studied, such as acceptance of pain and values-based action, among others, and a wider process called psychological flexibility (e.g., Vowles and McCracken 2008). The point is that the PASS-20 and its focus on fear and avoidance remains relevant and the field is also evolving so that these process are being examined in a broader and well-integrated cognitive behavioral framework. These theoretical and treatment developments may be important to those who are hoping to assess pain-related fear and avoidance and may be seeking to use an instrument such as the PASS-20.

Cross-References

▶ Chronic Pain
▶ Cognitive Behavior Therapy

References and Readings

Abrams, M. P., Carleton, R. N., & Asmundson, G. J. G. (2007). An exploration of the psychometric properties of the PASS-20 with a nonclinical sample. *The Journal of Pain, 8*, 879–886.

Hayes, S. C., Strosahl, K. D., & Wilson, K. G. (1999). *Acceptance and commitment therapy: An experiential approach to behavior change*. New York: Guilford Press.

Larsen, D. K., Taylor, S., & Asmundson, G. J. G. (1997). Exploratory factor analysis of the Pain Anxiety Symptoms Scale in patients with chronic pain complaints. *Pain, 69*, 27–34.

McCracken, L. M., & Dhingra, L. (2002). A short version of the Pain Anxiety Symptom Scale (PASS-20): Preliminary development and validity. *Pain Research & Management, 7*, 45–50.

McCracken, L. M., & Gross, R. T. (1998). The role of pain-related anxiety reduction in the outcome of multidisciplinary treatment for chronic low back pain: Preliminary results. *Journal of Occupational Rehabilitation, 8*, 179–189.

McCracken, L. M., Zayfert, C., & Gross, R. T. (1992). The Pain Anxiety Symptoms Scale: Development and validation of a scale to measure fear of pain. *Pain, 50*, 67–73.

Roelofs, J., McCracken, L., Peters, M. L., Crombez, G., van Breukelen, G., & Vlaeyen, J. W. S. (2004). Psychometric evaluation of the Pain Anxiety Symptoms Scale (PASS) in chronic pain patients. *Journal of Behavioral Medicine, 27*, 167–183.

Vlaeyen, J. W. S., & Linton, S. J. (2000). Fear-avoidance and its consequences in chronic musculoskeletal pain: A state of the art. *Pain, 85*, 317–332.

Vowles, K. E., & McCracken, L. M. (2008). Acceptance and values-based action in chronic pain: A study of treatment effectiveness and process. *Journal of Consulting and Clinical Psychology, 76*, 397–407.

Pain Management/Control

Michael James Coons
Department of Preventive Medicine, Feinberg School of Medicine, Northwestern University, Chicago, IL, USA

Synonyms

Pain, psychosocial aspects

Definition

Pain is a multidimensional phenomenon. Pain management refers to the physiological (i.e., pharmacological, surgical), psychological, and behavioral interventions that are aimed at minimizing pain perception and alleviating pain-related interference and disability.

Description

Historically, pain was conceptualized using a disease model and was considered to be a purely sensory experience resulting from injury, inflammation, or tissue damage. However, limitations to this model became evident after observing diverse responses to pain across individuals despite objectively similar physical stimuli or trauma. In 1965, Melzack and Wall published a seminal paper in *Science* that outlined a revolutionary theory of pain (Melzack and Wall 1965).

Gate Control Theory

The Gate Control Theory emphasized central neural mechanisms at the level of the spinal cord that modulate afferent signals from peripheral nerves en route to the brain. This sensory modulation and subsequent pain perception is influenced by sensory input, cognitive processing, affective states, neural inhibitory capacities, activities of the stress-regulation system, and subsequent behavioral responses. Therefore, interventions targeting these multiple mechanisms provide opportunity to achieve effective pain management.

Pharmacological and Surgical Interventions

Pharmacological interventions are often the first-line treatments for pain. Systemic analgesics are the focus of both acute and persistent pain management and include nonsteroidal anti-inflammatory drugs (NSAIDs), including acetaminophen (ASA), and opioid analgesics (pure or in combination with NSAIDs). Combination opioid analgesics are typically administered orally; however, other routes of administration include rectal and sublingual. Pure opioids can be administered through the skin (with a transdermal patch), subcutaneously, or intravenously. These latter routes of administration are typically used when adequate pain relief is not achieved with the use of NSAIDs or combination opioids. In cases of neuropathic pain (i.e., pain due to dysfunction of the nervous system, in the absence of tissue damage), antiepileptic medications are often used (e.g., pregabalin). In light of their misuse and abuse potential of opioids, individuals with persistent pain should be evaluated to determine if chronic opioid management is clinically appropriate. Individuals with a history of medical non-adherence or individuals with severe axis I or axis II pathology may require close monitoring if opioid medications are prescribed.

Surgical procedures for pain management range in their degree of invasiveness. Minimally invasive procedures include steroidal injections and nerve blocks (of the peripheral and sympathetic nerves). Maximally invasive procedures include radiofrequency ablations (for the local destruction of nervous tissue), spinal cord stimulator implantation (for the neuromodulation of afferent pain signals), and intrathecal pump implantations (for the direct administration of opioids and other analgesics into the cerebral spinal fluid when pain relief using other modalities has been unsuccessful). Particularly with these more invasive surgical interventions, individuals must adhere to medical recommendations to avoid potentially life-threatening adverse medical events. Consequently, candidates for these procedures also require careful evaluation and selection by qualified professionals to ensure patient safety.

Cognitive Behavioral Interventions

Cognitive behavioral interventions focus on developing adaptive pain coping skills to minimize the experience of pain, prevent long-term exacerbations in pain, and minimize pain-related disability. For individuals with persistent pain (either intermittent-recurrent pain or unremitting pain), they often become anxious and fearful of the pain experience and avoid engaging in physical activity to minimize the experience of pain. However, over time, this behavioral avoidance contributes to the loss of physical strength, physical deconditioning, and muscular atrophy (i.e., loss of muscle mass) that exacerbates pain perception. In essence, the avoidance of physical activity *because* of pain results in pain intensification. This behavioral avoidance reinforces the fear of pain, resulting in greater anxiety and propensity to avoid physical activity. Furthermore, avoidance of pain often leads to avoidance of activities through which individual's derive meaning and value (e.g., participation in one's profession, spending time with family/friends). Over time, avoidance may contribute to a sense of isolation, undermine one's confidence in their ability to manage their pain, and increase the focus of their attention to the perception of pain. This process contributes the development or exacerbation of depression, the intensification of pain, and pain-related interference and disability.

Components of cognitive behavioral interventions for persistent pain include psychoeducation and introduction, demonstration, and practice of a variety of adaptive coping skills (i.e., progressive muscle relaxation, diaphragmatic breathing, mental imagery, behavioral activation and pleasant activity scheduling, activity-rest cycling, physical therapy/exercise, problem-solving, cognitive restructuring, and calming self-statements). Within a CBT protocol, the relaxation procedures reduce sympathetic arousal to both "close the gate" to minimize the transmission of afferent pain signals to the brain and reduce muscle tension associated with pain. The attention procedures (i.e., mental imagery, pleasant activity scheduling) function to distract individuals from their pain experience and facilitate positive experiences and positive affect. The behavioral interventions (i.e., activity-rest cycling, behavioral activation, physical therapy/exercise) are intended to help individuals learn how to engage in activities despite experiencing pain and to both minimize pain-related interference and maintain their physical conditioning. While initial behavioral engagement often results in pain exacerbations, and over time, it is associated with reductions in pain intensity. In cases where individuals experience high degrees of pain-related fear and anxiety, graded exposure in vivo to physical movement may be required to minimize their affective response. Cognitive interventions (i.e., cognitive restructuring, calming self-statements, problem-solving) are intended to address pain catastrophizing (e.g., "This pain is so horrible I *cannot* do anything"), maladaptive pain beliefs (e.g., "Walking *should not* be painful"), and enable adaptive problem-solving skills. These cognitive behavioral interventions can be effectively delivered in individual or group formats, can be modified for family or system-based interventions, and can be augmented with the use of biofeedback equipment (e.g., superficial electromyography and monitoring of heart rate, respiration rate, peripheral temperature, and skin conductance). These applications are intended to provide individuals with physiological data that is used to help modulate sympathetic nervous system arousal using the coping skills outlined above.

Pain is a complex and multidimensional experience. In cases of persistent pain, individuals may benefit from clinical management by interdisciplinary teams. Although in some cases complete pain relief is not feasible, a combination of the approaches described above can minimize pain-related interference, disability, and the impact and potential for comorbid psychiatric conditions to maximize the quality of life experienced by individuals.

Cross-References

▶ Pain
▶ Pain Anxiety

► Pain, Psychosocial Aspects
► Pain-Related Fear

References and Readings

Asmundson, G. J. G., Norton, P. J., & Norton, G. R. (1999). Beyond pain: The role of fear and avoidance in chronicity. *Clinical Psychology Review, 19*, 97–119.

Asmundson, G. J. G., Norton, P. J., & Vlaeyen, J. W. S. (2004). Fear-avoidance models of chronic pain: An overview. In G. J. G. Asmundson, J. W. S. Vlaeyen, & G. Crobez (Eds.), *Understanding and treating fear of pain* (pp. 3–24). New York: Oxford University Press.

Bajwa, Z. H., & Ho, C. (2004). Antiepileptics for pain. In C. A. Warfield & Z. H. Bajwa (Eds.), *Principles and practice of pain medicine* (2nd ed., pp. 649–654). New York: McGraw Hill.

Day, M., & Anderson, S. (2004). Cryoanalgesia and radiofrequency. In C. A. Warfield & Z. H. Bajwa (Eds.), *Principles and practice of pain medicine* (2nd ed., pp. 751–764). New York: McGraw Hill.

DeSio, J. M. (2004). Epidural steroid injections. In C. A. Warfield & Z. H. Bajwa (Eds.), *Principles and practice of pain medicine* (2nd ed., pp. 655–661). New York: McGraw Hill.

Du Pen, S. L., & Du Pen, A. (2004). Neuraxial drug delivery. In C. A. Warfield & Z. H. Bajwa (Eds.), *Principles and practice of pain medicine* (2nd ed., pp. 720–739). New York: McGraw Hill.

Keefe, F. J., Beaupre, P. M., & Gil, K. M. (2002). Group therapy for patients with chronic pain. In R. J. Gatchel & D. C. Turk (Eds.), *Psychological approaches to pain management: A practitioner's handbook* (pp. 234–255). New York: Guilford.

Lamer, L. J. (2004). Intra-articular injections and facet blocks. In C. A. Warfield & Z. H. Bajwa (Eds.), *Principles and practice of pain medicine* (2nd ed., pp. 667–683). New York: McGraw Hill.

Lehmann, L. J. (2004). Peripheral nerve blocks. In C. A. Warfield & Z. H. Bajwa (Eds.), *Principles and practice of pain medicine* (2nd ed., pp. 684–695). New York: McGraw Hill.

Lipman, A. G., & Jackson, K. C. (2004). Opioid pharmacotherapy. In C. A. Warfield & Z. H. Bajwa (Eds.), *Principles and practice of pain medicine* (2nd ed., pp. 583–600). New York: McGraw Hill.

Melzack, R. (1999). From the gate to the neuromatrix. *Pain, 82*(Suppl 6), S121–S126.

Melzack, R., & Wall, P. D. (1965). Pain mechanisms: A new theory. *Science, 150*, 971–979.

Simon, L. S. (2004). Nonsteroidal anti-inflammatory drugs. In C. A. Warfield & Z. H. Bajwa (Eds.), *Principles and practice of pain medicine* (2nd ed., pp. 616–626). New York: McGraw Hill.

Turk, D. C. (2002). A cognitive-behavioral perspective on treatment of chronic pain patients. In R. J. Gatchel & D. C. Turk (Eds.), *Psychological approaches to pain management: A practitioner's handbook* (pp. 138–158). New York: Guilford.

Turk, D. C., Meichenbaum, D., & Genest, M. (1983). *Pain and behavioral medicine: A cognitive-behavioral perspective*. New York: Guilford.

Vlaeyen, J. W. S., de Jong, J., Sieben, J., & Crombez, G. (2002). Graded exposure in vivo for pain-related fear. In R. J. Gatchel & D. C. Turk (Eds.), *Psychological approaches to pain management: A practitioner's handbook* (pp. 210–233). New York: Guilford.

Pain Perception

► Gate Control Theory of Pain

Pain Recovery Inventory of Concerns and Expectations (PRICE) Questionnaire

William S. Shaw and Glenn Pransky
Center for Disability Research, Liberty Mutual Research Institute for Safety, Hopkinton, MA, USA
University of Massachusetts Medical School, Worcester, MA, USA

Definition

The Pain Recovery Inventory of Concerns and Expectations (PRICE) is a 46-item self-report questionnaire that was developed to identify individuals with acute low back pain (LBP) who are at greatest risk of transitioning to chronic back pain and disability and to match them to one of three early intervention strategies (Shaw et al. 2013). The items were selected from existing research measures and chosen based on their ability to discriminate patient subgroups and to predict 3-month outcomes of pain, function, and return to work (Shaw et al. 2007). The questionnaire includes items relating to pain and pain beliefs, function, psychological well-being, recovery expectations, and workplace support. The PRICE was designed for working adults with acute LBP and for administration within the first 2 weeks of pain onset. For each item, respondents are asked to indicate their level of agreement, their level of difficulty, or the frequency of their feelings and behaviors.

Description

Acute LBP is a common presenting complaint in primary care and other medical settings, and this painful condition often remits over time with little or no treatment. Approximately half of patients report a full recovery within 30 days. However, a significant number of acute cases transition to chronic pain and disability. One third of patients report lingering pain, functional impairment, or difficulties at work after 3 months, and 5–10% of patients will go on to experience long-term disability and work absence. Workplace and psychosocial variables have been shown to be important prognostic factors in LBP research (Shaw et al. 2006), and most clinical treatment guidelines for acute LBP have accordingly emphasized the need to take these issues into account when making early treatment decisions. However, few assessment tools are available to screen patients for elevated risk of disability and assign matching strategies for early intervention.

The PRICE measure was developed for both research and clinical applications. In clinical applications, the PRICE can be used to screen patients with acute LBP for risk of long-term disability and then match and prioritize early intervention strategies according to PRICE group designations: (a) cluster A, low risk (for whom only usual advice and reassurance is needed); (b) cluster B, *psychological distress* is the predominant risk factor for LBP disability; (c) cluster C, *workplace concerns* are the predominant risk factors for LBP disability; and (d) cluster D, *activity limitation* is the predominant risk factor for LBP disability.

The PRICE measure assesses eight core psychosocial constructs that are predictors of LBP recovery: (a) pain intensity rating, (b) pain catastrophizing, (c) pain recovery expectations, (d) perceived life impact of pain to family and career, (e) ratings of restricted physical function, (f) fears that activity will increase pain or result in a more serious injury, (g) perceptions of workplace organizational support, and (h) depressive mood symptoms. The 46 questions included in the final PRICE measure were selected from a larger pool of 159 items comprised of eight existing scale measures (Reme et al. 2012). For each of the eight scales, a sensitivity analysis was conducted to determine how many items could be excluded while still retaining 90% of the scale's association with 3-month outcomes of function and return to work.

PRICE total scores and group designations are associated with 3-month outcomes of pain duration, functional improvement, and return to work. The eight existing scale measures that provided the initial pool of items for the PRICE have already undergone considerable testing with evidence of good reliability and validity. Total scores and group designations generated by the PRICE are reasonably stable from the first to second week of acute LBP. Proportions of cluster membership do not vary by gender.

A total PRICE score is based on the equally weighted average of seven subscale scores. Group classifications are based on the similarity of an individual scoring profile to four research prototypes: a low-risk group (40%), a high-risk group with elevated psychological distress (20%), a moderate-risk group with elevated workplace concerns (20%), and a moderate-risk group with elevated physical activity concerns (20%). A data dictionary and scoring algorithm for the PRICE can be obtained at no charge from the authors.

The PRICE was derived from a US cohort of 496 workers who were referred to occupational health clinics by their employers for evaluation of work-related acute low back pain and assessed within 14 days from pain onset. Patients in this clinical care setting may vary from those in primary care and other medical care settings. The

PRICE was designed as an early screening measure for acute low back pain (LBP); thus, the measure has not been validated for use with other patient populations. Also, inclusion of workplace support in the formulation of the PRICE may limit its applicability for those who are not in a traditional employment arrangement. The PRICE was intended to augment, not replace, standard medical intake and evaluation procedures including assessment of medical "red flags" that might signal the need for other diagnostic evaluations and specialty care.

The PRICE was constructed from existing scales and measures, some of which represent previously copyrighted materials. However, the authors of those measures have given their express permission to allow these items to be freely circulated as part of the PRICE measure as long as no fee is charged. There is no fee for photocopying or administering the PRICE measure, but the authors request notification of its use in research and clinical practice to aid in tracking and further evaluation of the measure.

References and Further Readings

Reme, S. E., Shaw, W. S., Steenstra, I. A., Woiszwillo, M. J., Pransky, G., & Linton, S. J. (2012). Distressed, immobilized, or lacking employer support? A sub-classification of acute work-related low back pain. *Journal of Occupational Rehabilitation, 22*, 541–552.

Shaw, W. S., Linton, S. J., & Pransky, G. (2006). Reducing sickness absence from work due to low back pain: How well do intervention strategies match modifiable risk factors? *Journal of Occupational Rehabilitation, 16*, 591–605.

Shaw, W. S., Pransky, G., Patterson, W., Linton, S. J., & Winters, T. (2007). Patient clusters in acute, work-related back pain based on patterns of disability risk factors. *Journal of Occupational & Environmental Medicine, 49*, 185–193.

Shaw, W. S., Reme, S. E., Pransky, G., Woiszwillo, M. J., Steenstra, I. A., & Linton, S. J. (2013). The pain recovery inventory of concerns and expectations: A psychosocial screening instrument to identify intervention needs among patients at elevated risk of back disability. *Journal of Occupational & Environmental Medicine, 55*(8), 885–894.

Pain Self-Management at Work

William S. Shaw and Glenn Pransky
Center for Disability Research, Liberty Mutual Research Institute for Safety, Hopkinton, MA, USA
University of Massachusetts Medical School, Worcester, MA, USA

Definition

Pain self-management at work is the ability of individuals to master issues of communication, job modification, pacing, and problem-solving to overcome health challenges at work. For workers with chronic pain problems, this approach can improve workplace function, coping, job satisfaction, social relations at work, and organizational support.

Description

One significant trend in the workforce is the advancing median age of workers and the growing prevalence of chronic medical conditions that can contribute to workplace pain, fatigue, task limitations, and reduced productivity. Approximately 40% of working adults report persistent or recurrent musculoskeletal pain conditions or other chronic health conditions that limit their ability to work (Burton et al. 2004). Because of aging trends in the workforce, the prevalence of chronic medical conditions, especially musculoskeletal conditions, will increase in coming years, and this may lead to productivity losses for employers (van Leeuwen et al. 2006). The inability of workers to successfully manage chronic pain and fatigue in the workplace may not only reduce workforce productivity but also increase business costs through higher turnover rates, absenteeism, retraining, and healthcare expense. This also represents a serious quality-of-life issue for workers who are struggling to maintain employment and risking disability. Being able to continue to function at work has been shown to be a primary concern for aging workers with chronic health conditions (Peterson and Murphy 2010).

Despite having functional limitations, the majority of working-age adults with chronic musculoskeletal conditions are gainfully employed and continue full-time work without the need for formal job accommodations or physician-ordered restrictions. Qualitative research with workers suggests that the ability to continue working is possible by leveraging available job leeway and flexibility, by careful planning and decision-making with regard to work, by obtaining job assistance and social support in and out of work, and by communicating needs effectively and judiciously with peers and supervisors (Tveito et al. 2010). Past research has highlighted the importance of both organizational support and individual coping and problem-solving strategies to overcome health-related challenges at work, but there are only recent efforts to develop and test psychoeducational programs intended to improve coping and self-management strategies at work. What has not been studied is whether specific employer-supported organizational or educational interventions might help workers to improve coping and overcome health-related workplace challenges. More research is needed to assess pain and illness self-management interventions in the workplace.

One ongoing research trial is the "Manage at Work" study, a randomized trial of a five-session group intervention program targeting workers ($n = 240$) with chronic health concerns (Clinicaltrials.gov: NCT01978392). The Manage at Work study applies psychoeducational techniques borrowed from principles of cognitive behavioral therapy to enhance coping skills and provide individualized plans for problem-solving and dealing with temporary setbacks. The self-management approach to recurrent or persistent medical problems involves redefining health symptoms and functional challenges as subject to personal control and mastery and through the encouragement of an active, problem-solving perspective. Identification and modification of negative cognitions related to the health complaint is also emphasized. SM interventions have been shown to consistently reduce the experience of pain, fatigue, functional limitations, and distress in clinical trials, but these programs have included no attention to workplace problems (Shaw et al. 2012). The primary outcomes being assessed in the study are work limitations and work engagement measured at baseline, 6 months, and 12 months follow-up. Secondary outcomes include turnover intention, sickness absence, job satisfaction, and healthcare utilization. Process variables and covariates include assessment of self-efficacy, work-related fatigue, emotional distress, work characteristics, general health status, and basic demographic variables. A parallel process evaluation is also being conducted to address issues of feasibility, recruitment, reach, and uptake. The study will be an important first step toward employer-sponsored programs involving psychological coping of workers with chronic health conditions that can impair workplace function.

References and Further Readings

Burton, W. N., Pransky, G., Conti, D. J., Chen, C. Y., & Edington, D. W. (2004). The association of medical conditions and presenteeism. *Journal of Occupational and Environmental Medicine, 46*(6 Suppl), S38–S45.

Peterson, C. L., & Murphy, G. (2010). Transition from the labor market: Older workers and retirement. *International Journal of Health Services, 40*(4), 609–627.

Shaw, W. S., Tveito, T. H., Geehern-Lavoie, M., Huang, Y. H., Nicholas, M. K., Reme, S. E., Wagner, G., & Pransky, G. (2012). Adapting principles of chronic pain self-management to the workplace. *Disability and Rehabilitation, 32*(24), 2035–2045.

Tveito, T. H., Shaw, W. S., Huang, Y. H., Nicholas, M., & Wagner, G. (2010). Managing pain in the workplace: A focus group study of challenges, strategies and what matters most to workers with low back pain. *Disability and Rehabilitation, 32*(24), 2035–2045.

van Leeuwen, M. T., Blyth, F. M., March, L. M., Nicholas, M. K., & Cousins, M. J. (2006). Chronic pain and reduced work effectiveness: The hidden cost to Australian employers. *European Journal of Pain, 10*(2), 161–166.

Pain Sensitivity

▶ Gate Control Theory of Pain

Pain Threshold

Michael James Coons[1] and Jeremy Steglitz[2]
[1]Department of Preventive Medicine, Feinberg School of Medicine, Northwestern University, Chicago, IL, USA
[2]Department of Psychiatry and Behavioral Sciences, Clinical Psychology Division, Feinberg School of Medicine, Northwestern University, Chicago, IL, USA

Definition

Pain threshold is defined as the minimum intensity of a stimulus that is perceived to be painful. Previously, this threshold was believed to be uniform across individuals, such that given intensity of a stimulus was thought to produce a given pain response. However, it is now understood that the experience of pain is a subjective phenomenon, which is influenced by a complex interaction of biopsychosocial factors.

Historically, Specificity Theory and Pattern Theory posit that pain results from the direct transmission of peripheral stimuli to the brain, and stimulus response occurs in a reproducible relationship. However, limitations to these theories became evident after observing divergent responses to pain across individuals despite objectively similar physical stimuli or trauma. Consequently, Melzack and Wall proposed the Gate Control Theory of pain, which revolutionized our understanding of this phenomenon.

According to this theory, peripheral small diameter nerve fibers (i.e., pain receptors) and peripheral large diameter nerve fibers (i.e., normal receptors) project to the substantia gelatinosa (SG) in the dorsal horn of the spinal cord. The SG serves an inhibitory or gating function that modulates signal transduction. The SG also projects afferent fibers to the first transmission (T) cells. Activation of the T cells "activates the neural system" via the spinothalamic tract to facilitate pain perception.

In part, pain perception is determined by this bottom-up process. In the absence of sensory input, inhibitory neurons in the SG prevent projection neurons from transducing signals to the brain (i.e., maintaining a closed gate). When there is a preponderance of stimulation of pain receptors, the inhibitory neurons in the SG becomes inactivated (opening the gate), permitting the afferent projection neurons to transduce pain signals to the T cells and to the brain. However, pain perception is also influenced by top-down processes that include cognitive processes (e.g., attention), neural inhibitory capacities, affective states, and activities of the stress-regulation system. These processes transduce efferent signals to the dorsal horn in the spinal cord that further modulate the spinal gate and subsequent pain perception. Pain threshold is determined by variation in spinal gate modulation from both bottom-up and top-down processes that facilitate pain perception.

Cross-References

▶ Pain
▶ Pain Management/Control
▶ Pain, Psychosocial Aspects

References and Readings

Melzack, R. (1999). From the gate to the neuromatrix. *Pain, 82*(Suppl. 6), S121–S126.
Melzack, R., & Wall, P. D. (1965). Pain mechanisms: A new theory. *Science, 150*, 971–979.
McMahon, S. B., & Koltzenburg, M. (Eds.). (2006). *Melzack & Wall's textbook of pain*. London: Elsevier.

Pain, Psychosocial Aspects

Michael James Coons
Department of Preventive Medicine, Feinberg School of Medicine, Northwestern University, Chicago, IL, USA

Synonyms

Pain anxiety; Pain management/control; Pain-related fear

Definition

Researchers and clinicians have begun to map the trajectory of pain from acute to persistent states. These outcomes are influenced by a complex interaction of biological, psychological, behavioral, and social components, which can be clustered into intrapersonal factors (factors affecting the level of the individual) and interpersonal factors (factors affecting the interaction between the individual and their environment). These factors influence both pain perception and responses to treatment.

Description

Pain is a universal phenomenon experienced by most individuals. However, pain sometimes persists beyond a reasonable time during which tissue typically heals following injury. Several researchers have developed and articulated conceptual models to understand how and why for some individuals pain transitions from acute to persistent states.

Fear-Avoidance Models of Pain

Fear-Avoidance Models posit that following the onset of pain (from injury or disease process), individuals appraise and evaluate their experience (see Fig. 1 Norton and Asmundson 2003). For those who perceive their pain in a realistic manner, they do not experience excessive fear of pain, are able to engage in activities following a reasonable healing period, and subsequently recover from their experience. However, for others, a more complicated course of recovery ensues triggering a variety of cognitive, physiological, and behavioral symptoms. For those that progress to develop persistent pain (either recurrent intermittent pain or unremitting pain), they interpret their pain to be catastrophic in nature (e.g., "This pain is so excruciating I cannot function"). This overinterpretation triggers a state of autonomic arousal and pain-

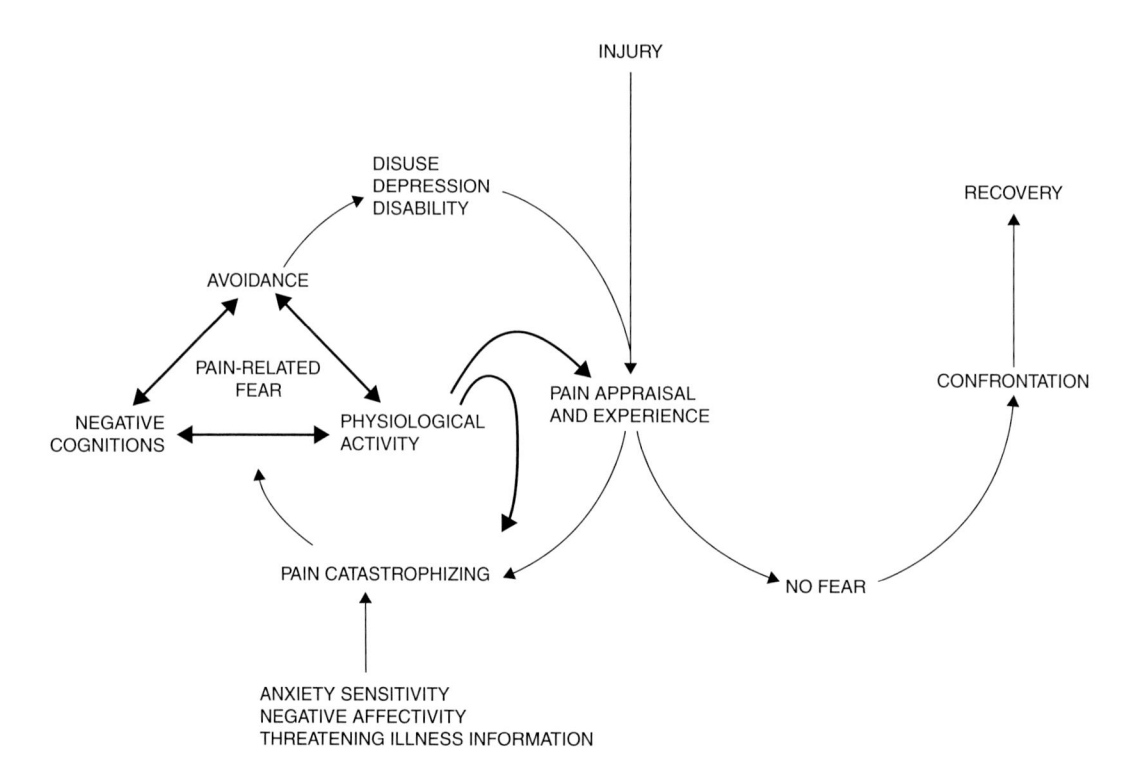

Pain, Psychosocial Aspects, Fig. 1 Amended fear-avoidance model of chronic pain (Copyright (2011) by the Association for Behavioral and Cognitive Therapies. Reprinted by permission of the publisher)

related fear. This fear is accompanied by a variety of somatic symptoms and negative cognitions about pain that motivates are variety of escape-avoidance behaviors (e.g., prolonged periods of rest, avoidance of physical activity). Over time, the anticipation of experiencing pain in the future motivates continued avoidance of activity, which in turn, leads to loss of physical strength, physical deconditioning, and muscle atrophy. These consequences result in increases in pain intensity, which continues to fuel this fear-avoidance cycle. Several individual difference variables have been identified that seem to place individuals at risk for developing persistent pain and include negative affectivity (i.e., trait experiences of negative emotions) and anxiety sensitivity (i.e., the propensity to experience fear of somatic sensations). Individuals that experience higher levels of these traits have been shown to be at greater risk for developing persistent pain conditions.

Intrapersonal Factors in Persistent Pain
Regardless of the nature of the pain experience (i.e., headache pain; orofacial pain), psychosocial factors have been shown to moderate pain intensity and progression. Specifically, depression, anxiety disorders (e.g., post-traumatic stress disorder, panic disorder, generalized anxiety disorder), substance use disorders, and somatoform pain disorders commonly co-occur with persistent pain conditions and are significantly higher than rates found in the general population. Furthermore, personality disorders also appear to occur more frequently among patients with persistent pain than among the general population; however, precise estimates in the general population are not available. These psychiatric phenomenon may share similar underlying processes to pain (that may account for their co-occurrence), are associated with more negative perceptions of pain, and influence individual's behavioral responses (e.g., are associated with greater pain-related avoidance). It has also been shown that heightened emotional reactivity, particularly when coupled with concurrent psychosocial stressors, further exacerbates negative perceptions of pain and predisposes individuals to pain-related disability. Furthermore, active coping skills (e.g., continuing to engage in activities, distraction from pain) are associated with lower pain intensity and minimize the risk of pain persistence. In contrast, passive coping skills (e.g., pain-related avoidance behavior, reliance on others) are associated with higher pain intensity and increase the risk of pain persistence.

Interpersonal Factors in Persistent Pain
Beyond the individual, several interpersonal factors are associated with pain severity, persistence, and pain-related disability. Within the context of intimate relationships, displays of pain-related behavior solicit responses from others that become reinforced over time and may perpetuate negative outcomes. For instance, an individual with persistent low back pain may display grimacing and guarding behaviors in response to pain experienced while attempting to dress them self. However, their partner may respond by providing physical assistance to help this individual put on their clothes. Although this physical assistance helps to minimize the pain experienced, and facilitates the timely completion of this task, it reinforces the need for assistance contributing to more significant pain-related disability. Over time, such pain-related behaviors become negatively reinforced (since the assistance provided minimizes the experience of pain), which increases the likelihood of similar future behavioral responses. Furthermore, the need for assistance may undermine an individual's self-efficacy (i.e., their confidence in their ability to manage pain) and contribute to greater pain intensity, more frequent pain-related behavior, physical inactivity, and pain-related disability.

Psychosocial Factors and Treatment Response
Following the progression from acute to persistent pain, psychosocial factors have also been shown to influence responses to a variety of treatments. Across different categorical subtypes (i.e., low back pain; headache pain), the presence of axis I pathology (e.g., depression, anxiety, somatization) is associated with lower response to treatment (i.e., greater frequency and intensity of pain reports, greater perceived functional impairment), and may interfere with individual's ability to

engage in the treatment process (e.g., depression interferes with treatment attendance and adherence to interventions). Furthermore, it has been shown that the continued use of maladaptive coping skills (i.e., pain-related avoidance behaviors), positive attitudes and expectations about pain and disability (i.e., pain facilitates the maintenance of supportive relationships; pain prevents the return to unsatisfactory employment), and unresolved worker's compensation/personal injury cases are further associated with lower treatment response. Therefore, a comprehensive assessment of these psychosocial factors is imperative at the outset of any pain-related intervention. This can be accomplished by obtaining a detailed medical and psychosocial history, conducting semi-structured clinical and diagnostic interviews with both patients and their caregivers, the administration of self-report instruments, and consultation with current and past health-care providers.

Considered together, persistent pain conditions arise from a complex interaction of biological, psychological, social, and environmental factors. Understanding these relationships will help to identify factors that maintain and reinforce persistent pain across time and will provide insight into the development of effective pain management interventions.

Cross-References

▶ Pain
▶ Pain Anxiety
▶ Pain Management/Control
▶ Pain-Related Fear

References and Readings

Asmundson, G. J. G., Norton, P. J., & Norton, G. R. (1999). Beyond pain: The role of fear and avoidance in chronicity. *Clinical Psychology Review, 19*, 97–119.

Asmundson, G. J. G., Norton, P. J., & Vlaeyen, J. W. S. (2004). Fear-avoidance models of chronic pain: An overview. In G. J. G. Asmundson, J. W. S. Vlaeyen, & G. Crobez (Eds.), *Understanding and treating fear of pain* (pp. 3–24). New York: Oxford University Press.

Gatchel, R. J., & Dersh, J. (2002). Psychological disorders and chronic pain: Are there cause-and-effect relationships? In D. C. Turk & R. J. Gatchel (Eds.), *Psychological approaches to pain management: A practitioner's handbook* (2nd ed., pp. 30–51). New York: Guilford Press.

Gatchel, R. J., & Epker, J. (1999). Psychosocial predictors of chronic pain and response to treatment. In R. J. Gatchel & D. C. Turk (Eds.), *Psychosocial factors in pain: Critical perspectives* (pp. 412–434). New York: Guilford Press.

Goubert, L., Crombez, G., & Peters, M. (2004). Pain-related fear and avoidance: A conditioning perspective. In G. J. G. Asmundson, J. W. S. Vlaeyen, & G. Crobez (Eds.), *Understanding and treating fear of pain* (pp. 25–50). New York: Oxford University Press.

Keogh, E., & Asmundson, G. J. G. (2004). Negative affectivity, catastrophizing, and anxiety sensitivity. In G. J. G. Asmundson, J. W. S. Vlaeyen, & G. Crobez (Eds.), *Understanding and treating fear of pain* (pp. 91–116). New York: Oxford University Press.

Linton, S. J., & Boersma, K. (2004). The role of fear-avoidance in the early identification of patients risking the development of disability. In G. J. G. Asmundson, J. W. S. Vlaeyen, & G. Crobez (Eds.), *Understanding and treating fear of pain* (pp. 213–235). New York: Oxford University Press.

Norton, P. J., & Asmundson, G. J. G. (2003). Amending the fear-avoidance model of chronic pain: What is the role of physiological arousal? *Behavior Therapy, 34*, 17–30.

Sanders, S. H. (2002). Operant conditioning with chronic pain: Back to basics. In D. C. Turk & R. J. Gatchel (Eds.), *Psychological approaches to pain management: A practitioner's handbook* (2nd ed., pp. 128–137). New York: Guilford Press.

Turk, D. C., & Flor, H. (1999). Chronic pain: A biobehavioral perspective. In R. J. Gatchel & D. C. Turk (Eds.), *Psychosocial factors in pain: Critical perspectives* (pp. 18–34). New York: Guilford Press.

Turk, D. C., & Gatchel, R. J. (1999). Psychosocial factors and pain: Revolution and evolution. In R. J. Gatchel & D. C. Turk (Eds.), *Psychosocial factors in pain: Critical perspectives* (pp. 481–494). New York: Guilford Press.

Pain-Related Fear

Michael James Coons
Department of Preventive Medicine, Feinberg School of Medicine, Northwestern University, Chicago, IL, USA

Synonyms

Pain anxiety; Pain, psychosocial aspects

Definition

It is an affective manifestation of the fight-or-flight system in response to pain perception. The sympathetic nervous system becomes activated by the amygdala, resulting in cognitive, physiological, and behavioral symptoms. Following pain perception subsequent to injury or pain-inducing stimuli, pain is interpreted catastrophically by inferring more harmful or life-threatening outcomes to its underlying cause. For instance, when an individual experiences acute pain after rolling over on their ankle, they might infer that the pain is caused by a broken bone, rather than by a sprain. This negative cognitive bias is predisposed by trait-like factors including anxiety sensitivity (i.e., fear of interoceptive experiences) and negative affectivity (i.e., the propensity toward experiencing negative emotions). This cognitive process prompts hypervigilance toward interoceptive cues (e.g., pain or muscle tension consequent to their injury) and illness information in the internal of external environment (continued or exacerbated pain). This motivates a constellation of defensive behaviors (e.g., guarding, rest) that are intended to provide relief or escape from the pain-inducing state. Fear-avoidance models of pain, and the empirical evidence supporting such models, suggest that pain-related fear is a predisposing factor to the development of persistent pain conditions.

Assessment of Pain-Related Fear

The most common mode of assessment of pain-related fear involves the administration of well-validated self-report instruments. Several published scales are available including the Fear of Pain Questionnaire-III (FPQ-III) and the Fear-Avoidance Beliefs Questionnaire (FABQ). These measures assess the nature and extent of pain-related fear by asking individuals to rate how much they fear the pain associated with a variety of situations (e.g., "having someone slam a heavy car door on your hand," "biting your tongue while eating") or the nature and extent of a variety of pain-related beliefs (e.g., "Physical activity might harm my back," "I should not do physical activities that (might) make my pain worse"). Alternative modes of assessing pain-related fear include semi-structured clinical interviews and the direct observation of patient behavior.

Treatment of Pain-Related Fear

Cognitive behavior therapy (CBT) is a mainstay in the treatment of pain-related fear. Treatment components include psychoeducation, and introduction, demonstration, and practice of a variety of adaptive coping skills (i.e., progressive muscle relaxation, diaphragmatic breathing, mental imagery, behavioral activation and pleasant activity scheduling, activity-rest cycling, physical therapy/exercise, problem-solving, cognitive restructuring, and calming self-statements). In treating pain-related fear, special emphasis is placed on graded in vivo exposure with behavioral experiments. These latter components allow individuals to construct situations in which they collect information to test and challenge their distorted pain-related cognitions.

Cross-References

▶ Pain Anxiety
▶ Pain, Psychosocial Aspects

References and Readings

Asmundson, G. J. G., Norton, P. J., & Vlaeyen, W. S. (2004). Fear-avoidance models of chronic pain: An overview. In G. J. G. Asmundson, J. W. S. Vlaeyen, & G. Crombez (Eds.), *Understanding and treating fear of pain* (pp. 3–24). New York: Oxford University Press.

de Williams, A. C., & McCracken, L. M. (2004). Cognitive behavioral therapy for chronic pain: An overview with specific reference to fear avoidance. In G. J. G. Asmundson, J. W. S. Vlaeyen, & G. Crobez (Eds.), *Understanding and treating fear of pain* (pp. 293–312). New York: Oxford University Press.

McNeil, D. W., & Vowles, K. E. (2004). Assessment of fear and anxiety associated with pain: Conceptualization, methods, and measures. In G. J. G. Asmundson, J. W. S. Vlaeyen, & G. Crombez (Eds.), *Understanding and treating fear of pain* (pp. 189–211). New York: Oxford University Press.

Palliative Care

Satoru Iwase and Chica Mori
Department Of Palliative Medicine, The University of Tokyo Hospital, Tokyo, Japan

Synonyms

Hospices; Palliative medicine; Supportive care; Terminal care

Definition

The World Health Organization (WHO) defines palliative care as "an approach that improves the quality of life of patients and their families facing the problems associated with life-threatening illness, through the prevention and relief of suffering by means of early identification and impeccable assessment and treatment of pain and other problems, physical, psychological and spiritual" (World Health Organization 2002).

Description

The goal of palliative care is to achieve the best possible quality of life for both the patients and their families.

Palliative care:

- Is a multidisciplinary task and uses a team approach by physicians, nurses, psychologists, social workers, and other health professionals to address the needs of patients and their families
- Offers a support system to help patients and their families in the community
- Is applicable at any age and at any stage in the course of illness, in conjunction with other therapies such as chemotherapy or radiation therapy which may prolong life
- Provides relief from distressing symptoms such as pain, shortness of breath, depression, drowsiness, and nausea
- Alleviates the adverse side effects, such as relieving the nausea related to chemotherapy
- Influences positively in the course of illness (Temel et al. 2010.

Dying is a normal event; however, many people feel uncomfortable discussing their own death as well as the death of someone close. A book "Hagakure," written by a samurai warrior, who was keenly aware of the events of the day, teaches us how to cope with spiritual pain within the framework of our own insight. "There is something to be learned from a rainstorm. When meeting with a sudden shower, you try not to wet and run quickly along the road. But doing such things as passing under the eaves of houses, you still get wet. When you are resolved from the beginning, you will not be perplexed, though you still get the same soaking. This understanding extends to everything" (Yamamoto 2005).

Perception of physical, psychological, and spiritual pain may differ in various countries with different cultures and religions; nonetheless, we all aim for the same goal in palliative care.

Cross-References

▶ End-of-Life
▶ Religion/Spirituality
▶ World Health Organization (WHO)

References and Readings

Temel, J. S., Greer, J. A., Muzikansky, A., Gallagher, E. R., Admane, S., Jackson, V. A., et al. (2010). Early palliative care for patients with metastatic non-small-cell lung cancer. *New England Journal of Medicine, 363*(8), 733–742. Retrieved August 19, 2010, from https://www.nejm.org.

World Health Organization. (2002). *WHO definition of palliative care*. Retrieved September 28, 2009, from http://www.who.int/cancer/palliative/definition/en/

Yamamoto, T. (2005). *Hagakure: The book of the samurai* (W. S. Wilson, Trans.). Tokyo: Kodansha International.

Palliative Medicine

▶ Palliative Care

Panic Attack

Michael James Coons
Department of Preventive Medicine, Feinberg School of Medicine, Northwestern University, Chicago, IL, USA

Synonyms

Panic disorder

Definition

Panic attacks are a state of sympathetic nervous system arousal that results in a discrete episode of intense fear or discomfort in the absence of objective danger. This fear is accompanied by a host of somatic and cognitive symptoms. Symptoms include tachycardia (i.e., racing heart), sweating, palpitations, trembling, dyspnea (i.e., shortness of breath), feelings of being smothered or feelings of choking, nausea, chest pain, abdominal distress, dizziness, light headedness, derealization or depersonalization, numbness or tingling in the face or extremities, chills or hot flushes, fear of "going crazy," fear of losing control, or fear of death from such an episode. Individuals must report experiencing at least 4 of the 13 possible somatic and cognitive symptoms. These aforementioned symptoms typically peak in intensity over a short period of time (i.e., 10 min or less). If individuals report experiencing excessive fear but manifest fewer than four symptoms, it is considered to be a limited-symptom panic attack. Panic attacks are classified into three main subtypes: cued panic attacks (i.e., panic attacks can occur in response to a specific situation or event), uncued panic attacks (i.e., panic attacks that occur "out of the blue" in the absence of a discernable trigger), or situationally predisposed panic attacks (i.e., panic attacks that occur immediately on exposure to or in anticipation of a specific situational cue or trigger). The experience of at least two *uncued* panic attacks is a prerequisite for the diagnosis of panic disorder. However, panic attacks can occur in the context of any other anxiety disorder (e.g., generalized anxiety disorder, social anxiety disorder) when cued by situational events or triggers (e.g., in response to excessive worry; during a social interaction). The possible consequences of such episodes make panic attacks of interest to behavioral medicine.

Cross-References

▶ Panic Disorder

References and Readings

American Psychiatric Association. (2000). *Diagnostic and statistical manual for mental disorders (Revised)* (4th ed.). Washington, DC: APA.

Antony, M. M., & Swinson, R. P. (2000). *Phobic disorder and panic in adults: A guide to assessment and treatment*. Washington, DC: American Psychological Association.

McCabe, R. (2001). Panic disorder and agoraphobia: A brief overview and guide to assessment. In M. M. Antony, S. M. Orsillo, & L. Roemer (Eds.), *Practitioner's guide to empirically based measures of anxiety* (pp. 87–94). New York: Kluwer Academic/Plenum.

Panic Disorder

Michael James Coons
Department of Preventive Medicine, Feinberg School of Medicine, Northwestern University, Chicago, IL, USA

Synonyms

Panic attack

Definition

According to the Diagnostic and Statistical Manual for Mental Disorders, Fourth Edition (DSM-IV-TR), panic disorder (PD) is an anxiety disorder that is defined by the experience of recurrent (two or more) uncured panic attacks. Following these attacks and for a period of at least 1 month, individuals must report experiencing concern about either having additional attacks, concern about the potential implications of having panic attacks (e.g., death), or significantly change their behavior because of the experience of panic attacks (e.g., avoidance of certain situations). In this context, panic attacks cannot occur in response to the physiological effects of a substance (e.g., caffeine, marijuana), cannot be due to a general medical condition, and cannot be better accounted for by another mental disorder (e.g., generalized anxiety disorder). PD can occur in isolation, or in the presence of agoraphobia (i.e., anxiety about particular places or situations in which individuals fear experiencing a panic attack). According to the DSM-IV-TR, PD occurs in approximately 1–2% of the general population. The onset of PD typically occurs between late adolescence and mid-30s. Researchers have shown that anxiety sensitivity (i.e., an individual difference variable involving the fear of anxiety-related somatic symptoms) is a robust predictor of the development of PD. However, PD (with or without agoraphobia) is diagnosed more commonly among women than among men.

Cognitive Behavioral Models

Theoretical models of PD suggest that among individuals who are predisposed to being fearful of somatic cues (i.e., having high levels of anxiety sensitivity), they catastrophically misinterpret physiological sensations when they occur (e.g., "my heart is racing, I *must* be having a heart attack"). Such distorted cognitions motivate a series of maladaptive behaviors (e.g., escaping the current situation to prevent the catastrophic outcome, avoiding situations because of the fear of experiencing a future panic attack, not leaving the house alone in the event of a panic attack). Over time and across situations, these escape-, avoidance-, and safety-seeking behaviors become negatively reinforced, resulting in a reliance on engaging in these behaviors to either prevent a panic attack from occurring, or in minimizing the potential (perceived) negative and catastrophic outcome(s). Together, these maladaptive cognitions and behaviors contribute to greater sympathetic arousal that results in a host of somatic symptoms (e.g., racing heart, dyspnea, nausea, shaking/trembling), which perpetuates the cycle of panic.

Assessment

Prior to commencing any pharmacological or psychological intervention, it is essential to establish a differential diagnosis to determine if PD is the most appropriate diagnosis. This can be accomplished through the administration of structured clinical interviews, the completion of various self-report instruments, and if necessary, a thorough medical evaluation. The Structured Clinical Interview for DSM-IV (SCID-IV) and the Anxiety Disorders Interview Schedule IV (ADIS-IV) are the two "gold standard" clinical interviews for the anxiety disorders. These interviews are modeled after diagnostic criteria from the DSM-IV and assess the presence of all anxiety disorders, along with a variety of potentially comorbid axis I conditions (e.g., mood disorders, substance use disorders, somatoform disorders, psychotic disorders, and adjustment disorders). In conjunction with structured clinical interviews, a variety of well-validated self-report instruments are available to assess the nature, extent, and risk for PD symptoms. These include the Anxiety Sensitivity Index, Revised (ASI-R), the Panic Disorder Severity Scale (PDSS), and the Agoraphobic Cognitions Questionnaire (ACQ). If there is potential for a patient's panic symptoms to be caused by an underlying medical condition (e.g., atrial fibrillation), a thorough medical evaluation is required before a diagnosis of PD can be established.

Treatment of PD

Efficacious treatments for PD include both pharmacological and psychological interventions. Both selective serotonin reuptake inhibitors (SSRIs) and benzodiazepines are used in the treatment of PD. However, it is recommended that benzodiazepines be prescribed using a scheduled dose, as opposed to an "as needed" basis (i.e., PRN). This helps to minimize the risk of the benzodiazepine use becoming a maladaptive safety behavior that may exacerbate PD-related cognitive distortions. Cognitive behavior therapy (CBT) remains as the front-line psychological intervention for PD. Treatment components include psychoeducation (around the fight-or-flight system, CBT model of panic), identification and restructuring of cognitive distortions, and graded exposure (cognitive, in vivo, and interoceptive). Recent technological advancements permit the augmentation of exposure-based interventions with virtual reality equipment.

Cross-References

▶ Panic Attack

References and Readings

American Psychiatric Association. (2000). *Diagnostic and statistical manual for mental disorders* (Revised 4th ed.). Washington, DC: Author.

Antony, M. M., & Swinson, R. P. (2000). *Phobic disorder and panic in adults: A guide to assessment and treatment*. Washington, DC: American Psychological Association.

Taylor, S. (2000). *Understanding and treating panic disorder: Cognitive-behavioral approaches*. New York: Wiley.

Paradoxal Sleep

▶ REM Sleep

Parallel Group Design

J. Rick Turner
Campbell University College of Pharmacy and Health Sciences, Buies Creek, NC, USA

Synonyms

Independent treatments group design

Definition

A parallel group design is an experimental study design in which each subject is randomized to one of two or more distinct treatment/intervention groups. Those who are assigned to the same treatment are referred to as a treatment group.

While the treatments that these groups receive differ, all groups are treated as equally as possible in all other regards, and they complete the same procedures during the study. This parallel activity on the part of the groups of individuals is captured in the term "parallel group design."

The term controlled study is often heard in this context. One group will receive the treatment of interest and another group a control treatment, against which responses during and at the end of the treatment intervention are compared. Going one step further, the term concurrently controlled study makes clear that the different groups take part in their respective treatment arms at the same time. If all of the subjects in one treatment group completed their participation first, and then all of the other subjects completed their participation at some later time, it is quite possible that other factors could confound the results.

Cross-References

▶ Crossover Design
▶ Randomization

Parasympathetic

▶ Autonomic Balance
▶ Heart Rate Variability

Parasympathetic Nervous System (PNS)

Michael Richter[1] and Rex A. Wright[2]
[1]Department of Psychology, University of Geneva, Geneva, Switzerland
[2]Department of Psychology, College of Arts and Sciences, University of North Texas, Denton, TX, USA

Definition

The parasympathetic nervous system (PNS) is one of two main branches or subsystems of the autonomic nervous system (ANS). It originates in the brain stem and sacral spinal cord and commonly – but not always – yields peripheral adjustments that are complementary to those produced by its counterpart, the sympathetic nervous system (SNS).

Description

The parasympathetic nervous system is one of two main branches or subsystems of the autonomic nervous system, the physical system responsible for nonconsciously maintaining bodily homeostasis and coordinating bodily responses. Working with the second main branch, the sympathetic nervous system, the parasympathetic nervous system regulates a wide range of functions such as blood circulation, body temperature, respiration, and digestion. Parasympathetic activation commonly leads to adjustments on organs and glands that are complementary to those produced by sympathetic activation and suitable for low activity and bodily restoration ("rest and digest" as opposed to "fight and flight"). Examples of low activity and restorative adjustments are constriction of blood vessels in the lungs, increased gastric secretion, and decreased heart rate and contraction force. Although parasympathetic adjustments tend to complement sympathetic adjustments, they do not always. For example, both parasympathetic nervous system arousal and sympathetic nervous system arousal increase salivary flow, although to different degrees and yielding different compositions of saliva.

Basic functional units of the parasympathetic nervous system are preganglionic and postganglionic neurons. Preganglionic neurons have cell bodies in the brainstem or sacral spinal cord and axons that extend to cell bodies of postganglionic neurons. Postganglionic neurons have cell bodies that are clustered in so-called ganglia and relatively short axons that innervate target organs and glands.

The major neurotransmitter of the parasympathetic nervous system is acetylcholine. It is the neurotransmitter of all preganglionic and postganglionic neurons. Stimulation of the cholinergic receptors of the nicotinergic subtype located on the cell bodies of the postganglionic neurons by acetylcholine leads to an opening of nonspecific ion channels. This opening permits the transfer of potassium and sodium ions, which depolarizes the postganglionic cell and initiates an action potential in the postganglionic cells. Muscarinic cholinergic receptors are located on target organs and glands. Stimulation of muscarinic receptors by acetylcholine activates G-proteins, which trigger the effector response via a second-messenger pathway. Specific effects depend on the innervated visceral structure. For instance, activation of the muscarinic receptors of the heart muscle leads to reduced heart rate and heart contraction force. Stimulation of muscarinic receptors of the salivary glands increases salivary flow.

In working jointly with the sympathetic nervous system, the parasympathetic nervous system does not function in an all-or-none fashion, but rather activates to different degrees. Depending on the affected visceral structure and situation, it may be more or less active than the sympathetic nervous system. Shifts in the magnitude of sympathetic and parasympathetic influence can occur locally within a single visceral structure (e.g., the eye) or across visceral structures, with local shifts occurring to meet highly specialized demands (e.g., a change in ambient light) and global shifts adapting the body to large-scale environmental changes (e.g., the appearance of a substantial physical threat). Autonomic control is maintained by structures in the central nervous system that receive visceral information from an afferent (incoming) nervous system. A key central nervous system structure is the hypothalamus, which integrates autonomic, somatic, and endocrine responses that accompany different organism states.

Cross-References

- ▶ Acetylcholine
- ▶ Autonomic Activation
- ▶ Autonomic Balance
- ▶ Autonomic Nervous System (ANS)
- ▶ Epinephrine
- ▶ Sympathetic Nervous System (SNS)

References and Readings

Berne, R. M., Levy, M. N., Koeppen, B. M., & Stanton, B. A. (2004). *Physiology* (5th ed.). St. Louis: Mosby.
Cacioppo, J. T., & Tassinary, L. G. (1990). *Principles of psychophysiology: Physical, social, and inferential elements*. New York: Cambridge University Press.
Cacioppo, J. T., Tassinary, L. G., & Berntson, G. G. (2000). *Handbook of psychophysiology* (2nd ed.). New York: Cambridge University Press.
Ganong, W. F. (2005). *Review of medical physiology* (22nd ed.). New York: McGraw-Hill.
Levick, J. R. (2009). *An introduction to cardiovascular physiology* (5th ed.). London: Hodder.

Paraventricular Nucleus

- ▶ Hypothalamus

Parent-Child Concordance

- ▶ Family Aggregation

Parent-Rated Life Orientation Test of Children (P-LOT)

- ▶ Optimism and Pessimism: Measurement

Parietal

- ▶ Brain, Cortex

Parkinson's Disease

- ▶ Parkinson's Disease: Psychosocial Aspects

Parkinson's Disease: Psychosocial Aspects

Shawn McClintock, Matthieu Chansard and Mustafa M. Husain
Department of Psychiatry, The University of Texas Southwestern Medical Center at Dallas
Columbia University/New York State Psychiatric Institute, Dallas, TX, USA

Synonyms

Degenerative parkinsonism; Parkinson's disease; Parkinsonism; PD; Secondary parkinsonism

Definition

Parkinson's disease (PD) is the second most common neurodegenerative disorder and is characterized by motoric symptoms of resting tremor, rigidity, bradykinesia, and gait disturbance. The psychosocial aspects of PD involve the interaction of PD symptomatology, psychological development and function, personal relationships, and environmental factors.

Description

Parkinson's disease (PD) is a common neurodegenerative disorder that affects approximately between 500,000 and a million Americans of all races and ethnic groups, and 0.3% (5 million) of the world's population. Pathologically, PD is an inexorably progressive disorder of unknown cause in which neurons of the substantia nigra progressively degenerate resulting in greater degrees of brain dopamine deficiency. In addition, a number of other neuronal pathways degenerate including cholinergic, noradrenergic, and serotonergic pathways. Primary motor manifestations of PD include resting tremor, bradykinesia (e.g., slowed motor ability), rigidity, and gait disturbance. Important clinical features to establish the diagnosis of PD include asymmetric symptom onset and responsiveness to levodopa, a commonly used medication to treat PD symptoms. Due to a combination of endogenous and exogenous factors, a significant proportion of patients with PD also suffer from comorbid medical and psychiatric illnesses. This can include pain, insomnia, autonomic dysfunction, as well as sensory and cognitive difficulties.

There has been a primary use of a biomedical approach to inform PD that has focused on the physical, neurological, and medical PD symptoms. A biopsychosocial approach may inform other domains, particularly psychosocial function. Psychosocial aspects of PD revolve around three broad domains including (1) personal relationships, (2) psychological function, and (3) environmental factors (see Fig. 1). These domains are all impacted by the progression and severity of PD symptomatology and age. As patients progress through different disease stages, psychosocial aspects will be relatively affected. There are approximately five stages of PD. In stage 1, the PD symptoms are minimal and may have some impact on activities

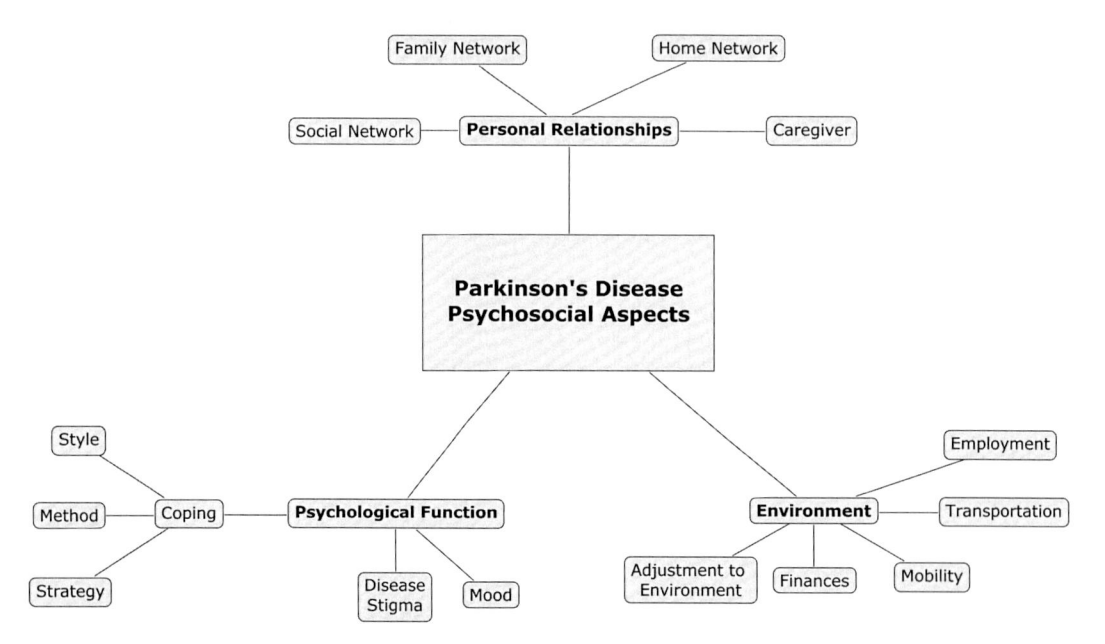

Parkinson's Disease: Psychosocial Aspects, Fig. 1 Three global domains of psychosocial aspects relevant to persons with Parkinson's disease (PD) including psychological function, personal relationships, and the environment. These three domains, independently or collectively, may be impacted by the progression and severity of PD symptomatology

of daily living, though by stage 2, the PD symptoms are more noticeable and begin to interfere with routine physical tasks. At stage 3, the PD symptoms may be more severe and impede most physical activities. At stages 4 and 5, the PD symptoms may be of such severity that the person is unable to live independently. Thus, greater PD disease severity is associated with greater adverse impact on psychosocial functions. For instance, late-stage PD decreases mobility and communication, thus limiting patients' ability to care for themselves and resulting in greater reliance upon others for activities of daily living. Decreased processing speed, medical problems, and other normal effects of aging exacerbated by PD factors limit self-care behaviors, which further impact psychosocial functioning.

Personal relationships are a tremendous resource for patients with PD. These relationships include many integrated networks of family and friends, and most importantly, caregivers. The size and quality of the social network as well as the subjective viewpoint of the patient all determine a social network's ability to assist patients with PD. A larger and higher quality network may be able to provide more resources than one that is small and of poor quality. The network's quality can be determined by its ability to provide resources for the PD patient in terms of physical and emotional support. Adequate relationship networks are essential to patient well-being, and patients should be encouraged to engage in activities that foster and enhance supportive relational networks. Importantly, should a professional caregiver be unavailable, family and friends may serve dual roles as caregivers, which can complicate the interpersonal relationship. The role of the caregiver may be minimal at the early stages of PD, but increases proportionately to the disease stage, as does stress and strain. Thus, it is important for caregivers to practice healthy stress management techniques.

The psychological functions domain includes mood and affect, personal view of self, and coping. There is a complex interaction between PD and psychological functions. For example, intact psychological functions before the onset of PD can help mitigate the onset of psychiatric illnesses such as depression and decreased self-worth. On the other hand, PD has been associated with an increase in depression and decrease quality of life. Regarding personal perception, patients may be burdened by disease stigma and see themselves as impaired, incapable to care for themselves, and less worthy than others. These negative personal perceptions can be changed with therapeutic management, which can then have positive impacts on overall health. Coping functions can be subdivided into coping style (active, passive), coping method (problem-solving, emotional focused), and coping strategies (cognitive, behavioral, cognitive-behavioral). Adaptive coping functions can help minimize the impact of PD symptoms, decrease poor health burden, and increase psychosocial function. Patients and caregivers should work together when implementing coping strategies in order to ensure that they are in sync and achieve maximal benefit.

The environmental domain includes areas that involve patients with PD to interact with others. This includes such areas as finances, employment and occupational performance, and transportation and mobility. Physical PD symptoms (e.g., tremor, postural instability) can affect safety as well as employment and occupational performance. Patients may be unable to perform certain job duties due to PD symptoms or may be embarrassed by some symptoms such as tremors. This can impede work performance for those who are employed or limit others from seeking employment. Mobility and transportation difficulties can decrease self-reliance and increase dependency on others, which can then impact psychological functions. The adverse impact on environmental factors is related to the age of PD onset. Early PD onset tends to have a more marked adverse impact on multiple domains including employment, marital status, and quality of life. Some patients may view early PD onset as premature aging, with profound negative psychosocial consequences.

Parkinson's disease impacts not only motoric function but also psychosocial function. Given its progressive, degenerative nature, it can negatively affect psychosocial domains of personal relationships, psychological function, and environmental factors. These domains are interrelated and are further associated with PD disease severity, age, and age of illness onset. A biopsychosocial approach to therapeutic management will help to inform these domains.

Cross-References

▶ Coping
▶ Family Social Support

References and Reading

Ellgring, H., Seiler, S., Perleth, B., Frings, W., Gasster, T., & Oertel, W. (1993). Psychosocial aspects of Parkinson's disease. *Neurology, 43*(Suppl. 6), S41–S44.

Imke, S. C. (2010). *Psychosocial care for Parkinson patients and care partners*. New York: Springer.

Olanow, C. W., Stern, M. B., & Sethi, K. (2009). The scientific and clinical basis for the treatment of Parkinson disease. *Neurology, 72*(Suppl. 4), S1–S136.

Tagliati, M., Guten, G., & Horne, J. (2007). *Parkinson's disease for dummies*. Hoboken: Wiley.

Parkinsonism

▶ Parkinson's Disease: Psychosocial Aspects

Paroxetine

▶ Selective Serotonin Reuptake Inhibitors (SSRIs)

Partial Sleep Deprivation

▶ Sleep Restriction

Participation

▶ Occupational Therapy

Participation Bias

▶ Bias

Participation Restrictions

▶ Disability

Participatory Research

Sheryl Zimmerman
School of Social Work, The University of North Carolina at Chapel Hill, Chapel Hill, NC, USA

Synonyms

Community-based participatory research

Definition

Participatory research is an approach to research that emphasizes equitable involvement and shared decision making of community members, organizational representatives, and researchers in all aspects of the research process, ranging from the choice of research question through the interpretation, dissemination, and application of results (Israel et al. 2005). While there has been longstanding recognition that meaningful, ongoing collaboration between communities and researchers is essential to the design and conduct of research that will ethically address community concerns and translate research findings into sustainable public health gains, there has been a resurgence of interest in the participatory approach to health research due to the confluence of two trends. First, researchers have faced the disconcerting fact that many promising findings published in the academic literature are never translated into behavior change by the target populations and therefore do not result in health improvement. Second, potential participants have grown tired of being viewed as the "subjects" of research, and some feel that there has been little benefit to their communities in return for their participation even while they recognize the need for information-gathering. This convergence has led to a restriking of the power balance between the observers and the observed, and the promotion of participatory research.

Cross-References

▶ Community-Based Participatory Research

References and Readings

Israel, B. A., Eng, E., Schulz, A. J., & Parker, E. A. (Eds.). (2005). *Methods in community-based participatory research for health*. San Francisco: Josey-Bass.

Lantz, P. M., Israel, B. A., Schultz, A. J., & Reyes, A. (2005). *Community-based participatory research: Rationale and relevance for social epidemiology*. San Francisco: Josey-Bass.

Minkler, M., & Wallerstein, N. (Eds.). (2003). *Community based participatory research for health*. San Francisco: Josey-Bass.

Passive Coping Strategies

Linda Carroll
Department of Public Health Sciences, University of Alberta, Edmonton, AB, Canada

Synonyms

Avoidance; Helplessness

Definition

Coping is the set of intentional, goal-directed efforts people engage in to minimize the physical, psychological, or social harm of an event or situation (Lazarus and Folkman 1984; Lazarus 1999). There are many different theoretical and empirical frameworks for understanding coping and many different ways of classifying coping strategies, but one such classification is "passive coping."

Passive coping refers to feeling of helplessness to deal with the stressor and relying on others to resolve the stressful event or situation (Zeidner and Endler 1996). Those engaging in passive coping relinquish to others the control of the stressful situation and of their reaction to that situation, or allow other areas of their lives to be adversely affected by the stressful event or situation (Field, McCabe, & Schneiderman, 1985). This reliance on external resources is contrasted with "active coping," in which the individual is relying upon their own resources to cope with the stressor. Passive coping is associated with depression and poor psychological adjustment, as well as a poor outcome.

Passive coping generally involves avoidance, withdrawal, and wishful thinking. Examples of passive coping strategies are such cognitions as "it's awful and I feel that it overwhelms me," "I pray to God it won't last long," and "I know someday someone will be here to help me and it will go away for a while." Behavioral examples of passive coping strategies include talking (complaining) to others about the situation either to ventilate feelings, get sympathy or elicit their help, withdrawing from social and other activities, or relying on medication to cope with the situation. Catastrophization (e.g., thinking "it's terrible and I think it's never going to get better") is sometimes considered a passive coping strategy.

Cross-References

▶ Active Coping
▶ Coping

References and Readings

Field, T., McCabe, P. M., & Schneiderman, N. (1985). *Stress and coping*. Hillsdale: Erlbaum.

Lazarus, R. S. (1999). *Stress and emotion: A new synthesis*. New York: Springer.

Lazarus, R. S., & Folkman, S. (1984). *Stress, appraisal and coping*. New York: Springer.

Moos, R. H. (1986). *Coping with life crises: An integrated approach*. New York: Plenum Press.

Zeidner, M., & Endler, N. S. (1996). *Handbook of coping: Theory, research, applications*. New York: Wiley.

Passive Sensing

Mashfiqui Rabbi
Harvard University, Cambridge, MA, USA

Definition

Passive sensing is a data collection method that requires no or minimal interactions from humans. Examples of passive sensing are location tracking, physical activity recognition, conversation detection, etc.

Description

Passive sensing is a data collection method that requires no or minimal interactions from humans. A familiar example of passive sensing is location tracking, where a mobile app continuously tracks an individual's location in the background. Passive sensing, however, is not limited to location tracking. Other forms of passive sensing include tracking steps, physical activity (Lu et al. 2010), sleep (Lane et al. 2011), heart rate (Hovsepian et al. 2015), electrodermal response (Sano and Rosalind 2011), nonverbal speech patterns (Rabbi et al. 2011), app usage (Gordon et al. 2019), etc. Typically, passive sensing is done via smartphones, wearables (e.g., smartwatches), or implantable devices in the environment (e.g., Amazon Echo), but custom-made devices can empower novel ways to passively sense (Rahman et al. 2016).

A broad variety of data can be passively sensed. The most common form of passive sensing uses *physical sensors* (accelerometer, microphone, GPS, ECG) on the phones or wearables. However, passive sensing can include *derived streams* from sensor data; for example, physical activity data is a continuous stream that uses accelerometer and GPS sensors to recognize walking, running, sitting still, etc. Passive sensing is not done by physical sensors only; for example, we can capture app usage or typing speed. Such information can be used to assess cognitive decline (Gordon et al. 2019) and Parkinson's symptoms (Arroyo-Gallego et al. 2017).

Passive sensing is rapidly growing in popularity in healthcare. The main advantage of passive sensing is that it can continuously and objectively monitor fine-grained human behavior in real-world settings. Prior to passive sensing, clinic visits in which patients recall their past behavior were the primary source of patient data. Such self-reporting is not only error-prone (people often cannot fully recall past events in their entirety), but it is also subjective and sporadic. It cannot capture human behavior between clinic visits or provide information like step counts or whether someone's blood pressure level falls outside of recommended ranges. Ecological momentary assessments (EMAs), in which people fill out surveys one or more times a day, can mitigate the lack of data between clinic visits. However, EMA data is not as fine-grained as passive sensing, and EMAs are prone to high-attrition rates because they interrupt users to ask for self-reports. Passive sensing, on the other hand, is usually an unobtrusive and low-burden method of data collection.

Research is ongoing on how passive sensing can make a difference in healthcare. Passive sensing has already made significant headway in some areas. For example, the electrocardiogram (ECG) feature in the latest smartwatches from Apple, Samsung, and Omron received FDA clearance for diagnostic purposes. Several devices for step count, actigraphy, and fall detection also received FDA clearance. Passive sensing technology to monitor sleep is also swiftly maturing – various sleep-tracking technologies using Doppler radar or Wi-Fi are quite promising. Mental health is another area where passive sensing has much potential (Cornet and Holden 2018). Researchers hypothesize that passive sensing can detect behavioral anomalies or biomarkers of a mental health decline at an early stage. Recent work with smartphone sensing, for example, suggests that depressive symptoms are correlated with lack of movement variability (Saeb et al. 2015) and lack of face-to-face conversation (Rabbi et al. 2011). People are working on using passive sensing in other areas too, notably for substance abuse among younger adults (Bae et al. 2017) or cognitive decline among older adults (Gordon et al. 2019).

Passive sensing research needs to advance in several key areas in order to be more useful:

(i) *Subjective Measures and Engagement*: Passive sensing is limited in capturing subjective data (e.g., mood, loneliness, helplessness, etc.). EMAs can capture subjective data, but they can cause disengagement due to their high burden (Rabbi et al. 2018). Passive sensing may be able to reduce the need for EMAs; if people behave differently in different subjective states, passive sensing might be able to pick up on these behavioral anomalies. For such a hybrid sensing approach, active learning and transfer learning from the artificial intelligence literature can be useful.

(ii) *Clinically Relevant End-Points*: Clinical or behavioral science literature often describe abstract constructs (e.g., self-efficacy, barrier, lack of sleep) to predict health behavior and then define treatments based on these abstract constructs (Michie et al. 2014). Thus, predicting these abstract constructs could be more useful because clinicians find them more familiar and actionable. Furthermore, predicting these abstract constructs using machine learning is more feasible, since the risk of relapse and decline of health conditions often mediate through these constructs. For example, predicting mental health decline is harder than predicting sleep variability which often is a precursor to mental health decline.

(iii) *Larger-Scale Deployment and Deep Learning*: Existing passive sensing studies are small, and they primarily focused on the feasibility of the technology. Unsurprisingly these feasibility results lack inconsistencies. Large-scale deployments are needed for more generalizable results. Larger deployments can also create big data for deep learning models which showed remarkable performance in other areas.

(iv) *Privacy, Low Latency, and Poor Connectivity*: Passively sensing data are inherently personal and private. An open question is how to make this private data publicly available for research. Research on privacy and cryptography (differential privacy (Dwork 2011), multiparty authentication (Bater et al. 2017), etc.) can be useful to enable privacy-sensitive access to data even when the data is located at different sites. Processing data on-device can improve privacy as well as enable low latency service in poor connectivity environments. Low latency can provide real-time feedback, and poor connectivity can be useful for low SES. Google's TensorFlow Lite (https://www.tensorflow.org/lite) and Apple's Core ML (https://developer.apple.com/documentation/coreml) initiatives are taking steps to put sophisticated machine learning models on low-power devices like phones or wearables.

(v) *Just-in-Time Adaptive Interventions*: A compelling application of passive sensing is to use the continuously monitored data to provide the right intervention at the right time (Nahum-Shani et al. 2017). Passive sensing can play a significant role in such timely interventions because it can pinpoint the right intervention for the right context.

In summary, passive sensing can continuously monitor and provide feedback on health behavior. Once passive sensing technologies mature, they will enable low-burden objective data collection outside of clinic visits, and their continuous monitoring capability will pave ways to provide the right intervention when people can benefit from it the most.

References and Further Reading

Arroyo-Gallego, T., et al. (2017). Detection of motor impairment in Parkinson's disease via mobile touchscreen typing. *IEEE Transactions on Biomedical Engineering, 64*(9), 1994–2002.

Bae, S., et al. (2017). Detecting drinking episodes in young adults using smartphone-based sensors. *Proceedings of the ACM on Interactive, Mobile, Wearable and Ubiquitous Technologies, 1*(2), 5.

Bater, J., et al. (2017). SMCQL: Secure querying for federated databases. *Proceedings of the VLDB Endowment, 10*(6), 673–684.

Cornet, V. P., & Holden, R. J. (2018). Systematic review of smartphone-based passive sensing for health and wellbeing. *Journal of Biomedical Informatics, 77*, 120–132.

Dwork, C. (2011). Differential privacy. *Encyclopedia of cryptography and security* (pp. 338–340).

Gordon, M. L., et al. (2019). App usage predicts cognitive ability in older adults. In: *Proceedings of the 2019 CHI conference on human factors in computing systems*, ACM.

Hovsepian, K., et al. (2015). cStress: Towards a gold standard for continuous stress assessment in the mobile environment. In: *Proceedings of the 2015 ACM international joint conference on pervasive and ubiquitous computing*, ACM.

Lane, N. D., et al. (2011). Bewell: A smartphone application to monitor, model and promote wellbeing. In: *5th international ICST conference on pervasive computing technologies for healthcare*.

Lu, H., et al. (2010). The Jigsaw continuous sensing engine for mobile phone applications. In: *Proceedings of the 8th ACM conference on embedded networked sensor systems*, ACM.

Michie, S. F., et al. (2014). *ABC of behaviour change theories*. London: Silverback Publishing.

Nahum-Shani, I., et al. (2017). Just-in-time adaptive interventions (JITAIs) in mobile health: Key components and design principles for ongoing health behavior support. *Annals of Behavioral Medicine, 52*(6), 446–462.

Rabbi, M., et al. (2011). Passive and in-situ assessment of mental and physical well-being using mobile sensors. In: *Proceedings of the 13th international conference on ubiquitous computing*, ACM.

Rabbi, M., et al. (2018). Toward increasing engagement in substance use data collection: Development of the substance abuse research assistant app and protocol for a microrandomized trial using adolescents and emerging adults. *JMIR Research Protocols, 7*(7), e166.

Rahman, T., et al. (2016). Nutrilyzer: A mobile system for characterizing liquid food with photoacoustic effect. In: *Proceedings of the 14th ACM conference on embedded network sensor systems CD-ROM*, ACM.

Saeb, S., et al. (2015). Mobile phone sensor correlates of depressive symptom severity in daily-life behavior: An exploratory study. *Journal of Medical Internet Research, 17*(7), e175.

Sano, A., & Rosalind, W. (2011). Picard. Toward a taxonomy of autonomic sleep patterns with electrodermal activity. In: *2011 annual international conference of the IEEE engineering in medicine and biology society*, IEEE.

Passive Smoking

▶ Secondhand Smoke

Past Smokers

▶ Ex-Smokers

Pastors

▶ Williams LifeSkills Program

Pathophysiology

Michael Witthöft
Psychologisches Institut Abteilung Klinische Psychologie und Psychotherapie, Johannes Gutenberg Universität Mainz, Mainz, Germany

Definition

Pathophysiology (consisting of the Greek origin words "pathos" = suffering; "physis" = nature, origin; and "logos" = "the study of") refers to the study of abnormal changes in body functions that are the causes, consequences, or concomitants of disease processes. Studies of pathophysiology are concerned with the investigation of *biological* processes that are directly related to disease processes of physical, mental, or psychophysiological conditions and disorders (e.g., alterations in the endocrine system, in certain neurotransmitters, or inflammatory parameters related to the activity of the immune system). Thus, pathophysiological research aims at identifying biological markers and mechanisms for predicting and explaining disease processes in terms of *etiology* and *pathogenesis*. Pathophysiology is formally considered as a subdiscipline within physiology.

Description

The fundamental aim of the domain of pathophysiology is to unravel the altered biological (i.e., physical and chemical) processes in our organism that precede, accompany, or follow certain disorders or diseases. In this regard, pathophysiological research aims at identifying factors and mechanisms that are relevant for answering questions of *why* and *how* certain disorders and diseases develop (i.e., questions about *etiology* and *pathogenesis*). Pathophysiological mechanisms of mental, physical, and psychophysiological disorders are rather complex. Yet, many pathophysiological findings and models are incomplete, preliminary, and speculative. However, research into the biological mechanisms of conditions in behavioral medicine is growing rapidly.

Methods and Designs in Pathophysiology Research

Since *pathophysiology* is mainly concerned with indentifying objective, biological factors that are relevant for certain disease processes, *quantitative methods* and *experimental* research designs are typically used. Current examples of research methods used in *pathophysiological* research in behavioral medicine are brain imaging techniques (i.e., (functional) magnetic resonance or positron emission tomography) to explore altered patterns of brain morphology and neural activity associated with certain disorders. Another example of pathophysiological research represents studies that aim at quantifying the amount of stress hormones (e.g., corticosteroids) in the blood and saliva (either in a resting state or after acute stress induction). In addition, *electroencephalography* and *electrocardiography* are typical diagnostic tools in pathophysiology research. In addition to studies with human patients and control participants, animal models (e.g., mouse and rat models) are also routinely used to test predictions of *pathophysiological* hypotheses relevant for our understanding of complex medical, psychological, and psychophysiological conditions in humans (e.g., stroke, schizophrenia).

Examples of Pathophysiological Research

As examples of *pathophysiological* investigations and findings relevant to the field or *behavioral medicine*, three examples from the realm of *obesity*, *chronic pain*, and *stress-related disorders* will be outlined briefly.

Pathophysiology of Obesity: The Metabolic Syndrome

Obesity is associated with an increased risk to develop numerous chronic and life-threatening diseases (e.g., cardiovascular diseases, type-2 diabetes, stroke). Several *pathophysiological* factors have been identified that frequently co-occur with obesity and that are suspected to mediate between *obesity* and severe medical diseases. In this regard, the following physiological abnormalities have been identified and termed "the metabolic syndrome" (Cornier et al. 2008): abdominal obesity, insulin resistance, dyslipidemia (i.e., abnormal amount of lipids in the blood), and hypertension. Among these four defining features, abdominal obesity and insulin resistance appear as the core factors in the *pathophysiology* of the *metabolic syndrome*. The *etiology* of the *metabolic syndrome* has to be considered as complex and multifactorial and is still widely unknown. As interventions aiming at treating and preventing the *metabolic syndrome*, lifestyle modifications and weight loss (e.g., via increased physical activity) are recommended.

Pathophysiology of Chronic Pain

Pain is considered as a highly adaptive sensation that effectively signals dangers in terms of threats to our body integrity and helps to avoid injuries. *Pain* is the result of a complex interplay between neurobiological and psychological processes, both in the peripheral and central nervous system. Although acute *pain* is highly adaptive, *chronic pain* typically lacks this adaptive purpose. Regarding chronic pain conditions, the mechanism of "central sensitization" (Woolf 2011) has been proposed to account for the phenomenon of ongoing pain in the absence of sufficient "objective" *nociceptive* stimulation. Accordingly, changes in the excitability of spinal cord neurons are responsible for reductions in pain thresholds, and prolonged neuronal responses to certain stimuli explain why stimuli that are generally considered as non-noxious and non-painful become pain-eliciting stimuli in patients with *chronic pain*. The concept of *central sensitization* rests on the principle of *neural plasticity* of the nociceptive system and a cascade of molecular and biochemical processes has been observed to be involved in *central sensitization* (e.g., Latremoliere and Woolf 2009).

Pathophysiology of Stress Related Disorders

Ongoing and severe stress represents a threat to one's mental and physical well-being. Regarding the *pathophysiology* of the stress response, a chronic state of uncontrollable, stressful life circumstances has been linked to alterations in the function of the hormonal stress system. Qualitatively different alterations are thereby observed in certain mental and psychophysiological disorders: In the *pathophysiology* of depressive disorders, the hormonal stress system (in terms o the *hypothalamic-pituitary-adrenocortical* system; *HPA*) has been observed to be hyperactive which is reflected in increased *cortisol* secretion of the adrenal glands (e.g., Müller and Holsboer 2004). This *hypercortisolism* is the direct consequence of increased secretion of the corticotrophin releasing hormone (CRH) (from the paraventricular nucleus of the hypothalamus) and the release of the adrenocorticotropic hormone (ACTH) via stimulation of the anterior pituitary gland (Ehlert et al. 2001). The *hypercortisolism* observed in depression is most likely attributable to dysfunctions in HPA-axis feedback mechanisms that are responsible for the downregulation of the cortisol release (via CRH and ACTH). It has to be acknowledged that the phenomenon of *hypercortisolism* only occurs in certain subtypes of depression (e.g., melancholic depression).

Interestingly, the opposite phenomenon of a reduced activity of the *HPA* system resulting in a state of *hypocortisolism* is observed in patients with atypical depression, and patients with complex stress-related disorders. Regarding the latter group of disorders, reduced levels of cortisol indicative of lower HPA-axis reactivity have been observed in patients with *posttraumatic stress disorder*, *chronic fatigue syndrome*, *chronic pain disorders*, *fibromyalgia*, *irritable bowel syndrome* and other *functional somatic syndromes* and *somatoform disorders*. Childhood traumas have also been linked to *hypocortisolism* as evidence for early life stress-induced dysregulation of the *HPA* axis (Heim et al. 2009). Moreover, *hypocortisolism* was detected in people with rheumatoid arthritis and asthma.

Cross-References

▶ Functional Magnetic Resonance Imaging (FMRI)
▶ Functional Somatic Syndromes
▶ Homeostasis
▶ Inflammation
▶ Psychopathology
▶ Somatoform Disorders

References

Cornier, M.-A., Dabelea, D., Hernandez, T. L., Lindstrom, R. C., Steig, A. J., Stob, N. R., et al. (2008). The metabolic syndrome. *Endocrine Reviews, 29*, 777–822.

Ehlert, U., Gaab, J., & Heinrichs, M. (2001). Psychoneuroendocrinological contributions to the etiology of depression, post-traumatic stress disorder, and stress related bodily disorders: The role of the hypothalamus-pituitary-adrenal axis. *Biological Psychology, 57*, 141–152.

Heim, C., Ehlert, U., & Hellhammer, D. H. (2000). The potential role of hypocortisolism in the pathophysiology of stress-related bodily disorders. *Psychoneuroendocrinology, 25*, 1–35.

Heim, C., Nater, U., Maloney, E., Boneva, R., Jones, J. F., & Reeves, W. C. (2009). Childhood trauma and risk for chronic fatigue syndrome. *Archives of General Psychiatry, 66*, 72–80.

Latremoliere, A., & Woolf, C. J. (2009). Central sensitization: A generator of pain hypersensitivity by central neural plasticity. *The Journal of Pain, 10*, 895–926.

Lautenbacher, S., & Fillingim, R. B. (2004). *Pathophysiology of pain perception*. New York: Kluwer Academic/Plenum.

Müller, M., & Holsboer, F. (2004). Hormones, stress and depression. In C. Kordon, R.-C. Gaillard, & Y. Christen (Eds.), *Hormones and the brain*. Berlin: Springer.

Steptoe, A. (2010). *Handbook of behavioral medicine – methods and application*. New York: Springer.

Woolf, C. J. (2011). Central sensitization: Implications for the diagnosis and treatment of pain. *Pain, 152*, 2–15.

Patient Complexity

▶ Comorbidity

Patient Compliance

▶ Adherence

Patient Control

Yori Gidron
SCALab, Lille 3 University and Siric Oncollile, Lille, France

Definition

This is a central issue in behavior medicine, since it relates to models of stress and to patient behaviors and outcomes and has vast clinical implications. Patient control (PC) can reflect both subjective or perceived control and objective control. Perceived control can be understood as one's subjective appraisal of the ability to influence the causes or outcomes of a situation. Perceived control reflects a secondary appraisal process in general stress models (Lazarus and Folkman 1984; Taylor 1995). In contrast, objective control reflects the externally determined and externally validated level of control over a situation. Thus, objective PC is accurate, while subjective PC refers to subjective levels of control and, thus, could also be inaccurate. Subjective PC is a crucial predictor of health behaviors in the theory of planned behavior, showing a relation to behavior either directly or via intentions. For example, subjective PC has been shown to be important in choice over food types (Lawrence and Barker 2009), of relevance to overweight. Subjective PC is strongly related to the broader concept of self-efficacy, the belief that one can carry out a certain behavior despite the existence of barriers. Subjective PC could be affected by objective control but also by past experiences with similar or different stressful situations. Overgeneralizing the lack of control from an uncontrollable to a controllable situation reflects the core of "learned helplessness," which has vast implications for multiple outcomes including depression (Abramson et al. 1989) and possibly even acceleration of tumors (Palermo-Neto et al. 2003). In pain patients, subjective PC is positively correlated with engagement in activity, of clinical relevance to daily functioning (Chiros and O'Brien 2011). Subjective PC can also be an important moderating variable in the detrimental effect of various factors on health or well-being. For example, Tovbin et al. (2003) found that low albumin (reflecting poor nutritional status) was related to poorer quality of life in dialysis patients, but only in those with low, but not high, subjective control. Objective PC is important in "patient-controlled analgesia" (PCA), where patients control the amount and timing of receiving analgesics during treatment for pain. A meta-analysis of 55 studies found that PCA led to less pain and greater patient satisfaction than did conventional analgesic regiments given by a health professional (Hudcova et al. 2006). Importantly, the subjective and objective aspects of PC are interrelated and are related to another related concept called locus of control. In patients receiving PCA, those with an external locus of control (thinking outcomes are due to chance or powerful others) had more pain and less satisfaction with this treatment. In contrast, an internal locus of control (thinking outcomes are due to one's own efforts, thus reflecting greater perceived control) was predictive of lower pain and greater satisfaction from PCA (Johnson et al. 1989). Taken together, PC is an important predictor of patient outcomes and can be a moderator of the effects of other factors or treatments on health outcomes. It is thus of great importance to assess and consider PC in behavior medicine research and clinical practice.

Cross-References

▶ Perceived Control

References and Further Readings

Abramson, L. Y., Metalsky, G. I., & Alloy, L. B. (1989). Hopelessness depression: A theory-based subtype of depression. *Psychological Review, 96*, 358–372.

Chiros, C., & O'Brien, W. H. (2011). Acceptance, appraisals, and coping in relation to migraine headache: An evaluation of interrelationships using daily diary methods. *Journal of Behavioral Medicine, 34*, 307–320.

Hudcova, J., McNicol, E., Quah, C., Lau, J., & Carr, D. B. (2006). Patient controlled opioid analgesia versus conventional opioid analgesia for postoperative pain. *Cochrane Database of Systematic Reviews, 18*, CD003348.

Johnson, L. R., Magnani, B., Chan, V., & Ferrante, F. M. (1989). Modifiers of patient-controlled analgesia efficacy. I. Locus of control. *Pain, 39*, 17–22.

Lawrence, W., & Barker, M. (2009). A review of factors affecting the food choices of disadvantaged women. *Proceedings of the Nutrition Society, 68*, 189–194.

Lazarus, R. S., & Folkman, S. (1984). *Stress, appraisal, and coping*. New York: Springer.

Palermo-Neto, J., de Oliveira, M. C., & Robespierre de Souza, W. (2003). Effects of physical and psychological stressors on behavior, macrophage activity, and Ehrlich tumor growth. *Brain, Behavior, and Immunity, 17*, 43–54.

Taylor, S. E. (1995). *Health psychology* (3rd ed.). New York: McGraw-Hill.

Tovbin, D., Jean, T., Schnieder, A., Granovsky, R., & Gidron, Y. (2003). Psychosocial correlates and moderators of QOL in hemodialysis. *Quality of Life Research, 12*, 709–717.

Patient Decision Aid

▶ Decision Aid

Patient Decision Support Technology

▶ Decision Aid

Patient Education

▶ Diabetes Education
▶ Health Education

Patient Health/Engagement

▶ Consumer Health Informatics

Patient Privacy

▶ Confidentiality

Patient Protection

▶ Health Insurance Portability and Accountability Act (HIPAA)

Patient Safety

▶ Human Factors/Ergonomics

Patient-Centered Care

Cassie Cunningham
College of Public Health, University of Iowa, Liberty, IA, USA

Definition

Patient-centered care is a term that is becoming widely used in medical practice. It is typically described in the context of patient-practitioner communication. In contrast to provider-centered care, which places control and decision-making power almost solely in the hands of the healthcare provider, is patient-centered. Patient-centered care promotes active participation on the part of the patient decisions regarding their health and health care. Moreover, patient-centered care requires practitioners to provide care concordant with the patient's values as well as account for the patient's desire for information provision and for shared decision-making responsibilities. Patient-centered care has been shown to be associated with increased patient satisfaction and adherence and may also enhance the relationship between the patient and the health-care provider.

References and Readings

Mead, N., & Bower, P. (2000). Patient-centredness: A conceptual framework and review of the empirical literature. *Social Science Medicine, 51*, 1087–1110.

Stewart, M. (2001). Towards a global definition of patient-centered care. *British Medical Journal, 233*, 444–445.

Patient-Reported Outcome

Hiroe Kikuchi
Department of Psychosomatic Medicine, Center Hospital, National Center for Global Health and Medicine, Tokyo, Japan

Definition

Patient-reported outcomes (PROs) are responses to questions or statements about their perceptions or activities, such as symptoms, capabilities, or performance of roles or responsibilities (Revicki et al. 2008).

Description

PROs are typically measured by self-completed questionnaires and combined in some way to create summary scores that can be used to measure concepts such as physical, psychological, or social functioning and well-being or symptom burden or severity. Symptoms can be rated based on frequency, severity, duration, degree of bother, or impact on patient activities. PROs are increasingly accompanying the traditional clinical ways of measuring health and the effects of treatment on the patient, both nationally and internationally, in order to make a more comprehensive evaluation. According to this context, The Patient-Reported Outcomes Measurement Information System (PROMIS®) initiative, funded by National Institutes of Health (NIH), began in 2004 with six primary research sites and a statistical coordinating center in the USA. The aims of PROMIS® are to use measurement science to create a state-of-the-art assessment system for self-reported health and to provide clinicians and researchers access to a national resource for precise and efficient measurement of patient-reported symptoms, functioning, and health-related quality of life, appropriate for patients with a wide variety of chronic disease conditions (Cella et al. 2010). In addition, the US Food and Drug Administration (FDA) guidance on "Patient-Reported Outcome Measures: Use in Medical Product Development to Support Labeling Claims" (2009) has engendered wide discussion about PRO domains that should be endpoints in clinical trials (Cleeland et al. 2010). In the guidance, reducing the severity and impact of symptoms is considered as a natural intervention endpoint for cancer, a condition associated with considerable symptom burden. Because symptoms are best described by patients who have them, PROs as measures of treatment effectiveness or the differences among treatments provide essential information about the efficacy and toxicity of a treatment and its effects on function. The FDA guidance provides a framework for addressing such issues as clinical significance, study design, and statistical methods. However, there are some problems to be solved. In the guidance, no set of recommended approaches for assessing specific symptoms by patient report in clinical trials exists, other than for pain. Recommendations about the best approach for evaluating responsiveness and determining minimally important differences for PRO instruments are still needed (Revicki et al. 2008). With regard to PROMIS®, there are many sets of items including physical health, mental health, social health, and global health for adult and pediatric measures (Batterham et al. 2015). In addition, it has both versions of paper-and-pencil and computer adaptive tests and translations in Spanish and many other languages (Sung et al. 2016).

Cross-References

► Cancer, Types of
► National Institutes of Health
► Pain

References and Further Reading

Batterham, P. J., Brewer, J. L., Tjhin, A., Sunderland, M., Carragher, N., & Calear, A. L. (2015). Systematic item selection process applied to developing item pools for assessing multiple mental health problems. *Journal of Clinical Epidemiology, 68*, 913–919.

Boers, M. (2010). Standing on the promises: First wave validation reports of the patient-reported outcome measurement information system. *Journal of Clinical Epidemiology, 63*, 1167–1168.

Cella, D., Riley, W., Stone, A., Rothrock, N., Reeve, B., Yount, S., et al. (2010). Initial adult health item banks and first-wave testing of the Patient-Reported Outcomes Measurement Information System Network: 2005–2008. *Journal of Clinical Epidemiology, 63*, 1179–1194.

Cleeland, C. S., Sloan, J. A., & ASCPRO Organizing Group. (2010). Assessing the symptoms of Cancer using patient-reported outcomes (ASCPRO): Searching for standards. *Journal of Pain and Symptom Management, 39*, 1077–1085.

Revicki, D., Hays, R. D., Cella, D., & Sloan, J. (2008). Recommended methods for determining responsiveness and minimally important differences for patient-reported outcomes. *Journal of Clinical Epidemiology, 61*, 102–109.

Sung, V. W., Griffith, J. W., Rogers, R. G., Raker, C. A., & Clark, M. A. (2016). Item bank development, calibration and validation for patient-reported outcomes in female urinary incontinence. *Quality of Life Research, 25*, 1645–1654.

Patients

▶ Care Recipients

Pavlovian Conditioning

▶ Classical Conditioning

Paxil®

▶ Selective Serotonin Reuptake Inhibitors (SSRIs)

PCP

▶ Primary Care Physicians

PD

▶ Parkinson's Disease: Psychosocial Aspects

Pediatric Psychology

▶ Child Development

Pediatric Quality of Life Inventory (PedsQL)

Meghan L. Marsac[1] and Melissa A. Alderfer[2]
[1]Department of Pediatrics, Kentucky Children's Hospital and College of Medicine, University of Kentucky, Lexington, PA, USA
[2]Division of Oncology, The Children's Hospital of Philadelphia, Philadelphia, PA, USA

Synonyms

PedsQL 4.0

Definition

The Pediatric Quality of Life Inventory or PedsQL™, now in its fourth version, is a series of assessment instruments designed to measure the health-related quality of life. The authors of the measure conceptualize health-related quality of life as physical, psychological, and social functioning. The PedsQL 4.0 provides an opportunity for the assessment of both overall (generic) quality of life and disease-specific quality of life.

The PedsQL 4.0 Generic Core Scales are appropriate for assessing health-related quality of life in both healthy and chronically ill children. The four scales making up this generic battery include Physical Functioning (8 items), Emotional Functioning (5 items), Social Functioning (5 items), and School Functioning (5 items). From these four core scales, three standardized summary scores can be calculated: a Total Quality of Life Score, a Physical Health Summary Score (based on the physical functioning items), and a Psychosocial Health Summary Score (combining emotional, social, and school items). In addition to these generic core scales, condition-specific modules have been developed for children with arthritis, asthma, brain tumors, cancer, cardiac conditions, cerebral palsy, diabetes, Duchenne muscular dystrophy, end-stage renal disease, eosinophilic esophagitis, neuromuscular disorders, pain, gastrointestinal diseases, sickle cell disease, rheumatological diseases, and transplant.

On each of the PedsQL 4.0 scales, the respondent is asked to indicate how much of a problem each item has been in the past month with response options of 0 = never, 1 = almost never, 2 = sometimes, 3 = often, and 4 = almost always. Item scores are reverse coded, linearly converted to a 100-point scale, and averaged to form scale and summary scores with higher scores indicating better quality of life. Parent-completed versions of the scales, reporting on their child's health-related quality of life, are available for infants (aged 1–12 months, 13–24 months), toddlers (aged 2–4 years), young children (aged 5–7 years), children (aged 8–12 years), and adolescents (aged 13–18 years). Parallel, developmentally appropriate, child self-report versions of the scales are available for young children (5–7 years), children (8–12 years), adolescents (13–18 years), young adults (18–25 years), and adults (>25 years). The PedsQL 4.0 is available in many languages including Spanish, French, German, Italian, Hebrew, Portuguese, and Russian. In addition, authors provide a guide for a linguistic validation process, if the language desired is not yet available. Authors of the PedsQL have chosen to allow organizations to build their own online version of the measure per their licensing agreement; the organization must agree to allow the online version of the measure to be reviewed by measure authors.

The psychometric properties of the PedsQL 4.0 are generally good. Adequate internal consistency has been demonstrated for the scales with most researchers reporting coefficient alphas greater than .70. As evidence of validity, scores on the scales have been shown to correlate with other measures of health-related quality of life and to functional indices of health such as the number of days the child was ill, the number of school days missed by the child, the number of work days missed by the parent, and objective measures of disease severity. The generic core scales have also been found to distinguish between children with chronic health conditions and those who are healthy.

Further information regarding the PedsQL™ 4.0 including access to the measures can be obtained at www.pedsql.org.

Cross-References

▶ Quality of Life
▶ Quality of Life: Measurement

References and Further Readings

Desai, A. D., Zhou, C., Stanford, S., Haaland, W., Varni, J. W., & Mangione-Smith, R. M. (2014). Validity and responsiveness of the Pediatric Quality of Life Inventory (PedsQL) 4.0 Generic Core Scales in the pediatric inpatient setting. *JAMA Pediatrics, 68*, 1114–1121.

Franciosi, J. P., Hommel, K. A., Bendo, C. B., King, E. C., Collins, M. H., Eby, M. D., Marsolo, K., Abonia, J. P., von Tiehl, K. F., Putnam, P. E., Greenler, A. J., Greenberg, A. B., Bryson, R. A., Davis, C. M., Olive, A. P., Gupta, S. K., Erwin, E. A., Klinnert, M. D., Spergel, J. M., Denham, J. M., Furuta, G. T., Rothenberg, M. E., & Varni, J. W. (2013). PedsQL™ Eosinophilic Esophagitis Module: Feasibility, reliability and validity. *Journal of Pediatric Gastroenterology & Nutrition, 57*, 57–66.

Palermo, T. M., Long, A. C., Lewandowski, A., Drotar, D., Quittner, A. L., & Walker, L. S. (2008). Evidence-based assessment of health-related quality of life and functional impairment in pediatric psychology. *Journal of Pediatric Psychology, 33*, 983–996.

Panepinto, J. A., Torres, S., Bendo, C. B., McCavit, T. L., Dinu, B., Sherman-Bien, S., Bemrich-Stolz, C., &

Varni, J. W. (2014). PedsQL™ Multidimensional Fatigue Scale in sickle cell disease: Feasibility, reliability and validity. *Pediatric Blood & Cancer, 61*, 171–177.

Varni, J. W., Limbers, C. A., & Burwinkle, T. M. (2007). Impaired health-related quality of life in children and adolescents with chronic conditions: A comparative analysis of 10 disease clusters and 33 disease categories/severities utilizing the PedsQL 4.0 Generic Core Scales. *Health and quality of life outcomes, 5*, 43. http://www.hqlo.com/content/5/1/43

Varni, J.W., Bendo, C.B., Denham, J., Shulman, R.J., Self, M.M., Neigut, D.A., Nurko, S., Patel, A.S, Franciosi, J. P., Saps, M., Yeckes, A., Langseder, A., Saeed, S., & Pohl, J.F. (2015). PedsQL™ Gastrointestinal Symptoms Scales and Gastrointestinal Worry Scales in pediatric patients with functional and organic gastrointestinal diseases in comparison to healthy controls. Quality of Life Research, 24, 363–378.

Varni, J. W., Seid, M., & Kurtin, P. S. (2001). PedsQL™4.0: Reliability and validity of the Pediatric Quality of Life Inventory™ Version 4.0 generic core scales in healthy and patient populations. *Medical Care, 39*, 800–812.

PedsQL 4.0

▶ Pediatric Quality of Life Inventory (PedsQL)

Peer Coaches

▶ Promotoras

Peer Health Educators

▶ Promotoras

Peer Health Promoters

▶ Promotoras

Penetrance

Rong Jiang
Department of Psychiatry and Behavioral Sciences, Duke University, Durham, NC, USA

Definition

Penetrance in genetics is the proportion of individuals carrying a particular gene variant (allele or genotype) that also possess an associated trait (phenotype). If penetrance of a disease allele is 100%, then all individuals carrying that allele will have the associated disease. Penetrance only considers whether individuals express the trait or not. This differs from expressivity, which characterizes qualitatively or quantitatively the extent of phenotypic variation given a particular genotype. Penetrance is age related (Bessett et al. 1998) and is affected by environmental and behavioral factors such as diet and smoking. It is also modified by other genes and epigenetic regulation.

Cross-References

▶ Allele
▶ Epigenetics
▶ Genotype
▶ Phenotype

References and Further Readings

Bessett, J. H., Forbes, S. A., Pannett, A. A. J., Lloyd, S. E., Christie, P. T., Wooding, C., et al. (1998). Characterization of mutations in patients with multiple endocrine neoplasia type 1. *American Journal of Human Genetics, 62*(2), 232–244.

Pepper

▶ Capsaicin

Peptic Ulcer

▶ Gastric Ulcers and Stress

Perceived Behavioral Control

▶ Perceived Control

Perceived Benefits

Yvonne Leung
Department of Psychosocial Oncology and Palliative Care, Princess Margaret Hospital, University Health Network/University of Toronto, Toronto, ON, Canada

Synonyms

Benefit finding; Flourishing; Positive by-products; Positive changes; Positive meaning; Posttraumatic growth; Stress-related growth; Thriving

Definition

Perceived benefit refers to the perception of the positive consequences that are caused by a specific action. In behavioral medicine, the term perceived benefit is frequently used to explain an individual's motives of performing a behavior and adopting an intervention or treatment. Researchers and theorists attempt to measure positive perceptions because they believe that a behavior is driven by an individual's cognition in terms of acceptability, motives, and attitudes toward such behavior, especially if positive.

In psychology, five models may explain the performance of health behavior related to the construct of perceived benefit. First, the Health Belief Model (Becker 1974) describes that the perceived benefit is one of the four major predictors of health-related behavior. Second, the Transtheoretical Model (Prochaska and DiClemente 1986) posits that the progress of change depends upon the decisional balance weighting between perceived benefits and barriers. Third, the Protection Motivation Theory (Rogers 1983) puts forward that the intention to protect oneself depends upon four cognitions among which is the perceived efficacy (inlcuding benefits) of the recommended preventive behavior. Finally, the Theory of Reasoned Action (Fishbein and Ajzen 1975) and its extension the Theory of Planned Behavior (Ajzen 1985) both suggest that a person's behavior is driven by the persons' attitude about the behavior, which consists of beliefs about the consequences of performing the behavior multiplied by his or her valuation of these consequences.

In trauma literature, perceived benefits essentially mean the perceptions of positive psychological changes as a result of coping with a trauma or a highly stressful event (McMillen and Fisher 1998). For example, after struggling with a highly stressful event, an individual may experience increases in personal strength, relatedness to others, and one's appreciation of life. In particular, McMiller and Fisher have developed the Perceived Benefit Scales (PBS) to assess several commonly reported positive by-products of adversity. On the PBS, respondents rate 30 positive by-product items on how similar they were to their own experiences by using a 5-point scale. The PBS has eight subscales: increased self-efficacy, increased faith in people, increased compassion, increased spirituality, increased community closeness, increased family closeness, lifestyle changes, and material gain. This concept is a form of cognitive coping strategy often associated with improved outcomes including participation in cancer screening tests.

Cross-References

▶ Benefit Finding
▶ Coping Strategies
▶ Positive Psychology
▶ Posttraumatic Growth

References and Readings

Ajzen, I. (1985). From intentions to actions: A theory of planned behavior. In J. Kuhl & J. Beckmann (Eds.), *Action control: From cognition to behavior.* Berlin/Heidelberg/New York: Springer.

Ajzen, I., & Fishbein, M. (1980). *Understanding attitudes and predicting social behavior.* Englewood Cliffs: Prentice-Hall.

Becker, M. H. (Ed.). (1974). The health belief model and personal health behavior. *Health Education Monographs, 2,* 324–473.

Fishbein, M., & Ajzen, I. (1975). *Belief, attitude, intention, and behavior: An introduction to theory and research.* Reading: Addison-Wesley.

McMillen, J. C., & Fisher, R. H. (1998). The perceived benefit scales: Measuring perceived positive life changes after negative events. *Social Work Research, 22,* 173–186.

Prochaska, J. O., & DiClemente, C. C. (1986). Toward a comprehensive model of change. In W. R. Miller & N. Heather (Eds.), *Treating addictive behaviors: Processes of change* (pp. 3–27). New York: Plenum Press.

Rogers, R. W. (1983). Cognitive and physiological processes in fear appeals and attitude change: A revised theory of protection motivation. In J. Cacioppo & R. Petty (Eds.), *Social psychophysiology.* New York: Guilford Press.

Perceived Control

Peter A. Hall[1] and Chris Zehr[2]
[1]Faculty of Applied Health Sciences, University of Waterloo, Waterloo, ON, Canada
[2]Department of Health Studies and Gerontology, University of Waterloo, Waterloo, ON, Canada

Synonyms

Perceived behavioral control

Definition

Perceived behavioral control is the extent to which an individual perceives that they are in control of a given target behavior. It is considered a core construct in the theory of planned behavior.

Description

Perceived behavioral control (PBC) was included in the theory of planned behavior (TPB; Ajzen 1991) in order to predict/explain behaviors that are not entirely under the volitional control of the individual. According to the TPB, PBC is determined by beliefs regarding factors that may act to facilitate or inhibit successful behavioral performance (Ajzen 1991; Conner and Armitage 1998). For example, a belief that exercising after work is associated with intractable barriers (i.e., cold weather, icy sidewalks, limited schedule) may lead to low perceived behavioral control over exercise, in turn leading to less frequent exercise during winter months. However, a belief that there are few barriers to exercising (i.e., favorable weather, few other time commitments) may result in greater perceived behavioral control over exercise, which in turn may lead to more frequent exercising during summer months. Importantly, control beliefs may concern factors external to the individual (e.g., weather conditions) or internal (e.g., innate ability; Conner and Armitage 1998).

In the context of the TPB, PBC is thought to influence behavioral performance in two ways: directly and indirectly. PBC affects behavioral performance indirectly by influencing behavioral intentions to perform a particular behavior (Armitage and Connor 2001). Those who perceive that they are in greater control of a given behavior may have stronger intentions to act compared to those who perceive less control over the behavior. That is, the influence of PBC on behavior is mediated through intentions.

PBC can affect behavioral performance directly (Armitage and Connor 2001). Given that perceptions of behavioral control may reflect actual behavioral control, PBC may influence behavioral performance as an immediate antecedent under conditions where there is little volitional control (Ajzen 1991). For example, if an individual does not have access to a fitness facility or equipment, low PBC for engaging in resistance training would accurately reflect the individual's actual (low) control over the behavior.

References and Further Readings

Ajzen, I. (1991). The theory of planned behavior. *Organizational Behavior and Human Decision Processes, 50*(2), 179–211.

Ajzen, I. (2002). Perceived behavioral control, self-efficacy, locus of control, and the theory of planned behavior. *Journal of Applied Social Psychology, 32*(4), 665–683.

Armitage, C. J., & Connor, M. (2001). Efficacy of the theory of planned behavior: A meta-analytic review. *British Journal of Social Psychology, 40*(4), 471–499.

Conner, M., & Armitage, C. J. (1998). Extending the theory of planned behavior: A review and avenues for further research. *Journal of Applied Social Psychology, 28*(15), 1429–1464 Special issue: Expectancy-value models of attitude and behavior.

Godin, G., & Kok, G. (1996). The theory of planned behaviour: A review of its application to health-related behaviors. *American Journal of Health Promotion, 11*(2), 87–98.

Perceived Risk

Yori Gidron
SCALab, Lille 3 University and Siric Oncollile, Lille, France

Definition

This term refers to an individual's subjective evaluation of his or her risk of an illness or an adverse outcome, often in relation to performing a certain risky behavior. This term maps onto the Health Belief Model (Rosenstock 1966), which tries to model why people use health services or adhere to medically advocated healthy behaviors. Perceived risk, for example, can be in relation to having a myocardial infarction due to smoking or having skin cancer due to sun exposure or having an accident due to risk taking on the road. Relevant to perceived risk, Weinstein (1982) coined the terms "unrealistic optimism" and "unrealistic pessimism," where people are asked to estimate their risk of having a disease or an adverse outcome, compared to people of their age and sex. Answers are rated on a Likert scale ranging, for example, from -5 (far below others' risk) through 0 (same as others' risk) to $+5$ (far above others' risk). Levels of perceived risk could be related to prior exposure to a condition, one's knowledge of such a condition, exposure to one of a condition's risk factors, and personality aspects. For example, in a recent review of 53 studies on risk perception among people at high risk for cancer, Tilburt et al. (2011) found that family cancer history, previous tests and treatments, younger age, believing in cancer's preventability and severity, monitoring coping style, distress, and the ability to process numbers all correlated with cancer risk perceptions. Concerning prediction, many studies have shown that perceived risk is related to various behavioral and health outcomes. For example, Mann et al. (2007) found that the level of perceived risk was one of several predictors of adherence to prescribed statins, which are used to treat hypercholesterolemia and prevent cardiac events. An older study found that young male drivers estimated their chance of having an accident as lower than their peers and as lower than older male drivers' estimates, when viewing various traffic scenarios (Finn and Bragg 1986). These incorrect perceptions of risk were interpreted as one of the reasons for the overrepresentation of young male drivers in fatal accidents. Knowing one's levels of perceived risk can help predicting his or her adherence to an advocated health behavior or to stopping an unhealthy behavior. Furthermore, perceived risk, if unrealistic, can be a target of brief cognitive restructuring, in the service of healthier behaviors, disease prevention, and treatment.

References and Further Readings

Finn, P., & Bragg, B. W. (1986). Perception of the risk of an accident by young and older drivers. *Accident Analysis and Prevention, 18*, 289–298.

Mann, D. M., Allegrante, J. P., Natarajan, S., Halm, E. A., & Charlson, M. (2007). Predictors of adherence to

statins for primary prevention. *Cardiovascular Drugs and Therapy, 21*, 311–316.
Rosenstock, I. M. (1966). Why people use health services. *The Milbank Memorial Fund Quarterly, 44*, 94–124.
Tilburt, J. C., James, K. M., Sinicrope, P. S., Eton, D. T., Costello, B. A., Carey, J., et al. (2011). Factors influencing cancer risk perception in high risk populations: A systematic review. *Hereditary Cancer in Clinical Practice, 19*, 2.
Weinstein, N. D. (1982). Unrealistic optimism about susceptibility to health problems. *Journal of Behavioral Medicine, 5*, 441–460.

Perceived Stress

Anna C. Phillips
School of Sport, Exercise and Rehabilitation Sciences, University of Birmingham, Edgbaston, Birmingham, UK

Synonyms

Stress

Definition (and Description)

Perceived stress is the feelings or thoughts that an individual has about how much stress they are under at a given point in time or over a given time period.

Perceived stress incorporates feelings about the uncontrollability and unpredictability of one's life, how often one has to deal with irritating hassles, how much change is occurring in one's life, and confidence in one's ability to deal with problems or difficulties. It is not measuring the types or frequencies of stressful events which have happened to a person, but rather how an individual feels about the general stressfulness of their life and their ability to handle such stress. Individuals may suffer similar negative life events but appraise the impact or severity of these to different extents as a result of factors such as personality, coping resources, and support. In this way, perceived stress reflects the interaction between an individual and their environment which they appraise as threatening or overwhelming their resources in a way which will affect their well-being (Lazarus and Folkman 1984). Perceived stress is commonly measured as the frequency of such feelings via a questionnaire such as the Perceived Stress Scale (Cohen et al. 1983).

Cross-References

▶ Life Events
▶ Negative Thoughts
▶ Perceived Stress Scale (PSS)
▶ Stress

References and Further Readings

Cohen, S., Kamarck, T., & Mermelstein, R. (1983). A global measure of perceived stress. *Journal of Health and Social Behavior, 24*, 385–396.
Lazarus, R. S., & Folkman, S. (1984). *Stress, coping and adaptation*. New York: Springer.

Perceived Stress Scale (PSS)

Sherilynn F. Chan[1] and Annette M. La Greca[2]
[1]Cincinnati Children's Hospital Medical Center, University of Cincinnati College of Medicine, Cincinnati, OH, USA
[2]Department of Psychology, University of Miami, Miami, FL, USA

Definition and Description

The Perceived Stress Scale (PSS) is one of the most widely used instruments to measure stress perceptions. The original PSS is a 14-item self-report measure designed to assess "the degree to which situations in one's life are appraised as stressful" (Cohen et al. 1983, p. 385). It is a global measure of stress, rather than a measure of specific stressful life events. Specifically, items assess the extent to which one's life is perceived as "unpredictable, uncontrollable, and overloading" (Cohen et al. 1983, p. 387). The measure was intended for use with community samples of adolescents or adults with an educational level of junior high school or more. Sample items include the following: "In the last month...how often have you been upset because of something that happened unexpectedly?," "...how often have you felt that you were unable to control the important things in your life?," and "...how often have you felt confident about your ability to handle your personal problems?" (Cohen et al. 1983). Half of the questions are positively stated and reverse coded. Each item is rated on a 5-point scale (0 = Never, 1 = Almost Never, 2 = Sometimes, 3 = Fairly Often, 4 = Very Often) and summed to create a total score. Ten-item (PSS-10) and four-item (PSS-4) versions of this measure have been developed (Cohen and Williamson 1988; Cohen et al. 1983).

Both the 14- and 10-item versions have good psychometric properties. In studies of adults, the PSS-14 has strong internal consistency ($\alpha = 0.84$ to 0.86) and good test-retest reliability ($r = 0.85$ over a 2-day period, $r = 0.55$ over a 6-week period; Cohen et al. 1983). In terms of concurrent validity, the PSS-14 is positively related to the number and perceived impact of life stressors ($r = 0.17$ to 0.35; Cohen et al. 1983). With regard to predictive validity, PSS scores predict depressive symptoms ($r = 0.65$ to 0.76), social anxiety ($r = 0.37$ to 0.48), and various health-related outcomes ($r = 0.52$ to 0.65) (Cohen et al. 1983). Factor analyses conducted with psychiatric inpatients revealed two factors: perceived distress and perceived coping (Hewitt et al. 1992; Martin et al. 1995).

Psychometric data also support the reliability and validity of the PSS-10 (Roberti et al. 2006), and an exploratory factor analysis revealed two factors: perceived helplessness and perceived self-efficacy (Roberti et al. 2006). Measurement invariance across gender and a 2-year time frame for the two-factor model has been demonstrated (Barbosa-Leiker et al. 2013). The PSS-4 can be a useful measure when an abridged version is needed; however, its internal reliability ($\alpha = 0.72$) and test-retest reliability ($r = 0.55$) are lower than that for the longer versions (Cohen et al. 1983). The PSS-14 and PSS-10 have been translated into many languages, including Spanish, Portuguese, Italian, German, Danish, Norwegian, Swedish, Finnish, Polish, Hungarian, Bulgarian, Serbian, Turkish, Greek, Hebrew, Russian, Arabic, Chinese, Korean, Japanese, and Thai. While some of these translated versions have been validated, the psychometric properties for many of them have not yet been evaluated ("Dr. Cohen's Scales" 2015).

The PSS has been used to assess perceived stress among many different populations including college, graduate, and medical students, nurses, physicians, athletes, pregnant and postpartum women, and the elderly. The PSS can be used to examine the role of appraised stress in physiological and behavioral disorders and can also be employed in research and clinical settings as an outcome variable (Cohen et al. 1983). Furthermore, this measure can be used as a screening device to identify individuals at risk for certain psychiatric disorders such as depression (Cohen et al. 1983) and may be a valuable tool for use within clinical settings to aid treatment planning and monitor treatment response (Roberti et al. 2006).

Cross-References

▶ Perceived Stress
▶ Psychological Stress

References and Further Reading

Barbosa-Leiker, C., Kostick, M., Lei, M., McPherson, S., Roper, V., Hoekstra, T., & Wright, B. (2013). Measurement invariance of the perceived stress scale and latent mean differences across gender and time. *Stress and Health, 29*, 253–260.

Cohen, S., & Williamson, G. (1988). Perceived stress in a probability sample of the United States. In S. Spacapam & S. Oskamp (Eds.), *The social psychology of health: Claremont symposium on applied social psychology*. Newbury Park: Sage.

Cohen, S., Kamarck, T., & Mermelstein, R. (1983). A global measure of perceived stress. *Journal of Health and Social Behavior, 24*, 385–396.

Dr. Cohen's Scales. (2015, February 19). Retrieved August 9, 2019, from https://www.cmu.edu/dietrich/psychology/stress-immunity-disease-lab/scales/index.html

Hewitt, P. L., Flett, G. L., & Mosher, S. W. (1992). The perceived stress scale: Factor structure and relation to depression symptoms in a psychiatric sample. *Journal of Psychopathology and Behavioral Assessment, 14*, 247–257.

Martin, R. A., Kazarian, S. S., & Brieter, H. J. (1995). Perceived stress, life events, dysfunctional attitudes, and depression in adolescent psychiatric inpatients. *Journal of Psychopathology and Behavioral Assessment, 17*, 81–95.

Roberti, J., Harrington, L., & Storch, E. (2006). Further psychometric support for the 10-item version of the perceived stress scale. *Journal of College Counseling, 9*(2), 135–147.

Perception of Internal Noise (False)

▶ Tinnitus and Cognitive Behavior Therapy

Perceptions of Stress

Kristen Salomon[1] and Mardís Karlsdóttir[2]
[1]Department of Psychology, University of South Florida College of Arts and Sciences, Tampa, FL, USA
[2]Department of Psychology, The University of Iceland School of Health Sciences, Reykjavík, Iceland

Synonyms

Stress appraisals

Definition

The construals or appraisals of an event that result in the experience of stress. Major theoretical definitions of stress emphasize perception as an important component responsible for the experience of stress. According to Lazarus and Folkman (1984), events are perceived as stressful if they are perceived as (1) relevant to one's well-being and (2) having the potential for harm or loss. Primary appraisals of demand, difficulty, and/or uncertainty when weighed against secondary appraisals of coping resources and abilities may result in further perceptions of stress as a challenge to be met and overcome (resources outweigh demands) or as a threat to be endured (demands outweigh resources). These resultant perceptions can influence the psychological and physiological responses to the stressor (Tomaka et al. 1993). Perceptions of a stressful event's duration (chronic vs. acute), severity, controllability, and predictability can also influence responses to the stressor. According to Hobfoll (1989), stress results from the perceived potential loss of resources. As a result, perceptions of current resources and the potential to gain resources are involved in perceiving an event as stressful.

Cross-References

▶ Mental Stress
▶ Stress
▶ Stress Responses

References and Readings

Hobfoll, S. E. (1989). Conservation of resources: A new attempt at conceptualizing stress. *American Psychologist, 44*, 513–524.

Lazarus, R. S., & Folkman, S. (1984). *Stress, appraisal and coping*. New York: Springer.

Tomaka, J., Blascovich, J., Kelsey, R. M., & Leitten, C. L. (1993). Subjective, physiological, and behavioral effects of threat and challenge appraisals. *Journal of Personality and Social Psychology, 65*, 248–260.

Performance Anxiety

▶ Anxiety

Peripheral Arterial Disease (PAD)/Vascular Disease

Leah Rosenberg
Department of Medicine, School of Medicine, Duke University, Durham, NC, USA

Synonyms

Complications of atherosclerosis; Intermittent claudication; Rest pain

Definition

Peripheral arterial disease is the mismatch of blood flow supply and demand in the distal arteries.

Description

Peripheral arterial disease (PAD) is a common manifestation of atherosclerosis and is often a complication of hypertension and/or diabetes. It is estimated that PAD affects more than eight million Americans. PAD, or the accumulation of atherosclerotic plaques leading to narrowing in noncardiac vasculature, can affect renal arteries, carotid arteries, or any other branch vessels from the aorta like the subclavian artery or iliacs. When patients with PAD become symptomatic, there is a mismatch between the metabolic supply and demand of a tissue. When an upper or lower extremity is involved, PAD may starve the affected muscle of oxygenated blood flow and causes discomfort or pain, usually exacerbated by increased activity of the affected limb. In the lower extremity, this mismatch generally presents as intermittent claudication, commonly referred to as "walking pain," where patients develop lower extremity discomfort while ambulating. While there are anatomical entrapment syndromes, deep venous thromboses, and other neurological entities that must be ruled out, PAD is a significant cause of morbidity and mortality (American Heart Association 2011).

PAD may present before arteriosclerotic disease of the great vessels, or heart becomes clinically relevant. Signs of lower extremity PAD on physical exam include shiny, tight, and hairless skin on the lower leg. Other signs of PAD include ischemic nonhealing leg ulcers and gangrene. The limb temperature often feels cool to the touch and has decreased sensation on examination. Most patients do not perceive the rest pain of intermittent claudication. In fact, only approximately 10% of patients with measurable PAD present to physicians complaining of the typical activity-related symptoms of PAD. Early signs of PAD include erectile dysfunction, leg cramps, or muscle fatigue that exceeds the expected effects of normal exertion.

The ankle-brachial index (ABI) is an excellent screening test for PAD of the distal extremity, although direct arteriography is the gold standard. Measuring a patient's ABI is a relatively low-cost, noninvasive diagnostic test that uses the systolic blood pressure readings of the brachial, posterior tibial, and dorsalis pedis arteries. Each lower extremity is examined separately. The formula involves by dividing the maximal ankle pressure in each lower extremity by the higher of the two brachial artery pressures.

The symptoms of PAD may be modifiable through lipid management and behavioral change. While not life threatening, moderate-to-severe PAD and claudication can have a serious impact on a patient's quality of life. Treatment for PAD may be behavioral (i.e., physical activity, smoking cessation), medication-based (statins and antiplatelet agents), or interventional (angioplasty, stent implantation, or bypass surgery).

References and Reading

Statistical Fact Sheet. (2011). Peripheral arterial disease. American Heart Association. http://www.americanheart.org. Accessed 9 Oct 2011.

Perseverative Cognition

J. F. Brosschot[1], Bart Verkuil[1] and Julian F. Thayer[2]
[1]Clinical, Health and Neuro Psychology, Leiden University, Leiden, The Netherlands
[2]Department of Psychology, The Ohio State University, Columbus, OH, USA

Synonyms

Intrusive thoughts; Repetitive thinking; Rumination; Worry

Definition

Perseverative cognition is defined as "the repeated or chronic activation of the cognitive representation of one or more psychological stressors" (Brosschot et al. 2006). Stressful events, or stressors, can make people "linger on" mentally. Humans, unlike animals, can make mental representations of stressors, long before and long after these events occur or are believed to occur. This continued cognitive representation of stressful events, before or after their occurrence, and even regardless of their actual occurrence, is called perseverative cognition. It can take the form of worry, rumination, angry brooding, etc., but also, for example, as mind wandering about negative topics. Perseverative cognition appears to play a causal or sustaining role in several major psychopathologies (anxiety disorders, depression, post-traumatic disorder) (Watkins 2008) – indeed, worry is the hallmark of general anxiety disorder – as well as in somatic disease, including subjective bodily complaints as well as cardiovascular disease (Verkuil et al. 2010).

During perseverative cognition, physiological activity can be increased. The "perseverative cognition hypothesis" (Brosschot et al. 2006) holds that the health damage due to stress is actually caused ("mediated") by perseverative cognition, because the latter prolongs the physiological responses to stressors. It has been suggested that perseverative cognition may partly be unconscious, while it still has physiological effects (Brosschot et al. 2010). This possibility, or the more general possibility of unconscious stress having health impacts, has the potential to open a new area in stress research.

There are several ways to reduce perseverative cognition. The most direct way is "postponing" or "scheduling" worrying or rumination, that is, limiting it to small daily time periods to obtain control over it. More indirect interventions are mediation mindfulness and computer-based attentional training techniques (Verkuil et al. 2010).

Cross-References

▶ Intrusive Thoughts
▶ Worry

References and Readings

Brosschot, J. F., Gerin, W., & Thayer, J. F. (2006). The perseverative cognition hypothesis: A review of worry, prolonged stress-related physiological activation, and health. *Journal of Psychosomatic Research, 60*, 113–124.

Brosschot, J. F., Verkuil, B., & Thayer, J. F. (2010). Conscious and unconscious perseverative cognition: Is a large part of prolonged physiological activity due to unconscious stress? *Journal of Psychosomatic Research, 69*(4), 407–416.

Verkuil, B., Brosschot, J. F., Gebhardt, W., & Thayer, J. F. (2010). When worries make you sick: A review of perseverative cognition, the default stress response and somatic health. *Journal of Experimental Psychopathology, 1*(1), 87–118.

Watkins, E. R. (2008). Constructive and unconstructive repetitive though. *Psychological Bulletin, 134*(2), 163–206.

Persistent Depressive Disorder

▶ Unipolar Depression

Persistent Pain

▶ Chronic Pain Patients

Personal Data Analytics

▶ Quantified Self

Personal Health Informatics

▶ Consumer Health Informatics

Personal Health Record

▶ Electronic Health Record

Personality

Matthew Cribbet and Paula Williams
Department of Psychology, University of Utah, Salt Lake City, UT, USA

Synonyms

Disposition; Individual Difference Factors; Traits

Definition

Although definitions may vary across the theoretical and methodological approaches, the term *personality* generally refers to stable patterns in how people think, act, and feel that make them unique.

Description

The study of personality has been guided by two major themes: (a) the study of individual dimensions along which people differ (i.e., nomothetic approaches) and (b) the study of individuals as unique and integrated people (i.e., idiographic approaches). Diverse theoretical and methodological approaches that have guided research in these two major domains have also contributed to controversies that have waxed and waned throughout the history of this discipline. In addition, research focused on explicating the relative role of the person versus the situation, as well as biology versus environment has been central to this area of psychology; however, in recent years, the focus on such false dichotomies has yielded to more integrated theoretical perspectives on personality. Emerging personality research ranges from the study of genetics and biological systems to the influence of culture on personality development and expression. An overview of the prominent theoretical approaches to the study of personality is provided below, including psychoanalytic, trait, social-cognitive, and interpersonal approaches.

Psychoanalytic Approaches to the Study of Personality

Although less prominent in current personality research, it is important to describe the psychoanalytic perspective on the development and manifestation of personality. Specifically, psychoanalytic approaches assert that stable personality patterns develop in childhood. According to this perspective, early childhood experiences are important, because they shape how individuals relate to others as adults. As individuals develop into mature adults, mental processes not only guide interpersonal interactions, but may also operate in parallel so that people can feel conflicted about the same person or situation. According to this perspective and start the sentence with Personality develops as individuals learn to relate to others by regulating tension associated with sexual and aggressive drives. Finally, psychoanalytic theory emphasizes the role of mental representations of the self, others, and relationships as a framework for how people interact with one another. Psychoanalytic approaches have emphasized that behavior arises from thoughts, feelings, and motives that are outside of awareness. This reliance on unconscious mental processes separates psychoanalytic approaches from other perspectives on personality development.

Early psychoanalytic writing placed motivation at the center of theories of personality.

According to this perspective, human motives could be grouped into two broad classes: life instincts (that include self-preservation and sexual motives) and death instincts or aggressive motives. This dualistic approach to personality was criticized for being overly simplistic. Subsequent research efforts expanded upon these two instincts by creating a more extensive catalog of "needs" or motives. These attempts to reformulate the psychoanalytic concept of instincts and motives stimulated a great deal of empirical research. Despite stark criticism, research on unconscious motives on adult behavior has provided the foundation for several important developments in the study of personality. For example, empirical work on unconscious motives has stimulated the fields of cognitive information processing, including research on implicit psychological mechanisms that have made the study of the unconscious more scientifically acceptable.

An important criticism of the psychoanalytic approach to personality is that the operationalization of key theoretical constructs has proven difficult. Assessments of unconscious motives and thoughts through the traditional psychoanalytic methods of free association, the unpacking of defense mechanisms, the analysis of transference processes, and dream interpretation have generally failed to hold up to minimal standards of reliability and validity necessary for empirical investigation.

Among the many attempts to operationalize psychoanalytic constructs for empirical investigation of personality, the Thematic Apperception Test (TAT) is perhaps the most well known and widely used. The popularity of the TAT as a measure of unconscious motives greatly diminished due to early criticisms of low internal consistency, temporal reliability, and a lack of correlation with self-reported measures of motives.

Trait Approaches to the Study of Personality

Trait theories of personality have typically used three different strategies to study the number, nature, and organization of dimensions along which people differ. One trait approach uses statistical techniques, such as factor analysis, to identify underlying personality dimensions applicable to all people. Another approach is to construct typologies based on a priori theories that are applicable to subgroups of people. Finally, idiographic approaches to the study of personality reject the search for basic traits common to all people, and instead focus on patterns of behavior that are unique to an individual.

The *lexical hypothesis* has been central to trait approaches to personality. The *lexical hypothesis* states that most of the descriptors that distinguish one individual from another have become embedded in our natural language. If the *lexical hypothesis* is correct, the basic dimensions of personality can be discovered, because all important individual differences will be spoken and eventually encoded into trait descriptors. Early work guided by the *lexical hypothesis* provided some initial structure, but did not provide a framework for distinguishing, naming, and ordering individual differences in behavior and experience. Early taxonomic efforts paired down initial attempts to derive personality traits from large lists of terms, but were limited by data-analytic techniques that were not sophisticated enough to handle large and complex data sets. With statistical advancements, research focused on examining the factor structure of personality descriptors in the lexicon grew considerably. Proponents of this approach debated about the number of factors sufficient to describe personality (with 16, 5, and 3 being the predominant models) and the applicability of applying a group of factors to all people. Critics of the trait approach argued that these individual difference factors lacked consistency across situations and were poor at actually predicting specific behavior.

Following a brief period of relative dormancy in the 1970s and 1980s, due in part to the above-stated criticisms, research on the trait structure of personality increased dramatically during the mid-1980s. By the early 1990s, many personality psychologists reached a general (though still not unanimous) consensus that the trait domains could be described most broadly by five orthogonal factors, or clusters of traits. This five-factor trait model has been typically measured with self-report questionnaires and includes the following factors: neuroticism – hostility, depression, and anxiety; extraversion – warm, active, and assertive; openness to experience – open to ideas, values, and fantasy; agreeableness – modest, straightforward, and altruistic; and conscientiousness–dutiful, self-disciplined, and ordered. Yet, some psychologists have maintained that three factors, not five, characterized as neuroticism, extraversion, and psychoticism – a dimension characterized by low agreeableness and low conscientiousness – account for a majority of the variance. Despite criticism regarding the underlying assumptions of factor-analytic techniques, the five-factor model approach to the study of personality has proven to be a useful model for predicting outcomes at the individual, interpersonal, and social levels of analysis.

Beyond factor-analytic approaches, some trait theorists propose that personality is based on bundles of trait-like characteristics that can be classified as types or typologies presumed to cover all people. Recent statistical advancements (e.g., multilevel modeling techniques) have greatly increased our understanding of individual differences by allowing for the examination of the trajectory and rate at which people change. These approaches tend to focus on limited subgroups by examining combinations of personality variables as well as other variables such as intelligence, conduct, and externalizing behavior. These statistical and methodological advances have allowed researchers to examine more variables and the ability to account for interactions among those variables when describing what constitutes personality. Whereas these approaches to the study of personality are innovative, they are not without flaw. Specifically, critics have noted that this approach dissembles people into component parts that results in "types" that account for a limited amount of the variance in whatever outcome is under investigation.

Finally, the idiographic approach to the study of personality rejects the search for underlying personality traits common to all people, and instead focuses on identifying central themes in an individual's life. The idiographic approach is also concerned with describing the patterning of traits within an individual and using that pattern to predict future behavior. Research advocating for an idiographic approach claims that factor-analytic approaches might not account for the full range of personality characteristics within a person.

Social-Cognitive Approaches to the Study of Personality

Personality psychology was greatly influenced by the cognitive revolution in psychology that occurred during the late 1950s and early 1960s. This early research rejected the construct of motivation and focused on the complexity of cognitive processes. Importantly, the cognitive revolution in psychology spurred interest in the importance of "the self," leading to the examination of constructs such as self-esteem, self-schema, self-monitoring, and self-regulation. Research on the self broadened the view of personality by considering not only conceptions of what constitutes "the self," but also the ways in which our self-concept reflects our perceptions of how others view and respond to us.

More broadly, the concept of self-identity has spawned research endeavors aimed at creating a conceptual bridge between the self and the role that social variables such as gender, race, class, and nationality play in the development of personality. Recent theoretical models of self-identity emphasize a "life story" approach to the study of personality. According to this perspective, personality is constructed by an individual through self-defining life narratives. These life narratives are created with the intent of describing individuals as integrated, whole people.

During the late 1960s and early 1970s, critiques of personality psychology produced a major crisis within the field, and led to an in-depth examination of many of the fundamental theories and methods used by personality psychologists. This perspective placed emphasis on situations, claiming that the examination of broad dispositional personality variables was unnecessarily overemphasized.

This approach advocated the notion that it is difficult to demonstrate the consistency of individual difference factors from one situation to the next and that individual difference factors rarely predict specific behaviors. This assertion not only challenged the basic premise of personality psychology, but also generated a paradigmatic crisis, resulting in an ideological split between those who study individual difference factors and those who examine the effect of situations on people. Those psychologists who advocate for a situationist approach construe personality as an organized system of goals, motives, and expectancies that mediate psychological processes that occur across situations. Proponents of this approach maintain that this characterization of personality accounts for both stability within the person as well as adaptive behavior across situations.

The response to this critique was to improve measurement techniques and to conduct studies demonstrating the consistency of personality over time. Yet, other researchers responded by examining how moderator variables, such as gender, interact with situational factors and with traditional trait descriptors. Those who emphasize the importance of context or situation maintain that dispositional traits are manifest as affective and cognitive processes that become activated during a distinct situation. Over time, these situation-by-behavior profiles are thought to shape who we are as individuals, leading to "dispositional signatures" that distinguish us as unique individuals.

Interpersonal Approaches to the Study of Personality

From an interpersonal perspective, personality is considered to be expressed in interactions with other people. Interpersonal theories of personality development do not merely emphasize observable behavior between individuals. Instead, interpersonal theories extend beyond personality development to include personality structure, function, and even pathology. According this perspective, interpersonal interactions support the development and maintenance of personality as patterns of interpersonal interactions give rise to lasting concepts of the self and others.

There have been two distinct empirical traditions to describe interpersonal functioning – the individual differences approach and the dyadic approach. The individual differences approach focuses on the qualities of an individual that are assumed to give rise to behavior that is consistent over time. This perspective led to various formulations of a structural model of interpersonal traits, actions, and problems often referred to as the interpersonal circle or circumplex. Circumplex models of behavior are used to anchor descriptions of theoretical concepts. Circumplex models of personality maintain that individual differences can be described as combinations of the circle's two underlying dimensions of dominance/submission and warmth/hostility. Interpersonal qualities close to one another on the perimeter of the circle are conceptually and statistically similar, qualities 90° apart are conceptually independent, but related, whereas qualities located 180° apart on the circle are considered conceptual and statistical opposites. This model of interpersonal functioning is not typically tied to interactions with a specific person or context, but rather is most often used to describe qualities of an individual interacting with a generalized other person.

In contrast, the dyadic approach assumes that two people comprise a basic unit of analysis for understanding personality. Accordingly, the interpersonal learning of social behaviors and self-concept is based on a variety of interpersonal situations. Interpersonal learning occurs across situations when interactions with others shape, refine, and maintain lasting conceptions of the self and others in relation to the self. In addition, this perspective on personality emphasizes that interpersonal behavior does not occur at random; instead, reciprocal relational patterns between two or more people help to define an interpersonal field. Within this interpersonal field, behavior from one individual pulls for responses from another, creating a dynamic, transactional process that leads to a conceptualization of the self. Interpersonal theories also include aspects of other theories of personality, but uniquely contribute to personality psychology by combining structural models that describe behavior with an examination of interpersonal situations.

Emerging Approaches to the Study of Personality

In recent years, the study of personality has benefited from advances in molecular genetics and functional imaging techniques. Within the domain of molecular genetics, research has focused on identifying specific biological pathways that contribute to complex cognitive and emotional behaviors. Advancements in the field of behavioral genetics may increase our understanding of the biological underpinnings of how individual differences in personality emerge and how those individual differences confer risk or resilience for mental and physical health. Other approaches that apply molecular genetic techniques to the study of personality involve examining the association between a particular phenotype and a specific allele of a gene.

Functional neuroimaging techniques hold promise for understanding personality by examining brain activity among individuals with varying levels of individual difference factors. Emerging advances in neuroimaging techniques may also help to further refine our understanding of how people process emotional information, including social connections. Yet, examining a single variation in alleles or the functional contributions of one brain region will not hold much explanatory value for our understanding of individual differences in thought, behavior, and emotions. With advancing techniques, future research should involve the careful application of methods and concepts learned from decades of investigation in order to refine our understanding of personality.

Personality and Health: Implications for Behavioral Medicine

Theory and research examining the influence of personality on health and disease has been an influential force for the development of the fields of health psychology and behavioral medicine. Research in this domain has been concerned with understanding the effects of personality on both the development and trajectory of health and disease. Possible mechanisms linking personality and health include the psychophysiological effects of stress and the extent to which personality traits are related to specific behaviors that may either promote or compromise health. Of particular interest to behavioral medicine is research that examines how certain personality characteristics confer differential risk toward negative affective states and behavioral dysregulation that often accompanies the diagnosis of and adjustment to chronic illness. Evidence that personality is a powerful predictor of health and illness has not only contributed to the development of behavioral medicine and health psychology, but has also helped revitalize personality research by challenging the critique of personality traits as having limited predictive utility.

Cross-References

▶ Behavioral Medicine
▶ Character Traits
▶ Health Psychology
▶ Phenotype
▶ Trait Anger
▶ Trait Anxiety

References and Further Readings

Barenbaum, N. B., & Winter, D. G. (2009). History of modern personality theory and research. In O. P. John, R. W. Robins, & L. A. Pervin (Eds.), *Handbook of personality: Theory and research* (pp. 3–28). New York: Guilford Press.

McCrae, R. R., & John, O. P. (1992). An introduction to the five-factor model and its applications. *Journal of Research in Personality, 60*, 175–215.

Pincus, A. L., & Ansell, E. B. (2003). Interpersonal theory of personality. In T. Millon & M. Lerner (Eds.), *Comprehensive handbook of psychology (Personality and social psychology)* (Vol. 5, pp. 209–229). New York: Wiley.

Williams, P. G., Smith, T. W., & Cribbet, M. R. (2008). Personality and health: Current evidence, potential mechanisms, and future directions. In G. J. Boyle, G. Matthews, & D. H. Saklofske (Eds.), *Personality theory and assessment* (Vol. 1, pp. 635–658). Thousands Oaks: Sage.

Personality Hardiness

▶ Hardiness and Health

Pervasive Health

▶ Quality of Life Technologies

Pessimism

Ryan Garcia
University of Texas Southwestern Medical Center at Dallas, Dallas, TX, USA

Synonyms

Dispositional pessimism

Definition

Pessimism is a personality variable that reflects the generalized tendency for an individual to have negative expectations about the future. Its development emerged along with that of dispositional optimism from models of self-regulation and goal achievement. Originally, pessimism was construed to reflect low levels of optimism, but it has emerged as an independent construct as the field of research has developed and grown. It is associated with a coping style characterized by problem and emotion avoidance coping (Solberg Nes and Segerstrom 2006). Research suggests a pessimistic orientation places one at increased risk for depression and anxiety. Pessimism has also been associated with several different adverse health outcomes across a variety of settings, ranging from HIV + populations to increased mortality rates in individuals with cancer. The following terms are related to pessimism: defensive pessimism, unrealistic pessimism, and self-handicapping; however, these terms are not identical to pessimism, and have different associations with other variables.

Cross-References

- ▶ Attribution Theory
- ▶ Avoidance
- ▶ Dispositional Optimism
- ▶ Explanatory Style
- ▶ Life Orientation Test (LOT)
- ▶ Negative Thoughts
- ▶ Optimism and Pessimism: Measurement
- ▶ Optimism, Pessimism, and Health
- ▶ Self-Regulation Model

References and Further Readings

Abela, J. R. Z., Auerbach, R. P., & Seligman, M. E. P. (2008). Dispositional pessimism across the lifespan. In K. S. Dobson & D. J. A. Dozois (Eds.), *Risk factors in depression* (pp. 195–220). San Diego: Academic Press.

Cantor, N., & Norem, J. K. (1989). Defensive pessimism and stress and coping. *Social Cognition, 7*, 92–112.

Carver, C. S., & Scheier, M. F. (2002). Optimism, pessimism, and self-regulation. In E. C. Chang (Ed.), *Optimism & pessimism: Implications for theory, research, and practice* (pp. 31–51). Washington, DC: American Psychological Association.

Norem, J. K. (2002). Defensive pessimism, optimism, and pessimism. In E. C. Chang (Ed.), *Optimism & pessimism: Implications for theory, research, and practice* (pp. 77–100). Washington, DC: American Psychological Association.

Scheier, M. F., & Carver, C. S. (1985). Optimism, coping, and health: Assessment and implications of generalized outcome expectancies. *Health Psychology, 4*(3), 219–247.

Scheier, M. F., & Carver, C. S. (1987). Dispositional optimism and physical well-being: The influence of generalized outcome expectancies on health. *Journal of Personality, 55*(2), 169–210.

Scheier, M. F., & Carver, C. S. (1992). Effects of optimism on psychological and physical well-being: Theoretical overview and empirical update. *Cognitive Therapy and Research, 16*(2), 201–228.

Solberg Nes, L., & Segerstrom, S. C. (2006). Dispositional optimism and coping: A meta-analytic review. *Personality and Social Psychology Review, 10*(3), 235–251.

Pew Internet and American Life Project

Chad Barrett
Department of Psychology, University of Colorado, Denver, CO, USA

Definition

The Pew Internet and American Life Project is part of the Pew Research Center and is a nonpartisan and nonprofit organization that conducts research in order to provide information on the issues, attitudes, and trends that influence America and the world. According to their website, The Pew Internet and American Life Project examines "the impact of the internet on families, communities, work and home, daily life, education, health care, and civic and political life" (Pew Internet and American Life Project website). Each year, The Pew Internet and American Life Project releases 15–20 reports of research that address "how Americans use the internet and how their online activities affect their lives" (Pew Internet and American Life Project website n.d.). Data collection methods typically involve nationwide random phone surveys, online surveys, and qualitative research. In addition, data collection efforts are often augmented by research conducted by government agencies, technology firms, academia, and by various other expert researchers. Pew Internet and American Life Project aims to provide authoritative reports while maintaining neutral positions on policy issues and abstaining from providing endorsements of specific technologies, industries, organizations, companies, and individuals.

Description

The website for the Pew Internet and American Life Project provides a brief summary of highlights from their research related to health and health care (Fox 2011). Such highlights include the following findings from recent surveys. Seventy-eight percent of adults in the USA use the internet and 83% own a cell phone. Eighty percent of internet users, or 59% of all US adults, use the internet to search for health or medical information. Seventeen percent of cell phone owners, or 15% of all US adults, have used their cell phones to look up health or medical information. Fox notes that since young people, Latinos, and African Americans are more likely than other groups to access the internet through their cell phones, this finding is of particular interest for studies targeting trends in these groups. Internet users most commonly search for health and medical information related to specific diseases or conditions, treatments or procedures, and doctors or other health professionals.

Another line of research has been examining the trends in how the internet influences people's relationships with health and medical information and with each other. As summarized by Fox (2011), many people use the internet to search for health information from other people's personal health-related experiences or to connect with others with similar conditions. Thirty-four percent of internet users, 25% of adults in the USA, have read about another person's experience with health or medical related issues by visiting an online news group, a website, or a blog. Twenty-four percent of internet users, or 18% of adults in the USA, have read online reviews of particular drugs or medical treatments. Eighteen percent of internet users, or 13% of adults in the USA, have used the internet to connect with other people who share similar health concerns. People with rare or chronic conditions are especially likely to attempt to connect with others through the internet. Twenty-seven percent of internet users, or 20% of adults in the USA, have used online applications to monitor their weight, diet, exercise routine, or some other health indicators or symptoms. Six percent of internet users, or 4% of adults in the USA, have visited one or more websites in order to post comments or questions concerning health or medical issues. Four percent of internet users, 3% of adults in the USA, have posted comments or discussions about their experiences with a particular drug or treatment.

In addition to such highlighted findings, the website of the Pew Internet and American Life Project provides links to relevant study reports. The Pew Internet and American Life Project collects a variety of data that could be relevant to the field of behavioral medicine. The Project's website provides access to various studies and raw data sets dating back to 2000.

Cross-References

▶ eHealth and Behavioral Intervention Technologies

- Health Care
- Health Care Access
- Health Care Utilization
- Home Health Care
- Internet-Based Interventions
- Internet-Based Studies
- Public Health
- Social Capital and Health
- Telehealth

References and Further Reading

Fox, S. (2011). *Pew internet: Health*. Retrieved November 25, 2011 from http://www.pewinternet.org/Commentary/2011/November/Pew-Internet-Health.aspx

Pew Internet and American Life Project website. (n.d.). Retrieved November 25, 2011 from http://pewinternet.org/About-Us.aspx

PGD

- In Vitro Fertilization, Assisted Reproductive Technology

Pharmaceutical Industry: Research and Development

J. Rick Turner
Campbell University College of Pharmacy and Health Sciences, Buies Creek, NC, USA

Synonyms

Drug development; New drug development

Definition

Contemporary research and development within the pharmaceutical industry is best described employing a lifecycle perspective. Four components of this are: drug discovery and drug design; nonclinical development; clinical development; and postmarketing surveillance (Turner 2010).

Description

Drug Discovery and Drug Design

Drug discovery can be thought of as the work done from the time of the identification of a therapeutic need in a particular disease area to the time the drug candidate deemed most likely to safely affect the desired therapeutic benefit is identified. This drug candidate may be a small molecule or a biological macromolecule such as a protein or nucleic acid. The traditional mode of drug discovery is a long iterative process in which each molecule more closely approximates the ideal drug candidate. The modern discipline of drug design is much quicker. Computer simulation modeling examines the "docking" of the drug molecule with the drug receptor and identifies the most likely chemical structure that will best dock with the receptor. The science of molecular engineering is then used to create the molecule suggested by the computer simulation.

Nonclinical Development

Nonhuman animal research is currently necessary before regulatory permission will be given to test a new drug in humans. Since part of the overall nonhuman animal testing is done before the drug is first given to humans, the term "preclinical" has a certain appeal and is used by many authors in place of nonclinical. However, a significant amount of nonhuman animal testing is typically conducted after the first administration of the drug to humans. Some of the more lengthy, more complex, and more expensive nonhuman animal testing is typically not started until initial human testing reveals that the drug has a good safety profile in humans and therefore has a reasonable chance of being approved for marketing if it also proves to be effective in later clinical trials. In this entry, therefore, the term "nonclinical" has been adopted for research involving nonhuman animals.

While human pharmacological therapy is the ultimate goal, understanding nonclinical drug safety and efficacy is critical to subsequent rationally designed, ethical human trials. Nonclinical research gathers critical information concerning safety, drug dose, and route and frequency of administration. It involves in vitro, ex vivo, and in vivo testing. For example, when investigating the cardiac safety of noncardiac drugs (drugs for noncardiac indications are not supposed to influence the heart's activity, and if they do it is likely to be in a deleterious manner), the following progression of levels of testing occurs: subcellular (investigation of individual ion channels within cardiac cell muscles or cardiomyocytes); cellular; isolated cardiac tissue; isolated heart; anesthetized intact animal; and conscious animal.

Preapproval Clinical Development and Postmarketing Trials and Surveillance

Pharmaceutical clinical trials are often categorized into various phases, with any given trial being identified as belonging to one of them. These categories traditionally include Phase I, Phase II, Phase III, and Phase IV, described as follows:

- Phase I. Pharmacologically oriented studies that typically look for the best dose to employ. Comparison to other treatments is not typically built into the study design.
- Phase II. Trials that look for evidence of activity, efficacy, and safety at a fixed dose. Again, comparison to other treatments is not typically built into the study design.
- Phase III. Trials in which comparison with another treatment (e.g., placebo, an active control) is a fundamental component of the design. These trials are undertaken if Phase I and Phase II studies have provided preliminary evidence that the investigational drug is safe and effective.
- Phase IV. These are postmarketing trials, conducted once the drug has been approved and in therapeutic use. There are various sorts of Phase IV trials. Some can be quite similar in design and conduct to preapproval therapeutic confirmatory trials. Other kinds include open-label trials, when both investigators and subjects know what treatment subjects are receiving, and large simple trials.

However, while commonly employed, these designations are not always used consistently. Accordingly, two studies with the same aims may be classified into different phases, and two studies classified into the same phase may have different aims. This nomenclature, therefore, can be confusing, and alternate systems of categorization are arguably more informative. One such system is presented in Table 1. The four categories correspond closely to Phase I to Phase IV, respectfully, but are more descriptive.

Among the goals of clinical development are:

- Estimation of the investigational drug's safety and tolerance in healthy adults.
- Determination of a safe and effective dose range, safe dosing levels, and the preferred route of administration.
- Investigation of pharmacokinetics and pharmacodynamics following a single dose and a multiple-dose schedule.
- Establishment and validation of biochemical markers in accessible body fluids that may permit the assessment of the desired pharmacological activity.
- Identification of metabolic pathways.
- Evaluation of the drug's safety and efficacy in a relatively small group of subjects with the disease or condition of clinical concern (the targeted therapeutic indication).
- Selection and optimization of final formulations, doses, regimens, and efficacy endpoints for larger scale, multicenter studies. Efficacy endpoints should be able to be measured reliably and should quantitatively reflect clinically relevant changes in the disease or condition of clinical concern.
- Evaluation of the drug's comparative efficacy (measured against placebo or an active comparator) in larger scale, multicenter studies, and collection of additional safety data.

Pharmaceutical Industry: Research and Development, Table 1 Classifying clinical studies according to their objectives. (Based on ICH E8: General considerations for clinical trials)

Objective of trials	Study examples
Human pharmacology Assess tolerance Describe or define pharmacokinetics (PK) and pharmacodynamics (PD) Explore drug metabolism and drug interactions Estimate (biological) activity	Dose-tolerance studies Single- and multiple-dose PK and/or PD studies Drug interaction studies
Therapeutic exploratory Explore use for the targeted indication Estimate dosage for subsequent studies Provide basis for confirmatory study design, endpoints, methodologies	Earliest trials of relatively short duration in well-defined narrow populations with the disease or condition of clinical concern, using surrogate of pharmacological endpoints or clinical measures Dose-response exploration studies
Therapeutic confirmatory Demonstrate/confirm efficacy Establish safety profile Provide an adequate basis for assessing benefit/risk relationship to support licensing (market approval) Establish dose-response relationship	Adequate and well-controlled studies to establish efficacy Randomized parallel dose-response studies Clinical safety studies Studies of mortality/morbidity outcomes Large simple trials Comparative studies
Therapeutic use Refine understanding of benefit-risk relationship in general or special populations and/or environments Identify less common adverse drug reactions Refine dosing recommendations	Comparative effectiveness studies Studies of mortality/morbidity outcomes Studies of additional endpoints Large simple trials Pharmacoeconomic studies

Cross-References

▶ Comparative Effectiveness Research
▶ Efficacy
▶ Metabolism
▶ Placebo and Placebo Effect

References and Further Readings

ICH E8. (1997). *General considerations for clinical trials*. Accessed 09 Apr 2011, from http://www.ich.org/fileadmin/Public_Web_Site/ICH_Products/Guidelines/Efficacy/E8/Step4/E8_Guideline.pdf.
Turner, J. R. (2010). *New drug development: An introduction to clinical trials*. New York: Springer.

Pharmacological Challenge Tests

▶ Pharmacological Stress Tests

Pharmacological Stress Tests

Beate Ditzen[1], Urs M. Nater[2] and Christine Heim[3]
[1]Department of Psychosocial Medicine, Heidelberg University, Heidelberg, Germany
[2]Department of Psychology, University of Vienna, Vienna, Austria
[3]Institute of Medical Psychology, Charité University Medicine Berlin, Berlin, Germany

Synonyms

HPA axis stimulation tests; Pharmacological challenge tests

Definition

The Hypothalamic-Pituitary-Adrenal (HPA) axis is the major neuroendocrine stress system in humans. Appropriate functioning of this highly dynamic multilevel system and its feedback mechanisms are assumed to modulate psychophysiological adaptation to all major and minor challenges in life. In line with this, profound HPA axis alterations have been found in psychiatric disorders (most prominently affective disorders), in chronic medical disorders (e.g., cardiovascular disease), and in unexplained medical symptoms (e.g., chronic fatigue, Nater et al. 2008). Furthermore, it has been suggested that restoration of glucocorticoid receptor functioning and thereby improvement of HPA axis integrity might mediate treatment outcome in some disorders (such as depression) (Holsboer 2000).

In order to assess the functional integrity of the HPA axis and its feedback mechanisms, standard pharmacological challenge tests have been developed. Targeting different levels of the axis, these tests meet two main goals: (a) to stimulate the HPA axis in order to assess its top-down reactivity, and (b) to stimulate negative feedback mechanisms of the HPA axis in order to test its feedback sensitivity.

Description

In general, HPA axis functioning can be assessed with repeated measures of its unstimulated effector steroids, that is, corticotropin-releasing hormone (CRH), adrenocorticotropic hormone (ACTH), and cortisol.

CRH is best measured in the cerebrospinal fluid (CSF). Plasma levels do not seem to reflect hypothalamic CRH secretion because (1) in addition to the CNS, many tissues in the periphery (such as the placenta) produce CRH and (2) the relatively high concentrations of CRH from the hypothalamic-hypophyseal portal venous blood are bound by CRH-binding protein until they reach the peripheral veins (Cunnah et al. 1987).

ACTH can be assessed in blood. Because the analysis of ACTH concentrations from blood plasma is relatively expensive, the number of repeated measures is usually limited. With a short plasma half-life and episodic secretion, ACTH levels in plasma have shown wide fluctuations and should be assessed in combination with repeated cortisol measures in order to increase reliability.

Cortisol can be measured in plasma (unbound and bound cortisol fraction), in saliva (unbound cortisol fraction), and in urine (unbound fraction).

Note that single measures of CRH, ACTH, or cortisol do not give a valid picture of HPA axis integrity, and more information is obtained by repeated testing.

Besides psychological challenge tests of HPA axis activity (Dickerson and Kemeny 2004), highly standardized pharmacological challenge tests have also been developed. Among others, the administration of Insulin, Naloxone, Fenfluramine, Alprazolam, synthetic CRH, synthetic ACTH, Metyrapone, and Dexamethasone have been used to provoke changes in HPA axis activity. In the following, the most widely used HPA axis challenge tests will be briefly characterized. Note that all challenge tests need to be employed under standardized conditions in a clinical setting.

CRH Stimulation Test

CRH stimulates ACTH secretion. Accordingly, administration of CRH is used to assess information about HPA axis dysregulation occurring down from the level of the pituitary (ACTH and cortisol).

Following one or two blood draws in order to assess ACTH and cortisol baseline levels, an IV bolus of 1 μg/kg of body weight CRH is administered. Repeated blood sampling at min 15, 30, 60, 90, and 120 will show a rapid rise and subsequent gradual decline in ACTH and cortisol following CRH administration.

In healthy subjects, the cortisol response in plasma after 30–60 min following injection is higher than 10 μg/dL (276 nmol/L). Usually, the test is well tolerated, with transient facial flushing in about 20% of the participants, occasional shortness of breath, or rare tachycardia, and hypotension.

ACTH Stimulation Test

With the ACTH stimulation test, the acute adrenal response to ACTH can be assessed. Before and following administration of 0.25 mg synthetic human α1–24-ACTH (tetracosactrin, cosyntropin, or "Synacthen") intramuscularly or intravenously, cortisol levels are measured repeatedly (e.g., baseline, 30, 45, and 60 min after injection). Due to ACTH administration, plasma cortisol rapidly increases within 30 min to at least 18–20 μg/dL (496–552 nmol/L), with peak responses at 30–60 min. Interestingly, substantially lower doses of ACTH were associated with the same endocrine response as the above-described high dosage. Consequently, the so-called low-dose ACTH test (1 μg) is gaining greater importance in endocrine research (Dickstein et al. 1991). Possible adverse side effects of this test include bradycardia, tachycardia, hypertension, peripheral edema, and rash. These side effects should disappear within a few hours after testing.

Dexamethasone Suppression Test

The synthetic corticosteroid Dexamethasone (Dex) binds to glucocorticoid receptors and thereby mimics the effects of cortisol. Consequently, researchers employ the Dexamethasone Suppression Test (DST) in order to assess HPA axis feedback sensitivity with an expected reduction in cortisol secretion following the administration of Dex.

In the standard DST procedure, 1 mg Dex is administered orally at 11:00 p.m. The following morning (8:00 a.m.), cortisol levels are determined in blood, saliva, or urine and may be again measured at 4:00 p.m. In healthy subjects, the standard DST will minimize cortisol secretion with plasma cortisol levels less than 2 μg/dL (50 nmol/L) at both measure time points. In depressed patients, the DST is thought to show non-suppression of cortisol due to *reduced* feedback sensitivity. However, studies on this test in depression have not shown high sensitivity and specificity (APA Task Force on Laboratory Tests in Psychiatry 1987), with only about 40–60% of patients demonstrating a failure to suppress cortisol in response to the standard DST (Yehuda 2006). In disorders characterized by *increased* HPA axis feedback sensitivity (such as Post-traumatic Stress Disorder, PTSD), the low-dose DST (0.5 mg or 0.25 mg) is preferably used. Following this test, normal cortisol suppression results in values around 5 μg/dL. The low-dose DST has been widely used in PTSD research, with PTSD subjects having been exposed to traumas (e.g., childhood abuse, combat, or Holocaust exposure) showing hyperresponsiveness (= lower post-DST cortisol) in this test (Yehuda 2006). No adverse side effects have been reported for the DST.

Dex-CRH Test

In order to more precisely characterize underlying mechanisms of non-suppression in the Dex test, the combined Dex-CRH test has been developed, and improved sensitivity of this test compared to the Dex test has been shown in depression (Heuser et al. 1994). With the Dex-CRH test, the oral administration of Dexamethasone (1.5 mg) at 11:00 p.m. is combined with the intravenous administration of 100 μg CRH the following day in the afternoon (between 2:00 p.m. and 3:00 p.m.). Blood samples will be repeatedly collected before CRH administration, and again at 15, 30, 60, 90, and 120 min after administration.

In healthy individuals, ACTH and cortisol will be suppressed prior to CRH administration. After CRH injection, ACTH and cortisol levels are first increasing and then decreasing (Carroll et al. 1981). Patients suffering from current major depression, but also from other psychiatric and medical conditions, show increased sensitivity, with markedly elevated ACTH and cortisol levels following the Dex-CRH test (Ising et al. 2005). Particularly in depression, repeated Dex-CRH testing has been discussed as a surrogate marker for drug efficacy (Ising et al. 2007). Adverse side effects following the combined Dex-CRH test are identical to those following CRH administration alone.

Metyrapone Test

Metyrapone is a method for assessing ACTH secretory reserve via the interruption of the negative feedback on the HPA axis. The drug inhibits P450c11 (11β-hydroxylase), the enzyme that catalyzes the final step in cortisol biosynthesis. The inhibition of cortisol secretion interrupts negative feedback of the HPA axis, which results in a compensatory increase in ACTH. This increase in ACTH secretion then stimulates biosynthesis in the cortisol precursor steroid (11-deoxycortisol) in plasma.

The overnight metyrapone test is used in order to test whether altered cortisol secretion is a function of increased/decreased ACTH drive from the pituitary or a result of adrenal alterations. A quantity of 30 mg/kg of metyrapone is administered orally, preferably at midnight. Plasma 11-deoxycortisol is then determined the following morning at 8 a.m. In healthy subjects, 11-deoxycortisol levels in plasma rise to more than 7 μg/dL (0.2 μmol/L) and plasma ACTH levels rise to greater than 100 pg/mL (22 pmol/L) the following morning. The test has been used in PTSD research (for a review see Yehuda 2006) as well as in depression research (Young et al. 2007). Possible adverse side effects include gastrointestinal symptoms, headaches, dizziness, hypotension, and allergic skin reactions.

Summary and Outlook

The investigation of neuroendocrine alterations in psychiatric and medical disorders has largely improved our knowledge of the pathophysiology of these disorders. The next steps will be to further improve the sensitivity, specificity, and thereby validity of HPA axis challenge tests. Note that so far, reliable results can only be obtained with repeated application of challenge tests and repeated HPA axis assessment. Confounding factors, such as eating disorders, restrictive dieting, diabetes, gender, and alcohol consumption have been discussed in the literature with mixed results (e.g., APA Task Force on Laboratory Tests in Psychiatry 1987; Ising et al. 2005; Young et al. 2007). This is particularly relevant, as oftentimes these factors might be substantially altered in psychiatric and medical conditions.

A variety of CNS processes can trigger or dampen HPA activation. Among others, these mechanisms may include alterations in levels vasopressin, serotonin, endorphins, oxytocin, neuropeptide Y, substance P, and cytokines. So far, on the level of HPA axis dynamics alone, we are not able to trace back specifically involved CNS mechanisms; in other words, the specificity of HPA axis challenge tests cannot exceed the specificity of the HPA axis itself. Future studies should combine imaging data, administration of centrally active substances (e.g., intranasal administration of vasopressin and oxytocin), in combination with HPA axis challenge tests, thus providing further insights into the specificity of the involved mechanisms in healthy as well as in pathological endocrine functioning.

Cross-References

▶ Adrenal Glands
▶ Hypothalamic-Pituitary-Adrenal Axis
▶ Pituitary-Adrenal Axis

References and Readings

APA Task Force on Laboratory Tests in Psychiatry. (1987). The dexamethasone suppression test: An overview of its current status in psychiatry. The APA task force on laboratory tests in psychiatry. *American Journal of Psychiatry, 144*(10), 1253–1262.

Carroll, B. J., Feinberg, M., Greden, J. F., Tarika, J., Albala, A. A., Haskett, R. F., et al. (1981). A specific laboratory test for the diagnosis of melancholia. Standardization, validation, and clinical utility. *Archives of General Psychiatry, 38*(1), 15–22.

Cunnah, D., Jessop, D. S., Besser, G. M., & Rees, L. H. (1987). Measurement of circulating corticotrophin-releasing factor in man. *Journal of Endocrinology, 113*(1), 123–131.

Dickerson, S. S., & Kemeny, M. E. (2004). Acute stressors and cortisol responses: A theoretical integration and synthesis of laboratory research. *Psychological Bulletin, 130*(3), 355–391.

Dickstein, G., Shechner, C., Nicholson, W. E., Rosner, I., Shen-Orr, Z., Adawi, F., et al. (1991). Adrenocorticotropin stimulation test: Effects of basal cortisol level, time of day, and suggested new sensitive low dose test. *Journal of Clinical Endocrinology and Metabolism, 72*(4), 773–778.

Felitti, V. J., Anda, R. F., Nordenberg, D., Williamson, D. F., Spitz, A. M., Edwards, V., et al. (1998). Relationship of childhood abuse and household dysfunction to many of the leading causes of death in adults. The Adverse Childhood Experiences (ACE) Study. *American Journal of Preventive Medicine, 14*(4), 245–258.

Heuser, I., Yassouridis, A., & Holsboer, F. (1994). The combined dexamethasone/CRH test: A refined laboratory test for psychiatric disorders. *Journal of Psychiatric Research, 28*(4), 341–356.

Holsboer, F. (2000). The corticosteroid receptor hypothesis of depression. *Neuropsychopharmacology, 23*(5), 477–501.

Ising, M., Kunzel, H. E., Binder, E. B., Nickel, T., Modell, S., & Holsboer, F. (2005). The combined dexamethasone/CRH test as a potential surrogate marker in depression. *Progress in Neuro-Psychopharmacology & Biological Psychiatry, 29*(6), 1085–1093.

Ising, M., Horstmann, S., Kloiber, S., Lucae, S., Binder, E. B., Kern, N., et al. (2007). Combined dexamethasone/corticotropin releasing hormone test predicts treatment response in major depression – a potential biomarker? *Biological Psychiatry, 62*(1), 47–54.

Nater, U. M., Maloney, E., Boneva, R. S., Gurbaxani, B. M., Lin, J. M., Jones, J. F., et al. (2008). Attenuated morning salivary cortisol concentrations in a population-based study of persons with chronic fatigue syndrome and well controls. *Journal of Clinical Endocrinology and Metabolism, 93*(3), 703–709.

Yehuda, R. (2006). Advances in understanding neuroendocrine alterations in PTSD and their therapeutic implications. *Annals of the New York Academy of Sciences, 1071*, 137–166.

Young, E. A., Ribeiro, S. C., & Ye, W. (2007). Sex differences in ACTH pulsatility following metyrapone blockade in patients with major depression. *Psychoneuroendocrinology, 32*(5), 503–507.

Pharmacotherapy for Depression

▶ Depression: Treatment

Phasic REM

▶ REM Sleep

Phenotype

Jeanette McCarthy
Community and Family Medicine, Duke University Medical Center, Durham, NC, USA

Definition

The term phenotype refers to an organism's outward appearance and characteristics. This contrasts with the individual's genotype, the set of alleles that an offspring inherits from both parents. In the behavioral sciences, including Behavioral Medicine, the fundamental issue of heredity is the extent to which differences in genotype account for differences in phenotype, i.e., observed differences among individuals (Plomin et al. 1997).

In contrast to single-gene disorders such as Huntington's disease and phenylketonuria (PKU), complex dimensions, disorders, and conditions of clinical concern in Behavioral Medicine are influenced by heredity, but not by one gene alone. Multiple genes are typically involved, and so too are multiple environmental influences, and phenotypes are often the result of the combined effects of both genotype and environmental factors.

Cross-References

▶ Allele
▶ Genotype

References and Further Readings

Plomin, R., DeFries, J. C., McClearn, G. E., & Rutter, M. (1997). *Behavioral genetics* (3rd ed.). New York: W.H. Freeman and Company.

Physical Ability/Disability

▶ Activities of Daily Living (ADL)

Physical Activity

▶ Benefits of Exercise
▶ Exercise

Physical Activity and Cancer

▶ Cancer and Physical Activity

Physical Activity and Health

M. Bernardine[1] and Georita Marie Frierson[2]
[1]Centers for Behavioral and Preventive Medicine, Brown University, Providence, RI, USA
[2]Department of Psychology, Southern Methodist University, Dallas, TX, USA

Synonyms

Assessment; Exercise

Definition

Physical activity (PA) is any body movement that leads to skeletal muscle contraction and noticeable increases in energy expenditure (US Department of Health and Human Services [USDHHS] 2008). Such activities can be walking, washing windows, or gardening.

Description

Introduction

There is strong evidence that there are greater physical, physiological, and possibly mental health benefits from a lifestyle that includes more occupational and leisure-time physical activity (PA) than a predominantly sedentary (inactive or underactive) lifestyle (USDHHS 2008). These benefits include a risk reduction for type 2 diabetes, overweight/obesity, cardiovascular disease, stroke, high blood pressure, an adverse lipid profile, osteoporosis, sarcopenia, and loss of function and autonomy in older age. There is also a great interest in the benefits of PA for mitigating and possibly preventing cancer and its significant morbidity and mortality rates: the evidence is strongest for the prevention of colon and breast cancer. Regular PA can also help in weight loss (when combined with reduced calorie intake) and is associated with reduced depression and better cognitive functioning (among older adults) (USDHHS).

On the negative end, there is low risk of adverse events such as injuries, when generally healthy people engaged in moderate-intensity activity. However, when performing the same activity, people who are less fit are more likely to be injured than those who are fitter. The risk of cardiac events such as heart attacks during PA is rare. But there is a risk of such events when an individual suddenly becomes much more active than usual (e.g., shoveling snow). When both the benefits and risks of PA are considered, it is clear that the health benefits of PA far outweigh the risks of adverse events for a majority of people.

Given the overwhelming evidence for substantial benefits from PA, *physical inactivity* is a national public health problem. Recent data from the 2009 National Health Interview Survey (NHIS) indicates that 35% of US adults report engaging in regular leisure-time PA, 33% reported some leisure-time PA, and 33% report no participation in leisure-time PA (http://www.cdc.gov/nchs/fastats/exercise.htm.) NHIS data for 2005–2007 showed that 30.7% of US adults engaged in PA sufficient in frequency and duration to be classified as regular and 39.7% report no leisure-time PA (Schoenborn and Adams 2010). Men (61.9%) were more likely than women (58.9%) to engage in at least some leisure-time activity. The percentage of adults who engage in at least some leisure PA increased with education and with family income but decreased with increasing age. Married adults were more likely than those in other marital status groups to engage in at least some leisure-time PA. White adults (61.9%) and Asian adults (60.3%) were more likely than black adults (48.8%) to engage in at least some leisure-time PA. Finally, adults living in the US South (27.4%) were least likely to engage in regular leisure-time PA compared with adults living in any other region.

What Is Physical Activity?

Body movement for the purposes of health benefits can be defined by multiple constructs. Some of these constructs are similar but are still distinct. *PA* is any body movement that leads to skeletal muscle contraction and noticeable increases in energy expenditure (USDHHS 2008). Such activities can be walking, washing windows, or gardening. To assess how much PA someone has to engage in for a specific health outcome, the term "dose response" is used (USDHHS). Dose response refers to the frequency, intensity, duration, and type of PA needed for a certain health outcome (i.e., fitness). Typically, PA is measured in kilocalorie (kcal), metabolic equivalent (MET), minutes, or MET-minutes per day or week (USDHHS). Such measurements occur through various assessment methods that will be addressed below.

A construct that can be seen as interchangeable with PA is exercise, but these terms are not identical. *Exercise*, a subset of PA, is planned, structured, and repetitive bodily movement (such as participating in an aerobics class) with the goal of improving or maintaining physical fitness (USDHHS 2008). *Physical fitness* primarily consists of aerobic power or cardiorespiratory fitness measured by maximal and submaximal stress testing or a field test (USDHHS). PA is something an individual does which can help to achieve greater physical fitness. In addition to PA, various factors such as age, sex, health status, and genetics can also affect physical fitness. In *aerobic activity* or endurance activity, the body's large muscles move in a rhythmic manner for a sustained period of time as in brisk walking, biking, or swimming. *Resistance training* (or strength training) consists of repetitive movements geared toward greater skeletal muscle strength, power, endurance, and mass (USDHHS). *Flexibility training* refers to repetitive activities to improve the movement of joints through their full range of motion (USDHHS).

Assessment of Physical Activity

Reliable and valid measures of PA are essential to understand energy expenditure in various populations. There are three common ways to assess PA: (1) criterion methods, (2) objective measures, and (3) subjective/self-reports. The selection of any of these three methods can be based on feasibility, cost, the specific research or clinical setting, and type of population.

Criterion methods such as doubly labeled water and indirect calorimetry are the gold standards for measuring PA (Vanhees et al. 2005). Doubly labeled water (DWL) measures total energy expenditure and does not require individuals to log their daily activity because it uses the body's water to record metabolic rates. Thus, this technique is objective and requires little participant burden. Even with these advantages, various factors that lead to changes in energy expenditure such as PA, basal metabolic rate, and diet-induced energy expenditure cannot be teased apart from each other (Vanhees et al. 2005). Another important criterion method is indirect calorimetry. Energy expenditure is measured by oxygen consumption and carbon dioxide production through collected respiratory gases or in a respiration chamber (Vanhees et al. 2005). Both DWL and indirect calorimetry are expensive and have limited usability. They are less feasible in studies where participants have to monitor their daily PA in the community or home setting or over multiple assessments or over extended periods.

The objective measures of PA include fitness testing, accelerometers, and pedometers. As mentioned earlier, aerobic capacity is measured through fitness testing conducted on a treadmill, stationary bike, or a field test. These tests yield levels of peak oxygen consumption (VO_2 peak) which is an index of cardiorespiratory capacity (Gelibeter et al. 1997). These treadmill or bike tests must be overseen by a physician and are expensive but are used to assess fitness in clinical and research studies.

Accelerometers and pedometers are more commonly seen in the literature because they are relatively inexpensive ($10–$450 and above) and participants can be taught how to use them without extensive training. Accelerometers and pedometers are motion sensors but with different purposes. Accelerometers measure all body movement and physical activities and can yield the dose of PA (e.g., Fogelholm et al. 1998). Thus, accelerometers are significantly more expensive than pedometers due to their use of technology (Vanhees et al. 2005).

Pedometers are battery-operated step counters that are worn on the waist and measure steps when engaging in PA (Vanhees et al. 2005). They are efficient in monitoring steps but may produce inaccurate readings due to inadvertent body movements. Activities such as biking and other activities where the body torso is stationary are not suitable for pedometers as are water activities. The reliability and validity of pedometers have been addressed in the literature (e.g., Vanhees et al.). It is anticipated that the next generation of pedometers will yield information on the "dose" of PA (i.e., intensity, frequency, and duration).

The third category of assessments is the subjective, self-report measures which include diaries, interviews, and questionnaires (e.g., Van Poppel et al. 2010). These subjective methods are inexpensive and generally do not take significant time. The measures are commonly used when assessing PA of large numbers of individuals. As with all self-report measures, problems with recall, over-estimation, and interviewer skill limit the validity of these instruments.

Physical Activity Guidelines

There are various PA guidelines for public health benefits, weight loss, or weight management and for patients treated for diseases such as cancer (Schmitz et al. 2010; USDHHS 2008). For the purposes of this chapter, PA guidelines for improving general health for adults will be discussed.

In the 1960s and 1970s, the PA literature provided information that many health benefits could be achieved through vigorous intensity or high levels of PA. Since then, a large research base led to the first public health and PA guidelines issued in 1995 by the American College of Sports Medicine (ACSM) and Centers for Disease Control and Prevention (CDC) (Pate et al. 1995). These guidelines recommended that "every US adult should accumulate 30 min or more of moderate-intensity PA on most, preferably all, days of the week." The guidelines were based on evidence that moderate-intensity PA accumulated in short bouts could lead to improved health outcomes.

Due to further advances in understanding the health benefits of PA, misunderstanding of the prior 1995 ACSM and CDC PA guidelines, and continued physical inactivity of many Americans, a new set of PA guidelines were issued in 2007 by the ACSM and American Heart Association (AHA) (Haskell et al. 2007). These 2007 guidelines were tailored for children, healthy adults between the ages of 18–65, and older adults over age 65. For healthy adults, the guidelines recommend moderate-intensity aerobic PA for at least 30 min on 5 days each week or vigorous-intensity aerobic activity for at least 20 min on 3 days each week (Haskell et al. 2007). These guidelines also clarified that (a) 30 min of aerobic or endurance activity can be achieved in at least 10-min bouts, (b) resistance training should be performed at least twice a week, and (c) individuals who wish to engage in more activity to improve health or reduce risk of disease could surpass the minimum recommendations (Haskell et al.).

In 2008, the US Department of Human and Health Services (USDHHS) released PA guidelines for health benefits and recommended a minimum of 150 min of moderate-intensity PA, 75 min of vigorous-intensity PA, or 500–1000 MET min of PA per week. A combination of moderate- and vigorous-intensity activity could be used to achieve these recommendations. These guidelines did not provide an empirically supported dose response prescription that included frequency of PA (i.e., number of days a week) because of insufficient evidence. On the other hand, the guidelines did clarify that the upper limit of MET values for moderate activity is 5.9 and the lower limits of vigorous activity are 6 METs. In the past, 6 METs overlapped as the highest and lowest values for moderate and vigorous PA, respectively (USDHHS 2008).

Finally, there are other PA guidelines such as those related to the number of steps per day needed to achieve health benefits. It is commonly known that 2000 steps equal 1 mile. Current PA guidelines suggest that accumulating at least 10,000 steps and greater per day indicates that one is active, and accumulating at least 12,500 steps per day indicates that an individual is very active (e.g., Tudor-Locke and Bassett 2004).

Theories and Interventions

To respond to the challenge of reducing sedentary behavior, numerous interventions have been developed and tested for specific patient populations (e.g., individuals with diabetes, cardiovascular disease, osteoarthritis, cancer), individuals with specific risk factors (high cholesterol, hypertension), and the general population at various phases of the lifespan (young children, school-aged, college-level, middle-aged, and older adults). The interventions have been offered at schools, work sites, and in communities. PA has also been targeted to reduce other risk behaviors (e.g., smoking, alcohol, and other drug addiction). More recently, PA has been emphasized as part of the initiatives to combat the obesity epidemic in the USA. The interventions have yielded varying degrees of success. The Task Force on Community Preventive Services (Kahn et al. 2002) concluded that there are six types of interventions that have been shown to increase PA and cardiorespiratory fitness: point-of-decision prompts, community-wide education, school physical education and community social support, individual health behavior, and enhanced access to places for PA combined with informational outreach activities. Interventions have been offered using various modalities (in-person, by telephone, web-based, and more recently, using mobile technology such as palmtop computers and mobile phones) with varying degrees of "reach" to modify sedentary behavior.

In developing interventions, there is growing interest in *community-based participatory research* especially to reach subgroups that are more challenging to reach but are characterized by sedentary lifestyles. This type of research addresses predictors of health at the community and individual levels and includes the community of interest in the whole research enterprise. Thus, the participants or community are commonly involved with all areas of research conceptualization, development, and data collection. Furthermore, culturally relevant strategies and theories and social marketing principles are integrated a priori in the study to enhance recruitment and retention efforts. Community-based participatory research is gaining popularity given the public health epidemic of obesity and physical inactivity in diverse populations (Yancey et al. 2004).

PA interventions have been based on theories of behavior change. One of the more commonly used theories is *Social Cognitive Theory* (SCT) (Bandura 1986) which posits that behavior, environmental factors, and personal factors of the individual, such as cognitions, emotions, and physical characteristics, are mutually influential. Interventions based on SCT focus on the importance of individuals' ability to control their behavior and how changes in the individual or the environment can produce changes in behavior. Success in being able to initiate and maintain the behavior change is determined by an individual's ability to regulate his or her own behavior through personal strategies (e.g., setting PA goals, monitoring progress toward goals), as well as environmental approaches (e.g., using social support or environmental prompts).

The *Theory of Planned Behavior* (Tpb) (Ajzen 1991) is another widely used theory that proposes that behavior is directly predicted by intention, which in turn, is directly predicted by attitude, subjective norm, and perceived control. Perceived control is the belief that a behavior can be performed with ease or difficulty and it may directly predict the behavior, attitude is the personal evaluation of performing the behavior, and subjective norm is the perceived normative beliefs of relevant others regarding the behavior. Thus, according to the theory, individuals will intend, and be motivated to, perform a behavior such as PA when they view it favorably, believe that important others think they should be physically active, and believe that PA is under their control and can be carried out.

The *Transtheoretical Model* (TTM) of health behavior change (Prochaska and DiClemente 1983) postulates that individuals move through a series of six stages of motivational readiness while making a behavior change (i.e., precontemplation, contemplation, preparation, action, maintenance, and termination), and this approach has been applied to PA (Marcus and Simkin 1993). While progressing through these stages, the individual engages in ten different cognitive and behavioral processes of change that are important in the adoption and maintenance of a new behavior. For example, research suggests that cognitive processes of change (e.g., setting realistic goals) should be encouraged among those in precontemplation and contemplation, while behavioral processes (e.g., placing reminders to exercise at work or home) should be promoted among those in the more advanced stages of motivational readiness. TTM-based interventions attempt to tailor PA programs to a participant's motivational readiness to change and utilize the processes of change to encourage progression in motivational readiness for PA.

The *Self-Determination Theory* (SDT) posits that behaviors are regulated by motives that range on a continuum from highly controlled (extrinsically motivated) to fully autonomous (intrinsically motivated). Extrinsically motivated behaviors arise to avoid negative emotions, a threat or a demand. Extrinsic motivation is also involved when an individual performs a behavior that he or she feels is valuable (but not necessarily inherently enjoyable; Ryan and Deci 2000). Intrinsically motivated behaviors are those that are done to provide the individual inherent enjoyment, satisfaction, or pleasure. It is thought that intrinsic motivation for behaviors such as PA leads to greater interest, more confidence, and longer persistence of the behavior.

The *Protection Motivation* Theory (Rogers 1983) emphasizes threat and coping appraisal. Threat appraisal consists of perceived severity (estimated threat of disease) and perceived vulnerability (estimate of chance of developing the disease), and coping appraisal consists of response efficacy (expectancy that the recommended behavior, i.e., PA, can remove the threat) and self-efficacy (belief that one can carry out the recommended behavior successfully, i.e., adopt and maintain PA). Both threat and coping appraisal affect intention to be physically active and PA behavior.

Theories that focus on the individual (e.g., beliefs, attitudes) have led to the development of various interventions to promote PA. However, variables based on these theories do not explain more than a relatively small percentage of the variance in PA levels. *Ecological models* have become increasingly popular in acknowledging multiple levels of influence on PA: individual, social/cultural, organizational, community, physical environment, and policy. They are "macro" in the sense that they go beyond the individual-level choices and decisions to become active in an effort to reduce sedentary lifestyles (King et al. 2002). Such models focus on the environmental variables, the related type of PA (e.g., transit vs. recreational), and the extent to which specific environmental conditions (e.g., built environment) can facilitate or constrain recreational activity, transit activities, or both. For example, availability of playgrounds, sidewalks, biking, or walking trails is likely to facilitate PA. Conversely, unsafe neighborhoods and lack of sidewalks are likely to hinder PA.

To achieve widespread adoption of physically active lifestyles, much needs to be done to determine what models will facilitate dissemination of PA interventions and which approaches will help adapt interventions for culturally diverse subgroups. The costs and benefits of such interventions also require attention. Finally, sustaining PA over time will require change at the policy and legislative levels as has been the case with smoking cessation.

Conclusions

PA has an important role to play in the prevention and management of many chronic diseases. Although there has been improvement in the overall prevalence of regular PA in the USA, a large subgroup does not engage in regular PA. Efforts to promote PA have focused on individual-level factors and, to a lesser extent, factors at the community and population level. New technologies can help extend the reach of interventions. However, addressing the barriers to adopting and maintaining PA in the twenty-first century will require efforts at the individual, community, population, and policy levels.

References and Readings

Ajzen, I. (1991). The theory of planned behavior. *Organization Behavior and Human Decision Processes, 50*, 179–211.

Bandura, A. (1986). *Social foundations of thought and action: A social cognitive theory.* Englewood Cliffs: Prentice-Hall.

Fogelholm, M., Hilloskorpi, H., Laukkanen, R., Oja, P., Van Marken, L. W., & Westerterp, K. (1998). Assessment of energy expenditure in overweight women. *Medicine and Science in Sports and Exercise, 30,* 1191–1197.

Gelibeter, A., Maher, M. M., Gerace, L., Gutin, B., Heymsfield, S. B., & Hashim, S. A. (1997). Effects of strength of aerobic training on body composition, resting metabolic rate, and peak oxygen consumption in obese dieting subjects. *American Journal of Clinical Nutrition, 66*(3), 557–563.

Haskell, W. L., Lee, I.-M., Pate, R. R., Powell, K. E., Blair, S. N., Franklin, C. A., et al. (2007). Physical activity and public health: Updated recommendation for adults from the American College of Sports Medicine and the American Heart Association. *Medicine and Science in Sports and Exercise, 39*(8), 1423–1434.

Kahn, E. B., Ramsey, L. T., Brownson, R. C., Heath, G. W., Howze, E. H., Powell, K. E., et al. (2002). The effectiveness of interventions to increase physical activity: A systematic review. *American Journal of Preventive Medicine, 22*(4S), 73–107.

King, A. C., Stokols, D., Talen, E., Brassington, G. S., & Killingsworth, R. (2002). Theoretical approaches to the promotion of physical activity. *American Journal of Preventive Medicine, 23*(2), 15–25.

Marcus, B. H., & Simkin, L. R. (1993). The stages of exercise behavior. *Journal of Sports Medicine and Physical Fitness, 33*(1), 83–88.

Pate, R. R., Pratt, R. M., Blair, S. N., Haskell, W. L., Macera, C. A., Bouchard, C., et al. (1995). Physical activity and public health: A recommendation from the Centers for Disease Control and Prevention and the American College of Sports Medicine. *Journal of the American Medical Association, 273,* 402–407.

Prochaska, J. O., & DiClemente, C. C. (1983). Stages and processes of self-change of smoking: Toward an integrative model of change. *Journal of Consulting & Clinical Psychology, 51*(3), 390–395.

Rogers, R. W. (1983). Cognitive and physiological process in fear appeals and attitude change: A revised theory of protection motivation. In J. R. Cacioppo & R. E. Petty (Eds.), *Social psychology: A source book* (pp. 153–176). New York: Guildford Press.

Ryan, R. M., & Deci, E. L. (2000). Self-determination theory and the facilitation of intrinsic motivation, social development, and well-being. *American Psychologist, 55*(1), 68–78.

Schmitz, K. H., Courneya, K. S., Matthews, C. M., Demark-Wahnefried, W., Galvao, D. A., Pinto, B. M., et al. (2010). American College of Sports Medicine roundtable on exercise guidelines for cancer survivors. *Medicine & Science in Sports and Exercise, 42,* 258–266.

Schoenborn, C. A., & Adams, P. F. (2010). Health behaviors of adults: United States 2005–2007. National Center for Health Statistics. *Vital and Health Statistics, 10*(245), 1–132.

Tudor-Locke, C., & Bassett, D. R. (2004). How many steps/day are enough? Preliminary pedometer indices for public health. *Sports Medicine, 34,* 1–8.

U.S. Department of Health and Human Services. (2008). *Physical Activity Guidelines Advisory Committee report, 2008.* Washington, DC: U.S. Department of Health and Human Services.

Van Poppel, M. N., Chinapaw, M. J., Mokkink, L. B., van Mechelen, W., & Terwee, C. B. (2010). Physical activity questionnaires for adults: A systematic review of measurement properties. *Sports Medicine, 440*(7), 565–600.

Vanhees, L., Lefevre, J., Philippaerts, R., Martens, M., Huygens, W., Troosters, T., et al. (2005). How to assess physical activity? How to assess physical fitness? *European Journal of Cardiovascular Prevention and Rehabilitation, 12,* 102–114.

Yancey, A. K., Kumanyika, S. K., Ponce, N. A., McCarthy, W. J., Fielding, J. E., Leslie, J. P., et al. (2004). Population-based interventions engaging communities of color in healthy eating and activity living: A review. *Preventing Chronic Disease, 1,* A09.

Physical Activity Change in Healthcare Settings

Mark Stoutenberg
Department of Kinesiology, Temple University, Philadelphia, PA, USA

Synonyms

Exercise is medicine; Exercise prescription; Physical activity counseling

Definition

Clinicians and other health personnel can influence public health outcomes through physical activity counseling in health settings. However, counseling alone is often not sufficient for the adoption of sustained, long-term physical activity habits. A more comprehensive framework is needed for implementing behavior change strategies throughout the entire patient visit to a healthcare setting. This framework provides an organized, systems-change approach for busy clinicians and their healthcare teams who may have had little formal training in physical activity counseling and face multiple institutional barriers. This approach is guided by lessons learned from decades of experience integrating of physical activity counseling in health settings around the world.

Description

The engagement of our health systems and healthcare providers in promoting physical activity is one potential strategy for increasing physical activity levels at a population level (Patrick et al. 2009). Healthcare providers see a large portion of the general population, often several times throughout the year. These ongoing, multiple contacts, offer the ideal opportunity to provide brief, impactful physical activity counseling to patients. Comprehensive strategies exist for conducting physical assessment and counseling as part of a normal clinic visit (Lobelo et al. 2014, 2018). Assessing patient physical activity levels, providing brief counseling, writing customized prescriptions, and referring patients to existing community resources can all be completed in a matter of minutes when done in a coordinated manner by the entire healthcare team.

Two of the earliest trials examining physical activity counseling in health settings were the Physician-based Assessment and Counseling for Exercise (PACE) (Calfas et al. 1996) and the Activity Counseling Trial (ACT) (Simons-Morton et al. 2001). In PACE, physicians spent 3–5 min of the office visit discussing information and strategies based on patient level of readiness for becoming more active, followed by a phone counseling session with a health educator to reinforce information provided during the clinic visit. A significantly greater proportion of patients who visited physicians in the PACE intervention arm reported being regularly active, increasing their walking time by 40 min a week. In ACT, investigators examined the effectiveness of three different physical activity counseling interventions compared to current practices in the primary care setting. Inactive adults received either advice (information only), assistance (behavioral counseling), or counseling (behavioral counseling + biweekly phone counseling). Patients in both the assistance and the counseling interventions significantly increased their physical fitness by 5%, with a significantly greater proportion of patients in the counseling group achieving national physical activity guidelines 24 months after the beginning of the trial. Together, these two trials demonstrated that physical activity counseling in the healthcare setting is feasible without unduly burdening healthcare providers, leading to multiple calls of action urging healthcare providers to provide brief physical activity counseling to all of their inactive patients (McPhail and Schippers 2012; Vuori et al. 2013; Berra et al. 2015).

A necessary first step to effectively providing physical activity counseling is to determine the current physical activity level of patients (Greenwood et al. 2010). Assessing patient physical activity levels is the cornerstone to any subsequent behavior change counseling (Stoutenberg et al. 2017). As with other clinical indicators, the initial diagnosis sends a crucial message to patients that physical activity is of equal importance to traditional vital signs, such as bodyweight and blood pressure, while emphasizing the importance of maintaining favorable activity levels to achieve optimal health. When incorporated as a vital sign in the electronic medical record, the simple act of assessing physical activity levels has shown to effectively increase discussion and documentation of physical activity habits, as well as provision of physical activity referrals, while resulting in small but significant reductions in bodyweight and hemoglobin A1c levels (Grant et al. 2014). The assessment of physical activity levels identifies inactive individuals and serves as the initial catalyst in a physical activity "counseling cascade."

Once a patient's current activity level is identified, the next step is to understand the patient's readiness to change their physical activity behavior. Readiness for change is a component of the transtheoretical model, a theory which emerged from psychotherapy to treat addictive behaviors

(Prochaska and Velicer 1997), but has since been adapted to help understand readiness to engage in physical activity (Hutchinson et al. 2009). The transtheoretical model is a dynamic model that facilitates behavior change through a series of stage-specific strategies and processes of change. Individuals are characterized into one of five "stages of change" (pre-contemplation, contemplation, preparation, action, and maintenance) with specific behavior change strategies customized to facilitate transition to a higher stage of change. Strategies for individuals at lower levels of readiness include the provision of information about physical activity and its benefits, discussion of perceived barriers, and advocating for small changes. Individuals at higher levels of readiness may be engaged in goal setting, developing a specific physical activity plan to achieve their goals, creating a supportive environment for being active, and self-monitoring techniques (Riebe 2018).

Armed with knowledge of the patient's physical activity levels and readiness to change, the provider is now positioned to engage their patient in behavior change strategies. One model commonly used in healthcare settings to facilitate physical activity behavior change is the 5As model (Pinto et al. 2005; Carroll et al. 2011, 2012). The 5As (assess, advise, agree, assist, arrange) is a proven framework for providers to assess current physical activity levels; advise on the benefits of becoming more physically active; collaboratively agree on physical activity goals based on the patient's desires and needs; assist the patient in utilizing problem-solving techniques, overcoming barriers, and identifying supportive resources; and arrange a specific plan for future follow-up. Another proven physical activity counseling technique that is widely used in health setting is the use of motivational interviewing (VanBuskirk and Wetherell 2014). Motivational interviewing is a method for approaching patients, who are ambivalent about making a health behavior change, and is considered to be more effective than traditional, advice giving, counseling strategies (Rubak et al. 2005; Miller and Rollnick 2013). The goal of motivational interviewing is to encourage patients to express their own reasons for behavior change by fostering internal motivation. Motivational interviewing has proven to be effective in promoting physical activity in breast cancer survivors (Pudkasam et al. 2018), as well as in adults with type 2 diabetes (Soderlund 2018), obesity (Burgess et al. 2017), and chronic health conditions (O'Halloran et al. 2014).

After behavioral counseling, patients should receive both a customized physical activity "prescription" and a referral to community-based physical activity resources. The physical activity prescription is a reinforcing behavioral strategy encouraging patients to become more physically active (Thornton et al. 2016). Physical activity prescriptions can be provided through a number of different written or electronic formats, such as simple, customized prescription pads or handouts with information about being active with specific health conditions. The "Green Prescription" in New Zealand is an example of a successful, nationally coordinated effort to provide patients with a basic physical activity prescription (Swinburn et al. 1998). When delivering the physical activity prescription, it is important for providers to be mindful of their scope of practice and, potentially, a lack of formal physical activity training.

The last step in the clinic setting – providing patients with a physical activity referral – is critically important in supporting their efforts to become more physically active, especially when considering that effective physical activity counseling conducted by healthcare providers may be unfeasible given the lack of time to engage patients in preventive counseling (Lamming et al. 2017). Given that the most common barrier to providing physical activity counseling in the clinic setting is a limited amount of time providers have with their patients, physical activity counseling needs to be very brief (<5 min). The referral connects patients to supportive resources for becoming more physically active in their local community setting. These resources may include certified exercise professionals, recognized places for being physically active (i.e., local park systems, community recreation centers), and evidence-based programs (i.e., Matter of Balance,

EnhanceFitness). Physical activity referral schemes have been used with great success throughout Europe (Leijon et al. 2009; Campbell et al. 2015) and are a valuable primary care intervention for promoting physical activity.

Employing specific behavior change strategies with patients is an essential component of increasing patient physical activity levels. The optimal way to intervene and encourage patients to be physically active is still unknown but likely varies across a number of different factors, such as gender, socioeconomic status, education level, and neighborhood characteristics of the patient. Implementation of the steps discussed in this entry need not be the responsibility of any one person. Multiple members of the healthcare team, such as medical assistants during the assessment of traditional vital signs, can assess physical activity levels and readiness to change, while discharge nurses or front desk personnel can provide the final referral. While healthcare providers cannot single-handedly solve the epidemic of physical inactivity, they have a special opportunity to be an important part of the solution by integrating physical activity as a part of routine care.

Cross-References

▶ Benefits of Exercise
▶ Exercise
▶ Motivational Interviewing
▶ Physical Activity and Health
▶ Primary Care
▶ Primary Care Physicians
▶ Primary Care Providers
▶ Stages-of-Change Model
▶ Transtheoretical Model of Behavior Change

References and Further Reading

Berra, K., Rippe, J., & Manson, J. E. (2015). Making physical activity counseling a priority in clinical practice: The time for action is now. *JAMA, 314*(24), 2617–2618.

Burgess, E., Hassmén, P., Welvaert, M., & Pumpa, K. L. (2017). Behavioural treatment strategies improve adherence to lifestyle intervention programmes in adults with obesity: A systematic review and meta-analysis. *Clinical Obesity, 7*(2), 105–114.

Calfas, K. J., Long, B. J., Sallis, J. F., Wooten, W. J., Pratt, M., & Patrick, K. (1996). A controlled trial of physician counselling to promote the adoption of physical activity. *Preventive Medicine, 25*, 225–233.

Campbell, F., Holmes, M., Everson-Hock, E., Davis, S., Woods, H. B., Anokye, N., et al. (2015). A systematic review and economic evaluation of exercise referral schemes in primary care: A short report. *Health Technology Assessment, 19*(60), 1–110.

Carroll, J. K., Antognoli, E., & Flocke, S. A. (2011). Evaluation of physical activity counseling in primary care using direct observation of the 5as. *Annals of Family Medicine, 9*(5), 416–422.

Carroll, J. K., Fiscella, K., Epstein, R. M., Sanders, M. R., & Williams, G. C. (2012). A 5a's communication intervention to promote physical activity in underserved populations. *BMC Health Services Research, 12*, 374.

Grant, R. W., Schmittdiel, J. A., Neugebauer, R. S., Uratsu, C. S., & Sternfeld, B. (2014). Exercise as a vital sign: A quasi-experimental analysis of a health system intervention to collect patient-reported exercise levels. *Journal of General Internal Medicine, 29*(7), 1081.

Greenwood, L. J., Joy, E. A., & Stanford, J. B. (2010). The physical activity vital sign: A primary care tool to guide counseling for obesity. *Journal of Physical Activity and Health, 7*, 571–576.

Hutchinson, A. J., Breckon, J. D., & Johnston, L. H. (2009). Physical activity behavior change interventions based on the transtheoretical model: A systematic review. *Health Education & Behavior, 36*(5), 829–845.

Lamming, L., Pears, S., Mason, D., Morton, K., Bijker, M., Sutton, S., et al. (2017). What do we know about brief interventions for physical activity that could be delivered in primary care consultations? A systematic review of reviews. *Preventive Medicine, 99*, 152–163.

Leijon, M. E., Bendtsen, P., Nilsen, P., Festin, K., & Ståhle, A. (2009). Does a physical activity referral scheme improve the physical activity among routine primary health care patients? *Scandinavian Journal of Medicine & Science in Sports, 19*(5), 627–636.

Lobelo, F., Stoutenberg, M., & Hutber, A. (2014). The exercise is medicine global health initiative: A 2014 update. *British Journal of Sports Medicine, 48*(22), 1627–1633.

Lobelo, F., Rohm Young, D., Sallis, R., Garber, M. D., Billinger, S. A., Duperly, J., et al. (2018). Routine assessment and promotion of physical activity in healthcare settings: A scientific statement from the American Heart Association. *Circulation, 137*(18), e495–e522.

McPhail, S., & Schippers, M. (2012). An evolving perspective on physical activity counselling by medical professionals. *BMC Family Practice, 13*, 31.

Miller, W. R., & Rollnick, S. (2013). *Motivational interviewing: Helping people change*. New York: Guilford Press.

O'Halloran, P. D., Blackstock, F., Shields, N., Holland, A., Iles, R., Kingsley, M., et al. (2014). Motivational interviewing to increase physical activity in people with chronic health conditions: A systematic review and meta-analysis. *Clinical Rehabilitation, 28*(12), 1159–1171.

Patrick, K., Pratt, M., & Sallis, R. E. (2009). The healthcare sector's role in the U.S. national physical activity plan. *Journal of Physical Activity & Health, 6*(Suppl 2), S211–S219.

Pinto, B. M., Goldstein, M. G., Ashba, J., Sciamanna, C. N., & Jette, A. (2005). Randomized controlled trial of physical activity counseling for older primary care patients. *American Journal of Preventive Medicine, 29*(4), 247–255.

Prochaska, J. O., & Velicer, W. F. (1997). The transtheoretical model of behavior change. *American Journal of Health Promotion, 12*(1), 38–48.

Pudkasam, S., Polman, R., Pitcher, M., Fisher, M., Chinlumpraseert, N., & Apostolopopoulos, V. (2018). Physical activity and breast cancer survivors: Importance of adherence, motivational interviewing and psychological health. *Maturitas, 116*, 66–72.

Riebe, D. (2018). *ACSM's guidelines for exercise testing and prescription* (10th ed.). Philadelphia: Wolters Kluwer.

Rubak, S., Sandbæk, A., Lauritzen, T., & Christensen, B. (2005). Motivational interviewing: A systematic review and meta-analysis. *British Journal of General Practice, 55*(513), 305–312.

Simons-Morton, D. G., Blair, S. N., King, A. C., Morgan, T. M., Applegate, W. B., O'Toole, M., et al. (2001). Effects of physical activity counseling in primary care: The activity counseling trial: A randomized controlled trial. *JAMA, 286*(6), 677–687.

Soderlund, P. D. (2018). Effectiveness of motivational interviewing for improving physical activity self-management for adults with type 2 diabetes: A review. *Chronic Illness, 14*(1), 54–68.

Stoutenberg, M., Shaya, G. E., Feldman, D. I., & Carroll, J. K. (2017). Practical strategies for assessing patient physical activity levels in primary care. *Mayo Clinic Proceedings. Innovations, Quality & Outcomes, 1*(1), 8–15.

Swinburn, B. A., Walter, L. G., Arroll, B., Tilyard, M. W., & Russell, D. G. (1998). The green prescription study: A randomized controlled trial of written exercise advice provided by general practitioners. *American Journal of Public Health, 88*(2), 288–291.

Thornton, J. S., Frémont, P., Khan, K., Poirier, P., Fowles, J., Wells, G. D., & Frankovich, R. J. (2016). Physical activity prescription: A critical opportunity to address a modifiable risk factor for the prevention and management of chronic disease: A position statement by the Canadian Academy of Sport and Exercise Medicine. *British Journal of Sports Medicine, 50*, 1109–1114.

VanBuskirk, K. A., & Wetherell, J. L. (2014). Motivational interviewing with primary care populations: A systematic review and meta-analysis. *Journal of Behavioral Medicine, 37*(4), 768–780.

Vuori, I. M., Lavie, C. J., & Blair, S. N. (2013). Physical activity promotion in the health care system. *Mayo Clinic Proceedings, 88*(12), 1446–1461.

Physical Activity Counseling

▶ Physical Activity Change in Healthcare Settings

Physical Activity Intensity

▶ Non-exercise Behavior
▶ Physical Activity/Inactivity: Objective Measurement of

Physical Activity Monitors

Danielle Arigo and Kristen Pasko
Department of Psychology, Rowan University, Glassboro, NJ, USA

Synonyms

Activity trackers; Wearable fitness trackers

Definition

Physical activity monitors are technological devices that provide objective assessment of physical activity engagement, including parameters such as frequency, intensity (type) of activity (e.g., steps, light intensity, aerobic intensity), length of time in specific types of activity, and energy expenditure.

Description

Regular engagement in physical activity (PA) can lower risk for several of the leading causes of death in the USA (e.g., cardiovascular disease, cancer) and shows unique benefits for weight control, mood disorders, and overall well-being (Penedo and Dahn 2005; Warburton and Bredin 2017). As a result, PA engagement is a key outcome of interest in behavioral medicine research, practice, and policy, and decisions about how best to measure PA in behavioral medicine work are critical to the success of the field's PA promotion efforts. Self-reports of PA engagement are useful for some purposes. Given that people tend to overestimate the length of time and intensity of their PA (Garriguet et al. 2015; Steene-Johannessen et al. 2016), however, objective measures of PA are preferable to maximize the reliability and validity of PA outcomes (Ong et al. 2011). A wide range of PA monitoring devices is available for this purpose, differing in measurement method, price, and strengths/limitations. Popular devices for collecting ambulatory PA (i.e., in individuals' natural environments) in research and practice include:

1. **Pedometers** are worn on the waist or hip to capture accumulated steps (e.g., per day, within a specific time frame), measured from vertical pelvic displacements. Pedometers are inexpensive, inconspicuous, and easy to use, making them accessible to a wide range of populations (Ong et al. 2011). Limitations include lack of information about activity intensity, timing, or energy expenditure and modest reliability among individuals with BMIs >30 (Berlin et al. 2006; Shepherd et al. 1999; Vanhees et al. 2005).
2. **Research-grade accelerometers** measure change in speed with respect to time in gravitational acceleration units, typically for multiple spatial axes (Berlin et al. 2006). Many stand-alone devices are worn on the wrist, waist, or ankle and collect information about steps, activity intensity (including sedentary time), episodes ("bouts") of sedentary and moderate- or vigorous-intensity activity, timing of activity, and energy expenditure. These devices also can be used to estimate sleep parameters and can be integrated with geolocation (GPS). Related technology provides additional information about body posture (i.e., thigh-worn inclinometers such as activPAL), which increases the accuracy of sedentary activity measurement. Some devices require a hard line connection to download data, whereas others sync data wirelessly. Research-grade devices have high accuracy and often high cost to purchase, and some have proprietary software required to download and/or calculate desired outcome estimates (e.g., ActiGraph, activPAL). The use of device-specific software necessitates additional skills to calculate and interpret data. These devices usually do not provide real-time feedback to users, which is useful for observational studies or PA promotion programs for which the device itself is not intended to change behavior.
3. **Commercially available accelerometers** (e.g., Fitbit, Apple Watch, Samsung Gear Fit) use similar technology to research-grade devices; they are most often worn on the wrist and provide real-time feedback, offering the consistent self-monitoring that facilitates health behavior change (Lewis et al. 2015; Teixeira et al. 2015). Many commercially available devices have associated webpages and/or smartphone apps that can sync data wirelessly and display (or output to data files) PA parameters in attractive user interfaces. Parameters include steps per day and minutes in different activity intensities, and some models also monitor and display/output sleep and heart rate data. These are lower in cost than research-grade tools and show somewhat lower accuracy (Evenson et al. 2015), and it may be difficult for some users to maximize their benefit without technical assistance (e.g., setting up profiles, syncing devices with apps, or interpreting feedback). Accelerometers also come embedded in many available smartphones (e.g., iPhone) with associated apps that display PA engagement. This technology is not likely to require costs beyond the smartphone hardware and may be easiest for smartphone users to incorporate, as it does not require a separate device. However, smartphone accelerometers show variable accuracy when used to measure daily activities in the natural environment – particularly for women, who often do not carry phones in their pockets (Brodie et al. 2018).
4. **Heart rate (HR) monitors** approximate energy expenditure via heart rate, which is

associated with oxygen consumption (Freedson and Miller 2000). Early HR monitors used a transmitter belt (worn around the chest) and a receiver watch; commercial devices worn on the wrist are now used more often (e.g., Fitbit, portable navigation devices, smartwatches; Dooley et al. 2017). Strengths of modern HR devices include low cost and ease of wear; given that many factors influence HR (e.g., emotional state, temperature, humidity, body position, food intake; Livingstone 1997; Tapia et al. 2007), however, these monitors provide limited accuracy for PA parameters.

5. **Portable indirect calorimeters** measure energy expenditure via inhalation of oxygen and exhalation of carbon dioxide, which are used to calculate metabolic rate. This method requires users to breathe into a device (e.g., bag or mask); modern handheld models have reduced the cost, size, and difficulty of data collection with this method, though it remains fairly costly and requires considerable training to maximize accuracy (Haugen et al. 2007; Ndahimana and Kim 2017). Consequently, indirect calorimetry is most often used in clinical settings among patients with specific health conditions (Frankenfield et al. 2005; Haugen et al. 2007).

6. **Smart clothing** embeds sensor technology into fabrics or between layers of fabric, to collect information about electrocardial activity, respiration, acceleration, and heart rate (Lymberis and Paradiso 2008). Commercially available smart clothing often connects to smartphone applications that display parameters such as steps and activity intensity (e.g., Sensoria Fitness Socks). These devices are expensive and not yet routinely used in PA research or practice, but may become more common in these settings as cost and functionality improve.

Decisions about the use of ambulatory PA monitoring devices in research, practice, or policy should be informed by several situational factors, including:

1. The purpose of a given program (e.g., observation vs. intervention via device)
2. The specific parameters and level of accuracy needed to achieve this purpose (e.g., accurately quantifying the proportion of a population who engages in recommended levels of PA per week)
3. Availability of resources (e.g., funds to purchase devices, skill required to train device users or interpret PA data)

Cross-References

▶ Ambulatory Monitoring
▶ Behavior Change
▶ Physical Activity
▶ Self-monitoring

References and Further Reading

Berlin, J. E., Storti, K. L., & Brach, J. S. (2006). Using activity monitors to measure physical activity in free-living conditions. *Physical Therapy, 86*, 1137–1145.

Brodie, M. A., Pliner, E. M., Ho, A., Li, K., Chen, Z., Gandevia, S. C., & Lord, S. R. (2018). Big data vs accurate data in health research: Large-scale physical activity monitoring, smartphones, wearable devices and risk of unconscious bias. *Medical Hypotheses, 119*, 32–36.

Dooley, E. E., Golaszewski, N. M., & Bartholomew, J. B. (2017). Estimating accuracy at exercise intensities: A comparative study of self-monitoring heart rate and physical activity wearable devices. *JMIR mHealth and uHealth, 5*, 1–12.

Edwardson, C. L., Winkler, E. A., Bodicoat, D. H., Yates, T., Davies, M. J., Dunstan, D. W., & Healy, G. N. (2017). Considerations when using the activPAL monitor in field-based research with adult populations. *Journal of Sport and Health Science, 6*, 162–178.

Evenson, K. R., Goto, M. M., & Furberg, R. D. (2015). Systematic review of the validity and reliability of consumer-wearable activity trackers. *International Journal of Behavioral Nutrition and Physical Activity, 12*, 1–22.

Frankenfield, D., Roth-Yousey, L., & Compher, C. (2005). Comparison of predictive equations for resting metabolic rate in healthy nonobese and obese adults: A systematic review. *Journal of the American Dietetic Association, 105*, 775–789.

Freedson, P. S., & Miller, K. (2000). Objective monitoring of physical activity using motion sensors and heart rate. *Research Quarterly for Exercise and Sport, 71*, 21–29.

Garriguet, D., Tremblay, S., & Colley, R. C. (2015). Comparison of physical activity adult questionnaire results with accelerometer data. *Statistics Canada, 26*(7). Retrieved from https://www150.statcan.gc.ca/n1/pub/82-003-x/2015007/article/14205-eng.pdf.

Haugen, H. A., Chan, L. N., & Li, F. (2007). Indirect calorimetry: A practical guide for clinicians. *Nutrition in Clinical Practice, 22*, 377–388.

Jagim, A. R., Camic, C. L., Kisiolek, J., Luedke, J., Erickson, J., Jones, M. T., & Oliver, J. M. (2018). Accuracy of resting metabolic rate prediction equations in athletes. *The Journal of Strength & Conditioning Research, 32*, 1875–1881.

Lewis, Z. H., Lyons, E. J., Jarvis, J. M., & Baillargeon, J. (2015). Using an electronic activity monitor system as an intervention modality: A systematic review. *BMC Public Health, 15*, 1–15.

Livingstone, M. B. E. (1997). Heart-rate monitoring: The answer for assessing energy expenditure and physical activity in population studies? *British Journal of Nutrition, 78*, 869–871.

Lymberis, A., & Paradiso, R. (2008). Smart fabrics and interactive textile enabling wearable personal applications: R&D state of the art and future challenges. In *2008 30th annual international conference of the IEEE engineering in medicine and biology society* (pp. 5270–5273). IEEE.

McArdle, W. D., Katch, F. I., & Katch, V. L. (2010). *Exercise physiology: Nutrition, energy, and human performance* (7th ed.). Philadelphia: Lippincott Williams & Wilkins.

Ndahimana, D., & Kim, E. K. (2017). Measurement methods for physical activity and energy expenditure: A review. *Clinical Nutrition Research, 6*, 68–80.

Ong, L., & Blumenthal, J. A. (2010). Assessment of physical activity in research and clinical practice. In *Handbook of behavioral medicine* (pp. 31–48). New York: Springer.

Penedo, F. J., & Dahn, J. R. (2005). Exercise and well-being: A review of mental and physical health benefits associated with physical activity. *Current Opinion in Psychiatry, 18*, 189–193.

Shepherd, E. F., Toloza, E., McClung, C. D., & Schmalzried, T. P. (1999). Step activity monitor: Increased accuracy in quantifying ambulatory activity. *Journal of Orthopaedic Research, 17*, 703–708.

Steene-Johannessen, J., Anderssen, S. A., Van der Ploeg, H. P., Hendriksen, I. J., Donnelly, A. E., Brage, S., & Ekelund, U. (2016). Are self-report measures able to define individuals as physically active or inactive? *Medicine and Science in Sports and Exercise, 48*, 235–244.

Tapia, E. M., Intille, S. S., Haskell, W., Larson, K., Wright, J., King, A., & Friedman, R. (2007). Real-time recognition of physical activities and their intensities using wireless accelerometers and a heart rate monitor. In *2007 11th IEEE international symposium on wearable computers* (pp. 37–40).

Teixeira, P. J., Carraça, E. V., Marques, M. M., Rutter, H., Oppert, J. M., De Bourdeaudhuij, I., ... & Brug, J. (2015). Successful behavior change in obesity interventions in adults: A systematic review of self-regulation mediators. *BMC Medicine, 13*, 1–16.

Vanhees, L., Lefevre, J., Philippaerts, R., Martens, M., Huygens, W., Troosters, T., & Beunen, G. (2005). How to assess physical activity? How to assess physical fitness? *European Journal of Cardiovascular Prevention & Rehabilitation, 12*, 102–114.

Warburton, D. E., & Bredin, S. S. (2017). Health benefits of physical activity: A systematic review of current systematic reviews. *Current Opinion in Cardiology, 32*, 541–556.

Physical Activity/Inactivity: Objective Measurement of

Sophia Brady[1], Jet J. C. S. Veldhuijzen van Zanten[1], Joan L. Duda[1], George D. Kitas[2] and Sally A. M. Fenton[1]
[1]School of Sport, Exercise and Rehabilitation Sciences, University of Birmingham, Birmingham, UK
[2]Russells Hall Hospital, The Dudley Group NHS Foundation Trust, Dudley, UK

Synonyms

Non-exercise physical activity; Physical activity intensity

Definition

Device-based assessments of physical activity, including pedometers, accelerometers, and multi-sensor devices.

Description

Background

Unequivocal evidence exists for the association between physical activity (PA) and health. Consequently, the promotion of PA is a global public health priority, with intervention efforts increasing exponentially worldwide. In developing and evaluating interventions, the accurate surveillance of free-living PA is critical for several reasons: first to be able to examine dose-response relationships between PA and health to optimize the potential efficacy of interventions, second to determine adherence to (a) current PA recommendations (e.g., 150 min of moderate-intensity PA/week) and/or (b) doses of PA evidenced to produce meaningful changes in health outcomes, and third to establish whether interventions to promote PA are effective at bringing about change in behavior.

Until recently, self-report measures (e.g., questionnaires, proxy reports, diaries) have been extensively used to estimate and quantify levels of PA, due to their low cost and ease of administration. However, self-report measures are prone to recall bias, with participants overreporting and misinterpreting the frequency, intensity, and duration of their PA. By comparison, device-based (objective) assessments of PA – such as pedometers and accelerometers – offer a relatively more valid and reliable means of assessing PA (1). Consequently, these instruments are increasingly considered the preferred method for quantifying PA in both large-scale epidemiological research and smaller observational and experimental studies. Below, we describe the most commonly used objective methods to assess "free-living PA" (PA accumulated as part of normal daily activity), highlighting advantages and limitations of each method.

Pedometers

Pedometers assess free-living PA via recording daily step counts, to provide an estimate of total PA accumulated across a specific time period (e.g., days, weeks). Typical study protocols require participants to wear pedometers during waking hours for 5–7 days, to obtain a reliable estimate of daily physical activity. Pedometers are small and inexpensive and do not require any skill or training of the participant. As a result, they are frequently used to provide objective estimates of free-living PA in large-scale, cohort studies.

Advantages and Limitations: Pedometers are valid and reliable measures of PA in adults (2), yielding a percentage error of only ±3% and correlations of >0.89, when compared to direct observation. However, some studies suggest pedometers lack sensitivity when used to assess PA in specific populations. For example, pedometers demonstrate 56% error where participants had a step cadence of 50 steps/min, leading to significant inaccuracies and misestimations in measurements of PA in older, less mobile populations (3). In addition, non-ambulatory activities cannot be assessed with pedometers (e.g., swimming and cycling), and pedometers do not afford the ability to measure frequency, intensity, and duration of PA. As such, pedometers are particularly limited in their application to research which seeks to understand the dose-response relationship between PA and health, as well as estimate adherence to PA recommendations concentrated on specific doses of PA. Even so, pedometers offer a useful alternative to self-report when seeking to determine changes in PA over time (e.g., epidemiology, in response to intervention) or to examine incidental, less structured PA (e.g., housework or gardening), as well as differences in total levels of PA engagement between individuals.

Accelerometers

Accelerometers are small, lightweight devices which measure the accelerations of body movements to which they are attached (e.g., the torso or wrist). To reliably assess free-living PA, protocols require that accelerometers are worn for at least 7 days (1). Devices record accelerations resulting from body movement continuously, and data is stored within the device for subsequent download and interpretation. Accelerometer data can be extracted as raw data (i.e., gravity-based acceleration units (g-units), where $1 \text{ g} = 9.81 \text{ m/s}^2$) or "count-based" data. The latter involves raw data being compressed (using manufacturers software) and time-stamped, to provide an "accelerometer count" per unit of time (i.e., per epoch). Epochs are user-specified and can range from 1 to 60 s.

Both raw and count-based accelerometer data can be interpreted to quantify frequency, intensity, and duration of free-living PA. Specifically, accelerometer output (raw or count-based data) can be calibrated against energy expenditure (EE) (measured by indirect calorimetry), to identify thresholds at which accelerometer data corresponds to different intensities of PA. These thresholds are determined according metabolic equivalents (METS) and referred to as "cut-points."

Advantages and Limitations: Accelerometers have been widely validated among healthy adults and children, in controlled laboratory conditions and free-living settings. Studies demonstrate correlations of 0.88 between counts/minute measured by accelerometer and indirect calorimetry during treadmill walking in an adult population (4), as well as high inter-instrument reliability in free-living settings (5). As such, the superior validity of accelerometers relative to self-report, and their ability to accurately measure frequency, intensity, and duration of PA (which pedometers cannot assess), is the main advantage of these devices and offers the ability to more accurately establish dose-response associations between PA and health, estimate population prevalence of physical inactivity and/or adherence to physical activity recommendations, and measure response to interventions targeting increasing PA. Consequently, accelerometers are viewed as the most promising tool for accurately assessing free-living PA, particularly in large-scale epidemiological and intervention studies.

However, many complex methodological and analytical decisions are required to deal with accelerometer data. Consequently, measurement protocols (e.g., number of days wear, epoch length) and analysis approaches (e.g., cut points used) are highly heterogenous across studies, even where similar research questions are being asked in comparable populations (6). This absence of a "gold standard recommendation," for analysis of accelerometer data, results in subjective interpretation of what is advocated to be "objective data" (7).

A further notable drawback of accelerometry is the inability of these devices to accurately assess activities that require increased EE, but no (or little) whole-body movement (e.g., weight-lifting, cycling). In addition, accelerometers underestimate the energy cost of stair climbing, as they are unable to capture the energy cost of lifting body weight against gravity. Nevertheless, engagement in such behaviors can be captured via other means (e.g., self-report), to give an indication of the contributions of these activities toward daily PA. Thus combining accelerometry with self-report is recommended.

With that said, where studies are conducted on smaller scale, and with sufficient financial resource, more expensive "multi-sensor devices" – which combine physiological parameters (e.g., heart rate) with accelerometer data – may offer a more valid and reliable alternative to PA measurement.

Multi-sensor Activity Monitors

Multi-sensor activity monitors are combined sensors that measure and integrate data from two sources: physiological data collected in response to activity (e.g., heart rate, skin temperature) and movement data captured with accelerometry. Examples include the ActiHeart™ monitor (heart rate + accelerometery) and the SenseWear Armband (galvanic skin response + accelerometry).

Advantages and Limitations: Multi-sensor activity monitors overcome the key limitation of accelerometry; namely, dual input from both accelerometry and a physiological parameter not only enhances their validity and accuracy for measuring PA EE but also means these devices are less likely to misclassify low acceleration-high intensity behaviors (e.g., weight lifting) as low-intensity activities. For example, studies have shown that multi-sensor devices give more accurate estimations of EE during cycling, non-weight bearing activities, low intensity activities, and stair climbing, when compared to accelerometers. However, due to (a) increased complexity of data recorded and analytical approaches required and (b) the necessity for multi-sensor devices to be individually calibrated, these dual-input monitors are particularly time-consuming for use in research. They are also more expensive than accelerometers, therefore typically used in small-scale experimental/intervention studies which require precise estimates of PA, rather than population-based studies of PA behavior.

A rise in the popularity of multi-sensor PA monitoring has been observed in the commercial market. Currently, several "fitness trackers" have been developed, employing accelerometry and heart rate to estimate free-living PA and quantify daily EE. However, recent research has indicated most commercially available activity trackers significantly underestimate free-living EE, when compared to the research grade monitors (e.g., the ActiHeart and SenseWear Armband) (8). Consequently, commercial physical activity devices are not currently considered appropriate for use in research.

Conclusion

Assessment of PA using pedometers, accelerometers, and multi-sensor devices enables more accurate and valid assessment of free-living PA, relative to traditional self-report methods. Pedometers offer large-scale, cheap, and reliable measurements of daily physical activity; however they lack the ability to measure the frequency, intensity, and duration of PA. Accelerometers are able to capture these different dimensions of PA, but the manner in which the data gathered is analyzed to provide estimates regarding frequency, intensity, and duration of PA requires a degree of subjective interpretation (e.g., which cut points to use, cut-based vs. raw data) (1). As a result, while accelerometers are termed objective devices, it would be more accurate to refer to them as "device-based assessments of PA." Multi-sensor activity monitors currently provide more valid means of quantifying PA intensity, frequency, and duration, but researchers should consider the "trade-off" between precision vs. ease of assessment and cost.

Cross-References

▶ Exercise
▶ Exercise Testing
▶ Interventions and Strategies to Promote Physical Activity
▶ Physical Activity
▶ Physical Activity and Health
▶ Physical Inactivity

References and Further Readings

Chowdhury, E. A., Western, M. J., Nightingale, T. E., Peacock, O. J., & Thompson, D. (2017). Assessment of laboratory and daily energy expenditure estimates from consumer multi-sensor physical activity monitors. *PLoS One, 12*(2), e0171720.

Dowd, K. P., Szeklicki, R., Minetto, M. A., Murphy, M. H., Polito, A., Ghigo, E., et al. (2018). A systematic literature review of reviews on techniques for physical activity measurement in adults: A DEDIPAC study. *The International Journal of Behavioral Nutrition and Physical Activity, 15*(1), 15.

Freedson, P., Bowles, H. R., Troiano, R., & Haskell, W. (2012). Assessment of physical activity using wearable monitors: Recommendations for monitor calibration and use in the field. *Medicine and Science in Sports and Exercise, 44*(1 Suppl 1), S1–S4.

Kelly, L. A., McMillan, D. G., Anderson, A., Fippinger, M., Fillerup, G., & Rider, J. (2013). Validity of actigraphs uniaxial and triaxial accelerometers for assessment of physical activity in adults in laboratory conditions. *BMC Medical Physics, 13*(1), 5.

Liu, S., Brooks, D., Thomas, S., Eysenbach, G., & Nolan, R. P. (2015). Lifesource XL-18 pedometer for measuring steps under controlled and free-living conditions. *Journal of Sports Sciences, 33*(10), 1001–1006.

Martin, J., Krc, K., Mitchell, E., Eng, J., & Noble, J. (2012). Pedometer accuracy in slow walking older adults. *International Journals of Therapeutic Rehabilitation, 19*(7), 387–393.

Troiano, R. P., McClain, J. J., Brychta, R. J., & Chen, K. Y. (2014). Evolution of accelerometer methods for physical activity research. *British Journal of Sports Medicine, 48*(13), 1019–1023.

Vanhelst, J., Baquet, G., Gottrand, F., & Beghin, L. (2012). Comparative interinstrument reliability of uniaxial and triaxial accelerometers in free-living conditions. *Perceptual and Motor Skills, 114*(2), 584–594.

Physical Capacity

▶ Physical Fitness

Physical Condition

▶ Physical Fitness

Physical Environment

▶ Built Environment

Physical Exam

▶ Physical Examination

Physical Examination

Margaret Hammersla
University of Maryland School of Nursing,
Baltimore, MD, USA

Synonyms

Health assessment; Physical exam

Definition

Physical examination, assessment, is the systematic process of collecting data about a patient or client using the techniques of inspection, palpation, percussion, and auscultation to guide a clinician in the process of diagnosis of pathological states as well as developing a plan of care (Fennessey and Wittmann-Price 2011). Physical assessment is an ongoing process that enables the clinician to continuously evaluate a patient's signs and symptoms, to monitor effectiveness of treatment, and to make adjustments in the plan of care as required (Zambas 2010). This physical assessment is conducted in a systematic manner that is comfortable to both the patient and clinician; typically this is done using a head-to-toe approach.

Physical assessment is done for one of two reasons. The first reason is to conduct a complete physical exam of the entire body in order to screen the patient for potential health problems that have not yet manifested symptoms (Bickley and Szilagy 2008) and monitor chronic health concerns. This exam is traditionally categorized based on body system (e.g., cardiovascular, respiratory, gastrointestinal). Each body system has its own set of unique advanced assessment procedures that allow the clinician to make a judgment about physical function based on what he or she sees, hears, and feels.

The second reason is to investigate a patient's chief complaint or follow-up on a current health problem such as hypertension or diabetes (Stern et al. 2009). For this more focused exam the clinician makes a determination of what body systems and exam components need to be conducted based on the differential diagnosis and/or the pathophysiology of the current health problem. This more focused exam typically utilizes more advanced techniques to obtain a deeper understanding of the physical changes that may be occurring due to disease process (Bickley and Szilagy 2008).

Physical assessment, along with health history, is the first and most vital step in diagnosing and planning care for patients. A skilled clinician will be able to utilize findings from the physical exam to both support and rule out diagnoses.

Cross-References

▶ Clinical Settings
▶ Diabetes
▶ Hypertension
▶ Primary Care
▶ Primary Care Physicians

References and Readings

Bickley, L. S., & Szilagy, P. G. (2008). *Bates' guide to physical examination and history taking* (10th ed.). Philadelphia: Lippincott Williams and Wilkins.

Fennessey, A., & Wittmann-Price, R. A. (2011). Physical assessment: A continuing need for clarification. *Nursing Forum, 46*(1), 45–50.

Stern, S. D. C., Cifu, A. S., & Altkorn, D. (2009). *Symptom to diagnosis: An evidence based guide* (2nd ed.). New York: McGraw-Hill Medical.

Zambas, S. I. (2010). Purpose of the systematic physical assessment in everyday practice: Critique of a "sacred cow". *Journal of Nursing Education, 49*(6), 305–310.

Physical Fitness

Nerissa Campbell[1], Stefanie De Jesus[1] and Harry Prapavessis[2]
[1]Exercise and Health Psychology Laboratory, The University of Western Ontario, London, ON, Canada
[2]Faculty of Health Sciences, The University of Western Ontario, London, ON, Canada

Synonyms

Functional health; Habitual performance; Physical capacity; Physical condition

Definition

Physical fitness is one's ability to execute daily activities with optimal performance, endurance, and strength with the management of disease, fatigue, and stress and reduced sedentary behavior.

Description

Physical fitness has multiple components and is conceptualized as either performance- or health-related. The specificity of performance-related fitness regarding one's athletic skill best relates to an individual's athletic performance. Conversely, health-related fitness is generalized to health status and is affected positively or negatively by one's habitual physical activity habits. Given the complexity of physical fitness and the epidemiological analysis taken presently, health-related fitness will be the focus of this discussion.

There are five major components of health-related fitness: morphological, muscular, motor, cardiorespiratory, and metabolic (see below), with muscular and cardiorespiratory fitness being the two primary facets assessed in research. As outlined in Fig. 1, a complex relationship exists among the five biological traits, physical activity level, and health outcome.

There are numerous methods to assess the different components of health-related physical fitness, ranging in feasibility and utility for a laboratory versus field-based testing. Morphology is typically assessed using body mass index (BMI, expressed as kg/m^2), a crude measure of body composition. More

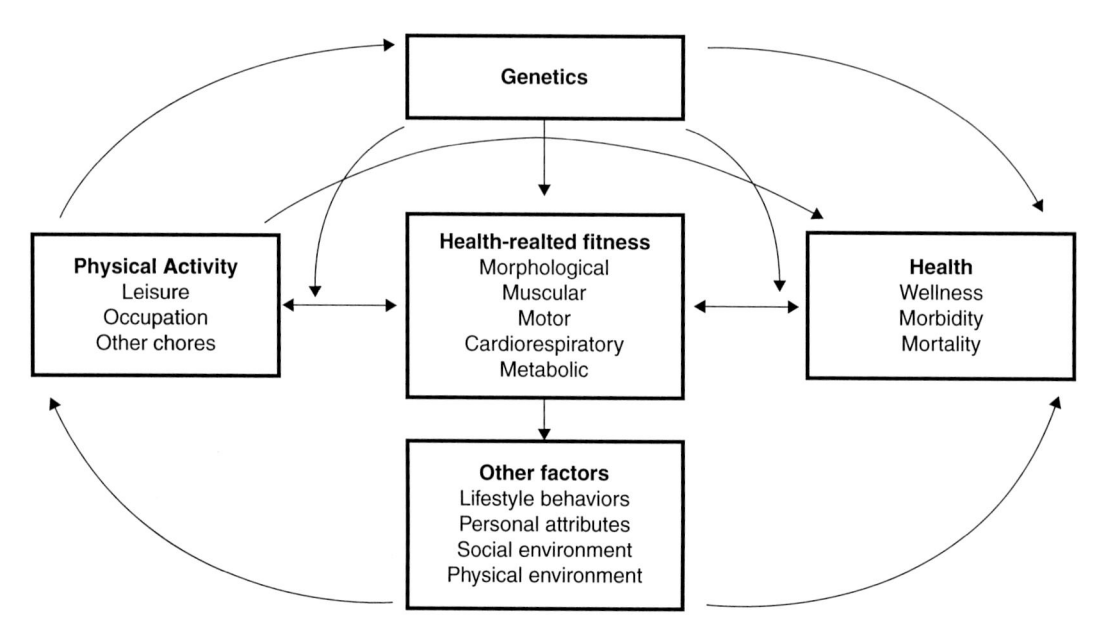

Physical Fitness, Fig. 1 Bouchard et al. (2006), p. 17

objective measures of body composition include skinfold technique, bioelectrical impedance, and dual-energy x-ray absorptiometry. Muscular strength can be evaluated by tensiometers, handgrip dynamometers, and strength gauges. Conversely, muscular endurance is measured by performing the maximum number of repetitions of common body movements, such as sit-ups or push-ups. Motor skills involve fine and gross motor skills and are most commonly assessed by a battery of tests that target balance, speed, control precision, reaction time, aim, and coordination. Cardiorespiratory fitness is the ability of the cardiovascular and respiratory systems to deliver oxygen to working muscles, in addition to the ability of those tissues to utilize that oxygen to produce energy. Peak VO_2, a reflection of cardiorespiratory fitness, is the highest rate of oxygen consumption by muscles during exercise and can be directly assessed by a maximal exercise test. Alternatively, peak VO_2 can be measured indirectly using a submaximal exercise test or timed distance run/walk protocol. Finally, to determine metabolic health, blood pressure and biochemical analyses of blood triglycerides and fasting plasma glucose are examined.

Natural differences exist in health-related physical fitness across the life span and by sex and ethnicity. The extent of the difference is dependent on the specific component of fitness. In general, level of physical fitness declines with age. Age-related decreases in peak VO_2 and muscular strength make even the simplest tasks physically demanding for the elderly compared to younger people. Sex differences in physical fitness are primarily attributed to differences in absolute muscle mass and morphology between males and females. Males generally tend to have higher levels of cardiorespiratory fitness and strength and decreased flexibility compared to females. Similarly, differences in cardiorespiratory fitness have been found between white and black individuals. On average, white males and females are found to have higher maximal VO_2 values compared to black males and females. It is important to keep in mind that depending on the population of interest, different approaches may be needed in order to appropriately assess physical fitness. For example, a maximal VO_2 exercise test may be appropriate for healthy adults or the fit elderly, whereas a different approach for assessing VO_2 in obese individuals or frail older persons may be required.

A multidisciplinary approach is necessary to achieve and maintain physical fitness. Specifically, meeting recommended physical activity and nutrition guidelines as well as acquiring adequate rest are each important components to overall functional health. Not surprisingly, cardiovascular disease, diabetes, cancer, obesity, depression, osteoporosis, and premature death are associated with inadequate physical activity and hence poor physical fitness.

Health-Related Fitness Components and Traits

Morphological component	Body mass for height
	Body composition
	Subcutaneous fat distribution
	Abdominal visceral fat
	Bone density
	Flexibility
Cardiorespiratory component	Submaximal exercise capacity
	Maximal aerobic power
	Heart functions
	Lung functions
	Blood pressure
Muscular component	Power
	Strength
	Endurance
Motor component	Agility
	Balance
	Coordination
	Speed of movement
Metabolic component	Glucose tolerance
	Insulin sensitivity
	Lipid and lipoprotein metabolism
	Substrate oxidation characteristics

Bouchard et al. (2006), p. 17.

Cross-References

▶ Body Composition
▶ Body Mass Index
▶ Exercise Testing
▶ Handgrip Strength
▶ Maximal Exercise Stress Test
▶ Physical Activity and Health

References and Readings

Bouchard, C., Blair, S. N., & Haskell, W. L. (2006). *Physical activity and health*. Champaign: Human Kinetic.

Bouchard, C., & Shephard, R. J. (1994). Physical activity, fitness and health: The model and key concepts. In C. Bouchard, R. J. Shephard, & T. Stephens (Eds.), *Physical activity, fitness and health, International Proceedings and concensus statement* (pp. 77–88). Champaign: Human Kinetics.

Caspersen, C. J., Powell, K. E., & Christenson, G. M. (1985). Physical activity, exercise, and physical fitness: Definitions and distinctions for health-related research. *Public Health Reports, 100*(2), 126–131.

Larson, L. A. (1974). *Fitness, health, and work capacity: International Standards for assessment*. New York: Macmillan.

Warburton, D. E. R., Nicol, C. W., & Bredin, S. S. D. (2006). Health benefits of physical activity: The evidence. *Canadian Medical Association Journal, 174*(6), 801–809.

Physical Fitness Testing

▶ Exercise Testing

Physical Illness

▶ Psychosocial Work Environment

Physical Inactivity

Tyler Clark
School of Psychology, The University of Sydney, Sydney, NSW, Australia

Definition

Physical inactivity is the failure to meet the minimum recommended physical activity guidelines (i.e., 30-min moderate-intensity exercise on at least 5, although preferably all, days of the week or 75-min vigorous-intensity exercise to be undertaken in no less than 20-min increments thrice a week). Physical inactivity is one of the World Health Organization's (WHO) 12 leading risks to health. Physical inactivity is widespread and associated with increases in all causes of mortality and is an independent risk factor for chronic diseases.

Physical inactivity differs from sedentary behavior (e.g., sitting and not moving); physical inactivity refers to not meeting the aforementioned guidelines.

Description

Prevalence

The American Heart Association estimates that 60% of the world population does not meet recommended physical activity guidelines (American Heart Association 2001). The American Centre for Disease Control (CDC) estimates 25% of adults are not active at all.

Risk Factors

Physical inactivity increases with age. While physical activity typically peaks in early adolescence, it then begins to decline, regardless of gender (World Health Organization 2011a). Other demographic risk factors include low income and less education.

Behavioral correlates of physical inactivity include a reduction in leisure-time physical activity and the inclusion of more sedentary occupational and domestic activities (Healey 2007).

Other environmental correlates of physical activity include population overcrowding, increased levels of crime, high-density traffic, low air quality, and a lack of parks, sidewalks, and sports/recreation facilities (WHO 2011a).

Health Risks

Physical inactivity increases all cause mortality (World Health Organization 2011b). The WHO estimates as many as two million deaths worldwide as attributable to physical inactivity. It is also an independent risk factor for chronic diseases such as ischemic heart disease, stroke, type 2 diabetes, breast cancer, colon cancer, and depression. Physical inactivity is also a leading cause of falls and fall-related injuries, particularly in older populations.

Physical inactivity has indirect health burdens as well, which include pain, disability, anxiety, and increased suffering due to medical conditions. These indirect burdens often lead to a reduction in an individual's quality of life, as well as shorter life expectancy, less workforce participation, decreased bone and functional health, and weight gain (Taylor 2009).

Cross-References

▶ Chronic Disease or Illness
▶ Lifestyle, Sedentary
▶ Physical Activity
▶ Quality of Life
▶ Risk Factors and Their Management
▶ Sedentary Behaviors

References and Readings

American Heart Association. (2009). Physical inactivity. Available at americanheart.org. Accessed 8 Dec 2010.
Fletcher, G. F., Balady, G. J., Amsterdam, E. A., et al. (2001). Exercise standards for testing and training: A statement for healthcare professionals from the American Heart Association. *Circulation, 104*, 1694–1740.
Healey, J. (2007). *Physical activity*. Thirroul: Spinney Press.
Taylor, S. E. (2009). *Health psychology* (7th ed.). New York: McGraw Hill. International Edition.
World Health Organization. (2011a). Global strategy on diet, physical activity and health. Available at http://www.who.int/dietphysicalactivity/pa/en/index.html. Accessed 8 Jan 2011.
World Health Organization. (2011b). Physical activity. Available at: http://www.who.int/topics/physical_activity/en/. Accessed 8 Jan 2011.

Physical Therapy

Marilyn Moffat
Department of Physical Therapy, New York University, New York, NY, USA

Synonyms

Kinesiotherapy; Physiotherapy; Therapy, Physical

Definition

Physical therapy is a health service concerned with identifying and maximizing quality of life and movement potential within the spheres of promotion, prevention, intervention/treatment, habilitation, and rehabilitation. The spheres of practice are aimed at physical, psychological, emotional, and social well-being of a patient/client. Physical therapy involves the interaction between physical therapists and patients/clients, other health professionals, families, caregivers, and communities in a process where movement potential is assessed, goals are agreed upon, and interventions carried out using knowledge and skills unique to physical therapists (World Confederation for Physical Therapy 2011a, b).

Description

Physical therapy is the service provided only by, or under the direction and supervision of, physical therapists to people and populations to develop, maintain, and restore maximum movement and functional ability throughout the lifespan. Physical therapist practice includes the provision of services in circumstances where movement and function are threatened by the process of aging or by injury, diseases, disorders, or other conditions of health. Functional movement and physical activity are central to physical therapist practice since they are at the core of what it means to be healthy. Physical therapists are guided in their practice by the professional behaviors of accountability, altruism, compassion/caring, cultural competence, ethical behavior, integrity, personal/professional development, professional duty, and social responsibility and advocacy. Physical therapist education consists of university-based education leading to entry-level qualifications that range internationally from bachelors to masters or doctorate entry qualifications.

Physical therapist practice follows a patient/client management model that includes examination/assessment, evaluation, diagnosis, prognosis, plan of care, intervention/treatment, and reexamination (World Confederation for Physical Therapy 2011a, b).

Examination by the physical therapist involves history taking, screening of the patient's/client's systems (cardiovascular/pulmonary, musculoskeletal, neuromuscular, and integumentary) and the use of specific tests and measures, the results of which are evaluated within a process of evidence-based clinical reasoning to determine the facilitators and barriers to optimal human functioning. The tests and measures used by physical therapists include any of the following: aerobic capacity/endurance; anthropometric characteristics; assistive technology; balance; circulation (arterial, venous, lymphatic); community, social, and civic life; cranial and peripheral nerve integrity; education life; environmental factors; gait; integumentary integrity; joint integrity and mobility; mental functions; mobility (including locomotion); motor function; muscle performance (including strength, power, endurance, and length); neuromotor development and sensory integration; pain; posture; range of motion; reflex integrity; self-care and domestic life; sensory integrity; ventilation and respiration; and work life.

Based upon the examination results, physical therapists evaluate the findings from the examination (history, systems review, and tests and measures) to make clinical judgments regarding patients/clients. Physical therapists formulate the diagnosis(es) that results in the identification of existing or potential impairments, activity limitations, and participation restrictions and then determine patient/client prognoses and identify the most appropriate intervention/treatment strategies for the patient/client management. The plan of care is developed that is consistent with legal, ethical, and professional obligations and administrative policies and procedures of the practice environment. Specific interventions/treatments are determined with measurable outcomes and goals associated with the plan of care and with the involvement of the person and their care providers, both professional and personal. Plans may include referral to other agencies and service delivery providers.

Physical therapists provide, whenever possible, evidence-based physical therapy interventions to achieve patient/client goals and outcomes. These interventions/treatment encompass the following major areas:

1. Patient/client-related instruction.
2. Therapeutic exercise (including aerobic capacity/endurance conditioning or reconditioning, flexibility exercises, neuromotor development training, relaxation, and strength, power, and endurance training for head, neck, limb, pelvic-floor, trunk, and ventilatory muscles).
3. Functional training in self-care and domestic life, work, community, social and civic life; (including activities of daily living training, barrier accommodations or modifications, developmental activities, device and equipment use and training, functional training programs, instrumental activities of daily living training, and injury prevention or reduction).
4. Airway clearance techniques (including breathing strategies, manual/mechanical techniques, and positioning).
5. Assistive technology (including aids for locomotion, orthoses, prostheses, seating and positioning technologies, and devices to improve safety, function, and independence).
6. Biophysical agents (including forms of energy to assist muscle force generation, decrease

unwanted muscular activity, increase wound healing, modulate or decrease pain, reduce or eliminate edema, improve circulation, and decrease inflammation and connective tissue extensibility or restriction);
7. Integumentary repair and protection techniques (including techniques to enhance wound perfusion and facilitate healing, biophysical agents, debridement, dressings, and topical agents);
8. Manual therapy techniques (including manual lymphatic drainage, manual traction, massage, mobilization/manipulation, neural tissue mobilization, and passive range of motion);
9. Motor function training (including balance training, gait and locomotion training, and posture training).

Interventions/treatment are aimed at prevention of impairments, activity limitations, participation restrictions, and injury. Interventions provided by physical therapists also include prevention, health promotion, and fitness for individuals of all ages and for groups and communities.

Reexamination by physical therapists occurs throughout the episode of service delivery to evaluate the effectiveness of interventions/treatment and outcomes and to adjust the plan of care in response to findings. Outcomes monitoring is part of building the evidence base for modifying the patient/client plan, as well as for the research underpinning professional physical therapy practice.

Physical therapy is an essential part of the health and community/welfare services delivery systems. Professional education prepares physical therapists to practice independently of other health service delivery providers as autonomous practitioners and also within interdisciplinary rehabilitation/habilitation programs to prevent, gain, maintain, or restore optimal function and quality of life in individuals with loss and disorders of movement. Physical therapists may act as first contact practitioners, and patients/clients may seek direct services without referral from another health professional. Physical therapists provide consultation within their expertise and determine when patients/clients need to be referred to other professional providers.

Physical therapists are guided by their own code of ethical principles. Thus, they may be concerned with any of the following purposes:

- Promoting the health and well-being of individuals and the general public/society, emphasizing the importance of physical activity and exercise.
- Preventing impairments, activity limitations, participatory restrictions and disabilities in individuals at risk of altered movement behaviors due to health or medically related factors, socioeconomic stressors, environmental factors, and lifestyle factors.
- Providing interventions/treatment to restore integrity of body systems essential to movement, maximize function and recuperation, minimize incapacity, and enhance the quality of life, independent living, and workability in individuals and groups of individuals with altered movement behaviors resulting from impairments, activity limitations, participatory restrictions, and disabilities.
- Modifying environmental, home, and work access and barriers to ensure full participation in one's normal and expected societal roles.

Physical therapists also contribute to the development of local, national, and international health policies and public health strategies. Physical therapists may also have roles in management, administration, supervision of personnel, education, research, and consultation to businesses, schools, government agencies, other organizations, or individuals.

Physical therapy services may be provided to individuals or populations and in a wide range of service settings, including but not limited to: community-based rehabilitation programs;

community settings including primary health care centers; individual homes; field settings (including in response to disasters); educational and research centers; fitness centers; health clubs; gymnasia and spas; hospices; hospitals; nursing homes; occupational health centers; out-patient clinics; physical therapist private offices and clinics; prisons; public settings (e.g., shopping malls) for health promotion; rehabilitation centers; residential homes; schools including pre-schools and special schools; senior citizen centers; sports centers/clubs; and workplaces/companies.

Cross-References

▶ Activities of Daily Living (ADL)
▶ Activity Level
▶ Aerobic Exercise
▶ Back Pain
▶ Cancer and Physical Activity
▶ Cardiac Rehabilitation
▶ Cardiovascular Disease Prevention
▶ Chronic Disease Management
▶ Exercise
▶ Exercise Testing
▶ Exercise, Benefits of
▶ Interventions and Strategies to Promote Physical Activity
▶ Lifestyle, Active
▶ Lifestyle, Healthy
▶ Massage Therapy
▶ Physical Activity and Health
▶ Physical Fitness
▶ Vocational Assessment

References and Further Reading

World Confederation for Physical Therapy. (2007). Description of physical therapy. https://www.wcpt.org/policy/ps-descriptionPT. Accessed 5 Aug 2018.
World Confederation for Physical Therapy. (2011a). Policy statement: Description of physical therapy. https://www.wcpt.org/policy/ps-descriptionPT. Accessed 5 Aug 2018.
World Confederation for Physical Therapy. (2011b). Policy statement: Protection of title. http://www.wcpt.org/sites/wcpt.org/files/files/PS_Protection_Title_Sept 2011.pdf. Accessed 5 Aug 2018.

Physical Well-Being

▶ Happiness and Health

Physician-Assisted Suicide

▶ Euthanasia

Physiological Reactivity

Kristen Salomon
Department of Psychology, University of South Florida College of Arts and Sciences, Tampa, FL, USA

Synonyms

Stress reactivity; Stress responses

Definition

Physiological reactivity involves bodily changes in response to stressful stimuli or events. The classic features of physiological reactivity are increases in sympathetic nervous system and hypothalamic-pituitary-adrenal axis (HPA) activity, often referred to as the "fight-or-flight" response (Cannon 1932). These responses include increases in heart rate, blood pressure, cardiac contractility, and cortisol. Changes in parasympathetic nervous system activity, immune function (Cacioppo 1994), and non-HPA endocrine function (Taylor et al. 2000) can also occur. For reactivity to serve as a meaningful metric, stress responses must be compared to an unstressed resting state, or baseline, to control for wide individual differences in resting levels (Jennings et al. 1992). Physiological reactivity is most often assessed in response to acute stressors on the order of minutes (Steptoe and Vögele 1991).

Cross-References

▶ Mental Stress
▶ Perceptions of Stress
▶ Stress
▶ Stress Responses

References and Readings

Cacioppo, J. T. (1994). Social neuroscience: Autonomic, neuroendocrine, and immune responses to stress. *Psychophysiology, 31*, 113–128.
Cacioppo, J. T., Tassinary, L. G., & Berntson, G. G. (2007). *Handbook of psychophysiology*. New York: Cambridge University Press.
Cannon, W. B. (1932). *The wisdom of the body*. New York: Norton.
Jennings, J. R., Kamarck, T., Stewart, C., Eddy, M., & Johnson, O. (1992). Alternate cardiovascular baseline assessment techniques: Vanilla or resting baseline. *Psychophysiology, 29*, 742–750.
McEwen, B. S. (1998). Stress, adaptation, and disease: Allostasis and allostatic load. *Annals of the New York Academy of Sciences, 840*, 33–44.
Sapolsky, R. M. (1994). *Why zebras don't get ulcers*. New York: Holt.
Steptoe, A., & Vögele, C. (1991). Methodology of mental stress testing in cardiovascular research. *Circulation, 83*, II-14–II-24.
Stern, R. M., Ray, W. J., & Quigley, K. S. (2001). *Psychophysiological recording*. New York: Oxford University Press.
Taylor, S. E., Klein, L. C., Lewis, B. P., Gruenewald, T. L., Gurung, R. A., & Updegraff, J. A. (2000). Biobehavioral responses to stress in females: Tend-and-befriend, not fight-or-flight. *Psychological Review, 107*, 411–429.

Physiotherapy

▶ Physical Therapy

Pickering, Thomas G.

Eoin O'Brien
The Conway Institute, University College Dublin, Belfield, Dublin, Ireland

Biographical Information

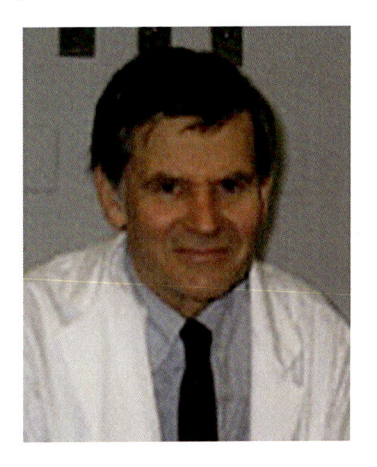

Dr. Thomas George Pickering

Thomas George Pickering was born in the United Kingdom in 1940. He was educated at Bryanston School in Blandford, England, and went on to study medicine at Trinity College, Cambridge, and the Middlesex Hospital Medical School, London, where he graduated in 1966.

Pickering's early postgraduate years were spent at the Middlesex and the Radcliffe Infirmary. He became a member of the Royal College of Physicians of London in 1968, becoming a fellow in 1980. He received a Ph.D. degree from Oxford University in 1970. In 1972, he went to New York to take up appointments as Associate Physician at the Rockefeller University Hospital and Assistant Professor at Cornell University. He spent 2 years as Assistant Professor at the Rockefeller University working with Neal Miller on biofeedback mechanisms. He was appointed Assistant Physician to the New York Hospital in

Editors' Note: Dr. Pickering passed away in 2009. The American Society of Hypertension has established the Thomas Pickering Memorial Lecture, the first of which was delivered at the Scientific Meeting in May 2012.

1974. He returned to theRadcliffe Infirmary in 1974 to work with Peter Sleight.

Pickering's earliest hypertension research at Oxford focused on baroreceptor function, the autonomic nervous system, and the emerging class of cardiovascular medications known as the adrenoreceptor blockers. Although he remained in Oxford from 1974 to 1976, the possibility of being able to work as both a practicing physician and a clinical investigator drew him back to New York City and Cornell University Medical College, where he spent more than 20 years in a productive career in cardiovascular behavioral medicine, clinical hypertension, and blood pressure measurement research. In 2000, he became Director of Behavioral Cardiovascular Health and the Hypertension Program at the Cardiovascular Institute of Mount Sinai Medical Center, and in 2003 he moved to Columbia University Medical College as Professor of Medicine and Director of the Behavioral Cardiovascular Health and Hypertension Program.

Major Accomplishments

Pickering practiced "translational research" long before the term became fashionable, translating his clinical observations in medical practice to research endeavors throughout his career. He made important observations on the relationship between renovascular disease and cardiovascular complications, and the impact of renal revascularization. He also observed that anxiety, perceived stress, job strain, and the medical care environment itself induced hypertension in some individuals who otherwise would not have been classified as hypertensive. He had a deep belief that psychosocial mechanisms played an important role in the pathogenesis of cardiovascular disorders.

Pickering's research interests also focused on new methods of blood pressure measurement, particularly the use of 24-h ambulatory monitoring and self monitoring. His identification of the importance of the circadian variability of blood pressure led to the study of the psychological influences of work and stress in hypertension and heart disease, a field in which he was regarded as the world authority. At a clinical level he studied the influence of sleep in hypertension and methods of improving adherence to medication in order to obtain better control of elevated blood pressure. Pickering also studied the application of non-pharmacological approaches to the management of hypertension, publishing prolifically in these areas. He published a total of almost 500 original research articles in a clear and concise manner. Several highly acknowledged experts acknowledge his leadership in coining the terms "white-coat hypertension" and "masked hypertension," conditions which he not only described, but did much to explain with well-designed studies. This work systematically investigated whether white-coat hypertension was benign, and whether masked hypertension enhanced risk.

Pickering served on many governmental and academic bodies including the American Society of Hypertension; the National Heart, Lung, and Blood Institute; the International Society of Hypertension; the American Heart Association; the US Cardiorenal Advisory Committee; the US Food and Drug Administration; and the Committee on Gulf War and Stress of the Institute of Medicine. As a senior editor of the Journal of Clinical Hypertension he wrote numerous editorials. In his later years he came to feel strongly that self-monitoring of blood pressure, as well as ambulatory blood pressure monitoring, should be covered by third-party insurance companies for patient hypertension care. In 2002, after 19 years of lobbying, a scientific meeting of the Center for Medicare and Medicaid Services was established to develop a national policy for coverage of ambulatory blood pressure monitoring for patients with white-coat hypertension. At Pickering's suggestion, not only was evidence of the benefits of ambulatory monitoring presented at this meeting but the patients who had benefited gave testimony. The patients' stories had a substantial impact, and the meeting voted unanimously to approve national coverage for ambulatory monitoring.

Cross-References

▶ Adherence
▶ Hypertension

References and Reading

Devereux, R. B., Pickering, T. G., Harshfield, G. A., Kleinert, H. D., Denby, L., Clark, L., et al. (1983). Left ventricular hypertrophy in patients with hypertension: Importance of blood pressure response to regularly recurring stress. *Circulation, 68*, 470–476.

O'Brien, E. (2009). In memoriam. *Journal of Hypertension, 27*, 1715–1716.

O'Brien, E., & White, W. B. (2010). Thomas George Pickering, 1940–2009. Special memorial tribute issue. *Blood Pressure Monitoring, 15*, 67–114.

Pickering, T. G. (1992). The ninth Sir George Pickering memorial lecture: Ambulatory monitoring and the definition of hypertension. *Journal of Hypertension, 10*, 401–409.

Pickering, T. G., & White, W. B. (2008). American Society of Hypertension position paper: Home and ambulatory blood pressure monitoring-when and how to use self (home) and ambulatory blood pressure monitoring. *Journal of Clinical Hypertension, 10*, 850–855.

Pickering, T. G., Harshfield, G. A., Kleinert, H. D., Blank, S., & Laragh, J. H. (1982). Blood pressure during normal daily activities, sleep, and exercise: Comparison of values in normal and hypertensive subjects. *Journal of the American Medical Association, 247*, 992–996.

Pickering, T. G., Sos, T. A., Vaughan, E. D., Case, D. B., Sealey, J. E., Harshfield, G. A., et al. (1984). Predictive value and changes in renin secretion in hypertensive patients with unilateral renovascular disease undergoing successful renal angioplasty. *The American Journal of Medicine, 76*, 398–404.

Pickering, T. G., Herman, L., Devereux, R. B., Sotelo, J. E., James, G. D., Sos, T. A., et al. (1988a). Recurrent pulmonary oedema in hypertension due to bilateral renal artery stenosis: Treatment by angioplasty or surgical revascularization. *Lancet, 2*, 551–552.

Pickering, T. G., James, G. D., Boddie, C., Harshfield, G. A., Blank, S., & Laragh, J. H. (1988b). How common is white coat hypertension? *Journal of the American Medical Association, 259*, 225–228.

Pickering, T. G., Coats, A., Mallion, J. M., Mancia, G., & Verdecchia, P. (1999). Blood pressure monitoring: Task force V-white-coat hypertension. *Blood Pressure Monitoring, 4*, 333–341.

Pickering, T. G., Hall, J. E., Appel, L. J., Falkner, B. E., Graves, J., Hill, M. N., et al. (2005). Recommendations for blood pressure measurement in humans and experimental animals: Part 1-blood pressure measurement in humans: A statement for professionals from the Subcommittee of Professional and Public Education of the American Heart Association Council on High Blood Pressure Research. *Hypertension, 45*, 142–161.

Pickering, T. G., Shimbo, D., & Haas, D. (2006). Ambulatory blood pressure monitoring. *The New England Journal of Medicine, 354*, 2368–2374.

Pickering, T. G., Miller, N. H., Ogedegbe, G., Krakoff, L. R., Artinian, N. T., & Goff, D. (2008). Call to action on use and reimbursement for home blood pressure monitoring: Executive summary-a joint scientific statement from the American Heart Association, American Society of Hypertension, and Preventive Cardiovascular Nurses Association. *Hypertension, 26*, 2259–2267.

White, W. B. (2009). In memoriam. Thomas G. Pickering 1940–2009. *Hypertension, 54*, 917–918.

Pilot Study

J. Rick Turner
Campbell University College of Pharmacy and Health Sciences, Buies Creek, NC, USA

Synonyms

Exploratory study; Feasibility study

Definition

An initial, relatively small-scale study that tests the methods and procedures that researchers are considering using in a larger-scale study, which may be a randomized concurrently controlled clinical trial.

Description

When researchers have identified a potential intervention for a disease or condition of clinical concern and are considering conducting a large clinical trial to determine if there is compelling evidence of the intervention's likely usefulness in clinical practice, designing and conducting a smaller-scale pilot study can be very informative. Most large-scale clinical trials are expensive to conduct and take a long time to complete. So, if a pilot study reveals that the likely success of such a trial is unacceptably low, the researchers may decide that their resources may be better directed toward another potential intervention.

At the point in time when a large-scale clinical trial is designed, a research question, a null hypothesis, and a research hypothesis need to be determined and hypothesis testing undertaken. However, formalized hypothesis testing is not the goal of a pilot study. A pilot study's purpose is to assess the feasibility and acceptability of the approach being considered for a subsequent clinical trial.

Questions a pilot study can answer include, but are not limited to, the following: Are there sufficient individuals with the disease or condition of clinical concern in the geographic region(s) in which the clinical trial would be conducted, i.e., is recruitment of an appropriately large number of trial participants feasible? Once participants have been recruited, is the nature of the trial sufficiently amenable to participants for them to remain in the trial, i.e., is retention going to be adversely affected by burdensome requirements of participating in the trial? Can the intended trial treatments actually be delivered per protocol at the investigational sites conducting the trial? Will trial participants actually do what they are required to do by the study protocol, i.e., will treatment-specific adherence rates be sufficiently high? For each of these feasibility measures, clear quantitative benchmarks for evaluating successful or unsuccessful feasibility should be determined in advance of conducting the pilot study.

Pilot studies can be nonrandomized or randomized in nature. Nonrandomized studies may be designed as open-label studies, where participants, and others involved in running the trial, know what treatment they are receiving. At the other end of the study design spectrum, some pilot studies may be randomized, double-blind studies, where neither the participants nor the investigators at the clinical sites conducting the trial know what treatment each participant is receiving.

As noted, hypothesis testing is not a component of pilot studies, which should be thought of as a means of determining whether or not it is feasible to design and conduct a large-scale clinical trial that will incorporate hypothesis testing.

That said, researchers should take equal care in the design, conduct, interpretation, reporting, and transparency of pilot studies as they do in later confirmatory studies.

Cross-References

▶ Adherence
▶ Double-Blind Study
▶ Public Health
▶ Randomization
▶ Randomized Clinical Trial
▶ Study Protocol

References and Further Reading

Craig, P. (2017). A new CONSORT extension should improve the reporting of randomized pilot and feasibility trials. *Journal of Clinical Epidemiology, 84*, 30–32.

Eldridge, S. M., Chan, C. L., Campbell, M. J., et al. (2016). CONSORT 2010 statement: Extension to randomised pilot and feasibility trials. *Pilot Feasibility Studies, 2*, 64.

Enrique, A., Mooney, O., Salamanca-Sanabria, A., Lee, C. T., Farrell, S., & Richards, D. (2019). Assessing the efficacy and acceptability of an internet-delivered intervention for resilience among college students: A pilot randomised control trial protocol. *Internet Interventions, 17*, 100254.

Kaur, N., Figueiredo, S., Bouchard, V., Moriello, C., & Mayo, N. (2017). Where have all the pilot studies gone? A follow-up on 30 years of pilot studies in clinical rehabilitation. *Clinical Rehabilitation, 31*, 1238–1248.

Kistin, C., & Silverstein, M. (2015). Pilot studies: A critical but potentially misused component of interventional research. *Journal of the American Medical Association, 314*, 1561–1562.

National Institutes of Health. National Center for Complementary and Integrative Health. Pilot studies: common uses and misuses. Available at: https://nccih.nih.gov/grants/whatnccihfunds/pilot_studies. Accessed 23 July 2019.

Pitocin

▶ Oxytocin
▶ Oxytocin, Social Effects in Humans

Pituitary-Adrenal Axis

Jennifer Heaney
Clinical Immunology Service, The University of Birmingham, Birmingham, UK

Definition

The pituitary-adrenal axis comprises the pituitary gland (located at the base of the brain) and adrenal glands (located on top of the kidneys). The main interactions that take place between these two endocrine glands are part of the hypothalamic-pituitary-adrenal (HPA) axis. Corticotrophin-releasing hormone (CRH) stimulates the secretion of adrenocorticotropic hormone (ACTH) from the anterior pituitary; this in turn stimulates the release of cortisol from the adrenal cortex (Martin et al. 1997). More detail on the pituitary-adrenal axis and its function in the HPA axis can be found in Widmaier et al. (2004), O'Riordan et al. (1988), and Greenspan and Forsham (1983).

Cross-References

▶ ACTH
▶ Adrenal Glands
▶ Corticotropin-Releasing Hormone (CRH)
▶ Energy: Expenditure, Intake, Lack of
▶ Hypothalamic-Pituitary-Adrenal Axis
▶ Hypothalamus

References and Further Reading

Greenspan, F. S., & Forsham, P. H. (1983). *Basic and clinical endocrinology*. Los Altos: Lange Medical Publications.
Martin, J. B., Reichlin, S., & Brown, G. M. (1997). *Clinical neuroendocrinology*. Philadelphia: F.A. Davis.
O'Riordan, F. L. H., Malan, P. G., & Gould, R. P. (1988). *Essentials of endocrinology* (2nd ed.). Oxford: Blackwell.
Widmaier, E. P., Raff, H., & Strang, K. T. (2004). *Vander, Sherman, and Luciano's human physiology: The mechanism of body function*. New York: McGraw-Hill.

Placebo and Placebo Effect

Magne Arve Flaten[1] and Mustafa Al'absi[2]
[1]Department of Psychology, University of Tromsø, Tromsø, Norway
[2]University of Minnesota Medical School, School of Medicine, University of Minnesota, Duluth, MN, USA

Synonyms

Conditioned response; Context effect; Expectancy effect

Definition

A placebo is any inert substance, procedure, apparatus, or similar, that alone has no effect in the body. The placebo effect is the psychological and/or physiological response to the placebo when it is administrated with a suggestion that the substance, procedure, apparatus, or similar will have an effect in the individual.

Description

Placebo comes from the Latin word "placere" which means "I shall please" and has been used in medicine to describe treatments that pleases the patient, but that has no specific effect on the symptom.

A placebo effect may occur when a substance, procedure, or other stimulus is administrated to a person, together with a suggestion that this will reduce or heal a symptom. The placebo effect may occur whether the substance or procedure is effective in reducing the symptom or not, as effective treatments may also induce placebo effects. Both the substance or procedure and the suggestion are necessary to produce a placebo effect. Administration of a pill without the suggestion, or the suggestion without the pill, will not generate a placebo effect. Thus, a placebo alone is not sufficient to generate a placebo effect, as it must be accompanied by a suggestion. The suggestion can be in the form of verbal information, e.g., "this capsule may contain a painkiller," that induces an expectation that the treatment will reduce the symptom. The expectation has been found to be correlated to the actual placebo response. Thus, it could be argued that the term "expectancy effect" should replace the vague and often misinterpreted term "placebo effect." Placebo effects may also be implicit and communicated through contextual factors. For example, a "pill" provided by a physician may have a stronger "placebo" effect than a pill provided by a nonmedical professional.

Placebo effects may also occur as a result of a conditioning process. For example, after the individual has been subject to effective treatment, an association between treatment and its outcome may develop. The shape or color of tablets the patient has taken in the past to reduce pain or other problems may be associated with the drug effect, since the shape or color of the tablet (the conditioned stimulus) is reliably followed by reduction in the symptom (the unconditioned response). The features of the tablet can be associated with the effect of the drug in the central nervous system (the unconditioned stimulus) and come to elicit conditioned decreases in the symptom. Placebo effects induced by actual experience with the drug effect are stronger than placebo effects induced by verbal information alone (Flaten et al. 1999). For some symptoms, the conditioned stimulus exerts its effect by inducing an expectation, for other symptoms unconscious, automatic processes seem to be responsible for the placebo effect (Benedetti et al. 2003).

The placebo effect is observed as a reduction in a symptom in a group that receives placebo treatment with suggestion, compared to a natural history control group that receives no treatment and no suggestion. The natural history group controls for normal variations in the symptom due to normal healing processes or other changes that are not due to expectations of treatment effects. Response bias is serious problem, as subjects may feel obliged or may have a tendency to report on the symptom in accordance with the suggestion provided by the experimenter, without there being any improvement in the symptom, and studies must control for demand characteristics. Placebo analgesia, a reduction in pain due to expectations of having received a painkiller, is the most studied form of placebo effect. Pain is accompanied by changes in autonomic function, by well-defined changes in the event-related potential to painful stimulation, and by a cerebral response reliably involving the somatosensory cortex, the anterior cingulate cortex, and the insula. Placebo analgesia is accompanied by reduction in these correlates to the reported pain, indicating that the placebo effect is due to changes in the brain's response to the pain signal and not solely to a response bias, although this may contribute.

Multiple neurobiological pathways are thought to be involved in mediating effects of placebo, including those related to the endogenous opioid system and stress response systems. Placebo analgesia has been found to be reversible or partly reversible by the opioid antagonist naloxone. This is further evidence that the placebo effect is not due to a response bias, and indicates that expectations of pain relief activate the mid-brain descending pain inhibitory system. Wager et al. (2004) found that expectations of pain relief were associated with increased activity in the periaqueductal gray in the midbrain, a nucleus that controls pathways descending to the rostral ventral medulla and the dorsal horn. There, this pathway inhibits pain transmission, resulting in a reduced pain signal to the brain areas mentioned above, with a consequent reduction in pain sensation. Injections of opioids into the periaqueductal gray and the ventral medulla reduce pain, suggesting that endogenous opioids reduce pain via the same descending system. Eippert et al. (2009) furthermore showed that placebo analgesia involved dorsal horn activity, indicating that placebo analgesia is due to expectation of pain relief that in turn activates the descending endorphin-mediated pain inhibitory system.

In addition to pain, placebo effects are documented in, e.g., Parkinson's disease, depression, cardiac heart disease, sexual function, and airway resistance in asthmatic patients. This implies that there are several placebo effects with different underlying mechanisms. In Parkinson's disease, placebo treatment has been found to increase dopamine release in the basal ganglia, thereby improving motor function. Increased dopamine release has also been implicated in placebo analgesia. Most studies have found only a partial reversal of placebo analgesia by naloxone, whereas some studies have found no effect of naloxone on the placebo analgesic response. Thus, non-opioid mechanisms play a role in placebo analgesia. It has been hypothesized that placebo treatment leads to reduced anxiety or negative emotions, that could be a common factor across placebo effects, and that different placebo treatments could activate additional disease-specific mechanisms.

Placebo effects can also be observed in the response to drugs of habitual use or abuse. Caffeine, e.g., increases arousal and decreases reaction time and fatigue, and habitual coffee drinkers who believe they receive caffeine but get a placebo, respond with caffeine-like reactions of increased alertness and faster reaction times, and increased dopamine release in areas associated with reinforcement. Subjects who believe they drink alcohol but receive placebo drinks report symptoms of intoxication and display deteriorated performance on cognitive and motor tasks. Likewise, subjects who believe they receive amphetamine but receive a placebo still report amphetamine-like effects.

Placebos are used as controls in randomized clinical trials, where the effect of the intervention is defined as the improvement over placebo. Since the participant does not know to which arm of the trial he or she has been randomized to, expectations of drug effects are the same in both arms, and expectations of receiving effective treatment are lower than in ordinary clinical practice or in experimental studies on the placebo effect. Thus, placebo effects are smaller or absent in clinical trials (Hróbjartsson and Gøtzscke 2001). Drugs or other treatments may have noticeable subjective effects like drowsiness or nausea that may inform the participant that he or she has received active medication, thereby unblinding the trial for the participants in the active arm. To solve this problem active placebos are used, i.e., drugs that have similar subjective effects to the tested drug, but that have no effect on the symptom, instead of inactive placebos.

Cross-References

▶ Functional Magnetic Resonance Imaging (fMRI)
▶ Pain
▶ Randomized Controlled Trial

References and Readings

Benedetti, F., Pollo, A., Lopiano, L., Lanotte, M., Vighetti, S., & Rainero, I. (2003). Conscious expectation and unconscious conditioning in analgesic, motor, and hormonal placebo/nocebo responses. *Journal of Neuroscience, 23*(10), 4315–4323.

Eippert, F., Finsterbusch, J., Bingel, U., & Buchel, C. (2009). Direct evidence for spinal cord involvement in placebo analgesia. *Science, 326*(5951), 404–404.

Flaten, M. A., Simonsen, T., & Olsen, H. (1999). Drug-related information generates placebo and nocebo responses that modify the drug response. *Psychosomatic Medicine, 61*(2), 250–255.

Hróbjartsson, A., & Gøtzscke, P. C. (2001). Is the placebo powerless? *The New England Journal of Medicine, 344*(21), 1594–1602.

Wager, T. D., Rilling, J. K., Smith, E. E., Sokolik, A., Casey, K. L., Davidson, R. J., et al. (2004). Placebo induced changes in fMRI in the anticipation and experience of pain. *Science, 303*(5661), 1162–1167.

Plain Tobacco Packaging

Melanie Wakefield
Centre for Behavioural Research in Cancer, Cancer Council Victoria, Melbourne, VIC, Australia

Synonyms

Standardized tobacco packaging

Definition

Plain tobacco packaging is a legislative measure that requires the removal of branding from tobacco packages (including colors, imagery, corporate logos, and trademarks) and permits manufacturers to print only the brand name on packages in a mandated location, font size, and style. Plain tobacco packs may contain health warnings and other government-mandated information, but pack appearance, including color, is otherwise standardized.

Description

Plain tobacco packaging is one of the measures in tobacco control that forms a broader comprehensive suite of strategies (involving tobacco taxation, regulation, and education) that are designed to lower population demand for tobacco and ultimately reduce tobacco's harmful consequences. Plain packaging provides an incremental step that builds upon other tobacco control policies.

Tobacco marketing has been dominated by three themes: promoting satisfaction with the product (taste, freshness, mildness), assuaging concerns about the harms of smoking, and creating associations between smoking and desirable outcomes (such as independence, social success, sexual attraction, thinness, etc.) (National Cancer Institute 2008). Traditional avenues for tobacco marketing have included advertising on television, radio, magazines, billboards, transit signage, and at the point of sale. With strong evidence that tobacco advertising and promotion is causally related to increased tobacco use (National Cancer Institute 2008), governments have increasingly banned traditional avenues for promoting tobacco. In response, tobacco companies have gradually placed much greater reliance on promotion through tobacco packaging.

It is notable that compared to most other consumer packaging that is discarded after purchase, tobacco packaging remains with the product and is therefore taken out and may be displayed whenever tobacco is used. Internal tobacco company documents made public as a result of litigation demonstrate how companies used package design and branding to reassure consumers of harms and increase appeal, including to targeted population groups such as youth and women (Wakefield et al. 2002; Kotnowski and Hammond 2013), and to reduce the salience of health warnings (Chapman and Carter 2003).

Recognizing the enormous global burden of harm caused by tobacco, the Framework Convention on Tobacco Control (FCTC), which was adopted by the World Health Organization in 2003 (World Health Organization 2003) and has been ratified by some 180 countries, provides guidelines for policy action to reduce the demand for and supply of tobacco. FCTC Articles 11 (packaging and labeling) and 13 (tobacco advertising, promotion, and sponsorship) provide relevant guidelines for plain tobacco packaging implementation. In the context of FCTC Articles 11 and 13, plain packaging aims to reduce the attractiveness of tobacco products; reduce the effects of tobacco packaging as a form of advertising; address package design elements that may suggest some products are less harmful than others; and increase the noticeability and effectiveness of health warnings.

Plain packaging refers to the removal of branding from packs aside from the brand name, which, like other elements of the pack, must be standardized (Fig. 1). Australia was the first nation to fully implement plain packaging in December 2012, followed by France (2017), the United Kingdom (2017), New Zealand (2018), and Norway (2018). There has since been a great deal of momentum worldwide around the adoption of plain packaging, with some 25 countries and territories either having fully adopted the measure or working toward it by late 2018 (Canadian Cancer Society 2018). The growing momentum internationally for plain packaging implementation occurred despite the first plain packaging legislation in Australia being stridently opposed and challenged by tobacco companies and by certain nations under international trade law. For example, the Australian law was subject to a constitutional challenge in its High Court (dismissed in 2012), a challenge under a bilateral investment treaty between Australia and Hong Kong (dismissed in 2015) and a World Trade Organization challenge brought by four nations (dismissed 2018 (World Trade Organization 2018), under appeal). The tobacco industry also pursued unsuccessful challenges to plain packaging in the courts of the

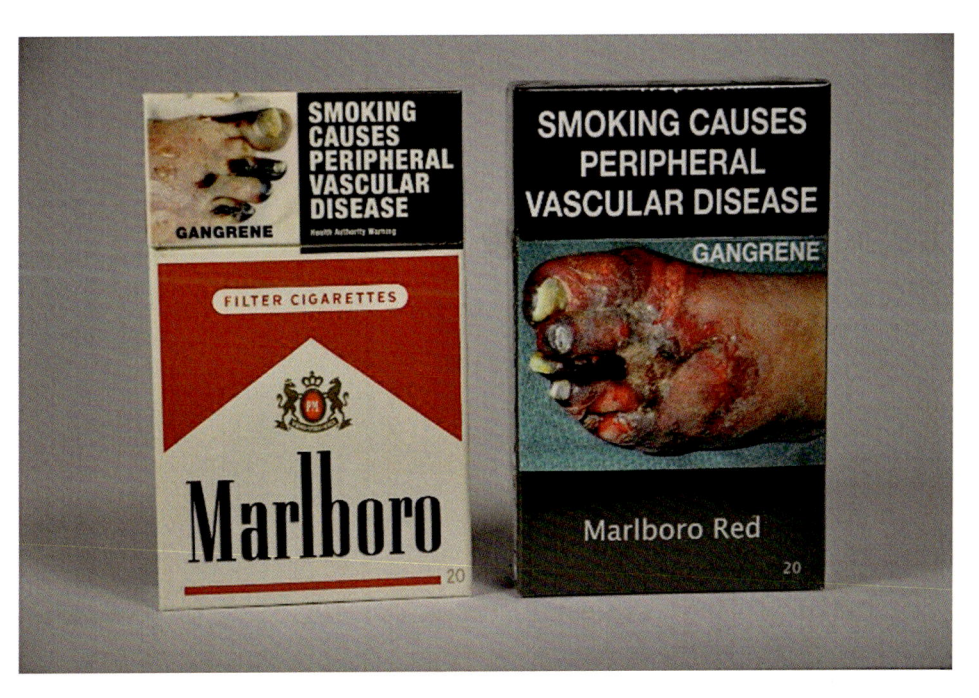

Plain Tobacco Packaging, Fig. 1 Cigarette packs in Australia before and after plain packaging. (Reproduced with permission of Quit Victoria)

United Kingdom, France, and Norway (World Health Organization Framework Convention on Tobacco Control; McCabe Centre for Law and Cancer 2019).

A comparison of the first five countries showed considerable variation in plain packaging implementation (Moodie et al. 2019). For example, in Australia and New Zealand, plain packaging applies to all tobacco products, whereas in the United Kingdom and France, the law applies only to cigarettes and rolling papers and excludes cigars and shisha tobacco. While all countries specify that cigarette sticks must have standard appearance with no marking other than the brand variant name (United Kingdom, Norway, France) or an alphanumeric code (Australia, New Zealand) appearing in a specified font size, type, and position, only New Zealand standardizes tobacco pack and pouch sizes and cigarette stick dimensions.

Most research to date has not aimed to measure the direct effectiveness of plain packaging on smoking prevalence, especially given its implementation in most countries is so recent. Rather, research has generally examined its impact on intermediate outcomes that are known to contribute to reducing smoking prevalence within a comprehensive tobacco control strategy. A recent systematic review concluded that plain packaging reduces product appeal, generally reduces expectations of taste and quality, reduces misperceptions that some cigarettes are less harmful than others (although only when plain packs are a uniformly dark color), and may reduce smoking prevalence (McNeill et al. 2017). A Post-Implementation Review of plain packaging legislation in Australia included analysis of smoking prevalence between 2001 and 2015. Controlling for the effects of tobacco tax increases and other tobacco policies over this period, the report concluded that plain packaging policy contributed approximately 0.55% of the 2.2% decline in smoking prevalence over the 34 months following implementation (Australian Government Department of Health 2016).

The tobacco industry has continued to pursue marketing strategies through packaging innovations that were not completely limited in nations that were early adopters of plain packaging. These strategies included a rapid increase in brand variant names and descriptors, cigarettes with varying filter types, and novel pack sizes. These marketing strategies influence product appeal and can create erroneous perceptions about the relative harms of different products and therefore undermine the intent of plain packaging. Researchers have encouraged subsequent countries to extend and strengthen plain packaging legislation by restricting or banning brand variant names and color descriptors (such as in Uruguay, where only one brand variant is permitted per brand family (DeAtley et al. 2018)); developing larger and more salient pack warnings; requiring cigarette sticks themselves to have a more dissuasive appearance (e.g., by being an unattractive color or featuring a health warning); and using package inserts to direct tobacco users to smoking cessation support (Hoek and Gendall 2017; Moodie et al. 2019).

Cross-References

▶ Tobacco Advertising
▶ Tobacco Control

References and Further Reading

Australian Government Department of Health. (2016). Tobacco plain packaging post–implementation review – Department of Health. Available from: https://ris.pmc.gov.au/2016/02/26/tobacco-plain-packaging. Accessed 27 Aug 2019.

Canadian Cancer Society. (2018). Cigarette packaging health warnings: International status report, 6th ed. Canada, Canadian Cancer Society. Available from: http://www.cancer.ca/~/media/cancer.ca/CW/for%20media/Media%20releases/2018/CCS-international-warnings-report-2018%2D%2D-English%2D%2D-2-MB.pdf?la=fr-CA. Accessed 27 Aug 2019.

Chapman, S., & Carter, S. M. (2003). "Avoid health warnings on all tobacco products for just as long as we can": A history of Australian tobacco industry efforts to avoid, delay and dilute health warnings on cigarettes. *Tobacco Control, 12*(Suppl 3), iii13–iii22. Available from: https://www.ncbi.nlm.nih.gov/pubmed/14645944.

DeAtley, T., Bianco, E., Welding, K., & Cohen, J. E. (2018). Compliance with Uruguay's single presentation requirement. *Tobacco Control, 27*(2), 220–224. Available from: http://tobaccocontrol.bmj.com/content/tobaccocontrol/27/2/220.full.pdf.

Hoek, J., & Gendall, P. (2017). Policy options for extending standardized tobacco packaging. *Bulletin of the World Health Organization, 95*(10), 726–728. Available from: https://www.ncbi.nlm.nih.gov/pubmed/29147047.

Kotnowski, K., & Hammond, D. (2013). The impact of cigarette pack shape, size and opening: Evidence from tobacco company documents. *Addiction, 108*(9), 1658–1668. https://doi.org/10.1111/add.12183. Available from: https://www.ncbi.nlm.nih.gov/pubmed/23600674.

McNeill, A., Gravely, S., Hitchman, S. C., Bauld, L., Hammond, D., et al. (2017). Tobacco packaging design for reducing tobacco use. *Cochrane Database of Systematic Reviews, 4*, CD011244. Available from: http://www.ncbi.nlm.nih.gov/pubmed/28447363. Accessed 27 Aug 2019.

Moodie, C., Hoek, J., Scheffels, J., Galopel-Morvan, K., & Lindorff, K. (2019). Plain packaging: Legislative differences in Australia, France, the UK, New Zealand and Norway, and options for strengthening regulations. *Tobacco Control, 28*, 485–492. https://doi.org/10.1136/tobaccocontrol-2018-054483. Available from: https://www.ncbi.nlm.nih.gov/pubmed/?term=moodie+scheffels.

National Cancer Institute. The Role of the Media in Promoting and Reducing Tobacco Use. Tobacco Control Monograph No. 19. Bethesda, MD: U.S. Department of Health and Human Services, National Institutes of Health, National Cancer Institute. NIH Pub, No. 07–6242, June 2008. (Chapter 1 Overview and Conclusions, pp 3–24).

Wakefield, M., Morley, C., Horan, J., & Cummings, K. M. (2002). The cigarette pack as image: New evidence from tobacco industry documents. *Tobacco Control, 11*(Suppl 1), i73–i80. https://www.ncbi.nlm.nih.gov/pubmed/11893817.

World Health Organization. (2003). Framework Convention on Tobacco Control. https://www.who.int/fctc/cop/about/en/ with FCTC Guidelines available from: https://www.who.int/fctc/treaty_instruments/adopted/en/. Accessed 27 Aug 2019.

World Health Organization. (2016). Plain packaging of tobacco products: Evidence, design and implementation. Geneva, World Health Organization. Available from: https://apps.who.int/iris/bitstream/handle/10665/207478/9789241565226_eng.pdf;jsessionid=6F11C5FF4131C1609BC38DA04E54FC65?sequence=1. Accessed 27 Aug 2019.

World Trade Organization. Reports of the panels, Australia – certain measures concerning trademarks, geographical indications and other plain packaging requirements applicable to tobacco products and packaging. WTO docs WT/DS435/R,WT/DS441/R, WT/DS458/R, WT/DS467/R. June 28, 2018. Available from: https://www.wto.org/english/tratop_e/dispu_e/435_441_458_467r_e.pdf. Accessed 27 Aug 2019.

World Health Organization Framework Convention on Tobacco Control; McCabe Centre for Law and Cancer. Challenges in domestic courts to plain (standardized) packaging (WHO FCTC Articles 11 and 13). Available from: https://untobaccocontrol.org/kh/legal-challenges/domestic-courts/plain-packaging/. Accessed 27 Aug 2019.

Plasma Lipid

▶ Lipid

Plasminogen Activator Inhibitor (PAI-1)

Jonathan Newman
Columbia University, New York, NY, USA

Definition

The rupture of an atherosclerotic plaque is a recognized key event in acute ischemic syndromes, such as myocardial infarctions. The intravascular thrombotic response to a ruptured plaque is a complex cascade of thrombogenic (clot-forming) and thrombolytic (clot-dissolving) mechanisms. A key component of the thrombotic cascade is plasminogen activator inhibitor type 1 (PAI-1). PAI-1 inhibits the activation of plasminogen by tissue plasminogen activator (tPA) and urokinase (uPA) and, hence, inhibits clot lysis.

PAI-1 is a single-chain glycoprotein composed of nearly 380 amino acids. It is a member of the serine proteases family and is synthesized by vascular endothelium and smooth muscle cells in both normal and atherosclerotic arteries. By synthesizing molecules like PAI-1, arterial smooth muscle cells can prevent bleeding from small vascular injuries; congenital deficiencies of PAI-1 are a rare cause of abnormal bleeding.

Associations between PAI-1 and incident or recurrent coronary heart disease (CHD) have been demonstrated, but not definitively proven. While circadian variation in PAI-1 levels (highest in the morning) may correlate to circadian patterns of myocardial infarction (highest in the morning), the relationship of PAI-1 to CHD, independent of other prothrombotic risk factors for coronary heart disease, such as diabetes or insulin resistance, has not been clearly shown. Additionally, individuals with specific genetic variations leading to increased PAI-1 production have not been clearly shown to have an increased risk of CHD. Lastly, while important in constitutive pathways of fibrinolysis, it is not clearly known whether the increased PAI-1 expression seen following plaque rupture and thrombosis is a causal pathway or an effect of the inciting event.

References and Readings

Humphries, S. E., Panahloo, A., Montgomery, H. E., Green, F., & Yudkin, J. (1997). Gene-environment interaction in the determination of levels of haemostatic variables involved in thrombosis and fibrinolysis. *Thrombosis and Haemostasis, 78*(1), 457–461.

Juhan-Vague, I., Pyke, S. D., Alessi, M. C., Jespersen, J., Haverkate, F., & Thompson, S. G. (1996). Fibrinolytic factors and the risk of myocardial infarction or sudden death in patients with angina pectoris. ECAT Study Group. European Concerted Action on Thrombosis and Disabilities. *Circulation, 94*(9), 2057–2063.

Lee, M. H., Vosburgh, E., Anderson, K., & McDonagh, J. (1993). Deficiency of plasma plasminogen activator inhibitor 1 results in hyperfibrinolytic bleeding. *Blood, 81*(9), 2357–2362.

Platelet Plug

▶ Fibrinogen

Pleasant Affect

▶ Positive Affectivity

PMD

▶ Primary Care Physicians

Polymorbidity

▶ Comorbidity

Polymorphism

J. Rick Turner
Campbell University College of Pharmacy and Health Sciences, Buies Creek, NC, USA

Definition

The term "polymorphism" refers to a locus with two or more alleles. The translation from Latin is "multiple forms." It is therefore a difference in DNA sequence at a particular locus.

Cross-References

▶ Allele
▶ DNA
▶ Locus
▶ Single Nucleotide Polymorphism (SNP)

References and Further Readings

Britannica. (2009). *The Britannica guide to genetics (Introduction by Steve Jones)*. Philadelphia: Running Press.

Polysomnogram

▶ Polysomnography

Polysomnography

Christopher E. Kline
Department of Health and Physical Activity, University of Pittsburgh, Pittsburgh, PA, USA

Synonyms

Polysomnogram; Sleep study

Definition

Polysomnography is the simultaneous recording of numerous physiological signals during attempted sleep, including activity of the brain, heart, eyes, and muscles. Polysomnography is considered the gold standard for the objective assessment of sleep and diagnosis of many clinical sleep disorders.

Description

Polysomnography (PSG), termed as such because of the multiple physiological signals that are recorded during attempted sleep, has been employed for the characterization of sleep/wake status since the early 1900s. Measurement of brain electrical activity, or electroencephalography (EEG), is the primary physiological signal assessed during PSG. Concurrent measurement of eye movement (electrooculography, or EOG), submentalis muscle activity (electromyography, or EMG), and cardiac activity (electrocardiography, or ECG) is essential for the discrimination of specific stages of sleep. Besides the basic recording montage of EEG, EOG, EMG, and ECG, supplemental measures can be added to PSG for the assessment of respiratory and limb movement activity during sleep (Fig. 1).

Polysomnography is most commonly performed in a sleep laboratory. However, due to digitization of sleep signals, portability of data collection units, and increased data storage capacities, full-scale polysomnography is now able to be performed in the home. Home-based PSG allows for a more

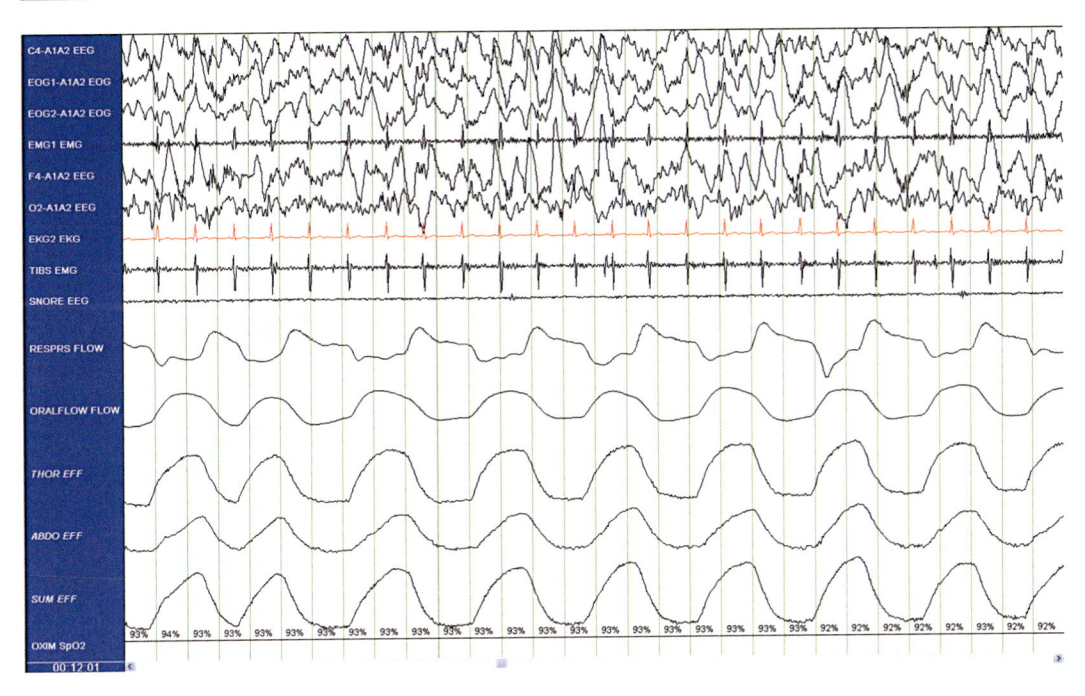

Polysomnography, Fig. 1 A 30-s epoch of a standard clinical polysomnogram. Channels are listed on the left column. Electroencephalographic (C4-A1A2, F4-A1A2, O2-A1A2), electrooculographic (EOG1-A1A2, EOG2-A1A2), and electromyographic (EMG1) channels are shown here and are needed for identification of sleep stages. Additional channels are included here for monitoring leg movements (TIBS; anterior tibialis EMG activity), cardiac activity (EKG2), snoring (SNORE), breathing patterns (RESPRS, nasal pressure; ORALFLOW, oronasal thermistor), respiratory effort (THOR EFF, thoracic effort; ABDO EFF, abdominal effort; SUM EFF, sum of thoracic and abdominal effort channels), and oxyhemoglobin saturation (OXIM SpO2)

ecological assessment of sleep, since patients often report altered sleep due to the artificial sleep laboratory environment (Edinger et al. 2001).

Indications

Polysomnography can be conducted for the objective assessment of sleep for any individual, regardless of whether a sleep disorder is suspected. However, PSG is indicated for the diagnosis of sleep-disordered breathing, narcolepsy, certain types of parasomnias (e.g., seizure disorders), and periodic limb movement disorder (Kushida et al. 2005).

Preparation

Prior to electrode placement, sites should be briefly cleaned with alcohol and an abrasive skin preparation to minimize impedance levels. Electrode cups are then filled with conducting paste and affixed to the proper site with medical tape or electrode paste backed by gauze. Alternatively, some sleep laboratories attach scalp electrodes with collodion glue. Electrode position for the EEG follows the International 10–20 system (Harner and Sannitt 1974). A typical EEG montage for sleep includes bilateral electrodes in the occipital, central, and frontal regions, with bilateral mastoid process electrodes as reference electrodes (Iber et al. 2007).

For the electrooculogram, electrodes should be placed 1 cm lateral to and above the outer canthus of the right eye and 1 cm lateral to and below the outer canthus of the left eye. For the electromyogram, electrodes are placed to assess the activity of the submentalis muscle of the chin; when limb movements need to be assessed, EMG activity of the anterior tibialis is measured with two electrodes on each leg. A basic electrocardiogram lead, with torso electrodes corresponding to right arm and left leg placement, provides an assessment of cardiac activity. When sleep-disordered breathing is suspected, an oronasal thermal sensor and nasal cannula pressure transducer are used to detect airflow, respiratory effort is assessed with either esophageal manometry or (more commonly) inductance plethysmography belts around the thorax and abdomen, and measurement of oxyhemoglobin saturation is obtained with finger pulse oximetry. Sensors that measure snoring intensity and track body position through the night are commonly added to the recording montage.

Recording and Analysis

Following patient preparation, impedance checks and biocalibrations are performed to assure signal quality. Ideally, the electrode impedance for facial and scalp electrodes should not exceed 5 kilohms (Iber et al. 2007). Biocalibrations are a set of instructions delivered to the patient to verify signal quality. Recording system calibration is also undertaken before commencement of the sleep study.

With EEG, EOG, EMG, and ECG, changes in electrical potential are detected from electrodes at the skin surface, with the electrical potential at one site measured in relation to its referent electrode. Physiological signals are amplified, digitized, and then displayed for inspection and analysis. During digitization, signals are sampled at a specific rate (a minimum of 200 Hz is recommended for the recording of EOG, EEG, EMG, and ECG), with low- and high-frequency filter settings used to reduce signal artifact. For EOG, EEG, and EMG, signals are measured and displayed in microvolts, whereas millivolts are used to display ECG signals.

Standardized scoring guidelines for sleep were first established in 1968 (Rechtschaffen and Kales 1968), updated in 2007 (Iber et al. 2007) and continue to be modified periodically (Berry et al. 2018). Separate guidelines for scoring pediatric sleep were included in the 2007 update (Grigg-Damberger et al. 2007; Iber et al. 2007). Sleep stage scoring occurs in 30-s epochs, with each epoch assigned a specific sleep stage that occupies the majority of the epoch.

Electroencephalographic activity is the primary characteristic that distinguishes sleep stages, with EOG and EMG being essential for the detection of rapid eye movement (REM) sleep. In adults, five distinct stages can be scored: wakefulness (W), stage 1 non-REM sleep (N1), stage 2 non-REM sleep (N2), stage 3 non-REM sleep (N3), and REM sleep (R). Stage W is characterized by a predominance of low-voltage, high-frequency EEG (most often alpha and beta frequency) and eye blinks, with elevated chin EMG activity. In stage N1 sleep, alpha EEG activity transitions to slightly lower-frequency EEG (typically theta frequency), often accompanied by slow rolling eye movements, vertex sharp waves (sharply negative, transient waveforms distinguishable from background activity), and an attenuation of chin EMG from stage W. Stage N2 sleep is characterized by the presence of K complexes (high-amplitude biphasic waveforms typically ≥ 0.5 s in duration) or sleep spindles (rhythmic bursts of sigma-frequency EEG for ≥ 0.5 s) over a background of low-voltage, high-frequency EEG, along with a lack of EOG activity and further attenuation of chin EMG activity. Sleep is considered to be stage N3 sleep, also known as slow-wave sleep, when $\geq 20\%$ of an epoch contains slow-wave activity (delta EEG frequency with amplitude >75 μV). Finally, stage R sleep is characterized by low-amplitude, high-frequency EEG activity similar to wakefulness and N1 sleep but with irregular rapid eye movements and minimal chin EMG activity (Iber et al. 2007).

The duration, percentage of total sleep time, and distribution of sleep stages across the night are typically retained for analysis. In addition, typical parameters measured from PSG-scored sleep include sleep onset latency (i.e., the length of time it takes to fall asleep), wakefulness after sleep onset (i.e., the amount of wakefulness that occurs after initially falling asleep), total sleep time (i.e., the total amount of sleep obtained), and sleep efficiency (i.e., the ratio of time spent asleep to the total duration of attempted sleep). In addition to these traditional measures of sleep, quantitative assessment of the sleep EEG is possible, in which the spectral content of the sleep

EEG is decomposed to reveal the power of specific EEG frequency bands (Vasko et al. 1997).

Additional guidelines are present when assessing respiratory events and periodic limb movements (Berry et al. 2018). An apnea is characterized by a $\geq 90\%$ reduction in airflow for at least 10 s. A hypopnea is typically defined as $\geq 30\%$ reduction in airflow for ≥ 10 s with a $\geq 3\%$ decrease in oxyhemoglobin saturation or an arousal, although alternative (older) scoring rules are sometimes used that can significantly impact the total number of hypopneas detected (e.g., $\geq 50\%$ airflow reduction, $\geq 4\%$ oxyhemoglobin desaturation; Hirotsu et al. 2019). An apnea that is accompanied by inspiratory effort is considered to be obstructive, whereas an apnea without inspiratory effort is classified as a central apnea. An apnea that is without inspiratory effort initially but resumes in the latter portion of the event is considered a mixed apnea. Significant leg movements during sleep are characterized by elevated tibialis anterior EMG activity that lasts for 0.5–10 s that is not immediately preceded or followed by a respiratory event (Berry et al. 2018).

Limitations

Despite its recognition as the gold standard for the objective assessment of sleep, there are many situations in which PSG might not be desirable and/or feasible. These include assessment of sleep across multiple nights, 24-h recording of sleep/wake activity, and assessment of a large cohort of patients. Under these conditions, PSG may be excessive in cost, labor, or patient burden. Wrist actigraphy may be an acceptable alternative in these situations.

In addition, the "first night effect" is a well-documented phenomenon in which disturbed sleep is reported when assessed by PSG, presumably due to the discomfort and burden imposed by the numerous wires and electrodes and, if conducted in the laboratory, unfamiliar environment. Although this sleep disturbance has been shown to take multiple nights of PSG recording before resolution in some studies, most address the first night effect by conducting at least two consecutive nights of PSG recording and discarding the data from the first night in subsequent analyses.

Although considered an objective measure of sleep, the scoring of PSG is subject to human influence and therefore some degree of subjectivity. Although most sleep laboratories employ trained polysomnographic technicians to evaluate sleep studies, significant between-technician variation is possible (Rosenberg and Van Hout 2013). Automated sleep stage scoring systems have the potential to remove the variability in manual sleep stage scoring and greatly reduce labor costs, but these are still in development (Sun et al. 2017).

Cross-References

▶ Actigraphy (Wrist, for Measuring Rest/Activity Patterns and Sleep)
▶ Brain Wave
▶ Non-REM Sleep
▶ Quantitative EEG Including the Five Common Bandwidths (Delta, Theta, Alpha, Sigma, and Beta)
▶ REM Sleep
▶ Sleep
▶ Sleep and Health
▶ Sleep Apnea
▶ Sleep Architecture
▶ Slow-Wave Sleep

References and Further Reading

Berry, R. B., Albertario, C. L., Harding, S. M., Lloyd, R. M., Plante, D. T., Quan, S. F., ... Vaughn, B. V. (2018). *The AASM manual for the scoring of sleep and associated events: Rules, terminology and technical specifications (version 2.5)*. Darien: American Academy of Sleep Medicine.

Butkov, N., & Lee-Chiong, T. (Eds.). (2007). *Fundamentals of sleep technology*. Philadelphia: Lippincott Williams & Wilkins.

Edinger, J. D., Glenn, D. M., Bastian, L. A., Marsh, G. R., Daile, D., Hope, T. V., ... Meeks, G. (2001). Sleep in the laboratory and sleep at home II: Comparisons of middle-aged insomnia sufferers and normal sleepers. *Sleep, 24*, 761–770.

Grigg-Damberger, M., Gozal, D., Marcus, C. L., Quan, S. F., Rosen, C. L., Chervin, R. D., ... Iber, C. (2007). The visual scoring of sleep and arousal in infants and children. *Journal of Clinical Sleep Medicine, 3*, 201–240.

Harner, P. F., & Sannitt, T. (1974). *A review of the international ten-twenty system of electrode placement*. Quincy: Grass Instrument Company.

Hirotsu, C., Haba-Rubio, J., Andries, D., Tobback, N., Marques-Vidal, P., Vollenweider, P., ... Heinzer, R. (2019). Effect of three hypopnea scoring criteria on OSA prevalence and associated comorbidities in the general population. *Journal of Clinical Sleep Medicine, 15*, 183–194.

Iber, C., Ancoli-Israel, S., Chesson, A., & Quan, S. F. (2007). *The AASM manual for the scoring of sleep and associated events: Rules, terminology and technical specifications* (1st ed.). Westchester: American Academy of Sleep Medicine.

Keenan, S., & Hirshkowitz, M. (2017). Sleep stage scoring. In M. H. Kryger, T. Roth, & W. C. Dement (Eds.), *Principles and practice of sleep medicine* (6th ed., pp. 1567–1575). Philadelphia: Elsevier.

Kushida, C. A., Littner, M. R., Morgenthaler, T., Alessi, C. A., Bailey, D., Coleman, J., Jr., ... Wise, M. (2005). Practice parameters for the indications for polysomnography and related procedures: An update for 2005. *Sleep, 28*, 499–521.

Rechtschaffen, A., & Kales, A. (Eds.). (1968). *A manual of standardized terminology, techniques and scoring system for sleep stages in human subjects*. Los Angeles: UCLA Brain Information Service/Brain Research Institute.

Rosenberg, R. S., & Van Hout, S. (2013). The American Academy of Sleep Medicine inter-scorer reliability program: Sleep stage scoring. *Journal of Clinical Sleep Medicine, 9*, 81–87.

Sun, H., Jia, J., Goparaju, B., Huang, G. B., Sourina, O., Bianchi, M. T., & Westover, M. B. (2017). Large-scale automated sleep staging. *Sleep, 40*, zsx139.

Vasko, R. C., Jr., Brunner, D. P., Monahan, J. P., Doman, J., Boston, J. R., el-Jaroudi, A., ... Kupfer, D. J. (1997). Power spectral analysis of EEG in a multiple-bedroom, multiple-polygraph sleep laboratory. *International Journal of Medical Informatics, 46*, 175–184.

Polyunsaturated Fats

▶ Fat, Dietary Intake

Polyunsaturated Fatty Acids

▶ Fat: Saturated, Unsaturated

Population Health

Peter A. Hall[1] and Chris Zehr[2]
[1]Faculty of Applied Health Sciences, University of Waterloo, Waterloo, ON, Canada
[2]Department of Health Studies and Gerontology, University of Waterloo, Waterloo, ON, Canada

Definition

Population health is a general approach to assessing and managing health at the level of the whole population. Reduction of healthcare inequities, prevention of illness, and ecological improvement are all central objectives of the population health approach.

Description

Population health is an approach that aims to improve the health of entire population with an emphasis on understanding and decreasing health inequities among groups of people within the population (Hertzman et al. 1994). This approach deviates from a traditional biomedical approach that focuses treatment at an individual level and instead targets group-level phenomena through the implementation of broad-based and widely diffusible health interventions (Jeffery 1989; Rose 1985). Rather than focusing on treating illnesses after they emerge, population health interventions are characterized by a strong emphasis on primary prevention or preventing illness before it develops. As such, modifiable risk factors for illness are a common focus of population health intervention such as smoking, obesity, high blood pressure, physical inactivity, and unhealthy diet as well as preventable disease such as heart disease, stroke, preventable cancers, and diabetes (Wanless 2003).

A defining feature of the population health approach is an emphasis on upstream determinants of illness rather than proximal causes

(Hawe 2007; Link and Phelan 1995). For example, it has been established that cigarette smoking is associated with myriad negative health consequences. A population health approach seeks to elucidate the conditions and factors that put individuals at greater risk of smoking uptake (e.g., low education levels, low income levels, peer group influence). By identifying such upstream determinants of illness, population health interventions are developed to target these.

The population health approach considers health status as a product of a diverse range of factors that include, but are not limited to, individual behavior and lifestyle; biological and genetic factors; early development; the physical, social, and economic environment; and the nature of the healthcare system itself (Evans and Stoddart 1990; Kindig and Stoddart 2003). Rather than viewing these influences as distinct and individual causes of illness and/or health, these and any other health-determining factors are viewed to interact with each other to determine the health status of the population as a whole.

Population health research has highlighted social conditions as a particularly important determinant of health (Link and Phelan 1995; Marmot 2003). Socioeconomic status (SES), a measure of income and social position, has received a significant amount of attention. For example, those living higher on the socioeconomic gradient tend to experience better health outcomes and a longer life expectancy than those lower on the gradient (Hertzman et al. 1994; Lynch et al. 2000). Due to the emphasis on minimizing inequities, a central focus of population health has been to determine the nature of the SES-longevity relationship and how to mitigate it.

Because population health research seeks to impact the greatest number of people possible, interventions based on population health research are often implemented through policy, but also include media campaigns that serve to educate and make individuals aware of certain health-protective behaviors while warning of health-risk behaviors (Hawe 2007). Population health interventions can also be delivered as programming in settings such as schools, churches, and workplaces. Moreover, when considering the diverse array of determinants of health, population health interventions have the potential to span different sectors not traditionally associated with health intervention (i.e., public transportation, education, agriculture, urban planning) to address a particular health issue.

A criticism of the population health approach is that while biomedical approaches to health care provide tailored treatment for individuals with specific health conditions, population health interventions generally work in a broad stroke manner targeting groups of individuals for whom intervention may not be necessary or beneficial. For example, using data from the Framingham Heart Study, Rose (1985) calculated that even a 10 mmHg lowering of the blood pressure distribution of a population could result in 30% reduction in mortality attributed to blood pressure. Though this may be potentially beneficial for the overall health of a population, this may provide little personal benefit to each individual. This has been termed the "prevention paradox" (Rose 1985).

Despite this, Rose (1985) notes that population strategies can be powerful in their influence. Given that population health approaches are concerned with affecting large groups of people, they have the capacity to change social norms so that a health-risk behavior becomes less socially acceptable or, alternatively, that a health-protective behavior becomes more accepted.

Cross-References

▶ Health Promotion
▶ Public Health

References and Further Reading

Evans, R. G., & Stoddart, G. L. (1990). Producing health, consuming health care. *Social Science & Medicine, 31*(12), 1347–1363.

Evans, R. G., Barer, M. L., & Marmor, T. R. (Eds.). (1994). *Why are some people healthy and others are not? The determinants of health of populations*. Hawthorne: Aldine De Gruyter.

Frankish, C. J., Green, L. W., Ratner, P. A., Chomik, T., & Larsen C. (1996). *Health impact assessment as a tool for population health promotion and public policy*. A Report Submitted to the Health Promotion Division of Health Canada. Institute of Health Promotion Research, University of British Columbia.

Glouberman, S., & Miller, J. (2003). Evolution of the determinants of health, health policy, and health information systems in Canada. *American Journal of Public Health, 93*(3), 388–392.

Hawe, P. (2007). What is population health? Retrieved from http://www.ucalgary.ca/PHIRC/pdf/Hawe_2007-PopHealth.pdf.

Health, S. (1999). *A population health framework for Saskatchewan regional health authorities*. Regina: Saskatchewan Health.

Hertzman, C., Frank, J., & Evans, R. G. (1994). Heterogeneities in health status and the determinants of population health. In R. G. Evans, M. L. Barer, & T. R. Marmor (Eds.), *Why are some people healthy and others not?* (pp. 67–92). New York: Walter de Gruyter.

Jeffery, R. W. (1989). Risk behaviors and health: Contrasting individual and population perspectives. *American Psychologist, 44*(9), 1194–1202.

Kindig, D., & Stoddart, G. (2003). What is population health? *American Journal of Public Health, 93*(3), 380–383.

Link, B. G., & Phelan, J. (1995). Social conditions as fundamental causes of disease. *Journal of Health and Social Behavior, 35*, 80–94.

Lynch, J. W., Smith, G. D., Kaplan, G. A., & House, J. S. (2000). Income inequality and mortality: Importance to health of individual income, psychosocial environment, or material conditions. *British Medical Journal, 320*(7243), 1200–1204.

Marmot, M. G. (2003). Understanding social inequalities in health. *Perspectives in Biology and Medicine, 46*(3), S9–S23.

Public Health Agency of Canada. (1996). *Towards a common understanding: Clarifying the core concepts of population health approach*. Discussion paper. Cat. No. H39-391/1996E. ISBN 0-662-25122-9. Retrieved from: http://www.phac-aspc.gc.ca/ph-sp/docs/common-commune/index-eng.php

Rose, G. (1985). Sick individuals and sick populations. *International Journal of Epidemiology, 14*(1), 32–38.

Wanless, D. (2003). *Securing good health for the whole population: Population health trends*. London: HM Treasury.

Population Health Monitoring or Tracking

▶ Mental Health Surveillance

Population Stratification

Abanish Singh
Duke University Medical Center, Durham, NC, USA

Definition

Often an apparently homogenous population group contains subgroups that are genetically distinct. These subgroups may have allele frequency differences due to systematic ancestry differences. Such population structure is known as population stratification.

Description

The mixture of groups of individuals with different allele frequency, i.e., heterogeneous genetic backgrounds, undermines the reliability of association testing results. The assumption of population homogeneity in association studies may not always be true, and violation of the assumption can result in statistical errors. Genetically distinct population subgroups, possibly resulted from interbreeding of two different population groups, can exhibit disequilibrium between pairs of unlinked loci which may create confounding or spurious associations. Therefore, it becomes important to find and quantify genetically distinct subgroups within a population group. Various techniques including principal component analysis have been successfully used to quantify population stratification.

Cross-References

▶ Allele
▶ Gene
▶ Genetics
▶ Genome-Wide Association Study (GWAS)

References and Further Readings

Cardon, L. R., & Palmer, L. J. (2003). Population stratification and spurious allelic association. *The Lancet, 361*, 598–604.

Engelhardt, B. E., & Stephens, M. (2010a). Analysis of population structure: A unifying framework and novel methods based on sparse factor analysis. *PLoS Genetics, 6*(9), 1–12. https://doi.org/10.1371/journal.pgen.1001117. e1001117.

Engelhardt, B. E., & Stephens, M. (2010b). Analysis of population structure: A unifying framework and novel methods based on sparse factor analysis. *PLoS Genetics, 6*, 1–12. e1001117.

Patterson, N., Price, A. L., & Reich, D. (2006). Population structure and eigenanalysis. *PLoS Genetics, 2*(12), 2074–2093. https://doi.org/10.1371/journal.pgen.0020190. e190.

Price, A. L., Patterson, N. J., Plenge, R. M., Weinblatt, M. E., Shadick, N. A., & David, R. (2006). Principal components analysis corrects for stratification in genome-wide association studies. *Nature Genetics, 38*(8), 904–909.

Tiwari, H. K., Barnholtz-Sloan, J., Wineinger, N., Padilla, M. A., Vaughan, L. K., & Allison, D. B. (2008). Review and evaluation of methods correcting for population stratification with a focus on underlying statistical principles. *Human Heredity, 66*, 67–86. https://doi.org/10.1159/000119107.

Wacholder, S., Rothman, N., & Caporas, N. (2000). Population stratification in epidemiologic studies of common genetic variants and cancer: quantification of bias. *Journal of the National Cancer Institute, 92*(14), 1151–1158. https://doi.org/10.1093/jnci/92.14.1151.

Population-Based Study

Roselind Lieb
Department of Psychology, Division of Clinical Psychology and Epidemiology, Basel, Switzerland

Definition

Population-based studies aim to answer research questions for defined populations. Answers should be generalizable to the whole population addressed in the study hypothesis, not only to the individuals included in the study. This point addresses the point of external validity of research findings. Therefore, the valid definition as well as the reliable and valid identification of populations in which research questions for specific populations can be studied is the most important issue in population-based studies.

Population-based studies may include a variety of study types. They may include case-control studies, cross-sectional studies, twin studies, or prospective and retrospective cohort studies. The important issue is the selection of the individuals that are included into the study – they should be representative of all individuals in the a priori defined specific population.

For example, in a population-based prospective cohort study, in which an association between a specific exposure and a specific outcome (i.e., the onset of a certain disease) is studied, all individuals sampled for the study should be representative for the addressed population. This means that the individuals under exposure and non-exposure should be identified within the same population. They should differ only on the exposition factor. Likewise, in a population-based case-control study, cases and controls should be also identified in the same population. Otherwise, differences between cases and controls can be attributed to different population characteristics.

Cross-References

▶ Cohort Study
▶ Follow-Up Study

References and Further Reading

Rothman, K. J., Greenland, S., & Lash, T. L. (2012). *Modern epidemiology* (3rd ed.). Philadelphia: Lippincott Williams & Wilkins.

Susser, E., Schwartz, S., Morabia, A., & Bromet, E. J. (2006). *Psychiatric epidemiology*. Oxford: Oxford University Press.

Szklo, M. (1998). Poplation-based cohort studies. *Epidemiologic Reviews, 20*, 81–90.

Positive Affect

▶ Happiness and Health

Positive Affect Negative Affect Scale (PANAS)

Vincent Tran
Southwestern Medical Center, University of Texas, Dallas, TX, USA

Synonyms

Positive and negative affect schedule

Definition

The Positive and Negative Affect Schedule (PANAS) (Watson et al. 1988) is one of the most widely used scales to measure mood or emotion. This brief scale is comprised of 20 items, with 10 items measuring positive affect (e.g., excited, inspired) and 10 items measuring negative affect (e.g., upset, afraid). Each item is rated on a five-point Likert Scale, ranging from 1 = *Very Slightly or Not at all* to 5 = *Extremely*, to measure the extent to which the affect has been experienced in a specified time frame. The PANAS was designed to measure affect in various contexts such as at the present moment, the past day, week, or year, or in general (on average). Thus, the scale can be used to measure state affect, dispositional or trait affect, emotional fluctuations throughout a specific period of time, or emotional responses to events.

The PANAS is based on a two-dimensional conceptual model of mood, where the full range of affective experiences are reflected along two broad dimensions of positive mood (i.e., extent to which one is experiencing a positive mood such as feelings of joy, interest, and enthusiasm) and negative mood (i.e., extent to which one is generally experiencing a negative mood such as feelings of nervousness, sadness, and irritation). Importantly, the PANAS was developed to provide a brief scale that measures positive and negative affect as separate and largely uncorrelated constructs, such that one can experience both positive and negative emotions simultaneously. Both the positive and negative affect scales have good internal consistency, with Chronbach's alpha $\geq .84$ for each scale across multiple time frames. The scales also demonstrate good convergent and discriminant validity. The two-factor structure of the PANAS has been examined extensively and appears to be robust across different populations and temporal instructions.

Other versions of the PANAS have been developed. The PANAS-X is an extended version of the PANAS that may be used when more discrete measures of specific affective experiences are necessary. The PANAS-X includes 60 items that measure not only the two higher order scales (positive affect and negative affect), but also specific affects (joviality, self-assurance, attentiveness, fear, hostility, guilt, sadness, shyness, fatigue, serenity, and surprise). The I-PANAS-SF (International-PANAS-Short Form) contains 10 items to measure positive and negative affect, and was developed to reduce redundancy or eliminate ambiguous meanings of some of the original PANAS terms. The PANAS-C is a child version of the PANAS; emotion terms were altered and instructions were simplified for use in childhood populations. Finally, the PANAS has also been translated into other languages, such as Japanese and Spanish.

Cross-References

▶ Affect
▶ Emotions: Positive and Negative
▶ Mood

References and Further Readings

Eid, M., & Diener, E. (Eds.). (2006). *Handbook of multi-method measurement in psychology.* Washington, DC: American Psychological Association.

Joiner, T. E., Sandín, B., Chorot, P., Lostao, L., & Marquina, G. (1997). Development and factor analytic validation of the SPANAS among women in Spain: (More) cross-cultural convergence in the structure of mood. *Journal of Personality Assessment, 68,* 600–615.

Kaplan, R. M., & Saccuzzo, D. P. (2008). *Psychological testing: Principles, applications, and issues* (7th ed.). Belmont: Wadsworth.

Laurent, J., Catanzaro, S. J., et al. (1999). A measure of positive and negative affect for children: Scale development and preliminary validation. *Psychological Assessment, 11*(3), 326–338.

McDowell, I. (2006). *Measuring health: A guide to rating scales and questionnaires* (3rd ed.). New York: Oxford University Press.

Thompson, E. R. (2007). Development and validation of an internationally reliable short-form of the positive and negative affect schedule (PANAS). *Journal of Cross-Cultural Psychology, 38*(2), 227–242.

Watson, D., & Clark, L. A. (1994). *The PANAS-X: Manual for the positive and negative affect schedule-expanded form*. Iowa City: University of Iowa.

Watson, D., & Clark, L. A. (1997). The measurement and mismeasurement of mood: Recurrent and emergent issues. *Journal of Personality Assessment, 68*, 267–296.

Watson, D., Clark, L. A., & Tellegen, A. (1988). Development and validation of brief measures of positive and negative affect: The PANAS scales. *Journal of Personality and Social Psychology, 54*(6), 1063–1070.

Positive Affectivity

Katherine T. Fortenberry[1], Kate L. Jansen[2,3] and Molly S. Clark[4]
[1]Department of Family and Preventative Medicine, The University of Utah, Salt Lake City, UT, USA
[2]Behavioral Health, Midwestern University, Glendale, AZ, USA
[3]Department of Family Medicine, University of Mississippi Medical Center, Jackson, MS, USA
[4]Midwestern University College of Health Sciences, Clinical Psychology, Glendale, AZ, USA

Synonyms

Pleasant affect; Positive emotion

Definition

Positive affect can be described as the experience of a set of emotions reflecting pleasurable engagement with the environment. Positive affect reflects neither a lack of negative affect nor the opposite of negative affect, but is a separate, independent dimension of emotion (Watson and Tellegen 1985). It may be exhibited as either a trait-like variable, typically referred to as *positive affectivity*, or as a state-like variable (Watson 2002). Research on positive affectivity has focused on associations with beneficial coping mechanisms, increased cognitive flexibility, and certain health benefits and improved outcomes.

Description

Watson and Tellegen (1985) presented a two-factor model of mood and affect, in which high levels of positive affect reflect enthusiastic, active, and alert mood states. They contrast this to negative affect, which includes aversive mood states, such as anger, guilt, nervousness, and fear. They suggest that a lack of positive affect reflects sadness and lethargy, whereas a lack of negative affect reflects calmness and serenity. Alternately, positive affect has been conceptualized to include positive emotions that reflect both high and low levels of energy and activation, including joy, interest, contentment, and love (Fredrickson 1998; Fredrickson and Losada 2005). Positive affectivity (i.e., the trait-like disposition to experience positive affect) has been found to relate to the personality variable of extraversion (Finch et al. 2012), which is one broad factor in the Five Factor Model of personality. This trait is frequently measured via the Positive and Negative Affect Schedule (PANAS; Watson et al. 1988; see also Tuccito et al. (2010) for more information regarding measurement validation). Lack of positive affect is considered central in the development and maintenance of depressive disorders (Watson et al. 1995); individuals with major depression have more difficulty experiencing and maintaining positive affect in response to a pleasant experience than would an individual without depression (Horner et al. 2014). An effective treatment for depression utilizes behavioral activation to target anhedonia and induce positive experiences, which is thought to increase experience of positive affect (Dimidjian et al. 2011).

Fredrickson's (1998) *broaden and build model* of positive affect posits that positive emotion broadens individuals' awareness, encouraging creative, flexible, and exploratory thoughts and actions. She suggests that positive emotions serve an evolutionary function by expanding physical, intellectual, and social resources, enhancing overall well-being and health. Empirical research finds that individuals with induced positive, but not negative, affect experienced broader scope of attention and more a varied repertoire of potential action (Fredrickson and Branigan 2005). Neuropsychological research has supported positive affect's beneficial influence on cognition. Specifically, positive affect enhances consolidation of long-term memory, working memory, and creative problem solving, potentially via an increase in brain dopamine levels (Ashby et al. 2002).

The influence of positive affectivity on health and health processes has been extensively examined (see Pressman and Cohen 2005). Positive affectivity is consistently and prospectively linked to lower reports of pain, fewer symptoms, and better self-rated heath. Positive affectivity is also associated reduced risk of stroke incidence (Ostir et al. 2001), reduced risk of infection in healthy adults (Cohen et al. 2003), and improved cognitive functioning in older adults (Allerhand et al. 2014). However, less consistent evidence has been found in mortality and survival studies (Freak-Poli et al. 2015). Positive affectivity is thought to influence health either through a main effect model, in which positive affect directly affects physiological processes and/or coping behavior, or through a stress-buffering model, in which positive affectivity influences health by ameliorating potentially harmful influences of stressful life events on health (see Dockrey and Steptoe 2010; Ong et al. 2011).

The research on positive affectivity can be associated with the rise of interest in Positive Psychology, which examines the science of positive human functioning and its association with health outcomes (see Seligman and Csikszentmihalyi 2000; Seligman 2008).

Cross-References

▶ Emotions: Positive and Negative
▶ Negative Affectivity
▶ Positive Affect Negative Affect Scale (PANAS)
▶ Positive Psychology

References and Further Readings

Allerhand, M., Gale, C. R., & Deary, I. J. (2014). The dynamic relationship between cognitive functioning and positive well-being in older people: A prospective study using the English Longitudinal Study of Aging. *Psychology and Aging, 29*, 306–318.

Ashby, F. G., Valentin, V. V., & Turken, A. U. (2002). The effects of positive affect and arousal and working memory and executive attention: Neurobiology and computational models. In S. C. Moore & M. Oaksford (Eds.), *Emotional cognition: From brain to behavior* (pp. 245–287). Amsterdam: John Benjamins Publishing Company.

Cohen, S., Doyle, W. J., Turner, R. B., Alper, C. M., & Skoner, D. P. (2003). Emotional style and susceptibility to the common cold. *Psychosomatic Medicine, 65*, 652–657.

Dimidjian, S., Barrera, M., Martell, C., Munoz, R. F., & Lewinsohn, P. M. (2011). The origin and current status of behavioral activation treatments for depression. *Annual Review of Clinical Psychology, 7*, 1–38.

Dockrey, S., & Steptoe, A. (2010). Positive affect and psychobiological processes. *Neuroscience and Biobehavioral Reviews, 35*, 69–75.

Finch, J. F., Baranik, L. E., Lui, Y., & West, S. G. (2012). Physical health, positive and negative affect, and personality: A longitudinal analysis. *Journal of Research in Personality, 46*, 537–545.

Freak-Poli, R., Mirza, S. S., Franco, O. H., Ikram, M. A., Hofman, A., & Tiemeier, H. (2015). Positive affect is not associated with incidence of cardiovascular disease: A population-based study of older persons. *Preventive Medicine, 74*, 14–20.

Fredrickson, B. L. (1998). What good are positive emotions? *Review of General Psychology, 2*, 300–319.

Fredrickson, B. L., & Branigan, C. (2005). Positive emotions broaden the scope of attention and thought-action repertoires. *Cognition and Emotion, 19*, 313–332.

Fredrickson, B. L., & Losada, M. F. (2005). Positive affect and the complex dynamics of human flourishing. *American Psychologist, 60*, 678–686.

Horner, M. S., Siegle, G. J., Schwartz, R. M., Price, R. B., Haggerty, A. E., Collier, A., & Friedman, E. S. (2014). C'mon get happy: Reduced magnitude and duration of response during a positive-affect induction in depression. *Depression and Anxiety, 31*, 952–960.

Ong, A. D., Mroczek, D. K., & Riffin, C. (2011). The health significance of positive emotions in adulthood and later life. *Social and Personality Psychology Compass, 5*(8), 538–551.

Ostir, G. V., Markides, K. S., Peek, K., & Goodwin, J. S. (2001). The associations of emotional well-being and the incidence of stroke in older adults. *Psychosomatic Medicine, 63*, 210–215.

Pressman, S. D., & Cohen, S. (2005). Does positive affect influence health? *Psychological Bulletin, 131*, 925–971.

Seligman, M. E. P., & Csikszentmihalyi, M. (2000). Positive psychology: An introduction. *American Psychologist, 55*, 5–14.

Seligman, M. E. P. (2008). Positive health. *Applied Psychology: An international review, 57*, 3–18.

Tuccito, D. E., Giacobbi, P. R., & Leite, W. L. (2010). The internal structure of positive and negative affect: A confirmatory factor analysis of the PANAS. *Educational and Psychological Measurement, 70*, 125–141.

Watson, D. (2002). Positive affectivity: The disposition to experience pleasurable emotional states. In C. R. Snyder (Ed.), *Handbook of Positive Psychology* (pp. 106–119). New York: Oxford.

Watson, D., Clark, L. A., & Tellegen, A. (1988). Development and validation of brief measures of positive and negative affect: The PANAS Scales. *Journal of Personality and Social Psychology, 54*, 1063–1070.

Watson, D., & Tellegen, A. (1985). Toward a consensual structure of mood. *Psychological Bulletin, 98*, 219–235.

Watson, D., Weber, K., Assenheimer, J. S., Clark, L. A., Strauss, M. E., & McCormick, R. A. (1995). Testing a tripartite model: I. *Evaluating the convergent and discriminant validity of anxiety and depression symptom scales. Journal of Abnormal Psychology, 104*, 1–14.

Positive Aging

Susan J. (Sue) Ferguson
Department of Psychology, Macquarie University, Sydney, NSW, Australia

Synonyms

Active aging; Proactive aging; Productive aging; Resilient aging

Definition

Positive aging incorporates concepts and research from developmental psychology, gerontology, and positive psychology to understand and improve the health and broader well-being of older adults (usually defined as those over 65 years old). It is the ability to adapt positively to and make the best of the experiences of aging, including maintaining well-being in the face of age-related events and transitions (such as multiple chronic illnesses and disabilities, sensory decline, caregiving duties, and bereavement). The term positive aging developed out of dissatisfaction with the term successful aging, which (at least initially) required the absence of both chronic illnesses and cognitive decline. Many older adults describe themselves as aging successfully despite having chronic illnesses and functional decline, and their own definitions of successful aging include not merely health, but also activity, happiness and contentment, relationships, and independence.

Positive aging thus involves keeping as healthy as possible, while maintaining positive attitudes, and continuing to engage socially and meaningfully in life despite the challenges of aging. As an extension of positive psychology, positive aging emphasizes strengths acquired throughout the life span which help older adults optimize their well-being while dealing with the transitions occurring in later life (Hill and Smith 2015).

Description

Older adults typically report higher levels of subjective well-being (such as positive affect) and lower rates of mental illnesses (except dementia), at least until around age 75 years, compared to other age groups. Thus, a sizable proportion of older adults are aging positively. This higher *positive affect* may contribute to better physical health outcomes through a range of pathways including promoting health behaviors, reducing physiological reactivity to stress, and enhancing recovery from stress. There is promising evidence that positive affect may have its effect on physical health through the immune system and HPA axis and that the effects of these pathways may be strongest among older adults (Ong et al. 2011). Conversely, other evidence suggests that the effects of positive affect on health are most likely bidirectional. Similarly, having high *purpose or meaning in life* is another aspect of positive aging, and predicts a range of health behavior and health outcomes over time, including mortality, health-related quality of life, less frequent heart attacks, and less physical decline in older adults (Krause and Hayward 2012).

Other developmental and positive psychological *strengths* linked to positive aging (e.g., social support, forgiveness, hope and optimism, gratitude, self-compassion, positive attitudes to aging, mindfulness, and wisdom) have also been associated with various measures of physical health (subjective health, health behaviors, functional limitations, physiological measures, and in some cases longevity) in older adults. For example, a review by Westerhof et al. (2014) concluded that subjective aging (how people view their own aging process) had a small but significant effect on health behaviors, health, and even survival. Positive aging constructs are also linked to better quality of life outcomes in those older adults who have chronic illnesses. For example, optimism is associated with improved well-being in individuals diagnosed with cancer, and in cardiovascular disease (CVD) patients, optimism even prospectively predicted fewer readmissions to hospital (Huffman et al. 2016).

Interventions

Several approaches have been taken to enhance the aging experience through psychosocial intervention. One area with promising evidence of potential health improvements is gratitude interventions. For example, in heart failure patients (with a mean age of 66 years), a gratitude journaling intervention led to reduced inflammatory markers and improved heart rate variability responses (Redwine et al. 2016). A review of mindfulness interventions has also demonstrated improvements by alleviating mental symptoms and improving physical functioning in individuals diagnosed with CVD, and chronic pain (Greeson and Chin 2019). While this review was not specific to older adults, encouraging findings from recent small studies (e.g., Perez-Blasco et al. 2016) suggest the findings also apply to this age group. Unfortunately, positive psychology interventions in older adults are still rare and most have not yet been subject to efficacy and effectiveness investigations in terms of physical health outcomes. Qualitative research suggests that wisdom acquired in dealing with other challenges earlier in life helps older adults deal with self-management of new chronic illnesses later in life (Perry et al. 2015). This suggests that health professionals should develop interventions that build on pre-existing skills, rather than assuming that self-management skills or psychosocial resources or strengths need to be taught/developed from scratch.

Cross-References

▶ Aging
▶ Emotions: Positive and Negative
▶ Forgiveness
▶ Gerontology
▶ Hope
▶ Optimism
▶ Positive Psychology
▶ Successful Aging
▶ Well-Being

References and Further Reading

Greeson, J. M., & Chin, G. R. (2019). Mindfulness and physical disease: a concise review. *Current Opinion in Psychology, 28*, 204–210. https://doi.org/10.1016/j.copsyc.2018.12.014.

Hill, R. D., & Smith, D. J. (2015). Positive aging: At the crossroads of positive psychology and geriatric medicine. In P. A. Lichtenberg, B. T. Mast, B. D. Carpenter, & J. Loebach Wetherell (Eds.), *APA handbook of clinical geropsychology, vol 1: History and status of the field and perspectives on aging* (pp. 301–329). Washington, DC: American Psychological Association.

Huffman, J. C., Beale, E. E., Celano, C. M., Beach, S. R., Belcher, A. M., Moore, S. V., ... Januzzi, J. L. (2016). Effects of optimism and gratitude on physical activity, biomarkers, and readmissions after an acute coronary syndrome.: The gratitude research in acute coronary events study, *Circulation: Cardiovascular Quality and Outcomes, 9*(1), 55–63. https://doi.org/10.1161/circoutcomes.115.002184.

Krause, N., & Hayward, D. (2012). Religion, meaning in life, and change in physical functioning during late adulthood. *Journal of Adult Development, 19*, 158–169. https://doi.org/10.1007/s10804-012-9143-5.

Ong, A. D., Mroczek, D. K., & Riffin, C. (2011). The health significance of positive emotions in adulthood and later life. *Social and Personality Psychology Compass, 5*(8), 538–551. https://doi.org/10.1111/j.1751-9004.2011.00370.x.

Perez-Blasco, J., Sales, A., Meléndez, J. C., & Mayordomo, T. (2016). The effects of mindfulness and self-compassion on improving the capacity to adapt to stress situations in elderly people living in the community. *Clinical Gerontologist, 39*(2), 90–103. https://doi.org/10.1080/07317115.2015.1120253.

Perry, T. E., Ruggiano, N., Shtompel, N., & Hassevoort, L. (2015). Applying Erikson's wisdom to self-management practices of older adults: Findings from two field studies. *Research on Aging, 37*(3), 253–274. https://doi.org/10.1177/0164027514527974.

Redwine, L. S., Henry, B. L., Pung, M. A., Wilson, K., Chinh, K., Knight, B., . . . Mills, P. J. (2016). Pilot randomized study of a gratitude journaling intervention on heart rate variability and inflammatory biomarkers in patients with stage B heart failure. *Psychosomatic Medicine, 78*(6), 667–676. https://doi.org/10.1097/PSY.0000000000000316.

Westerhof, G. J., Miche, M., Brothers, A. F., Barrett, A. E., Diehl, M., Montepare, J. M., . . . Wurm, S. (2014). The influence of subjective aging on health and longevity: A meta-analysis of longitudinal data. *Psychology & Aging, 29*(4), 793–802. https://doi.org/10.1037/a0038016.

Positive and Negative Affect

▶ Emotions: Positive and Negative

Positive and Negative Affect Schedule

▶ Positive Affect Negative Affect Scale (PANAS)

Positive By-Products

▶ Perceived Benefits

Positive Changes

▶ Perceived Benefits

Positive Emotion

▶ Happiness and Health
▶ Positive Affectivity

Positive Emotions

▶ Well-Being: Physical, Psychological, and Social

Positive Meaning

▶ Perceived Benefits

Positive Psychology

Lisa G. Aspinwall[1] and Watcharaporn Pengchit[2]
[1]Department of Psychology, The University of Utah, Salt Lake City, UT, USA
[2]Faculty of Psychology, Chulalongkorn University, Bangkok, Thailand

Definition

Positive psychology, the scientific study of positive phenomena from the neurobiology of positive emotions to application in the clinic and in everyday life, encompasses multiple efforts to understand and promote well-being and health (Aspinwall and Staudinger 2003; Aspinwall and Tedeschi 2010; Lopez and Snyder 2009; Ryff and Singer 1998; Seligman and Csikszentmihalyi 2000). Key elements include (a) the identification of human strengths (qualities and processes that allow people to navigate adversity, pursue their goals, and make the most of life) and (b) empirical research directed toward understanding the diverse conditions that create and sustain such strengths. These processes have been investigated in a wide variety of domains, including education, social development, close relationships, aging, work, and health.

Description

Core Concerns of Positive Psychology and Health

Positive psychology is an active and growing field, with thousands of published articles in the last decade, two major handbooks, a new *Encyclopedia of Positive Psychology*, a specialized journal (the *Journal of Positive Psychology*), and several edited volumes, journal special issues, and international conferences devoted to this topic. Within this voluminous literature, there are three main areas that examine the relationship of positive phenomena to physical health: (a) psychological adaptation to illness, (b) the impact of positive phenomena, such as positive mood, optimism, and hope, on physical health, and (c) interventions that use insights from this research to improve well-being in general and among people managing serious illness.

Understanding Psychological Adaptation to Illness

Multiple lines of research have examined the impact of negative life events, including serious illness, on people's beliefs about themselves, the benevolence of others, personal control, and views of the future. In general, research suggests that people who have experienced serious illness or other forms of adversity frequently report *both* positive and negative life changes. Frequently reported positive changes include a better sense of one's values and priorities, stronger social relationships, and an enhanced appreciation for life. Negative changes include fears for the future and feelings of personal vulnerability. Such changes are understood by many researchers to be the product of active efforts to manage and derive meaning and/or benefit from one's circumstances (Folkman 2011; Taylor 1983). Exciting developments in this line of research have related finding meaning and/or benefit to subsequent physical health outcomes, such as immune function (Park et al. 2009; Taylor et al. 2000).

As exciting as these findings are, it is important to understand their boundary conditions. In particular, not all events produce benefits or growth or do so for all people. Some particularly challenging events (severe interpersonal stressors, wartime experiences) seem to defy meaning-making coping. Further, large-scale longitudinal panel studies of life satisfaction following long-term unemployment and divorce suggest that people may not, on average, fully adjust to these events. Finally, there appear to be multiple "normal" responses to adversity. A recent advance in this area – made possible by rigorous prospective longitudinal studies of bereavement (Bonanno 2004) – is the recognition that there may be multiple trajectories of mental health outcomes following adversity, with many respondents reporting stable good or even improving outcomes and a subset of respondents reporting either enduring preexisting distress or new elevations in distress. These different patterns of adjustment over time highlight the need to understand the antecedents and processes that account for them. The finding that there is considerable variation in response to adversity also suggests that global positive outcomes (e.g., "Cancer was the best thing that ever happened to me") may be true for some people, but may grossly misrepresent the experiences of others.

Understanding the Relation of Positive Phenomena to Physical Health

Although most research in positive psychology focuses on psychological well-being, there is increasing interest in the relation of such concepts as optimism, hope, positive affect, gratitude, benefit finding, and growth to physical health. Several recent meta-analyses suggest that positive phenomena show a reliable prospective beneficial relationship to multiple health outcomes, including longevity, in both healthy and ill samples (Diener and Chan 2011; Howell et al. 2007;

Pressman and Cohen 2005; Rasmussen et al. 2009). Importantly, this relationship is (a) not explained by the detrimental effects of either negative emotions or pessimistic expectations and (b) comparable in magnitude to that of these more widely studied negative phenomena. At present, the findings seem to be stronger for healthy samples than among people managing illness, and the strength of the findings varies by disease, with stronger and more encouraging findings for cardiovascular disease and HIV than for cancer mortality.

Researchers have examined multiple complementary pathways through which positive phenomena are related to health outcomes (Aspinwall and Tedeschi 2010). Five sets of pathways are shown in Fig. 1. The first set of pathways involves direct relations to neuroendocrine and immune functions implicated in the etiology and progression of disease, as well as physiological reactivity to laboratory stressors. A second and third set of pathways involve the relation of positive phenomena to multiple aspects of attending to, appraising, and coping with health-risk information and the demands of serious illness, including the benefit-finding and meaning-making processes described earlier. A fourth set of pathways involves the relationship between positive phenomena and the development and maintenance of supportive social ties, especially during times of illness or other adversity. The fifth pathway represents the relationship of positive phenomena to the practice of preventive health behaviors, such as good nutrition, exercise, and sleep; the decreased practice of risk behaviors, such as substance abuse; and improved medical adherence.

Recent findings from the Women's Health Initiative illustrate the multiple pathways through which positive phenomena may influence health outcomes. In an 8-year prospective study of coronary heart disease in a sample of more than 97,000 US women, ages 50–79 (Tindle et al. 2009), dispositional optimism was found to prospectively predict decreased risk for coronary heart disease and all-cause mortality in the overall

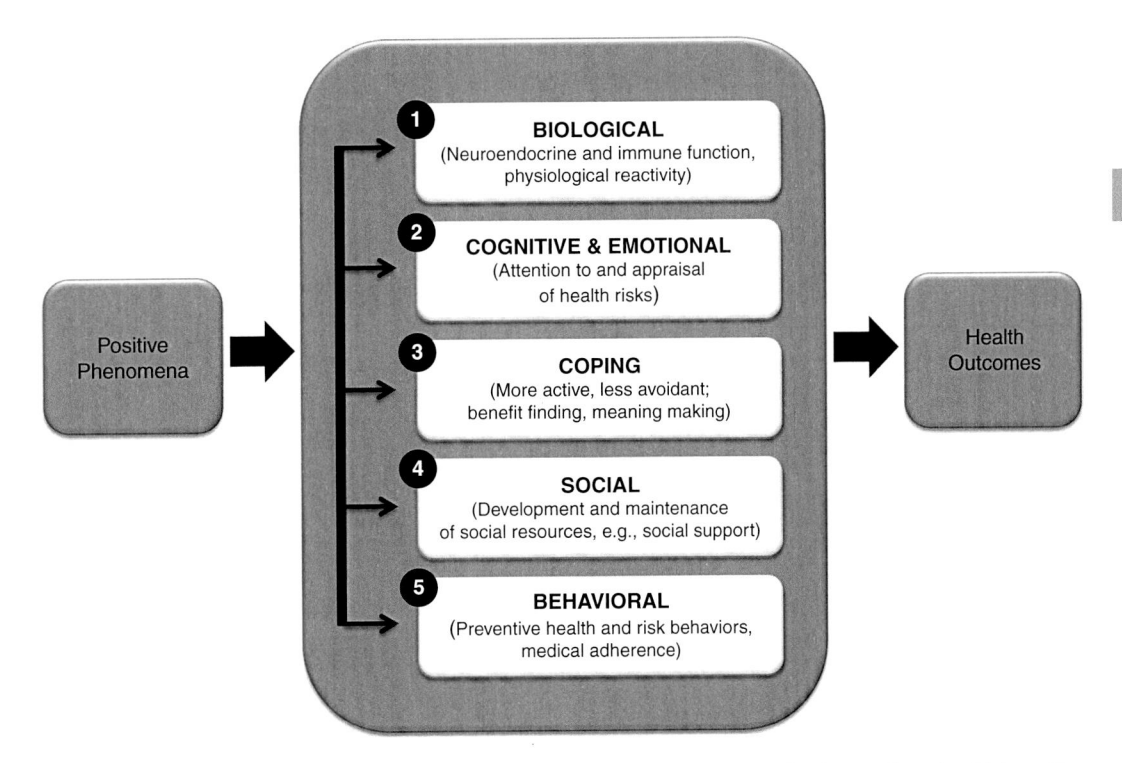

Positive Psychology, Fig. 1 Five mutually interactive and complementary sets of pathways through which positive phenomena, such as positive mood and optimism, may influence human health

sample. Optimism also predicted lower cancer-related mortality for African-American women, but not Caucasian women. Compared to pessimists, optimists were less likely to have diabetes, hypertension, high cholesterol, or depressive symptoms; they were less likely to smoke, be sedentary, or be overweight; and they reported higher education and income, greater employment and health insurance, and greater religious attendance. However, the real kicker is that controlling for *all* of the above factors, optimism still predicted better health outcomes. These findings suggest that there is much that remains to be understood about the relationship of positive beliefs to important health outcomes and that the multiple pathways outlined in Fig. 1 and described in the following sections may be implicated in such findings.

1. *Biological pathways*. At present, more is known about the prospective relationship of positive phenomena to diverse health outcomes than about the specific pathways through which these outcomes are realized. Most studies have focused on cardiovascular, neuroendocrine, and immune function. Both experimental laboratory studies and field experiments link the induction of positive self-beliefs to reduce cardiovascular and neuroendocrine reactivity to evaluative stressors and to more rapid recovery from induced negative states among healthy young adults. Recent reviews link optimism to improved immune function, both among healthy people managing naturalistic stressors such as law school entry and among people managing HIV infection. These lines of research have also identified some potential short-term physiological costs associated either with optimists' active coping efforts or with the relatively intense positive affect inductions used to study physiological outcomes in laboratory settings (Pressman and Cohen 2005). However, these authors also noted that these costs were not seen in naturalistic ambulatory studies where positive affect was associated with health-protective responses. Many researchers have attributed the health-protective findings of optimism and positive mood to reductions in perceived stress, highlighting the importance of such appraisals in understanding how positive phenomena are related to health outcomes.

2. *Attention to and appraisal of threatening health information*. In contrast to the idea that being happy or optimistic reduces awareness of negative realities (e.g., seeing one's world through "rose-colored glasses"), several experiments have demonstrated that induced positive affect or positive self-beliefs (e.g., through self-affirmation or success manipulations) promote constructive attention to negative information about health risks and personal weaknesses when the information is relevant to the self and said to be useful (Aspinwall and Tedeschi 2010). Similar findings have been obtained for dispositional optimism. Interestingly, this greater attention to negative information does not appear to be in the service of downplaying its negativity or relevance to the self, but instead appears to be strongly responsive to its potential value in warding off or managing future negative events. The ability to adaptively confront, manage, and remember such information may have beneficial links to both coping and health behavior.

3. *Coping with serious illness*. A large literature suggests that positive affect and optimism promote constructive methods of coping with adversity, involving planning, information-seeking, suppression of competing activities, and seeking both instrumental and emotional social support (Aspinwall and Tedeschi 2010). Notably, positive beliefs are consistently inversely associated with deleterious forms of avoidant coping, such as denial, mental and behavioral disengagement, and substance use. Researchers have argued that the tendency toward active, engaged forms of coping with adversity shown in pathway #3 and the ability to attend to negative information shown in pathway #2 may work together to promote a more informed understanding of actual or potential stressors. The term "upward spiral" has been used to characterize such processes.

4. *Development and maintenance of social resources.* Recent meta-analytic evidence suggests that positive affect plays a major role in the maintenance of satisfying social relationships (Lyubomirsky et al. 2005). Specifically, people who report frequent positive affect also report a greater number of – and more satisfying – social relationships. Similarly, college students who reported greater optimism on arrival to college reported both greater initial friendship network size and greater increases in perceived social support over the course of their first semester, and these social ties buffered distress at the end of the semester. Existing evidence suggests that there may be more at work in such findings than the idea that it is pleasant to be around people in a good mood. People in a good mood seem better able to understand the goals and priorities of their interaction partners, to express more gratitude, and to be more likely to help others than people in a neutral mood. These particular processes suggest that an important direction for future research and intervention might be to examine these processes among people managing illnesses and other demands such as caregiving that are known to tax social resources over time.

5. *Health behaviors and medical adherence.* An emerging literature suggests that positive beliefs and states are robust prospective predictors of better health behavior, including diet, exercise, and sleep, and lower practice of risk behaviors, such as substance abuse (Aspinwall and Tedeschi 2010). These findings have been obtained both in healthy community samples, including large samples of older adults, and among people managing serious illnesses, such as HIV infection. In contrast, prospective studies link negative beliefs, such as pessimism and fatalism, to the practice of a wide range of health-risk behaviors, including substance abuse and high-risk sexual behavior. Understanding how positive beliefs like hope and optimism are related to the practice of inherently forward-looking behaviors, like preventive health behavior, remains an important research question. Researchers are also starting to examine how positive phenomena may be related to behavior change and medical adherence. Although it is well known that negative affect and interpersonal stressors contribute to relapse from behavior change efforts in multiple domains, the question of whether and how positive phenomena may have facilitative effects needs further investigation. With respect to medical adherence, randomized controlled trials of interventions in hospital settings demonstrate that increasing patients' optimism about the success of cardiac rehabilitation improves outcomes like angina symptoms and return to work.

Summary and Remaining Conceptual Questions. This section outlined five sets of pathways through which positive feelings and beliefs may influence physical health. These multiple pathways are complementary, rather than competing, and are likely to work in concert (Aspinwall and Tedeschi 2010). Specifically, the ability to maintain attention to negative information about health risks may work in tandem with more active forms of coping that are more likely to elicit information about one's situation and support for managing it. Similarly, finding benefits and growth in one's experience and maintaining supportive social ties may each be related to subsequent health behaviors in important ways. Research that examines the interplay of these different pathways will likely yield not only a more complex account of the ways in which positive phenomena may be linked to human health but also an understanding of some of the cumulative benefits that may result.

Interventions to Promote Health and Well-Being

Interventions derived from the principles and pathways reviewed here have been employed to promote well-being in healthy samples, as well as psychosocial adjustment to chronic illness (Folkman 2011; Park et al. 2009). For example, a burgeoning literature on the kinds of experiences that make people happy and the processes that contribute to hedonic adaptation both to positive and negative events have been usefully employed in interventions to improve daily positive affect, primarily in healthy samples. For people living with chronic illnesses like diabetes, various interventions ranging from writing about one's positive experiences to multiple-component programs have proved effective in enhancing positive affect, at least in laboratory settings. Experimental interventions to increase hope and gratitude have also been shown to improve reported pain tolerance and physical symptoms, respectively. Finally, although they were not conducted under the rubric of positive psychology, psychosocial interventions to provide social support and reduce stress among people managing serious illness suggest that such interventions reliably reduce pain and anxiety and improve quality of life (Aspinwall and Tedeschi 2010; Park et al. 2009). Understanding how the various pathways suggested here may be implicated in such effects – and used to enhance them – among people managing serious illness remains an important goal for future research.

Controversies with Respect to Both Theory and Application

The study of how positive phenomena – especially positive thinking – are related to health has generated both academic and cultural controversies (Aspinwall and Staudinger 2003; Aspinwall and Tedeschi 2010; Becker and Marecek 2008; Lazarus 2003). Researchers have questioned whether the focus on positive or optimal human functioning is new or sufficiently distinctive or developed to merit a special name as a new field; whether separating positive phenomena from negative phenomena is practicable, desirable, or meaningful (e.g., coping with adversity may inherently involve both); and whether the field focuses too much on the individual as the unit of analysis at the neglect of important social, cultural, economic, structural, and environmental determinants of health and well-being. With respect to positive psychology and health, critics have questioned (a) whether the field is too narrowly focused on individual positive feelings and self-beliefs as the primary outcomes of optimal human functioning; (b) whether the promotion of positive thinking among those managing serious illness may be trivial, distracting, and ultimately useless; and (c) whether positive thinking might actually be actively harmful if it impairs attention to negative aspects of experience or contributes to a culture of blame for individual misfortune.

Several critics (as well as the present authors) have traced the history of these ideas to the New Thought movement and subsequent popular efforts to promote health, well-being, and financial success through positive thinking (e.g., *The Power of Positive Thinking, The Secret*; see Aspinwall and Tedeschi 2010, for discussion). With respect to the application of positive psychology to understanding health and illness, a primary concern – reflected more in critiques of the popular self-help literature on positive thinking than in scientific discourse on these issues – is the potential misuse of findings suggesting that positive emotions and beliefs may predict physical health and recovery from illness. Specifically, the demonstration that a positive attitude (e.g., optimism or hope) is linked to better health outcomes for some people in some situations may create, or be used to promote, unrealistic expectations about the ability to cure disease through positive thinking. Similarly, the demonstration that some people with serious illness report benefits and growth can be misconstrued to suggest that all people should do so, all of the time and regardless of circumstance. These pressures to maintain uniformly positive thoughts and feelings and to ascribe deteriorating health to failures of positive attitude have been described as "saccharine terrorism" and the "tyranny of optimism." While researchers have in general been quite careful not to mandate positive feelings among people dealing with adversity (and in fact have documented the presence of both positive and negative life changes and multiple trajectories of adjustment), various popular treatments have promoted the notion that an exclusive focus on positive thoughts and feelings will cure illness. Some critics aptly note that this approach is particularly prevalent – and pernicious – in popular treatments of cancer survivorship (Aspinwall and Tedeschi 2010).

Conclusion

As scientific research on the relationship of positive phenomena to health proceeds, rigorous process-oriented research should dispel the notion that there is some kind of magic bullet to be found in positive thinking. Continued examination of the multiple biological, cognitive, emotional, social, and behavioral pathways linking positive phenomena to health is essential. Further, researchers interested in a balanced understanding of the link between positive phenomena and health outcomes should continue to design studies that are sensitive to both potential benefits and liabilities of particular kinds of positive (and negative) thoughts and feelings in different situations (Aspinwall and Staudinger 2003; Aspinwall and Tedeschi 2010). Indeed, what the study of health and illness has to offer positive psychology is the opportunity to examine the multiple ways in which positive and negative phenomena may go hand in hand as people manage serious illness and its treatment.

Cross-References

▶ Adherence
▶ Aging
▶ Behavior Change
▶ Benefit Finding
▶ Bereavement
▶ Cancer Survivorship
▶ Cardiac Rehabilitation
▶ Cardiovascular Disease
▶ Coping
▶ Coronary Heart Disease
▶ Denial
▶ Diabetes
▶ Exercise
▶ Fatalism
▶ Hypertension
▶ Immune Function
▶ Longevity
▶ Meta-analysis
▶ Mortality
▶ Nutrition
▶ Optimism
▶ Overweight
▶ Perceived Benefits
▶ Pessimism
▶ Physiological Reactivity
▶ Sexual Risk Behavior
▶ Sleep
▶ Stressor
▶ Substance Abuse
▶ Well-Being

References and Readings

Aspinwall, L. G., & Staudinger, U. M. (Eds.). (2003). *A psychology of human strengths: Fundamental questions and future directions for a positive psychology.* Washington, DC: APA Books.

Aspinwall, L. G., & Tedeschi, R. G. (2010). The value of positive psychology for health psychology: Progress and pitfalls in examining the relation of positive phenomena to health. *Annals of Behavioral Medicine, 39,* 4–15.

Becker, D., & Marecek, J. (2008). Dreaming the American dream: Individualism and positive psychology. *Social and Personality Psychology Compass, 2,* 1767–1780.

Bonanno, G. A. (2004). Loss, trauma, and human resilience: Have we underestimated the human capacity to thrive after extremely aversive events? *American Psychologist, 59,* 20–28.

Diener, E., & Chan, M. Y. (2011). Happy people live longer: Subjective well-being contributes to health and longevity. *Applied Psychology: Health and Well-being, 3*(1), 1–43.

Folkman, S. (Ed.). (2011). *The Oxford handbook of stress, health, and coping.* New York: Oxford University Press.

Howell, R. T., Kern, M. L., & Lyubomirsky, S. (2007). Health benefits: Meta-analytically determining the impact of well-being on objective health outcomes. *Health Psychology Review, 1,* 1–54.

Lazarus, R. S. (2003). Does the positive psychology movement have legs? *Psychological Inquiry, 14,* 93–109.

Lopez, S. J., & Snyder, C. R. (Eds.). (2009). *Oxford handbook of positive psychology* (2nd ed.). New York: Oxford University Press.

Lyubomirsky, S., King, L., & Diener, E. (2005). The benefits of frequent positive affect: Does happiness lead to success? *Psychological Bulletin, 131,* 803–855.

Park, C. L., Lechner, S. C., Antoni, M. H., & Stanton, A. L. (Eds.). (2009). *Medical illness and positive life change.* Washington, DC: American Psychological Association.

Pressman, S. D., & Cohen, S. (2005). Does positive affect influence health? *Psychological Bulletin, 131,* 925–971.

Rasmussen, H. N., Scheier, M. F., & Greenhouse, J. B. (2009). Optimism and physical health: A meta-analytic review. *Annals of Behavioral Medicine, 37*, 239–256.

Ryff, C. D., & Singer, B. (1998). The contours of positive human health. *Psychological Inquiry, 9*, 1–28.

Seligman, M. E. P., & Csikszentmihalyi, M. (2000). Positive psychology: An introduction. *American Psychologist, 55*, 1–54.

Taylor, S. E. (1983). Adjustment to threatening events: A theory of cognitive adaptation. *American Psychologist, 38*, 1161–1173.

Taylor, S. E., Kemeny, M. E., Reed, G. M., Bower, J. E., & Gruenewald, T. L. (2000). Psychological resources, positive illusions, and health. *American Psychologist, 55*, 99–109.

Tindle, H. A., Chang, Y.-F., Kuller, L. H., Manson, J. E., Robinson, J. G., et al. (2009). Optimism, cynical hostility, and incident coronary heart disease and mortality in the women's health initiative. *Circulation, 120*, 656–662.

Positron Emission Tomography (PET)

▶ Brain, Imaging
▶ Neuroimaging

Post Traumatic Stress Disorder

Cortney Taylor Zimmerman[1], Whitney M. Herge[2] and Annette M. La Greca[3]
[1]Department of Pediatrics, Baylor College of Medicine/Texas Children's Hospital, Houston, FL, USA
[2]Department of Psychology, Texas Scottish Rite Hospital for Children, Dallas, TX, USA
[3]Department of Psychology, University of Miami, Miami, FL, USA

Definition (and Description)

A majority of adolescents have been exposed to a potentially traumatic event in their lifetime (61.8%; McLaughlin et al. 2013), and a significant percentage of trauma-exposed youth develop post-traumatic stress disorder (PTSD) (Alisic et al. 2014). PTSD is a debilitating condition that is associated with several poor mental and physical health outcomes. As such, it is imperative to understand the development and course of PTSD, including its prevalence, comorbid conditions, assessment, treatment, and prognosis.

Diagnostic Criteria

PTSD is listed under trauma- and stressor-related disorders in the DSM-5 (American Psychiatric Association 2013). Criteria for diagnosis includes (A) direct or indirect *exposure* to actual or threatened death, serious injury, or sexual violence as well as symptoms from the following clusters; (B) one or more *intrusion* symptoms following the event; (C) persistent *avoidance* of stimuli (i.e., memories, thoughts, feelings, or external reminders) associated with the traumatic event; (D) two or more indications or *negative alterations* in cognition and mood; and (E) two or more symptoms of marked alterations in *arousal and reactivity* following the event (APA DSM-5 2013, pp. 271–272). The disturbances in criteria B-E must last more than 1 month. These symptoms must cause clinically significant distress or impaired functioning in the individual and cannot be accounted for by another disorder.

Some of these criteria represent a change from DSM-IV-TR (American Psychiatric Association 2010). For example, criterion A expanded to include direct and *indirect* exposure to trauma. The other criteria expanded as well to include (B) *intrusion*, (C) *avoidance* of stimuli, (D) two or more indications or *negative alterations* in cognition and mood, and (E) two or more symptoms of marked alterations in *arousal and reactivity* following the event.

Further, the DSM-5 accounts for the differences in symptom presentation between young children (6 years and younger) and older children and adults who experience PTSD. Criterion A changed to reflect direct exposure, in-person witnessing of the event, and learning the event occurred to a *parent or caregiving figure*. Within Category B (intrusion), DSM-5 notes that children may have *repetitive play* reflecting the traumatic event, or trauma-specific *reenactment during play*, whereas adults may have recurrent, involuntary, or intrusive memories of the event. Category C was modified for young children to reflect *both the avoidance and the negative alterations* in cognitions (which are Categories C and D in older children and adults). Further, DSM-5 specifies a different number of symptoms required to meet criteria for children than adults. For example, children are required to evidence one or more symptoms of avoidance or negative alterations in cognitions, whereas adults are required to exhibit one symptom of avoidance and two symptoms of negative alterations in cognitions. Importantly, studies suggest that the DSM-5 criteria for young children also may be a good fit for preadolescent youth and identify about twice as many children with PTSD as the adult-based criteria (Danzi and La Greca 2017). Also noteworthy is the fact that DSM-5 and the new ICD-11 criteria identify different children as meeting criteria for PTSD (La Greca et al. 2017).

Prevalence

Prevalence rates for PTSD vary greatly depending on the severity, type, and length of exposure or repeated exposure to traumatic events, as well as other demographic factors (Alisic et al. 2014). In the United States, 62% of adolescents surveyed reported experiencing at least one traumatic event, and 19% reported experiencing three or more traumatic events (McLaughlin et al. 2013). Reported lifetime DSM-IV PTSD prevalence in the same sample was 4.7% and was higher among females than males (McLaughlin et al. 2013). Recent meta-analyses suggest that 15.9% of trauma-exposed youth develop post-traumatic stress disorder (PTSD) and the rate is twice as high in girls as in boys (Alisic et al. 2014). Also, rates of PTSD are typically highest with events that involve interpersonal violence, such as sexual abuse or the unexpected death of a loved one (Alisic et al. 2014; Kessler et al. 2017). Per the APA, US Latinos, African Americans, and American Indians tend to have higher rates of PTSD than US non-Latino whites. Lower SES, lower education, and childhood adversity such as family dysfunction or parental separation are all risk factors for development of PTSD following a traumatic event.

Course of Disorder over Time

Individuals who experience PTSD symptoms less than 1 month from the traumatic event may meet criteria for a diagnosis of acute stress disorder; if symptoms persist for more than 1 month, then the diagnosis is changed to PTSD. Child physical or sexual abuse is often associated with a more chronic course of PTSD from childhood through adulthood. Finally, individuals who initially present with subsyndromal PTSD, but meet the full criteria at six months or more posttrauma, are considered to have PTSD *with delayed expression*. Some resilient individuals present with only a few symptoms of traumatic stress that never reach clinical thresholds and remit over time.

Common Comorbidities

People with PTSD are 80% more likely than those without PTSD to have symptoms that meet criteria for at least one other mental disorder (APA 2013). Further, 70–90% of the time, PTSD has been found to be comorbid with at least one other disorder in adolescents (Fan et al. 2011) and young children (Scheeringa et al. 2003). Depression, anxiety, and substance use are common comorbid diagnoses (Bonanno et al. 2010). Substance use disorder and conduct disorder are more common among males than females. Among young children, oppositional defiant disorder and separation anxiety disorder are the most common comorbidities (APA 2013).

It is unclear whether PTSD plays a casual role in the development of additional comorbid conditions or whether preexisting psychological conditions predispose a person to develop

PTSD following a trauma (Perrin et al. 2000). In one study with adult flood survivors, authors concluded PTSD lead to some psychiatric disorders (McMillen et al. 2002), and that concept was replicated in another study with young children following a hurricane (Scheeringa and Zeanah 2008). It is also possible that a broader underlying factor leads to the development of both PTSD and other conditions, which would account for the high rate of comorbidity (Perrin et al. 2000). Additional research is necessary to better understand the directionality of these comorbid relationships, which would also advance the conceptualization and treatment of PTSD.

Measures

There are several measures used in the assessment and diagnosis of PTSD in children and adults. The type of measure chosen depends on many factors, including the availability of a trained clinician, the individual's time and presenting condition(s), and the cost of the measure.

Clinician-administered interviews are the most thorough tools available and include (1) the Structured Clinical Interview for DSM-5 (Clinician Version), used with adolescents and adults (SCID-5-CV; First et al. 2016), and (2) the Kiddie-Schedule for Affective Disorders and Schizophrenia, used with children and adolescents and revised to be compatible with DSM-5 diagnoses (K-SADS-PL DSM-5; Kaufman et al. 2016). Each of these interviews includes a PTSD-specific module for assessing the presence of a traumatic event and any resulting symptoms required for diagnosis (American Psychiatric Association 2013). Although clinician-administered interviews are the most thorough diagnostic tool, they are also the most time-consuming as well as the most expensive option.

Self-report measures of PTSD for adults include the PTSD Checklist for DSM-5 (PCL-5; Weathers et al. 2013). For school-aged children and adolescents, the Child PTSD Symptom Scale for DSM-5 (CPSS-5; Foa et al. 2018) and the UCLA PTSD Reaction Index for DSM-5 (PTSD-RI-5; Steinberg and Beyerlein 2014) are the most widely used measures. Although these measures are easy to administer and do not require a trained clinician, the measures provide only a screening for elevated PTSD symptoms and require follow-up evaluations for a formal diagnosis.

Treatment and Prognosis

Several treatment options are available for individuals with PTSD. Trauma-focused cognitive behavioral therapy (TF-CBT) for children and adults has the strongest evidence as an effective treatment; prolonged exposure is also effective for adults and promising for youth (Courtois et al. 2017; La Greca and Danzi 2019). Eye movement desensitization and reprocessing (EMDR) is probably efficacious for adults and youth with PTSD (Courtois et al. 2017; Diehle et al. 2015; La Greca and Danzi 2019). Trauma and Grief Component Therapy for Adolescents (TGCTA) is another newer therapy option with strong initial support (Saltzman et al. 2017). Another treatment option, sometimes utilized in conjunction with psychotherapy, is medication. However, there is not strong research support for utilization of SSRIs or SNRIs, especially in children (La Greca and Danzi 2019).

Typically, PTSD symptoms decline substantially over the first year posttrauma (Bonanno et al. 2010), after which symptoms are chronic and further declines are more gradual (e.g., La Greca et al. 2010; Shaw et al. 1996). The prognosis for individuals with PTSD varies greatly depending on whether the individual has any comorbid conditions, their level of social support, or whether they have received treatment. Individuals with comorbid conditions (such as depression or substance use), poor social support, and who do not seek treatment have a poorer prognosis than those without these concerns. For individuals who do receive treatment, some evidence a decrease in symptoms after only four sessions of CBT, while others may require a longer course of treatment (Foa et al. 2008).

References and Further Reading

Alisic, E., Zalta, A. K., van Wesel, F., Larsen, S. E., Hafstad, G. S., Hassanpour, K., & Smid, G. E. (2014). Rates of post-traumatic stress disorder in trauma-exposed children and adolescents: Meta-analysis. *The British Journal of Psychiatry, 204*, 335–340.

American Psychiatric Association. (2010). DSM-5 development. Downloaded from http://www.dsm5.org/ProposedRevisions/Pages/proposedrevision.aspx?rid=165

American Psychiatric Association. (2013). *Diagnostic and statistical manual of mental disorders* (5th ed.). Arlington: American Psychiatric Association.

Bisson, J., & Andrew, M. (2007). Psychological treatment of post-traumatic stress disorder (PTSD). *Cochrane Database of Systematic Reviews, 3*, CD003388. https://doi.org/10.1002/14651858.CD003388.pub3.

Bonanno, G. A., Brewin, C. R., Kaniasty, K., & La Greca, A. M. (2010). Weighing the costs of disaster: Consequences, risks, and resilience in individuals, families, and communities. *Psychological Science in the Public Interest, 11*(1), 1–49. https://doi.org/10.1177/1529100610387086.

Cohen, J. A., Berliner, L., & Mannarino, A. (2010). Trauma focused CBT for children with co-occurring trauma and behavior problems. *Child Abuse and Neglect, 34*, 215–224.

Copeland, W. E., Keeler, G., Angold, A., & Costello, E. J. (2007). Traumatic events and posttraumatic stress in childhood. *Archives of General Psychiatry, 64*, 577–584.

Costello, E. J., Erkanli, A., Fairbank, J. A., & Angold, A. (2002). The prevalence of potentially traumatic events in childhood and adolescence. *Journal of Traumatic Stress, 15*, 99–112.

Courtois, C. A., Sonis, J., Brown, L. S., Cook, J., Fairbank, J. A., & Friedman, M. et al. (2017). Clinical practice guidelines for the treatment of posttraumatic stress disorder (PTSD) in adults. Retrieved from https://www.apa.org/ptsd-guideline/ptsd.pdf

Danzi, B. A., & La Greca, A. M. (2017). Optimizing clinical thresholds for PTSD: Extending the DSM-5 preschool criteria to school-age children. *International Journal of Clinical and Health Psychology, 17*(3), 234–241. https://doi.org/10.1016/j.ijchp.2017.07.001.

Diehle, J., Opmeer, B. C., Boer, F., Mannarino, A. P., & Lindauer, R. J. (2015). Trauma-focused cognitive behavioral therapy or eye movement desensitization and reprocessing: what works in children with post-traumatic stress symptoms? A randomized controlled trial. *European Journal of Child and Adolescent Psychiatry, 24*(2), 227–236.

Fan, F., Zhang, Y., Yang, Y., Mo, L., & Liu, X. (2011). Symptoms of posttraumatic stress disorder, depression, and anxiety among adolescents following the 2008 Wenchuan earthquake in China. *Journal of Traumatic Stress, 24*(1), 44–53.

First, M. B., Williams, J. B., Karg, R. S., & Spitzer, R. L. (2016). *Structured clinical interview for DSM-5 disorders-clinician version (SCID-5-CV)*. Arlington: American Psychiatric Association Publishing.

Foa, E. B., Johnson, K. M., Feeny, N. C., & Treadwell, K. R. (2001). The child PTSD symptom scale: A preliminary examination of its psychometric properties. *Journal of Clinical Child Psychology, 30*(3), 376–384. https://doi.org/10.1207/S15374424JCCP3003_9.

Foa, E. B., Keane, T. M., Friedman, M. J., & Cohen, J. (Eds.). (2008). *Effective treatments for PTSD: practice guidelines from the International Society for Traumatic Stress Studies* (2nd ed.). New York: Guilford Press.

Foa, E. B., Asnaani, A., Zang, Y., Capaldi, S., & Yeh, R. (2018). Psychometrics of the child PTSD symptom scale for *DSM-5* for trauma-exposed children and adolescents. *Journal of Clinical Child & Adolescent Psychology, 47*(1), 38–46. https://doi.org/10.1080/15374416.2017.1350962.

Kaufman, J., Birmaher, B., Brent, D., Rao, U., Flynn, C., Moreci, P., et al. (1997). Schedule for affective disorders and schizophrenia for school-age children-present and lifetime version (K-SADS-PL): Initial reliability and validity data. *Journal of the American Academy of Child and Adolescent Psychiatry, 36*, 980–988.

Kaufman, J., Birmaher, B., Axelson, D., Perepletchikova, F., Brent, D., & Ryan, N. (2016). K-SADS-PL DSM-5. Retrieved from https://www.kennedykrieger.org/sites/default/files/library/documents/faculty/ksads-dsm-5-screener.pdf

Kessler, R. C., Aguilar-Gaxiola, A., Alonso, J., Benjet, C., Bromet, E. J., Cardoso, G., ... Koenen, K. C. (2017). Trauma and PTSD in the WHO world mental health surveys. *European Journal of Psychotraumatology, 8*(5). https://doi.org/10.1080/20008198.2017.1353383

La Greca, A. M., & Danzi, B. A. (2019). Posttraumatic stress disorder. In M. J. Prinstein, E. A. Youngstrom, E. J. Mash, & R. A. Buckley (Eds.), *Treatment of childhood disorders* (4th ed.). New York: Guilford Press.

La Greca, A. M., Silverman, W., Lai, B., & Jaccard, J. (2010). Hurricane-related exposure experiences and stressors, other life events, and social support: Concurrent and prospective impact on children's persistent posttraumatic stress. *Journal of Consulting and Clinical Psychology*, (6), 78. https://doi.org/10.1037/a0020775.

La Greca, A. M., Taylor, C. J., & Herge, W. (2012). Traumatic stress disorders in children and adolescents. In G. Beck & D. Sloan (Eds.), *Oxford handbook of traumatic stress disorders*. Oxford: Oxford University Press.

La Greca, A. M., Danzi, B. A., & Chan, S. F. (2017). DSM-5 and ICD-11 as competing models of PTSD in preadolescent children exposed to a natural disaster: Assessing validity and co-occurring symptomatology. *European Journal of Psychotraumatology, 8*(1), 1310591. https://doi.org/10.1080/20008198.2017.1310591.

McLaughlin, K. A., Koenen, K. C., Hill, E. D., Petukhova, M., Sampson, N. A., Zaslavsky, A. M., & Kessler, R. C. (2013). Trauma exposure and posttraumatic stress

disorder in a national sample of adolescents. *Journal of the American Academy of Child and Adolescent Psychiatry, 52*(8), 815–830.e14.
McMillen, C., North, C., Mosley, M., & Smith, E. (2002). Untangling the psychiatric comorbidity of post-traumatic stress disorder in a sample of flood survivors. *Comprehensive Psychiatry, 43*(6), 478–485.
Perrin, S., Smith, P., & Yule, W. (2000). Practitioner review: The assessment and treatment of post-traumatic stress disorder in children and adolescents. *Journal of Child Psychology and Psychiatry, 41*(3), 277–289.
Saltzman, W. R., Layne, C. M., Pynoos, R. S., Olafson, E., Kaplow, J. B., & Boat, B. (2017). *Trauma and grief component therapy for adolescents: A modular approach to treating traumatized and bereaved youth*. Cambridge: Cambridge University Press.
Scheeringa, M. S., & Zeanah, C. H. (2008). Reconsideration of harm's way: Onsets and comorbidity patterns of disorders in preschool children and their caregivers following Hurricane Katrina. *Journal of Clinical Child and Adolescent Psychology, 37*(3), 508–518.
Scheeringa, M. S., Zeanah, C. H., Myers, L., & Putnam, F. W. (2003). New findings on alternative criteria for PTSD in preschool children. *Journal of the American Academy of Child and Adolescent Psychiatry, 42*(5), 561–560.
Shaw, J. A., Applegate, B., & Schorr, C. (1996). Twenty-one-month follow-up study of school-age children exposed to Hurricane Andrew. *Journal of the American Academy of Child and Adolescent Psychiatry, 35*, 359–364.
Steinberg, A. M. & Beyerlein, B. (2014). UCLA PTSD reaction index: DSM-5 version. Retrieved from http://www.nctsn.org/nctsn_assets/pdfs/mediasite/ptsd-training.pdf
Steinberg, A. M., Brymer, M. J., Decker, K. B., & Pynoos, R. S. (2004). The University of California at Los Angeles post-traumatic stress disorder reaction index. *Current Psychiatry Reports, 6*(2), 96–100.
Weathers, F. W., Litz, B. T., Keane, T. M., Palmieri, P. A., Marx, B. P., & Schnurr, P. P. (2013). The PTSD checklist for DSM-5 (PCL-5). Scale available from the National Center for PTSD at www.ptsd.va.gov

Posterior Hypothalamic Area

▶ Hypothalamus

Postpartum Blues

▶ Postpartum Depression

Postpartum Depression

Michele L. Okun
Department of Psychology, University of Colorado Colorado Springs, Colorado Springs, CO, USA

Synonyms

Major depressive disorder; Postpartum blues

Definition

Postpartum depression is moderate to severe depression in a woman after she has given birth. It may occur soon after delivery or up to a year later. Most of the time, it occurs within the first 3 months after delivery.

Description

Major depressive disorder with a postpartum onset (PPMD) is a prevalent and serious disorder. Postpartum major depression (PPMD) is moderate to severe depression in a woman after she has given birth, clinically resembling major depression as described in DSM-IV. Feelings of anxiety, irritation, tearfulness, and restlessness are common in the week or two after pregnancy. These feelings are often called the postpartum blues or "baby blues." These symptoms almost remit without the need for treatment. Postpartum depression may occur when the baby blues do not fade away or when signs of depression start 1 or more months after childbirth. Up to 20% of women will have an initial major depressive episode within the first 3-month postpartum (Gavin et al. 2005; O'Hara and Wisner 2014), with the risk of suffering recurrent postpartum major depression (PPMD) at about 25% (Wisner et al. 2004) and up to 49.9% of indigent women (Mayberry et al. 2007). Women are at the highest risk during their lifetimes for depressive episodes during the childbearing years (O'Hara et al. 1990).

PPMD is considered a serious public health concern (Gaynes et al. 2005; Wisner et al. 2006). The maternal role, which is vital to the infant's safety, survival, and well-being (Logsdon et al. 2006), can be compromised by PPMD and result in impaired maternal-infant bonding. Children of mothers with PPMD are at an increased risk of impaired mental and motor development, poor self-regulation, and behavior problems (Moehler et al. 2006). Postpartum depression and its consequences can persist from months to years after childbirth, with lingering limitations in physical and psychological functioning after recovery from depressive episodes (Burt and Stein 2002; Marcus and Heringhausen 2009; McCarter-Spaulding and Horowitz 2007).

A myriad of factors contribute to the etiology of both incident and recurrent PPMD (Beck 2001; Bloch et al. 2003; Gaynes et al. 2005). Among the established risk factors, previous episodes of depression, family history of depression, and depressive symptomatology during pregnancy (O'Hara et al. 1991a, b) are the strongest predictors for both incident and recurrent episodes. Demographic variables, including marital status, race, age, and socioeconomic status, have also been implicated as risk factors (Beck 2001; Ross et al. 2006). Unfortunately, these recognized risk factors have proven inadequate at predicting which women will have a recurrent episode. Other risk factors that have been identified include the following: (1) age below 20 years; (2) currently abusing alcohol, taking illegal substances, or smoking (these also cause serious medical health risks for the baby); (3) having an unplanned pregnancy, or have mixed feelings about the pregnancy; (4) a stressful event during the pregnancy or delivery, including personal illness, death or illness of a loved one, a difficult or emergency delivery, premature delivery, or illness or birth defect in the baby; (5) little support from family, friends, or the significant other.

Disturbed sleep during late pregnancy represents another potential risk factor for PPMD. Several investigators report that disturbed sleep is a prodromal symptom of both first onset and recurrent depressive symptoms and/or episodes outside of the postpartum (Ford and Kamerow 1989) as well as during the postpartum (Coble et al. 1994; Wolfson et al. 2003). Okun and colleagues showed that poor sleep quality in late pregnancy (Okun et al. 2009) as well as in the first 8 weeks postpartum (Okun et al. 2011) significantly contributed to recurrent PPMD. Wolfson and colleagues noted that women reporting more sleep disturbances in late pregnancy are more likely to have clinically significant depressive symptomatology at 2–4 weeks postpartum than those with few sleep disturbances (Wolfson et al. 2003). Coble and colleagues found that women with a history of depression had more sleep disturbances throughout pregnancy and into the postpartum than women without a history of depression (Coble et al. 1994). Taken together, these findings suggest that sleep disturbances in late pregnancy increase vulnerability to PPMD, particularly in women who are susceptible, such as those with a history of PPMD (Wisner et al. 2002).

There are two identified biological systems attributed to have an effect on the risk of developing PPMD. First are endocrine factors. Hormones such as progesterone, estradiol, prolactin, and cortisol peak during the last few weeks of pregnancy, followed by a drastic drop in their levels following delivery and into the early postpartum period (Abou-Saleh et al. 1998). Dramatic drops in hormone concentrations, especially progesterone and the estrogens, likely contribute to postpartum depression (Abou-Saleh et al. 1998; Bloch et al. 2003); however, their specific role is unclear. Administration of estrogens to postpartum women appears to reduce depressive symptoms (Dennis 2004). However, the dramatic reduction in concentrations of gonadal steroids after delivery does not lead to PPMD in all women (Bloch et al. 2003).

The second pathway involves alterations in the cytokine milieu (Bloch et al. 2003; Maes et al. 2000). The "cytokine hypothesis of depression" states that both the etiology and pathophysiology of depression are linked to dysregulation of inflammatory cytokines (Maes 1994). Puerperal women may be particularly vulnerable because inflammatory cytokines increase significantly during the last trimester of pregnancy in preparation for delivery (Romero et al. 2006). Women who report increased depressive symptoms in pregnancy and the postpartum have corresponding higher levels of proinflammatory cytokines (Maes et al. 2000; Okun et al. 2013).

PPMD is a significant health concern. While there is no single test to diagnose PPMD, it is imperative for a woman to be evaluated if there is any indication that she has signs of depression or risk for depression. This will buttress not only her own mental and physical health but the health of her baby.

Cross-References

▶ Antidepressant Medications
▶ Women's Health

References and Further Reading

Abou-Saleh, M. T., Ghubash, R., Karim, L., Krymski, M., & Bhai, I. (1998). Hormonal aspects of postpartum depression. *Psychoneuroendocrinology, 23*, 465–475.

Beck, C. T. (2001). Predictors of postpartum depression: An update. *Nursing Research, 50*, 275–285.

Bloch, M., Daly, R. C., & Rubinow, D. R. (2003). Endocrine factors in the etiology of postpartum depression. *Comprehensive Psychiatry, 44*, 234–246.

Burt, V. K., & Stein, K. (2002). Epidemiology of depression throughout the female life cycle. *Journal of Clinical Psychiatry, 63*(Suppl 7), 9–15.

Coble, P. A., Reynolds, C. F., Kupfer, D. J., Houck, P. R., Day, N. L., & Giles, D. E. (1994). Childbearing in women with and without a history of affective disorder. II. Electroencephalographic sleep. *Comprehensive Psychiatry, 35*, 215–224.

Dennis, C. L. (2004). Preventing postpartum depression. Part I: A review of biological interventions. *Canadian Journal of Psychiatry, 49*(7), 467–475.

Ford, D. E., & Kamerow, D. B. (1989). Epidemiologic study of sleep disturbances and psychiatric disorders. An opportunity for prevention? *Journal of the American Medical Association, 262*, 1479–1484.

Gavin, N. I., Gaynes, B. N., Lohr, K. N., Meltzer-Brody, S., Gartehner, G., & Swinson, T. (2005). Perinatal depression: A systematic review of prevalence and incidence. *Obstetrics and Gynecology, 106*(5 Pt 1), 1071–1083.

Gaynes, B. N., Gavin, N., Meltzer-Brody, S., et al. (2005). Perinatal depression: Prevalence, screening accuracy, and screening outcomes. *Evidence Report/Technology Assessment, 119*, 1–8.

Logsdon, M. C., Wisner, K. L., & Pinto-Foltz, M. D. (2006). The impact of postpartum depression on mothering. *Journal of Obstetric, Gynecologic, and Neonatal Nursing, 35*, 652–658.

Maes, M. (1994). Cytokines in major depression. *Biological Psychiatry, 36*(7), 498–499.

Maes, M., Lin, A. H., Ombelet, W., et al. (2000). Immune activation in the early puerperium is related to postpartum anxiety and depressive symptoms. *Psychoneuroendocrinology, 25*, 121–137.

Marcus, S. M., & Heringhausen, J. E. (2009). Depression in childbearing women: When depression complicates pregnancy. *Primary Care, 36*, 151–165.

Mayberry, L. J., Horowitz, J. A., & Declercq, E. (2007). Depression symptom prevalence and demographic risk factors among U.S. women during the first 2 years postpartum. *Journal of Obstetric, Gynecologic, and Neonatal Nursing, 36*, 542–549.

McCarter-Spaulding, D., & Horowitz, J. A. (2007). How does postpartum depression affect breastfeeding? *American Journal of Maternal/Child Nursing, 32*, 10–17.

Moehler, E., Brunner, R., Wiebel, A., Reck, C., & Resch, F. (2006). Maternal depressive symptoms in the postnatal period are associated with long-term impairment of mother–child bonding. *Archives of Women's Mental Health, 9*(5), 273–278.

O'Hara, M. W., Zekoski, E. M., Philipps, L. H., & Wright, E. J. (1990). Controlled prospective study of postpartum mood disorders: Comparison of childbearing and nonchildbearing women. *Journal of Abnormal Psychology, 99*, 3–15.

O'Hara, M. W., Schlechte, J. A., Lewis, D. A., & Varner, M. W. (1991a). Controlled prospective study of postpartum mood disorders: Psychological, environmental, and hormonal variables. *Journal of Abnormal Psychology, 100*, 63–73.

O'Hara, M. W., Schlechte, J. A., Lewis, D. A., & Wright, E. J. (1991b). Prospective study of postpartum blues: Biologic and psychosocial factors. *Archives of General Psychiatry, 48*, 801–806.

O'Hara, M. W. & Wisner, K. L. (2014). Perinatal mental illness: definition, description and aetiology. Best. Pract. Res. Clin. Obstet. Gynaecol., 28, 3–12.

Okun, M. L., Hanusa, B. H., Hall, M., & Wisner, K. L. (2009). Sleep complaints in late pregnancy and the recurrence of postpartum depression. *Behavioral Sleep Medicine, 7*, 106–117.

Okun, M. L., Luther, J., Prather, A. A., Perel, J. M., Wisniewski, S., & Wisner, K. L. (2011). Changes in sleep quality, but not hormones predict time to postpartum depression recurrence. *Journal of Affective Disorders, 130*, 378–384.

Okun, M. L., Luther, J., Wisniewski, S., & Wisner, K. L. (2013). Disturbed sleep and inflammatory cytokines in depressed and nondepressed pregnant women: An exploratory analysis of pregnant outcomes. *Psychosomatic Medicine, 75*, 1–13.

Romero, R., Espinoza, J., Goncalves, L. F., Kusanovic, J. P., Friel, L. A., & Nien, J. K. (2006). Inflammation in preterm and term labour and delivery. *Seminars in Fetal and Neonatal Medicine, 11*(5), 317–326.

Ross, L. E., Campbell, V. L., Dennis, C. L., & Blackmore, E. R. (2006). Demographic characteristics of participants in studies of risk factors, prevention, and treatment of postpartum depression. *Canadian Journal of Psychiatry, 51*, 704–710.

Wisner, K. L., Parry, B. L., & Piontek, C. M. (2002). Clinical practice. Postpartum depression. *New England Journal of Medicine, 347*, 194–199.

Wisner, K. L., Perel, J. M., Peindl, K. S., & Hanusa, B. H. (2004). Timing of depression recurrence in the first year after birth. *Journal of Affective Disorders, 78*(3), 249–252.

Wisner, K. L., Chambers, C., & Sit, D. K. (2006). Postpartum depression: A major public health problem. *Journal of the American Medical Association, 296*, 2616–2618.

Wolfson, A. R., Crowley, S. J., Anwer, U., & Bassett, J. L. (2003). Changes in sleep patterns and depressive symptoms in first-time mothers: Last trimester to 1-year postpartum. *Behavioral Sleep Medicine, 1*, 54–67.

Posttraumatic Growth

Vincent Tran
Southwestern Medical Center, University of Texas, Dallas, TX, USA

Synonyms

Adversarial growth; Benefit finding; PTG; Stress-related growth; Transformational coping

Definition

Posttraumatic growth is the experience of positive change after a traumatic or negative life event. It is theorized to be the positive or adaptive outcome of a meaning-making process in which individuals are forced into a reevaluation process of their worldviews after experiencing a negative or life-changing event. Through this reevaluation process, some individuals may develop a more coherent understanding of themselves and the world. Common examples of growth after trauma include changes in life values, improved relationships with family and/or friends, growth in spiritual beliefs, and increased personal strength, empathy, or patience.

Description

The concept of growth from adversity is an ancient concept based in many religions and philosophical systems. However, it has been a formal focus of investigation in psychology only in the past few decades, coinciding with the development of psychometrically sound measures and the rise of positive psychology. The fields of health psychology and behavioral medicine, in particular, have latched onto the notion that one may experience positive change in response to adversity, including the adversity of coping with serious health threats and illnesses. For example, research on posttraumatic growth has been carried out in chronic illness populations such as patients with heart disease, cancer, rheumatoid arthritis, HIV/AIDS, and multiple sclerosis. It has also been studied in the context of veterans of war, victims of violence, bereavement, and family members/caregivers of those experiencing a negative life event.

Posttraumatic growth is conceptually very similar to benefit finding and stress-related growth, and these terms are often used interchangeably in the research literature. Multiple measures have been developed, which have facilitated the rigorous study of posttraumatic growth and related constructs. These scales include: benefit finding (Mohr et al. 1999; Tomich and Helgeson 2004); Stress-Related Growth Scale (Park et al. 1996); and the Posttraumatic Growth Inventory (Tedeschi and Calhoun 1996). Posttraumatic growth is differentiated from concepts such as resilience and hardiness, in which one may cope or adjust well in response to stress rather than experience positive transformation and an *improvement* in functioning, quality of life, or worldview. Posttraumatic growth is also conceptually differentiated from optimism because it reflects a change in experience rather than a dispositional trait, although the two constructs have been shown to be correlated.

Posttraumatic growth has been associated with adaptive coping processes including heightened problem-focused coping, social-support seeking, acceptance and positive reinterpretation, optimism, religion, cognitive processing, and positive affect. It has often been associated with better illness adjustment and health outcomes, less depression, and more positive well-being in chronic illness populations. Although the prevalence of posttraumatic growth varies widely from study to study, numerous studies suggest a majority of research participants endorse some type of growth from a negative or traumatic event.

Although research suggests that posttraumatic growth is associated with improved functioning and quality of life, there have been conflicting reports. Some studies report nonsignificant or even negative correlations between posttraumatic growth and well-being. These inconsistencies have driven researchers to more rigorously test proposed theories of posttraumatic growth and better clarify the processes by which posttraumatic growth occurs. More meticulous study has led to investigation of non-transformational change, mediators, moderators, and study of curvilinear associations between posttraumatic growth and well-being. Further elaboration on the theory of posttraumatic growth has led to studies on whether posttraumatic growth is the outcome of a series of life changes that have occurred or whether it is a cognitive process of reevaluation and understanding that unfolds over time. Researchers are also investigating whether posttraumatic growth reflects genuine changes in one's life (veridical growth) or whether it reflects perceptions of change or growth (non-veridical growth). Some have suggested that non-veridical growth may even reflect a maladaptive, defensive denial process, although others claim that perceptions of growth that do not reflect true life changes may promote well-being in response to a traumatic event.

Cross-References

▶ Benefit Finding
▶ Coping
▶ Defensiveness
▶ Hardiness
▶ Optimism
▶ Positive Psychology
▶ Perceived Benefits
▶ Resilience

References and Reading

Affleck, G., & Tennen, H. (1996). Construing benefits from adversity: Adaptational significance and dispositional underpinnings. *Journal of Personality, 64*(4), 899–922.

Calhoun, L. G., & Tedeschi, R. G. (Eds.). (2006). *Handbook of posttraumatic growth: Research & practice*. Mahwah: Lawrence Erlbaum.

Helgeson, V. S., Reynolds, K. A., & Tomich, P. L. (2006). A meta-analytic review of benefit finding and growth. *Journal of Consulting and Clinical Psychology, 74*(5), 797–816.

Joseph, S., & Linley, P. A. (Eds.). (2008). *Trauma, recovery, and growth: Positive psychological perspectives on posttraumatic stress*. Hoboken: Wiley.

Linley, P. A., & Joseph, S. (2004). Positive change following trauma and adversity: A review. *Journal of Traumatic Stress, 17*(1), 11–21.

Lopez, S. J., & Snyder, C. R. (Eds.). (2009). *Oxford handbook of positive psychology* (2nd ed.). New York: Oxford University Press.

Mohr, D. C., Dick, L. P., Russo, D., Pinn, J., Boudewyn, A. C., Likosky, W., et al. (1999). The psychosocial impact of multiple sclerosis: Exploring the patient's perspective. *Health Psychology, 18*(4), 376–382.

Park, C. L., & Helgeson, V. S. (2006). Growth following highly stressful life events: Current status and future directions. *Journal of Consulting and Clinical Psychology, 74*(5), 791–796.

Park, C. L., Cohen, L. H., & Murch, R. L. (1996). Assessment and prediction of stress-related growth. *Journal of Personality, 64*, 71–105.

Park, C. L., Lechner, S. C., Antoni, M. H., & Stanton, A. L. (Eds.). (2009). *Medical illness and positive life change: Can crisis lead to personal transformation?* Washington, DC: American Psychological Association.

Tedeschi, R. G., & Calhoun, L. G. (1996). The posttraumatic growth inventory: Measuring the positive legacy of trauma. *Journal of Traumatic Stress, 9*(3), 455–471.

Tedeschi, R. G., & Calhoun, L. G. (2004). Target article: Posttraumatic growth: Conceptual foundations and empirical evidence. *Psychological Inquiry, 15*(1), 1–18.

Tedeschi, R. G., Park, C. L., & Calhoun, L. G. (Eds.). (1998). *Posttraumatic growth: Positive changes in the aftermath of crisis*. Mahwah: Lawrence Erlbaum.

Tomich, P. L., & Helgeson, V. S. (2004). Is finding something good in the bad always good? Benefit finding among women with breast cancer. *Health Psychology, 23*, 16–23.

Potential Years of Life Lost (PYLL)

▶ Life Years Lost

Power Spectral Analysis

▶ Quantitative EEG Including the Five Common Bandwidths (Delta, Theta, Alpha, Sigma, and Beta)

Practice Guideline

▶ Clinical Practice Guidelines

Praise

▶ Prayer

Prayer

Donna C. Burdzy and Kenneth Pargament
Department of Psychology, Bowling Green State University, Bowling Green, OH, USA

Synonyms

Meditation; Praise; Supplication; Thanksgiving; Worship

Definition

Prayer in all of its variations can be defined by two fundamental principles: (1) prayer is a form of communication and (2) the exchange of communication takes place between the self and the transcendent, immanent, and numinous forces that represent human notions of the sacred. Defining prayer in this way broadens William James' classic conceptualization of prayer as "every kind of inward communion or conversation with the power recognized as divine" to include not only that which comes from God but everything that is imbued with the power of sacredness.

Description

Throughout history, humankind has manifested a yearning to communicate with the sacred through prayer. Expressed in vastly different cultures and religious traditions, prayer constitutes a universal phenomenon that plays a crucial role in humanity's religious experience. In fact, for many individuals, prayer is their primary religious practice.

Prayer, in the theocentric Judaic, Christian, and Islamic religious traditions, represents a way to express thanks to God, participate in God's will, and move closer to God. From a theocentric perspective, prayer is, simply put, communication with God. Prayer, however, is not limited to God-centered religions; it also features prominently in the practices of nontheistic religious traditions such as Zen and Theravada Buddhism, Jainism, and Taoism as well as animistic and pantheistic belief systems such as Shinto and the indigenous religions that feature the worship of nontheistic spiritual entities. Secular individuals without religious affiliations or theistic beliefs also pray regularly in a variety of ways.

Types of Prayer

Scholars have devised a number of classification schemes in an attempt to impose some order on the extraordinarily diverse modes of prayer expression. Traditional descriptive typologies have focused on the reasons people pray as well as on the content of prayers. Gill (1994) classified prayers according to their intent: petition, invocation, thanksgiving, dedication, supplication, intercession, confession, penitence, and benediction prayers. Heiler (1932) proposed a rich typology to capture the "astonishing multiplicity" of the forms of prayer: primitive; ritual; Hellenistic; philosophical; personal; mystical; prophetic; the prayers of great religious personalities; the prayers of great men, poets, and artists; prayer in public worship; and prayer as a law of duty and good works.

More recently, researchers have developed typologies by asking people what they pray about, when they pray, why they pray, and to whom or what they pray. Ladd and Spilka (2002) proposed a threefold scheme which distinguishes among recipients of prayer. Inward prayer is directed toward one's inner self, outward prayer represents a connection with another human, and upward prayer signifies sacred communication with the divine. Poloma and Pendleton (1991) classified prayer in terms of four concise categories. Petitionary prayer involves requests to fulfill one's own spiritual or material needs or those of others by asking for guidance, forgiveness, and physical well-being. Meditative prayer involves thinking about the divine, communicating with the sacred, or merely being in the presence of the sacred. Ritual prayer involves silent or verbal recitation of specific religious texts or mantras from memory or by reading scripture. Colloquial prayer, which takes the form of a conversation between individuals and their God or divine figure, may blend aspects of petitionary and meditative prayer. Poloma and Gallup (1991) found that while Americans most widely practice colloquial prayer, meditative prayer was associated with a closer relationship with God and higher levels of well-being.

Most prayer typologies have been created out of research involving individuals from predominantly Western cultures in which prayer is typically experienced in the context of organized, theistic religion. However, Banzinger et al. (2008) found that the prayer experiences of individuals from the Netherlands, a highly secularized society, also could be categorized using a typology similar to Poloma and Pendleton's scheme. While Banzinger et al. argued for the creation of a secular prayer type, their findings support the notion that some types of prayer experiences may be common to both secular and nonsecular individuals.

Prayer and Well-Being

The way that people communicate with the sacred can influence their physical and psychological health. Studies have linked prayer to better medical outcomes among patients dealing with cardiovascular disease, cancer, migraines, chronic pain post surgical recovery, and HIV.

Research studies have also shown that people who pray more frequently report a greater sense of well-being. More specifically, prayer has been associated with higher levels of overall mental health, lower levels of depression and anxiety, higher levels of self-esteem, and more positive mood among individuals with post-traumatic stress disorder ("PTSD"). How well prayer works may depend at least in part on how people perceive God. Bradshaw et al. (2008) found that frequency of prayer was positively correlated with higher rates of psychopathology among individuals who perceived God as remote or not loving. In contrast, among individuals who viewed God as close and loving, more prayer was tied to lower psychopathology. Other factors may also affect the relationship between prayer and well-being, including the content and intent of prayers, an individual's level of spiritual maturity, and the availability of additional coping resources.

Although studies have consistently demonstrated significant correlations between prayer and well-being, researchers have not yet identified the underlying psychological mechanisms that account for this relationship. Prayer may affect well-being indirectly by strengthening the relationships between individuals, God, and their faith community which may buffer the negative impact of stressors on health and well-being. Prayer may also manifest its effects through other psychological factors, such as increasing feelings of gratitude. Researchers have shown that greater frequency of prayer is associated with increased feelings of gratitude which are, in turn, correlated with lower rates of depression as well as higher levels of optimism and fewer negative health symptoms.

Prayer for one's own health and for the health of others represent the two most frequently used alternative health treatments in the United States. The proportion of Americans who pray to alleviate health problems increased from 43% in 2002 to 49% in 2007. This number may grow even further as the number of individuals who live with chronic physical or psychological illnesses rises. Many individuals who pray have also expressed a desire to integrate prayer practices into their medical treatment. In one study, 79% of critical care providers were asked by patients or their families to pray for them. In another survey, 48% of American patients indicated that they would like their doctor to pray for them. Over 90% of these patients felt that their doctor's prayers on their behalf had enhanced their health and aided in their recovery.

Some clinicians have begun to respond to the promising research findings and to the desires of many of their patients by considering how to incorporate prayer into specific treatments. Seventy-three percent of critical care nurses surveyed by Tracy et al. (2005) prayed while treating clients, and 81% of these nurses had recommended the use of prayer to their patients. Pargament et al. (1998) suggested that positive forms of religious coping such as seeking spiritual support through prayer could be successfully integrated into psychotherapy. The appropriateness of integrating spiritual practices such as prayer into treatment, however, remains a highly divisive topic within the health-care community.

Cross-References

▶ Meditation
▶ Religion
▶ Religious Ritual
▶ Spirituality

References and Readings

Bänzinger, S., Janssen, J., & Scheepers, P. (2008). Praying in a secularized society: An empirical study of praying practices and varieties. *The International Journal for the Psychology of Religion, 18*, 256–265.

Bradshaw, M., Ellison, C. G., & Flannelly, K. J. (2008). Prayer, god imagery, and symptoms of psychopathology. *Journal for the Scientific Study of Religion, 47*(4), 644–659.

Fincham, F. D., Beach, S. R. H., Lambert, N., Stillman, T., & Braithwaite, S. R. (2008). Spiritual behaviors and relationship satisfaction: A critical analysis of the role of prayer. *Journal of Social and Clinical Psychology, 27*(4), 362–388.

Gill, S. D. (1994). Prayer. In M. Eliade (Ed.), *The encyclopedia of religion* (Vol. 11, 2nd ed.). New York: Macmillan Reference.

Heiler, F. (1932). *Prayer: A study in the history and psychology of religion*. London: Oxford University Press.

Krause, N. (2009). Lifetime trauma, prayer and psychological distress in later life. *International Journal for the Psychology of Religion, 19*(1), 55–72.

Ladd, K. L., & Spilka, B. (2002). Inward, outward, upward: Cognitive aspects of prayer. *Journal for the Scientific Study of Religion, 41*(3), 475–484.

Levin, J. (1996). How prayer heals: A theoretical model. *Alternative Therapies in Health & Medicine, 2*(1), 66–73.

McCullough, M. E. (1995). Prayer and health: Conceptual issues, research review, and research agenda. *Journal of Psychology and Theology, 23*(1), 15–29.

Pargament, K. I. (1997). *The psychology of religion and coping: Theory, research, practice*. New York: The Guilford Press.

Pargament, K. I., Smith, B. W., Koenig, H. G., & Perez, L. (1998). Patterns of positive and negative religious coping with major life stressors. *Journal for the Scientific Study of Religion, 37*(4), 710–724.

Poloma, M. M., & Gallup, G. H., Jr. (1991). *Varieties of prayer: A survey report*. Philadelphia: Trinity Press International.

Poloma, M. M., & Pendleton, B. F. (1991). The effects of prayer and prayer experiences on general wellbeing. *Journal of Psychology and Theology, 19*, 71–83.

Tracy, M. F., Lindquist, R., Savik, K., Watanuki, S., Sendelbach, S., Kreitzer, M. J., et al. (2005). Use of complementary and alternative therapies: A national survey of critical care nurses. *American Journal of Critical Care, 14*, 404–414.

Prediabetes

▶ Hyperinsulinemia
▶ Impaired Glucose Tolerance

Pregnancy

▶ Coffee Drinking, Effects of Caffeine
▶ Gestation

Pregnancy Anxiety

Melissa Julian[1], Isabel F. Ramos[2], Nicole E. Mahrer[3] and Christine Dunkel Schetter[4]
[1]George Washington University, Washington, DC, USA
[2]Department of Psychology, UCLA, Los Angeles, CA, USA
[3]Department of Psychology, University of La Verne, La Verne, CA, USA
[4]Department of Psychology, University of California, Los Angeles (UCLA), Los Angeles, CA, USA

Synonyms

Pregnancy-related anxiety; *Pregnancy-specific anxiety*

Definition

Pregnancy anxiety is a situation-specific negative emotional state tied to pregnancy-specific concerns or worries.

Description

Pregnancy is the period from conception to childbirth and is divided into three trimesters, with an average gestational length of 40 weeks. While pregnancy can be a positive experience for many women and their families, it can also be a very stressful time. Some pregnant women become anxious about the health of their fetus, labor and delivery, and their ability to parent a new infant, among other concerns. *Pregnancy anxiety* (also referred to as *pregnancy-specific anxiety* or *pregnancy-related anxiety*) is a situation-specific negative emotional state tied to pregnancy-specific concerns or worries. *Anxiety* is defined as a negative emotional state characterized by worry, fear, and intrusive thoughts that are typically related to future events and often accompanied by somatic symptoms such as sweating and rapid heartbeat. Pregnancy anxiety is distinct from general anxiety in that the nature of the worries, fears, and thoughts are tied to pregnancy specifically. Research has documented that women who have higher pregnancy anxiety have higher risks of preterm birth and adverse developmental outcomes for their offspring. This entry will discuss the features of pregnancy anxiety, measures used to assess it, socioeconomic and personal factors associated with its development, potential mechanisms, and implications for infant and child developmental outcomes.

What Is Pregnancy Anxiety?

The worries and fears that underlie pregnancy anxiety usually focus on one's own health as a mother, the baby's health, labor, childbirth and hospital experiences, and parenting competence (Dunkel Schetter 2011). For example, anxiety about one's own health may include worries about high-risk medical conditions such as gestational diabetes or pregnancy-induced hypertension (preeclampsia) which can affect the mother's health. Some women worry that these conditions will hurt them and the baby. Women may also have significant concerns about the fetus in utero and about whether their baby will be healthy after birth. These particular fears are more frequent in women with previous miscarriages or difficulties with infertility (Guardino and Dunkel Schetter 2014). Concerns or worries about having a painful or traumatic birth experience also contribute to pregnancy anxiety, with many women being afraid that either they or their children will be harmed in the labor and delivery process. This occurs more often in women from countries with high rates of maternal mortality (Campos et al. 2007). Anxiety surrounding the ability to parent may take the form of worrying about finances, childcare, or breast-feeding.

While these fears may be present throughout pregnancy, the nature of the fears typically change over the course of pregnancy as particular pregnancy-specific concerns and worries shift. For example, fears about miscarriage are greater in the first trimester when risk is higher, whereas concerns about the labor process or parenting a newborn tend to become more salient toward the end of pregnancy. Research has found that pregnancy anxiety is highest in the first trimester, decreases in the second semester, and increases again in the third trimester (Guardino and Dunkel Schetter 2014).

Measuring Pregnancy Anxiety

A review of pregnancy anxiety measures indicates that there are at least 15 pregnancy anxiety instruments that have been used internationally (Alderdice et al. 2012). One pregnancy anxiety scale (Rini et al. 1999) includes ten items that inquire about each of the concerns noted above and has reliability and validity data in English and Spanish. Another measure, published by Roesch et al. (2004), is a checklist measure that asks participants how often they experienced specific emotions (anxious, concerned, afraid, and panicky) due to their pregnancy in the past week. In our work, both measures have predicted preterm birth (Kramer et al. 2009) and length of gestation in term births (Ramos et al. 2019).

What Are the Harmful Effects of Pregnancy Anxiety?

Pregnancy anxiety is one of the strongest predictors of adverse birth outcomes, namely, preterm birth (PTB), and there is growing evidence for adverse implications for infant and child development. Other forms of stress and anxiety have been associated with poor birth outcomes; however, studies have found that pregnancy anxiety emerges as a stronger predictor (Dunkel Schetter 2011). Pregnancy anxiety is also associated with less optimal developmental outcomes in children, even when controlling for medical risk during pregnancy. For example, pregnancy anxiety is associated with cognitive and motor performance in the infant's first year, including more behavioral reactivity, less cognitive development, and poorer attention regulation (Huizink et al. 2003). Many of these developmental difficulties can also persist into toddlerhood, childhood, and even preadolescence, with exposure to pregnancy anxiety in utero increasing risk for higher negative affectivity, greater anxiety, and impaired executive functioning in youth (Blair et al. 2011; Buss et al. 2011; Davis and Sandman 2012).

Why Is Pregnancy Anxiety Harmful?

The mechanisms through which pregnancy anxiety influences birth and developmental outcomes are being uncovered. Recent studies have focused on the effects of pregnancy anxiety on the intrauterine environment and ways in which fetal development is programmed by maternal influences. One important potential mechanism is the mother's physiological stress response system, which is activated with elevated levels of pregnancy anxiety. Evidence suggests that pregnancy anxiety is linked to elevated levels of a stress-responsive peptide, placental corticotropin-releasing hormone (CRH), which in turn is known to trigger the timing of delivery (Mancuso et al. 2004; Ramos et al. 2019).

Who Is Most Likely to Have Pregnancy Anxiety?

Several socioeconomic and personal characteristics are associated with higher pregnancy anxiety. In general, first-time mothers have higher levels of pregnancy anxiety than those who have given birth before. Women with greater medical risks or complications that develop during pregnancy also score higher on measures of pregnancy anxiety. Women with lower incomes have higher levels of pregnancy anxiety. Also, married women and women with more social support are lower in pregnancy anxiety. Women with lower self-esteem and mastery tend to have higher levels of pregnancy anxiety (Rini et al. 1999). Finally, women who are generally high in anxiety in their everyday lives or have anxiety disorders are more anxious in pregnancy as well.

In conclusion, pregnancy anxiety is a specific context-dependent form of anxiety characterized by concerns or worries surrounding pregnancy and childbirth. It is associated with serious birth complications and suboptimal developmental outcomes via effects on maternal physiology and fetal development. A better understanding of factors associated with the development of pregnancy anxiety may inform future interventions that prevent maternal and infant health risks. Models that explain pathways through which pregnancy anxiety influences birth and developmental outcomes are currently under investigation (Dunkel Schetter 2011).

Cross-References

▶ Anxiety
▶ Maternal Stress
▶ Postpartum Depression
▶ Women's Health

References and Further Reading

Alderdice, F., Lynn, F., & Lobel, M. (2012). A review and psychometric evaluation of pregnancy-specific stress measures. *Journal of Psychosomatic Obstetrics and Gynecology, 33*(2), 62–77. https://doi.org/10.3109/0167482X.2012.673040.

Blair, M. M., Glynn, L. M., Sandman, C. A., & Davis, E. P. (2011). Prenatal maternal anxiety and early childhood temperament. *Stress, 14*(6), 644–651. https://doi.org/10.3109/10253890.2011.594121.

Buss, C., Davis, E. P., Hobel, C. J., & Sandman, C. A. (2011). Maternal pregnancy-specific anxiety is associated with child executive function at 6–9 years age. *Stress, 14*(6), 665–676. https://doi.org/10.3109/10253890.2011.623250.

Campos, B., Schetter, C. D., Walsh, J. A., & Schenker, M. (2007). Sharpening the focus on acculturative change: ARSMA-II, stress, pregnancy anxiety, and infant birthweight in recently immigrated Latinas. *Hispanic Journal of Behavioral Sciences, 29*(2), 209–224. https://doi.org/10.1177/0739986307300841.

Davis, E. P., & Sandman, C. A. (2012). Prenatal psychobiological predictors of anxiety risk in preadolescent children. *Psychoneuroendocrinology, 37*(8), 1224–1233. https://doi.org/10.1016/j.psyneuen.2011.12.016.

Dunkel Schetter, C. (2011). Psychological science on pregnancy: Stress processes, biopsychosocial models, and emerging research issues. *Annual Review of Psychology, 62*, 531–558. https://doi.org/10.1146/annurev.psych.031809.130727.

Guardino, C. M., & Dunkel Schetter, C. (2014). Understanding pregnancy anxiety: Concepts, correlates and consequences. *Zero to Three, 34*(4), 12–21.

Huizink, A. C., Robles de Medina, P. G., Mulder, E. J., Visser, G. H., & Buitelaar, J. K. (2003). Stress during pregnancy is associated with developmental outcome in infancy. *Journal of Child Psychology and Psychiatry, 44*, 810–818. https://doi.org/10.1111/1469-7610.00166.

Kramer, M. S., Lydon, J., Séguin, L., Goulet, L., Kahn, S. R., McNamara, H., ... & Platt, R. W. (2009). Stress pathways to spontaneous preterm birth: The role of stressors, psychological distress, and stress hormones. *American Journal of Epidemiology, 69*(11), 1319–1326. https://doi.org/10.1093/aje/kwp061.

Mancuso, R. A., Schetter, C. D., Rini, C. M., Roesch, S. C., & Hobel, C. J. (2004). Maternal prenatal anxiety and corticotropin-releasing hormone associated with timing of delivery. *Psychosomatic Medicine, 66*(5), 762–769. https://doi.org/10.1097/01.psy.0000138284.70670.d5.

Ramos, I. F., Guardino, C. M., Mansolf, M., Glynn, L. M., Sandman, C. A., Hobel, C. J., & Dunkel Schetter, C. (2019). Pregnancy anxiety predicts shorter gestation in Latina and non-Latina white women: The role of placental corticotrophin-releasing hormone. *Psychoneuroendocrinology, 99*, 166–173. https://doi.org/10.1016/j.psyneuen.2018.09.008.

Rini, C. K., Dunkel-Schetter, C., Wadhwa, P. D., & Sandman, C. A. (1999). Psychological adaptation and birth outcomes: The role of personal resources, stress, and sociocultural context in pregnancy. *Health Psychology, 18*(4), 333–345. https://doi.org/10.1037/0278-6133.18.4.333.

Roesch, S. C., Dunkel Schetter, C., Woo, G., & Hobel, C. J. (2004). Modeling the types and timing of stress in pregnancy. *Anxiety, Stress & Coping, 17*(1), 87–102. https://doi.org/10.1080/1061580031000123667.

Pregnancy Complications

▶ Pregnancy Outcomes: Psychosocial Aspect

Pregnancy Outcomes: Psychosocial Aspect

Michele L. Okun
Department of Psychology, University of Colorado Colorado Springs, Colorado Springs, CO, USA

Synonyms

Depression; Pregnancy complications

Definition

For most women, pregnancy is viewed as a natural and joyful event. In more than 80% of pregnancies, the delivery process is unremarkable, with no physiological or psychological complications. Indeed, the most notable changes associated with pregnancy often occur in social and partner relations, as well as changes to one's lifestyle. For instance, sleep deprivation and disturbance are the most frequently reported pregnancy-related disturbances. Pregnancy-related sleep disturbances, in turn, impact numerous facets of life including mood, cognition, social functioning, and memory (Harding 1975).

For a small percentage of women, pregnancy and delivery are complicated by a variety of adverse outcomes. Preeclampsia, intrauterine growth restriction (IUGR), or preterm delivery can significantly affect the psychological health of women. Psychosocial aspects of pregnancy outcomes range along a continuum and are multidimensional. Psychosocial functioning in association with pregnancy complications may be a function of coping strategies, social support, and the overall emotional health of the mother and father. Sociodemographic factors including parental age, socioeconomic status, and relationship quality also influence parental response to pregnancy complications. In the wake of adverse outcomes, parents may feel guilt, depression, anger, resentment, or withdrawal. Parents of infants transferred to the neonatal intensive care unit (NICU) may experience additional psychological burden, sometimes altering relationship dynamics (Zager 2009) or mother-child bonding. Links between psychosocial factors and adverse pregnancy outcomes are currently underrecognized by health-care providers, which suggest that systematic prospective research is needed to more convincingly establish the significance of psychosocial factors and their potential for prevention.

Cross-References

▶ Psychosocial Factors

References and Further Reading

Harding, M. E. (1975). Maternity. In M. E. Harding (Ed.), *The way of all women* (pp. 160–170). New York: Harper and Row.
Lederman, R., & Weis, K. (2009). *Psychosocial adaptation to pregnancy: Seven dimensions of maternal role development* (3rd ed.). Dordrecht: Springer.
Zager, A. (2009). Women's Medicine. The Global Library of Women's Medicine. Ref Type: Online Source.

Pregnancy Spacing

▶ Family Planning

Pregnancy-Related Anxiety

▶ Pregnancy Anxiety

Pregnancy-Specific Anxiety

▶ Pregnancy Anxiety

Prehypertension

Jonathan Newman
Columbia University, New York, NY, USA

Description

In 2003, the seventh report of the Joint National Committee guidelines (JNC 7) proposed a classification for normal blood pressure (BP) and prehypertension based on the average of two more properly measured readings:

- Normal blood pressure: systolic < 120 mmHg and diastolic < 80 mmHg
- Prehypertension: systolic 120–139 mmHg or diastolic 80–89 mmHg

Compared to individuals with normal BP, prehypertensive individuals have a greater number of traditional cardiovascular disease (CVD) risk factors and have a greater risk of developing CVD independent of other CVD risk factors than individuals with BP < 120/80. Prehypertensive individuals also have a greater risk of developing hypertension than normotensive individuals. Therefore, prehypertension can be conceptualized as an intermediate phenotype at elevated risk of developing traditional risk factors for CVD (such as hypertension) and at independent risk of developing CVD itself.

However, the ideal surveillance and management strategies for patients with prehypertension have not been well defined. Due to the associations between prehypertension and the development of overt hypertension and CVD, in 2007, the United States Preventive Services Task Force (USPSTF) recommended yearly BP screening for prehypertensive individuals and every other year screening for those with normotension. It remains unclear, however, how much of the excess CVD risk associated with prehypertension is due to the BP itself and how much is related to associated CVD risk factors: some analyses have shown that the excess CVD risk associated with prehypertension is attenuated after controlling for concomitant CVD risk factors. A more concrete problem with the diagnosis of prehypertension, however, may be the number of people affected: a recent analysis of the US population found that 39% of adults were normotensive, 31% prehypertensive, and 29% hypertensive. This suggests only a minority of Americans have normal blood pressure and raises the question of whether prehypertension should be defined as a "disease" state.

While there is limited evidence to suggest that treatment of prehypertension may prevent the development of hypertension, JNC 7 recommends careful follow-up for the development of hypertension or signs of end-organ damage (e.g., renal dysfunction or left-ventricular hypertrophy). Without the presence of CVD or other CVD risk factors (such as diabetes), prehypertension is generally treated with nonpharmacologic therapies such as weight loss, sodium restriction, dietary modification, and exercise.

References and Readings

Greenlund, K. J., Croft, J. B., & Mensah, G. A. (2004). Prevalence of heart disease and stroke risk factors in persons with prehypertension in the United States, 1999–2000. *Archives of Internal Medicine, 164*(19), 2113–2118.

Julius, S., Nesbitt, S. D., Egan, B. M., Weber, M. A., Michelson, E. L., Kaciroti, N., Black, H. R., Grimm, R. H., Jr., Messerli, F. H., Oparil, S., & Schork, M. A. (2006). Trial of Preventing Hypertension (TROPHY) Study Investigators. Feasibility of treating prehypertension with an angiotensin-receptor blocker. *The New England Journal of Medicine, 354*(16), 1685–1697.

U.S. Preventive Services Task Force. (2007). Screening for high blood pressure: U.S. Preventive Services Task Force reaffirmation recommendation statement. *Annals of Internal Medicine, 147*(11), 783–786.

Zhang, Y., Lee, E. T., Devereux, R. B., Yeh, J., Best, L. G., Fabsitz, R. R., & Howard, B. V. (2006). Prehypertension, diabetes, and cardiovascular disease risk in a population-based sample: The strong heart study. *Hypertension, 47*(3), 410–414.

Preimplantation Genetic Diagnosis

▶ In Vitro Fertilization, Assisted Reproductive Technology

Prejudice

▶ Stigma

Premenstrual Headache

▶ Migraine Headache

Pressure

▶ Stress

Prevalence

Linda Carroll
Department of Public Health Sciences, University of Alberta, Edmonton, AB, Canada

Synonyms

Prevalence number; Prevalence rate

Definition

Prevalence is a measure of frequency of an illness, disease, or health conditions. Unlike incidence, which reflects new occurrences or changes in health states, prevalence is concerned with already existing health conditions, regardless of whether that health condition is of recent onset or is long-standing. Thus, prevalence of a particular condition refers to the proportion of the population which has that condition at a specified time. It is usually presented as x cases per 1000 (or 10,000 or 100,000) people in the population. There are two types of prevalence: point prevalence (the type of prevalence most commonly reported) and period prevalence. Consider the example of the common cold. The "point prevalence" of the common cold in New York City means the proportion of people in New York City with a cold at a given point in time, i.e., the number of New York City residents with a cold on a specific day divided by the total number of New York City residents on that day. It is like a "prevalence snapshot." A 1-month "period prevalence" means the proportion of people in New York City who have had a cold at any point within the past month. It is analogous to time-lapse photography, reflecting the health state that has existed over a set period of time. A variation is lifetime prevalence or the proportion of people who have had the condition at any point during their lifetime.

Prevalence is usually measured in surveys or cross-sectional studies and reflects the burden of disease, rather than risk (incidence) of disease, which must be measured in longitudinal studies. Because prevalence is a measure of existing health conditions, it is affected by both incidence of that health state (the rate at which new cases develop) and the duration of that health state. A health condition might have a short duration because it is rapidly fatal, for example, rabies or Ebola, or because recovery is rapid, such as the case in the "24-h flu." Prevalence of a particular health condition can increase because there is an increase in incidence (e.g., during an influenza epidemic) or because people with that health condition are living longer with that condition (e.g., treatments may have extended the lives of those who suffer from that health condition). Alternatively, more effective treatments may shorten the recovery time.

Because prevalence is affected by recovery or death, it is an unreliable estimate of disease risk. This can be illustrated in the following example. The Framingham Heart Study reported equal prevalence of coronary heart disease in men and women. This could lead to the mistaken conclusion that men and women are at equal risk of developing coronary heart disease. However, the follow-up studies demonstrated that men were at greater risk of developing coronary heart disease and also had a higher fatality rate; while women were less likely to develop heart disease, but when they did, it was also less likely to be fatal. Thus, the prevalence in men and women was roughly equal because a lower risk was coupled with a longer duration of disease in women.

References and Readings

Oleckno, W. A. (2002). *Essential epidemiology: Principles and applications*. Long Grove: Waveland Press.

Rothman, K. J., Greenland, S., & Lash, T. L. (2008). *Modern epidemiology* (3rd ed.). Philadelphia: Lippincott Williams & Wilkins.

Szklo, M., & Nieto, F. J. (2007). *Epidemiology: Beyond the basics* (2nd ed.). Sudbury: James and Bartlett.

Prevalence Number

▶ Prevalence

Prevalence Rate

▶ Prevalence

Prevention: Primary, Secondary, Tertiary

Linda C. Baumann[1] and Alyssa Ylinen[2]
[1]School of Nursing, University of Wisconsin-Madison, Madison, WI, USA
[2]Allina Health System, St. Paul, MN, USA

Synonyms

Levels of prevention

Definition

The natural history of disease is the course from onset to resolution (Last 2000). The goal of epidemiology is to identify and understand causal factors of disease, disability, and injury so that effective interventions can be implemented to prevent the occurrence of adverse processes before they begin or progress (Stanhope and Lancaster 2008). The definitions used in public health distinguish between primary prevention, secondary prevention, and tertiary prevention (Commission on Chronic Illness 1957).

Description

The term "primary prevention" refers to intervention measures to prevent the occurrence (incidence) of new disease, disability, or injury (Leavell and Clark 1965). This intervention must be implemented prepathogenesis and directed at individuals or groups at risk. Primary prevention efforts include health promotion and specific protection and are generally aimed at populations, not individuals (see Fig. 1). The application of primary prevention extends beyond medical problems and includes the prevention of other concerns that impact health and well-being, such as violence to environmental degradation. Education and public policy are major strategies for primary prevention.

Two other levels of prevention are termed secondary and tertiary prevention. Secondary prevention is a set of measures used for early detection and prompt intervention to control a problem or disease (prevalence) and minimize the consequences. Secondary prevention encompasses interventions that increase the probability that a person with a condition will have it diagnosed at a stage that treatment is likely to result in cure or reduction in the severity of a condition. Health screening is a major strategy of secondary prevention. Tertiary prevention focuses on the reduction of further complications of an existing disease, disability, or injury, through treatment and rehabilitation.

A landmark report published by the Institute of Medicine entitled *Reducing Risks for Mental Disorders* (IOM 1994) evaluated the body of research on the prevention of mental disorders. This report offered new definitions of prevention and provided recommendations on federal policies and programs. Levels of prevention across the natural

THE NATURAL HISTORY OF ANY DISEASE OF MAN					
Interrelations of Agent, Host, and Environmental Factors		Reaction of the HOST to the STIMULUS			
Production of STIMULUS		Early pathogenesis	Discernible Early Lesions	Advanced Disease	Convalescence
Prepathogenesis period		Period of Pathogenesis			
HEALTH PROMOTION	SPECIFIC PROTECTION	EARLY DIAGNOSIS and PROMPT TREATMENT	DISABILITY LIMITATION		REHABILITATION
Health education	Use of specific immunizations	Case-finding measures, individual and mass	Adequate treatment to arrest the disease process and to prevent further complications and sequelae		Provision of hospital and community facilities for retraining and education for maximum use of remaining capacities
Good standard of nutrition adjusted to developmental phases of life	Attention to personal hygiene	Screening surveys			
	Use of environmental sanitation	Selective examinations			Education of the public and industry to utilize the rehabilitated
Attention to personality development	Protection against occupational hazards	Objectives:	Provision of facilities to limit disability and to prevent death		
Provision of adequate housing, recreation and agreeable working conditions		To cure and prevent disease processes			As full employment as possible
	Protection from accidents				
	Use of specific nutrients	To prevent the spread of communicable diseases			Selective placement
Marriage counseling and sex education	Protection from carcinogens				Work therapy in hospitals
Genetics	Avoidance of allergens	To prevent complications and sequelae			Use of sheltered colony
Periodic selective examinations		To shorten period of disability			
Primary Prevention		Secondary Prevention		Tertiary Prevention
LEVELS of APPLICATION of PREVENTIVE MEASURES					

Prevention: Primary, Secondary, Tertiary, Fig. 1 Levels of application of preventive measures in the natural history of disease

disease history (Fig. 1) were defined as "prevention, treatment, and rehabilitation." Prevention, according to the IOM report (1994), is similar to the concept of primary prevention and refers to interventions to delay or avoid the initial onset of a disorder. Further, prevention has three types: universal, selective, and indicated, to reduce new cases. Universal efforts are directed to the entire population; selective prevention is for those at significant risk of a disorder due to biological, social, or psychological risk factors; and indicated prevention is for those with a mild disorder that has the potential to become more severe if not addressed in a timely manner.

Treatment refers to the identification of individuals with a disorder and providing treatment for those disorders, which includes interventions to reduce the likelihood of future co-occurring disorders. Maintenance refers to interventions that are oriented to reduce relapse and recurrence and to provide rehabilitation. Maintenance incorporates what public health defines as some forms of secondary and all forms of tertiary prevention.

The concepts of risk and protective factors, risk reduction, and enhancement of protective factors (also referred to as fostering resilience) are central to most evidence-based prevention programs. Risk factors are those characteristics, variables, or hazards that, if present for a given individual, make it more likely that this individual, rather than someone selected at random from the general population, will develop a disorder. Protective factors improve a person's response to an environmental hazard resulting in an adaptive outcome.

The Agency for Health Research and Quality (AHRQ) provides ongoing administrative, research, technical, and dissemination support to the US Preventive Services Task Force (USPSTF) (http://www.USPreventiveServicesTaskForce.org). The USPSTF is an independent panel of nonfederal experts in prevention and evidence-based medicine and is composed of an interdisciplinary mix of primary care providers (physicians, nurses, and health behavior specialists). The USPSTF conducts scientific evidence reviews of a broad range of clinical preventive healthcare services (such as screening, counseling, and preventive medications) and develops recommendations for primary care clinicians and health systems. These recommendations are published in the form of "Recommendation Statements."

References and Further Readings

Commission on Chronic Illness. (1957). *Chronic illness in the United States* (Vol. 1). Cambridge, MA: Harvard University Press.
Institute of Medicine. (1994). *Reducing risks for mental disorders*. Washington, DC: National Academy Press.
Last, J. M. (2000). *A dictionary of epidemiology* (4th ed.). New York: Oxford University Press.
Leavell, H. R., & Clark, E. G. (1965). *Preventive medicine for the doctor in his community* (3rd ed.). New York: McGraw-Hill.
Stanhope, M., & Lancaster, J. (2008). *Public health nursing: Population-centered health care in the community* (7th ed.). St. Louis, MO: Mosby Elsevier.

Preventive Care

Shannon Idzik
University of Maryland School of Nursing, Baltimore, MD, USA
University of Maryland Upper Chesapeake Health Comprehensive CARE Center, Bel Air, MD, USA

Synonyms

Preventive healthcare; Preventive medicine; Prophylactic care

Definition

Preventive care is the segment of health care that strives to prevent mental and physical illness. Many members of the health care team partner together to achieve proper preventive care. Preventive care is divided into three levels of care: primary prevention, secondary prevention, and tertiary prevention.

Description

Primary preventive care is the prevention of disease in a susceptible population through health promotion, education, and protective efforts. Ensuring adequate nutrition, advising patients about skin protection from ultraviolet radiation, educating about seat belt use, promoting safe home and work environments, prescribing oral fluoride supplementation in children with fluoride-deficient water, and administering immunizations are all examples of primary preventive care.

Secondary preventive care is the prevention of disease through screening and early detection. Early recognition of disease through health care screening allows treatment to occur early in the course of the disease and may decrease complications. Examples of screening procedures that lead to the prevention of disease include fecal occult blood testing for detecting colon cancer, Pap smear for detecting early cervical cancer, routine mammography for early breast cancer, blood pressure and blood cholesterol measurement, oral examinations for early dental caries, and use of screening tools for depression.

Tertiary preventive care is the prevention of disease progression and disease sequelae after a chronic or irreversible disease diagnosis has been made. Limiting disability and promoting rehabilitation are important in tertiary prevention. Examples of tertiary prevention efforts include prescribing anticlotting agents such as aspirin in patients who have cardiovascular disease, physical rehabilitation in patients who have suffered a stroke, and endodontic therapy in patients with severe dental decay.

Cross-References

▶ Prevention: Primary, Secondary, Tertiary

References and Further Readings

Partnership for Prevention. (2016). *Clinical prevention*. Retrieved September 4, 2016 from http://www.prevent.org/Publications-and-Resources.aspx

Patient Protection and Affordable Care Act (PPACA). Pub. L. No. 111-148, 124 Stat. 119 (2010). Retrieved October 20, 2011 from http://www.gpo.gov/fdsys/pkg/PLAW-111publ148/pdf/PLAW-111publ148.pdf

Preventive Services – HealthCare.gov Glossary. (2016). *HealthCare.gov*. Retrieved September 4, 2016, from https://www.healthcare.gov/glossary/preventive-services/

U.S. Preventive Services Task Force. (2016). *Recommendations*. Retrieved September 4, 2016 from http://www.uspreventiveservicestaskforce.org/Page/Name/recommendations

Preventive Healthcare

▶ Preventive Care

Preventive Medicine

▶ Preventive Care

Preventive Medicine Research Institute (Ornish)

Manjunath Harlapur[1] and Daichi Shimbo[2]
[1]Center of Behavioral Cardiovascular Health, Division of General Medicine, Columbia University, New York, NY, USA
[2]Center for Behavioral Cardiovascular Health, Columbia University, New York, NY, USA

Synonyms

Dean Ornish

Definition

Preventive Medicine Research Institute (PMRI) is a nonprofit research institute located in Sausalito, California, and founded by Dr. Dean Ornish. The mission of PMRI is to conduct scientific research examining the effects of diet and lifestyle choices on health outcomes.

Description

PMRI is a nonprofit research institute that is involved with scientific research studying the effects of diet and lifestyle choices on health and diseases. PMRI was founded by Dr. Dean Ornish, a leading researcher and physician advocating this type of prevention. The mission of PMRI is to conduct scientific research examining the effects of diet and lifestyle choices on health outcomes. In addition to research, another emphasis of PMRI is to educate health professionals and the lay public about the importance of preventive medicine and the benefits of lifestyle changes including diet, exercise, and stress management.

Cross-References

▶ Coronary Artery Disease

References and Further Reading

http://www.pmri.org/

Previous Smokers

▶ Ex-Smokers

Pride

▶ Self-esteem

Primary Care

Shannon Idzik
University of Maryland School of Nursing, Baltimore, MD, USA
University of Maryland Upper Chesapeake Health Comprehensive CARE Center, Bel Air, MD, USA

Synonyms

Primary health care

Definition

Primary care is a component of integrated health care in which comprehensive and accessible care is provided to a defined population. It is not disease or organ specific but rather examines a person's overall state of health and well-being. Primary care is often the first point of contact into a health system for persons with a health concern including those with acute and chronic physical, mental, and social health issues. Primary care is a longitudinal and continuous approach to health maintenance including health promotion, disease prevention, health education, and counseling and includes diagnosis, treatment, and management of acute and chronic conditions. Primary care focuses on the provision of primary, secondary, and tertiary prevention measures, such as screenings, immunizations, and prevention of disease progression or sequelae. In primary care, the patient is seen as a partner in their health and health decisions. The primary care provider partners with the patient to coordinate other health services which includes collaboration with and referral to other members of the health-care team. Continuity in primary care is essential to develop and establish a patient-provider relationship. Primary care is not setting specific and can be provided across a continuum of health settings such as the patient's private residence, provider office, hospital, or long-term care facility.

Cross-References

▶ Clinical Settings
▶ Family Practice/Medicine
▶ Primary Care
▶ Primary Care Physicians
▶ Primary Care Provider

References and Further Reading

American Academy of Family Physicians. (2016). Primary care. Retrieved from http://www.aafp.org/online/en/home/policy/policies/p/primarycare.html#Parsys0002. Accessed 4 Sept 2016.
Patient Protection and Affordable Care Act (PPACA), Pub. L. No. 111–148, 124 Stat. 119. (2010). Retrieved from http://www.gpo.gov/fdsys/pkg/PLAW-111publ148/pdf/PLAW-111publ148.pdf. Accessed 4 Sept 2016.
Primary Care – HealthCare.gov Glossary. (2016). Health*Care.gov*. Retrieved September 4, 2016, from https://www.healthcare.gov/glossary/primary-care/

Primary Care Nurse Practitioner

▶ Primary Care Providers

Primary Care Physicians

Steven Gambert
Department of Medicine, School of Medicine, University of Maryland, Baltimore, MD, USA

Synonyms

Family physician; General internist; PCP; PMD; Primary care provider; Primary medical doctor

Definition

A primary care physician is the physician who provides primary care, the physician selected to be the first doctor contacted for any medical condition. The physician acts as the patient's "gatekeeper," providing ongoing medical care, preventive services, medical counseling, and referrals to specialists as needed. Examples of physicians who may be considered to be primary care physicians include family medicine physicians, internal medicine physicians, OB/GYN physicians, pediatricians, and at times emergency medicine physicians. The number of primary care physicians has been declining in recent years with more physicians seeking careers as subspecialists or pursuing specialty care with financial rewards and increasing demands on time being major reasons for this change (Bodenheimer 2006).

Cross-References

▶ Primary Care Providers

References and Readings

Bodenheimer, T. (2006). Primary care – will it survive? *New England Journal of Medicine, 355*(9), 861–864.

Primary Care Provider

▶ Primary Care Physicians
▶ Primary Care Providers

Primary Care Providers

Shannon Idzik
University of Maryland School of Nursing, Baltimore, MD, USA
University of Maryland Upper Chesapeake Health Comprehensive CARE Center, Bel Air, MD, USA

Synonyms

Family nurse practitioner: Family physician; General internist; General practitioner (GP); Internist; Primary care nurse practitioner; Primary care provider; Primary medical doctor

Definition

Primary care providers are generalist clinicians who provide integrated accessible health care to a defined population. Nurse practitioners, physicians, and physicians' assistants who provide primary care are specially trained to provide primary care services. The primary care provider develops a sustained relationship with the patient and oversees all aspects of the patient's health. The primary care provider partners with the patient to coordinate other health services which include collaboration with and referral to other members of the health-care team. Primary care providers are advocates for the patient throughout the entire health-care system.

Cross-References

▶ Primary Care
▶ Primary Care Physicians
▶ Primary Care Provider

References and Further Readings

American Academy of Family Physicians. (2016). *Primary care*. Retrieved 4 Sept 2016, from http://www.aafp.org/online/en/home/policy/policies/p/primarycare.html#Parsys0002
Patient Protection and Affordable Care Act (PPACA), Pub. L. No. 111-148, 124 Stat. 119. (2010). Retrieved 4 Sept 2016, from http://www.gpo.gov/fdsys/pkg/PLAW-111publ148/pdf/PLAW-111publ148.pdf
Primary Care Provider – HealthCare.gov Glossary. (2016). *HealthCare.gov*. Retrieved 4 Sept 2016, from https://www.healthcare.gov/glossary/primary-care-provider/

Primary Health Care

▶ Primary Care

Primary Medical Doctor

▶ Primary Care Physicians
▶ Primary Care Providers

Primary Raynaud's Phenomenon

▶ Raynaud's Disease and Stress
▶ Raynaud's Disease: Behavioral Treatment

Principle of Equipoise

J. Rick Turner
Campbell University College of Pharmacy and Health Sciences, Buies Creek, NC, USA

Synonyms

Clinical equipoise; Equipoise

Definition

Clinical equipoise exists when all of the available evidence about a new intervention/treatment does not show that it is more beneficial than an alternative and, equally, does not show that it is less beneficial than the alternative. For example, to be able to conduct a clinical trial that involves administering an investigational treatment that may confer therapeutic benefit to subjects for whom such benefit is desirable to some individuals, and to administer a control intervention treatment that is not capable of conferring therapeutic benefit to others, there cannot be any evidence that suggests that the investigational intervention shows greater efficacy than the control treatment or that it leads to greater side effects than the control treatment.

When individuals agree to participate in a clinical study, they do so with the understanding that all of the treatments are assumed to be of equal value. By the end of the trial, there may be compelling evidence that the investigational intervention is acceptably safe and statistically significantly more effective than the control intervention, but the study must be started with a good faith belief that the two treatments are of equal merit.

Treating subjects in clinical studies (trials) in an ethical manner is of paramount importance. Clinical equipoise is a cornerstone of such ethical conduct. Other fundamental ethical principles include respect for persons, beneficence, and justice (see Turner 2010).

Derenzo and Moss (2006) commented as follows:

Each study component has an ethical aspect. The ethical aspects of a clinical trial cannot be separated from the scientific objectives. Segregation of ethical issues from the full range of study design components demonstrates a flaw in understanding the fundamental nature of research involving human subjects. Compartmentalization of ethical issues is inconsistent with a well-run trial. Ethical and scientific considerations are intertwined.

Cross-References

▶ Clinical Trial
▶ Randomized Clinical Trial

References and Further Readings

Derenzo, E., & Moss, J. (2006). *Writing clinical research protocols: Ethical considerations.* San Diego: Elsevier.
Turner, J. R. (2010). *New drug development: An introduction to clinical trials.* New York: Springer.

Privacy

▶ Confidentiality

Proactive Aging

▶ Positive Aging

Probability

J. Rick Turner
Campbell University College of Pharmacy and Health Sciences, Buies Creek, NC, USA

Definition

In situations where certainty is not possible, it can be helpful to assess how likely it is that something will occur. Quantification of this likelihood is particularly helpful in statistical analysis. The concept of probability is used in everyday language, but more loosely than in statistics. The statement "I'll probably be there on Saturday" involves a probabilistic statement, but there is no precise degree of quantification. If you know the individual making this statement, past experience may lead you to an informed judgment concerning the relative meaning of probably, but this is still a subjective judgment, not a quantitative statement.

In statistics, a probability is a numerical quantity between zero (represented here as 0.00) and one (1.00) that expresses the likely occurrence of a future event. Past events cannot be associated with a probability of occurrence, since it is known in absolute terms whether they occurred or not. A probability of zero denotes that the event will not (cannot) occur. A probability of one denotes certainty that the event will occur. Any numerical value between zero and one expresses a relative likelihood of an event occurring. Additionally, the decimal expression of a probability value can be multiplied by 100 to create a percentage statement of likelihood. A probability of 0.50 would thus be expressed as a 50% chance that an event would occur. Similarly, and more relevantly to inferential hypothesis testing, probabilities of 0.05 and 0.01 would be expressed as a 5% chance and a 1% chance, respectively, that an event would occur.

Cross-References

▶ Hypothesis Testing
▶ Statistics

Problem Drinking

▶ Binge Drinking

Problem Solving

Seth A. Margolis[1], Patricia Osborne[1] and Jeffrey S. Gonzalez[2]
[1]Clinical Psychology, Health Emphasis, Ferkauf Graduate School of Psychology, Yeshiva University, Bronx, NY, USA
[2]Departments of Medicine and Epidemiology & Public Health, Albert Einstein College of Medicine, Bronx, NY, USA

Synonyms

Problem-solving skills training (PSST); Problem-Solving Therapy – Primary Care (PST-PC); Problem-Solving Therapy – SO (PST-SO); Social Problem-Solving Therapy (SPST)

Definition

Problem-solving therapy (PST) is a brief, empirically supported, cognitive-behavioral intervention aimed at training clients to identify, evaluate, and resolve everyday problems through the methodical application of problem-solving skills. In addition to teaching specific coping skills, PST emphasizes the importance of maintaining a positive *problem-solving orientation* and a rational *problem-solving style* (D'Zurilla and Nezu 2010).

An individual's *problem-solving orientation* encompasses how one perceives problems, to what/whom they attribute these problems, how they appraise problematic situations, and the degree to which they view their problems as under their control. A major goal of PST is to help clients view problems as solvable challenges instead of insurmountable impasses.

A person's *problem-solving style* addresses the characteristic way in which he or she attempts to manage problems in living. PST advocates a rational approach. This form of problem solving is taught through the use of four essential skills: defining the problem in precise and objective terms (i.e., problem definition and formulation), brainstorming potential solutions (i.e., generation of alternatives), weighing the pros and cons of each alternative and creating a plan of action (i.e., decision making), and implementing the most appropriate solution and evaluating the outcome (i.e., implementation and verification). In combination, these skills are meant to help individuals manage their problems in an organized and systematic manner.

Problem solving serves a critical function in the successful management of chronic medical conditions. PST has, therefore, been adapted for individuals affected by cancer, obesity, diabetes, cardiovascular disease, traumatic brain injury, stroke, as well as older adults, caregivers, and to promote treatment adherence.

PST has been successfully delivered in individual, group, and family formats by psychologists, psychiatrists, social workers, nurses, and graduate-level trainees. Most forms of PST are manual based and all make use of homework assignments. PST therapists tend to balance directive and collaborative treatment styles.

PST interventions have been implemented in primary care settings (Catalan et al. 1991; Mynors-Wallis and Gath 1997; Oxman et al. 2008; Areán et al. 2010), via telephone and in the home (Grant et al 2002), within community clinics and online (Wade et al. 2005, 2008).

Even though PST has been provided as both a stand-alone treatment and as a component of multifaceted interventions, more research is needed to adequately compare the two. Although some studies have addressed PST's applicability to minority groups (Sahler et al. 2005) and different age ranges (Areán et al. 2010), supplementary research is needed in these areas. Finally, given the evidence that PST can be a successful intervention for behavioral medicine settings, it would behoove future investigators to attempt to extend findings to other chronic health conditions.

Cross-References

▶ Cognitive Behavioral Therapy (CBT)
▶ Stroop Color-Word Test

References and Readings

Allen, S. M., Shah, A. C., Nezu, A. M., Ciambrone, D., Hogan, J., & Mor, V. (2002). A problem-solving approach to stress reduction among younger women with breast carcinoma: A randomized controlled trial. *Cancer, 94*(12), 3089–3100.

Arean, P. A., Perri, M. G., Nezu, A. M., Schein, R. L., Christopher, F., & Joseph, T. X. (1993). Comparative effectiveness of social problem-solving therapy and reminiscence therapy as treatments for depression in older adults. *Journal of Consulting and Clinical Psychology, 61*(6), 1003–1010.

Areán, P. A., Raue, P., Mackin, R. S., Kanellopoulos, D., McCulloch, C., & Alexopoulos, G. S. (2010). Problem-solving therapy and supportive therapy in older adults with major depression and executive dysfunction. *American Journal of Psychiatry, 167*, 1391–1398.

Catalan, J., Gath, D. H., Anastasiades, P., Bond, S. A., Day, A., & Hall, L. (1991). Evaluation of a brief psychological treatment for emotional disorders in primary care. *Psychological Medicine, 21*(4), 1012–1018.

Chang, E. C., D'Zurilla, T. J., & Sanna, L. J. (Eds.). (2004). *Social problem solving: Theory, research, and training.* Washington, DC: American Psychological Association.

D'Zurilla, T. J., & Nezu, A. M. (2010). Problem-solving therapy. In K. S. Dobson (Ed.), *Handbook of cognitive-behavioral therapies* (3rd ed., pp. 197–225). New York: Guilford Press.

Grant, J. S., Elliott, T. R., Weaver, M., Bartolucci, A. A., & Ginger, J. N. (2002). Telephone intervention with family caregivers of stroke survivors after rehabilitation. *Stroke, 33*(8), 2060–2065.

Hegel, M. T., Barrett, J. E., & Oxman, T. E. (2000). Training therapists in problem-solving treatment of depressive disorders in primary care: Lessons learned from the "treatment effectiveness project". *Families, Systems & Health, 18*, 423–435.

Houts, P. S., Nezu, A. M., Nezu, C. M., & Bucher, J. A. (1996). The prepared family caregiver: A problem-solving approach to family caregiver education. *Patient Education and Counseling, 27*, 63–73.

Mynors-Wallis, L., & Gath, D. (1997). Predictors of treatment outcome for major depression in primary care. *Psychological Medicine, 27*(3), 731–736.

Nezu, A. M., Nezu, C. M., Felgoise, S. H., McClure, K. S., & Hots, P. S. (2003). Project genesis: Assessing the efficacy of problem-solving therapy for distressed adult cancer patients. *Journal of Consulting and Clinical Psychology, 71*(6), 1036–1048.

Nezu, A. M., Nezu, C. M., & D'Zurilla, T. J. (2010). Problem-solving therapy. In N. Kazantzis, M. S. Reinecke, & A. Freeman (Eds.), *Cognitive and behavioral theories in practice* (pp. 76–114). New York: Guilford Press.

Oxman, T. E., Hegel, M. T., Hull, J. G., & Dietrich, A. J. (2008). Problem-solving treatment and coping styles in primary care for minor depression. *Journal of Consulting and Clinical Psychology, 76*(6), 933–943.

Perri, M. G., Nezu, A. M., McKelvey, W. F., Shermer, R. L., Renjilian, D. A., & Viegener, B. J. (2001). Individual versus group therapy for obesity: Effects of matching participants to their treatment preferences. *Journal of Consulting and Clinical Psychology, 69*(4), 722–726.

Sahler, O. J., Fairclough, D. L., Phipps, S., Mulhern, R. K., Dolgin, M. J., Noll, R. B., et al. (2005). Using problem-solving skills training to reduce negative affectivity in mothers of children with newly diagnosed cancer: Report of a multisite randomized trial. *Journal of Consulting and Clinical Psychology, 73*(2), 272–283.

Wade, S. L., Wolfe, C., Brown, T. M., & Pestian, J. P. (2005). Putting the pieces together: Preliminary efficacy of a web-based family intervention for children with traumatic brain injury. *Journal of Pediatric Psychology, 30*(5), 437–442.

Wade, S. L., Walz, N. C., Carey, J. C., & William, K. M. (2008). Preliminary efficacy of a web-based family problem-solving treatment program for adolescents with traumatic brain injury. *Journal of Head Trauma Rehabilitation, 23*(6), 369–377.

Problem-Focused Coping

Linda Carroll
Department of Public Health Sciences, University of Alberta, Edmonton, AB, Canada

Synonyms

Active coping

Definition

Coping refers to the intentional efforts we engage in to minimize the physical, psychological, or social harm of an event or situation. There are many different frameworks for understanding coping and many different ways of classifying coping strategies, but one such classification is problem-focused coping vs. emotion-focused coping. Problem-focused coping is that kind of coping aimed at resolving the stressful situation or event or altering the source of the stress. Coping strategies that can be considered to be problem-focused include (but are not limited to) taking control of the stress (e.g., problem solving or removing the source of the stress), seeking information or assistance in handling the situation, and removing oneself from the stressful situation.

Problem-focused coping is distinguished from emotion-focused coping, which is aimed at managing the emotions associated with the situation, rather than changing the situation itself. For example, when anxious about an upcoming exam, use of problem-focused coping strategies might involve checking with the teacher about material one is unsure of, or increasing the time spent studying, or even deciding not to take the exam (although removing oneself from the stressor might have other negative consequences in this particular example). In contrast, emotion-focused coping strategies might involve self-talk to increase one's confidence in one's test taking ability or using relaxation techniques to decrease fear and anxiety. Problem-focused coping works best when the source of the stress is potentially under an individual's control; however, when the source of the stress is beyond the individual's control, such strategies are not usually helpful. Examples are dealing with bereavement. In situations like this, problem-focused coping is less likely to be helpful than emotion-focused coping, for example, processing one's feelings or releasing one's feelings. Problem- and emotion-focused coping are not mutually exclusive, and individuals frequently use both problem- and emotion-focused coping strategies to deal with stress. For example, when feeling threatened, initial use of emotion-focused coping to gain control over the fear can facilitate the subsequent use of problem-focused coping. Problem- and emotion-focused coping are the two subscales that comprise the Ways of Coping Checklist.

Cross-References

▶ Active Coping
▶ Coping

References and Readings

Field, T., McCabe, P. M., & Schneiderman, N. (1985). *Stress and coping*. Hillsdale: Erlbaum.

Lazarus, R. S. (1999). *Stress and emotion: A new synthesis*. New York: Springer.

Lazarus, R. S., & Folkman, S. (1984). *Stress, appraisal and coping*. New York: Springer.

Moos, R. H. (1986). *Coping with life crises: An integrated approach*. New York: Plenum Press.

Zeidner, M., & Endler, N. S. (1996). *Handbook of coping: Theory, research, applications*. New York: Wiley.

Problem-Solving Skills Training (PSST)

▶ Problem Solving

Problem-Solving Therapy – Primary Care (PST-PC)

▶ Problem Solving

Problem-Solving Therapy – SO (PST-SO)

▶ Problem Solving

Productive Aging

▶ Positive Aging

Productivity

▶ Job Performance

Progress

▶ Aging

Promotoras

P. H. Amelie Ramirez[1] and Barbara Turner[2]
[1]Department of Epidemiology and Biostatistics, The University of Texas Health Science Center at San Antonio, San Antonio, TX, USA
[2]The University of Texas Health Science Center at San Antonio, San Antonio, TX, USA

Synonyms

Community health advisors; Community health representatives; Community health workers (CHW); Health navigators; Lay health advisors; Lay health advocates; Outreach educators; Peer coaches; Peer health educators; Peer health promoters

Definition

Promotoras (or *promotoras de salud*) are female community health workers who provide a variety of services in their role as liaison between underserved Hispanics and traditional health care services. Their male counterparts are *promotores*, although it is less common to have men serve in this role. These terms translate to "promoters" of health, in this case among Hispanics who have historically experienced challenges accessing health care services and deficiencies in outcomes of care. These individuals are either volunteers or employees of the local health care system or other entities administering community interventions. They typically live in the community or neighborhood that they serve and thus can better communicate and relate to their clients because of their shared community experiences.

Description

Essentially, the *promotora* concept is a form of community-based peer support: nonprofessionals helping others with various health needs. These needs include: culturally appropriate education, informal advice and counsel, social support and encouragement, interpretation and translation, advocacy for health needs, disease management and prevention, health care system navigation, and community resource guidance. Depending upon the community health priorities and the specific goals and objectives of particular programs, *promotoras* may provide one or a combination of these services.

Historically, *promotoras* are part of a long tradition of lay health workers who serve critical health care and disease prevention roles in cultures around the world. For example, in eighteenth century Russia, *feldshers* began providing medical assistance in urban hospitals and the army. In China, during the 1960s, farmworkers were trained as "barefoot doctors" to give first aid, immunizations, and health education in rural areas. In Haiti, village health workers known as *accompagnateurs* attended individuals suffering from tuberculosis and HIV/AIDS. In Africa, health care workers provide the main form of health care delivery and especially have served as the linchpin for HIV prevention and treatment. Origins of the *promotoras* can also be found in Latin American countries, where laymen and laywomen were trained by church groups and other organizations to give community health assistance.

Efforts to establish formal community health worker programs in this country can be traced back over a half-century. Such outreach was subsequently included in the federal Migrant Health Act of 1962 and the Economic Opportunity Act of 1964, mandating utilization of community health aides in many neighborhoods and migrant worker camps (Hill et al. 1996). The Affordable Care Act of 2010 provided a more recent endorsement of the concept, specifying community health workers as an integral component of the nation's health care workforce (Affordable Care Act of 2010). With the rise in health care costs in recent times and increased awareness of the scope and cost of health disparities in this country, the peer-support approach has gained increasing support as a viable and potentially cost-effective means of helping fill gaps in the health care system. However, the evidence so far is conflicting and comes from less than optimally designed studies.

In the USA today, the nomenclature for peer health promotion personnel is diverse, including: community health workers (CHW), community health advisors, lay health advisors, lay health advocates, peer coaches, outreach educators, health navigators, peer health promoters, peer health educators, community health representatives, and, in Hispanic communities, *promotoras*. Often, some of these terms, including CHW and *promotoras*, are used interchangeably or in combination.

Surveys have found that these community health workers operate in all 50 states (U.S. Department of Health and Human Services Health Resources and Services Administration 2007). Programs utilizing *promotoras* have flourished especially in states with large Hispanic populations such as California and along the USA-Mexico border. In 2009, Hispanics represented 16% of the US population (U.S. Census Bureau News 2010) and this proportion is expected to rise dramatically in the coming decades. With the growing number of Hispanics, the peer-assistance concept has been incorporated into health programs and interventions across the country. This model has been evaluated in large cities, mid-size and smaller communities, as well as agricultural areas (working with farmworkers and their families), with favorable results in many studies.

Promotora involvement has been found to be useful in a broad range of needs, such as management of diabetes and other health conditions prevalent among Hispanics, screening for cancer and other diseases, and access to health care overall. They also can focus on addressing specific needs such as prenatal care, or healthy lifestyle behaviors in general (e.g., proper diet and exercise). In addition to working with diabetes and cancer patients, survivors, and at-risk individuals, *promotoras*/CHW have been involved in interventions targeting cardiovascular disease,

HIV/AIDS, high blood pressure, asthma, mental illness, and other diseases.

Firsthand knowledge of the local Hispanic community and the personal and institutional barriers that residents of the community face in attaining adequate health care uniquely prepares *promotoras* for their liaison role. As Spanish speakers and residents of the neighborhoods they serve, *promotoras* offer assistance to reduce or remove linguistic and cultural barriers for segments of the population that have historically been difficult to reach for local health care agencies and services. At the same time, *promotoras* can provide assistance to professional health care personnel by educating providers and their staff about sociocultural factors that influence the health knowledge, beliefs, and attitudes, as well as the values and behaviors, of their Hispanic patients.

Among the strengths of the *promotora*/CHW models employed in various community health programs is the broad diversity of services peer health workers have been able to deliver. For example, as liaisons between health providers and underserved Hispanics, *promotoras* sometimes serve as interpreters as well as health system navigators, assisting in identification of benefits that clients are eligible to receive, and helping them complete necessary applications and forms. As case managers, *promotoras* typically facilitate contacts of health care providers with community members by maintaining accurate contact information and a record of interactions. As community organizers, *promotoras* have been called upon to motivate and encourage members of the community to participate actively in efforts to improve neighborhood living conditions. And as health educators, *promotoras* distribute and explain print and other informative materials aimed at promoting screening, preventing disease, discouraging smoking, managing chronic diseases, and other health promotion purposes. In addition, interventions have utilized *promotoras* in various other roles, including as group presentation leaders; role models; and guides to community social, transportation, childcare, and other services and resources.

Promotoras are typically respected and trusted members of the community they serve. Due to their familiarity with their community and neighborhood, *promotoras* can move freely within the community and engage with various sectors. They provide their services in convenient locations, including homes, schools, churches, clinics, hospitals, community centers, job sites, and other locales. In many programs, they also participate in community events, such as health fairs.

In the past, *promotoras* and other community health workers have typically been trained on the job. With the increased utilization of peer-support models over the years, concerns about the quality of this training and the need for more standard certification of these workers have been increasingly raised. However, as of 2010, only a handful of states had taken steps to address these issues. In 1999, Texas was the first state to legislate voluntary training and certification for *promotoras* and community health workers (Nichols et al. 2005). In Minnesota, select community colleges offer a standardized curriculum for community health worker certification, with completion required for a worker to be eligible as a Medicaid provider (Rosenthal et al. 2010). In numerous states, certificates are being awarded, typically by community colleges and other programs, for completion of a course of community health worker studies. Proponents of required certification or credentialing note potential benefits, including offering assurance that workers possess basic competencies and promoting perceived legitimacy within health/human services fields. Others, however, contend that requiring certification may have a detrimental effect on the number of peer health workers from poor, minority neighborhoods and communities that most need to be served (Family Strengthening Policy Center 2006).

From the substantial experience with *promotora*/CHW program implementation and research, the evidence is growing that peer support offers unique benefits to improve health care delivery and outcomes. This is particularly relevant, given rapidly expanding lower-socio economic status (SES) racial/ethnic segments of the population (particularly Hispanics), growing numbers of patients with chronic diseases, and spiraling health care costs. Systematic reviews of the benefit of peer support currently find that the evidence lacks sufficient rigor. Consequently, much more research needs to be conducted to define roles and scope of activities, determine effectiveness, develop consistent and adequate training, provide fair compensation, and, via certification and/or similar means, define a universally accepted and respected niche for *promotoras* among the nation's health care workforce.

Cross-References

▶ Health Disparities
▶ Health Education
▶ Health Literacy

References and Readings

Balcazar, H. G., Byrd, T. L., Ortiz, M., Tondapu, S. R., & Chavez, M. (2009). A randomized community intervention to improve hypertension control among Mexican Americans: Using the *promotoras de salud* community outreach model. *Journal of Health Care for the Poor and Underserved, 20*(4), 1079–1094.

Boothroyd, R. I., & Fisher, E. B. (2010). Peers for progress: Promoting peer support for health around the world. *Family Practice, 27*(Suppl. 1), i62–i68.

Centers for Disease Control and Prevention (2011). Community health workers/*Promotores de Salud*: Critical connections in communities. Accessed online from http://www.cdc.gov/diabetes/projects/comm.htm

Doull, M., O'Connor, A. M., Welch, V., Tugwell, P., Wells, G. A. (2008). Peer support strategies for improving the health and well-being of individuals with chronic diseases (Protocol). Copyright © 2008 The Cochrane Collaboration. Published by Wiley.

Family Strengthening Policy Center. (2006). *Community health workers: Closing gaps in families' health resources* (Policy Brief No. 14). Accessed online from http://www.nydic.org/fspc/practice/documents/Brief14.pdf

Hill, M. N., Bone, L. R., & Butz, A. M. (1996). Enhancing the role of community health workers in research. *Image, 28*, 221–226.

Kumar, P. (2007). Providing the providers – Remedying Africa's shortage of health care workers. *The New England Journal of Medicine, 356*, 2564–2567.

Nichols, D. C., Berrios, C., & Samar, H. (2005). Texas' community health workforce: from state health promotion policy to community-level practice. *Preventing Chronic Disease, 2*(Special Issue), A13. Published online 2005 October 15.

O'Brien, M. J., Halbert, C. H., Bixby, R., Pimentel, S., & Shea, J. A. (2010). Community health worker intervention to decrease cervical cancer disparities in Hispanic women. *Journal of General Internal Medicine, 25*(11), 1186–1192. Epub 2010 July 7.

Patient Protection and Affordable Care Act, PL111-148, § 5101, 5102, 5313, 5403, and 3509 (2010).

Rosenthal, E. L., Brownstein, J. N., Rush, C. H., Hirsch, G. R., Willaert, A. M., Scott, J. R., et al. (2010). Community health workers: Part of the solution. *Health Affairs, 29*(7), 1338–1342.

U.S. Census Bureau News, U.S. Department of Commerce. (2010, July 15). Facts for Features CB10-FF.17. Accessed online from http://www.census.gov/newsroom/releases/pdf/cb10ff-17_hispanic.pdf

U.S. Department of Health and Human Services Health Resources and Services Administration. (2007, March). Community health workers national workforce study. Accessed online from http://bhpr.hrsa.gov/healthworkforce/chw/default.htm#preface

Vargas, R. B., & Cunningham, W. E. (2006). Evolving trends in medical care-coordination for patients with HIV and AIDS. *Current HIV/AIDS Reports, 3*(4), 149–153.

Viswanathan, M., Kraschnewski, J., Nishikawa, B., Morgan, L. C., Thieda, P., Honeycutt, A., et al. (2009). *Outcomes of community health worker interventions* (Evidence Report/Technology Assessment No. 181, Prepared by the RTI International-University of North Carolina Evidence-based Practice Center under Contract No. 290 2007 10056 I, AHRQ Publication No. 09-E014). Rockville, MD: Agency for Healthcare Research and Quality.

Prophylactic Care

▶ Preventive Care

Prophylactic Use

▶ Condom Use

Prospective Study

▶ Follow-Up Study

Prostate

Marc A. Kowalkouski[1,2], Heather Honoré Goltz[1,2], Stacey L. Hart[3] and David Latini[4]
[1]HSR&D Center of Excellence, Michael E. DeBakey VA Medical Center (MEDVAMC 152), Houston, TX, USA
[2]Department of Social Sciences, University of Houston-Downtown, Houston, TX, USA
[3]Department of Psychology, Ryerson University, Toronto, ON, Canada
[4]Scott Department of Urology, Baylor College of Medicine, Houston, TX, USA

Synonyms

Prostate gland

Definition

Prostate Anatomy
The prostate is a walnut-sized gland that functions in the male reproductive system. It is positioned in front of the rectum and directly below the bladder, which stores urine. The prostate also encircles the proximal urethra, the canal which carries urine from the bladder and through the penis.

Three distinct zones of glandular tissue make up the prostate: the peripheral zone, central zone, and transition zone. Additionally, there is an area of fibromuscular tissue on the anterior surface. Each anatomic zone is uniquely affected by different disease processes. The majority of prostate cancers develop in the peripheral zone, the largest zone by volume, while benign prostatic hyperplasia originates in the transition zone.

Description

Prostate Function
The prostate produces the thick, milky-white alkaline fluid that forms part of semen. The fluid provides nourishment to sperm and, along with fluid from the bulbourethral (Cowper's) glands, helps to neutralize the acidity of the urine residue in the male urethra and of the female vaginal canal, increasing the life span of sperm. During ejaculation, contraction of smooth muscles moves the fluid from the prostate into the urethral tract where it mixes with the sperm produced by the testicles and additional fluid from the bulbourethral glands and seminal vesicles. The resulting mixture, semen, passes from the urethra and out through the penis.

Common Disorders of the Prostate
There are three common conditions of the prostate: prostatitis, benign prostatic hyperplasia, and prostate cancer. Generally, older men are more susceptible to prostate disease. However, prostatitis can affect men at any age. Prostatitis is a benign infection of prostatic tissue, usually caused by bacteria. Inflammation can result in urine retention in the bladder, resulting in bladder distention (i.e., enlargement) and exposing the bladder to additional risk for infection. Additionally, prostatitis can trigger several urinary problems (e.g., pain or burning upon urination, urgency, and trouble voiding). Benign prostatic hyperplasia, or BPH, is another common prostatic condition caused by the noncancerous enlargement of the prostate gland in aging men. As the prostate enlarges, it compresses the urethra and irritates the bladder. Obstruction of the urethra, as well as gradually diminishing bladder function, results in the symptoms of BPH including dribbling after urination or a need to urinate often, especially at night. Some men also experience urinary incontinence, the involuntary discharge of urine. BPH symptoms can severely affect a man's, as well as his partner's, quality of life and can be further compounded by psychological factors (e.g., depression and anxiety) associated with BPH symptoms. Prostate cancer is the most common malignancy and the second most common cause of cancer death among men in the United States. Response to treatment is best when the disease is caught early. However, prostate cancer is generally asymptomatic when the disease is

localized to the prostate. Screening for prostate cancer includes serum prostate-specific antigen (PSA) testing and digital rectal examination. There are many treatment options available to men diagnosed with prostate cancer (e.g., active surveillance, radiotherapy, and surgery). However, there is currently no consensus regarding the optimal treatment.

Cross-References

▶ Prostate-Specific Antigen (PSA)

References and Readings

Gacci, M., Bartoletti, R., Figlioli, S., Sarti, E., Eisner, B., Boddi, V., et al. (2003). Urinary symptoms, quality of life and sexual function in patients with benign prostatic hypertrophy before and after prostatectomy: A prospective study. *British Journal of Urology International, 91*, 196.

Mitropoulos, D., Anastasiou, I., Giannopoulou, C., Nikolopoulos, P., Alamanis, Z., & Dimopoulos, C. (2002). Symptomatic benign prostatic hyperplasia: Impact on partners' quality of life. *European Urology, 41*, 240–245.

Ramakrishnan, K., & Salinas, R. C. (2010). Prostatitis: Acute and chronic. *Primary Care, 37*, 547–563, vii–ix.

Tanagho, E. A., & McAninch, J. W. (Eds.). (2008). *Smith's general urology* (17th ed.). New York: McGraw-Hill.

Wein, A. J., Coyne, K. S., Tubaro, A., Sexton, C. C., Kopp, Z. S., & Aiyer, L. P. (2009). The impact of lower urinary tract symptoms on male sexual health: EpiLUTS. *British Journal of Urology International, 103*(Suppl. 3), 33–41.

Prostate Gland

▶ Prostate

Prostatectomy

▶ Radical Prostatectomy, Psychological Impact

Prostate-Specific Antigen (PSA)

Marc A. Kowalkouski[1,2], Heather Honoré Goltz[1,2], Stacey L. Hart[3] and David Latini[4]
[1]HSR&D Center of Excellence, Michael E. DeBakey VA Medical Center (MEDVAMC 152), Houston, TX, USA
[2]Department of Social Sciences, University of Houston-Downtown, Houston, TX, USA
[3]Department of Psychology, Ryerson University, Toronto, ON, Canada
[4]Scott Department of Urology, Baylor College of Medicine, Houston, TX, USA

Synonyms

Kallikrein-3; P-30 antigen; Semenogelase; Seminin

Definition

Prostate-specific antigen (PSA) is a protein produced by cells of the prostate gland. PSA functions in male fertility, and most of it gets expelled from the body in semen. However, low levels circulate in the blood. Elevated serum PSA levels often indicate the presence of prostate cancer and other prostate disorders.

Description

Measuring PSA
The PSA screening test measures the total level of PSA circulating in the blood serum. PSA levels above 4 ng per milliliter are considered above normal. However, total PSA does not offer a definitive diagnosis for cancer or other prostate disease. Therefore, additional measures of PSA have been integrated to depict a more comprehensive profile of prostate disease characteristics. For example, PSA velocity measures the rate of increase in PSA over time. Generally, larger PSA velocity is associated with prostate cancer. Free

PSA is the percentage of circulating PSA that is not bound to other proteins. On average, men with a low percentage of free PSA are more likely to have cancer. PSA density is the PSA level divided by prostate volume. The likelihood of cancer is increased when PSA density is high.

PSA Testing and Current Guidelines

PSA testing has become increasingly popular because it allows detection of prostate cancer at early stages, before palpable detection during digital rectal examination. However, PSA testing also presents a high rate of false-positive and false-negative results, which has generated substantial controversy with regard to whether or not PSA screening is effective at reducing cancer deaths. Two large, randomized clinical trials are currently evaluating the efficacy of PSA screening. Preliminary findings indicate modest reductions in cancer deaths in the screening group but also note over-detection and potential overtreatment of clinically insignificant cancers in the same group. Accounting for these complex issues, the American Cancer Society (ACS) has revised its recommendations regarding routine PSA screening. The revised guidelines now recommend that doctors initiate comprehensive discussions with patients about their options for screening and that men use decision-making tools to make an informed choice about testing. The ACS suggests these guidelines are appropriate for patients over age 50 who are in good health with greater than 10 years of life expectancy. For men at higher risk (e.g., African American men and men with a positive family history), ACS guidelines suggest that discussions about screening begin earlier. The ACS does not endorse screening for men with several comorbid conditions or for men with less than 10 years of life expectancy. In response to the preliminary findings from the previously mentioned studies, the American Urological Association (AUA) also revised its screening recommendations, which suggest extending screening to younger men. The AUA advises that PSA screening should be offered to well-informed men aged 40 years or older who have a life expectancy of at least 10 years. Additionally, AUA guidelines emphasize a shift away from using a single PSA threshold to determine whether to proceed to additional diagnostics. Instead, the combination of many factors (e.g., PSA profile over time, family history, race, age) should be considered.

References and Readings

American Cancer Society. (2010). *Cancer facts and figures 2010*. Atlanta, GA: Author.

American Urological Association. (2009). *Prostate-specific antigen best practice statement: 2009 Update*. Washington, DC: American Urological Association Education and Research.

Andriole, G. L., Grubb, R. L., Buys, S. S., Crawford, E. D., Chia, D., Church, T. R., et al. (2009). Mortality results from a randomized prostate-cancer screening trial. *The New England Journal of Medicine, 360*, 1310–1319.

Carroll, P. R., Whitson, J. M., & Cooperberg, M. R. (2010). Serum prostate-specific antigen for the early detection of prostate cancer: Always, never, or only sometimes? *Journal of Clinical Oncology, 28*, 1–3.

Jacobsen, S. J., Katusic, S. K., Bergstralh, E. J., Oesterling, J. E., Ohrt, D., Klee, G. G., et al. (1995). Incidence of prostate cancer diagnosis in the eras before and after serum prostate-specific antigen testing. *Journal of the American Medical Association, 274*, 1445–1449.

Schroder, F. H., Hugosson, J., Roobol, M. J., Tammela, T. L., Ciatto, S., Nelen, V., et al. (2009). Screening and prostate-cancer mortality in a randomized European study. *The New England Journal of Medicine, 360*, 1320–1328.

Tanagho, E. A., & McAninch, J. W. (Eds.). (2008). *Smith's general urology* (17th ed.). New York: McGraw-Hill.

Vickers, A. J., Savage, C., O'Brien, M. F., & Lilja, H. (2008). Systematic review of pretreatment prostate-specific antigen velocity and doubling time as predictors for prostate cancer. *Journal of Clinical Oncology, 27*, 398–403.

Prostatic Adenocarcinoma

▶ Cancer, Prostate

Protected Sex

▶ Condom Use

Protection of Human Subjects

Marianne Shaughnessy
School of Nursing, University of Maryland,
Baltimore, MD, USA

Synonyms

Human subjects protections

Definition

The organized oversight of research to ensure the rights and well-being of participants.

Description

The protection of human subjects in clinical research evolved in response to conditions surrounding medical research that were deemed unacceptable in the early to mid-twentieth century. In December 1946, an American military tribunal opened criminal proceedings against 23 German physicians who conducted medical experiments on thousands of concentration camp prisoners without their consent. Most of the subjects of these experiments died or were permanently disabled as a result. The Nuremberg Code of 1948 resulted, stating that "voluntary consent of a human subject is absolutely essential" and that "the benefits of research must outweigh the risks" (NIH). In 1964, the World Medical Association published recommendations for research involving human subjects, and the Declaration of Helsinki governs international research ethics and defines rules for "research combined with clinical care" and "non-therapeutic research." This declaration was revised in 1975, 1983, 1989, and 1996 and remains the basis for Good Clinical practices used today (WMA).

In the United States, the Tuskeegee Syphilis Study (1932–1972) described the natural history of syphilis in 600 low-income African American males, 400 of whom were infected. Over 40 years, researchers provided medical examinations, but infected subjects were never told of their disease nor offered treatment, even after a known cure became available in 1947. Many of the subjects died from syphilis-related causes during the study. The study was stopped in 1973 by the U.S. Department of Health, Education and Welfare after its existence was publicized (CDC). The publicity generated by the Nuremberg trials, the Tuskeegee study, and other studies created a mistrust of medical researchers and a demand for a standards and guidelines for the ethical conduct of research. On July 12, 1974, the National Research Act (Pub. L. 93–348) was signed into law, creating the National Commission for the Protection of Human Subjects of Biomedical and Behavioral Research. This commission generated the Belmont Report in 1976, a summary of the ethical principles identified by the Commission that should be used to guide human subjects research. These principles include (1) respect for persons, (2) beneficence, and (3) justice. The application of these general principles is further described in specific guidance for obtaining informed consent, complete assessment of risks, and benefits and selection of research subjects.

Medical research is conducted in a variety of academic and corporate settings, but all human subjects research studies should be evaluated by an Institutional Review Board or similar research oversight committee prior to initiation. This is a requirement for all federally funded research in the United States. These oversight boards are responsible for the review of each proposed study to ensure that the principles of the Belmont Report are applied and that the rights of potential and actual participants are respected. The Association for the Accreditation of Human Research Protection Programs (AAHRPP) reviews the processes established by these research oversight bodies and grants accreditation for such programs that meet general requirements and demonstrate processes geared toward continual improvement of research and the protection of human subjects.

Cross-References

▶ Research Participation, Risks and Benefits of

References and Readings

Association for the Accreditation of Human Research Protection Programs. Retrieved May 18, 2011 from http://www.aahrpp.org
Center for Information and Study on Clinical Research Participation (CISCRP). Retrieved May 18, 2011 from http://www.ciscrp.org/
Centers for Disease Control and Prevention (CDC). Retrieved May 18, 2011 from http://www.cdc.gov/tuskegee/timeline.htm
NIH Office of Human Subjects Research. Retrieved May 18, 2011 from http://ohsr.od.nih.gov/guidelines/nuremberg.html
The Belmont report. Retrieved May 18, 2011 from http://ohsr.od.nih.gov/guidelines/belmont.html
The Hastings Center. Retrieved May 18, 2011 from http://www.thehastingscenter.org
World Medical Association (WMA). Retrieved May 18, 2011 from http://www.wma.net/en/30publications/10policies/b3/

Protective Factors

▶ Cardiovascular Risk Factors

Protein Methylation

▶ Methylation

Proteomics

J. Rick Turner
Campbell University College of Pharmacy and Health Sciences, Buies Creek, NC, USA

Definition

Proteomics is the study of all of a genome's putative proteins and involves the systematic analysis of proteins to determine their identity, quantity, and function (Soloviev et al. 2004).

Description

The Human Genome Project and related work have focused considerable attention on sequencing aspects of genomic research. However, as Holmes et al. (2005) noted, "The eventual goal of these projects is actually to determine how the genome builds life through proteins. DNA has been the focus of attention because the tools for studying it are more advanced and because it is at the heart of the cell, carrying all the information – the blueprint – for life. However, a blueprint without a builder is not very useful, and the proteins are the primary builders within the cell."

It is of interest to characterize the complement of expressed proteins from a single genome. Monitoring the expression and properties of a large number of proteins provides important information about the physiological state of a cell and, by extension, an organism. Cells can express very large numbers of different proteins, and the "expression profile" (the number of proteins expressed and the expression level of each of them) can vary in different cell types. Given that each cell contains all genomic material and hence information, this differential expression of proteins explains why cells perform different functions (Soloviev et al. 2004).

The 20,000–25,000 genes in the human genome actually generate many more than the commensurate number of proteins, with estimates as high as one million appearing in the literature (Augen 2005). This huge number results from the observation that multiple, distinct proteins can result from a single gene. Consider the following steps in the journey from the genome to the proteome (Holmes et al. 2005):

- DNA replication results in many gene forms.
- Ribonucleic acid (RNA) transcription leads to pre-messenger RNA.
- RNA maturation results in mature messenger RNA.
- Protein translation results in an immature protein.

- Protein maturation results in a mature protein in the proteome (posttranslational modifications are possible here).

The tremendous diversity of proteins in the proteome is facilitated by multiple possible means of protein expression. At each stage of the multistep process just described, alternate mechanisms produce variants of the "standard" protein, resulting in a proteome that is far greater than the genome that generates it. Posttranslational modifications play a considerable part in this creation of diversity. These modifications include, for example, the process of glycosylation in which proteins are glycosylated and hence become glycoproteins, which act as receptors and enzymes.

Nobel Laureate James Watson commented as follows with regard to the fields of proteomics and transcriptomics (Watson 2004): "In the wake of the Human Genome Project, two new post-genomic fields have duly emerged, both of them burdened with unimaginative names incorporating the '-omic' of their ancestor: proteomics and transcriptomics. Proteomics is the study of the proteins encoded by genes. Transcriptomics is devoted to determining where and when genes are expressed – that is, which genes are transcriptionally active in a given cell."

Cross-References

- ▶ DNA
- ▶ Genomics
- ▶ Human Genome Project

References and Further Readings

Augen, J. (2005). *Bioinformatics in the post-genomic era: Genome, transcriptome, proteome, and information-based medicine*. Boston: Addison-Wesley.
Holmes, M. R., Ramkissoon, K. R., & Giddings, M. C. (2005). Proteomics and protein identification. In A. D. Baxevanis & B. F. F. Ouellette (Eds.), *Bioinformatics: A practical guide to the analysis of genes and proteins* (3rd ed.). Hoboken: Wiley-Interscience.
Soloviev, M., Barry, R., & Terrett, J. (2004). Chip-based proteomics technology. In R. Rapley & S. Harbron (Eds.), *Molecular analysis and genome discovery*. Hoboken: Wiley.
Watson, J. D. (2004). *DNA: The secret of life*. New York: Alfred A Knopf.

Prototyping

▶ Agile Science

Proxy

▶ Surrogate Decision Making

Prozac®

▶ Selective Serotonin Reuptake Inhibitors (SSRIs)

Psychiatric Diagnosis

Toru Okuyama
Division of Psycho-oncology and Palliative Care, Nagoya City University Hospital, Nagoya, Aichi, Japan

Synonyms

Diagnostic criteria; Psychiatric disorder

Definition

Psychiatric diagnosis defines a psychiatric disorder which causes subjective distress and disability and can be conceptualized based on symptomatology, epidemiology, and pathophysiology. The primary purpose of the psychiatric diagnosis is to distinguish a certain condition from non-disease conditions or other disease conditions and to make health providers communicate better with each other by using shared concepts and languages. Psychiatric diagnosis facilitates researches by maintaining the internal validity of each psychiatric disease and is important for examining the external validity of findings when applying research evidences into individual patients.

Description

The top two most important and frequently used psychiatric diagnoses classification systems are the International Classification of Disease (ICD) by World Health Organization (WHO) and the Diagnostic and Statistical Manual of Mental Disorders (DSM) edited by the American Psychiatric Association.

The ICD is the international standard diagnostic classification of physical and psychiatric diseases and other health conditions, defined by WHO. It has been developed for the purpose of international use since the beginning, and WHO Member States compile national mortality and morbidity statistics based on this diagnostic system. The tenth revision was published in 1992. The classification of mental and behavioral disorders is included in Chap. F. ICD-10 consists of Clinical Descriptions and Diagnostic Guidelines and Diagnostic Criteria for Research. The former provides clinical descriptions detailing the principal signs and symptoms of each disorder. The latter is intended to help those researching specific disorders to maximize the homogeneity of study groups.

The latest version of DSM is the fourth edition text revision published in 2000 (DSM-IV-TR), in which several important features are included. First, it adopts the descriptive approach: the diagnoses criteria are defined based on the symptomatology, rather than the underlying causes. Secondly, clearly defined diagnostic criteria are provided for each specific disorder. These criteria include lists of features that must be present for diagnoses to be made. Thirdly, DSM-IV-TR is a multidimensional evaluation system (Axis I: clinical disorders and other conditions that may be a focus of clinical attention, Axis II: personality disorders and mental retardation, Axis III: any physical disorder or general medical condition, Axis IV: the psychosocial and environmental problems that contribute significantly to the development or exacerbation of the current disorder, Axis V: a global assessment of functioning). The codes and terms used in the DSM-IV are designed to correspond with the codes used in the ICD-10.

It is also important how to apply these diagnostic criteria into each actual patient, in order to maximize the reliability of psychiatric diagnosis. Structured interviews were developed for this purpose. In structured interviews, the procedures for interviews including how to ask about the presence or absence of certain symptom and how to categorize patients' responses are strictly defined so that high inter-rater reliability of the diagnosis can be achieved. Since currently there are no gold standard objective diagnostic tests for psychiatric diagnosis, structured interviews are considered to be gold standard.

A clinical diagnosis includes the whole process of diagnostic formulation in addition to a psychiatric diagnosis based on the diagnostic criteria. A diagnostic formulation is an attempt to understand each patient comprehensively and individually by describing what has been influencing the feeling and behavior of the patient and what relationship might exist between the patient's life situation/background and the psychiatric illness.

Cross-References

▶ Diagnostic Interview Schedule

References and Readings

American Psychiatric Association. (2000). *Diagnostic and statistical manual of mental disorders (Text revision)* (4th ed.). Washington, DC: Author.

World Health Organization. (1992). *ICD-10: The ICD-10 classification of mental and behavioural disorders: Clinical descriptions and diagnostic guidelines*. Geneva: Author.

Zimmerman, M., & Spitzer, R. L. (2009). Classification in psychiatry. In B. J. Sadock, V. A. Sadock, & P. Ruiz (Eds.), *Comprehensive textbook of psychiatry* (pp. 1003–1052). Philadelphia: Lippincott Williams & Wilkins.

Psychiatric Disorder

- Psychiatric Diagnosis
- Psychiatric Illness
- Psychological Disorder

Psychiatric Illness

Maxine Holmqvist
Clinical Health Psychology, University of Manitoba, Winnipeg, MB, Canada

Synonyms

Mental illness; Psychiatric disorder; Psychological disorder

Definition

A condition or syndrome with distinctive cognitive, affective, and/or behavioral symptoms, arising from underlying psychobiological dysfunction and causing significant distress, impairment, or an increased risk of death, pain, disability, or an important loss of freedom (American Psychiatric Association [APA] 2000).

Description

Psychiatry is a branch of medicine that focuses on the diagnosis and treatment of mental illness. It did not emerge as an independent discipline until the late 1800s; however, the roots of psychiatric assessment and treatment extend back to the ancient Greeks and Egyptians (for a comprehensive overview of the history of psychiatry, see Wallace and Gach 2008). Psychiatric illnesses are currently diagnosed with reference to either the Diagnostic and Statistical Manual of Mental Disorders, 4th edition (DSM-IV; APA 2000) or the International Classification of Disease, 10th revision (ICD-10; for more information on these systems, see *Psychological Disorders*, this volume). Psychiatric diagnoses are descriptive, and with few exceptions, they convey very little about etiology. McHugh and Slavney (McHugh and Slavney 1998) identify different perspectives that psychiatrists use to conceptualize cases and plan interventions. Disease reasoning presupposes that a patients' condition is the result of changes or defects in brain functioning. In contrast to this, behavioral reasoning presupposes that a patient's condition is the result of dysfunctional behavior. These two perspectives suggest different interventions; where the presumed cause is pathology of the brain, it follows that the appropriate treatment would likely involve medical intervention (e.g., pharmaceutical drugs, surgery, transcranial magnetic stimulation), while a behavioral disorder would respond best to behavioral treatment (e.g., attention to antecedents and consequences, behavior modification, exposure therapy). The use of the word "illness" in the term "psychiatric illness" implies that disease reasoning is being used; an illness is something a patient *has* rather than something that they are *doing* (McHugh and Slavney 1998). Therefore, this term may be more commonly used to refer to psychoses and disorders with known biological pathophysiology (e.g., Huntington's disease) and less commonly used to refer to conditions where symptoms are primarily behavioral or appear more voluntary (e.g., gambling, anorexia nervosa).

Regardless of their presumed origin, psychiatric illnesses such as depression and post-traumatic stress disorder are risk factors for the onset of complex medical conditions like coronary heart disease. Furthermore, psychiatric illnesses may develop as a consequence of disease processes, and can be significant independent predictors of poor prognosis in several conditions, including heart disease and end-stage renal disease.

Cross-References

- Mental Illness
- Psychiatric Diagnosis
- Psychiatric Disorder
- Psychological Disorder

References and Readings

American Psychiatric Association. (2000). *Diagnostic and statistical manual of mental disorders, Fourth Edition, Text Revision*. Washington, DC: American Psychiatric Association. See also http://www.psych.org/mainmenu/research/dsmiv.aspx.

Lippi, G., Montagnana, M., Favaloro, E. J., & Franchini, M. (2009). Mental depression and cardiovascular disease: A multifaceted, bidirectional association. *Seminars in Thrombosis and Hemostasis, 35*, 325–336.

McHugh, P. R., & Slavney, P. R. (1998). *The perspectives of psychiatry*. Baltimore: Johns Hopkins University Press.

Wallace, E. R., & Gach, J. (Eds.). (2008). *History of psychiatry and medical psychology: With an epilogue on psychiatry and the mind-body relation*. New York: Springer.

World Health Organization. (2007). *International statistical classification of diseases and related health problems, 10th revision, version for 2007*. Retrieved 1 Jan 2011 from http://apps.who.int/classifications/apps/icd/icd10online/

Psychiatric Surgery

▶ Psychosurgery

Psychoeducation

Shin-ichi Suzuki[1] and Asuka Tanoue[2]
[1]Faculty of Human Sciences, Graduate School of Human Sciences, Waseda University, Tokorozawa-shi, Saitama, Japan
[2]Advanced Research Center for Human Science, Waseda University, Tokorozawa, Saitama, Japan

Synonyms

Health Education

Definition

Psychoeducation is a method of providing patients/clients and their families a theoretical and practical approach to understanding and coping with the consequences of their psychological disorders/problems or physical illnesses/responses.

The main goals of psychoeducation are the enhancement of adherence; improvement of illness management or stress control skills, such as early recognition of episode recurrence and development of strategies for effective coping with symptoms; improvement of social and occupational functions; and quality of life.

The role of psychoeducation encompasses not only imparting knowledge and information regarding treatment/psychological support through media such as leaflets or information web sites or feedback to individuals based on test results, but it is also characterized by active cooperation such as intervention exercises with patients and their families.

Psychoeducation may be conducted in a group including individuals with similar problems (e.g., chronic diseases such as diabetes, HIV/AIDS, and PTSD) and individual therapy sessions. Group therapy is also expected to foster support among patients/clients. Thus, the psychoeducational approach has a lot in common with general psychosocial support for schizophrenia, mood disorders, eating disorders, and drug addiction, but it can also be applied to further the field of education.

Particularly, in the context of a medical setting, the therapists will try to explain the normal reactions of symptoms related to each psychological disorder or physical illness at the beginning. This will prevent any misinformation from being circulated among the patients and expand their understanding of the intervention, and it will lead to an improvement in the interactions of patients/clients in the treatment. Evidence from systematic reviews has reinforced the effect of these treatments stating that psychoeducational interventions for unipolar depression are effective, can prevent the worsening of depression, and be used as a preventive instrument (e.g., Cuijpers 1997).

As mentioned above, psychoeducation is a treatment that is routinely practiced in a number of fields, and it will continue to be considered essential in terms of the treatment and prevention of relapses.

Cross-References

▶ Health Education

References and Further Reading

Cuijpers, P. (1997). Bibliotherapy in unipolar depression: A meta-analysis. *Journal of Behavior Therapy and Experimental Psychiatry, 28*, 139–147.

Psychological and Social Conditions People Experience in the Workplace

▶ Psychosocial Work Environment

Psychological and Social Effects

▶ Psychosocial Impact

Psychological Disorder

Maxine Holmqvist
Clinical Health Psychology, University of Manitoba, Winnipeg, MB, Canada

Synonyms

Behavioral disorder; Emotional disorder; Mental disorder; Psychiatric disorder; Psychiatric illness

Definition

A distinctive pattern of cognitive, and/or behavioral symptoms in an individual, arising from underlying psychobiological dysfunction and causing significant distress, impairment, or an increased risk of death, pain, disability, or an important loss of freedom (American Psychiatric Association 2000). Psychological disorders do not include culturally sanctioned responses to life events (e.g., feeling sad after a significant loss).

Description

The term "psychological disorder" is often used interchangeably with similar terms, including "mental disorder" and "psychiatric illness." It may be a preferable term to "mental disorder," which evokes a mind/body dualism that is inconsistent with modern theories that emphasize the biopsychosocial origins of disease (Fulford et al. 2006). The term "psychological disorder" is broad, encompassing both disorders that manifest primarily with dysfunctional behaviors (e.g., anorexia nervosa, alcohol dependence) and disorders that manifest primarily with involuntary symptoms (e.g., schizophrenia, depression; McHugh and Slavney 1998). In contrast, the term "psychiatric illness" more typically refers to the latter category, assuming that these disorders are more rooted in brain dysfunction (see *Psychiatric Illness*, this volume). To date, genetic studies have not supported this distinction (e.g., Bienvenu et al. 2011).

Historical Background

Psychological disorders are cultural constructs, created through a variety of social processes, including debate, voting, and expert consensus (Raskin and Lewandowski 2000). Classifying psychological symptoms into disorders allows service providers to communicate with one another and for evidence-based knowledge to be accumulated and shared. It can enhance treatment planning and is critical for health care management (e.g., allowing governments to monitor the incidence and prevalence of various conditions in the population and allocate resources appropriately). While modern classification systems are empirically informed, current diagnostic categories are heavily influenced by historical forces (Kendler 2009). Today, the two most common classification systems for psychological disorders are the Diagnostic and Statistical Manual of Mental Disorders, 4th edition (DSM-IV), and the International Statistical Classification of Diseases and Related Health Problems, 10th revision (ICD-10). Both the DSM-IV and the ICD-10 are categorical systems that enable the user to record the presence or absence of a condition or disease according to certain standardized rules; in contrast to this, dimensional systems of classification are quantitative and are more likely to utilize psychometric measures and statistical procedures. In addition to more closely mirroring theoretical models of psychological pathology that characterize symptoms on a continuum with normal functioning (see "Psychological Pathology", this volume), these systems can be helpful in providing additional information that is likely to be important clinically. The importance of dimensional assessment to treatment planning and monitoring in particular has also been highlighted, and several proposed dimensional assessments are being evaluated for feasibility during the upcoming DSM-V field trials (Stein et al. 2010).

The Diagnostic and Statistical Manual of Mental Disorders (DSM)

The DSM is published by the American Psychiatric Association (APA). Its aim is to provide common language and standard criteria for the classification of mental disorders, and it is the primary system used in North America. There have been five revisions since the DSM was first published in 1952 (APA 2000). The current edition is the 4th edition, text revision (DSM-IV-TR); the fifth edition (DSM-V) is due to be published in May 2013 (American Psychiatric Association 2011). The DSM describes how qualified individuals can assign diagnoses based on predetermined criteria. Diagnoses are recorded using a multiaxial system, with different disorder subtypes coded on different axes. While efforts have been made to keep the diagnostic codes in the DSM consistent with the ICD, this has not always been possible due to the differing revision cycles. Primary goals for the DSM-V include improving diagnostic validity and reliability and enhancing clinical utility.

International Statistical Classification of Diseases and Related Health Problems (ICD)

The ICD originated in the 1850s, when medical statisticians identified the need for a standard nomenclature to record cause of death and other important health statistics. Originally published as the International List of Causes of Death by the International Statistical Institute in 1893, responsibility for the ICD was taken over by the World Health Organization (WHO) when it was created in 1948 (World Health Organization 2007). Currently, the ICD is the international standard diagnostic classification system for epidemiological reporting and research among WHO member states (e.g., monitoring the incidence and prevalence of diseases in a population, recording national mortality and morbidity statistics); it also aims to provide useful information for health management and clinical purposes. The scope of the ICD has increased with each revision and update. In the early 1960s, a series of meetings were held with the aim of improving the diagnosis and classification of mental health disorders. The current edition, the ICD-10, was completed in 2007 and contains a comprehensive listing of "mental and behavioral disorders," which are coded on axis V (F00-F99).

As with psychiatric illnesses, psychological disorders can often predict the risk of developing complex medical conditions (e.g., heart disease); the reverse is also true. Furthermore, psychological disorders have prognostic value in some illnesses, including cancer, heart disease and renal failure.

Cross-References

▶ Mental Illness
▶ Psychiatric Disorder

▶ Psychiatric Illness
▶ Psychological Pathology

References and Readings

American Psychiatric Association. (2000). *Diagnostic and statistical manual of mental disorders, Fourth Edition, Text revision*. Washington, DC: American Psychiatric Association. See also http://www.psych.org/mainmenu/research/dsmiv.aspx.

American Psychiatric Association. (2011). DSM-5 Development Page. Retrieved from http://www.dsm5.org/Pages/Default.aspx

Bienvenu, O. J., Davydow, D. S., & Kendler, K. S. (2011). Psychiatric 'diseases' versus behavioral disorders and degree of genetic influence. *Psychological Medicine, 41*, 33–40.

Fulford, K. W. M., Thornton, T., & Graham, G. (2006). *Oxford textbook of philosophy and psychiatry*. Oxford: Oxford University Press.

Kendler, K. S. (2009). An historical framework for psychiatric nosology. *Psychological Medicine, 39*, 1935–1941.

Ladwig, K. H., Baumert, J., Marten-Mittag, B., Kolb, C., Zrenner, B., & Schmitt, C. (2008). Posttraumatic stress symptoms and predicted mortality in patients with implantable cardioverter-defibrillators: Results from the prospective living with an implanted cardioverter-defibrillator study. *Archives of General Psychiatry, 65*, 1324–1330.

McHugh, P. R., & Slavney, P. R. (1998). *The perspectives of psychiatry* (2nd ed.). Baltimore: The Johns Hopkins University Press.

Raskin, J. D., & Lewandowski, A. M. (2000). The construction of disorder as human enterprise. In R. A. Neimeyer & J. D. Raskin (Eds.), *Constructions of disorder: Meaning-making frameworks for psychotherapy* (pp. 15–40). Washington, DC: American Psychological Association.

Stein, D. J., Phillips, K. A., Bolton, D., Fulford, K. W. M., Sadler, J. Z., & Kendler, K. S. (2010). What is a mental/psychiatric disorder? From DSM-IV to DSM-V. *Psychological Medicine, 40*, 1759–1765.

World Health Organization. (2007). *International statistical classification of diseases and related health problems, 10th Revision, version for 2007*. Retrieved 1 Jan 2011 from http://apps.who.int/classifications/apps/icd/icd10online/

Psychological Factors

▶ Psychosocial Factors

Psychological Factors and Health

Jane Upton
Department of Psychology, William James College, Newton, MA, USA

Synonyms

Psychological variables; Psychosocial factors

Definition

Thoughts, feelings, and attitudes that influence behavior

Description

Behavioral medicine incorporates not only the effect of individual's actions on their health but also how psychological factors affect the physical body. This is a progression from traditional biomedicine, which conceptualizes the mind and the body as separate entities. Behavioral medicine has started to break down this artificial boundary, illuminating the close relationship between mind and body, and therefore the role that psychological factors play in disease.

A key psychological factor is stress, which is known to affect many systems of the body. This summary will focus on the immune system, a system once thought to be independent of psychological factors. Research investigating the effect of stress on vaccinations generally indicates that chronic psychological stress impacts on the immune response. In a study conducted by Cohen and colleagues, 394 healthy individuals completed a questionnaire to assess degree of psychological stress and were then given nasal drops containing a respiratory virus (Cohen et al. 1991). The rates of respiratory infection increased in a dose-response manner with increases in psychological stress. This relationship was not altered when the researchers controlled for variables that might affect this relationship (e.g., the infectious status of subjects in close vicinity to each other). The level of psychological stress reported by the individuals prior to exposure to the virus was therefore directly related to the level of infection. This relationship has been consistently duplicated; for example, Phillips and colleagues found that the stress of bereavement in the year prior to influenza vaccination was associated with a poorer antibody response (Phillips et al. 2006).

However, it is too simplistic to conclude that stress suppresses the immune system. Different types of psychological stress have different effects on the immune system. It is therefore important to differentiate between acute, short-term stress and long-term chronic stress. It has generally been found that long-term stress suppresses the immune system (Bauer et al. 2000), whereas acute stress potentiates it (Herbert et al. 1994).

It is important to note though that the effect of psychologically stressful events varies between individuals based on how they evaluate the event and their coping strategies (Lazarus and Folkman 1984). Pettingale and colleagues investigated the effect of coping strategy on recovery from cancer (Pettingale et al. 1985). Fifty-seven women who had recently undergone mastectomy were interviewed 4 months after their operation. They were categorized in to four groups dependent on coping strategy: stoic acceptance, denial, fighting spirit, and helplessness/hopelessness. They found that coping strategy was related to 10-year disease-free survival; those women who adopted denial or fighting spirit coping strategies tended to survive longer.

The level of chronic stress and coping styles may interact to affect the immune system. Stowell and colleagues found that under conditions of high chronic stress, people who had active coping styles had higher proliferation of leukocytes to stimulation by mitogens than people who had avoidance coping mechanisms (Stowell et al. 2001). However, they also found that when experiencing low levels of chronic stress, people that used avoidance mechanisms to cope had higher proliferation levels of leukocytes than those that used more active mechanisms to cope. The relationships between certain coping methods and immune function may therefore depend on perceived stress levels.

Immune response may also be affected by personality traits such as neuroticism (Phillips et al. 2005), internalization in adolescents (Morag et al. 1999), and trait negative affect (Marsland et al. 2001). More widely, it has been suggested that a constellation of personality traits such as high levels of anxiety, neuroticism, depression, anger, and hostility may be linked with a range of diseases (Friedman and Booth-Kewley 1987). However, prospective studies are required to confirm that these traits contribute to the etiology and progression of disease.

Schnurr and colleagues investigated the effect of post-traumatic stress disorder (PTSD) in 605 veterans of World War II and the Korean conflict (Schnurr and Avion 2000). They controlled for age, smoking, alcohol use, and body weight at study entry. They found that PTSD symptoms were associated with increased onset of arterial lower gastrointestinal dermatologic and musculoskeletal disorders. The authors state that it is premature to draw firm conclusions from their study about the relationship of PTSD to these disorders. However, their findings were very similar to those reported by Boscarino and colleagues in their study of Vietnam War veterans (Boscarino 1997).

Less dramatically, it has also been found that daily hassles affect the physical body. In a study of 48 undergraduate students, levels of daily hassles correlated with the General Health Questionnaire somatic symptoms scale (Sheffield et al. 1996). Daily hassles have also been linked with fluctuations in blood pressure. Steptoe and colleagues (1996) recorded the blood pressure (BP) hourly from 49 male firefighters on work and nonwork days (Steptoe et al. 1996). They found that systolic BP readings accompanied by feelings of anger and stress were significantly greater than those without negative moods in both work and nonwork settings. They concluded that the raised systolic BP during working hours observed was affected both by physical activity and concurrent mood and that stress and anger were particularly influential.

Cross-References

▶ Psychosocial Predictors
▶ Psychosocial Variables

References and Further Reading

Bauer, E., Vedhara, K., Perks, P., Wilcock, G. K., Lightman, S. L., Shanks, N., et al. (2000). Chronic stress in caregivers of dementia patients is associated with reduced lymphocyte sensitivity to glucocorticoids. *Journal of Neuroimmunology, 103*, 84–92. https://doi.org/10.1016/S0165-5728(99)00228-3.

Boscarino, J. (1997). Diseases among men 20 years after exposure to severe stress: Implications for clinical research and medical care. *Psychosomatic Medicine, 59*(6), 605–614.

Cohen, S., Tyrrell, D., & Smith, A. (1991). Psychological stress and susceptibility to the common cold. *The New England Journal of Medicine, 325*, 606–612.

Friedman, H., & Booth-Kewley, S. (1987). The "disease-prone personality": A meta-analytic view of the construct. *The American Psychologist, 42*, 539–555. https://doi.org/10.1037/0003-066X.42.6.539.

Herbert, T., Cohen, S., Marsland, A. L., Bachen, E., Rabin, B., Muldoon, M., et al. (1994). Cardiovascular reactivity and the course of immune response to an acute psychological stressor. *Psychosomatic Medicine, 56*(4), 337–344.

Lazarus, R., & Folkman, S. (1984). *Stress, appraisal and coping*. New York: Springer.

Marsland, A. L., Cohen, S., Rabin, B., & Manuck, S. (2001). Associations between stress, trait negative affect, acute immune reactivity, and antibody response to hepatitis b injection in healthy young adults. *Health Psychology, 20*, 4–11. https://doi.org/10.1037/0278-6133.20.1.4.

Morag, M., Morag, A., Reichenberg, M., Lerer, B., & Yirmiya, R. (1999). Psychological variables as predictors of rubella antibody titers and fatigue – A prospective double blind study. *Journal of Psychiatric Research, 33*, 389–395.

Pettingale, K., Morris, T., Greer, S., & Haybittle, J. (1985). Mental attitudes to cancer; an additional prognostic factor. *Lancet, 1*(8431), 750.

Phillips, A. C., Carroll, D., Burns, V. E., & Drayson, M. (2005). Neuroticism, cortisol reactivity, and antibody response to vaccination. *Journal of Personality, 42*, 232–238. https://doi.org/10.1111/j.1469-8986.2005.00281.x.

Phillips, A. C., Carroll, D., Burns, V. E., Ring, C., Macleod, J., Drayson, M., et al. (2006). Bereavement and marriage are associated with antibody response to influenza vaccination in the elderly. *Immunity, 20*, 279–289. https://doi.org/10.1016/j.bbi.2005.08.003.

Schnurr, P. P., & Avion, S. (2000). Physician-diagnosed medical disorders in relation to PTSD symptoms in older male military veterans. *Health Psychology, 19*(1), 91–97. https://doi.org/10.1037//0278-6133.19.1.91.

Sheffield, D., McVey, C., & Carroll, D. (1996). Daily events and somatic symptoms: Evidence of a lagged relationship. *The British Journal of Medical Psychology, 69*, 267–269.

Steptoe, A., Roy, M., & Evans, O. (1996). Psychosocial influences on ambulatory blood pressure over working and non-working days. *Journal of Psychophysiology, 10*(3), 218–227.

Stowell, J. R., Kiecolt-glaser, J. K., & Glaser, R. (2001). Perceived stress and cellular immunity: When coping counts. *Journal of Behavioral Medicine, 24*(4), 323–339.

Psychological Pathology

Maxine Holmqvist
Clinical Health Psychology, University of Manitoba, Winnipeg, MB, Canada

Synonyms

Abnormal psychology; Psychopathology

Definition

The scientific study of psychological disorders and their causes.

Description

Psychological pathology is the study of the causes, components, course, and consequences of psychological disorders. These are characterized by *abnormality* and *dysfunction*.

Abnormality

Psychological disorders are defined by diagnostic criteria, like those outlined in the Diagnostic and Statistical Manual of Mental Disorders (DSM; American Psychiatric Association [APA] 2000) or the International Statistical Classification of Diseases and Related Health Conditions (ICD; World Health Organization 2007). These criteria are composed of "marker symptoms," or thoughts, feelings, and/or behaviors identified as abnormal for a variety of reasons (e.g., because they cause distress, disadvantage, or disability or are highly inflexible or irrational; Stein et al. 2010). Symptoms can be understood as qualitatively different from normal or as extreme variants of common traits. Some symptoms are abnormal because they deviate significantly from a statistical mean. The notion of deviance from the mean is the underlying rationale for many commonly used psychometric tests, but is perhaps most clearly illustrated using the concept of intelligence. It is assumed that intelligence is normally distributed in the population; thus, individuals whose scores on a standardized test of intelligence fall below a specific cutoff may be diagnosed with mental retardation. It is important to note that even in this circumstance, meeting this cutoff is not sufficient for a diagnosis; there must be additional evidence of dysfunction (e.g., deficits in self-care and academic performance; APA 2000). Thus, a trait or behavior is not necessarily "pathological" simply because it is highly unusual – high intelligence may be equally rare, but is not usually debilitating. Similarly, some characteristics that are presumed to be dysfunctional may be quite common (e.g., depressive thoughts, binge drinking). Importantly, abnormality can only be defined in reference to a given population; thus, the boundaries between normal and abnormal will shift over time and across cultures.

Dysfunction

Symptoms that cause significant impairment in important life domains may also be considered "pathological." Accordingly, dysfunction is often assessed with reference to the consequences of the symptom or disorder. Increasingly, psychological research is providing evidence of dysfunction by showing that certain psychological traits or behavioral patterns (e.g., perfectionism, type "A" personality, avoidance of feared stimuli) are reliably associated with undesirable physiological, social, and occupational outcomes (e.g., procrastination, chronic hypertension, strengthening of a phobic response). Dysfunction is also sometimes assessed in evolutionary terms, with symptoms referred to as "maladaptive," suggesting that they deviate from functioning that would have led to survival and reproductive success in the past.

Cross-References

▶ Psychiatric Disorder
▶ Psychiatric Illness
▶ Psychological Disorder

References and Readings

American Psychiatric Association. (2000). *Diagnostic and statistical manual of mental disorders, text revision* (4th ed.). Washington, DC: Author.
Stein, D. J., Phillips, K. A., Bolton, D., Fulford, K. W. M., Sadler, J. Z., & Kendler, K. S. (2010). What is a mental/psychiatric disorder? from DSM-IV to DSM-V. *Psychological Medicine, 40*, 1759–1765.
World Health Organization. (2007). *International statistical classification of diseases and related health problems, 10th revision, version for 2007*. Retrieved 1 Jan 2011 from http://apps.who.int/classifications/apps/icd/icd10online/

Psychological Predictors

▶ Psychosocial Predictors

Psychological Researcher

▶ Psychologist

Psychological Science

Peter A. Hall
Faculty of Applied Health Sciences, University of Waterloo, Waterloo, ON, Canada

Synonyms

Scientific psychology

Definition

The term *psychological science* refers to the accumulated body of psychological knowledge (i.e., pertaining to brain, behavior, social, or mental processes) that has been generated through the systematic application of the scientific method. The term *psychological science* may also refer to the process of conducting psychological research through the use of the scientific method.

Description

The scientific approach to studying social, mental, and behavioral phenomena has existed for the full history of the field of psychology. Though some have questioned the applicability of scientific methods to the exploration of mental phenomena for at least as long as its existence, psychological science has always been at the core of psychology as a field, and scientific rigor has been an aspiration even within the applied subdisciplines of psychology, including clinical psychology, health psychology, and behavioral medicine. Psychology as a discipline has stricter adherence to the scientific method than most social sciences, and so the nature of accumulated knowledge within psychology in the first century of its existence can be largely described as "scientific" in nature.

Commitment to the scientific method in psychological research is traceable back to William James (1842–1910) in North America and Wilhelm Wundt (1832–1920) in Europe, though its roots likely extend even earlier than these two individuals. Notably, both James and Wundt were trained initially as physicians, highlighting the long-standing interconnectedness of psychological science and medical science from the time that psychology emerged as a legitimate area of scientific inquiry. Psychological knowledge aims to be scientifically grounded by following basic scientific criteria of empiricism, replicability of a method, and the testing of generalizable hypotheses and models which eventually explain psychological phenomena.

In 1989, the inaugural issue of *Psychological Science* was published by the Association for Psychological Science (formerly named the American Psychological Society). This flagship journal was intended to be a showcase for leading psychological research conducted with rigorous adherence to the scientific method. The prominence of *Psychological Science* has grown steadily from its inception to present, and it is currently the highest ranking empirical journal in the field of psychology (Association for Psychological Science 2015).

Cross-References

▶ Behavioral Sciences at the Centers for Disease Control and Prevention
▶ Health Psychology

References and Further Readings

Association for Psychological Science. (2015). *Psychological Science (journal home page)*. http://www.psychologicalscience.org/index.php/publications/journals/psychological_science

Psychological Scientist

▶ Psychologist

Psychological Stress

Shin-ichi Suzuki[1] and Daisuke Ito[2]
[1]Faculty of Human Sciences, Graduate School of Human Sciences, Waseda University, Tokorozawa-shi, Saitama, Japan
[2]Department Clinical Psychology, Graduate School of Education, Hyogo University to Teacher Education, Kato, Hyogo, Japan

Synonyms

Distress; Strain; Stress; Stressor

Definition

H. Selye (1936) defined stress as "nonspecific responses that be resulted from a variety of different kinds of stimuli." However, Selye's stress theory has only focused on physiological stress, and psychological factors have not been considered. Research on life stress examined the relationship between diseases and life events. Many studies were conducted for clarifying the psychological factors related to stress, and the results revealed that psychological factors play a significant role in the occurrence of physiological and psychological stress responses. Lazarus and Folkman (1984) proposed that stress occurs when people perceived that the demands from external situations were beyond their coping capacity. Today, the definition "stress is the process of interaction from resolution requests from the environment (known as the *transactional* model)" is widely accepted.

From the perspective of psychological stress research, the ambiguous elements related to stress have distinguished two aspects of stress. One is called "stressors," which cause stress (e.g., interpersonal problem, hard work, noise, and trauma). Another is called "stress responses," which are nonspecific physical and mental changes induced by stressors (e.g., frustration, depression, anxiety, and stomachache). Psychological stress responses that caused by various daily experiences are emotional, cognitive, and behavioral changes; their degrees have also become main factors affecting physical and mental health. However, as mentioned in the definition of Lazarus and Folkman (1984), psychological stressors are related to one's cognition and coping process rather than induced stress responses directly. Therefore, an effective approach for reducing psychological stress responses should include not only the removal of stressors but also enhancing the cognitive and behavioral coping capability. A number of studies have demonstrated the effectiveness of cognitive–behavioral stress management in influencing psychological and physiological parameters.

Cross-References

▶ Cognitive Appraisal
▶ Coping
▶ Mental Stress
▶ Stress
▶ Stress Responses
▶ Stress, Emotional
▶ Stressor

References and Further Reading

Lazarus, R. S., & Folkman, S. (1984). *Stress, appraisal, and coping.* New York: Springer.
Selye, H. (1936). A syndrome produced by diverse nocuous agents. *Nature, 138,* 32.

Psychological Stress Task

▶ Stress Test

Psychological Stressor

▶ Stress Test

Psychological Testing

▶ Assessment

Psychological Variables

▶ Psychological Factors and Health
▶ Psychosocial Variables

Psychologist

Vincent Tran
Southwestern Medical Center, University of Texas, Dallas, TX, USA

Synonyms

Mental health professional; Psychological researcher; Psychological scientist

Definition

A psychologist is a professional who has earned a doctoral degree in psychology at a regionally accredited university or professional school. Some psychologists are primarily involved in conducting research and contributing to the scientific body of knowledge in psychology, while others use this scientific knowledge in applied settings. Psychologists work in several different work sectors, including clinical practice settings, academic and research settings, and consultation to apply psychological principles in private or public industries. Major settings in which psychologists work include universities and medical schools, private practice, clinics and counseling centers, industry and government, hospitals, and school districts. In recent decades, psychologists have increasingly focused their work on health-related research and with patients in medical settings. This is evidenced in the rapid growth of the membership in the Health Psychology Division of the American Psychological Association (Division 38), and in the fact that psychologists comprise 73% of the interdisciplinary membership of the Society of Behavioral Medicine.

Although psychologists often enjoy a variety of professional roles, some psychologists (e.g., clinical and counseling psychologists) are primarily involved in the practice of psychology. Applied psychologists focus on the identification, assessment, treatment, and/or consultation related to psychological issues impacting human behavior in applied settings. Interventions may include individual, group, or family psychotherapy, as well as consultation with community and private organizations. In order to regulate the practice of psychology and to ensure mental and behavioral health services are provided by qualified professionals, psychologists must obtain a professional license. Each state has its own requirements for licensure; in addition to the doctoral degree, states commonly require additional postdoctoral training and passing scores on national and state licensure exams.

Other psychologists primarily conduct basic or applied research and/or teach in academic or university settings. Psychological science uses statistical and empirical methods of measurement to understand mental processes and behavior, which can be at the social, cognitive, biological, and/or emotional level. Major specialty areas studied in psychology include clinical, counseling, educational, experimental, industrial/organizational, developmental, social, personality, physiological, and quantitative psychology. The American Psychological Association, an organization representing psychologists in the United States, has 54 divisions and interest groups, demonstrating the range and variety of subdisciplines or specialty interest areas of psychologists. The Association for Psychological Science is an organization dedicated to promoting scientifically oriented psychologists and psychology as a scientific discipline.

Cross-References

▶ Health Psychology
▶ Medical Psychology
▶ Psychological Science

References and Further Readings

APA. (2011a). *American Psychological Asssociation*. Retrieved 13 Dec 2011, from http://www.apa.org/.
APA. (2011b). *What is APA's definition of a psychologist?* American Psychological Asssociation. Retrieved 11 Jan 2011, from http://www.apa.org/support/about/apa.
APS. (2011). *Association for Psychological Science*. Retrieved 13 Dec 2011, from http://www.psychologicalscience.org.
Keefe, F., Portner, L., & Somers, T. (2010). The SBM career trajectories survey: Findings and next steps. Society of Behavioral Medicine. Retrieved 13 Dec 2011, from http://www.sbm.org/about/councils/education-training-and-career-development/career-trajectories.
Smith, M. W., & Passer, R. E. (2001). *Psychology: Frontiers and applications*. New York: McGraw-Hill.
Stricker, G., Widiger, T. A., & Weiner, I. B. (Eds.). (2003). *Handbook of psychology: Clinical psychology* (Vol. 8). Hoboken: Wiley.

Psychometric Properties

Annie T. Ginty
School of Sport and Exercise Sciences,
The University of Birmingham, Edgbaston,
Birmingham, UK

Synonyms

Psychometrics

Definition

Psychometrics is the construction and validation of measurement instruments and assessing if these instruments are reliable and valid forms of measurement. In behavioral medicine, psychometrics is usually concerned with measuring individual's knowledge, ability, personality, and types of behaviors. Measurement usually takes place in the form of a questionnaire, and questionnaires must be evaluated extensively before being able to state that they have excellent psychometric properties, meaning a scale is both reliable and valid.

Description

A reliable scale consistently measures the same construct. This can occur across testing sessions, individuals, and settings. A valid measure measures what it says it is going to measure. If something is valid, it is always reliable. However, something can be reliable without being valid.

For example (see Fig. 1), if someone has five darts and is told to hit the bull's eye every time, their ideal aim is to be both reliable (consistent) and valid (accurate) with their throws. In part 1, the throws are neither reliable nor valid because their efforts are scattered across the board. In part 2, the throws were reliable, hitting the same spot every time. However, they did not hit the targeted spot of the bull's eye so they were not valid. Part 3 shows the perfect example of being both reliable and valid. The throws hit the spot they intended to hit and did so consistently. This same concept is applied to questionnaire measurements.

If a researcher is trying to create a new scale to measure depression, they want to make sure the scale reliably measures depression in someone with depression. For example, if the same individual filled out the questionnaire three times in the same day, they would produce the same score each time. The researcher also wants to make sure the scale is valid, which means that the scale is actually measuring depressive symptoms and not some other mood or behavior.

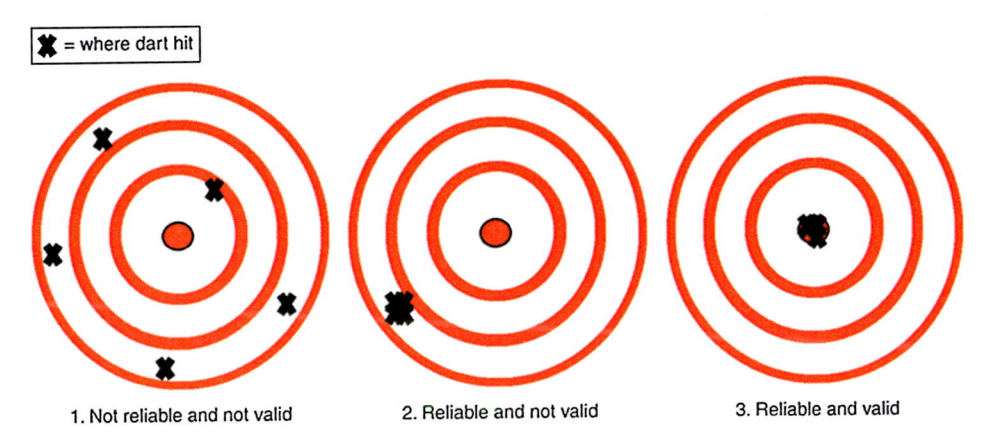

Psychometric Properties, Fig. 1 An example of reliability and validity

Cross-References

▶ Construct Validity
▶ Validity

References and Further Reading

DeVellis, R. F. (2003). *Scale development: Theory and applications* (2nd ed.). London: Sage.
Grimm, G. L., & Yarnold, P. R. (2000). *Reading and understanding more multivariate statistics*. Washington, DC: American Psychological Association.

Psychometric Theory

▶ Psychometrics

Psychometrics

J. Rick Turner
Campbell University College of Pharmacy and Health Sciences, Buies Creek, NC, USA

Synonyms

Psychometric theory

Definition

Psychometric theory is a well-recognized approach for developing psychological measurement and standardized education tests (Kim-O and Embretson 2010). It can be divided into two categories: classical test theory (CTT) and item response theory (IRT). CTT was pioneered a century ago by Spearman, while IRT developed in the 1950s and 1960s.

Kim-O and Embretson (2010) provided a thorough discussion of IRT and why it has become the preferred approach. In the CTT model, estimates of examinees' true test scores are often linear transformations of the raw test score, and are related to relevant normative populations by the transformation. Alternative test forms can be used to estimate true scores if the forms are parallel tests with the same expected true scores and error distributions. Psychometric indices for items in CTT are related to the properties of the test scores, particularly reliability and variance. In other words, item difficulty is defined as the proportion of persons passing or endorsing an item, while item discrimination is defined as the correlation of the item with the total test score.

The CTT approach, however, has several limitations. An examinee's true score depends on the difficulty level of a test, i.e., it is test-dependent: Scores will not be comparable between easy and hard tests. Second, the item characteristics depend on the ability of examinees, i.e., they are sample-dependent. Item difficulty, for example, will vary substantially if the true score distributions vary between populations. Third, one of the key assumptions, that two true test scores and two error variances are identical in the two tests (the parallel test assumption), is never fully met in practice. Therefore, it becomes difficult to compare examinees who take different tests, and to contrast items whose characteristic indices are computed using different groups of examinees.

In contrast, in the IRT approach the examinee's true score is not test-dependent, the item parameters are not sample-dependent, and the parallel test assumption is not needed. See Kim-O and Embretson (2010) for further discussion of this approach.

Psychometric theory is used extensively in behavioral medicine research. As two examples, Kiernan et al. (2011) assessed the psychometric properties, initial levels, and predictive validity of a measure of perceived social support and sabotage from friends and family for healthy eating and physical activity. Second, Lo et al. (2011) introduced the Death and Dying Distress Scale (DADDS), a new, brief measure developed to assess death-related anxiety in advanced cancer and other palliative populations. Their paper described its preliminary psychometrics based on a sample of 33 patients with advanced or metastatic cancer. Additional examples are provided in the "References and Readings" section of this entry.

Cross-References

▶ Psychometric Properties
▶ Validity
▶ Variance

References and Further Reading

Kiernan, M., Moore, S. D., & Schoffman, D. E. (2011). Social support for healthy behaviors: Scale psychometrics and prediction of weight loss among women in a behavioral program. *Obesity (Silver Spring, MD)*. Oct 13th [Epub ahead of print].

Kim-O, M.-A., & Embretson, S. E. (2010). Item response theory and its application to measurement in behavioral medicine. In A. Steptoe (Ed.), *Handbook of behavioral medicine: Methods and applications* (pp. 113–123). New York: Springer.

Kowalchuk Horn, K., Jennings, S., Richardson, G., et al. (2012). The patient-specific functional scale: Psychometrics, clinimetrics, and application as a clinical outcome measure. *The Journal of Orthopaedic and Sports Physical Therapy, 42*(1), 30–42.

Lo, C., Hales, S., Zimmermann, C., et al. (2011). Measuring death-related anxiety in advanced cancer: Preliminary psychometrics of the death and dying distress scale. *Journal of Pediatric Hematology/Oncology, 33* (Suppl. 2), S140–S145.

Maddux, R. E., Lundh, L. G., & Bäckström, M. (2011). The Swedish depressive personality disorder inventory: Psychometrics and clinical correlates from a DSM-IV and proposed DSM-5 perspective. *Nordic Journal of Psychiatry*. Sept 22nd [epub ahead of print].

Robinson, D. W., Jr., Cormier, J. N., Zhao, N., et al. (2012). Health-related quality of life among patients with metastatic melanoma: Results from an international phase 2 multicenter study. *Melanoma Research, 22*(1), 54–62.

Psychoneuroendocrinology

Jutta M. Wolf[1] and Eve Saucier[2]
[1]Department of Psychology, Brandeis University, Waltham, MA, USA
[2]Brandeis University, Waltham, MA, USA

Synonyms

Behavioral endocrinology

Definition

Psychoneuroendocrinology (PNE) is an interdisciplinary field of research integrating psychology, endocrinology, and neuroscience to study the interactions between mind, brain, and hormonal function (Dantzer 2010).

More specifically, PNE focuses on the way psychological factors influence neuroendocrine functions and, conversely, the way hormones influence higher brain functions. As such, PNE is not only interested in hormone synthesis, release, transport, breakdown, and feedback control but in the interaction of hormones with their target tissues (e.g., the immune system), including the molecular mechanisms of their action.

PNE research is often concerned with health implications associated with even subtle chronic changes in hormonal patterns. While sex is one of the biggest factors influencing the body's neuroendocrine state, other factors of interest include health effects of age-related changes and changes observed in the context of diseases such as the metabolic syndrome or mood and anxiety disorders. By far, the most intensely studied area, however, is PNE of stress, which aims at describing and understanding neuroendocrine changes associated with acute as well as chronic physiological and especially psychological stress and how stress-related changes in turn impact behavior, cognition, affect, and health (for a review, see Dantzer 2010).

Cross-References

▶ Behavioral Immunology
▶ Behavioral Medicine
▶ Psychoneuroimmunology
▶ Stress
▶ Sympathetic Nervous System (SNS)
▶ Sympatho-adrenergic Stimulation

References and Further Reading

Dantzer, R. (2010). Psychoneuroendocrinology of stress. In F. K. George, M. Le Michel, & F. T. Richard (Eds.), *Encyclopedia of behavioral neuroscience* (pp. 126–131). Oxford: Academic.

Psychoneuroimmunology

Jutta M. Wolf and Kirsten Rene
Department of Psychology, Brandeis University, Waltham, MA, USA

Synonyms

Behavioral immunology

Definition

Psychoneuroimmunology (PNI) is the study of the functional relationships between central nervous system, behavior, and immune system.

These relationships have been documented to be multidirectional. For example, while behavior can influence immune processes through changes in nervous system signals, immune signals have been shown to alter the function of the central nervous system, thereby influencing behavior. Further, all systems exert regulatory control over each other, forming a complex communication network.

PNI research aims at describing this network and thus to contribute to the understanding of the behavioral and biological mechanisms underlying the links between psychosocial factors and health as well as disease development and progression. Psychosocial factors studied in PNI thereby range from negative psychological states such as depression and anxiety, to social support, interpersonal relationships, and personality factors. Disease-related processes investigated include cancer, susceptibility to infection, wound healing, HIV/AIDS, autoimmune diseases, and cardiovascular diseases. One important PNI branch focuses on how stress and stress-related neuroendocrine processes (see "▶ Psychoneuroendocrinology") affect health as well as disease development and progression.

As such, PNI is truly interdisciplinary, integrating not only knowledge from immunology, neuroscience, and psychology but also from areas such as psychiatry, endocrinology, physiology, and pharmacology.

Cross-References

▶ Behavioral Immunology
▶ Behavioral Medicine
▶ Cytokines
▶ Immune Responses to Stress
▶ Inflammation
▶ Psychoneuroendocrinology
▶ Sickness Behavior
▶ Wound Healing

References and Further Reading

Ader, R. (2001). Psychoneuroimmunology. *Current Directions in Psychological Science, 10*(3), 94–98.

Cohen, S., & Herbert, T. B. (1996). Health psychology: Psychological factors and physical disease from the perspective of human psychoneuroimmunology. *Annual Review of Psychology, 47*, 113–142.

Maier, S. F., Watkins, L. R., & Fleshner, M. (1994). Psychoneuroimmunology: The interface between behavior, brain, and immunity. *American Psychologist, 49*(12), 1004–1017.

Schedlowski, M., & Tewes, U. (Eds.). (1996). *Psychoneuroimmunology: An interdisciplinary introduction*. New York/Boston/Dordrecht/London/Moscow: Kluwer Academic/Plenum.

Vedhara, K., & Irwin, M. (Eds.). (2007). *Human psychoneuroimmunology*. New York: Oxford University Press.

Psycho-oncology

▶ Cancer: Psychosocial Treatment

Psychopathology

▶ Psychological Pathology

Psychophysiologic Disorders

▶ Psychosomatic Disorder

Psychophysiologic Reactivity

Mark Hamer
Epidemiology and Public Health, Division of Population Health, University College London, London, UK

Synonyms

Stress response

Definition

Psychophysiologic reactivity refers to cardiovascular and biological responses to situations that are perceived as stressful, threatening, and/or physically harmful. Reactivity is defined as the response with respect to resting values. Some of the stressors that are commonly used in laboratory-based psychophysiological studies are designed to replicate real life, such as problem solving and public speaking tasks (Kamarck and Lovallo 2003). It is, however, often advantageous to use novel stressors, such as the Stroop word-color conflict task and mirror tracing, in order to remove the potential confounding influences of education and work experience. Psychophysiologic stress testing allows individual differences in responses to standardized stress to be evaluated and related to psychosocial factors and health outcomes (Chida and Hamer 2008). Behaviorally evoked psychophysiological responses are a relatively stable individual trait, consistent across time and stressor type. The magnitude or pattern of an individual's stress response is largely augmented by the immediate actions of the autonomic nervous system and delayed response of the hypothalamic-pituitary-adrenal axis, which releases various hormones (i.e., catecholamines, cortisol, etc.) into the circulation. These systems drive specific responses that include an increase in blood pressure and heart rate, changes in cardiac sympatho-vagal balance, skeletal muscle vasodilatation, the release of hemostatic and inflammatory markers, and activation of various immune cells. Although psychophysiologic reactivity is beneficial for maximizing performance, excessive and enduring responses are also relevant to health and well-being and are thought to contribute to underlying disease pathology.

Cross-References

▶ Blood Pressure Reactivity or Responses
▶ Heart Disease and Cardiovascular Reactivity
▶ Psychophysiologic Recovery
▶ Stroop Color-Word Test

References and Readings

Chida, Y., & Hamer, M. (2008). Chronic psychosocial factors and acute physiological responses to laboratory-induced stress in healthy populations: A quantitative review of 30 years of investigations. *Psychological Bulletin, 134*(6), 829–885.

Kamarck, T. W., & Lovallo, W. R. (2003). Cardiovascular reactivity to psychological challenge: Conceptual and measurement considerations. *Psychosomatic Medicine, 65*(1), 9–21.

Psychophysiologic Recovery

Mark Hamer
Epidemiology and Public Health, Division of Population Health, University College London, London, UK

Synonyms

Relaxation; Return to baseline; Rumination

Definition

Psychophysiologic recovery is defined as the rate at which a cardiovascular or biological variable returns to resting levels following a stressor. It is not uncommon to observe prolonged elevation in blood pressure following induction of mental stress, and this might last for up to an hour or so following the cessation of the stressor. This has also been observed in naturalistic settings, for example, in teachers, blood pressure has been shown to remain elevated throughout the evening following a stressful working day at school. A slower rate of psychophysiologic recovery has been linked to several risk factors and poorer health outcomes (Brosschot 2010). One difficulty with isolating the predictive value of recovery is that those taking the longest time to return to baseline are likely to be those who showed the greatest reactivity. Nevertheless, recent evidence suggests that poor recovery and heightened reactivity are in fact independent predictors of health outcomes. The mechanisms underlying poorer psychophysiologic recovery are incompletely understood, although various psychological factors such as rumination and coping strategies have been implicated.

Cross-References

▶ Cardiovascular Recovery
▶ Psychophysiologic Reactivity

References and Readings

Brosschot, J. F. (2010). Markers of chronic stress: Prolonged physiological activation and (un)conscious perseverative cognition. *Neuroscience and Biobehavioral Reviews, 35*(1), 46–50.

Psychophysiological

Douglas Carroll
School of Sport and Exercise Sciences,
The University of Birmingham, Edgbaston, Birmingham, UK

Definition

Psychophysiology is an interdisciplinary science concerned with the impact of psychological exposures and behavioral challenges on physiological systems. The adjective "psychophysiological" describes this impact. For example, the effect on blood pressure of exposure to a mental stress task would be described as a psychophysiological effect.

Cross-References

▶ Psychophysiology: Theory and Methods

Psychophysiology: Theory and Methods

William R. Lovallo[1] and Tony W. Buchanan[2]
[1]Department of Psychiatry and Behavioral Sciences, University of Oklahoma Health Sciences Center and VA Medical Center, Oklahoma City, OK, USA
[2]Department of Psychology, Saint Louis University, Saint Louis, MO, USA

Synonyms

Psychophysiological

Definition

How does our mental and emotional life tie in with the workings of the body? Psychophysiology is the branch of psychology that studies the behavior of the individual in a biological context. It is an attempt to chart the mutual interactions between psychological processes and the workings of the body, giving equal emphasis to both.

Description

A fundamental principle of psychophysiology is that thoughts and feelings cannot exist apart from the body – here we include the brain as part of the body. It follows that a full understanding of psychological processes depends on understanding the biological context from which they proceed. Due to its emphasis on integrating our understanding of mental and physiological processes, psychophysiology has contributed to research methods and theory building in behavioral medicine and also to the neurosciences of cognition and emotion. Psychophysiology finds its place in behavioral medicine by providing a theoretical basis and a set of measurement methods that help to disentangle relationships between psychology and biology and between our thoughts and emotional experiences in relation to good and poor health. From this perspective, psychophysiologists bring a physiological emphasis to the study of behavior relative to mental processes including the measurement of cognitive functions and emotional states. As a result of this effort, psychophysiology has contributed to the science of the physiology of emotions and the impact of these psychophysiological interactions on good and poor health. Although it is accepted in psychophysiology that thoughts and feelings do not exist without the brain and the body, it is necessary to emphasize that the thoughts and feelings of interest are not to be seen as equivalent to, or directly reducible to, these physiological processes.

Importantly, behavioral medicine focuses on the feelings, behaviors, and physiological responses in response to stressors as situated (a) in a person and (b) in a particular environmental context. Behavioral medicine as a field may focus on both the person and the influence of contextual factors such as socioeconomic status or race/ethnicity on stress-related illnesses. The emphasis of psychophysiology, by contrast, is primarily on the person and specifically the functions of organ systems, such as the cardiovascular system, endocrine system, or immune system, in the course of psychophysiological investigations. This calls for a methodology that allows cognitive processes and emotional experience to be studied simultaneously with physiological functioning in ways that are unobtrusive and minimally invasive. This ensures that the person being studied is behaving in a normal manner, as in everyday life, and is not reacting unduly to the apparatus or laboratory setting. Psychophysiological techniques used to study cognitive processes include extensive use of scalp recordings of the electroencephalogram (EEG) accompanied by increasingly sophisticated processing of the measured waveforms. A related method for the study of cognitive processes and emotional states is the use of functional magnetic resonance imaging (fMRI). The fMRI signal is frequently processed to study momentary activity of brain regions in persons performing specific psychological tasks.

Statistical mapping of activity in the cortex and subcortical structures can then allow comparison of task-related activation with activation during appropriate control tasks. This method allows inferences about specific psychological processes and simultaneous activation of discrete brain regions to be mapped spatially and in real time. Together these methods permit a degree of temporal and spatial resolution of generalized activity in relation to specific regions of the cortex as well as processing of specific sensory events relative to cognitive processes.

Recent work using these combined methods has allowed for a better understanding of the bidirectional relationships between brain activity and physical health, whereby specific brain activity may lead to poor physical health, or vice versa. For example, stressor-evoked activity in particular brain regions is positively related to both markers of inflammation and risk for cardiovascular disease. Such findings point to several potential targets for treatment: psychotherapy for changing brain responses to stress, immunotherapy, and therapies targeting the cardiovascular system. The inclusion of measures of brain function in the psychophysiological toolbox of behavioral medicine represents an important advance toward understanding and ultimately improving the well-being of the whole person.

In the area of behavioral medicine, a primary emphasis has been placed on psychophysiological principles to study responses to stress in the laboratory, responses to stressors in daily life, and individual differences in such responses. Behavioral medicine is both a science and an approach to clinical practice. These two parts are concerned with the influence of behavioral factors on health and disease. Behavioral medicine holds that states of health can be influenced by overt behaviors, such as dietary habits, and by covert behaviors, such as emotional states and stress responses. This perspective leads behavioral medicine researchers to ask questions about the ways that emotional states and stress responses can affect health through their influence on physiology. The goal is to bring to light how our behaviors and our ways of perceiving and reacting to the world may affect our well-being for better or worse. Such research addresses questions in several major areas, including (1) how the body responds during positive and negative emotional states, (2) how a given person's stress reactivity may vary over time, (3) the ways in which persons differ from one another in their stress responses, and (4) on the positive side, to establish the behavioral and physiological patterns that lead to good health and longevity. To carry out such research, behavioral medicine draws in part on the theory and methods developed in the field of psychophysiology. Psychophysiology, then, serves as a way of thinking and a set of methods that connect emotional and societal influences acting on an individual to physical health outcomes via measures of physiology that may impact such outcomes.

In laboratory studies, people are often exposed to stressors to determine how they react to such challenges both emotionally and physiologically. The results are thought to indicate how emotionally relevant events can affect physiology in daily life and whether they may contribute to disease. As one example, a commonly used stressor is public speaking. This challenges the subject to make up a short speech and deliver it without notes and to do so in a fluent and convincing manner. Public speaking is stressful because most people wish to avoid the embarrassment of doing poorly and to be seen as masterful and competent by observers in the laboratory. Using this method, the social evaluation and uncontrollability of the real world can be modeled in a small way in the laboratory, and the participant's ego is invoked to produce a stress response. During public speaking, this process of social evaluation, along with the resulting fear and anxiety, produces substantial increases in heart rate, blood pressure, and stress hormones, including catecholamines and cortisol. The person's mood states are assessed at rest before the task begins and again at the end using paper-and-pencil measures or brief interviews. Similarly, cardiovascular reactions are measured at rest and during stress using automated blood pressure monitors and impedance cardiographs, and endocrine responses may be collected using saliva or blood sampling. In this manner, the person's psychological, cardiovascular, and endocrine reactions may be measured to provide a picture of how physiological reactions are set off by psychologically meaningful events.

This research strategy can then be extended to compare different kinds of people for potential differences in their physiological reactivity to stress. One common example is for the researcher to identify young, healthy individuals who have a family history of high blood pressure and also to find those with no such history. These family history groups can then be compared in the laboratory for differences in their stress responses, perhaps using the public speaking stressor or some other method. This allows potential differences in stress reactivity to be assessed in relation to a family history of this prevalent cardiovascular disease. It is then possible to follow such people for a period of years to establish who among them will become hypertensive and who will retain a normal blood pressure. Do people from the family history group have a greater likelihood of becoming hypertensive in middle age? Are people with greater reactions to stress more likely to become hypertensive, regardless of family history? Such studies therefore allow potential interactions between family history and stress reactivity to be studied. If people with a family history of hypertension who are also highly reactive to social stress are much more likely to become hypertensive, then we would conclude that the family history constituted a biologically based risk factor that was enhanced by an elevated level of stress responsivity. In contrast, should risk of hypertension be increased equally by high reactivity in people with and without a family history of hypertension, we would conclude that family history and reactivity tendencies contribute to hypertension risk in an additive manner.

Although the laboratory provides a well-controlled environment with an extensive range of measurement techniques, ambulatory methods have been used with increasing frequency outside the laboratory to document how challenges in persons' daily lives can affect cardiovascular, endocrine, or immune systems. Such methods measure the person's responses to naturalistic stressors, such as work stress, or challenges in the home, such as family conflict or the stress of caring for a chronically ill spouse. Such studies rely on small, lightweight monitors that can be worn comfortably as persons go about their daily routines. These monitors can make reliable measurements in a wide range of circumstances. Such systems are able to track heart rate, blood pressure, and physical activity, as well as other indices. In addition, the person usually reports on their subjective state using smartphone-based measures. As in laboratory studies, this ambulatory method may be used to estimate the interaction of stress responses and disease risk. People with and without a family history of hypertension may be compared as they go about their daily lives. As in the laboratory, people with the largest or most prolonged reactions to stress at home or at work are suspected of having greater risk of future disease, and again, they may be followed up for actual occurrence of hypertension in future years. Ambulatory systems currently in use include traditional Holter electrocardiographs, blood pressure monitors, and impedance cardiographs. The success of these systems along with the increasing ubiquity of smartphone and smartwatch technology has led several commercial companies to develop reliable products for research and clinical use.

Although some research focuses on family history of disease in studying individual differences, other work seeks to connect psychological dispositions, such as hopelessness, depression, or temperament traits such as hostility to disease risk. Studies using this strategy may compare those who are highly hostile with nonhostile people using a specific hostility-provoking interaction, such as harassing comments during work on a difficult task. By measuring physiological reactions to such specific challenges in people with different psychological characteristics, a clearer picture may be developed of the psychological and physiological interplay that is suspected of contributing to disease.

Studies of genetic characteristics have recently yielded another influential method for establishing individual difference groups. In turn these genetically identified groups may be compared using psychophysiological methods. The availability of powerful genotyping technology on commercially available arrays and scanners has allowed large numbers of people to be classified with up to a million single nucleotide polymorphisms (SNPs). These SNPs are then taken to represent spontaneous mutations in functional genes that contribute to measurable differences in cognitive and emotional processes and ultimately health outcomes. For example, recent work has shown that variation in a SNP of the central catecholamine system is related to differences in stress hormone response, especially in people who have experienced early life stress. Such interactions among genetics, physiology, and life history demonstrate the complex patterns that may be addressed via psychophysiological research.

While much of this research focuses on negative emotional states, stress responses, and risk of disease, there is a growing interest in the relation between positive emotional states and resilience against disease. As in the above examples, such persons can be selected for their emotional traits using a combination of self-report techniques and in laboratory tests of brain function. Health outcomes can then be compared between people high in positive affect versus those reporting low positive affect.

The research examples listed above all depend on testing people while they are relaxed and resting, as well as when they are under stress or perhaps in a pleasurable mood. For these reasons, it is desirable to use measurement methods that do not cause discomfort or distress. Behavioral medicine research has therefore relied on methods of psychophysiological measurement that are noninvasive or minimally invasive and cause the volunteer no discomfort. Many of the examples above focused on the cardiovascular system which can be studied using noninvasive methods such as the electrocardiogram, blood pressure monitoring, and impedance cardiography to measure pumping action of the heart and constriction of the blood vessels and, occasionally, fluid output to assess kidney function. Stress research often uses additional methods to track responses of the endocrine system, involving collection of urine, blood, or saliva for measurement of stress hormones and other substances associated with stress and pain. Still, other studies examine the immune system using minimally invasive techniques in the collection of blood for later measurement of the numbers of immune system cells and their biological activity. The application of techniques such as EEG and fMRI are similarly noninvasive, requiring no exposure to radioactivity and allowing for at least a semblance of normal behavior. Finally, the application of such psychophysiological techniques calls for appropriate selection of tasks and ways to analyze the data.

Psychophysiology provides both an important way of thinking as well as a set of tools in the larger field of behavioral medicine. The advent of new technologies including smartphone applications, new methods of ambulatory monitoring, and functional neuroimaging adds to the psychophysiological toolkit to better address the relationships between our psychology and our health. Future directions for this work include addressing how the brain takes in information – both from the external world and from the body – and translates this into stress responses. In addition to the sensory role played by the brain, new questions focusing on how brain responses may mitigate or exacerbate a person's response to stress will be important to tackle. Ultimately, the methods of psychophysiology will enable researchers and clinicians to better understand how psychological variables translate into health, for better or for worse.

Cross-References

▶ Ambulatory Blood Pressure
▶ Ambulatory Monitoring
▶ Blood Pressure
▶ Blood Pressure Reactivity or Responses
▶ Heart Rate
▶ Hypertension

- ▶ Magnetic Resonance Imaging (MRI)
- ▶ Psychophysiological
- ▶ Psychosocial Factors
- ▶ Psychosocial Predictors
- ▶ Psychosocial Variables
- ▶ Stress Test
- ▶ Systolic Blood Pressure (SBP)

References and Further Readings

Buchanan, T., & Lovallo, W. R. (2019). The role of genetics in stress effects on health and addiction. *Current Opinion in Psychology, 27*, 72–76.

Carroll, D., Ginty, A. T., Whittaker, A. C., Lovallo, W. R., & de Rooij, S. R. (2017). The behavioural, cognitive, and neural corollaries of deficient biological reactions to acute psychological stress. *Neuroscience and Biobehavioral Reviews, 77*, 74–86.

Cohen, S., Gianaros, P. J., & Manuck, S. B. (2016). A stage model of stress and disease. *Perspectives on Psychological Science, 11*, 456–463.

Erickson, K. I., Creswell, J. D., Verstynen, T. D., & Gianaros, P. J. (2014). Health neuroscience: defining a new field. *Current Directions in Psychological Science, 23*, 446–453.

Gerin, W. (2010). Laboratory stress testing methodology. In A. Steptoe (Ed.), *Handbook of behavioral medicine: Methods and applications* (pp. 633–648). New York: Springer.

Gianaros, P. J., & Jennings, J. R. (2018). Host in the machine: A neurobiological perspective on stress and cardiovascular disease. *American Psychologist, 73*, 1031–1044.

Gianaros, P. J., Marsland, A. L., Kuan, D. C.-H., Schirda, B. L., Jennings, J. R., Sheu, L. K., Hariri, A., Gross, J. J., & Manuck, S. B. (2014). An inflammatory pathway links atherosclerotic cardiovascular disease risk to neural activity evoked by the cognitive regulation of emotion. *Biological Psychiatry, 75*, 738–745.

Lovallo, W. R. (2016). *Stress and health* (3rd ed.). Sage.

Obrist, P. A. (1981). *Cardiovascular psychophysiology: A perspective*. New York: Plenum Press.

Steptoe, A., & Poole, L. (2010). Use of biological measures in behavioral medicine. In A. Steptoe (Ed.), *Handbook of behavioral medicine: Methods and applications* (pp. 619–632). New York: Springer.

Turner, J. R. (1984). *Cardiovascular reactivity and stress: Patterns of physiological response*. New York: Plenum Press.

Psychosocial Adaptation

- ▶ Psychosocial Adjustment

Psychosocial Adjustment

Fong Chan[1], Elizabeth da Silva Cardoso[2], Julie Chronister[3] and Emma Hiatt[4]
[1]Department of Rehabilitation Psychology and Special Education, University of Wisconsin-Madison, Madison, WI, USA
[2]Department of Educational Foundations and Counseling Programs, The City University of New York-Hunter College, New York, NY, USA
[3]Department of Counseling, San Francisco State University, San Francisco, CA, USA
[4]Rehabilitaion Psychology and Special Education, University of Wisconsin-Madison, Madison, WI, USA

Synonyms

Psychosocial adaptation; Rehabilitation psychology; Response to disability

Definition

Chronic illness and disability profoundly impacts the lives of many individuals. For example, approximately one in five Americans has physical, sensory, psychiatric, or cognitive impairments that affect their daily activities. Psychosocial adaptation entails the integration of illness or disability into the individual's life, identity, self-concept, and body image. Psychosocial adaptation is defined as the process in which a person with a disability moves from a state of disablement to a state of enablement and is characterized by the transformation from negative to positive well-being (Livneh and Antonak 2005). Observed across disability groups, psychosocial adaptation occurs as the individual moves toward a state of optimal person-environment congruence. The final stage of psychosocial adaptation, known as adjustment, represents maximum congruence between the individual's subjective experience and his or her external environment.

Description

Introduction

Psychosocial adjustment to chronic illness and disability (CID) is a long-term, dynamic process influenced by intrinsic and extrinsic variables within a specific context (Chan et al. 2009a; Livneh and Antonak 2005). There are several terms used to describe the adjustment to disability process. Specifically, *adjustment, adaptation*, and *acceptance* of disability are concepts commonly used to describe the process and outcome of coping with CID. *Adaptation* has been defined as the dynamic process a person with CID experiences in order to achieve the final state of optimal person-environment congruence known as *adjustment* (Smedema et al. 2009). The term *acceptance* was coined by Beatrice Wright (1983) who defined *disability acceptance* as an outcome in which the disability is incorporated as part of the individual's self-concept and is accepted as nondevaluing. Today, *response to disability* is a widely accepted terminology considered to most accurately describe the adjustment process, because it fully conveys response to disability as a subjective experience that is not necessarily negative. Furthermore, response to disability involves a dynamic process as opposed to a one-time event (Smart 2009). The response to disability process reaches beyond psychological aspects of adjustment to include a complex and dynamic interaction of a wide variety of psychological, societal, environmental, and personal factors. This entry will provide readers with a review of the prominent psychological, social, environmental, and personal factors that interact to influence the individual process.

Psychological Factors

Somatopsychology. Psychological aspects of CID have been most broadly explored in the context of *somatopsychology*, the study of the physique's influence on behavior and how that relationship is mediated by the effectiveness of the body as a tool for actions. The emphasis of somatopsychology is on the meaning of disability that is unique to the individual, as well as the value the disability holds for other individuals in a person's life (Smedema et al. 2009). The theory considers self-concept, body image, and coping to be psychological schemas and functions crucial to successful adaptation. Specifically, *self-concept* and *body image* represent mental schemas by which humans perceive and identify themselves. An individual with CID must alter one's body image and self-concept to incorporate the physical changes into one's daily life. Therefore, reorganization of these mental schemas is critical to successful adaptation (Livneh and Antonak 2005).

Coping. Coping strategies also affect the response to disability process. Coping requires the individual draw on some personal or environmental resource to reduce the negative impact of a stressor (Chronister et al. 2009), including both adaptive and maladaptive strategies. In the context of disability adjustment, coping generally refers to cognitions, emotions, or behaviors that mediate the relationship between disability-related stressors (i.e., nature, type, duration, prognosis, perception, and severity) and the response to disability. Coping strategies associated with response to disability can be divided into three psychological categories: cognitive, behavioral, and affective (Smart 2009). *Cognitive* response refers to how an individual chooses to think about or view the disability. *Behavioral* response refers to actions taken to manage the disability, including compliance to treatment recommendations, seeking social support, returning to work, and using self-advocacy strategies to manage the impact of stigma and prejudice. *Affective* response refers to how the individual feels about the disability and how he or she manages the emotions associated with the disability (Smart 2009). A positive coping strategy within the context of disability may include having a realistic view of the disability and awareness of limitations without exaggerating them. Conversely, a negative coping strategy may involve substance use or self-blame. The coping strategies employed strongly influence the response to disability. For example, healthy coping strategies, such as seeking out social support or redefining life goals, may improve body image and quality of life while decreasing social isolation and feelings of helplessness.

Based upon the disability acceptance theory (Wright 1983), Wright developed a cognitive restructuring framework known as the *coping versus succumbing* model. In this model, a person said to be *succumbing* to disability overemphasizes negative effects of impairment and neglects the challenge for change and meaningful adaptation. Conversely, a person said to be *coping* with disability is able to focus on personal assets and is oriented to activities that are within the individual's physical capabilities (Smedema et al. 2009). Wright (1983) proposed four primary value changes that reflect the *coping* perspective including (a) *Enlargement of the scope of values*, which requires the individual recognize that values beyond those presumed lost can be achieved despite limitations of CID; (b) *Subordination of the physique* occurs when the individual changes the cognitive belief that physical is a true representation of one's worth, desirability, or competency; (c) *Containment of disability effects* occurs when the individual recognizes disability as limited to the impact of the actual impairment, rather than being globally debilitating; and (d) *Transformation from comparative status to asset values*, which occurs when the individual avoids comparing oneself to a nondisabled standard and focuses attention on his or her assets (Smart 2009). The four primary value changes challenge each of the previously held beliefs, resulting in acceptance of disability (Wright 1983). Conversely, signs of the *succumbing* perspective include (a) denial or acting as if the disability does not exist; (b) idolizing normal standards or applying old values to the new situation; (c) failure to modify previous aspirations within the context new situations; (d) eclipsing behavioral possibilities and limiting one's opportunity to learn new skills to address the new situations more effectively; and (e) overcompensation of perceived deficiencies in one area by exaggerated striving in another area (Wright 1983).

Stage model. The response to disability process has also been conceptualized as a sequence of psychological stages, similar to those experienced during grief (Smedema et al. 2009). Stage models typically describe the process of adjustment as a linear series of psychological stages, requiring the completion of previous stages before the final stage of adjustment. Many stage models have been proposed to describe stages of adjustment. Livneh and Antonak (2005) concluded that the numerous stage models may be described within these five broad categories: (a) initial impact, which includes shock and anxiety; (b) defense mobilization, which includes bargaining and denial; (c) initial realization, which includes mourning, depression, and internalized anger; (d) retaliation, which includes externalized anger or aggression; and (e) reintegration or reorganization, which includes acknowledgment, acceptance, and final adjustment. The stage models provide a structure for understanding and predicting the course and outcome of an individual's response process (Smart 2009). Nonetheless, the applicability of the stage theory to persons with CID has been criticized for the following three reasons: (a) "stages" are not universally experienced; (b) a state of final adjustment (e.g., resolution, acceptance, assimilation) is not always achieved; and (c) psychological recovery does not follow an orderly sequence of reaction phases (Livneh and Antonak 2005). Finally, the existence of a universal, progressive, phase-like, orderly sequence of predetermined psychosocial reactions to disability has not been adequately supported by empirical research (Livneh & Antonak).

Ecological model. The most contemporary approach to conceptualizing and understanding the response to disability process is the *ecological* approach. Considered atheoretical, this approach incorporates components of somatopsychology and stage theory, while emphasizing the interaction of personal *and* contextual variables (social/environmental and personal factors) on psychosocial adaptation (Smedema et al. 2009). This approach also adopts a comprehensive and holistic approach to outcome measurement beyond that of acceptance or adjustment to CID, encompassing a person's overarching quality of life (Livneh and Antonak 2005). As such, understanding response to disability beyond the psychological processes described above is critical in developing a full perspective of an individual's response to disability. Below is a review of key contextual variables important to consider in the response process.

Societal Factors

Societal definitions of disability. The manner in which society defines CID influences the adjustment to process. Definitions of disability help to identify the location of the problem and who is held responsible for the solution (Smart 2009). Four of the most popular models of disability include the (a) biomedical model; (b) environmental model; (c) functional model; and (d) sociopolitical model. The biomedical model has the longest history. This model defines disability as pathology located within the individual and represents a deviation from the norm. Therefore, treatment is focused solely on "fixing" the individual. The environmental model suggests that the individual's environment may cause, define, or exaggerate the disability. For example, if a person with paraplegia does not have a wheelchair, then the impairment is worsened. The functional model posits that the functions of the individual influence the definition of the disability. For example, an individual who is physically active would be much more affected by mobility impairments. Finally, the sociopolitical model, also known as the Minority Group Model or the Independent Living Model, proposes that disability is not a personal attribute, but caused by society, and thus society should bear the responsibility for dealing with disability (Smart 2009). *Self-advocacy* is a critical component of the sociopolitical model of disability. Self-advocacy is rooted in the American ideals of autonomy and self-determination. In contrast to consequences of the medical model, including dependency, marginality, and social exclusion, self-advocacy refers to persons with disabilities taking control of their own lives, speaking up for themselves, being in control of their own resources, and having the right to make life decisions without undue influence or control from others.

The World Health Organization International Classification of Functioning, Disability and Health (WHO 2001) is a contemporary, biopsychosocial approach to defining disability that considers the biomedical, environmental, functional, and social models in its explanation of disability. This model conceptualizes disability along five major domains: (a) body functions and structures; (b) activities; (c) participation; (d) personal factors; and (e) environmental factors (Chan et al. 2009b). The ICF recognizes disability as an interaction between all of these factors and cannot be defined apart from the individual's context.

Societal attitudes. Negative attitudes toward persons with disabilities are well documented in the literature (Chan et al. 2009c). Negative attitudes or unfavorable evaluative statements related to a person, object, or event are considered *invisible barriers* that arise from the environment and impact the response process by limiting opportunities, access, and help-seeking behaviors, as well as reducing overall quality of life (Chan et al. 2009c). Related concepts include *prejudice, discrimination*, and *stigma*. Prejudice is a negative generalization toward a group of people and the assumption that an individual belonging to that group has the characteristics based on the generalization. For example, "all persons with CID are intellectually inferior." *Discrimination* is the action carried out based upon prejudice. For example, an employer who does not hire a person with CID because he or she believes persons with CID are "unsafe." Finally, *stigma* is a term that encompasses the problems associated with stereotyping, prejudice, and discrimination; it is the chain of events resulting from negative attitudes and beliefs, resulting in discrimination. Persons with disabilities often have limited access to work, housing, and other community resources because of stigmatizing attitudes that have led to discriminatory behavior (Chan et al.).

Commonly cited sources of negative attitudes and stereotypical views regarding persons with CID include the *safety threat*, the *ambiguity of disability*, the *salience of the disability, spread or overgeneralization, moral accountability for the cause and management of the disability, inferred emotional consequences of the disability*, and the *fear of acquiring a disability* (Smart 2009). Cook (1998) indicated that the general public also exhibits a "hierarchy of preferences" for specific groups of persons with CID; for example, people hold more favorable attitudes toward persons with physical disabilities than individuals with mental disabilities and persons tend to have more positive attitudes toward persons with intellectual disabilities than those with psychiatric disabilities.

Environmental Factors

A large majority of persons with CID live at or below the poverty level (Smart 2009). Although most persons with CID report they want to work (Louis Harris Associate Inc. Polls 1994), and despite protections afforded by the Americans with Disabilities Act, persons with CID have greater difficulty finding or maintaining work, and unemployment and underemployment rates of persons with disabilities are high (Smart 2009). This is due in part to prejudice and discrimination, worksite inaccessibility, and financial disincentives built into many disability benefits programs (e.g., SSI/SSDI). Other environmental factors that influence the response process include limited mobility and access to transportation, architectural barriers, frequency and duration of hospitalizations, lack of institutional support (medical services, educational programs and technological supports; political and religious groups), poor living conditions, limited availability of job opportunities, and inadequate accessibility of worksites (Livneh and Antonak 2005).

Personal Factors

Age and developmental status. Age and developmental stage, such as those identified by Erikson (1968), interact with CID to influence the response process. For example, the process of adaptation differs significantly between individuals born with CID and those who acquire CID later in life. Developmentally speaking, for an *infant* with a congenital disability, the primary task of establishing trust in the world through the relationship with mother or primary caregiver may be compromised if the infant is hospitalized for long periods and is cared for by multiple health professionals (Smart 2009), whereas during *early adulthood*, the tasks of establishing a family and beginning a career are important and may be impacted by CID. For *older adults*, the resulting impact of CID on independence and functioning is variable, ranging from minimal impact to substantial lifestyle change. While functional loss and disability may be a normal part of aging for some, social isolation, dependence, restricted activities and participation, and the loss of loved ones surrounding the individual can impact quality of life. Indeed, with disability, older adults face multiple life transitions in later years of life.

Gender. Gender is important to consider in the response process. Patterson et al. (2005) suggest that men and women respond differently to various CIDs. For example, in the area of spinal cord injury, men experience greater difficulties related to sexual functioning than women, resulting in feelings of loss of "manhood" or "masculinity." With respect HIV/AIDS, women are more socially isolated than men because of cultural backgrounds commonly associated with females with HIV/AIDS, and because rates of transmission are lower and occur through a different mode. Furthermore, a woman with HIV/AIDS experiences issues related to pregnancy, including potential transmission from mother to infant. Women and men also respond differently following myocardial infarction, such that men return to work sooner and are more likely to participate in physical activity to cope with stressors related to the condition.

Culture. Culture involves the beliefs, customs, practices, social behaviors, and set of attitudes of a particular nation or group of people (Chronister and Johnson 2009), and *worldview* is the framework of ideas and beliefs through which an individual interprets the world and interacts with it according to their philosophy, values, emotions, and ethics. Culture and worldview inform how disability is defined and experienced, and both aspects contribute to the response to disability process. For example, in contrast to the explanation of disability perpetuated by the medical model, some cultures perceive the origin of disability to be of the metaphysical-spiritual realm. For other cultures, disability is a condition that should not be altered, because it is considered to be predetermined by fate and not amenable to adaptive intervention. For example, the deaf culture rejects the notion that group members have a disability and identify as individuals with a different communication modality that live in a hearing world. Furthermore, the number of persons from culturally diverse backgrounds in the USA with CID is disproportionate, and these individuals are often at risk for experiencing multiple negative experiences or "double" discrimination and stigmatization, barriers that are likely to influence response to CID (Chronister and Johnson 2009).

Disability. Disability characteristics are also important to consider in the adjustment process and vary significantly across and within conditions. According to Smart (2009), there are ten disability factors that influence response to disability including time of onset (congenital, acquired), type of onset (insidious versus acute), course of disability (direction, pace of movement, degree of predictability), functions impaired (meaning of functioning, degree of intrusiveness, residual functioning and assistive technology), severity of the disability (number of disabilities experienced and areas of functioning affected, treatment necessary, and degree of stigma directed at the individual), visibility of the disability, degree of disfigurement, and prognosis (what is expected for the future).

Sexual orientation/identity. Sexual orientation is an important factor to consider in the response to disability process. Persons with CID that are identified with sexual orientations, such as lesbian, gay, bisexual, transgender, queer, questioning, intersex, and asexual (LGBTQQIA), are vulnerable to stereotypes, bigotry, abuse, bullying, and violence. They are subject to a complex array of prejudices by the mainstream population, including double prejudice for equal rights, higher rates of marginalization and discrimination, confusion in navigating identity development, and the prevailing view that persons with disability are asexual or unsuitable sexual partners (Miville et al. 2009).

Conclusion

Response to CID involves a complex and dynamic interaction of psychological, social, environmental, and personal variables. Somatopsychology and stage models provide a foundation for understanding the psychological processes of disability adjustment. The ecological approach builds upon this work to facilitate a broader conceptualization of psychosocial adjustment to address the importance of additional personal and contextual variables. Indeed, response to CID is a unique, personal experience that must be considered within the individual's context, including the sociocultural influences that contribute to how society defines and responds to CID. Contemporary definitions of disability conceptualize disability from a biopsychosocial perspective (i.e., WHO ICF model), recognizing body functioning and contextual factors as critical to disability determination and intervention planning. This framework, coupled with the ecological approach to adjustment to disability, replaces traditional approaches to yield a more holistic picture of adaptation.

Cross-References

▶ Attitudes
▶ Chronic Disease or Illness
▶ Coping
▶ Depression
▶ Disability
▶ Health Disparities

Acknowledgments The contents of this entry were developed with support through the *Rehabilitation Research and Training Center on Effective Vocational Rehabilitation Service Delivery Practices* (EBP-VR-RRTC) established at both the University of Wisconsin-Madison and the University of Wisconsin-Stout under a grant from the Department of Education, National Institute on Disability and Rehabilitation Research (NIDRR) grant number PR# H133B100034. However, those contents do not necessarily represent the policy of the Department of Education, and endorsement by the Federal Government should not be assumed.

References and Readings

Chan, F., Cardoso, E., & Chronister, J. A. (2009a). *Understanding psychosocial adjustment to chronic illness and disability: A handbook for evidence-based practitioners in rehabilitation*. New York: Springer Publishing.

Chan, F., Gelman, J. S., Ditchman, N. M., Kim, J. H., & Chiu, C. Y. (2009b). The World Health Organization ICF model as a conceptual framework of disability. In F. Chan, E. Cardoso, & J. Chronister (Eds.),

Psychosocial interventions for people with chronic illness and disability: A handbook for evidence-based rehabilitation health professionals. New York: Springer.

Chan, F., Livneh, H., Pruett, S., Wang, C.-C., & Zheng, L. X. (2009c). Societal attitudes towards disability: Concepts, measurements, and interventions. In F. Chan, E. Da Silva Cardoso, & J. A. Chronister (Eds.), *Understanding psychosocial adjustment to chronic illness and disability: A handbook for evidence-based practitioners in rehabilitation* (pp. 333–367). New York: Springer.

Chronister, J., & Johnson, E. (2009). Multiculturalism and adjustment to disability. In F. Chan, E. Da Silva Cardoso, & J. A. Chronister (Eds.), *Understanding psychosocial adjustment to chronic illness and disability: A handbook for evidence-based practitioners in rehabilitation* (pp. 479–528). New York: Springer.

Chronister, J., Johnson, E., & Lin, C. P. (2009). In F. Chan, E. D. S. Cardoso, F. Chan, E. D. S. Cardoso, & J. A. Chronister (Eds.), *Understanding psychosocial adjustment to chronic illness and disability: A handbook for evidence-based practitioners in rehabilitation* (pp. 111–148). New York: Springer.

Cook, D. (1998). Psychosocial impact of disability. In R. M. Parker & E. M. Szymanski (Eds.), *Rehabilitation counseling: Basics and beyond* (3rd ed., pp. 303–326). Austin: Pro-Ed.

Erikson, E. H. (1968). *Identity: Youth and crisis.* New York: Norton.

Livneh, H., & Antonak, R. F. (2005). Psychosocial aspects of chronic illness and disability. In F. Chan, M. J. Leahy, & J. Saunders (Eds.), *Case management for rehabilitation health professionals* (Vol. 2, 2nd ed., pp. 3–43). Osage Beach: Aspen Professional Services.

Louis Harris Associate Inc. Polls. (1994). *N.O.D.L. Harris survey of disabled Americans.* Washington, DC: National Organization of Disability.

Miville, M. L., Romero, L., & Corpus, M. J. (2009). Incorporating affirming, feminist and relational perspectives: The case of Juan. In M. E. Gallardo & B. W. McNeil (Eds.), *Intersections of multiple identities: A casebook of evidence-based practices with diverse populations* (pp. 175–201). New York: Routledge.

Patterson, J. B., DeLaGarza, D., & Schaller, J. (2005). Rehabilitation counseling practice: Considerations and interventions. In R. M. Parker, E. M. Szymanski, & J. B. Patterson (Eds.), *Rehabilitation counseling, basics and beyond* (4th ed., pp. 155–186). Austin: ProEd.

Smart, J. (2009). *Disability, society, and the individual* (2nd ed.). Austin: Pro-Ed.

Smedema, S. M., Bakken-Gillen, S. K., & Dalton, J. (2009). Psyhosocial adaptation to chronic illness and disability: Models and measurement. In F. Chan, E. Da Silva Cardoso, & J. A. Chronister (Eds.), *Understanding psychosocial adjustment to chronic illness and disability: A handbook for evidence-based practitioners in rehabilitation* (pp. 51–73). New York: Springer.

World Health Organization. (2001). *International classification of functioning, disability, and health: ICF.* Geneva: World Health Organization. Retrieved November 28, 2008, from http://www.who.int/classification/icf.

Wright, B. A. (1983). *Physical disability: A physical approach* (2nd ed.). New York: Harper and Row.

Psychosocial Aspects

▶ Psychosocial Characteristics

Psychosocial Benefits and Aspects of Physical Activity

Rick LaCaille[1] and Elaine Marshall[2]
[1]Psychology Department, University of Minnesota Duluth, Duluth, MN, USA
[2]University of Minnesota Duluth, Duluth, MN, USA

Definition

Numerous aspects of psychological well-being related to physical activity (PA) have been examined using epidemiological, cross-sectional, and experimental research strategies, including depression, anxiety, mood/affect, stress, self-perception, cognitive performance, and quality of life. These aspects have been considered in terms of acute bouts and chronic exercise/PA and potential underlying mechanisms. Moreover, personality correlates of PA as well as excessive engagement in exercise have been examined.

Description

The beneficial effects of PA for enhanced physical health and reduced risk of premature mortality are well known; however, notable psychological benefits have also been documented in the literature

(Reiner et al. 2013). Although exercise has been used for treating a variety of mental disorders, currently there is limited high-quality research to support it as a stand-alone intervention rather than an adjunctive treatment to pharmacotherapy or psychological therapy (Morgan et al. 2013). Some meta-analytic evidence suggests sufficient levels of exercise may improve functioning, comorbid disorders, and cognition for individuals with schizophrenia (Firth et al. 2015) as well as reduce the risk for comorbid physical health problems (Holley et al. 2011). Although additional randomized control trials are needed to evaluate interventions for treating psychological disorders, some data suggest psychosocial benefits in terms of alleviating both primary and secondary symptoms of psychological disorders, including body dissatisfaction and improved social functioning and mood.

Depression

The most well-established support for the beneficial associations between psychosocial functioning and PA comes from studies examining depression. Prospective epidemiological studies have found 20% to 33% lower odds of depression for physically active individuals (Dishman et al. 2013). A recent meta-analytic review of exercise interventions found large effects for individuals with major depressive disorder, versus no treatment controls, with the reduction in depression appearing for aerobic exercise at moderate-to-vigorous levels of intensity (Schuch et al. 2016). Unfortunately, long-term maintenance of the beneficial effects for MDD was not available. Some data also point to PA yielding effects comparable to antidepressant medications with the effects for exercise appearing less quickly than medications but exercise offering a reduced risk for relapse with depression (Barbour et al. 2007).

A recent meta-analysis of high-quality meta-analyses of PA interventions and depressive symptoms (i.e., nonclinical depression) has reinforced the previous findings but revealed somewhat smaller moderate effects with subclinical depressed individuals (Rebar et al. 2015). Given that the severity of depression is greater in clinical populations and has more possibility for larger decreases than in nonclinical populations, the differences in effect sizes may be attributable to potential floor effects with the subclinical samples. Taken together, the findings from these systematic reviews establish that PA has noteworthy effects for reducing depression.

Anxiety and Stress Reactivity

Another noteworthy area of well-documented salutary effects of PA includes decreased anxiety for both clinical and nonclinical samples. Studies of individuals without an anxiety disorder have shown reductions in state anxiety immediately following single bouts of exercise as well as more sustained PA (Ensari et al. 2015; Rebar et al. 2015). A recent qualitative review of exercise intervention studies with individuals with elevated levels of anxiety or anxiety disorders concluded that small-to-medium effect sizes were evident, with exercise equally effective as established treatments for anxiety (cognitive behavioral therapy and medication; Stonerock et al. 2015). Paralleling the findings with depressive disorders, anxiety reduction resulting from PA appears to be stable but more delayed. Generally, PA interventions with clinical samples yield anxiolytic effects, and these effects appear more substantial than observed with nonclinical samples (Conn 2010). No consistent differential effect appears evident for aerobic versus non-aerobic forms of PA, though greater anxiety reduction typically results with moderate-to-vigorous intensity levels of exercise.

Acute exercise initially stimulates the same cardiovascular responses as psychosocial stressors; however, different mechanisms (e.g., parasympathetic withdrawal vs. sympathetic activity) are engaged through exercise, which contribute to both its beneficial health effects and reduction in reactivity to stressors. Some evidence suggests increased fitness and chronic exercise lessen physiological reactivity and improve recovery from psychosocial stressors (Forcier et al. 2006). A more recent meta-analysis of both animal and human controlled aerobic exercise programs observed moderate effects for reductions in stress reactivity (Ramirez sand Wipfli 2013). Data from the animal studies indicated that hormone and catecholamine reductions were the major variables of influence for reactivity to stressors following habitual exercise, whereas for the human studies, lowered blood pressure reactivity appeared an important outcome with chronic exercise. In addition to the beneficial effects of habitual PA, a meta-analytic review of acute aerobic exercise controlled trials revealed reduced stress reactivity for diastolic and systolic blood pressure with the stronger effects evident with moderate-to-vigorous exercise intensity lasting from 20 min to 2 h with stressors administered up to 30 min following exercise (Hamer et al. 2006).

Affective Response

While mood and affect have, at times, been used interchangeably, efforts have been made within the PA/exercise literature to elucidate these constructs (e.g., Ekkekakis and Petruzzello 2000). Moods are emotion-related expressions (e.g., anxious mood, depressed mood) that are multifaceted, spanning brief moments to days, and possibly developing without an identifiable event. Although affect is also viewed as an emotion-related expression, it is more basic and varies along the dimensions of activation-deactivation and the subjective experience of valence (i.e., pleasant-unpleasant). That said, following a single bout of exercise, affect has been found to increase in positive engagement and diminish in terms of physical exhaustion (Masters et al. 2011). Data have also suggested that exercise may result in greater vigor, relaxation, and tranquility and reduced tension, irritability, and fatigue. Exercise intensity strongly influences affective responses, with clearer positive affectivity occurring with low-to-moderate intensity exercise. Acute low-to-moderate exercise enhances affect for 30 min following an exercise session (Reed and Ones 2006). However, as intensity increases, more interindividual variability occurs in affective responses and may result in higher levels of negative/unpleasant affect. Research has indicated that the ventilatory threshold (i.e., near maximal level of intensity and transition from aerobic to anaerobic metabolic supplementation) appears to be the point at which pleasant affective responses diminish while exercising, with affective response almost entirely negative at intensities that exceed the threshold (Ekkekakis et al. 2011). Importantly, research has also examined the bidirectional nature of PA and affect and generally observed higher positive affect predicted PA over the next few hours, though negative affect appears more inconsistently predictive of subsequent PA (e.g., Schwerdtfeger et al. 2010). Cognitive variables (e.g., attentional focus) appear to influence affective responses with intensities below or near the threshold; however, physiological/interoceptive variables (e.g., muscular or respiratory cues) come to play a more dominant role in influencing the affective response as the threshold is approached or exceeded. An important implication of this line of investigation lies in the potential to improve adherence to a PA program for exercisers by developing self-monitoring skills and cognitive strategies (e.g., attentional distraction vs. association) while exercising to maximize reinforcing positive affective responses (e.g., Gillman and Bryan in press).

Self-Perception

Self-perception is a multifaceted construct within which lie several related subjective attitudes and beliefs about one's self (e.g., self-esteem, self-concept) that may be organized in hierarchical levels (e.g., global self-esteem, physical self-esteem domain, situation-specific efficacy). Data suggests concerns with body image increase from adolescence through adulthood for both males and females, although females are at a higher risk overall. Exercise interventions have been shown to improve body image concerns, especially for older populations who report greater dissatisfaction (Campbell and Hausenblas 2009). Reviews of PA interventions reinforce this pattern of improved self-perceptions with the greatest improvements occurring for individuals with lower self-esteem. Some data also suggest that females may benefit more from participation in an exercise program than their male counterparts in terms of increased body image, physical self-esteem, and self-efficacy for exercise (Hausenblas and Fallon 2006). Importantly, global self-esteem has been shown to improve with participation in

PA as well, especially when this results in lower BMI and a change in physical fitness (Elavsky 2010; Reddon et al. 2017; Spence et al. 2005). Multiple studies have reported increased self-efficacy as a factor in overall global self-esteem (Babic et al. 2014; Elavsky 2010; Reddon et al. 2017). For instance, adult women who were initially sedentary or had low activity that engaged in a PA program reported increases in self-efficacy, which led to improved global self-esteem (Elavsky 2010). In a meta-analysis of children and adolescents of both sexes, participation in PA was strongly associated with perceived competence, although it should be noted that the study could not identify whether increased PA led to increased perceived competence or vice versa (Babic et al. 2014). This data indicates that improvements to self-esteem seem to be associated with by-products of PA, including reductions in BMI and increases in body image, self-efficacy, and fitness. Although both aerobic forms of PA and weight/resistance training seem beneficial, the combination of the two appears to offer greater improvements in body image and physical self-esteem.

Cognitive Performance

The effect of PA on cognitive functioning is an area with a rapidly growing body of research with evidence supporting the cognitive benefits for both adults and children (Clark and Williams 2011; Etnier et al. 2006). Because it is well understood that some amount of cognitive decline is normal with increased age, many studies focus on the aging population. Typically, studies with older adults have the most pronounced effects with simple reaction time/speed-based tasks and executive-control tasks (e.g., planning, response inhibition, task choice/switching). There is some evidence to support that PA improves cognitive performance for both cognitively normal and impaired adults, though research points to cognitively impaired adults showing more improvements with aerobic activity than those who are not impaired (Etnier 2017). Importantly, data also suggest that exercise may confer protective benefits with older adults, as those with higher levels of daily PA have been shown to be at less risk of developing Alzheimer's disease compared with less active adults when evaluated 4 years later (Buchman et al. 2012).

With regard to school-aged children, benefits associated with PA have been observed in several cognitive domains (e.g., attention, reaction time, time-on-task, and executive functioning) as well as improved academic performance (Donnelly et al. 2016). Although cross-sectional design studies have suggested moderate size effects favoring fitter participants, most randomized exercise interventions indicate a more modest effect on improved cognitive processes. Not all forms of exercise demonstrate equivalent effects, in that more complex and controlled movements appear to yield greater improvements on executive functioning than simple actions (Álvarez-Bueno et al. 2017). For both children and adults, improved cognitive processing has been seen with acute bouts of exercise and longer-term PA programs (Biddle et al. 2000). Generally, acute bouts of exercise have demonstrated larger effects when lasting 30–60 min; PA programs exceeding 6 months have also shown greater improvements than briefer interventions. Although the emphasis within the literature is usually on aerobic forms of PA, combining aerobic and resistive/weight training forms of exercise has demonstrated somewhat larger cognitive performance gains.

While more robust research is needed, multiple studies have indicated that increased PA may lead to brain structure changes in both children and adults (Álvarez-Bueno et al. 2017). Studies point to increased volume in the hippocampus, an important structure for memory, with PA (Donnelly et al. 2016; Etnier 2017). In addition, increases in exercise have been associated with increases in brain-derived neurotrophic factor, which plays a large role in neuroplasticity and neural growth (Etnier 2017). The data in this area point to promising benefits of PA on multiple facets of cognition, with rapidly expanding research on the mechanisms and reasons for this.

Quality of Life

Quality of life (QoL) is a multifaceted construct often encompassing physical (e.g., physical functioning, bodily pain), mental (e.g., vitality), and social components (e.g., role limitations, social functioning) or overall satisfaction with life and psychological well-being. In terms of PA, QoL has been studied mostly with older adults and/or those managing a chronic illness. A meta-analysis of older adults, without clinical disorders, found small-to-medium effects for PA on various aspects of quality of life/well-being, with aerobic forms of exercise and moderate intensity providing the greatest benefits (Netz et al. 2005). Another recent review examined the quality of life outcomes in the general adult population and reported consistently moderate-to-strong positive effects of PA in cross-sectional studies (Bize et al. 2007). More recently, Awick et al. (2017) examined the effects of changes in moderate-to-vigorous PA and psychological distress (i.e., depression, anxiety, stress, sleep dysfunction) on QoL in older adults enrolled in a 6-month exercise program. Reduced psychological distress mediated the relationship between increased PA and improved QoL. Importantly, the findings from this study help disentangle the benefits of PA and specify the direction of changes in PA, psychological distress, and QoL. However, given that considerably fewer investigations have employed randomized control trials to examine the effects of PA on QoL in healthy samples, the generalizability to the general population is limited at present.

Personality

There is a long history of examining potential associations between PA and personality characteristics, particularly traits (extraversion, conscientiousness, neuroticism, openness, and agreeableness) encapsulated within the Five-Factor Model (FFM). Systematic reviews have reported small positive associations with PA for extraversion and conscientiousness and a small negative association with neuroticism (Rhodes and Smith 2006; Sutin et al. 2016; Wilson and Dishman 2015). Of these associations, conscientiousness appears to have a more robust relationship with increased frequency of activity. Furthermore, time engaged in actual sedentary behaviors is related to higher neuroticism and lower conscientiousness (Sutin et al. 2016). While less consistently noted in the literature, PA appears to be positively related to openness and inversely associated with agreeableness. The negative association between agreeableness and PA, however, looks to be accounted for by increases in agreeableness and declines in activity levels as one ages (Wilson and Dishman 2015).

Beyond higher-order personality traits, facet-level traits appear to show larger associations with PA (Rhodes and Pfaeffli 2012). In particular, activity (extraversion) and self-discipline and industriousness/ambition (conscientiousness) have shown larger effects. Other non-FFM-specific aspects of personality (e.g., grit, mental toughness) have also shown an association with greater PA (Gerber et al. 2012; Reed et al. 2012). Some attention has also been directed toward examining personality traits such as sensation seeking and impulsivity and their presence within individuals engaging in adventure-based PA (e.g., rock climbing, skiing, snowboarding). Generally, sensation seeking has been associated with higher levels of physical risk-taking (Taylor et al. 2006), though may vary somewhat by the type of activity (e.g., scuba divers; Lee and Tseng 2015). The potential bidirectional associations between regular PA and personality traits have also been garnering attention. However, thus far the findings appear mixed (Allen et al. 2017; Stephan et al. 2014), and it seems that personality is more involved in shaping of PA engagement than PA is in influencing personality changes.

Compulsive Physical Activity

Although most literature points to the vast benefits of PA on psychological well-being, some reports suggest potentially harmful effects for certain individuals. The diagnostic validity of "exercise addiction" has been questioned by some investigators, and the incidence of such patterns are thought to be rare, though excessive PA/exercise has been more frequently reported as a secondary feature of some pre-existing clinical disorders (e.g., body/muscle dysmorphia). Even though exercise addiction has not been included in any previous version of the *Diagnostic and Statistical Manual of Mental Disorders*, some researchers contend that compulsive patterns of exercise can be understood as behavioral addictions (Berczik et al. 2014). By using Brown's components of addiction (Brown 1993), it has been asserted that because exercise can alter mood, lead to tolerance, create personal conflict, and result in withdrawal, it can be considered a behavioral addiction in certain cases (Berczik et al. 2014). Some researchers have also utilized the dualist model of passion (Vallerand et al. 2003) to differentiate between exercise engagement that may be construed as harmonious versus obsessive. For instance, Paradis et al. (2013) found that exercise dependence, as operationalized by the dimensions of time, tolerance, withdrawal, continuance, intention effects, lack of control, and reduction in other activities, was associated with high levels of obsessive passion. In contrast, harmonious passion only showed a positive association with the dimensions of time and tolerance, suggesting that for some individuals engaging in exercise is related to time spent exercising and increases in fitness, rather than a dependence (Paradis et al. 2013).

A notable negative effect of excessive exercise is risk for injury. Some research shows that individuals who exercise at high levels do so despite conflicts like injury or lack of time (Lichtenstein et al. 2017). In addition, while excessive exercise is typically seen as being related to eating disorders, some compulsive exercise is unrelated to weight loss and is done as a means to improve performance, yet is still associated with an unattainable body ideal (Lichtenstein et al. 2017). However, some data support the use of PA/exercise as an adjunctive treatment for eating disorders with improvements in reduced drive for thinness and binge eating (Stathopoulou et al. 2006). Of note, those at risk of engaging in excessive exercise may demonstrate high level of perfectionism, obsessive-compulsive traits, and neuroticism (Lichtenstein et al. 2017). This data suggests that some populations are at a greater risk for developing an unhealthy relationship with exercise due to maladaptive behavioral patterns, personality traits, and other variables.

Summary and Conclusions

In addition to numerous salutary effects for health, chronic disease management, and increased longevity, PA has clearly demonstrated psychosocial benefits. Notably, PA has a sizeable antidepressant effect, as well as several other psychosocial benefits such as reduced anxiety, improved body image and physical self-esteem, enhanced cognitive performance, and greater QoL. Affective responses preceding and following PA are associated with subsequent PA and appear to vary as a consequence of the intensity with higher levels often resulting in a diminished positive and increased negative affective responses. Helping exercisers self-identify and regulate the affect-intensity relationship may prove useful in maximizing the reinforcing positive affective responses and improving longer-term adherence to a healthier PA lifestyle. Some personality traits (e.g., conscientiousness, extraversion) have been shown to have consistent, but relatively small, associations with PA. The association is less evident with lower-intensity lifestyle activities (e.g., walking) than more vigorous PA. Although PA may be associated with some diminished psychological well-being for select individuals engaging in compulsive behavioral patterns, overall, it appears that the benefits of PA surpass the risks of excessive activity. Numerous mechanisms have been proposed in the literature to elucidate the effects of PA, including psychological/cognitive (e.g., self-efficacy/competence, autonomy and personal control, distraction) and physiological/biochemical changes (e.g., thermogenic, cerebral adaptations, monoamine, and endorphin levels). Research directed toward further clarifying the underlying mechanisms for PA engagement is warranted and may serve a critical role in assisting identification of more efficacious and tailored strategies for those at risk of insufficient PA.

Cross-References

▶ Benefits of Exercise
▶ Interventions and Strategies to Promote Physical Activity
▶ Physical Activity and Health
▶ Stress, Exercise

References and Further Readings

Allen, M. S., Magee, C. A., Vella, S. A., & Laborde, S. (2017). Bidirectional associations between personality and physical activity in adulthood. *Health Psychology, 36*(4), 332–336. https://doi.org/10.1037/hea0000371.

Álvarez-Bueno, C., Pesce, C., Cavero-Redondo, I., Sánchez-López, M., Martínez-Hortelano, J. A., & Martínez-Vizcaíno, V. (2017). The effect of physical activity interventions on children's cognition and metacognition: A systematic review and meta-analysis. *Journal of the American Academy of Child & Adolescent Psychiatry, 56*(9), 729–738. https://doi.org/10.1016/j.jaac.2017.06.012.

Awick, E. A., Ehlers, D. K., Aguiñaga, S., Daugherty, A. M., Kramer, A. F., & McAuley, E. (2017). Effects of a randomized exercise trial on physical activity, psychological distress and quality of life in older adults. *General Hospital Psychiatry, 49*, 44–50. https://doi.org/10.1016/j.genhosppsych.2017.06.005.

Babic, M. J., Morgan, P. J., Plotnikoff, R. C., Lonsdale, C., White, R. L., & Lubans, D. R. (2014). Physical activity and physical self-concept in youth: Systematic review and meta-analysis. *Sports Medicine, 44*(11), 1589–1601. https://doi.org/10.1007/s40279-014-0229-z.

Barbour, K. A., Edenfield, T. M., & Blumenthal, J. A. (2007). Exercise as a treatment for depression and other psychiatric disorders: A review. *Journal of Cardiopulmonary Rehabilitation and Prevention, 27*, 359–367. https://doi.org/10.1097/01.HCR.0000300262.69645.95.

Berczik, K., Griffiths, M. D., Szabó, A., Kurimay, T., Urban, R., & Demetrovics, Z. (2014). Exercise addiction. *Behavioral Addictions*, 317–342. https://doi.org/10.1016/b978-0-12-407,724-9.00013-6.

Biddle, S. J. H., Fox, K. R., & Boutcher, S. H. (Eds.). (2000). *Physical activity and psychological well-being*. London: Routledge.

Bize, R., Johnson, J. A., & Plotnikoff, R. C. (2007). Physical activity level and health-related quality of life in the general adult population: A systematic review. *Preventive Medicine, 45*, 401–415. https://doi.org/10.1016/j.ypmed.2007.07.017.

Brown, R. I. F. (1993). Some contributions of the study of gambling to the study of other addictions. In W. R. Eadington & J. Cornelius (Eds.), *Gambling behavior and problem gambling* (pp. 341–372). Reno: University of Nevada Press.

Buchman, A., Boyle, P., Yu, L., Shah, R., Wilson, R., & Bennett, D. (2012). Total daily physical activity and the risk of AD and cognitive decline in older adults. *Neurology, 78*(17), 1323–1329. https://doi.org/10.1212/wnl.0b013e3182535d35.

Campbell, A., & Hausenblas, H. A. (2009). Effects of exercise interventions on body image. *Journal of Health Psychology, 14*(6), 780–793. https://doi.org/10.1177/1359105309338977.

Clark, U. S., & Williams, D. (2011). Exercise and the brain. In R. A. Cohen & L. H. Sweet (Eds.), *Brain imaging in behavioral medicine and clinical neuroscience* (pp. 257–273). New York: Springer.

Conn, V. S. (2010). Anxiety outcomes after physical activity interventions: Meta-analysis findings. *Nursing Research, 59*, 224–231. https://doi.org/10.1097/NNR.0b013e3181dbb2f8.

Dishman, R. K., Heath, G. W., & Lee, I. M. (2013). *Physical activity epidemiology* (2nd ed.). Champaign: Human Kinetics.

Donnelly, J. E., Hillman, C. H., Castelli, D., Etnier, J. L., Lee, S., Tomporowski, P., Lambourne, K., & Szabo-Reed, A. N. (2016). Physical activity, fitness, cognitive function, and academic achievement in children. *Medicine & Science in Sports & Exercise, 48*(6), 1223–1224. https://doi.org/10.1249/mss.0000000000000966.

Ekkekakis, P., & Petruzzello, S. J. (2000). Analysis of the affect measurement conundrum in exercise psychology: I Fundamental issues. *Psychology of Sport and Exercise, 1*, 71–88. https://doi.org/10.1016/S1469-0292(00)00010-8.

Ekkekakis, P., Parfitt, G., & Petruzzello, S. J. (2011). The pleasure and displeasure people feel when they exercise at different intensities. *Sport Medicine, 41*(8), 641–671. https://doi.org/10.2165/11590680-000000000-00000.

Elavsky, S. (2010). Longitudinal examination of the exercise and self-esteem model in middle-aged women. *Journal of Sport and Exercise Psychology, 32*(6), 862–880. https://doi.org/10.1123/jsep.32.6.862.

Ensari, I., Greenlee, T. A., Motl, R. W., & Petruzzello, S. J. (2015). Meta-analysis of acute exercise effects on state anxiety: An update of randomized controlled trials over the past 25 years. *Depression & Anxiety, 32*, 624–634. https://doi.org/10.1002/da.22370.

Etnier, J. L. (2017). Physical activity, physical fitness, and cognition. In *Oxford research encyclopedia of psychology*. https://doi.org/10.1093/acrefore/9780190236557.013.198.

Etnier, J. L., Nowell, P. M., Landers, D. M., & Sibley, B. A. (2006). A meta-regression to examine the relationship between aerobic fitness and cognitive performance. *Brain Research Reviews, 52*, 119–130. https://doi.org/10.1016/j.brainresrev.2006.01.002.

Firth, J., Cotter, J., Elliott, R., French, P., & Yung, A. R. (2015). A systematic review and meta-analysis of exercise interventions in schizophrenia patients. *Psychological Medicine, 45*, 1343–1361. https://doi.org/10.1017/S0033291714003110.

Forcier, K., Stroud, L. R., Papandonatos, G. D., Hitsman, B., Reiches, M., Krishnamoorthy, J., & Niaura, R. (2006). Links between physical fitness and cardiovascular reactivity and recovery to psychological stressors: A meta-analysis. *Health Psychology, 25*, 723–739. https://doi.org/10.1037/0278-6133.25.6.723.

Gerber, M., Kalak, N., Lemola, S., Clough, P. J., Puhse, U., Elliot, C., & Brand, S. (2012). Adolescents' exercise and physical activity are associated with mental toughness. *Mental Health and Physical Activity, 5*, 35–42. https://doi.org/10.1016/j.mhpa.2012.02.004.

Gillman, A. S., & Bryan, A. D. (in press). Mindfulness versus distraction to improve affective response and promote cardiovascular exercise behavior. *Annals of Behavioral Medicine*.

Hamer, M., Taylor, A., & Steptoe, A. (2006). The effect of acute aerobic exercise on stress related blood pressure responses: A systematic review and meta-analysis. *Biological Psychology, 71*, 183–190. https://doi.org/10.1016/j.biopsycho.2005.04.004.

Hausenblas, H. A., & Fallon, E. A. (2006). Exercise and body image: A meta-analysis. *Psychology and Health, 21*, 33–47. https://doi.org/10.1080/14768320500105270.

Holley, J., Crone, D., Tyson, P., & Lovell, G. (2011). The effects of physical activity on psychological wellbeing for those with schizophrenia: A systematic review. *British Journal of Clinical Psychology, 50*, 84–105. https://doi.org/10.1348/014466510X496220.

Lee, T. H., & Tseng, C. H. (2015). How personality and risk-taking attitude affect the behaviour of adventure recreationists. *Tourism Geographies: An International Journal of Tourism, 17*, 307–331. https://doi.org/10.1080/14616688.2014.1000955.

Lichtenstein, M. B., Hinze, C. J., Emborg, B., Thomsen, F., & Hemmingsen, S. D. (2017). Compulsive exercise: links, risks and challenges faced. *Psychology Research and Behavior Management, 10*, 85–95. https://doi.org/10.2147/prbm.s113093.

Masters, K. S., Spielmans, G. I., LaCaille, R. A., Goodson, J. T., Larsen, B. T., Heath, E. M., & Knestel, A. (2011). Effects of home exercise on immediate and delayed affect and mood among rural individuals at risk for type 2 diabetes mellitus. *Journal of Social, Behavioral, and Health Sciences, 5*(1), 1–16.

Morgan, A. J., Parker, A. G., Alvarez-Jimenez, M., & Jorm, A. F. (2013). Exercise and mental health: An exercise and sports Science Australia commissioned review. *Journal of Exercise Physiology Online, 16*, 64–73.

Netz, Y., Wu, M. J., Becker, B. J., & Tenenbaum, G. (2005). Physical activity and psychological wellbeing in advanced age: A meta-analysis of intervention studies. *Psychology and Aging, 20*, 272–284. https://doi.org/10.1037/0882-7974.20.2.272.

Paradis, K. F., Cooke, L. M., Martin, L. J., & Hall, C. R. (2013). Too much of a good thing? Examining the relationship between passion for exercise and exercise dependence. *Psychology of Sport and Exercise, 14*(4), 493–500. https://doi.org/10.1016/j.psychsport.2013.02.003.

Ramirez, E., & Wipfli, B. (2013). Exercise and stress reactivity in humans and animals: Two meta-analyses. *International Journal of Exercise Science, 6*(2), 144–156.

Rebar, A. L., Stanton, R., Geard, D., Short, C., Duncan, M. J., & Vandelanotte, C. (2015). A meta-meta-analysis of the effect of physical activity on depression and anxiety in non-clinical adult populations. *Health Psychology Review, 9*(3), 366–378. https://doi.org/10.1080/17437199.2015.1022901.

Reddon, H., Meyre, D., & Cairney, J. (2017). Physical activity and global self-worth in a longitudinal study of children. *Medicine & Science in Sports & Exercise, 49*(8), 1606–1613. https://doi.org/10.1249/mss.0000000000001275.

Reed, J., & Ones, D. S. (2006). The effect of acute aerobic exercise on positive activated affect: A meta-analysis. *Psychology of Sport and Exercise, 7*, 477–514. https://doi.org/10.1016/j.psychsport.2005.11.003.

Reed, J., Pritschet, B. L., & Cutton, D. M. (2012). Grit, conscientiousness, and the transtheoretical model of change for exercise behaviour. *Journal of Health Psychology, 18*, 612–619. https://doi.org/10.1177/1359105312451866.

Reiner, M., Niermann, C., Jekuac, D., & Woll, A. (2013). Long-term health benefits of physical activity – a systematic review of longitudinal studies. *BMC Public Health, 13*, 813. https://doi.org/10.1186/1471-2458-13-813.

Rhodes, R. E., & Pfaeffli, L. A. (2012). Personality and physical activity. In E. O. Acevedo (Ed.), *The Oxford handbook of exercise psychology* (pp. 195–223). New York: Oxford University Press. https://doi.org/10.1093/oxfordhb/9780195394313.013.0011.

Rhodes, R. E., & Smith, N. E. I. (2006). Personality correlates of physical activity: A review and meta-analysis. *British Journal of Sports Medicine, 40*, 958–965. https://doi.org/10.1136/bjsm.2006.028860.

Schuch, F. B., Vancampfort, D., Richards, J., Rosenbaum, S., Ward, P. B., & Stubbs, B. (2016). Exercise as a treatment for depression: A meta-analysis adjusting for publication bias. *Journal of Psychiatric Research, 77*, 42–51. https://doi.org/10.1016/j.jpsychires.2016.02.023.

Schwerdtfeger, A., Eberhardt, R., Chmitorz, A., & Schaller, E. (2010). Momentary affect predicts bodily movement in daily life: An ambulatory monitoring study. *Journal of Sport & Exercise Psychology, 32*, 674–693.

Spence, J. C., McGannon, K. R., & Poon, P. (2005). The effect of exercise on global self-esteem: A quantitative review. *Journal of Sport and Exercise Psychology, 27*, 311–334. https://doi.org/10.1123/jsep.27.3.311.

Stathopoulou, G., Powers, M. B., Berry, A. C., Smits, J. A. J., & Otto, M. W. (2006). Exercise interventions for mental health: A quantitative and qualitative review. *Clinical Psychology: Science and Practice, 13*, 179–193. https://doi.org/10.1111/j.1468-2850.2006.00021.x.

Stephan, Y., Sutin, A. R., & Terracciano, A. (2014). Physical activity and personality development across adulthood and old age: Evidence from two longitudinal studies. *Journal of Research in Personality, 49*, 1–7. https://doi.org/10.1016/j.jrp.2013.12.003.

Stonerock, G. L., Hoffman, B. M., Smith, P. J., & Blumenthal, J. A. (2015). Exercise as treatment for anxiety: Systematic review and analysis. *Annals of Behavioral Medicine, 49*(4), 542–556. https://doi.org/10.1007/s12160-014-9685-9.

Sutin, A. R., Stephan, Y., Luchetti, M., Artese, A., Oshio, A., & Terracciano, A. (2016). The five-factor model of personality and physical inactivity: A meta-analysis of 16 samples. *Journal of Research in Personality, 63*, 22–28. https://doi.org/10.1016/j.jrp.2016.05.001.

Taylor, M. K., Gould, D. R., Hardy, L., Woodman, T., & LaCaille, R. (2006). Factors influencing physical risk taking in rock climbing. *Journal of Human Performance in Extreme Environments, 9*(1), 15–26. https://doi.org/10.7771/2327-2937.1044.

Vallerand, R. J., Blanchard, C., Mageau, G. A., Koestner, R., Ratelle, C., Leonard, M., et al. (2003). Les passions de l'âme: On obsessive and harmonious passion. *Journal of Personality and Social Psychology, 85*, 756–767. https://doi.org/10.1037/0022-3514.85.4.756.

Wilson, K. E., & Dishman, R. K. (2015). Personality and physical activity: A systematic review and meta-analysis. *Personality and Individual Differences, 72*, 230–242. https://doi.org/10.1016/j.paid.2014.08.023.

Psychosocial Characteristics

Adriana Dias Barbosa Vizzotto[1],
Alexandra Martini de Oliveira[2], Helio Elkis[3],
Quirino Cordeiro[4] and Patrícia Cardoso Buchain[1]
[1]Occupational Therapist of the Occupational Therapy Service, Institute of Psychiatry – Hospital das Clínicas University of São Paulo Medical School, São Paulo, SP, Brazil
[2]Occupational Therapy Service, Institute of Psychiatry – Hospital das Clínicas University of São Paulo Medical School, São Paulo, SP, Brazil
[3]Department and Institute of Psychiatry, University of São Paulo Medical School, São Paulo, SP, Brazil
[4]Department of Psychiatry and Psychological Medicine, Santa Casa Medical School, São Paulo, SP, Brazil

Synonyms

Psychosocial aspects; Psychosocial factors

Definition

Psychosocial characteristics is a term used to describe the influences of social factors on an individual's mental health and behavior.

Description

A psychosocial approach to human behavior involves the relation between intrapersonal psychological and environmental aspects. Psychosocial characteristics is commonly described as an individual's psychological development in relation to his/her social and cultural environment. "Psychosocial" means "pertaining to the influence of social factors on an individual's mind or behavior, and to the interrelation of behavioral and social factors" (Oxford English Dictionary 2012). Psychosocial factors, at least in the context of health research, can be defined as the mediation of the effects of social structural factors on individual health, conditioned and modified by the social structures contexts in which they exist (Martikainen et al. 2002). These statements raise the question of what the relevant broader social structural forces are and how such forces might influence health through their effects on individual features.

Psychosocial health is another term very important which includes four components of well-being: mental, emotional, social, and spiritual health. Their balance and interrelationships help a person lead a healthier life (Donatelle 2004).

Individual psychological and social aspects are related to individual's social conditions, mental, and emotional health. For example, the main factors that influence children's mental health are the social and psychological environment (Halpen and Figueiras 2004).

Environmental factors play an important role in the etiology of emotional problems in childhood. The cumulative risk effects from a "vulnerable environment," e.g., negligence, poverty, drug abuse, are more important in determining emotional problems in children than the presence of one single stressor, regardless of its magnitude. According to Barylnik (2003), the analysis of the characteristics of a juvenile delinquent's sample showed a high rate of psychiatric disorder and social phobia, alcoholism, organic brain dysfunctions, low intelligence quotients, and behavior problems.

The term "psychosocial" is widely used for determining an individual's health outcome. Psychological and social factors expressed as thoughts, expressive emotions, and behaviors are significant for human functioning and the occurrence of disease. Mentally healthy people tend to react in positive ways to negative situations, compared to emotional unstable people, who react negatively to similar situations. Hence, irrational thoughts may be a sign of bad psychosocial health. Therefore, for psychosocial instable people, it is preferable to have special social bonds with and social support from other people. On the other hand, prejudice from others is often a result of poor psychosocial health that causes poor social relations.

Hence it is understood that health is better understood in terms of a combination of biological, psychological, and social factors rather than only in biological terms (Santrock 2007). This is in contrast to the traditional and reductionist biomedical model of medicine which suggests that every disease process can be explained in terms of an underlying deviation from normal function such as a pathogen, genetic or developmental abnormality, or injury (Engel 1977).

The World Health Organization's (WHO 2001) definition of health is "a state of complete physical mental and social well-being, and not merely the absence of disease and infirmity." The concept of "psychosocial health," in some cases, may combine traditional medical definitions of disease and infirmity with measures that reflect individual responses to disease and even in some cases indicators of the social context itself. However, such measures have merit in recognizing individuals' experiences and quality of life, meaning an important outcome of individual's psychosocial condition (Martikainen et al. 2002).

Cross-References

▶ Psychosocial Impact

References and Further Reading

Barylnik, J. (2003). Psychopathology, psychosocial characteristics, and family environment in juvenile delinquents. *The German Journal of Psychiatry, 6*, 30–32. http://www.gjpsy.uni-goettingen.de. ISSN 1433-1055.

Donatelle, R. J. (2004). *Health: The basics*. 5E. Publication, March 2004 copyrights date. San Francisco: Pearson/Benjamin Cummings.

Engel, G. L. (1977). The need for a new medical model: A challenge for biomedicine. *Science, 196*, 129–136.

Halpen, R., & Figueiras, A. C. M. (2004). Environmental influences on child mental health. *Journal of Pediatrics, 80*(2 Suppl), S104–S110.

Martikainen, P., Bartley, M., & Lahelma, E. (2002). Psychosocial determinants of health in social epidemiology. *International Journal of Epidemiology, 31*, 1091–1093.

OED Online. (2012). Oxford University Press. Dictionary online http://www.oed.com/. Retrieved April 29, 2012.

Santrock, J. W. (2007). *A topical approach to human life-span development* (3rd ed.). St. Louis: McGraw-Hill.

World Health Organization (WHO). (2001). *The mental health report 2001: Mental health, new understanding hope*. Genebra: Author.

Psychosocial Factors

Jane Upton
Department of Psychology, William James College, Newton, MA, USA

Synonyms

Psychological factors; Psychosocial variables

Definition

Social factors include general factors at the level of human society concerned with social structure and social processes that impinge on the individual. Psychological factors include individual-level processes and meanings that influence mental states. Sometimes, these words are combined as "psychosocial." This is shorthand term for the combination of psychological and social, but it also implies that the effect of social processes are sometimes mediated through psychological understanding (Stansfeld and Rasul 2007).

Description

The relationship between psychological factors and the physical body can be influenced by social factors, the effects of which are mediated through psychological understanding. Examples of psychosocial factors include social support, loneliness, marriage status, social disruption, bereavement, work environment, social status, and social integration. To illustrate that the role psychosocial factors can play in physical disease, this entry will focus on the relationship between social support and mortality.

In 1979, Berkman and Syme conducted a prospective study to investigate the relationship between social support and mortality (Berkman and Syme 1979). The study included 6,928 adults from the general population of Alameda County, California. They recorded four sources of social contact: marriage, contacts with close friends and relatives, church membership, and informal and formal group associations; mortality was followed-up 9 years later. They found that respondents with each type of social tie had lower mortality rates than respondents lacking such connections. From these four variables, they then constructed a Social Network Index, which weighted intimate contacts more heavily than more superficial ones. Using this index, they found a consistent pattern of increased mortality rates with each decrease in social connection. Men who were the most isolated had an age-adjusted mortality rate 2.3 times higher than men with the most connections. This relationship was independent of self reported physical health status, year of death, socioeconomic status, and such health behaviors as smoking, alcohol ingestion, physical inactivity, obesity, and low utilization of preventive health services or health practices.

The effects of level of social support on mortality rates were investigated by Rosengren and colleagues (Rosengren et al. 1993). They invited half of all men in Gothenburg who were born in 1933 (then 50 years old) to have a health examination and complete a measures of emotional support and social integration. Seventy-six percent responded. These men were then followed-up after 7 years, and mortality ascertained. Their data indicated that emotional support may attenuate the impact of adverse life events, possibly by strengthening the psychobiological resistance to stress.

Frasure-Smith and colleagues found in their study of 887 post-myocardial infarction (MI) patients that depression, but not social support, was directly related to mortality (Frasure-Smith et al. 2000). However, very high levels of support protected patients from the negative prognostic consequences of depression. They found that three different measures of social support independently improved depression: higher scores on a measure of perceived social support, a greater number of close friends and relatives, and living with other people. They suggest that clinicians should ascertain patient's views of their social support in their assessments of post-MI depression.

Differences in health status between people with differing levels of social integration cannot simply be attributed to differences in health behaviors between the two groups. In two parallel studies, Cacioppo and colleagues investigated four mechanisms by which loneliness (a discrepancy between their desired and actual relationships) may negatively impact on morbidity and mortality (Cacioppo et al. 2002): (1) poorer health behaviors than nonlonely individuals, (2) altered cardiovascular activation, (3) elevated levels of hypothalamic pituitary adrenocortical activation, and (4) poorer sleep quality. Participants were 89 undergraduate students, and in a second study, 25 older adults (age range 53–78 years). They found that the health behaviors of lonely and nonlonely participants were similar. However, cardiovascular function differed between these groups in both the younger and older participants. They speculated that the differences they found in the hemodynamic function observed in the younger subjects may contribute to elevated blood pressure in lonely older adults. They also found that younger and older lonely adults suffered lower quality sleep, possibly leading to diminished health and well-being.

The plethora of research in this area, measuring different aspects of social relationships, led to uncertainty as to which aspect increased the risk of mortality. A recent meta-analytic review of 148 studies has revealed that stronger social relationships increased the likelihood of survival by 50% (Holt-Lunstad et al. 2010). They found that complex measures of social integration were better predictors of mortality than binary indicators of residential status (e.g., living alone or with others). This is partly because living in a negative social relationship can increase risk of mortality. However, they also caution against assuming causation, due to the difficulty of conducting randomized controlled trials to investigate this topic. They conclude that the data they present makes a compelling case for social relationship factors to be viewed as an important risk factor alongside factors such as smoking, diet, and exercise.

Cross-References

▶ Acute Myocardial Infarction
▶ Bereavement
▶ Cardiovascular Risk Factors
▶ Daily Stress
▶ Loneliness
▶ Psychological Factors and Health
▶ Psychosocial Characteristics
▶ Social Support

References and Further Reading

Berkman, L., & Syme, S. (1979). Social networks, host resistance, and mortality: A nine-year follow-up study of alameda county residents. *American Journal of Epidemiology, 109*(2), 186–204.

Cacioppo, J., Hawkley, L., Crawford, L., Ernst, F., Burleson, M., Kowalewski, R., et al. (2002). Loneliness and health: Potential mechanisms. *Psychosomatic Medicine, 64*, 407–417.

Frasure-Smith, N., Lesperance, F., Gravel, G., Masson, A., Juneau, M., Talajic, M., et al. (2000). Social support, depression, and mortality during the first year after myocardial infarction. *Circulation, 101*, 1919–1924.

Holt-Lunstad, J., Smith, T., & Layton, J. (2010). Social relationships and mortality risk: A meta-analytic review. *PLoS Medicine, 7*(7). https://doi.org/10.1371/journal.pmed.1000316.

Rosengren, A., Orth-Gomer, K., Wedel, H., & Wilhelmsen, L. (1993). Stressful life events, social support, and mortality in men born in 1933. *British Medical Journal, 307*, 1102–1105.

Stansfeld, S., & Rasul, F. (2007). Psychosocial factors, depression and illness. In A. Steptoe (Ed.), *Depression and physical illness* (pp. 19–52). Cambridge, UK: Cambridge University Press.

Psychosocial Factors and Traumatic Events

Shin-Ichi Suzuki[1] and Yuko Yanai[2]
[1]Faculty of Human Sciences, Graduate School of Human Sciences, Waseda University, Tokorozawa-shi, Saitama, Japan
[2]Department of Psycho-Oncology, National Cancer Center Japan, Chuo-ku, Japan

Synonyms

Interpersonal relationships; Psychosocial stress; Stressful life event

Definition

Psychosocial factors are influences that affect a person psychologically or socially. There are multidimensional constructs encompassing several domains such as mood status (anxiety, depression, distress, and positive affect), cognitive behavioral responses (satisfaction, self-efficacy, self-esteem, and locus of control), and social factors (socioeconomic status, education, employment, religion, ethnicity, family, physical attributes, locality, relationships with others, changes in personal roles, and status).

Description

Psychosocial Factors in Everyday Life

Psychosocial factors and influences differ across individuals and may contribute to the development or aggravation of mental and physical disorders. Previous studies have indicated that depression, anxiety, hostility, social isolation and lack of social support, work-related stress, and behavioral escape-avoidance coping were associated with the risk of mortality for patients with cardiac disease (Rozanski et al. 1999; Hemingway and Marmot 1999). A serious loss (bereavement, divorce, and disability), relationship problems, work-related stress, family crisis, financial setback, or any unwelcome life change can trigger depressive disorders (Meltzer et al. 1995). Furthermore, those disorders may negatively impact some psychosocial factors. For example, depressive disorders substantially reduce a person's ability to work effectively and personal and family income and increase the probability of unemployment (Ormel et al. 1999).

Psychosocial Factors in Natural and Technological Disasters

Repeated disasters in Japan such as the Great Hanshin Earthquake and the Great East Japan Earthquake showed us the importance of these psychosocial factors in life events. Furthermore, the Great East Japan Earthquake caused not only death and destruction but also secondary disasters such as the Fukushima nuclear accident. The severity of these natural and technological disasters (e.g., the extent of death and destruction, the length of exposure, evacuation, proximity to the epicenter, and contradictory media reports about the health effects of radiation) are likely to have an adverse impact on victims' mental health (Bromet et al. 2011).

In contrast, positive psychosocial factors in life events such as connectedness to others, the spirit of patience, politeness, and mutual aid may contribute to prevent an aggravation of the situation and change things for the better. In The Great Hanshin Earthquake and The Great East Japan Earthquake, Japanese people have handled their grief and loss and overcome numerous difficulties with mutual cooperation and the spirit of patience. Indeed, some survivors managed to endure the traumatic events relatively well, and resilience and social tie were significant protective factors in dealing with such events (Kukihara et al. 2014; Sugimoto et al. 2015). These psychosocial factors provide us the energy to recover from severe life events.

Cross-References

- ▶ Cardiovascular Disease
- ▶ Depression: Symptoms
- ▶ Life Events
- ▶ Religion/Spirituality
- ▶ Self-Esteem
- ▶ Socioeconomic Status (SES)

References and Further Reading

Bernard, L. B. (1988). *Health psychology: A psychosocial perspective*. Englewood Cliffs: Prentice Hall.

Bromet, E. J., Havenaar, M., & Guey, L. T. (2011). A 25 year retrospective review of the psychological consequences of the Chernobyl accident. *Clinical Oncology, 23*, 297–305.

Davison, L. M., Weiss, L., O'Keefe, M., & Baum, A. (1991). Acute stressors and chronic stress at Three Mile Island. *Journal of Traumatic Stress, 4*, 481–493.

Hemingway, H., & Marmot, M. (1999). Psychosocial factors in the aetiology and prognosis of coronary heart disease: Systematic review of prospective cohort studies. *British Medical Journal, 318*, 1460–1467.

Kukihara, H., Yamawaki, N., Uchiyama, K., Arai, S., & Horikawa, E. (2014). Trauma, depression and resiliene of earthquake/tsunami/nuclear disaster survivors of Hirono, Fukushima, Japan. *Psychiatry and Clinical Neurosciences, 68*, 524–533.

Meltzer, H., Gill, B., & Petticrew, M. (1995). *The prevalence of psychiatric morbidity among adults living in private households*, OPCS surveys of psychiatric morbidity, report 1. London: HMSO.

Ormel, J., Von Korff, M., Oldehinkel, T., Simon, G., Tiemens, B. G., & Ustrun, T. B. (1999). Onset of disability in depressed and non-depressed primary care patients. *Psychological Medicine, 29*, 847–853.

Rozanski, A., Blumenthal, J. A., & Kaplan, J. (1999). Impact of psychological factors on the pathogenesis of cardiovascular disease and implications for therapy. *Circulation, 99*, 2192–2217.

Sugimoto, T., Umeda, M., Shinozaki, T., Naruse, T., & Miyamoto, Y. (2015). Sources of perceived social support associated with reduced psychological distress at 1 year after the great East Japan earthquake: Nationwide cross-sectional survey in 2012. *Psychiatry and Clinical Neurosciences, 69*, 580–586.

Psychosocial Impact

Alexandra Martini de Oliveira[1], Patrícia Cardoso Buchain[2], Adriana Dias Barbosa Vizzotto[2], Helio Elkis[3] and Quirino Cordeiro[4]
[1]Occupational Therapy Service, Institute of Psychiatry – Hospital das Clínicas University of São Paulo Medical School, São Paulo, SP, Brazil
[2]Occupational Therapist of the Occupational Therapy Service, Institute of Psychiatry – Hospital das Clínicas University of São Paulo Medical School, São Paulo, SP, Brazil
[3]Department and Institute of Psychiatry, University of São Paulo Medical School, São Paulo, SP, Brazil
[4]Department of Psychiatry and Psychological Medicine, Santa Casa Medical School, São Paulo, SP, Brazil

Synonyms

Psychological and social effects

Definition

Psychosocial impact is defined as the effect caused by environmental and/or biological factors on individual's social and/or psychological aspects.

Several psychiatric disorders may affect psychological and social aspects of individual's lives. Examples are (a) obsessive-compulsive disorder (OCD), whereas these patients might present social marital disabilities, problems related to occupations and low income (Vikas et al. 2011), (b) people with cancer, who experienced negative psychological effect such as bad feelings and fears, as well as moderate to high levels of anxiety and psychological distress (Primo et al. 2000), (c) traumatic events such disasters, urban violence, and expose of terrorism may also impact on present psychosocial status (Eisenman et al. 2009). Natural disasters, like flooding, have been reported to cause a wide range of psychosocial impacts, leading the victims to present psychiatric symptoms (Paranjothy et al. 2011). For example, after the tsunami in Southern Thailand and Hurricane Katrina in the USA caused high levels of posttraumatic stress disorder (PTSD) among the victims. The prevalence of mental health disorders has been significantly higher among individuals who experienced floodwater in their houses compared to individuals who did not face this type of personal experience (Paranjothy et al. 2011). Individuals who are victims of these environmental phenomena might need more substantial and sometimes sustained intervention (de Zulueta 2007).

Cross-References

▶ Psychosocial Characteristics

References and Readings

de Zulueta, C. F. (2007). Mass violence and mental health: Attachment and trauma. *International Review of Psychiatry, 19*, 221–233.
Eisenman, D. P., Glik, D., Ong, M., Zhou, Q., Tseng, C. H., Long, A., et al. (2009). Terrorism-related fear and avoidance behavior in a multiethnic urban population. *American Journal of Public Health, 99*, 168–174.
Paranjothy, S., Gallacher, J., Amlôt, R., Rubin, G. J., Page, L., Baxter, T., et al. (2011). Psychosocial impact of the summer 2007 floods in England. *BMC Public Health, 11*, 145.
Primo, K., Compas, B. E., Oppedisano, G., Howell, D. C., Epping-Jordan, J. E., & Krag, D. N. (2000). Intrusive thoughts and avoidance in breast cancer: Individual differences and associations with psychological distress. *Psychology and Health, 14*, 1141–1153.
Vikas, A., Avasthi, A., & Sharan, P. (2011). Psychosocial impact of obsessive-compulsive disorder on patients and their caregivers: A comparative study with depressive disorder. *The International Journal of Social Psychiatry, 57*, 45–56.

Psychosocial Implications

▶ Genetic Testing, Psychological Implications

Psychosocial Intervention

▶ Cancer: Psychosocial Treatment

Psychosocial Oncology

▶ Cancer: Psychosocial Treatment

Psychosocial Predictors

Joanna Long and Jennifer Cumming
School of Sport and Exercise Sciences,
The University of Birmingham, Edgbaston,
Birmingham, UK

Synonyms

Health behavior predictors; Psychological predictors

Definition

Psychosocial variables which act as predictors either of other psychosocial variables or behaviors, cognitions, risk, severity, mortality, or a number of other factors which may relate to behavioral medicine research, such as health outcomes.

Description

Psychosocial variables encompass both the social and psychological aspects of someone's life and cover a broad range of both positive and negative factors often measured in behavioral medicine research. Social factors include quality of life, health behaviors (alcohol consumption, smoking status, drug use), physical activity level, and socioeconomic status, whereas personal factors include depressive symptoms, perceived stress levels, anxiety, and mood (see ▶ "Psychosocial Variables"). Psychosocial variables often interrelate and can be used to predict behavioral and/or health outcomes. These variables also act as risk factors for mental health and chronic conditions, such as rheumatoid arthritis, HIV, gastrointestinal disorders, and Parkinson's disease, among many others. For these reasons, psychosocial predictors are important to assess when investigating cofactors of disease and targeting interventions within a population.

Within cross-sectional research, psychosocial predictors may correlate with other psychosocial variables or the behavior and health outcomes investigated. Examples of cross-sectional studies using psychosocial predictors within behavioral medicine research include Ng and Jeffery (2003) who found an inverse relationship between perceived stress and exercise, and Blair and Church (2004) who investigated the link between physical activity status with obesity and health behaviors, such as smoking and diet. Although this design provides immediate research, it is limited to a particular time point for assessing relationships that may vary over time. Alternatively, longitudinal designs are used to study psychosocial predictors in a group of individuals over a period of time, perhaps for many years. This may permit researchers to predict future behaviors, risk, and health outcomes in research. For example, Leserman et al. (1999) investigated the relationship between perceived stress and AIDS diagnosis in HIV patients over 5.5 years. Also, Whooley et al. (2008) investigated the relationship between depressive symptoms and health behaviors such as physical activity levels, smoking status, and alcohol consumption with risk of cardiovascular events over 5 years in patients with existing coronary heart disease. Taking assessments at multiple time points permits researchers to examine whether changes in psychosocial factors relate to long-term disease or condition changes. Compared to cross-sectional research, a longitudinal study also provides a more accurate idea of the direction of the predictor's relationship. However, cross-sectional and longitudinal studies cannot infer causation or show the direction of the relationship.

Cross-References

▶ Psychosocial Variables

References and Further Reading

Blair, S. N., & Church, T. S. (2004). The fitness, obesity, and health equation: Is physical activity the common denominator? *Journal of the American Medical Association, 292*(10), 1232–1234.

Leserman, J., Jackson, E. D., Petitto, J. M., Golden, R. N., Silva, S. G., Perkins, D. O., et al. (1999). Progression to AIDS: The effects of stress, depressive symptoms, and social support. *Psychosomatic Medicine, 61*, 397–406.

Ng, D. M., & Jeffery, R. W. (2003). Relationships between perceived stress and health behaviors in a sample of working adults. *Health Psychology, 22*(6), 638–642.

Whooley, M. A., de Jonge, P., Vittinghoff, E., Otte, C., Moos, R., Carney, R. M., et al. (2008). Depressive symptoms, health behaviors, and risk of cardiovascular events in patients with coronary heart disease. *Journal of the American Medical Association, 300*(20), 2379–2388.

Psychosocial Stress

▶ Psychosocial Factors and Traumatic Events
▶ Trier Social Stress Test

Psychosocial Traits

▶ Character Traits

Psychosocial Variables

Joanna Long and Jennifer Cumming
School of Sport and Exercise Sciences,
The University of Birmingham, Edgbaston,
Birmingham, UK

Synonyms

Health behavior variables; Psychological variables

Definition

Variables encompassing psychological and social factors.

Description

The term "psychosocial" has a broad meaning when considering health research and social epidemiology. It is formed from two words: psychological and social. Psychological factors can be positive, such as happiness, affect, and vitality, or negative, such as anxiety, perceived stress, and depressive symptoms. These can also be split to distinguish between trait and state aspects. Personality traits, depressive factors, well-being, quality of life, and the impact of significant life events and trauma are less likely to fluctuate on a day-to-day basis (i.e., more trait-like or stable variables), whereas anxiety, perceived stress, mood, affect, happiness, and vitality are more unstable (i.e., more state-like). Furthermore, cognitive, behavioral, and affective facets within psychosocial factors can be identified. For example, someone may think about taking up smoking, and subsequently begin smoking, which in turn may lower perceived stress levels.

Social factors involve the relationship a person has with their environment, such as their age, sex, ethnicity, level, and perception of social support, socioeconomic status, neighborhood factors, family history, and health behaviors. The environment can also promote or hinder whether individuals engage in positive or negative health behavior. For example, certain behavioral factors, such as the likelihood of exercise participation, smoking, alcohol intake, and drug abuse may be influenced by the physical environment. If an individual lives within a community that is safe and accessible, for example, they may be more likely to engage in high levels of outdoor physical activity, such as walking around the neighborhood.

Psychosocial variables therefore encompass a large range of factors relating to an individual's psychological state and social environment and potentially have either positive and negative consequences for health and behavioral outcomes (see ▶ "Psychosocial Predictors"). These variables are also important to consider when investigating either the risk, or progression, of an illness or disease. For example, high perceived stress levels, anxiety, and depression may accelerate progression of HIV or coronary heart disease (Barefoot et al. 1996; Leserman 2008). Similarly, understanding of these variables allows researchers to examine developmental processes, such as healthy aging or the effects of a long-term intervention within the population.

There are two main ways of measuring psychosocial variables. Administering questionnaires is the most common method used in research. For example, the Perceived Stress Scale (PSS) (Cohen et al. 1983) assesses the degree to which situations in one's life are perceived as stressful, whereas the Centre for Epidemiological Studies Depression Scale (CES-D) (Kohout et al. 1993) measures current level of depressive symptomatology. The items making up the questionnaire are often summed together to create an overall score for the variable being measured (e.g., depression) and can be compared to norms generated for clinical and general populations. For example, the CES-D questionnaire has a range between 0 and 30, with a score of 10 or more indicating possible clinical depression. It is important that the questionnaires used are reliable, valid, and specific to the population which is being studied. Alternatively, researchers may choose to use structured or semistructured interviews to assess psychosocial variables. A structured interview involves asking respondents a predetermined and limited number of questions about a specific topic, whereas a semistructured interview is more flexible and allows new questions to be brought up or emerging topics to be explored. Interviews provide a qualitative aspect to the research, which is often used to complement the quantitative data provided by questionnaires when taking a mixed-methods approach.

Cross-References

▶ Psychosocial Factors
▶ Psychosocial Predictors

References and Further Reading

Barefoot, J. C., Helms, M. J., Mark, D. B., Blumenthal, J. A., Califf, R. M., Haney, T. L., O'Connor, C. M., Siegler, I. C., & Williams, R. B. (1996). Depression and long term mortality risk in patients with coronary heart disease. *American Journal of Cardiology, 78*, 613–617.

Cohen, S., Kamarck, T., & Mermelstein, R. (1983). A global measure of perceived stress. *Journal of Health and Social Behaviour, 24*, 385–396.

Kohout, F. J., Berkman, L. F., Evans, D. A., & Cornoni-Huntley, J. (1993). Two shorter forms of the CES-D depression symptoms index. *Journal of Aging and Health, 5*, 179–193.

Leserman, J. (2008). Role of depression, stress and trauma in HIV disease progression. *Psychosomatic Medicine, 70*, 539–545.

Psychosocial Work Environment

Karen Jacobs[1], Miranda Hellman[2], Jacqueline Markowitz[1] and Ellen Wuest[2]
[1]Occupational Therapy, College of Health and Rehabilitation Science, Sargent College, Boston University, Boston, MA, USA
[2]Boston University, Boston, MA, USA

Synonyms

Mental strain; Physical illness; Psychological and social conditions people experience in the workplace; Stress and occupational health

Definition

Psychosocial work environment pertains to interpersonal and social interactions that influence behavior and development in the workplace. Research has been conducted to determine the effects of the psychosocial work environment on stress levels and overall health. One study in particular found that low levels of support and control at work leads to increased rates of sickness absence (North et al. 1996). In other words, a positive and supportive psychosocial work environment is beneficial to employees in an occupational organization.

Cross-References

- Job Demand/Control/Strain
- Positive Affectivity
- Positive Psychology
- Psychological Factors
- Psychosocial Characteristics
- Psychosocial Impact

References and Readings

North, F. M., Syme, S. L., Feeney, A., Shipley, M., & Marmot, M. (1996). Psychosocial work-environment and sickness absence among British civil servants: The Whitehall II study. *American Journal of Public Health, 86*, 332–340.

Psychosomatic

Makiko Ito
Department of Stress Science and Psychosomatic Medicine, Graduate School of Medicine, The University of Tokyo, Bunkyo-ku, Tokyo, Japan

Definition

Psychosomatic is defined as one involving or depending on both the mind and the body as mutually dependent entities.

The term has been used to refer to the following:

1. Physical disorders, those caused or aggravated by psychological factors and, less often, to mental disorders caused or aggravated by physical factors
2. The branch of medicine concerned with the mind-body relations
3. The field of study, one sometimes designated "psychosomatics," concerned with the relationship between mind and body

Description

It is said that the foundation for psychosomatic movement was laid 2,500 years ago in ancient Greece.

In the fifth century BC, Hippocratic principles emphasized what we consider to be some of the basic tenets of psychosomatic medicine: concern about the relationship between the physician and the patient and about importance of the environment and of the adaptive factors in health and disease.

Francis Bacon advocated investigation of the mental faculties and of the interaction of body and mind by case studies and by study of the relationships between the individual and society. A passage written by Bacon in 1605 is the first explicit scientific statement about psychosomatic medicine in English.

Psychiatry and psychosomatic medicine owe an immense debt to Johann Reli, who was the first use the word psychiatry.

Another pioneer in German psychiatry was Johann Heinroth, who was the first to use the word psychosomatic in 1818. He insisted that the mind in health and disease was essential to the treatment of illness.

The significance of Freud's dynamic principles of psychological causality and of the unconscious is enhanced.

In the 1920s and 1930s, psychosomatic concepts were supported by two major advances in physiology as well as by psychoanalytic findings. Pavlov's discovery of the conditioned reflex furnished a tool for measuring emotional correlates of stress, and Cannon's work on adrenaline, the endocrine glands, and on the autonomic nervous system stimulated the development of research in psychophysiology.

Resurgent interest in psychosomatic medicine in the 1920s and the 1930s started with clinical work, initially case histories that described psychosomatic phenomena. Within a few years, Alexander and Dunbar proposed theories of psychosomatic illness.

In 1950s, Hans Selye advocated a concept that an external stressor had an influence on physical health, which is called "general adaptation syndrome." The theory of Selye contributed to mind and body medical advance greatly.

George L. Engel proposed that health is affected by a biological factor, a psychological factor, and the social support.

After that, including a famous Framingham study, a way of thinking that an unhealthy habit and action had an influence on health directly came to attract attention worldwide. Health and a complicated biological, psychological, and sociological health model about the disease came to be recognized in the medicine, and a field called the behavior medicine was born in this way. The current psychosomatic medicine regards this behavior medicine as the one of the important theoretical bases, but aims at the promotion of the medical care of all people while not only it but also psychology takes in various study.

Cross-References

▶ Psychosomatic Disorder

References and Readings

Kannel, W. B., & Eaker, E. D. (1986). Psychosocial and other features of coronary heart disease: Insight from Framingham study. *American Heart Journal, 112*(5), 1066–1073.
Lipowski, Z. J. (1984). What does the word "Psychosomatic" Really mean? A historical and semantic inquiry. *Psychosomatic Medicine, 46*(2), 153–171.
Schwab, J. J. (1985). Psychosomatic medicine: Its past and present. *Psychosomatics, 26*(7), 583–593.

Psychosomatic Diseases

▶ Psychosomatic Disorder

Psychosomatic Disorder

Tetusya Ando
Department of Psychosomatic Research, National Institute of Mental Health, National Center of Neurology and Psychiatry, Kodaira-shi, Tokyo, Japan

Synonyms

Psychophysiologic disorders; Psychosomatic diseases; Psychosomatic illness

Definition

1. Somatic diseases or disorders characterized by objective organic changes and/or functional changes that could be induced, progressed, aggravated, or exacerbated by psychological, social, and/or behavioral factors.
2. Physical illness or symptom believed to be caused by psychological factors.

Description

The term "psychosomatic" carries two connotations having an ancient tradition in Western thinking and medicine: psychogenesis of disease and holism. Psychogenesis is an etiologic hypothesis about the role of psychological factors in human disease. The core notion of holism is that mind and body is inseparable and mutually dependent aspects of man, and it implies a view of the human being as a whole.

The idea of psychogenesis resulted in the concept of psychosomatic disorder, a physical illness or symptoms believed to be caused by psychological factors. Notion of psychogenesis has been criticized because it is incompatible with current multifactorial view of diseases, and the term "psychosomatic disorder" is misleading since it implies a special class of disorders of psychogenic etiology and absence of psychosomatic interface in other diseases.

Holistic concept resulted in multifactorial model of illness called "biopsychosocial" model by Engel. In this model, illness is a result of interacting mechanisms at the cellular, tissue, organic, interpersonal, and environmental level. Biopsychosocial approach to illness and health covers the psychosomatic medicine, behavioral science, social science, neuroscience, stress physiology and epidemiology, psychoneuroendocrinology/immunology, psycho-oncology, and so on.

Psychosomatic medicine has focused on the study of the interaction of psychosocial and biological factors in health and disease. Psychosocial factors may induce, sustain, or modify the course of virtually all kind of diseases including infections and cancer, though their relative weight may vary from disease to disease and from patient to patient suffering from the same disease. Japanese Society of Psychosomatic Medicine defined psychosomatic disorders as somatic diseases "characterized by objective organic changes and/or functional changes that could be induced, progressed, aggravated, or exacerbated by psychological, social, and/or behavioral factors."

Psychosocial factors possibly affecting individual vulnerability, onset, course, and outcome of diseases are early and recent life events, chronic stress, personality variables, coping ability, social support, psychological state such as depression, anxiety, anger, hostility, irritability, psychological well-being, and abnormal illness behavior. Mechanisms through which psychosocial factors could influence health and disease are mediated by central and autonomic nervous systems, neuroendocrine systems, and immune systems. Psychosocial stressors may also affect health and disease through changes in health-related habits and behaviors, such as smoking, eating, drinking, exercise, and drug use. Psychological factors may also play role in adjustment to disease, attitude to medical care, doctor-patient relationship, adherence to treatment, impairment in social functioning, and quality of life of patients.

For example, high levels of stress, low levels of social support or social isolation, low socioeconomic status, personality factors, and negative emotions such as anger or hostility, depression, and anxiety are associated with increased cardiovascular disease morbidity and mortality. These psychosocial factors have been associated with enhanced sympathetic nervous system activation, impaired parasympathetic activity, increased circulating levels of catecholamines and corticosteroid, enhanced blood coagulation and fibrinolysis, endothelial dysfunction, coronary vasospasm, and various inflammatory markers. Lifestyle modification (e.g., smoking cessation, diet, exercise) improves cardiovascular health. Psychological interventions, such as relaxation, stress management, cognitive, and behavior therapies may improve psychological distress and psychological functioning in cardiovascular patients.

As a summary, the term "psychosomatic disorders" is misleading and discouraged to be used at least in the sense of psychogenic disease. Holistic concept, another major connotation of "psychosomatic," resulted in biopsychosocial model of illness. Irrespective of whether the term "psychosomatic disorder" is used or not, it is important to perform research and medical practice of a disease from a multifactorial perspective.

Cross-References

▶ Psychoneuroendocrinology

References and Readings

Engel, G. L. (1977). The need for a new medical model: A challenge for biomedicine. *Science, 196*, 129–136.

Fava, G. A., & Sonino, N. (2000). Psychosomatic medicine: Emerging trends and perspectives. *Psychotherapy and Psychosomatics, 69*, 184–197.

Lipowski, Z. J. (1986). Psychosomatic medicine: Past and present. *Canadian Journal of Psychiatry, 31*, 2–21.

Psychosomatic Illness

▶ Psychosomatic Disorder

Psychosomatic Medicine

▶ Health Psychology

Psychosomatics

▶ Somatization

Psychosurgery

Douglas Carroll
School of Sport and Exercise Sciences,
The University of Birmingham, Edgbaston,
Birmingham, UK

Synonyms

Psychiatric surgery

Definition

Psychosurgery is brain surgery conducted explicitly to amend aspects of human behavior. As such, it can be distinguished from neurosurgery, where the aim is to address some specific and identifiable brain pathology such as a tumor. Although there are noticeable gray areas such as brain surgery for intractable pain or to halt the spread of epileptic seizures from one brain hemisphere to the other, the above distinction is important in differentiating between the primarily behavioral aims of psychosurgery and the primary aims of treating physical pathology that characterize neurosurgery.

Description

The first psychosurgical operation was undertaken on November 12, 1935 by Egas Moniz at the Neurological Institute of the University of Lisbon, Portugal. Moniz's surgery was conducted on severely disturbed psychiatric patients who had proved resistant to other forms of treatment. He called his operation the prefrontal leucotomy; a wire garrote inserted via a cannula or "leucotome" was used to severe connections between the prefrontal cortex and more posterior parts of the brain. In 1949, Moniz was awarded the Nobel Prize in Medicine "for his discovery of the therapeutic value of prefrontal leucotomy in certain psychoses." Moniz's activities in the field of psychosurgery were curtailed, though, when he was shot by one of his psychosurgical patients; the bullet lodged in his spine and he retired, a hemiplegic, in 1944.

However, Moniz's initiative was enthusiastically transported to the USA and UK, where the operation was re-branded: the frontal lobotomy was born. As indicated, the target patient group were psychiatric patients suffering from severe and intransigent psychoses. The Second World War through up a great number of such patients; the late 1940s and early 1950s were to prove the heyday of the frontal lobotomy. It has been estimated that between 40,000 and 50,000 operations were conducted in the USA during that period with a further 12,000 undertaken in the UK. From its outset, psychosurgery was subject to fierce controversy. Its opponents regarded it as a grievous, unjustified, and irreversible assault on the human personality. Its proponents, on the other hand, confidently testified that it was a valid and efficacious treatment for many seemingly intractable psychiatric disorders. Sober and objective assessment was difficult since the vast majority of psychosurgical data stem from uncontrolled observations where even the minimal attributes of good experimental design are absent: control groups, independent evaluation of treatment effects, lengthy follow-ups, etc. Accordingly, claims of efficacy based on data of such dubious scientific status can command little confidence.

By the late 1950s, psychosurgery was on the wane; the newly introduced major tranquilizers offered a seemingly easier and decidedly less contentious way of managing the behavior of severely disturbed psychiatric patients. Nevertheless, just as it seemed safe to go back into mental hospital, psychosurgery began to re-brand itself once more. By the late 1960s and early 1970s, psychosurgery was enjoying a modest renaissance. This time around, the operations were technically more sophisticated. The main differences, though, were the neural and behavioral targets. No longer was the prefrontal cortex the focus but rather structures that lay deep within the brain: components of the limbic system such as the amygdala, which is implicated in emotion and motivation. No longer was severe psychosis the sole or even main target; instead, the focus had shifted to vaguer and more diagnostically problematic behaviors such as aggression and hyperactivity. Deviance had replaced psychiatric disturbance. As before, the battle between opponents and proponents was enjoined, and as before, the available data did not afford anything like a proper scientific assessment. Again, its day in the sun was short-lived; psychosurgery had all but disappeared by the 1980s. This time, though, it was regulation and legislation that did the trick.

References and Further Reading

Valenstein, E. S. (1973). *Brain control: A critical examination of brain stimulation and psychosurgery.* New York: Wiley.

Psychotherapy for Depression

▶ Depression: Treatment

Psychotherapy for IBS

▶ Irritable Bowel Syndrome (IBS): Psychological Treatment

PTG

▶ Posttraumatic Growth

PTS

▶ Stress, Posttraumatic

Puberty

Adriana Carrillo and Carley Gomez-Meade
Department of Pediatrics, Miller School of Medicine, University of Miami, Miami, FL, USA

Synonyms

Menarche; Sexual maturation

Definition

Puberty is the transition from being sexually immature to sexual maturity and attainment of reproductive capacity. Complex interactions of hypothalamic-pituitary hormones and neuroendocrine factors take place to initiate puberty. Recent research indicates kisspeptin and its receptor GPR54 to play a key part in the initiation of puberty. Kisspeptin and GPR54 increase at the onset of puberty. Kisspeptin neurons innervate and stimulate hypothalamic gonadotropin releasing hormone (GNRH) neurons. In addition, kisspeptin neurons express estrogen and androgen receptors which may be important for the onset and tempo of puberty. The onset of puberty is also marked by increasing pulse and frequency of GNRH from the hypothalamus. GNRH then stimulates the pituitary to secrete gonadotropins (luteinizing hormone (LH) and follicle stimulating hormone (FSH)) which directly stimulates the ovaries or testes to produce sex steroids. The increase of sex steroids induces the physical changes of puberty. The progressive physical changes during puberty are described by the Tanner staging system. Both boys and girls have five stages. The first Tanner stage (Tanner stage I) is prepubertal or sexual immaturity and the fifth Tanner stage describes a sexually mature adult. Tanner stage II marks the beginning of sexual maturation (Lifshitz 2007; Oakley et al. 2009).

Puberty begins earlier in girls than boys. The normal range for the onset of puberty in females is 8–13 years of age. The first sign of puberty in girls is breast development at an average age of 10.4 years in Caucasian girls. African American girls begin puberty earlier at a mean age of 9.5 years. Tanner stages follow progress through puberty with changing contour of the breast. The development of pubic hair is not under the same control as the ovaries. Adrenarche is a result of increased adrenal androgens and occurs before breast development in 10% of girls. Pubic hair is also described by Tanner stages. Puberty is also marked by an increase in percent body fat, maturation of the vaginal mucosa, and uterine and endometrial growth. Accelerated growth begins early in puberty for girls with peak growth velocity during Tanner stage II– III. The average age of menarche for Caucasian girls is 12.5 years and 12 years for African American girls. Menarche is associated with a deceleration in growth and typically occurs during Tanner stage IV. Menarche occurs approximately 2 years after Tanner stage II breast development in normally maturing girls. Early menstrual cycles may be anovulatory and irregular with subsequent ovulation and development of regular cycles. Adult contour breast and adult pubic hair distribution marks Tanner stage V and the completion of puberty.

The normal age range for the onset of puberty in boys is 9–14 years. The average age for the development of Tanner stage II for Caucasian males is 12 years and 11.2 years for African American males. The first sign of puberty in boys is increased testicular volume. Puberty progresses with continued testicular enlargement and penile enlargement as described by the Tanner stages. Mid-puberty axillary hair and androgen sensitive hair on the face, chest and back begins. Also in mid-puberty, males have peak linear growth, voice change, and acne. There is a progressive increase in total bone mineral content and lean body mass and a decline in body fat. Spermarche is attained at Tanner stage III. Peak growth velocity occurs during Tanner stage IV in males. Puberty is complete at Tanner stage V with adult genitalia and adult distribution of pubic hair.

Deviations from normal in the onset of puberty and progression through puberty may represent normal variation or pathological disease. Normal variations include premature adrenarche, gynecomastia during male puberty, and premature thelarche in females. Precocious puberty or delayed puberty may represent abnormal pubertal development. It is important to recognize abnormal variations in puberty that may require intervention.

Premature adrenarche is the early development of pubic hair, typically after 6 years of age for males and females. It is more common in females and is usually benign. Females with a history of premature adrenarche have an increased risk of polycystic ovarian syndrome and insulin resistance. A bone age radiograph can be used to determine effects of sex steroids on skeletal maturation. The bone age in premature adrenarche is normal. In addition, gonadotropin hormones are normal and there is no breast development in females or testicular enlargement in males.

Gynecomastia is usually a self-limiting development of palpable breast tissue in 40% of males during puberty. It usually begins in early puberty and resolves within 2 years. It is typically minimal and does not require treatment. Some conditions are associated with excessive or prolonged gynecomastia including Klinefelter syndrome and other causes of decreased testosterone production. Other pathological causes of gynecomastia are some testicular tumors, liver failure, ketaconazole, spirinolactone, marijuana, and other medications.

In females, early benign breast development is called premature thelarche. It is usually present at birth and increases in size over the first 2 years of life. It may also occur around 6 years of age. It is nonprogressive and is not associated with accelerated growth, elevated pubertal hormones, or other changes associated with puberty. As with premature adrenarche, this is not associated with accelerated growth, normal bone age, or elevated pubertal hormones.

Precocious puberty is the abnormal development of secondary sexual characteristics before 7 years of age in Caucasian females, 6 years of age in African American females, and before 9 years of age in males. Precocious puberty in females is most commonly idiopathic premature activation of the hypothalamic-pituitary-gonadal axis, termed idiopathic central precocious puberty. Other causes of central precocious puberty include abnormalities of the central nervous system (CNS) such as brain tumors, intracranial irradiation, infections, or congenital malformations. CNS pathology is more common in males than in females. Outside of the CNS, estrogen or testosterone production may occur independent of gonadotropin secretion from the pituitary gland. In females, estrogen from ovarian cysts, ovarian tumors, or exogenous estrogen exposure may stimulate the onset of puberty. Rarely, genetic mutations can stimulate ovarian estrogen production. McCune Albright syndrome is due to an activating mutation of a signaling protein that results in café au lait spots, fibrous dysplasia, and precocious puberty in females. In males, androgen production stimulating penile growth and pubic hair can come from adrenal or testicular tumors. Congenital adrenal hyperplasia is due to a genetic mutation that leads to the overproduction of adrenal androgens that causes precocious puberty in males and virilization in females. Virilization in females includes clitoromegaly, hirsutism, and acne.

If puberty does not occur spontaneously prior to 14 years in males and 13 years in females it is considered delayed. In addition, puberty in males should be completed within 4.5 years after its onset. If a female has not menstruated by 16 years of age or 5 years after the onset of puberty it is termed primary amenorrhea. The most common reason for delayed puberty is constitutional delay of growth and puberty. Constitutional delay is characterized by a decline in growth velocity during early childhood followed by a normal growth velocity with a delayed bone age. Puberty occurs late and final height is normal. There is typically a family history of late puberty.

Pathologic causes of delayed puberty can be divided into those due to failure of the hypothalamus or pituitary to secrete gonadotropins and those due to failure of gonads to respond to gonadotropins. Delayed puberty with low gonadotropins can be secondary to chronic disease, genetic syndromes, gene mutations, or CNS pathology. Syndromes that are associated with low gonadotropins are Prader-Willi, Lawrence Moon, and Kallman syndromes. Anorexia, malnutrition, HIV, Crohn's disease and hemoglobinopathies are some of the chronic conditions that may cause delayed puberty. Endocrine disorders associated with delayed puberty are hypothyroidism and hyperprolactinemia. Tumors, radiation, infection, or congenital malformation can affect the production and secretion of gonadotropins.

Delayed puberty due to gonadal failure is most commonly due to sex chromosome abnormalities. Klinefelter syndrome males carry two X chromosomes and one Y chromosome. Klinefelter syndrome is characterized by testicular failure, disproportionate long limbs, poor musculature, and gynecomastia. In females, Turner syndrome is due to loss of genetic material from one X chromosome. Females with turners have ovarian failure, short stature, and a spectrum of other dysmorphisms. Gonadal failure can also be due to gonadal dysgenesis or direct damage to the gonads such as trauma, medication, radiation or infection (Lifshitz 2007; Sperling 2008).

References and Readings

Lifshitz, F. (2007). *Pediatric endocrinology* (5th ed.). New York: Informa Healthcare.
Oakley, A. E., Clifton, D. K., & Steiner, R. A. (2009). Kisspeptin signalling in the brain. *Endocrine Reviews, 30*(6), 713.
Sperling, M. (2008). *Pediatric endocrinology* (3rd ed.). Philadelphia: Suanders/Elsevier.

Public Health

Marc D. Gellman
Behavioral Medicine Research Center,
Department of Psychology, University of Miami,
Miami, FL, USA

Definition

Public health refers to activities by which a society attempts to increase life expectancy, decrease morbidity, and help improve health-related quality of life.

Description

An important cornerstone of public health is prevention. Primary prevention refers to measures taken to reduce the incidence of disease. In the case of CVD (cardiovascular disease), for example, people may be encouraged to quit smoking, decrease intake of dietary fat, and increase physical activity before diseases become evident. In contrast, secondary prevention involves reducing the prevalence of disease by shortening its duration. Mortality from certain cancers, for example, prostate cancer, is decreased by early detection of the cancers when they are still treatable. Still another form of prevention is tertiary prevention. This involves reducing the complications associated with chronic diseases reducing the complications associated with chronic diseases and minimizing disability and suffering. Medication adherence training in HIV/AIDS (human immunodeficiency virus/acquired immune deficiency syndrome) patients is a form of tertiary prevention.

There has often been a widespread misconception that public health is limited to "health care for low-income families." The Centers for Disease Control and Prevention created a list of the Ten Great Public Health Achievements in the twentieth century that remind us of how far we have come, how we got here, and exactly what public health is: the active protection of a nation's health and safety, credible information to enhance health decisions, and partnerships with local minorities and organizations to promote good health. The choices of topics for the following list were based on the opportunity for prevention and the impact on death, illness, and disability: they are not ranked by order of importance. The list includes the following: vaccination, motor vehicle safety, safer workplaces, control of infectious diseases, decline in deaths from coronary heart disease (CHD) and stroke, safer and healthier foods, healthier mothers and babies, family planning, fluoridation of drinking water, and, last but not least, the recognition of tobacco use as a health hazard.

During this period, the health and life expectancy of persons residing in the United States improved dramatically. Since 1900, their average lifespan lengthened by greater than 30 years, of which 25 years of this gain are attributable to advances in public health. The unprecedented increase in longevity seen during the first half of the twentieth century was also seen in other countries, primarily in economically advanced countries. The decrease in mortality rate was largely due to a decline in infectious diseases related to vaccination, decreased exposure to infection because of improved hygiene, improved nutrition, and the development of antibiotics to cope with bacterial infections. However, as infectious diseases declined as the leading cause of mortality in economically advanced countries, they were eclipsed by chronic diseases. By the middle of the twentieth century, CHD, cancer, and stroke accounted for more than 60% of the deaths in the United States.

Public health efforts to eradicate infectious diseases have successfully led to an increase in longevity in economically developed and even many less developed countries. Similarly, improvements in healthy lifestyle have led to decreases in morbidity and increases in longevity in these countries during the second half of the twentieth century. At the same time, the HIV/AIDS pandemic in sub-Saharan Africa has led to an even steeper decline in life expectancy. The growing spread of HIV/AIDS across the Asian continent is of considerable concern.

At this point, early in the twenty-first century, the major causes of death in the United States include (1) heart disease, (2) cancer, (3) stroke, (4) unintentional injuries, (5) chronic obstructive pulmonary disorder, (6) pneumonia and influenza, (7) diabetes, (8) suicide, (9) liver disease, (10) HIV/AIDS, and (11) homicide. Behavioral, psychosocial, and sociocultural factors associated with lifestyle contribute to virtually all of these causes of mortality. Even in the case of infectious disease such as pneumonia, risk factors can be related to disruptions of natural pulmonary host mechanisms related to lifestyle factors such as smoking and alcohol abuse. Similarly, infection from HIV is primarily spread through high-risk sexual practices and the sharing of contaminated drug paraphernalia.

As scientists attempted to find specific causal agents in the pathogenesis of cancer and CVD throughout most of the twentieth century, a new approach emerged. Unable to find single causes of diseases, attention shifted to the role of environment and host in the pathogenesis of chronic diseases. Whereas single cause-and-effect models proved successful in studying the genesis of infectious diseases, an understanding of the basis of chronic diseases turned to models based on the presence of risk factors. The identification of risk factors makes prediction of chronic diseases more likely, but individual risk factors cannot be identified as necessary and sufficient causes for many diseases. In this respect, interactions among agent, host, and the environment have now taken center stage.

At the beginning of the risk factor revolution, it was widely believed that the causes of chronic diseases such as CHD could be explained in terms of a few biological (e.g., high cholesterol, high blood pressure) and lifestyle (e.g., smoking) risk factors; this turned out not to be the case. Other variables contributing to CHD turned out to include physical inactivity, excess consumption of alcohol, and obesity. Still other factors under investigation include individual difference variables such as depression and hostility and sociocultural variables including low socioeconomic status, ethnic minority status, lack of social support, and occupational stress.

To achieve public health objectives, it is sometimes useful to deal with unyielding problems at multiple levels. Although behavioral interventions administered at the individual level tend to produce successful weight loss in the short term, few people maintain their weight loss over the long term. In order for individual-based interventions to succeed on a population basis, such interventions should take place in a sociocultural environment that is conducive to healthful eating and exercise. Improving the availability of healthy food choices, providing economic incentives for healthy eating by selective taxation, ensuring through the schools that children and adolescents get adequate exercise, enhancing accessibility of physical activity for the general public by providing bicycle paths and highway lanes, and initiating mass media campaigns supporting a healthy lifestyle could be useful for maintaining weight loss.

The recent successes in tobacco control in the United States provide a heartening example of how multilevel approaches to a major public health problem can lead to a decline in disease. In this case, the improvements have occurred in CVD, some cancers including lung and esophageal cancer, and respiratory diseases. At the interpersonal level, smoking cessation interventions, sometimes in conjunction with pharmacologic treatment, have been effective. At the organizational level, smoking cessation support groups, school campaigns against smoking, restrictions on smoking in restaurants and work sites, and reductions in health insurance premiums for nonsmokers have been established. Finally, at the societal level, laws against juvenile smoking, taxation of cigarettes, and government-sponsored antismoking campaigns have all been realized. These measures have led to a marked improvement in the nation's health.

A distinction is sometimes made between clinical or high-risk approaches to disease treatment and prevention versus population-based strategies. Although there is some value in differentiating between these approaches, they should be seen as complementary because neither strategy is effective for all behaviors or all target groups. Thus, an important public health task is to identify which risk behaviors are open to individual-based versus population-based interventions and how to make these interventions synergistic with one another. Application of the social and behavioral sciences to improve health and combat disease occurs at multiple levels and requires putting into practice different skills both within and across levels. Genetic counseling for those at familial risk of disease, family counseling to reduce substance abuse, and interfamilial violence and group counseling to help those living with HIV/AIDS are examples of interpersonal interventions at the individual level. At the organizational level, interpersonal interventions such as blood pressure screenings and smoking cessation programs, the provision of physical fitness facilities, and media communication have been used in schools, work sites, and community centers. Finally, societal-type interventions involving media and policy actions can occur at the community, state, or federal level. Seat belt laws, public service announcements about drunk driving, and taxation of cigarettes are examples of interventions at this level.

A recent concern within the field of public health is the impact climate change will have on health. A significant contribution to our understanding of the impact of climate change on health has come from the work of *The Lancet Countdown: Tracking Progress on Health and Climate Change*, an international, multidisciplinary research collaboration between academic institutions and experts across the world. The most recent report from this research collaboration, published in 2018, monitors progress on health and climate change across the domains of climate change impacts, exposures, and vulnerabilities; adaptation, planning, and resilience for health; mitigation actions and health co-benefits; finance and economics; and public and political engagement.

Widespread social disorganization and the growing disparity in income within and between nations also pose a global threat to public health. There is a strong association between socioeconomic status and health. This rise in income inequality has coincided with broadening inequalities in health and longevity. Poor people not only have lower incomes, they increasingly have shorter lives than do higher-income individuals.

Because public health is a global matter that is closely tied to international policies, hope for future improvements in public health will largely depend on global improvements in public policy.

Cross-References

▶ Cancer Prevention
▶ Cardiovascular Disease Prevention
▶ Cardiovascular Risk Factors
▶ Centers for Disease Control and Prevention
▶ HIV Prevention
▶ Multiple Risk Factors
▶ Prevention: Primary, Secondary, Tertiary
▶ Smoking Prevention Policies and Programs

References and Further Reading

Bor, J., Cohen, G. H., & Galea, S. (2017). Population health in an era of rising income inequality: USA, 1980–2015. *Lancet, 389*, 1475–1490. https://doi.org/10.1016/S0140-6736(17)30571-8.

Centers for Disease Control and Prevention. (1999). Achievements in public health, 1900–1999; Changes in the public health system. *Morbidity and Mortality Weekly Report, 48*, 1141–1147.

Institute of Medicine. (2001a). *Health and behaviour: The interplay of biological, behavioural and societal influences*. Washington, DC: National Academy Press.

Institute of Medicine. (2001b). *New horizons in health: An integrative approach*. Washington, DC: National Academy Press.

Kawachi, I. (1999). Social capital and community effects on population and individual health. *Annals of the New York Academy of Sciences, 896*, 120–130.

Posner, S. F. (2012). Advancing and improving preventing chronic disease: Public health research, practice and policy. *Preventing Chronic Disease, 9*, 110291. https://doi.org/10.5888/pcd9.110291.

Schneider, M. J. (2011). *Introduction to public health* (2nd ed.). Boston: Jones & Bartlett Learning.

Smedley, B. D., & Syme, S. L. (2000). *Promoting health: Intervention strategies from social and behavioral research*. Washington, DC: National Academy Press.

Turnock, B. J. (2012). *Essentials of public health* (2nd ed.). Boston: Jones & Bartlett Learning.

Watts, N., Adger, W. N., Ayeb-Karlsson, S., et al. (2016). The Lancet Countdown: Tracking progress on health and climate change. *Lancet, 389*, 1151–1164. https://doi.org/10.1016/S0140-6736(16)32124-9.

Watts, N., Amann, M., Arnell, N., et al. (2018). The 2018 report of the Lancet Countdown on health and climate change: Shaping the health of nations for centuries to come. *Lancet., 392*, 2479–2514. https://doi.org/10.1016/S0140-6736(18)32594-7.

World Health Organization. (2000). *The world health report 2000: Executive summary*. Geneva: World Health Organization.

Public Health Education

▶ MPH (Masters of Public Health)

Public Interest Advertising

▶ Social Marketing

Public Service Advertising

▶ Social Marketing

Puff Topography

▶ Smoking Topography

Pulmonary Disorders, COPD: Psychosocial Aspects

Akihisa Mitani
Department of Respiratory Medicine, The University of Tokyo Hospital, Tokyo, Japan

Synonyms

Chronic obstructive pulmonary disease

Definition

Patients with COPD often suffer from anxiety and depression. These psychological distresses cause low quality of life, social isolation, increased hospitalization rates, and might increase mortality. Treatments include pharmacotherapy, psychotherapy, and pulmonary rehabilitation.

Description

Patients pulmonary disorders are more likely to be of lower self-esteem and downgrade the significance of life in their depression, and chronic obstructive pulmonary disease (COPD) is no exception. However, in spite of the high prevalence of the disease, psychosocial aspects of COPD and other pulmonary diseases have not been fully investigated, compared to cancers or cardiovascular diseases (Hill and Geist 2008; Hynninen and Breitve 2005; Kaptein and Scharloo 2008; Kaptein and Scharloo 2009; Maurer and Rebbapragada 2008; von Leupoldt and Dahme 2007).

(COPD) is a disease characterized by airflow obstruction. The respiratory symptoms are dyspnea, chronic cough, and sputum production. The treatments of COPD include medications focusing on bronchodilators, pulmonary rehabilitation, and oxygen administration.

Psychiatric disorders often appear in patients with COPD. Among them, anxiety and depression are most frequent, but the accurate prevalence is hard to say. In previous reports, the prevalence of anxiety ranges between 10% and 100% and the prevalence of depression, between 10% and 80%. However, it is an indisputable fact that anxiety and depression are often underdiagnosed and/or undertreated. Other disorders include panic disorder, hypochondriasis, and hysteria.

Variables, such as physical disability, smoking, long-term oxygen therapy (LTOT), low body mass index, and severe dyspnea, are associated with anxiety and depression.

As for anxiety, major presumed underlying mechanisms are smoking and dyspnea. Smoking is the most important environmental risk factor for the development of COPD. Adolescents with high levels of anxiety tend to have smoking habits, and smokers with a history of an anxiety-related disorder also experience more symptoms of nicotine withdrawal on cessation of smoking, resulting in tendency to nicotine addiction. Therefore, patients with COPD caused by smoking are likely to show higher levels of anxiety than the general population. Dyspnea is the most common symptom of COPD. The severity of dyspnea changes in response to air temperature or exercise and notably increases during acute exacerbations. For the patients, such episodes of increased dyspnea during exacerbations are associated with anxious feelings, although dyspnea at rest or on exertion does not correlate so much with anxiety. Furthermore, anxiety, in turn, increases the sensation of dyspnea. These bidirectional relationships between dyspnea and anxiety contribute to the increased prevalence of anxiety-related disorders in COPD (Kaptein and Scharloo 2008).

Depression in COPD could be caused by various factors such as low body mass index. However, some of them are confounders, making the analysis difficult. The lack of social support for elderly people, their past medical history, and their low socioeconomic status are mixed as risk factors for depression. The use of systemic corticosteroids for treatment, although the long-term use of it is not a standard medication, might cause depression. In addition, there is a relationship between smoking and depression, but little is known about it. Cigarette smoking might prompt a feeling of relaxation for some patients, and smoking cessation could be associated with an increased rate of depression. Chronic hypoxemia and LTOT are also closely related to symptoms of depression, although the underlying mechanisms remain unclear. It is true that LTOT improves survival and exercise capacity, but it may, at the same time, reduce social interactions because the use of oxygen therapy makes the patients lose in several areas of their lives.

Psychological stress typically plays a considerable role in the life of COPD patients because of the interaction of somatic and psychological factors. The emotional response to chronic pulmonary disorders results in further inactivity and social isolation. The patient may feel useless and lose interest in future project. In addition, COPD patients with psychological disorder tend to feel fatigue and short of breath more than patients without such a distress, although psychological distress has not been proved to worsen objective measures of functional exercise capacity. Inadequate perception of dyspnea contributes to a progressive avoidance of activities, resulting in a vicious circle where a physical deconditioning leads to more dyspnea.

As a result, anxiety in COPD patients lowers quality of life and increases hospitalization rates and the economic burden. Intensities of anxiety are correlated with measures of social isolation, suggesting that COPD patients with anxiety have impaired social interactions. The impact of anxiety on the physical disability and mortality of COPD patients is less clear. Depression also causes low quality of life, decreased adherence to treatment, increased frequency of hospital admissions, and prolonged length of stay, resulting in higher medical cost. In addition, depression negatively affects physical function in COPD patients, and the mortality rate among depressed patients is increased. Furthermore, depressed patients tend to make a preference for "do not resuscitate" decisions.

Treatments of psychological distress in COPD patients consist of pharmacotherapy, psychotherapy, and pulmonary rehabilitation.

In pharmacological therapy, antidepressants are commonly used, although evidence for their use in COPD patients is inadequate. Still, they might benefit COPD patients with symptom of anxiety and depression. Selective serotonin reuptake inhibitors (SSRIs) are regarded as first-line therapy. Tricyclic antidepressants and low-dose benzodiazepines could be effective. Administration of benzodiazepines to COPD patients with hypercapnia demands extreme caution because of their respiratory depressant effect; needless to add, each drug has its own side effects and must be used carefully.

Many psychological aspects are relevant to a variety of treatments of COPD. One of the most recent focuses within behavioral treatment on COPD is on self-management. Self-management education is likely to be associated with a reduction in hospital admissions without any detrimental effects in other parameters. Other methods, such as relaxation and biofeedback training, also might have some good effect, although many questions are still not answered.

COPD patients with respiratory symptom should receive comprehensive pulmonary rehabilitation with or without psychological distress. There is growing evidence that it does improve depressive symptoms. However, there remain some questions to be solved. Further research should focus on finding effective and acceptable maintenance strategies. It also remains to be solved whether pulmonary rehabilitation is as effective in COPD patients with severe anxiety and depression. Above all, it is not clear which elements confer psychosocial benefits for COPD patients. Only improvements in exercise capacity may be associated with improvements in anxiety and depression, or it would be better to add a specific psychological component to pulmonary rehabilitation. At present, it is considered reasonable that a comprehensive pulmonary rehabilitation programs should include at least disease education or psychosocial components as the most effective formats.

Cross-References

▶ Chronic Obstructive Pulmonary Disease

References and Readings

Hill, K., & Geist, R. (2008). Anxiety and depression in end-stage COPD. *European Respiratory Journal, 31*(3), 667.

Hynninen, K. M., & Breitve, M. H. (2005). Psychological characteristics of patients with chronic obstructive pulmonary disease: A review. *Journal of Psychosomatic Research, 59*(6), 429.

Kaptein, A. A., & Scharloo, M. (2008). Illness perceptions and COPD: An emerging field for COPD patient management. *The Journal of Asthma, 45*(8), 625.

Kaptein, A. A., & Scharloo, M. (2009). 50 years of psychological research on patients with COPD–road to ruin or highway to heaven? *Respiratory Medicine, 103*(1), 3.

Maurer, J., & Rebbapragada, V. (2008). Anxiety and depression in COPD: Current understanding, unanswered questions, and research needs. *Chest, 134* (Suppl. 4), 43S.

von Leupoldt, A., & Dahme, B. (2007). Psychological aspects in the perception of dyspnea in obstructive pulmonary diseases. *Respiratory Medicine, 101*(3), 411.

Pulmonary Function

Valerie Sabol
School of Nursing, Duke University, Durham, NC, USA

Synonyms

Lung function

Definition

Pulmonary function testing (PFT) is a process for assessing functional status of the lungs, for screening obstructive and restrictive lung disease, and for evaluating treatment response (e.g., medications, chest physical therapy). Spirometry, using a spirometer, is the most common of the pulmonary function tests and measures the amount (volume) and the speed (flow) of air that can be inhaled and exhaled. It is designed to measure changes in lung volume and can only measure lung volume compartments that exchange gas with the atmosphere.

In preparation for PFT, bronchodilator medications are typically held so that bronchodilator response can be assessed after baseline spirometry. For example, short-acting inhaled bronchodilators should not be used for 4 h prior to testing; long-acting beta-agonist bronchodilators are typically held for 12 h prior to testing. Notably, the spirometry procedure is highly dependent on individual effort and cooperation and, to ensure reproducibility, is generally repeated three times.

The spirometry procedure measures the volume of air exhaled at specific time points (0.5, 1.0, 2.0, and 3.0 s) during a forceful and complete exhalation after a maximal inhalation. The total exhaled volume, known as the forced vital capacity (FVC), the volume exhaled in the first second, known as the forced expiratory volume in one second (FEV_1), and their ratio (FEV_1/FVC). The results are usually given in both raw data (liters per second) and percent predicted (i.e., the test result as a percent of the predicted values for the patients of similar characteristics). The FEV$_1$/FVC ratio is important for distinguishing obstructive airway disease and restrictive disease; a reduced ratio suggests obstructive airway disease. A reduced FVC in combination with a normal or increased ratio suggests restrictive disease (if accompanied by reduced lung volumes). Accordingly, spirometry is a key diagnostic test for asthma and chronic obstructive pulmonary disease (COPD) (when performed before and after bronchodilator) and is useful to assess for causes of airflow obstruction. It is also used to monitor management of a broad spectrum of respiratory and neuromuscular diseases (that affect respiratory muscles).

As a person ages, the natural elasticity of the lungs decreases, and this translates into smaller lung volumes and capacities. Males typically have a larger lung volume and capacity than females. Subsequently, PFT interpretation should be based on results of a normal person of the same age and gender. Body height and size also have an impact on PFT results. As an individual ages, their body mass may increase as the body fat to lean body mass ratio changes. For example, if an individual becomes overweight/obese, the abdominal mass limits diaphragm movement, and the PFT observed (measured) results will be less than predicted (from preestablished data tables of individuals with a normal body mass index). Ethnicity may also impact PFT results, and interpretation of observed data should be compared to data of similar ethnic groups.

Cross-References

▶ Bronchitis
▶ Chronic Obstructive Pulmonary Disease
▶ Emphysema
▶ Lung Function

References and Further Reading

Culver, B. H., Graham, B. L., Coates, A. L., Wanger, J., Berry, C. E., Clarke, P. K., Hallstrand, T. S., Hankinson, J. L., Kaminsky, D. A., MacIntyre, N. R., McCormack, M. C., Rosenfeld, M., Stanojevic, S., & Weiner, D. J. (2017). ATS Committee on proficiency standards for pulmonary function laboratories. Recommendations for a standardized pulmonary function report. An official American Thoracic Society technical statement. *American Journal of Respiratory and Critical Care Medicine, 196*(11), 1463.

Holland, A. E., Spruit, M. A., Troosters, T., Puhan, M. A., Pepin, V., Saey, D., McCormack, M. C., Carlin, B. W., Sciurba, F. C., Pitta, F., Wanger, J., MacIntyre, N., Kaminsky, D. A., Culver, B. H., Revill, S. M., Hernandes, N. A., Andrianopoulos, V., Camillo, C. A., Mitchell, K. E., Lee, A. L., Hill, C. J., & Singh, S. J. (2014). An official European Respiratory Society/American Thoracic Society technical standard: Field walking tests in chronic respiratory disease. *The European Respiratory Journal, 44*(6), 1428–1446.

Pellegrino, R., Viegi, G., Brusasco, V., Crapo, R. O., Burgos, F., Casaburi, R., Coates, A., van der Grinten, C. P., Gustafsson, P., Hankinson, J., Jensen, R., Johnson, D. C., MacIntyre, N., McKay, R., Miller, M. R., Navajas, D., Pedersen, O. F., & Wanger, J. (2005). Interpretative strategies for lung function tests. *The European Respiratory Journal, 26*(5), 948.

Pulse Rate

▶ Heart Rate

Purpose

▶ Meaning (Purpose)

Q

qEEG

▶ Quantitative EEG Including the Five Common Bandwidths (Delta, Theta, Alpha, Sigma, and Beta)

QTL

▶ Quantitative Trait Locus (QTL)

Qualitative Research Methods

J. Rick Turner
Campbell University College of Pharmacy and Health Sciences, Buies Creek, NC, USA

Definition

Qualitative research methods collect and analyze qualitative data, which are often expressed in words rather than numbers. Qualitative data can be distinguished from quantitative data, which are expressed in numbers (e.g., a systolic blood pressure of 120 mm of mercury [mmHg]).

One example of a qualitative characteristic is skin coloration (at least as traditionally described). While normal skin colors vary from pinkish white to black, medical conditions and diseases can cause alterations of an individual's skin color. Anemia can lead to a white color (in those not normally so white). Various inflammations can lead to a red color (e.g., a severe rash), and cyanosis resulting from cardiac failure or lung failure leads to a blue color. Such assessments are not recorded and reported in numbers but in descriptive text.

Some researchers regard categorical data as qualitative data, even though numerical representations do occur when presenting the data. Consider the variables sex and blood group. Each of us falls into a mutually exclusive category for each one, e.g., male or female, and O, A, B, and AB. None of us falls into more than one category in each case. Additionally, there is no order to the categories: blood group B neither comes before or after blood group O. In a group of individuals of interest, data could be presented as counts of the number of individuals falling into each category in each case, thereby using numbers.

There are categories that can be ordered. For example, ordered categories of a pain that is experienced would be mild, moderate, and severe. Again, for a group of individuals of interest (perhaps subjects undergoing mindful meditation therapy or another behavioral intervention for pain), it is possible to describe how many individuals reported a pain falling in each of the categories.

© Springer Nature Switzerland AG 2020
M. D. Gellman (ed.), *Encyclopedia of Behavioral Medicine*,
https://doi.org/10.1007/978-3-030-39903-0

Cross-References

► Data

References and Further Reading

Piantadosi, S. (2005). *Clinical trials: A methodologic perspective* (2nd ed.). Hoboken: Wiley-Interscience.

Quality of Life

Maartje de Wit and Tibor Hajos
Medical Psychology, VU University Medical Center, Amsterdam, North Holland, The Netherlands

Synonyms

Health-related quality of life

Definition

Quality of life (QoL) is a term used to refer to an individual's total well-being. There is disagreement between scientists, sociologists, and clinicians about the conceptualization of QoL, and hence, a clear definition is lacking (Hunt 1997). However, current definitions can be categorized into three types (Farquhar 1995): (1) global definitions, such as happiness/unhappiness; (2) definitions that break down QoL into a series of components or dimensions; and (3) focused definitions, which are often pragmatic approaches in which QoL is seen as synonymous with domains of the field of interest to the researchers (e.g., functional status is sometimes used as a measure of QoL by health researchers).

The first type of definitions has been researched since Aristotle, and still no consensus has been reached on how to define happiness and how to measure it (Fayers und Machin 2000). The second and third types of definitions have underlying assumptions for which consensus exists about the domains encompassed by QoL. These latter two types of definitions provide a more practical approach for research purposes.

Across all definitions, considerable agreement exists that QoL is conceptualized as a multidimensional construct incorporating primarily the person's evaluation of his/her own life. The World Health Organization (WHO) defines QoL as the individuals' perception of their position in life in the context of the culture and value systems in which they live and in relation to their goals, expectations, standards, and concerns. It is a broad-ranging concept affected in a complex way by the person's physical health, psychological state, level of independence, social relationships, personal beliefs, and their relationship to salient features of their environment (World Health Organization 1995).

The impact of health and illness on a person's QoL is referred to as health-related quality of life (HRQoL). QoL and HRQoL are often used interchangeably.

Cross-References

► Health-Related Quality of Life
► Multiple Sclerosis: Psychosocial Factors
► Quality of Life: Measurement

References and Readings

Farquhar, M. (1995). Definitions of quality of life: A taxonomy. *Journal of Advanced Nursing, 22*(3), 502–508.
Fayers, P., & Machin, D. (2000). *Quality of life assessment, analysis and interpretation*. Chichester: Wiley.
Hunt, S. M. (1997). The problem of quality of life. *Quality of Life Research, 6*(3), 205–212.
World Health Organization. (1995). The World Health Organization Quality of Life assessment (WHOQOL): Position paper from the World Health Organization. *Social Science and Medicine, 41*(10), 1403–1409.

Quality of Life Assessments

► Measures of Quality of Life

Quality of Life Instruments

▶ Measures of Quality of Life

Quality of Life Technologies

Katarzyna Wac
University of Copenhagen, Copenhagen, Denmark
QoL Lab, University of Geneva, Geneva, Switzerland

Synonyms

Health informatics; Health information systems; Pervasive health; Well-being technologies

Definition

Quality of Life Technologies (QoLT) refers to any technologies for assessment or improvement of the individual's QoL. QoLT leverage an increasing availability of miniaturized computing, storage, and communication sensor- and actuator-based, context-rich technologies that can be embedded within various personal devices, for example, smartphones and wearables. QoLT can rely on hardware technologies (i.e., devices or physical interaction elements) or software technologies (e.g., apps or web-based interfaces) or, most likely, a combination of both. QoLT on an increasing scale are personalizable to satisfy the intended needs of the user anywhere and anytime and can be used in a continuous and longitudinal yet minimally intrusive way, in the individual's daily life (Wac 2018). QoLT may interact with the user via visual, auditory, haptic, or olfactory interfaces. QoLT is usually always connected to the Internet via a wired (for stationary QoLT) or, on a growing scale, wireless technologies (e.g., WiFi, 4G), supporting its user's daily life mobility. QoLT designers and developers are continuously researching ways of understanding the appropriateness of the technology for its use and factors influencing their users' acceptance. QoLT ideally shall be evidence-based. However, many emerging technologies still lack evidence for their effectiveness and efficacy, especially in their early development stage.

Concerning the aims of QoLT, it may provide for the individual (Schulz et al. 2012):

(a) An objective, quantitative, embedded assessment of his/her QoL. Currently, QoL is assessed in individuals infrequently while relying on memory-based, context-poor approaches. These approaches are leveraging subjective self-reports via validated instruments to gather an individual's responses referred to as Patient-Reported Outcomes (PROs). The QoLT, as defined here, does not include ePROs, i.e., technologies for an assessment of PROs via electronic means, like a web or a mobile app (Jensen et al. 2015). For example, QoLT does not include a subjective assessment of physical activity via web-based self-report called IPAQ (Hagströmer et al. 2006).
(b) Maintenance or prevention of his/her QoL decline.
(c) Enhancement of his/her QoL.
(d) Compensation for his/her QoL loss.

The above-defined aims of QoLT may be redefined further. Namely, either QoLT focuses on enabling the specific external observable behaviors, e.g., physical activity, that contribute to the individual's QoL or it focuses on the assessment of the behaviors that are a result of the individual's QoL state. Therefore, given an example of physical activity in the context of the four aims (a–d), QoLT may:

(a) Enable an objective assessment of the individual QoL, e.g., an objective assessment of external observable physical activity via wearable actigraphy technologies or mobile apps embedded within a smartphone
(b) Enable physical activity maintenance or improvement toward predefined, evidence-based goals

(c) Enhance physical activity toward its optimization for athletes
(d) Enable physical activity via prosthetic limb or an exoskeleton

Concerning the types of QoLT users, a specific QoLT can be used (Chatterton and Wilson 2014):

(i) At the individual level
(ii) By an individual at the interpersonal, peer-to-peer level
(iii) At the community level
(iv) At the segment/group level
(v) At the population level, across socioeconomic, cultural, and environmental conditions

An example of wearable actigraphy technologies or mobile apps embedded within a smartphone for physical activity assessment can be applied at all levels (i–v): for an individual physical activity assessment, peer-based assessment, geographical community-based, a segment of the population, or whole population-based assessment of their physical activity.

Cross-References

▶ Patient-Reported Outcome
▶ Quality of Life
▶ Well-being

References and Further Reading

Chatterton, T., & Wilson, C. (2014). The '"Four Dimensions of Behaviour" framework: A tool for characterising behaviours to help design better interventions. *Transportation Planning and Technology, 37*(1), 38–61.
de Wit, M., & Hajos, T. (2013). Quality of life. In M. D. Gellman & J. R. Turner (Eds.), *Encyclopedia of behavioral medicine*. New York: Springer.
Hagströmer, M., Oja, P., & Sjöström, M. (2006). The International Physical Activity Questionnaire (IPAQ): A study of concurrent and construct validity. *Public Health Nutrition, 9*(6), 755–762.
Jensen, R. E., Rothrock, N. E., DeWitt, E. M., Spiegel, B., Tucker, C. A., Crane, H. M., ... Cella, D. (2015). The role of technical advances in the adoption and integration of patient-reported outcomes in clinical care. *Medical Care, 53*(2), 153.
Schulz, R., Beach, S. R., Matthews, J. T., Courtney, K. L., & Dabbs, A. J. D. V. (2012). Designing and evaluating quality of life technologies: An interdisciplinary approach. *Proceedings of the IEEE, 100*(8), 2397–2409.
Wac, K. (2018). From quantified self to quality of life. In *Digital health* (Health informatics). Dordrecht: Springer.
Wac, K., Fiordelli, M., Gustarini, M., & Rivas, H. (2015). Quality of life technologies: Experiences from the field and key research challenges. IEEE Internet Computing (IEEE IC), special issue on Personalized Digital Health, July 2015.
Wac, K., Rivas, H., & Fiordelli, M. (2017). *Guest editorial: Quality of life technologies*, special issue: IEEE Computer, March 2017.
WHO Working Group. (1998). The World Health Organization quality of life assessment (WHOQOL): Development and general psychometric properties. *Social Science & Medicine, 46*(12), 1569–1585.

Quality of Life: Measurement

Maartje de Wit
Medical Psychology, VU University Medical Center, Amsterdam, North Holland, The Netherlands

Definition

Subjective assessment of the various aspects of quality of life.

Description

Quality of Life (QoL) is considered an important outcome variable in health-care practice and research. Consideration of QoL provides health-care providers, researchers, and policy makers insight into how variables of interest (e.g., chronic disease, medication use, living environment) impact a person's subjective well-being, which is instrumental to improving health-care practice systems.

QoL measures may be of potential value in comparing outcomes in clinical trials, evaluating interventions, commissioning programs of care, assessing the outcomes of new treatments, and in audit work. Further on, measuring health-related QoL (HRQoL) can facilitate discussion between patients and professionals in health care and stimulate the dialogue between medical outcomes and patients' subjective views (de Wit et al. 2008; Detmar et al. 2002; Pouwer et al. 2001).

Measurement of QoL

Despite a clear definition of QoL, there is general agreement that health-related QoL (HRQoL) encompasses physical, cognitive, affective, psychological, social well-being, health perception, and disease- and treatment-related symptoms. Overall QoL expands upon this and incorporates non-medical-related aspects of a person's life such as the influence of work, spirituality, and other life circumstances (Koot 2001).

QoL can include both objective and subjective perspectives in each domain (Testa and Simonson 1996). The objective assessment of QoL focuses on what the individual can do, and is important in defining the degree of health. The subjective assessment of QoL includes the meaning to the individual; essentially it involves the translation or appraisal of the more objective measurement of health status into the experience of QoL. Differences in appraisal account for the fact that individuals with the same objective health status can report very different subjective QoL (Fayers and Machin 2000).

Generic and Disease Specific Instruments

There are a wide variety of instruments available to obtain information on QoL. These instruments can be divided into generic and disease-specific instruments. Generic measures attempt to measure all important domains of QoL. Generic measures are most useful when comparisons or decisions have to be made for large groups of patients with disparate conditions and backgrounds (Fayers and Machin 2000). For example, it gives the opportunity to compare the QoL of people with diabetes with their healthy peers or to people with asthma.

Disease-specific measures include domains that are designed to be valid only for a specified condition. Therefore they maximize content validity and support greater sensitivity and specificity (Guyatt et al. 1993), and may be particularly informative for disease management at the individual patient level. Advances in the development of QoL questionnaires for children resulted in generic questionnaires with complementary disease-specific modules (Bullinger 2005; Ravens-Sieberer et al. 2008; Varni et al. 1999, 2005). This measurement approach enables researchers and professionals to compare children with a specific disease to their healthy peers and also examine the impact of the disease at the same time.

QoL Measurement in Children

The development and validation of instruments for children have evolved over the past 30 years. Traditionally, parents have been the ones reporting on their child's HRQoL, because the child was seen as an unreliable respondent. When the child is very young or ill, the child may indeed be unable to complete questionnaires. However, relying on the parent as informant may result in incomplete assessment to the extent that the child's subjective experience and perceptions of HRQoL may be overlooked (Eiser and Morse 2001a). Especially as the child grows older and develops his/her own life, the HRQoL reports of parents become less informative. It has been shown that parents and children agree more on objective domains of HRQoL (i.e., physical functioning) than on subjective domains, like emotional and social functioning (Eiser and Morse 2001a; Janse et al. 2008).

As children and parents do not necessarily share similar views about the impact of illness, children are more directly involved in decisions about their own care and treatment as they mature. However, assessment of QoL in children poses unique problems (Eiser and Morse 2001a). Children do not share adult views about the cause, aetiology, and treatment of illness. They may interpret questions differently, and adopt a different time perspective. In addition, their abilitiy to use rating scales, understand the language, and generally complete lengthy questionnaires of the type used in adult work, may be compromised by age and cognitive development. These considerations have guided the development of QoL questionnaires especially for children (Eiser and Morse 2001a; Solans et al. 2008).

Choosing an Instrument

Because of the broad, multidimensional nature of QoL, it is advised that researchers who want to measure QoL define what they mean by "quality of life," or explain which domains of quality of life they want to measure using a specific instrument. For example, the terms "health-related QoL" (HRQoL), "functional status," and "health status" are often used interchangeably. However, although health or functional status can be part of HRQoL, it does not take the patient's perspective into account.

The Patient-Reported Outcome and Quality Of Life Instrument Database (PROQOLID) (www.proqolid.org, Mapi Research Institute 2001–2011) provides an outline of available instruments to measure patient-reported outcomes or QoL. It should be noted, however, that identification of an instrument in this database does not necessarily mean it is valid and reliable in view of the question at hand. Thus, instruments should be selected with care (Bradley 2001; Eiser and Morse 2001b; Fayers and Machin 2000; Koot and Wallander 2001; Solans et al. 2008).

Cross-References

▶ Health-Related Quality of Life
▶ Quality of Life

References and Readings

Bradley, C. (2001). *Handbook of psychology and diabetes*. Amsterdam: Harwood Academic.
Bullinger, M. (2005). *Translations DISABKIDS*. Retrieved February, 2006, from http://kidscreen.diehauptstadt.de/disabkids/master/translations/index.html
de Wit, M., Delemarre-van de Waal, H. A., Bokma, J. A., Haasnoot, K., Houdijk, M. C., Gemke, R. J., et al. (2008). Monitoring and discussing health-related quality of life in adolescents with type 1 diabetes improve psychosocial well-being: A randomized controlled trial. *Diabetes Care, 31*(8), 1521–1526.
Detmar, S. B., Muller, M. J., Schornagel, J. H., Wever, L. D., & Aaronson, N. K. (2002). Health-related quality-of-life assessments and patient-physician communication: A randomized controlled trial. *Journal of the American Medical Association, 288*(23), 3027–3034.
Eiser, C., & Morse, R. (2001a). Can parents rate their child's health-related quality of life? Results of a systematic review. *Quality of Life Research, 10*(4), 347–357.
Eiser, C., & Morse, R. (2001b). A review of measures of quality of life for children with chronic illness. *Archives of Disease in Childhood, 84*(3), 205–211.
Fayers, P., & Machin, D. (2000). *Quality of life. Assessment, analysis and interpretation*. Chichester: Wiley.
Guyatt, G. H., Feeny, D. H., & Patrick, D. L. (1993). Measuring health-related quality of life. *Annals of Internal Medicine, 118*(8), 622–629.
Janse, A. J., Sinnema, G., Uiterwaal, C. S., Kimpen, J. L., & Gemke, R. J. (2008). Quality of life in chronic illness: Children, parents and paediatricians have different, but stable perceptions. *Acta Paediatrica, 97*, 1118–1124.
Koot, H. M. (2001). The study of quality of life: Concepts and methods. In J. L. Wallander & H. M. Koot (Eds.), *Quality of life in child and adolescent illness. Concepts, methods and findings* (pp. 3–17). East Sussex: Brunner-Routledge.
Koot, H. M., & Wallander, J. L. (2001). Challenges in child and adolescent quality of life research. In H. M. Koot & J. L. Wallander (Eds.), *Quality of life in child and adolescent illness. Concepts, methods and findings* (pp. 431–456). East Sussex: Brunner-Routledge.
Mapi Research Institute. (2001–2011). *PROQOLID*. Retrieved January 25, 2011, from www.proqolid.org
Pouwer, F., Snoek, F. J., van der Ploeg, H. M., Ader, H. J., & Heine, R. J. (2001). Monitoring of psychological well-being in outpatients with diabetes: Effects on mood, HbA(1c), and the patient's evaluation of the quality of diabetes care: A randomized controlled trial. *Diabetes Care, 24*(11), 1929–1935.
Ravens-Sieberer, U., Gosch, A., Rajmil, L., Erhart, M., Bruil, J., Power, M., et al. (2008). The KIDSCREEN-52 quality of life measure for children and adolescents: Psychometric results from a cross-cultural survey in 13 European countries. *Value in Health, 11*(4), 645–658.
Solans, M., Pane, S., Estrada, M.-D., Serra-Sutton, V., Berra, S., Herdman, M., et al. (2008). Health-related quality of life measurement in children and adolescents: A systematic review of generic and disease-specific instruments. *Value in Health, 11*(4), 742–764.
Testa, M. A., & Simonson, D. C. (1996). Assessment of quality-of-life outcomes. *The New England Journal of Medicine, 334*(13), 835–840.
Varni, J. W., Seid, M., & Rode, C. A. (1999). The PedsQL: Measurement model for the pediatric quality of life inventory. *Medical Care, 37*(2), 126–139.

Varni, J. W., Burwinkle, T. M., & Seid, M. (2005). The PedsQL™ as a pediatric patient-reported outcome: Reliability and validity of the PedsQL™ Measurement Model in 25,000 children. *Expert Review of Pharmacoeconomics & Outcomes Research, 5*, 705–719.

Quality of Work

▶ Job Performance

Quality-Adjusted Life Years (QALYs)

M. Bryant Howren
Department of Psychology, The University of Iowa and Iowa City VA Healthcare System, Iowa City, IA, USA

Definition

The *quality-adjusted life year* (QALY) is a standardized measure of disease burden which combines both survival and health-related qualities of life into a single index. The QALY is primarily used in cost-effectiveness analyses to guide decisions regarding the distribution of limited healthcare resources among competing health programs or interventions for a population of interest but has also been used to aid decisions regarding clinical management and individual patient care.

Conceptually based in expected utility theory, the QALY rests on the assumption that preference-weighted values may be attached to specific health states relative to the time spent in those states. Because the QALY incorporates both quantity and quality of life, it therefore provides a reasonable estimate of the amount of quality time (i.e., health benefit) an individual may experience as a result of a particular health program or intervention. Furthermore, comparisons between programs or interventions may be made both within a single disease and across different diseases. Consequently, the QALY has been widely used as an outcome measure in medicine, psychology, public health, and economics.

Calculation of the QALY requires various health states be assigned a value ranging from zero to one, with zero representing death and one representing ideal health. Health states considered worse than death (i.e., a health state valuation less than zero) can also exist and are assigned a negative value. In order to determine the values of each particular health state, respondents are asked to rate them relative to one another or using an anchor point such as death. Several methods may be used to ascertain valuations, including preference measurement techniques such as the standard gamble or time trade-off, or through the use of rating scales, such as the EQ-5D, Health Utilities Index, Quality of Well-Being Scale, and SF-6D.

A number of limitations have been described with respect to the measurement and incorporation of QALYs. In particular, QALYs may be less useful in the context of preventive health programs (i.e., when health effects may not materialize for some time), or chronic diseases (i.e., where quality of life may be more important than survival). Other concerns include inconsistencies among valuations due to method variance, situations in which population-level preferences about a particular disease differ from preferences of the subgroup afflicted with the disease and, more generally, decisions regarding whose preferences should matter most when assigning values to specific health states. These limitations notwithstanding, the QALY serves as a straightforward, intuitive measure of disease burden and remains an important tool in healthcare decision-making.

Cross-References

▶ Benefit Evaluation in Health Economic Studies
▶ Clinical Decision-Making
▶ Health-Related Quality of Life

References and Further Readings

Drummond, M. F., Sculpher, M. J., Torrance, G. W., O'Brien, B. J., & Stoddart, G. L. (2005). *Methods for the economic evaluation of health care programmes*. Oxford: Oxford University Press.

Gold, M. R., Stevenson, D., & Fryback, D. G. (2002). HALYs and QALYs and DALYs, oh my: Similarities and differences in summary measures of population health. *Annual Review of Public Health, 23*, 115–134.

Kaplan, R. M., & Frosch, D. L. (2005). Decision making in medicine and health care. *Annual Review of Clinical Psychology, 1*, 525–556.

Kaplan, R. M., & Groessl, E. J. (2002). Applications of cost-effectiveness methodologies in behavioral medicine. *Journal of Consulting & Clinical Psychology, 70*, 482–493.

Kind, P., Lafata, J. E., Matuszewski, K., & Raisch, D. (2009). The use of QALYs in clinical and patient decision-making: Issues and prospects. *Value in Health, 12*, S27–S30.

Nord, E. (1999). *Cost-value analysis in health care: Making sense out of QALYs*. New York: Cambridge University Press.

Weinstein, M. C., Torrance, G., & McGuire, A. (2009). QALYs: The basics. *Value in Health, 12*, S5–S9.

Quantified Self

Melanie Swan
Philosophy Department, Purdue University, West Lafayette, IN, USA

Synonyms

Health self-management; Lifelogging; $n = 1$ science; Personal data analytics; Self-experimentation; Self-tracking

Definition

The Quantified Self is a social health movement that began in San Francisco, California, in 2007, led by Gary Wolf and Kevin Kelly from Wired magazine. The *Quantified Self* is an individual engaged in the self-tracking of any kind of biological, physical, behavioral, or environmental data. The attitude is a proactive stance toward obtaining information and acting on it, particularly to solve a problem. A variety of areas may be tracked and analyzed, for example, exercise, weight, energy level, mood, time usage, sleep quality, health, cognitive performance, and learning strategies (Fig. 1). Health is an important but nonexclusive focus, where objectives may include general tracking, pathology resolution, and peak performance. Regarding adoption, the quantified self is a broad phenomenon in the sense that 69% of US adults track a health indicator like weight, diet, exercise routine, or symptom (Fox 2013); and there are 25 million active worldwide Fitbit users (Fitbit 2018). In some sense everyone is already a self-tracker since many individuals measure something about themselves, and since humans have innate curiosity, tinkering, and problem-solving capabilities.

Description

Motivations for Quantified Self-Experimentation

In addition to immediate problem-solving, other motivations for self-tracking include collecting information about phenomena for greater understanding or longitudinal archiving, for example, to record and reference exercise histories on a scale of decades. The assumption is that the personalized informatics data streams that are now available bring visibility and quantification to a situation, such that different interventions might be tested, and problems resolved.

Genesis and Underpinnings

The Quantified Self is a modern phenomenon, emerging at the confluence of data science, wearable computing, and personalized medicine (the patient-centric Health 2.0 movement). The modern algorithmic society is one that tracks and surveils, including individuals that track and surveil themselves (Kelly 2016). This could have tyrannizing and detrimental effects, as in Foucault's panopticon concept, or an impact that is empowering and beneficial, as the Quantified Self movement promulgates. Wolf sees the

Self-Tracking Categories	Self-Tracking Variables
Physical activities	Sleep, exercise, distance (miles, steps), calories, repetitions, sets, heart rate, VO2 max, METs (metabolic equivalents), desk-sitting
Diet	Calories consumed (grams of carbs, fat, protein), ingredients, nutrients, glycemic index, satiety, portions, supplements, tastiness
Psychological states and traits	Health, energy, mood, happiness, irritation, emotions, anxiety, self-esteem, depression, confidence, engagement
Mental and cognitive states and traits	IQ, alertness, focus, attention, reaction, memory, verbal fluency, patience, creativity, reasoning, psychomotor vigilance
Environmental variables	Location, architecture, weather, noise, water, pollution, clutter, light, season, motivation, activity, surroundings
Episodic and situational variables	Context, situation, fulfillment, health status, time of day, day of week
Social variables	Influence, trust, values, role, community, recognition, support

Quantified Self, Fig. 1 Typical quantified self-tracking project categories and variables (Swan 2013, 86)

quantified self phenomenon as self-knowledge through self-tracking with technology (Wolf 2010).

Quantified Self Community and Tools

There is a worldwide Quantified Self Community which comes together in show-and-tell meetups and conferences. The typical format is presenting a self-tracking project and answering three questions in a simplified version of the scientific method: "What did you do?" "How did you do it?" and "What did you learn?" The tools used for quantified self-tracking include Fitbit smart watches, wearables, and apps, although Excel sheets and pen and paper are also not unusual. Data are typically analyzed with traditional techniques such as visualization and linear regression to establish correlations among the variables under investigation.

Quantified Self Research Studies

A study of quantified self-tracking projects found that the main motivation was to resolve or optimize a specific lifestyle issue such as sleep quality (Swan 2012). Another finding was that quantified self-experimenters often iterated through many different solutions, and kinds of solutions, before finding a final resolution point. The biggest area of self-experimentation was sleep quality, and of concern, its link to work productivity. For one individual, raising the bed mattress solved the problem, and for another, tracking and reducing caffeine consumption. Another finding was that there was not much introspection as to experimental results and their meaning, but rather a pragmatic attitude toward having a problem that needed solving. A benefit of self-experimentation projects was that the velocity of question-asking and experimental iteration could be much faster than with traditional methods. Further, it was not uncommon for study participants to forget the initial problem situation, once resolved.

Criticisms

Quantified self-experimentation has drawn critique regarding the scientific soundness of practitioner methods and conclusions. $N = 1$ science has so far not made a general contribution to scientific understanding, and some researchers wonder whether it is wise to conclude anything from $n = 1$ studies. One team points out that drawing additional attention to the self and personalized data may amplify a condition such as depression (Jarrold et al. 2011). Likewise, access to personalized data might increase cyberchondria (internet hypochondria). However, the main tenor of studies investigating the broad use of quantified self-experimentation has documented the overall benefits of self-tracking to life-long health and wellness outcomes, as well as the psychology of empowerment and responsibility-taking for health self-management (Meyer et al. 2014; Swan et al. 2010).

Quantified Self Data Rights and Health Policy

The Quantified Self movement raises important contemporary questions about a person's right to their own biological data, including ownership and monetization of these data, and who may legally interpret the data. Traditionally, there was not a clear business model for quantified self-tracking data; however, new technologies such as blockchain and deep learning could advance the possibility of new business models such as Data Markets. Financial incentives and tools might make it easier for individuals to self-assemble electronic medical records (EMRs) in an app with remunerated privacy-protected computation (blockchain) and medical diagnostic pattern recognition (deep learning). These kinds of Data Markets and quantified self-tracking applications could help link healthcare providers and individuals to realize the Meaningful Use provision regarding patient electronic data. This is part of the US American Reinvestment & Recovery Act of 2009, which includes the "Health Information Technology for Economic and Clinical Health (HITECH) Act" measure.

Quantified Self and the Scientific Method ($n = 1$ Studies)

The Quantified Self movement has made innovative contributions to the traditional scientific method. While not widely used or studied, the self-organized one-person study ($n = 1$ science) has nevertheless provided relevant results to some individuals for health self-management. Quantified self-experiments range in what professionals would gauge as their degree of rigor. One of the more exacting is Rosane Oliveira's multi-year investigation regarding diabetes and heart disease risk, using her identical twin sister as a control, and testing vegan dietary shifts and metabolism markers such as insulin and glucose (Oliveira 2016). Personal responsibility-taking is seen as a key element in health management, which can include an individual's data acquisition, interpretation, and self-experimentation activities. Movements like the Quantified Self could be helpful in the face of public health challenges such as the obesity epidemic.

The scientific method in turn provides quantified self-experimenters with useful tools for self-discovery. Interesting challenges arise regarding traditional features of the scientific method such as the placebo effect and the double-blind study. Self-experimenters have a conundrum in that they may forego any possible benefit of the placebo effect by being knowledgeable about their activity. Quantified self-experimentation might also provide new information about the placebo effect. For example, the individual could create (and measure) a different kind of placebo effect by mixing up the interventions, and remaining ignorant while recording data, until the conclusion of the experiment.

Health Social Networks and Preventive Medicine

The Quantified Self movement is characterized not only by $n = 1$ study but also by group study. Group health research studies could be a potential precursor and supplement to traditional clinical trials, which are expensive and time-consuming to run. The premise of preventive medicine is that conditions may not reach clinical detectability until they are 80% advanced in their lifecycle; however, having quantified self data might help predict and avoid condition onset. Persons engaged in Quantified Self data collection could be extremely helpful to the preventive medicine effort. Health Social Networks (such as Patients Like Me, TuDiabetes Inspire.com, and Facebook groups) are a mechanism for persons with similar conditions to meet and collaborate by joining condition-specific group studies.

Philosophy of Quantified Self and Behavior Change

To the extent that the stakes are improved health and well-being, for either the $n = 1$ Quantified

Self-tracker or the public health industry, quantified self methods could be helpful. The action-oriented component that seems to accompany quantified self data collection could be crucial to behavior change. Personalized data acquisition could be seen as the first step in any process that includes behavior change. The reason is because even merely having information, and being able to see the result of interventions, is an instigating tool that may prompt individuals to consider different courses of action. An analogy is available from the energy industry, in which studies found that having access to tracking data reduced electricity consumption by 10%, and 30% when financial incentives were added (Petersen et al. 2007).

The Quantified Self Becomes the Qualified Self

A salient philosophical aspect of quantified self activity is that it is fundamentally both a quantitative and a qualitative phenomenon. Quantified self-tracking includes both the collection of objective metrics data and the subjective experience of these data. The Quantified Self is becoming the Qualified Self in new ways. The individual body and mind becomes a more knowable, calculable, and administrable object through quantified self activity. Individuals are having an increasingly intimate relationship with data as it mediates the experience of the self and reality. The always-on data climate provides a new and objective fourth-person perspective from which to view the self and the world. The further impact of data-driven health social movements such as the Quantified Self could be having new ways of understanding and configuring human identity.

References and Further Reading

Fitbit. (Press Release, 2018) https://investor.fitbit.com/press/press-releases/press-release-details/2018/Fitbit-Community-Grows-to-More-Than-25-Million-Active-Users-in-2017/default.aspx. Accessed 4 Aug 2018.
Fox, S. (2013). Tracking for health. Pew Internet.
Jarrold, W., Javitz, H. S., Krasnow, R., et al. (2011). Depression and self- focused language in structured interviews with older adults. *Psychological Reports, 109*(2), 686–700.
Kelly, K. (2016). *The inevitable*. New York: Penguin Books.
Meyer, J., Simske, S., Siek, K. A., Gurrin, C. G., & Hermens, H. (2014). Beyond quantified self: Data for wellbeing. In: Proceedings: CHI EA '14 CHI '14 extended abstracts on human factors in computing systems, pp. 95–98.
Oliveira, R. (2016). My story: From vegetarian veterinarian to plant-based spokesperson. UC Davis Integrative Medicine.
Petersen, J. E., Shunturov, V., Janda, K., et al. (2007). Dormitory residents reduce electricity consumption when exposed to real-time visual feedback and incentives. *International Journal of Sustainability in Higher Education, 8*(1), 16–33.
Swan, M. (2012). Health 2050: The realization of personalized medicine through crowdsourcing, the quantified self, and the participatory biocitizen. *Journal of Personalized Medicine, 2*(3), 93–118.
Swan, M. (2013). The quantified self: Fundamental disruption in big data science and biological discovery. *Big Data, 1*(2), 85–99.
Swan, M., Hathaway, K., Hogg, C., McCauley, R., & Vollrath, A. (2010). Citizen science genomics as a model for crowdsourced preventive medicine research. *Journal of Participatory Medicine, 2*, e20.
Wolf, G. (2010). The data-driven life. *New York Times Magazine*.

Quantitative EEG Including the Five Common Bandwidths (Delta, Theta, Alpha, Sigma, and Beta)

Salvatore Insana
Western Psychiatric Institute and Clinic, Pittsburgh, PA, USA

Synonyms

Frequency analysis; Power spectral analysis; qEEG; Spectral analysis

Definition

Quantitative electroencephalography (qEEG) is an analytical technique that can be used to objectively describe the frequency and power of electroencephalography data.

Description

Quantitative electroencephalography (qEEG) can be used in any application where electroencephalography (EEG) is applied. In this entry, qEEG will be described in the context of its application in the measurement of brain activity patterns that can be used to infer sleep. Sleep can be measured with polysomnography (PSG), which is currently considered the "gold standard" measure of sleep-wake states. EEG is an integral component to PSG, along with electrooculography (EOG), and electromyography (EMG). In order to assure standardized PSG measurement procedures, there are uniform practice parameters established by the American Academy of Sleep Medicine (AASM [Iber et al. 2007]). The AASM sleep-monitoring practice parameters include specified criteria for electrode placement, equipment calibration, and PSG acquisition. Once PSG sleep signals (i.e., EEG, EOG, and EMG) are appropriately recorded, the signals can be used together for visual analyses; additionally or alternatively, EEG can be independently used for quantitative analyses.

Visual PSG Analyses: When sleep is measured with PSG, the measured signals are typically sectioned into consecutive 30-s intervals throughout the entire PSG recording period. These 30-s intervals are termed "epochs." Within each epoch, the PSG measured signals (i.e., EEG, EOG, and EMG) are cumulatively used to differentiate sleep from wake, and to further classify sleep into different categories that are known as sleep stages. According to the AASM (Iber et al. 2007), sleep can be classified into four stages that include N1, N2, N3, and Rapid Eye Movement (REM) sleep. Sleep stage scoring is completed by a trained technician who visually interprets the PSG signals in accordance with the aforementioned standard practice parameters. Once visually scored, sleep can be described by variables that include, but not limited to, time spent in particular stages, latency to particular stages, arousals from sleep, and specific physiological events during sleep. Visually scored sleep can be displayed on a hypnogram plot.

Quantitative EEG analyses: When sleep is measured with EEG, the measured signals can be analyzed and described quantitatively by their frequency and power. There are mathematically detailed components to quantitative EEG analysis; these components will be broadly described (see reviews, Campbell 2009; Thakor and Tong 2004). Preliminary processing includes digitization and prefiltering. Typically, EEG signals are digitized at a rate of 256 Hz, are band-limited using a low-frequency and high-frequency filters (e.g., signals ≤ 0.5 and ≥ 64 Hz are removed) to remove irrelevant signals, and are decimated (e.g., halved to 128 Hz) for the analyses. Low-frequency artifacts are removed; for example, epochs that were visually scored as wakefulness or movement artifact could be excluded. High-frequency EEG artifacts are removed; for example, an algorithm can be implemented that excludes a predetermined bin length (e.g., 4 s) if that bin exceeds a predetermined high-frequency threshold relative to the frequency in adjacent bins. Once artifacts are removed, a fast Fourier transformation (FFT) is implemented to analyze wave frequency (in Hertz) within the epochs; that is, epochs are analyzed according to moving windows that partially overlap with preceding and succeeding windows. For example, a 30-s epoch that is analyzed according to a 4-s window can have a 2-s overlap among windows, thus yielding 15 windows for the epoch. Common FFT window functions include Hanning, Hamming, Bartlett, and Welch; these functions differ in duration and window overlap lengths (Campbell 2009; Thakor and Tong 2004). Wave amplitude is sampled in microvolts and is squared to convert the wave amplitude to power; power is calculated within each frequency band, described below.

Power is grouped according to frequency within specific broad bands or frequency ranges. There are five commonly used frequency bands that are examined with spectral analysis. The frequency bands typically fall within the range of 0.5–32 Hz; however, these frequency bands can slightly vary by laboratory and can be further broken down into narrower components as guided by the research or clinical question. The behavioral functions that correspond to each frequency band during sleep have not been clearly elucidated; however, current theories are briefly mentioned. The delta band encompasses the frequency range of 0.5–4 Hz. Delta activity is positively associated with the homeostatic sleep drive in such a manner that delta activity increases in correspondence to increased awake time (Dijk et al. 1990). The theta band encompasses the frequency range of 4–8 Hz. Similar to delta activity, theta activity is positively associated with the homeostatic sleep drive (Dijk et al. 1990). The alpha band encompasses the frequency range of 8–12 Hz. Alpha activity is positively associated with relaxed wakefulness and drowsiness associated with sleep onset (Cantero et al. 2002). Alpha activity is also present during REM sleep and is theorized as being a micro-arousal that can then lead to a full arousal during sleep; the purpose(s) of alpha associated arousals during REM sleep is unknown (Cantero and Atienza 2000). The sigma band encompasses the frequency range of 12–16 Hz. Sigma activity is positively associated with sleep spindles and has been linked to learning, memory, and intelligence (Fogel and Smith 2011; Geiger et al. 2011). The beta band encompasses the frequency range of 16–32 Hz. Beta activity is positively associated with physiological arousal and psychological stress (Hall et al. 2007).

Spectral EEG power within particular bandwidths changes throughout development (Gaudreau et al. 2001). Spectral EEG power is highly variable across individuals, but demonstrates a trait-like "fingerprint" that is stable within individuals across nights (De Gennaro et al. 2005), as well as across both sleep and wake states (Ehlers et al. 1998). Spectral EEG power has been implicated in a wide range of sleep research topics including stress (Hall et al. 2000), intelligence (Geiger et al. 2011), memory (Fogel and Smith 2011), psychopathology (Tekell et al. 2005), and sleep disorders (Buysse et al. 2001; Krystal and Edinger 2010; Perlis et al. 2001).

Spectral power can be calculated for each EEG recording site (e.g., C3/M2, and C4/M1). Total, or absolute, power is the sum of all power frequencies, within each epoch, across all bandwidths analyzed. Relative power is the power per bandwidth divided by total power times 100. Relative power density can be used to describe individual differences in variability because it is standardized by an individual's total power. qEEG calculations are commonly paired with visually scored sleep stages; this pairing can yield power in particular bands during specific sleep stages (e.g., delta power during non-REM sleep [NREM]). Once analyzed, sleep power spectra can be visually displayed on modeled power frequency curves with frequency, in Hertz, on the X-axis and the logarithmic power transformation on the Y-axis. The modeled power frequency curve can represent the entire night, or a specified sleep state such as all NREM sleep, the first NREM sleep bout, all REM sleep, etc.

To date, neither qEEG standardized analyses nor practice parameters have been established; therefore, the qEEG techniques can vary by laboratory (e.g., Vasko et al. 1997). For instance, laboratories use different methods for identifying low- and high-frequency artifacts, choice of window for weighting epochs, definition of frequency broad band ranges, and the specific electrode placement used for analyses (e.g., C3/M2, C4/M1, or average of the two locations). Thus, when reporting qEEG values, a thorough description of the acquisition, processing, and interpretation techniques are of paramount importance.

Cross-References

▶ Non-REM Sleep
▶ Polysomnography
▶ REM Sleep
▶ Sleep
▶ Sleep Architecture

References and Reading

Buysse, D. J., Hall, M., Begley, A., Cherry, C. R., Houck, P. R., Land, S., et al. (2001). Sleep and treatment response in depression: New findings using power spectral analysis. *Psychiatry Research, 103*, 51–67.

Campbell, I. G. (2009). EEG recording and analysis for sleep research. *Current Protocols in Neuroscience, 49*, 10.2.1–10.2.19.

Cantero, J. L., & Atienza, M. (2000). Alpha burst activity during human REM sleep: Descriptive study and functional hypotheses. *Clinical Neurophysiology, 111*, 909–915.

Cantero, J. L., Atienza, M., & Salas, R. M. (2002). Human alpha oscillations in wakefulness, drowsiness period, and REM sleep: Different electroencephalographic phenomena within the alpha band. *Clinical Neurophysiology, 32*, 54–71.

De Gennaro, L., Ferrara, M., Vecchio, F., Curcio, G., & Bertini, M. (2005). An electroencephalographic fingerprint of human sleep. *NeuroImage, 26*, 114–122.

Dijk, D. J., Brunner, D. P., Beersma, D. G., & Borbély, A. A. (1990). Electroencephalogram power density and slow wave sleep as a function of prior waking and circadian phase. *Sleep, 13*, 430–440.

Ehlers, C. L., Kupfer, D. J., Buysse, D. J., Cluss, P. A., Miewald, J. M., Bisson, E. F., & Grochocinski, V. J. (1998). The Pittsburgh study of normal sleep in young adults: Focus on the relationship between waking and sleeping EEG spectral patterns. *Electroencephalography and Clinical Neurophysiology, 106*, 199–205.

Fogel, S. M., & Smith, C. T. (2011). The function of the sleep spindle: A physiological index of intelligence and a mechanism for sleep-dependent memory consolidation. *Neuroscience and Biobehavioral Reviews, 35*, 1154–1165.

Gaudreau, H., Carrier, J., & Montplaisir, J. (2001). Age-related modifications of NREM sleep EEG: From childhood to middle age. *Journal of Sleep Research, 10*, 165–172.

Geiger, A., Huber, R., Kurth, S., Ringli, M., Jenni, O., & Achermann, P. (2011). The sleep EEG as a marker of intellectual ability in school age children. *Sleep, 34*, 181–189.

Hall, M., Buysse, D. J., Nowell, P. D., Nofzinger, E. A., Houck, P., Reynolds, C. F., 3rd, & Kupfer, D. J. (2000). Symptoms of stress and depression as correlates of sleep in primary insomnia. *Psychosomatic Medicine, 62*, 227–230.

Hall, M., Thayer, J. F., Germain, A., Moul, D., Vasko, R., Puhl, M., Miewald, J., & Buysse, D. J. (2007). Psychological stress is associated with heightened physiological arousal during NREM sleep in primary insomnia. *Behavioral Sleep Medicine, 5*, 178–193.

Iber, C., Ancoli-Israel, S., Chesson, A., Quan, S. F., & American Academy of Sleep Medicine. (2007). *The AASM manual for the scoring of sleep and associated events: Rules, terminology and technical specifications* (1st ed.). Westchester: American Academy of Sleep Medicine.

Krystal, A. D., & Edinger, J. D. (2010). Sleep EEG predictors and correlates of the response to cognitive behavioral therapy for insomnia. *Sleep, 33*, 669–677.

Perlis, M. L., Smith, M. T., Andrews, P. J., Orff, H., & Giles, D. E. (2001). Beta/Gamma EEG activity in patients with primary and secondary insomnia and good sleeper controls. *Sleep, 24*, 110–117.

Tekell, J. L., Hoffmann, R., Hendrickse, W., Greene, R. W., Rush, A. J., & Armitage, R. (2005). High frequency EEG activity during sleep: Characteristics in schizophrenia and depression. *Clinical EEG and Neuroscience, 36*, 25–35.

Thakor, N. V., & Tong, S. (2004). Advances in quantitative electroencephalogram analysis methods. *Annual Review of Biomedical Engineering, 6*, 453–495.

Vasko, R. C., Brunner, D. P., Monhan, J. P., Doman, J., Boston, R. J., El-Jaroudi, A., et al. (1997). Power spectral analysis of EEG in a multiple-bedroom, multiple-polygraph sleep laboratory. *International Journal of Medical Informatics, 46*, 175–184.

Quantitative Trait Locus (QTL)

Matthew A. Simonson
Institute for Behavioural Genetics, Boulder, CO, USA

Synonyms

QTL

Definition

A quantitative trait locus (QTL) is a region of DNA that influences, or is otherwise associated with, a quantitative trait (Mackay 2001). Unlike "Mendelian" traits, most traits that vary within a population are influenced by a large number of genes. The genetic effects of Mendelian traits are predominantly influenced by a single genetic locus that is inherited through simple and predictable patterns. Some examples of such traits in humans include blood type, albinism, and Huntington's disease (Dipple and McCabe 2000). Alternatively, traits such as height, intelligence, risk for most forms of illness, as well as many others, are usually due to the combined effect of many genes and regulatory regions. Such traits vary over a continuous range and are quantifiable by the degree to which the trait is expressed (Weiss et al. 2006).

To identify genetic regions that harbor QTLs, genetic markers are first identified across an organism's chromosomes. By examining whether a marker co-segregates with a trait through a pedigree more often than expected by chance, the regions of the genome near those markers are thought to have some effect on the trait (Morgan 1911). This method of mapping traits to regions of genomes has been applied to several model organisms, both plant and animal, for roughly 100 years. The mapping of QTL regions, called "linkage analysis," has enabled the identification of genes and causal polymorphisms for several human traits (Almasy and Blangero 2009).

By locating which QTLs (and associated genes or regulatory regions) contribute to a trait, a better understanding of the genetic architecture of a phenotype is gained (Eaves 1994). Through an increased understanding of the genetic architecture of traits, more refined methods of analysis can be employed. By combining information from genome-wide linkage studies with genome-wide association studies (GWAS), susceptibility alleles that would have previously been overlooked can be identified (Howrigan et al. 2011). Also, if a region is identified as a QTL relevant to a phenotype, it can then be sequenced (Feltus et al. 2011). By analyzing the sequence in a region, a better understanding of the underlying biology of a trait can then be ascertained.

Cross-References

▶ Admixture
▶ Allele
▶ Benefit Evaluation in Health Economic Studies
▶ DNA
▶ Phenotype
▶ Single Nucleotide Polymorphism (SNP)

References and Further Reading

Almasy, L., & Blangero, J. (2009). Human QTL linkage mapping. *Genetica, 136*(2), 333–340.

Dipple, K. M., & McCabe, E. R. (2000). Phenotypes of patients with "simple" Mendelian disorders are complex traits: thresholds, modifiers, and systems dynamics. *American Journal of Human Genetics, 66*(6), 1729–1735.

Eaves, L. J. (1994). Effect of genetic architecture on the power of human linkage studies to resolve the contribution of quantitative trait loci. *Heredity, 72*(Pt 2), 175–192.

Feltus, F. A., Saski, C. A., Mockaitis, K., Haiminen, N., Parida, L., Smith, Z., et al. (2011). Sequencing of a QTL-rich region of the Theobroma cacao genome using pooled BACs and the identification of trait specific candidate genes. *BMC Genomics, 12*, 379.

Howrigan, D. P., Laird, N. M., Smoller, J. W., Devlin, B., & McQueen, M. B. (2011). Using linkage information to weight a genome-wide association of bipolar disorder. *American Journal of Medical Genetics. Part B, Neuropsychiatric Genetics, 156B*(4), 462–471.

Mackay, T. F. (2001). Quantitative trait loci in Drosophila. *Nature Reviews Genetics, 2*(1), 11–20.

Morgan, T. H. (1911). Random segregation versus coupling in mendelian inheritance. *Science, 34*(873), 384.

Weiss, L. A., Pan, L., Abney, M., & Ober, C. (2006). The sex-specific genetic architecture of quantitative traits in humans. *Nature Genetics, 38*(2), 218–222.

Questionnaire Development

▶ Scale Development

Quiet Sleep

▶ Non-REM Sleep

Quit Smoking

▶ Smoking Cessation

R

RA

▶ Degenerative Diseases: Joint
▶ Rheumatoid Arthritis: Psychosocial Aspects

Racial Inequality in Economic and Social Well-Being

Kristine M. Molina[1] and
Twyla Blackmond Larnell[2]
[1]Department of Psychological Sciences, University of California, Irvine, Irvine, CA, USA
[2]Loyola University Chicago, Chicago, IL, USA

Synonyms

Racial/ethnic disparities; Social health

Definition

Racial inequalities in economic and social well-being refer to disproportionate differences between as well as within racial/ethnic groups across areas of economic and social life (e.g., education, housing, and crime) that can fundamentally shape the life chances and opportunities for optimal health and functioning of individual persons and populations (Bambra et al. 2009; Blank 2001).

Description

Widely cited indicators of economic and social well-being include educational attainment, employment, marital status, income, wealth, housing, and crime. Wider economic and social indicators include broader conditions of living (e.g., physical infrastructure, sanitation), school (e.g., underperforming or dilapidated schools), and work environments (e.g., organizational and task structure), as well as access to resources (e.g., geographic access, paid sick time, and health insurance), services (e.g., language interpreters, transportation, and quality healthcare), and capital acquired through social, work, and community networks (Bambra et al. 2009; Blank 2001).

In the USA and other Western countries where the institutionalization of racism creates a socially stratified society, whites represent the dominant and privileged racial group whereas racial/ethnic minorities occupy subordinate positions in the social hierarchy; thus, inequalities in many indicators of economic and social well-being continue to be racially structured. Indeed, discriminatory policies as well as discrimination in the labor and housing markets contribute to concentration of certain racial/ethnic minority groups across geographic areas with high levels of poverty, underperforming schools, higher crime rates, and other social ills (Blank 2001; Brewer and Heitzeg 2008).

For example, on average, African Americans/Blacks, American Indian/Alaskan Natives, and

© Springer Nature Switzerland AG 2020
M. D. Gellman (ed.), *Encyclopedia of Behavioral Medicine*,
https://doi.org/10.1007/978-3-030-39903-0

Hispanics/Latinos continue to lag behind Whites on many economic indicators such as household income, wealth, and educational attainment (e.g., high school and college graduation rates). Further, Hispanics/Latinos have, on average, higher labor force participation rates than other racial/ethnic groups, yet tend to be overrepresented in low-wage (e.g., housekeeping and service sector jobs) and hazardous occupations (e.g., construction) (National Council of La Raza 2011). On the other hand, Asians are generally more likely to have rates of high socioeconomic status similar to Whites (CAP 2015). However, significant subgroup variation exists within racial/ethnic groups and by gender. For example, Pacific Islanders (e.g., Hmong, Laotian, and Cambodian) typically fare much worse than other Asian ethnic groups (Ramakrishnan and Ahmad 2014). Regarding some indicators of social well-being, compared to white women, women of color are more likely to be minimum-wage workers than any other group (Baron 2014). Further, men and women of color are more likely to encounter greater exposure to certain forms of violence, including state-sanctioned (e.g., police brutality) and community violence, to come into contact with the criminal justice system, and to be incarcerated (Brewer and Heitzeg 2008). Research that focuses on examining between as well as within-group variation across indicators of economic and social well-being is clearly warranted.

Racial inequalities in economic indicators are key contributors of inequalities in social well-being and vice-versa, both of which are fundamentally linked to the unequal burden of disease and increased mortality experienced by many racial/ethnic minority groups across every stage of life and worldwide (Bambra et al. 2009; Cheng et al. 2016). Racial inequalities experienced early in life (e.g., childhood and adolescence) across key indicators (e.g., poverty, parental education, household income, and incarceration) are known to contribute to accumulated economic and social disadvantages throughout the life-course and across generations – all of which can have significant effects on human development and quality of life (Cheng et al. 2016).

Eliminating existing disparities across economic and social indicators is critical to a nation's health. Given that racial inequalities in one area of well-being tends to be closely linked to inequalities in other areas, intergenerational (e.g., parents, youth, and families), multilevel (e.g., individual, schools, community, and policy), and intersectoral approaches (e.g., addressing health, educational, housing policies in concert) are sorely needed to reduce, and ultimately eliminate, the unequal distribution of economic and social inequalities that contribute to racial/ethnic health inequities.

Cross-References

▶ Racial/Ethnic Disparities
▶ Racism
▶ Socioeconomic Status (SES)

References and Further Reading

Bambra, C., Gibson, M., Sowden, A., Wright, K., Whitehead, M., & Petticrew, M. (2009). Tackling the wider social determinants of health and health inequalities: Evidence from systematic reviews. *Journal of Epidemiology and Community Health, 64*, 284–291.

Baron, S. (2014). *State of the states report 2014: Local momentum for national change to cut poverty and inequality.* Washington, DC: Center for American Progress.

Blank, R. M. (2001). An overview of trends in social and economic well-being, by race. In N. J. Smelser, W. J. Wilson, & F. Mitchell (Eds.), *America becoming: Racial trends and their consequences* (pp. 21–39). National Academies Press: National Research Council.

Brewer, R. M., & Heitzeg, N. A. (2008). The racialization of crime and punishment: Criminal justice, color-blind racism, and the political economy of the prison industrial complex. *American Behavioral Scientist, 51*, 625–644.

Center for American Progress. (2015). *Economic indicators and people of color.* Center for American Progress: Author. https://cdn.americanprogress.org/wp-content/uploads/2015/08/05075343/PeopleOfColor-Econ-FS.pdf

Cheng, T. L., Johnson, S. B., & Goodman, E. (2016). Breaking the intergenerational cycle of disadvantage: The three generation approach. *Pediatrics, 137*(6). https://doi.org/10.1542/peds.2015-2467.

National Council of La Raza. (2011). *We needed the work: Latino worker voices in the new economy.* Washington,

DC: National Council of La Raza. https://issuu.com/nclr/docs/jobquality_web

Ramakrishnan, K., & Ahmad, F.Z. (2014). Income and poverty. In *State of Asians Americans and Pacific Islanders*. Washington, DC: Center for American Progress. https://www.americanprogress.org/issues/race/reports/2014/04/23/87520/state-of-asian-americans-and-pacific-islanders-series/

Racial/Ethnic Discrimination

▶ Racism

Racial/Ethnic Disparities

▶ Racial Inequality in Economic and Social Well-Being

Racism

Twyla Blackmond Larnell[1] and
Kristine M. Molina[2]
[1]Loyola University Chicago, Chicago, IL, USA
[2]Department of Psychological Sciences, University of California, Irvine, Irvine, CA, USA

Synonyms

Racial/ethnic discrimination

Definition

Racism, rooted in the ideological belief that different phenotypic makeup (e.g., physical attributes) of racial groups makes them innately inferior or superior to others, is defined as a structured system that ranks groups based on their perceived value and used as a tool for justifying disparate treatment and allocation of resources, reinforcing unequal power relations, and maintaining structural inequalities (Golash-Boza 2016; Omi and Winant 2014; Wade 2014).

Description

Racism generates discriminatory practices and differential treatment toward those perceived as inferior (Golash-Boza 2016; Omi and Winant 2014). Historically, certain racial groups (e.g., Blacks, Hispanics/Latinos) have been regarded as biologically different compared to non-Hispanic/Latino whites, thereby *innately*, inferior (Golash-Boza 2016; Wade 2014). As a result, racial minorities are more likely to experience different forms of racism, including *institutional and structural, interpersonal, and internalized racism* (Jones 2000), and to bear the disproportionately associated economic, social, and health costs across the life span (Alvarez et al. 2016). Together, these varying forms of racism impact the health of different populations through a number of mechanisms and have thus been regarded as a fundamental cause of health and healthcare inequalities (Williams and Mohammed 2013).

Interpersonal discrimination involves discriminatory acts often based on biases and prejudices toward others, has generally been the most widely studied form of racism in health-related research, and is usually measured as a target's perceptions of unfair treatment (Kressin et al. 2008; Williams and Mohammed 2013). For example, racial biases held by healthcare professionals can shape their behavior, which can manifest as disparate treatment toward racial/ethnic minority patients, including inaccurate medical evaluations and assessments, less access to information and referrals, and lack of timely, appropriate, and quality provision of medical treatment (Feagin and Bennefield 2014; Williams and Mohammed 2013). Disparate treatment in the healthcare context has been shown to be associated with rising health and healthcare inequalities (Feagin and Bennefield 2014; Williams and Mohammed 2013). Research also shows that overt and subtle forms of interpersonal discrimination act as a psychosocial stressor that can engender pathogenic physiological responses (e.g., increased cortisol levels, inflammation), diminished cognition (e.g., impaired performance and self-regulation), health-damaging behavior (e.g., substance use, emotional eating), and negative emotions (e.g., sadness), thereby resulting in increased risk for a host of adverse health outcomes (e.g., chronic health conditions, psychiatric disorders, reduced health-related quality of life) (Alvarez et al. 2016; Williams and Mohammed 2013).

Second, institutional racism relates to discriminatory policies, practices, laws, social norms, and procedures embedded in the daily operations of institutional (e.g., healthcare system) and social structures – whether intentional or not – that systematically disproportionately adversely impact certain groups, including racial/ethnic minorities, by limiting their rights and privileges (Feagin and Bennefield 2014; Golash-Boza 2016; Omi and Winant 2014; Williams and Mohammed 2013). For example, racial/ethnic minority groups disproportionately experience structural racism as a result of discriminatory practices and policies in the housing and labor market, which have downstream effects that result in residential segregation – a key determinant of violent crime and incarceration rates, both of which have been shown to negatively impact the health of individuals, their families, and communities (Williams and Mohammed 2013). Further, racial/ethnic minority's overrepresentation in geographic areas with concentrated poverty, underperforming schools, higher crime rates, chemical pollutants, and other social issues can also directly or indirectly contribute to health (Alvarez et al. 2016; Feagin and Bennefield 2014; Jones 2000; Kressin et al. 2008; Williams and Mohammed 2013). Other manifestations of this form of racism include disparate access to goods and services (e.g., lack of access to health insurance or differential access to and quality of healthcare from preventative to end-of-life care) and opportunities, which can result in differential access to power (e.g., access to resources and knowledge) and limited economic and social mobility (Feagin and Bennefield 2014; Golash-Boza 2016; Jones 2000; Williams and Mohammed 2013). Limited access to societal resources positions racial/ethnic minorities to a host of downstream adverse outcomes across the life course. Overall, institutional racism – as systematic exclusion, segregation, and incarceration of racial "others" – contributes to the maintenance of the existing racial hierarchy and associated social and health inequalities across generations (Feagin and Bennefield 2014; Golash-Boza 2016; Omi and Winant 2014; Williams and Mohammed 2013).

Lastly, internalized racism has been neglected relative to other forms of racism, although it is now garnering greater attention given its harmful effects on the health of racial/ethnic minorities (Jones 2000; Williams and Mohammed 2013). This type of racism refers to the way people think and feel about themselves and toward members of their racial group. More specifically, it refers to the acceptance (i.e., internalization) by oppressed groups (e.g., racial/ethnic minorities) regarding negative stereotypes and prejudicial beliefs and attitudes held by the dominant group and society in general about one's own group (Jones 2000). The deleterious effects of internalizing societal beliefs of racial minority group's perceived inferiority and lack of value may indirectly impact health via the erosion of one's self-esteem and worth, engendering feelings of self-doubt, self-devaluation and self-blame, helplessness, and resignation – reinforcing the perceived superiority of the dominant group and sustaining unequal power relations and oppression (Jones 2000). Indeed, internalized racism has been shown to relate to greater engagement in health-damaging behaviors and poorer mental and physical health (Jones 2000; Williams and Mohammed 2013).

A growing body of research continues to document robust associations among different types of racism and a wide range of health indicators, finding support for their role in accounting for persistent disparities across different health indicators, even when controlling for the effect of other explanatory factors, including socioeconomic status (Williams and Mohammed 2013). Considering and addressing the role of racism on health thus remains an important area of scientific inquiry and a critical public health issue targeted at reducing risk of poor individual-level health and, ultimately, eliminating population-level health inequities (Williams and Mohammed 2013).

Cross-References

- Ethnicity
- Racial Inequality in Economic and Social Well-Being
- Racial/Ethnic Disparities
- Social Epidemiology
- Social Factors

References and Further Reading

Alvarez, A. N., Liang, C. T. H., & Neville, H. A. (2016). *The cost of racism for people of color: Contextualizing experiences of discrimination*. Washington, DC: American Psychological Association.

Feagin, J., & Bennefield, Z. (2014). Systemic racism and U.S. healthcare. *Social Science and Medicine, 103*, 7–14.

Golash-Boza, T. (2016). A critical and comprehensive sociological theory of race and racism. *Sociology of Race and Ethnicity, 2*(2), 129–141.

Jones, C. P. (2000). Levels of racism: A theoretical framework and a gardner's tale. *American Journal of Public Health, 90*(8), 1212–1215.

Kressin, N. R., Raymond, K. L., & Manze, M. (2008). Perceptions of race/ethnicity-based discrimination: A review of measures and evaluation of their usefulness for the health care setting. *Journal of Health Care for the Poor and Underserved, 9*(3), 697–730.

Omi, M., & Winant, H. (2014). *Racial formation in the United States: From the 1960s to the 1980s*. New York: Routledge.

Wade, N. (2014). *A troublesome inheritance: Genes, race, and human history*. New York: Penguin Press.

Williams, D. R., & Mohammed, S. A. (2013). Racism and health I: Pathways and scientific evidence. *American Behavioral Scientist, 57*(8), 1152–1173.

Racism and Health

- Discrimination and Health

Radiation Therapy

- Cancer Treatment and Management

Radical Prostatectomy, Psychological Impact

Heather Honoré Goltz[1,2],
Marc A. Kowalkouski[1,2], Stacey L. Hart[3] and David Latini[4]
[1]HSR&D Center of Excellence, Michael E. DeBakey VA Medical Center (MEDVAMC 152), Houston, TX, USA
[2]Department of Social Sciences, University of Houston-Downtown, Houston, TX, USA
[3]Department of Psychology, Ryerson University, Toronto, ON, Canada
[4]Scott Department of Urology, Baylor College of Medicine, Houston, TX, USA

Synonyms

Prostatectomy

Definition

Radical Prostatectomy

Radical prostatectomy (RP) is a technique used to surgically remove the prostate gland and, commonly, the seminal vesicles, lymph nodes, and surrounding tissue. Surgeons have used RP to treat benign and malignant prostate disease for over 100 years. Advances in knowledge of pelvic anatomy, technology, and surgical techniques have positioned RP as a definitive treatment for localized prostate cancer. Currently, RP refers to several surgical approaches that vary, based on site of surgical entry and whether the surgery is "open" or uses minimally invasive "laparoscopic" techniques. These options include open retropubic (RRP), perineal (RPP), and laparoscopic and robotic-assisted laparoscopic (LRP) surgical approaches. Additionally, RP approaches may be used as first-line treatment for prostate cancer or second treatment after "biochemical recurrence" (i.e., rising prostate-specific antigen levels posttreatment). Other options for treatment include radiation, hormone therapy, or surveillance instead of active treatment.

Factors Influencing Receipt of Radical Prostatectomy

A number of factors influence patients' decisions to undergo active prostate cancer treatment. Factors specifically influencing receipt of RP treatment include patients' age, comorbid conditions, prostate cancer stage and grade, and the presence of metastases. Men who are older, or who have poor health status (e.g., obesity, comorbidities) and advanced stage or grade at the time of diagnosis are more likely to receive treatment modalities other than RP. Research is divided on the association between race/ethnicity and receipt of RP. Some authors have reported that African Americans are less likely to receive RP, possibly because of more advanced disease at diagnosis; while others report no ethnic variations in treatment patterns.

Complications of Radical Prostatectomy

RP approaches produce similar cancer-control outcomes but vary in terms of peri- and postoperative complications. Perioperative complications include neurological, bowel, rectal, and bladder injuries; deep venous thrombosis; and pulmonary embolism. While there are less data for LRP, it appears that rates for many perioperative complications are low for LRP but somewhat higher than rates for RRP and RPP. More common perioperative complications include urine leakage into the abdominal cavity, restrictive narrowing of the bladder neck, and excessive blood loss requiring transfusion. Higher rates of complications occur during RRP and RPP than during LRP. Many perioperative complications can be corrected surgically after discovery. Patients opting for surgical intervention tend to experience postoperative complications at significantly higher rates than those opting for other prostate cancer treatment modalities (e.g., electron beam radiation).

Urinary and bowel incontinence and sexual dysfunction are well-documented postoperative complications of RP. For example, RP causes changes in urinary function (i.e., urgency, frequency, control, incomplete emptying), irrespective of surgical approach. Urinary effects are usually immediate, and recovery times may vary substantially for men who develop stress urinary incontinence. Men may take as long as 2–3 years before regaining some measure of continence after RP, though patients rarely experience continuous or complete incontinence. Post-RP continence rates at 12 months are between 40% and 95%, with patients at high-volume facilities achieving better continence rates. Hence, it is recommended that patients be monitored for 1 year post-RP before introducing medical or surgical interventions for urinary incontinence, as this issue may resolve with time. Findings from previous trials suggest that Kegel exercises and biofeedback prior to surgery may improve post-RP continence rates. In addition to provider- and facility-level factors, factors such as older age at the time of surgery, higher body mass index, higher prostate volume, perioperative RP bladder injury, and previous history of lower urinary tract symptoms or radiation therapy also contribute to post-RP urinary continence outcomes.

Post-RP sexual dysfunction is a complex phenomenon, with erectile dysfunction occurring in 25–85% of patients. This postoperative complication is more likely the result of a combination of the aging process, the disease itself, and RP treatment; but preoperative sexual function, comorbid health conditions, and lifestyle or behavioral factors (e.g., tobacco and alcohol use) are also contributing factors. Patients experiencing erectile difficulties immediately after surgery may gradually regain sexual function, particularly those with higher sexual functioning pre-RP; men have reported partial recovery of sexual function upwards of 2–4 years after surgery. Additional post-RP sexual effects include sterility, changes in penile length, and changes in orgasms resulting from concurrent removal of the prostate and seminal vesicles during RP.

Postoperative changes in bowel functioning are another potential complication of the RP surgical approach. Symptoms include increased frequency or urgency, diarrhea, and rectal bleeding. Men with post-RP bowel incontinence may report decline in bowel function at 4 months after surgery. As with urinary continence, many patients experiencing bowel dysfunction may recover function within the first year post-RP, while others may struggle with symptoms for years after treatment.

The Psychological Impact of Radical Prostatectomy

Advances in prostate cancer screening and detection are contributing to increasingly early prostate cancer diagnoses. A related trend concerns the often direct linkage between diagnosis and active treatment. Combined, these trends virtually ensure that younger men and those with low-risk prostate cancer will be offered treatment that they may or may not take and experience related side effects potentially for decades. In addition to medical complications, there are mental health and psychological complications.

A number of studies have examined psychosocial outcomes after prostate cancer treatment, including general, cancer-specific, and disease-specific health-related quality of life (HRQOL). General HRQOL encompasses a number of health domains related to mental/emotional, social, and physical/functional well-being. Cancer-specific instruments broadly assess the impact of having cancer across various health domains, while disease-specific instruments evaluate aspects of specific cancers. Commonly used general and cancer-specific HRQOL measures include the Medical Outcomes Survey Short Form-36 (or shorter versions) and the European Organization for Research and Treatment of Cancer Quality of Life Questionnaire (EORTC-QLQ-30), respectively. The Prostate Cancer Index (PCI) and Expanded Prostate Cancer Index: Composite (EPIC) are widely used disease-specific instruments.

Peer-reviewed literature provides strong evidence concerning the relationship between receiving RP and reduced HRQOL from chronic urinary, sexual, and bowel complications. Based on longitudinal studies, men receiving RP initially experience problems across general HRQOL domains, such as vitality/energy and role-physical well-being that substantially resolve over the course of the first year; most will return to preoperative general HRQOL levels across many domains during that time period. In terms of cancer-specific or disease-specific HRQOL, receiving RP is linked to immediate decrements in urinary and sexual function. Urinary function reaches its nadir around 3 months post-RP and gradually improves until years 2–3. At year 2, a substantial number of men's urinary function scores have not returned to preoperative levels, and they continue to report some degree of daily urine leakage. RP patients also experience decreased sexual functioning, reaching its nadir at 6 months post-RP and gradually improving through years 2–4. Yet return to presurgery levels of sexual function may not be possible for substantial numbers of patients; only about 34% of men undergoing RP return to preoperative levels by year 5. Men experiencing persistent erectile dysfunction may experience radical shifts in body image and confidence in initiating sexual intimacy, causing them to question their masculine and sexual identities.

Thus, post-RP complications cause a number of psychological, emotional, and social concerns that have lasting impact on men's HRQOL, including changes in masculine self-image and confidence and anxiety about cancer recurrence. The RP-HRQOL relationship is influenced by a number of demographic and psychosocial factors. Younger men undergoing RP experience greater recovery in terms of urinary and sexual function than their older male counterparts at 1-year post-prostatectomy. They also report lower urinary and sexual bother scores on average than older men. Men who are married or white are significantly more likely to return to pre-RP general HRQOL levels than their unmarried or racial/ethnic minority counterparts. Married men experience greater recovery in general health and social well-being domains; while those who are white experience gains in the physical, social well-being, and role-physical domains. Moderating or mediating psychosocial factors include health literacy, perceived stress, treatment satisfaction, and fear of recurrence.

Interventions exist that ameliorate many of the post-prostatectomy physical complications. For example, nonpharmacological interventions such as Kegel exercises or erectile aides (e.g., penile pumps) are available. Some RP patients may also experience enhanced sexual functioning with PDE-5 inhibitor usage; over one half of patients who initiate pharmacological penile rehabilitation recover natural erectile function by 18 months post-RP. Interestingly, a number of men with erectile difficulties will discontinue treatment after the first failed intervention, despite evidence suggesting that men attempting two or more options are more likely to find effective treatment.

A growing number of randomized controlled trial-tested interventions are targeting prostate cancer patients and caregivers in clinically modifiable areas, such as physical and psychological symptom management, literacy and culturally appropriate educational materials, decisional aids, marital communication and adjustment, and other areas. Integrative psychological and behavioral approaches to prostate cancer treatment-related complications are warranted for improving HRQOL after RP. Behavioral medicine researchers and clinicians will increasingly be called upon to lend their expertise as part of multidisciplinary teams or in disseminating study results within clinical settings.

References and Readings

Bokhour, B. G., Clark, J. A., Inui, T. S., Silliman, R. A., & Talcott, J. A. (2001). Sexuality after treatment for early prostate cancer: Exploring the meanings of "erectile dysfunction". *Journal of Internal Medicine, 16*, 649–655.

Cooperberg, M. R., Moul, J. W., & Carroll, P. R. (2005). The changing face of prostate cancer. *Journal of Clinical Oncology, 23*(32), 8146–8151.

Eton, D. T., & Lepore, S. J. (2002). Prostate cancer and health-related quality of life: A review of the literature. *Psycho-Oncology, 11*, 307–326.

Knight, S. J., & Latini, D. M. (2009). Sexual side effects and prostate cancer treatment decisions: Patient information needs and preferences. *Cancer Journal, 15*(1), 41–44.

Le, J. D., Cooperberg, M. R., Sadetsky, N., Hittleman, A. B., Meng, M. V., Cowan, J., et al. (2010). Changes in specific domains of sexual function and sexual bother after radical prostatectomy. *British Journal of Urology International, 106*(7), 1022–1029.

Michaelson, M. D., Cotter, S. E., Gargollo, P. C., Zietman, A. L., Dahl, D. M., & Smith, M. R. (2008). Management of complications of prostate cancer treatment. *CA: Cancer Journal for Clinicians, 58*, 196–213.

Muller, A., Parker, M., Waters, B. W., Flanigan, R. C., & Mulhall, J. P. (2009). Penile rehabilitation following radical prostatectomy: Predicting success. *Journal of Sexual Medicine, 6*(10), 2806–2812.

Namiki, S., & Arai, Y. (2010). Health-related quality of life in men with localized prostate cancer. *International Journal of Urology, 17*, 125–138.

Sandhu, J. S., & Eastham, J. A. (2010). Factors predicting early return of continence after radical prostatectomy. *Current Urology Reports, 11*, 191–197.

Schover, L. R., Fouladi, R. T., Warneke, C. L., Neese, L., Klein, E. A., Zippe, C., et al. (2002). The use of treatments for erectile dysfunction among survivors of prostate carcinoma. *Cancer, 95*(11), 2397–2407.

Shavers, V. L., & Brown, M. L. (2002). Racial and ethnic differences in the receipt of cancer treatment. *Journal of the National Cancer Institute, 94*(5), 334–357.

Sriprasad, S., Feneley, M. R., & Thompson, P. M. (2009). History of prostate cancer treatment. *Surgical Oncology, 18*, 185–191.

Wilt, T. J., MacDonald, R., Rutks, I., Shamliyan, T. A., Taylor, B. C., & Kane, R. L. (2008). Systematic review: Comparative effectiveness and harms of treatments for clinically localized prostate cancer. *Annals of Internal Medicine, 148*(6), 435–448.

Wittman, D., Northouse, L., Foley, S., Gilbert, S., Wood, D. P., Balon, R., et al. (2009). The psychosocial aspects of sexual recovery after prostate cancer treatment. *International Journal of Impotence Research, 21*, 99–106.

Wright, J. L., Lin, D. W., Cowan, J. E., Carroll, P. R., Litwin, M. S., & The CaPSURE Investigators. (2007). Quality of life in young men after radical prostatectomy. *Prostate Cancer and Prostatic Diseases, 11*(1), 67–73.

Random-Coefficient Model

▶ Hierarchical Linear Modeling (HLM)

Random-Coefficient Regression Modeling

▶ Multilevel Modeling

Random-Effects Modeling

▶ Multilevel Modeling

Randomization

J. Rick Turner
Campbell University College of Pharmacy and
Health Sciences, Buies Creek, NC, USA

Definition

Randomization is a process of randomly assigning experimental subjects to one of the treatment groups so that many potential influences that cannot be controlled for (e.g., height, weight) or cannot be determined by observation (e.g., specific metabolic pathway influences in pharmaceutical clinical trials) are likely to be as frequent in one treatment group as they are in the other. The goal of randomization is to eliminate bias.

Randomization occurs after a subject's eligibility for a clinical trial has been determined and before any experimental data are collected. The process facilitates the random assignment of subjects to different treatment groups with the intent of avoiding any selection bias in subject assignment.

As discussed in the entry titled ▶ "Hypothesis Testing," inferential statistics requires the random assignment of subjects to different treatment groups to allow differences in responses between treatment groups to be connected to the treatments received. Randomization means that other potential sources of influence on the data have been randomly allocated to each treatment group. That is, subjects have an independent (and usually, but not necessarily, equal) chance of being in the different groups. While subjects are typically randomized to two treatment groups in a 1:1 ratio, generating the same number of subjects in each group, other randomization ratios can be used. For example, a ratio of 2:1 for an active treatment versus a placebo treatment would mean that two thirds of the subjects would be randomized to the treatment group and one third to the placebo group. Such an unequal randomization ratio has various implications, including the consequence that the statistical power to detect a difference between the groups is not as high as it would be if the same number of subjects had been used and the number of subjects in each group had been equal.

As noted, the goal of randomization is to eliminate bias. This includes subject bias, based on their knowledge of which treatment group they have been assigned to (this is not possible on all occasions, and can be particularly difficult in studies of behavioral medicine interventions), and investigator bias. Investigator bias is eliminated by preventing researchers from deliberately assigning subjects to one treatment group or the other. Two possible unconscious or conscious biases on the part of the researcher that are thus removed are an inclination to place less healthy subjects in the treatment group receiving the intervention they believe to be most beneficial, and an inclination to place the more healthy subjects in the group receiving a "favored" intervention to demonstrate its superiority.

Cross-References

▶ Bias
▶ Hypothesis Testing
▶ Randomized Clinical Trial

Randomized Clinical Trial

J. Rick Turner
Campbell University College of Pharmacy and
Health Sciences, Buies Creek, NC, USA

Synonyms

Randomized concurrently controlled clinical trial; Randomized controlled clinical trial

Definition

A randomized clinical trial is one in which the subjects in each treatment group have been placed in that group by a randomization procedure. Randomization involves randomly assigning experimental subjects to one of the treatment groups so that many potential influences that cannot be controlled for (e.g., height, weight) or cannot be determined by observation (e.g., specific metabolic pathway influences that may be relevant to the efficacy or safety of interventions in the trial) are likely to be as frequent in one treatment group as they are in the other (Turner 2010).

Description

The fundamental goal of randomization is to eliminate bias (or, pragmatically, to reduce it as much as possible). This includes subject bias, based on their knowledge of which treatment/intervention group they have been assigned to, and investigator bias. Investigator bias is eliminated by preventing investigators from deliberately assigning patients to one treatment group or the other. Two possible unconscious or conscious biases on the part of the investigators that are thus removed are an inclination to place less healthy subjects in the treatment group receiving the intervention they believe to be most beneficial, and an inclination to place the more healthy subjects in the investigational intervention group to demonstrate its superiority.

Randomized concurrently controlled clinical trials are generally regarded as the "gold standard" for providing compelling evidence that an intervention is effective. The treatment can be of various kinds, including pharmacological and behavioral. In the realm of behavioral medicine, two examples of interventional treatments are physical exercise and cognitive behavioral therapy. These interventions would be tested against one or more control interventions. These can be "active controls," i.e., an intervention that is established to be efficacious in this context. They can also be "placebo controls," i.e., interventions that are not able to be efficacious in this context, but whose implementation involves as many as possible of the same demands and benefits that the interventional treatment makes on, and provides to, subjects in the interventional group. Matthews (2006) commented as follows:

"Over the last two to three decades randomized concurrently controlled clinical trials have become established as the method which investigators must use to assess new treatments if their claims are to find widespread acceptance. The methodology underpinning these trials is firmly based in statistical theory, and the success of randomized clinical trials perhaps constitutes the greatest achievement of statistics in the second half of the twentieth century."

Compelling evidence is sought that the investigational intervention is statistically significantly (and then clinically significantly) more effective than the comparator intervention. Such evidence is generated via the use of inferential hypothesis testing and a resultant p-value of less than 0.05. (Despite its attained prominence, the value of 0.05 was not ordained, but conceived by the renowned statistician Sir Ronald Fisher. Had he decided, for example, that odds of 1 in 25, with an analogous p-value of 0.04, were more suitable for this purpose than odds of 1 in 20, modern science might be held to a different standard.)

Randomization occurs after a subject's eligibility for a clinical trial has been determined and before any experimental data are collected. The process of randomization is facilitated by the generation of a randomization list. This list is generated (often by a random-number generator) in advance of recruiting the first subject. The list is generated under the direction of the trial statistician, but, to maintain confidentiality, is not released to the statistician until the completion of the study.

Inferential statistics requires the random assignment of subjects to different treatment groups to allow differences in responses between treatment groups to be connected to the treatments administered. Randomization means that other potential sources of influence on the data have been randomly allocated to each treatment group. That is, subjects have an independent (and usually, but not necessarily, equal) chance of receiving either the investigational intervention or a control intervention.

Kay (2007) highlighted several methods of randomization, including simple randomization, block randomization, and stratified randomization. Simple randomization involves assigning treatments to subjects in a completely random way. While this strategy is attractively simple, it is not advisable in the case of small trials. In the example of a trial involving 30 subjects randomized to two treatment groups, the probability of a 15–15 split, the most powerful from a statistical analysis point of view, is only 0.144, while the probability of a split of 11–19 or even more unbalanced is 0.20. While 30 subjects is a small number that is used for illustrative purposes here, some researchers advocate not using simple randomization schedules in trials with less than 200 participants. In such trials the stratified randomization approach is recommended. Many clinical trials in behavioral medicine are likely to involve such numbers of subjects, in contrast to therapeutic confirmatory trials in the pharmaceutical industry, where several thousands of subjects are typically employed.

Concurrent control is a critical feature of these trials. The term "control" has already been discussed here. The term "concurrent" simply means that the control treatment should be given at the same point in time (and also under the same conditions) as the intervention of interest.

Cross-References

▶ Mode

References and Further Reading

Kay, R. (2007). *Statistical thinking for non-statisticians in drug regulation*. Chichester: Wiley.
Matthews, J. N. S. (2006). *Introduction to randomized controlled clinical trials* (2nd ed.). Boca Raton: Chapman & Hall/CRC.
Turner, J. R. (2010). *New drug development: An introduction to clinical trials* (2nd ed.). New York: Springer.

Randomized Concurrently Controlled Clinical Trial

▶ Randomized Clinical Trial

Randomized Controlled Clinical Trial

▶ Randomized Clinical Trial

Randomized Controlled Trial

▶ Clinical Trial

Raynaud's Disease and Stress

Leah Rosenberg[1] and Sarah Piper[2]
[1]Department of Medicine, School of Medicine, Duke University, Durham, NC, USA
[2]Institute of Metabolic Science, Addenbrookes Hospital, Metabolic Research Laboratories, University of Cambridge, Cambridge, UK

Synonyms

Idiopathic Raynaud's Phenomenon; Primary Raynaud's Phenomenon

Definition

Raynaud's disease is a reversible vasospastic phenomenon triggered in susceptible patients by exposure to cold and/or emotional stress. The condition is characterized by arterial and arteriolar vasoconstriction, most commonly affecting the distal extremities such as the hands or, less commonly, the feet. The vasoconstriction produces a characteristic pallor and cyanosis of the involved digits (ischemic phase) followed by subsequent reperfusion and digit erythema, or redness.

Description

General Information

Raynaud's disease, or primary Raynaud's phenomenon, was first described in 1862 by Maurice

Raynaud, who observed the characteristic color changes of the hands of affected patients during episodes of vasospasm. Modern medicine differentiates Raynaud's disease, or primary Raynaud's phenomenon, which is an idiopathic disorder, from secondary Raynaud's phenomenon, which is commonly associated with rheumatologic or autoimmune causes and which often has a more severe clinical course.

Raynaud's disease predominantly affects females, with an estimated prevalence of 6–20% of women and 3–12.5% of men, and is more common in colder climates. The symptoms in Raynaud's disease typically begin prior to the age of 30, may involve associated pain or numbness during episodes of vasoconstriction, and tend to affect the extremities symmetrically. They can vary considerably in severity, with most individuals experiencing mild to moderate symptoms and others experiencing symptoms that are intermittently debilitating. Rarely, episodes of vasospasm in Raynaud's disease can progress to ulceration or necrosis of the involved digits.

Role of Stress

The exact relationship between emotional stress and Raynaud's disease is not clear. While most episodes of vasospasm in Raynaud's disease are caused by exposure to cold temperatures, emotional stress has long been thought to play a role in precipitating symptoms as well. In fact, management of Raynaud's disease during the mid-1900s fell under the purview and management of psychiatry and psychoanalysis, treated with questionable success with psychotherapeutic techniques. In more recent studies, patients have reported a role for stress in triggering Raynaud's attacks in up to 33% of episodes, experienced by a self-reported 21% of Raynaud's disease sufferers. Initially, it was hypothesized that Raynaud's patients who were susceptible to stress-triggered attacks may be more likely to manifest higher levels of anxiety in general, termed "trait anxiety," although the accuracy of this characterization is unclear. Studies in the 1980s failed to show any significant differences in measures of anxiety or "neuroticism" based on psychologic questionnaires. A study of the quality-of-life impact of primary Raynaud's phenomenon suggested that patients suffering from the disease reported worse quality of life than control subjects and were more likely to report the subjective experience of moderate to severe anxiety symptoms. It remains uncertain, however, whether these findings inform an underlying psychiatric predisposition among Raynaud's sufferers to stress-triggered episodes or if the results are simply commonly seen complications of long-standing chronic disease.

Suspected Pathogenesis

The proposed pathogenesis of Raynaud's disease is not fully elucidated but seems to be closely related to the sympathetic nervous system, a physiologic mechanism triggered frequently by physiologic or emotional stress. Scientists have found that Raynaud's disease sufferers show an increased peripheral responsiveness to circulating catecholamines, or stress hormones, which are increased in all individuals in response to cold temperatures or emotional stress. People diagnosed with Raynaud's disease have been shown to have an increased sensitivity of the alpha-2 adrenergic receptors in peripheral blood vessels that detect these hormones, perhaps either through altered characteristics of the receptors themselves or through an increased density of receptors. By this model, levels of circulating catecholamines caused by emotional stress that would not typically trigger vasoconstriction in normal individuals could understandably trigger vasospasm in patients who are more sensitive to their effects, either with or without a predisposition to higher anxiety states.

Researching Stress and Raynaud's Disease

Efforts to study the effects of stress in Raynaud's disease have frequently produced equivocal and at times conflicting results. Early research in the 1940s and 1950s focused on measuring finger temperature in relation to emotional states to determine if emotional distress could cause vasospasm. While some initial studies documented correlative evidence of markedly decreased finger temperatures in Raynaud's patients exposed to emotional stressors, this correlation was not consistently replicated over the next decades. Some studies even documented an increased finger temperature among Raynaud's sufferers in response to a provoked stress responses.

More recently, efforts to delineate the effect of stress in triggering Raynaud's attacks have revealed the possibility of a patient cohort that shows an increased susceptibility to emotional stress-triggered Raynaud's attacks, characterized by a higher trait anxiety scores than other Raynaud's sufferers. The Raynaud's Treatment Study in 2001 suggested that, while perceived stress alone did not seem to predict an increase in Raynaud's disease, increased anxiety scores were associated with more frequent attacks, particularly at warmer temperatures, as well as a higher reported severity of attacks at all temperatures and increased pain at temperatures greater than 40°. The observed effects were small but significant. It has been proposed that the effects of stress carry greater impact at higher temperatures than lower temperatures because of the absolute increase in cold-induced vasospasm below 40°. The effects of stress may only be observable at higher temperatures, where vasospasm is less universally triggering for Raynaud's sufferers.

Treatment

Understandably, the possible role of stress in triggering Raynaud's symptoms has led to the development and study of stress reduction-based interventions. Early recommendations of relaxation techniques have not shown any statistical benefit in studies. Cognitive-behavior treatments have been tested in small populations, again without any demonstrated benefit. Among non-pharmacologic treatments for Raynaud's disease, behavioral treatments seem to be the most effective in diminishing symptoms. For an in-depth discussion of behavioral treatments in Raynaud's disease, refer to "Raynaud's Disease and Behavioral Treatments."

References and Readings

Bakst, R., Merola, J. F., Franks, A. G., & Sanchez, M. (2008). Raynaud's phenomenon: Pathogenesis and management. *Journal of the American Academy of Dermatology, 49*(4), 633–653.

Brown, K. M., Middaugh, S. J., Haythornthwaite, J. A., & Bielory, L. (2001). The effects of stress, anxiety, and outdoor temperatures on the frequency and severity of Raynaud's attacks: The Raynaud's treatment study. *Journal of Behavioral Medicine, 24*(2), 137–153.

De Angelis, R., Salaffi, F., & Grassi, W. (2008). Health-related quality of life in primary Raynaud phenomenon. *Journal of Clinical Rheumatology, 14*(4), 206–210.

Goreczny, A. (Ed.). (1995). *Handbook of health and rehabilitative psychology*. New York: Plenum Press.

Mittelmann, B., & Wolff, H. G. (1939). Affective states and skin temperature: Experimental study on subjects with "Cold Hands" and Raynaud's syndrome. *Psychosomatic Medicine, 1*, 271–292.

Raynaud's Disease: Behavioral Treatment

Leah Rosenberg[1] and Sarah Piper[2]
[1]Department of Medicine, School of Medicine, Duke University, Durham, NC, USA
[2]Institute of Metabolic Science, Addenbrookes Hospital, Metabolic Research Laboratories, University of Cambridge, Cambridge, UK

Synonyms

Idiopathic Raynaud's Phenomenon; Primary Raynaud's Phenomenon

Definition

Raynaud's disease is a reversible vasospastic phenomenon triggered in susceptible patients by exposure to cold or emotional stress. The condition is characterized by arterial and arteriolar vasoconstriction, most commonly affecting the distal extremities, that produces a characteristic pallor and cyanosis of the involved digits (ischemic phase) followed by subsequent reperfusion and digit erythema, or redness.

Description

Symptoms of Raynaud's disease, including vasospasm and associated pain or numbness, are frequently amenable at least in part to conservative approaches to treatment. These initial approaches focus on avoidance of potential environmental triggers which can vary according to individual patients but most often relates to exposure to cold temperatures. To minimize the risk of cold exposure, patients are advised to practice full body insulation since other areas of exposed skin besides the hands can precipitate attacks. Patients are advised to avoid sudden changes in temperature as well. Discontinuation of known vasoconstrictive medications, smoking cessation, avoidance of vibration, and discontinuation of caffeine consumption have also been counseled. Some individuals also benefit from a swing-arm maneuver that causes pooling of blood in the distal extremities to counteract the effects of vasoconstriction, shown in some people to abort the onset of a Raynaud's attack. While a majority of Raynaud's disease sufferers respond well to these recommendations with at least some reduction in the severity and frequency of symptoms, others require more aggressive pharmacologic or even behavioral interventions, described below.

For patients who do not respond to conservative interventions, the next step in treatment is frequently the initiation of a medication to inhibit vasospasm, such as calcium channel blockers. This class of medication has been shown in multiple studies to help decrease the rate of Raynaud's attacks and to mitigate the severity of attacks in a significant number of patients. Reports of side effects from these medications are common, including orthostatic hypotension, edema, headache, tachycardia, and constipation. Given poor tolerance of pharmacotherapy in some patients, behavioral treatments have been concurrently developed and researched to provide an alternative to medications. These interventions, most notably thermal biofeedback, autogenic training, and classical conditioning, have been tested head to head with medical treatments in some studies and have been shown to have potential benefit.

Behavioral treatments have been developed alongside medical therapies in treating Raynaud's disease, in part due to the known side effects of many medications but also due to early evidence that principles of biofeedback may be very effective in controlling patient's symptoms.

Biofeedback is a behavioral technique developed in the last 40 years that links involuntary physiologic processes, such as heart rate, which often occur below the level of conscious awareness, to sensory stimuli that are easily perceptible and able to be tracked to note variations in these unconscious processes. Patients then use this information to manipulate the target physiologic response (e.g., slowing heart rate through conscious focus).

This technique has been applied to Raynaud's disease in several forms, the best-researched of which is thermal biofeedback. Thermal biofeedback (also called finger temperature biofeedback) is a behavioral treatment first studied in Raynaud's patients in the 1970s. The technique instructs individuals in the use of sensory feedback to convey an increase in finger temperature by facilitating peripheral vasodilation. This technique has been shown in several small studies to have strong efficacy in reducing Raynaud's attacks by up to 92.5%, particularly when the initial training was conducted during exposure to cold temperatures. Improvements in symptoms have been observed as long as 3 years from the time of initial training. Further studies, including those comparing the effectiveness of thermal biofeedback to standard medical therapies, have been inconclusive. The wide variability in study results is thought to be attributable to the underlying difficulty in teaching the technique, which often requires intensive instruction to achieve mastery. Patients who do achieve mastery are frequently able to facilitate hand rewarming through practiced conscious intervention in high-risk environments that would previously have triggered episodes of vasospasm. Despite these results, a recent head-to-head comparison of nifedipine, a standard medical treatment for Raynaud's, and thermal biofeedback was unimpressive, although authors highlighted the limitations in assessing the behavioral technique due to strong evidence that participants had not achieved mastery of the technique during the study, which likely significantly reduced its apparent effectiveness.

Another technique that may be in some part considered a relative of biofeedback is autogenic training. This technique was first introduced in the early 1930s within the mental health community to promote stress management and relief from somatic symptoms often related to anxiety. AT is a relaxation method consisting of passive self-monitoring of physiologic sensations such as heart rate to then inform self-initiated verbal cues intended to cause a desired change in physiologic effect or modification of the initial sensation. This technique has been applied to treatment models in Raynaud's disease through cultivation of an awareness of finger temperature and the application of cuing to trigger peripheral vasodilatation. The effectiveness of this technique is unclear. Some studies have shown an increase in finger temperature (often a measured outcome in Raynaud's research) that equals the observed efficacy of thermal biofeedback interventions, with reports of similar clinical efficacy. Combining the two techniques does not appear to convey any additional benefit, however.

Classical conditioning is a principle that pairs a behavior with a predictable outcome, such as salivation in response to the presentation of food, to an alternate stimulus to link the alternate stimulus with the outcome through repetitive training. In application to Raynaud's disease, Raynaud's disease sufferers have been conditioned to respond to exposure to cold temperatures with peripheral vasodilatation after serial exposures to cold ambient temperatures with concurrent immersion of the person's hands in warm water. Over time, patients were observed to have increased blood flow simply with exposure to cold temperatures even without the added exposure of warm water immersion. This technique, while not as well studied as thermal biofeedback, also has been shown to have a possible effect in decreasing the frequency and severity of Raynaud's attacks.

Less well-studied interventions have included progressive relaxation and guided imagery. These techniques focus on relieving emotional stress and providing improved relaxation. Progressive relaxation is a tool that involves the progressive contraction of muscle groups followed by sequential release of muscle tone to achieve a global state of relaxation. Guided imagery is a technique that teaches patients to directed imagining of calming or peaceful imagery to facilitate relief from anxiety and stress. Both techniques been studied in conjunction with other behavioral interventions such as thermal biofeedback, but not as a stand-alone treatment.

Behavioral treatments such as thermal biofeedback, autogenic training, and classical conditioning have been shown to have variable effects on the symptom frequency and severity of Raynaud's disease sufferers, although evidence overall is supportive for a role of these treatments among this patient population. Certainly, further research will help to clarify the role of these interventions and to elucidate the mechanism by which their effect is mediated.

Cross-References

▶ Raynaud's Disease and Stress

References and Readings

Bakst, R., Merola, J. F., Franks, A. G., & Sanchez, M. (2008). Raynaud's phenomenon: Pathogenesis and management. *Journal of the American Academy of Dermatology, 49*(4), 633–653.

Baum, A. (Ed.). (2001). *Handbook of health psychology.* Mahwah: Lawrence Erlbaum.

Freedman, R., Ianni, P., & Wenig, P. (1983). Behavioral treatment of Raynaud's disease. *Journal of Consulting and Clinical Psychology, 51,* 539–549.

Garcia-Carrasco, M., Jimenez-Hernandez, M., & Escarcega, R. (2008). Treatment of Raynaud's phenomenon. *Autoimmunity Reviews, 8,* 62–68.

Jobe, J. B., Sampson, J. B., Roberts, D. E., & Kelly, J. A. (1986). Comparison of behavioral treatments for Raynaud's disease. *Journal of Behavioral Medicine, 9*(1), 89–96.

Karavidas, M. K., Tsai, P. S., Yucha, C., McGrady, A., & Lehrer, P. M. (2006). Thermal biofeedback for primary Raynaud's phenomenon: A review of the literature. *Applied Psychophysiology and Biofeedback, 31*(3), 203–216.

Middaugh, S. J., Haythornthwaite, J. A., Thompson, B., Hill, R., Brown, K. M., Freedman, R. R., Attanasio, V., Jacob, R. G., Scheier, M., & Smith, E. A. (2001). The

Raynaud's treatment study: Biofeedback protocols and acquisition of temperature biofeedback skills. *Applied Psychophysiology and Biofeedback, 26*(4), 251–278.

Stetter, F., & Kupper, S. (2002). Autogenic training: A meta-analysis of clinical outcome studies. *Applied Psychophysiology and Biofeedback, 27*, 45–98.

Readiness for Return-to-Work (RRTW)

Timothy Wolf
Department of Occupational Therapy and Neurology, Program in Occupational Therapy, St. Louis, MO, USA

Synonyms

Vocational assessment

Definition

Readiness for return to work is the complex decision-making behavior related to returning to work after an injury or illness. In this process, individuals must consider their self-efficacy surrounding their ability to return to work; the interaction of the many third parties involved in returning to work including the employer and the healthcare and insurance providers; as well as the state of their disability as it interacts with the demands of the job. This term was originally conceived by Franche and Krause (2002) in their conceptual model for readiness for return to work.

Description

Work disability is often determined by an evaluation of impairments following injury or illness. This most often focuses on physical impairments which is apparent in most work evaluation methodologies, i.e., functional capacity evaluation. The limitation in this approach is that the healthcare community has long known that work disability involves a lot of factors beyond what impairment can explain. Workers who are seemingly more impaired may return to work very quickly and without difficulty while workers who are seemingly less impaired may struggle with returning to work or never attempt to return to work at all. The notion of readiness for return to work is used to help address this limitation in current work assessment methodologies. The concept for readiness for return to work was developed by Franche and Krause (2002) to provide a framework for work disability research and practice that would account for the multiple factors that influence work disability. These factors include physical (i.e., impairments), psychological (i.e., self-efficacy related to completing the demands of the job), and social (i.e., the employee's interactions in the work environment, with healthcare providers/health insurance companies). They developed the Readiness for Return to Work model in order to combine these factors to explain return to work behaviors. The Readiness for Return to Work model incorporates two well-known theoretical models to explain a work-disabled person's behavior regarding return to work. First, the Phase Model of Occupational Disability provides a framework for understanding the developmental component of disability (Krause and Ragland 1994). Second, the Readiness for Change Model provides a framework for understanding the motivation to change behavior relative to returning to work (Prochaska and Diclemente 1983).

Further work with the Readiness for Return to Work model has focused on the application of the Readiness for Change Model to work behavior to help understand work-disabled individuals' motivation to return to work following injury or illness. There are five stages within the Readiness for Change Model that an individual will progress through (Prochaska and Diclemente 1983):

- *Precontemplation*: Workers are not thinking about returning to work and are not making plans to do so either.
- *Contemplation*: Workers are considering return to work but are still not engaging in the planning process to do so.

- *Preparation for action*: Workers are seeking information about returning to work and are also looking for feedback on their ability to meet the demands of the workplace. In addition, workers are making plans to return to work.
- *Action*: Workers return to work in some capacity.
- *Maintenance*: Workers use their skills and social support to help cope with adversity they encounter in returning to work in order to maintain their ability to work.

Within this model, it is important to note that workers can relapse anytime and start regressing through these stages. The Readiness for Return-to-Work Scale (RRTW) (Franche et al. 2007) is used to determine the worker's present stage. The results might be helpful for healthcare providers to determine support and resources needed for the worker to be able to return to work. This information can also be used to tailor interventions for the worker in order to improve the effectiveness of rehabilitation efforts.

Cross-References

▶ Vocational Assessment

References and Further Reading

Franche, R. L., & Krause, N. (2002). Readiness for return to work following injury or illness: Conceptualizing the interpersonal impact of health care, workplace, and insurance factors. *Journal of Occupational Rehabilitation, 12*, 233–256.

Franche, R. L., Corbiere, M., Lee, H., Breslin, F. C., & Hepburn, C. G. (2007). The readiness for return-to-work (RRTW) scale: Development and validation of a self-report staging scale in lost-time claimants with musculoskeletal disorders. *Journal of Occupational Rehabilitation, 17*, 450–472.

Krause, N., & Ragland, D. R. (1994). Occupational disability due to low back pain: A new interdisciplinary classification based on a phase model of disability. *Spine, 19*, 1011–1020.

Prochaska, J. O., & Diclemente, C. C. (1983). Stages and process of self-change of smoking: Toward an integrative model of change. *Journal of Consulting and Clinical Psychology, 51*, 390–395.

Readiness for Return-to-Work (RRTW) Scale

Joanne Park[1,2], Douglas P. Gross[3], Shaniff Esmail[2] and Renée-Louise Franche[4,5,6]
[1]Workers' Compensation Board of Alberta Millard Health, Edmonton, AB, Canada
[2]Department of Occupational Therapy, University of Alberta, Edmonton, AB, Canada
[3]Department of Physical Therapy, University of Alberta, Edmonton, AB, Canada
[4]School of Population and Public Health, University of British Columbia, Vancouver, BC, Canada
[5]WorkSafe BC, Vancouver, BC, Canada
[6]Institute for Work and Health, Toronto, ON, Canada\

Definition

The Readiness for Return-To-Work (RRTW) scale assesses an individual's stage of readiness for return to work (RTW) among individuals off work due to a health condition and stage of readiness for work maintenance in those who have returned to work (Franche et al. 2007). Informed by the readiness for change model (Prochaska et al. 1994), the questionnaire categorizes respondents who are not working into four stages (*precontemplation, contemplation, prepared for action-self-evaluative,* or *prepared for action-behavioral*), while working respondents are categorized into either *uncertain maintenance* or *proactive maintenance*. The scale provides a final score for each readiness stage, calculated by taking the mean of items creating each factor. Higher scores within each stage indicate higher levels of beliefs associated with that stage. Questionnaire outcome can inform health-care providers and other stakeholders about how best to intervene (if at all) to facilitate sustainable RTW. The RRTW scale is relatively simple and straightforward to complete and freely available, making it attractive for use by clinicians in vocational and occupational

Description

The readiness for change model identifies individual and social factors that influence the initiation and maintenance of behavior change, such as RTW after injury (Franche and Krause 2002). This model conceptualizes the process of behavior change as the progression or relapse of an individual through the stages of change. A stage-based approach to RTW acknowledges that readiness for work varies across individuals off work due to a health condition. Some may be thinking about RTW, developing strategies for success, and actively planning their reintegration to the workforce. Others may not even be considering RTW. A developmental approach to RTW has been recommended (Pransky et al. 2005; Young et al. 2005). Although not yet widely adopted, evidence indicates that a phase-specific approach, or in this context stage-specific, offers a more complete and realistic understanding of the RTW process (Franche and Krause 2002).

The RRTW scale is one of the only tools measuring the construct of stage of readiness for RTW. The scale identifies four stages of change, informed by Prochaska's model, for those not working (Prochaska et al. 1994; Franche and Krause 2002). This includes:

(1) *Precontemplation*: the individual is not thinking about behaviors that would initiate RTW.
(2) *Contemplation*: the individual uses a decisional balance when considering RTW but is not actively engaging in behaviors involved in RTW.
(3) *Prepared for action-self-evaluative*: the individual participates in behaviors such as seeking information regarding RTW, testing their abilities for RTW, and making tangible plans.
(4) *Prepared for action-behavioral*: the individual engages in behaviors that put their RTW plan into action.

For those who are not working, the scale identifies two stages of change:

(1) *Uncertain maintenance*: characterized by higher levels of functional disability, fear avoidance, and experiencing challenges staying at work.
(2) *Proactive maintenance*: characterized by injured workers who utilize skills and social supports to manage high-risk situations that can lead to relapse and employ preventative strategies.

The RRTW scale was developed and validated in a Canadian study of workers' compensation claimants experiencing time loss from work due to musculoskeletal disorders (Franche et al. 2007). The 22-item tool consists of Scales A and B; Scale A contains 13 items for individuals who are not working, and Scale B includes nine items for individuals who are working. Each item is scored using a five-point Likert scale (1, strongly disagree; 5, strongly agree) representing characteristics of a specific readiness stage. For workers not working, 60% of the variance was explained by four factors: *precontemplation* (items a1, a2, a13), *contemplation* (items a9, a11, a12), *prepared for action-self-evaluative* (a4, a7 (item scale reversed), a8, a10), and *prepared for action-behavioral* (a3, a5, a6). For those working, 58% of the variance was explained by two factors: *uncertain maintenance* (b5, b6, b7, b8 (item scale reversed), b9) and *proactive maintenance* (b1, b2, b3, b4). Confirmatory factor analysis confirmed the initial model and had satisfactory fit indices. Concurrent validity of the RRTW scale was supported as relationships with other relevant constructs (i.e., depressive symptoms, fear avoidance, pain, and general health) were generally in the hypothesized direction.

The stability of the factorial structure of the RRTW scale remains to be established: The six stages initially identified (Franche et al. 2007) have not been consistently replicated in subsequent studies. The scale was tested in a Norwegian study evaluating a 5-day inpatient occupational rehabilitation program (Braathen et al. 2013). Unlike Franche et al., this study only found two stages for the not working group: *RTW inability* which corresponds to the *precontemplation* stage and *RTW uncertainty* which corresponds to the *contemplation* stage. However, like Franche et al., two stages were identified for the working group, corresponding to *uncertain maintenance* and *proactive maintenance*. In another study, Canadian injured workers with subacute (6–12 weeks) and chronic (+12 weeks) musculoskeletal disorders attending an outpatient rehabilitation program were enrolled (Park 2017). This study found three stages for the not working group, *contemplation*, *prepared for action-self-evaluative*, and *prepared for action-behavioral*, and two stages for the working group, *uncertain maintenance* and *proactive maintenance*. Across these three validation studies, there were differences in readiness factors identified for the not working group. However, all three studies consistently found two factors for those working in some capacity. Further evaluation and validation of the RRTW scale could provide valuable information for understanding what determinants contribute to factors identified for the not working group.

The RRTW scale has potential for facilitating stage-specific interventions tailored to the needs of injured workers. The RRTW scale could also be used as a screen to guide assessments, for goal-setting purposes, and to assist with RTW decision making. The only longitudinal study examining predictive validity of the scale found that three dimensions (*prepared for action-self-evaluative*, *prepared for action-behavioral*, and *uncertain maintenance*) were significantly associated with future RTW in a sample of sick-listed individuals in Norway (Aasdahl et al. 2017). However, issues were identified with stage allocation and more research is needed on factor structure. Although the development and validation of the RRTW scale have shown promise in work rehabilitation, further validation is required to examine the progression from one stage to another, to confirm readiness stages in different cultures and patient settings, and the utility of this scale in clinical settings.

Cross-References

▶ Cognitions
▶ Health Assessment Questionnaire
▶ Health Beliefs/Health Belief Model
▶ Pain, Psychosocial Aspects
▶ Psychosocial Factors
▶ Psychosocial Predictors
▶ Psychosocial Variables
▶ Stages-of-Change Model
▶ Transtheoretical Model of Behavior Change

References and Further Reading

Aasdahl, L., Pape, K., Jensen, C., et al. (2017). Associations between the readiness for return to work scale and return to work: A prospective study. *Journal of Occupational Rehabilitation*. Advanced online publication.

Braathen, T. N., Brage, S., Tellnes, G., & Eftedal, M. (2013). Psychometric properties of the readiness for return to work scale in inpatient occupational rehabilitation in Norway. *Journal of Occupational Rehabilitation, 23*, 371–380.

Franche, R. L., & Krause, N. (2002). Readiness for return to work following injury or illness: Conceptualizing the interpersonal impact of health care, workplace, and insurance factors. *Journal of Occupational Rehabilitation, 12*, 233–256.

Franche, R. L., Corbière, M., Lee, H., Breslin, F. C., & Hepburn, C. G. (2007). The Readiness for Return-To-Work (RRTW) scale: Development and validation of a self-report staging scale in lost-time claimants with musculoskeletal disorders. *Journal of Occupational Rehabilitation, 17*, 450–472.

Park J. (2017). *Motivational interviewing and injured workers: Facilitating behaviour change in work rehabilitation*. PhD thesis, University of Alberta.

Pransky, G., Gatchel, R., Linton, S. J., & Loisel, P. (2005). Improving return to work research. *Journal of Occupational Rehabilitation, 15*, 453–457.

Prochaska, J. O., Velicer, W. F., Rossi, J. S., et al. (1994). Stages of change and decisional balance for 12 problem behaviors. *Health Psychology, 13*, 39–46.

Young, A. E., Roessler, R. T., Wasiak, R., McPherson, K. M., van Poppel, M. N., & Anema, J. R. (2005). A developmental conceptualization of return to work. *Journal of Occupational Rehabilitation, 15*, 557–568.

RE-AIM Guidelines

Paul Estabrooks[1], Samantha M. Harden[2] and Kacie Allen Blackman[2]
[1]Department of Health Promotions, University of Nebraska Medical Center, Omaha, NE, USA
[2]Department of Human Nutrition, Foods, and Exercise, Virginia Tech, Blacksburg, VA, USA

Synonyms

Evaluation of potential public health impact; Implementation science; Internal and external validity issues; Translational research

Definition

RE-AIM is a planning and evaluation framework that addresses the five dimensions of **r**each, **e**ffectiveness, **a**doption, **i**mplementation, **m**aintenance (Glasgow et al. 1999). Interventions are defined broadly as community programs, clinical practices, environmental changes, and policy approaches. Reach is an individual-level measure and defined as the number, percent, and representativeness of participants, and in some cases, ongoing reach such as the dose or receipt of intervention components (c.f. Harden et al. 2014). Efficacy or effectiveness is defined as the individual-level change in the primary outcome, impact on quality of life, and assessment of potential negative outcomes. Adoption is a setting-level indicator and defined as the number, percent, and representativeness of settings and delivery personnel who agree to deliver an intervention. Setting-level implementation determines the cost of, and extent to which, the intervention is delivered as intended. Finally, maintenance is conceptualized at both the individual and setting level. At the individual level, maintenance is the degree to which behavior changes are sustained 6 months or longer after the intervention is complete. At the setting level, maintenance is the extent to which an intervention is sustained over time (c.f. Glasgow et al. 1999 and www.re-aim.org).

Description

The RE-AIM framework was developed to improve health behavior intervention reporting by also considering external validity during intervention planning and evaluation (Glasgow et al. 1999). The underlying proposition was that evidence that is contextual, practical, and robust is more likely to facilitate the translation of health behavior interventions into typical clinical or community practice. Further, considering each of the RE-AIM dimensions during the planning phase is hypothesized to result in interventions that can be widely adopted by different sites and personnel, have the ability for sustained and consistent implementation at a reasonable cost, reach large numbers of people (especially those who can most benefit), and produce replicable and long-lasting effects with minimal negative impacts (Glasgow and Emmons 2007; Harden et al. 2018; Klesges et al. 2005).

RE-AIM is one of the most frequently cited frameworks in dissemination and implementation grant applications at the National Institutes of Health (Kessler et al. 2013) and has been applied across a range of behavioral and health-related outcomes behavior interventions (Gaglio et al. 2013). Early reviews of the literature using the RE-AIM framework indicated that there was a paucity of focus on external validity-related dimensions (e.g., representativeness related to reach and adoption; Glasgow et al. 2004). More recently, reporting in these areas has improved, however, the degree to which RE-AIM dimensions have been consistently operationalized across studies is low (Harden et al. 2015). As a result, comparisons of relative reach, adoption, implementation, and maintenance are challenging (Harden et al. 2014). Most recently, a pragmatic focus on RE-AIM attempts to operationalize the framework using existing data and organizational goals to determine the relative value of assessment of each dimension for decision-making across a variety of settings (Estabrooks and Allen 2013; Glasgow and Estabrooks 2018; Harden et al. 2018). The remainder of this chapter will be dedicated to outlining pragmatic guidelines and operational definitions for each RE-AIM dimension.

Reach

Determining the number of individuals who participate in or are exposed to a given intervention is relatively straight forward. However, determining an appropriate denominator to calculate participation rate can be more difficult. In one study, investigators explored four indicators regarding reach of an older adult physical activity program that was delivered via DVD for 6-months (Harden et al. 2014). This study was conducted in a community where 105, 515 individuals may have been exposed to at least one of the recruitment strategies (e.g., newspaper, newsletter, radio announcement). During the intervention, 563 individuals responded to the recruitment strategies, 383 were determined to be eligible for intervention, and 307 individuals participated. In some cases, this would be reported as an 80% reach (307 of the 383). However, using the most conservative denominator, the total number exposed to recruitment was estimated at 105,515 with 307 final participants resulting in a study reach of 0.3%. The costs and types of recruitment strategies were deemed appropriate for this target audience, and the participants were representative (e.g., location in Illinois, race) of the target audience, with the exception of sex (participants were more likely to be female) and age (those who responded were more likely to be less than 65 years of age, and therefore ineligible). Finally, from months 1 to 6, DVD viewing *and* reporting decreased across the 6-month intervention. Taken together, ongoing reach data proved to be difficult to collect as it was participant self-reported, but costs and exposure data were more readily available via research records.

Efficacy or Effectiveness

Methods to determine the efficacy or effectiveness of a behavioral intervention have been exhaustively covered by other authors (e.g., Flay 1986). Briefly, a comparison of the ability of an intervention(s) to change a primary study outcome either under optimal or more real-world conditions provides estimates of efficacy or effectiveness, respectively. The comparison of changes in quality of life adds a dimension to effectiveness that allows a more patient-centered perspective and standardization for comparison across interventions targeting different primary outcomes. The focus on unintended negative consequences can range from issues related to safety or changes the reduction of one health behavior in favor of increasing another (e.g., adding a fruit and vegetable intervention to an ongoing physical activity intervention could reduce the effectiveness in terms of changes in physical activity (Doerksen and Estabrooks 2007)). Other issues related to improving the external validity of documenting effectiveness include assessment of differential attrition across participants with different demographic profiles and the use intention-to-treat analyses.

Adoption

A simple example of analyzing staff adoption rates can be found through an adoption randomized controlled trial in which county-based health educators (HEs) were assigned to deliver FitEx or Active Living Every Day (ALED). FitEx is a statewide walking program adapted specifically for the system in which the HEs worked, whereas ALED was developed by a research institute and packaged for translation in their system. Training contact and dose for each program was the same for all HEs. Fourteen of the 18 HEs assigned to FitEx (77%) adopted the program whereas only 2 of the 18 HEs assigned to ALED (11%) adopted the program. Furthermore, and in alignment with recommendations for fully employing RE-AIM (Kessler et al. 2014), qualitative data regarding adoption or non-adoption were collected (Johnson et al. 2015). This work complemented the quantitative data and found that HE perceived FitEx to be more adaptable to their county and needs.

Implementation

Implementation includes costs of and the degree to which the intervention was delivered as intended. Reilly et al. (2018) examined the degree to which a state policy to label food based on nutrient content as green, yellow, or red (i.e., traffic light approach; green go, yellow slow, red mostly no) was assessed. In the study, they examined three different implementation strategies and found that higher intensive implementation strategies trended towards higher adherence to the state level policy. When cost was considered more intensive, implementation strategies cost nearly twice the amount per school as the lower intensity option. However, when cost was considered relative to effectiveness in policy change, the lower intensity option was nearly twice the cost of the higher intensity option (Reilly et al. 2018).

Maintenance

It is recommended to gather data on individual- and system-level maintenance 6 months after the intervention ends. Perri et al. (2014) provide excellent examples of assessing individual level maintenance. In their studies, participants randomly assigned to different intensities of weight loss interventions delivered in rural sites were followed for 2 years (18 months after the initial 6-month weight loss intervention). They found that participants in medium and high intensity programs lost approximately 10 kg and sustained approximately two thirds of that weight loss 18 months later. They also examined cost effectiveness and found that the moderate intensity version was favored over low or high intensity versions of the intervention. Organizational level maintenance has been less studied to date, but Estabrooks and colleagues examined the potential to sustain physical activity programs for older adults to be more likely when the intervention strategies were integrated into organizational resources, job descriptions, and values (Estabrooks et al. 2011).

There is some interest in understanding how the dimensions of RE-AIM may interact to generate a significant public health impact (Glasgow et al. 2006). Specifically, it may be necessary to investigate the interplay between reach, effectiveness, and cost of adoption, implementation, and maintenance to inform public health practice related to multilevel health behavior/education interventions and policy decisions. The combination of Reach x Effectiveness measures the impact at the individual level primary outcome. A median effect size (ES) summary measure calculates an overall effectiveness score. The impact of an intervention treatment may vary between subgroups (e.g., gender, geographical location, and age). If the intervention effect is similar regardless of the participant characteristic of interest, the median $ES_{differential\ impact}$ will be low (close to zero) and specifies robust effectiveness. Next Intervention effectiveness can be calculated by identifying the median ES across primary outcome measure then subtracting the median ES for negative outcomes and the median $ES_{differential\ impact}$. Lastly, to calculate the composite estimate of individual level impact (RxE), multiply the composite estimate for reach x composite intervention effectiveness. For example, R × E = 100 participants/200 eligible and invited to participate × 0.2 effect size (ES) on total physical activity minutes, which is a RE of 0.1 which indicates that minimal or no difference across subgroups. To calculate the attributable population level impact of an intervention, multiply the individual level impact (RE) by the prevalence of a problem. For example, in a survey of 2000 women who gave birth in Wyoming in 2017, a total of 20 reported having gestational diabetes. Calculate the prevalence of gestational diabetes in this group (20 new and pre-existing cases)/(2000 US population) × 100 = 1%. If the individual level impact is 0.2, then multiply by 0.01 to yield an attributable individual level impact of 0.002. The RE "efficiency" assists decision makers in deciding on adopting a given program. It is calculated by dividing the cost of an intervention by its individual level impact. For example, RE "efficiency" would be calculated as the cost of an intervention ($5000) divided by individual level Impact (0.2) = 25,000. Glasgow and colleagues (2006) propose these types of interaction measurements for the other RE-AIM dimensions as well.

These operational definitions of constructs within the framework, examples across health promotion interventions, and suggested interaction calculations may lead to the pragmatic application of RE-AIM to inform decision-making and generalizability across practice settings and, ultimately, impact public health.

References and Further Reading

Almeida, F. A., Smith-Ray, R. L., Van Den Berg, R., Schriener, P., Gonzales, M., Onda, P., et al. (2005). Utilizing a simple stimulus control strategy to increase physician referrals for physical activity promotion. *Journal of Sport & Exercise Psychology, 27*(4), 505–514.

Doerksen, S. E., & Estabrooks, P. E. (2007). Brief fruit and vegetable messages integrated within a community physical activity program successfully change behavior. *International Journal of Behavioral Nutrition and Physical Activity, 4*, 12. https://doi.org/10.1186/1479-5868-4-12.

Estabrooks, P. A., & Allen, K. C. (2013). Updating, employing, and adapting: A commentary on what does it mean to "employ" the RE-AIM model. *Evaluation & the Health Professions, 36*(1), 67–72. https://doi.org/10.1177/0163278712460546. Epub 2012 Oct 8.

Estabrooks, P. A., & Gyurcsik, N. C. (2003). Evaluating the impact of behavioral interventions that target physical activity: Issues of generalizability and public health. *Psychology of Sport and Exercise, 4*(1), 41–55.

Estabrooks, P. A., Bradshaw, M., Dzewaltowski, D. A., & Smith-Ray, R. L. (2008). Determining the impact of Walk Kansas: Applying a team-building approach to community physical activity promotion. *Annals of Behavioral Medicine, 36*(1), 1–12.

Estabrooks, P. A., Smith-Ray, R. L., Dzewaltowski, D. A., Dowdy, D., Lattimore, D., Rheaume, C., et al. (2011). Sustainability of evidence-based community-based physical activity programs for older adults: Lessons from active for life. *Translational Behavioral Medicine, 1*(2), 208–215. https://doi.org/10.1007/s13142-011-0039-x.

Flay, B. R. (1986). Efficacy and effectiveness trials (and other phases of research) in the development of health promotion programs. *Preventive Medicine, 15*(5), 451–474.

Gaglio, B., Shoup, J. A., & Glasgow, R. E. (2013). The RE-AIM framework: A systematic review of use over time. *American Journal of Public Health, 103*(6), e38–e46. https://doi.org/10.2105/AJPH.2013.301299. Epub 2013 Apr 18.

Glasgow, R. E., & Emmons, K. M. (2007). How can we increase translation of research into practice? Types of evidence needed. *Annual Review of Public Health, 28*, 413–433.

Glasgow, R. E., & Estabrooks, P. E. (2018). Pragmatic applications of RE-AIM for health care initiatives in community and clinical settings. *Preventing Chronic Disease.* 2018, 15, 170271. https://doi.org/10.5888/pcd15.170271.

Glasgow, R. E., Vogt, T. M., & Boles, S. M. (1999). Evaluating the public health impact of health promotion interventions: The RE-AIM framework. *American Journal of Public Health, 89*(9), 1322–1327.

Glasgow, R. E., Klesges, L. M., Dzewaltowski, D. A., Bull, S. S., & Estabrooks, P. (2004). The future of health behavior change research: What is needed to improve translation of research into health promotion practice? *Annals of Behavioral Medicine, 27*(1), 3–12.

Glasgow, R. E., Klesges, L. M., Dzewaltowski, D. A., Estabrooks, P. A., & Vogt, T. M. (2006a). Evaluating the impact of health promotion programs: Using the RE-AIM framework to form summary measures for decision making involving complex issues. *Health Education Research, 21*(5), 688–694.

Glasgow, R. E., Nelson, C. C., Strycker, L. A., & King, D. K. (2006b). Using RE-AIM metrics to evaluate diabetes self-management support interventions. *American Journal of Preventive Medicine, 30*(1), 67–73.

Harden, S. M., Fanning, J. T., Motl, R. W., McAuley, E., & Estabrooks, P. A. (2014). Determining the reach of a home-based physical activity program for older adults within the context of a randomized controlled trial. *Health Education Research, 29*(5), 861–869. https://doi.org/10.1093/her/cyu049.

Harden, S. M., Smith, M. L., Ory, M. G., Smith-Ray, R. L., Estabrooks, P. A., & Glasgow, R. E. (2018). RE-AIM in clinical, community, and corporate settings: Perspectives, strategies, and recommendations to enhance public health impact. *Frontiers in Public Health, 6*, 71. https://doi.org/10.3389/fpubh.2018.00071.

Johnson, S. B., Harden, S. M., & Estabrooks, P. A. (2016). Uptake of evidence-based physical activity programs: Comparing perceptions of adopters and nonadopters. *Translational Behavioral Medicine, 6*(4), 629–637. https://doi.org/10.1007/s13142-015-0371-7.

Kessler, R. S., Purcell, E. P., Glasgow, R. E., Klesges, K. M., Benkeser, R. M., & Peek, C. J. (2013). What does it mean to "employ" the RE-AIM model? *Evaluation & the Health Professions, 36*(1), 44–66. https://doi.org/10.1177/0163278712446066.

Klesges, L. M., Estabrooks, P. A., Dzewaltowski, D. A., Bull, S. S., & Glasgow, R. E. (2005). Beginning with the application in mind: Designing and planning health behavior change interventions to enhance dissemination. *Annals of Behavioral Medicine, 29*, 66–75.

Perri, M. G., Limacher, M. C., von Castel-Roberts, K., Daniels, M. J., Durning, P. E., Janicke, D. M., et al. (2014). Comparative effectiveness of three doses of weight-loss counseling: Two-year findings from the rural LITE trial. *Obesity (Silver Spring), 22*(11), 2293–2300. https://doi.org/10.1002/oby.20832.

Reilly, K. L., Reeves, P., Deeming, S., Yoong, S. L., Wolfenden, L., Nathan, N., & Wiggers, J. (2018). Economic analysis of three interventions of different intensity in improving school implementation of a government healthy canteen policy in Australia: Costs, incremental and relative cost effectiveness. *BMC Public Health, 18*(1), 378. https://doi.org/10.1186/s12889-018-5315-y.

Schillinger, D., Handley, M., Wang, F., & Hammer, H. (2009). Effects of self-management support on structure, process, and outcomes among vulnerable patients with diabetes: A three-arm practical clinical trial. *Diabetes Care, 32*(4), 559–566.

Stetler, C. B., Mittman, B. S., & Francis, J. (2008). Overview of the VA Quality Enhancement Research Initiative (QUERI) and QUERI theme articles: QUERI series. *Implementation Science, 3*, 8. www.re-aim.org.

Real-Life Blood Pressure Monitoring

▶ Ambulatory Blood Pressure

Reasons

▶ Attribution Theory

Recessive Inheritance

Laura Rodriguez-Murillo[1] and Rany M. Salem[2,3]
[1]Department of Psychiatry, Columbia University Medical Center, New York, NY, USA
[2]Broad Institute, Cambridge, MA, USA
[3]Cambridge Center, Cambridge, MA, USA

Definition

A trait that is inherited in a recessive fashion only manifests phenotypically in homozygous individuals, i.e., when the individual has two copies of the same recessive allele. Humans have two versions of all autosomal genes, called alleles, one from each parent. The recessive trait is hidden in the heterozygous individual (Dd) if the other allele is inherited in a dominant fashion, and so this person is a called a "carrier" of the recessive allele, but does not manifest the disease or trait. A recessive trait can only be passed to the offspring if both parents carry (Dd or dd) and transmit the recessive allele to their offspring. In the scenario where both parents are heterozygous carriers of the recessive trait, the children have 25% chance of inheriting two copies (dd) of the recessive allele and exhibiting the recessive trait (see pedigree figure, Fig. 1). An example of a disease with a recessive inheritance is Tay-Sachs disease that occurs when a child has two defective copies of the HEXA gene, neither of which can be successfully transcribed and form a functional enzyme product (Myerowitz and Costigan 1988).

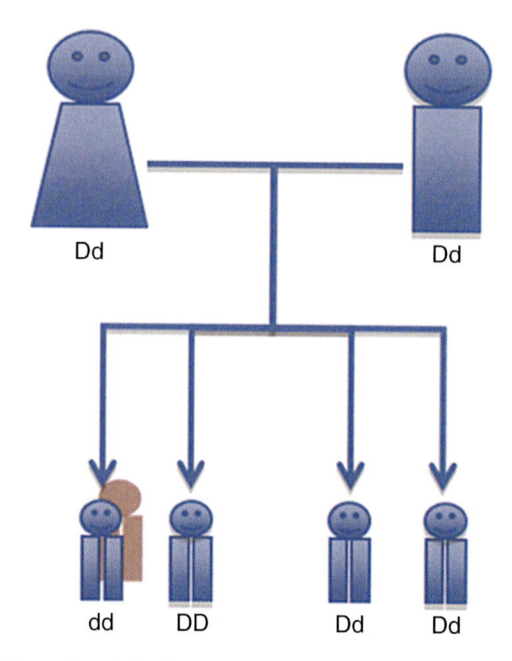

Recessive Inheritance, Fig. 1 Recessive inheritance diagram. Highlighted individuals are affected by the disease after inheriting one recessive allele from each carrier parent (dd)

Cross-References

▶ Allele
▶ Dominant Inheritance
▶ Gene
▶ Genotype
▶ Heterozygous
▶ Homozygous

References and Further Reading

Lewis, R. (2005). *Human genetics. Concepts and applications* (7th ed.). Boston: McGraw-Hill Science/Engineering/Math.
Myerowitz, R., & Costigan, F. C. (1988). The major defect in Ashkenazi Jews with Tay-Sachs disease is an insertion in the gene for the alpha-chain of beta-hexosaminidase. *Journal of Biological Chemistry, 263*(35), 18587–18589.
Strachan, T., & Read, A. P. (2003). *Human molecular genetics* (3rd ed.). London/New York: Garland Science/Taylor & Francis Group.

Recognition (Means of Acknowledgment)

▶ Respect

Recruitment and Retention of Research Subjects

J. Rick Turner
Campbell University College of Pharmacy and Health Sciences, Buies Creek, NC, USA

Synonyms

Recruitment of research participants

Definition

Recruitment of research subjects is the process by which individuals are recruited as potential subjects in a research study. Upon learning full details of the study by reading the Informed Consent Form, eligible individuals may or may not decide to participate: Nonetheless, they have participated in the process of recruitment.

Description

While individual investigators can play an important role in subject recruitment – their access to potential subjects likely having been a reason for their being selected to participate in the trial – the primary responsibility for subject recruitment can fall on the principal investigator/holder of the grant that is funding the behavioral medicine research study. For all but the smallest studies, creation and implementation of a recruitment strategy and plan is an important and potentially critical operational step. This plan should be a formal written document that carefully considers best-case and worst-case scenarios, takes into account various timing influences (e.g., national holidays and typical vacation periods, seasons of the year, likely onset of flu season), and has contingencies built in to address all anticipated potential recruitment barriers.

Spilker (2009) provided the following operational definition of recruitment:

- Identifying potential pools of subjects and specific individual subjects who may be eligible to enroll in the trial.
- Attracting those individuals to consider participation.
- Discussing the trial with them.
- Prescreening subjects.
- Having subjects read an informed consent form, answering any questions they may have, and then having the subjects sign the consent form.
- Conducting a more complete and formal screening procedure.
- Being able to state that subjects are now enrolled in the trial.

Recruitment is of ongoing interest to a principal investigator throughout a trial, and there are several common metrics addressing this. One is "first subject first visit," the date on which the first subject completes his or her first visit to the investigational site. In cases where there are multiple investigational sites another metric of interest is the date when 50% of the sites have each enrolled at least one subject.

Traditional subject recruitment strategies include the following:

- Advertisements on radio and television, and in print media.
- Mailing flyers to individuals and patient advocacy groups.
- Data mining from insurance company databases.
- Using web sites to publicize the trial.
- Posting information on a hospital's bulletin board.
- Hospital staff wearing lapel pins that bring attention to the trial.

Cabell (2009) recently discussed another approach that focuses on understanding and utilizing the "patient pathway," the route by which patients receive treatment. By understanding and documenting the pathway via which patients with the disease or condition of clinical concern receive their current medical care, it becomes possible for recruitment specialists to reach out to clinicians and other behavioral medicine specialists who provide the care. This allows the specialists to access the appropriate patients and, should they be willing, recruit them as subjects for the trial.

While this entry focuses primarily on subject recruitment, it has become widely accepted that principal investigators need to devote considerable resources to subject retention as well as recruitment: The ultimate goal is for an enrolled subject to complete participation in the trial. Many characteristics of a subject's participation in the trial can influence the likelihood that he or she will complete the trial, including:

- The length of the treatment period. All subjects have personal and professional lives, and events that preclude trial completion – personal or family illness, relocating, financial difficulties – do and will happen. Some trials have relatively long treatment periods, and the researcher cannot alter this, but the length should alert the researcher to the need for appropriate contingency plans.
- How onerous participation is. If the trial's protocol requires subjects to undergo many procedures at many visits, withdrawal rate may increase. The burden of the trial should be considered at the protocol development phase, with an eye to decreasing noncritical subject tasks, such as filling out a large number of questionnaires that do not address the primary objective.
- Ease of traveling to the investigational site(s). If many subjects participating at a given site have to travel a considerable distance, and/or at considerable expense, each time they visit the site, the PI is well advised to address this proactively.

Specific retention strategies include:

- Providing reimbursement for expenses such as parking, meals, and babysitting.
- Calling subjects shortly before each visit to remind and assure them that provisions for their attendance are in place.
- Paying for, or actually providing transportation to and from the site.
- Providing escorts from and back to a parking lot, particularly if it is not well lighted, and/or in bad weather.
- Optimizing the environment in the subject waiting area. This can include having sufficient and appropriate magazines that are not 5 years out of date, providing toys for children who accompany subjects out of necessity, and ensuring that all trial staff treat the subjects courteously at all times.
- Reminding the subjects throughout the trial that their participation is extremely valuable in evaluating a new behavioral medicine intervention that, if successful, may provide considerable benefit to many patients. This can be done verbally and also by sending out regular newsletters.

Cross-References

▶ Informed Consent

References and Further Reading

Cabell, C. (2009). Patient recruitment: Are we looking in the right place? *International Pharmaceutical Industry*, Summer issue, 38–41.

Spilker, B. (2009). *Guide to drug development: A comprehensive review and assessment*. Philadelphia: Wolters Kluwer/Lippincott Williams & Wilkins.

Recruitment of Research Participants

▶ Recruitment and Retention of Research Subjects

Recurrence Risk Ratio

Jennifer Wessel
Public Health, School of Medicine, Indiana University, Indianapolis, IN, USA

Definition

Recurrence risk ratio is a measure of familial aggregation of disease. When a genetic factor(s) cannot be measured directly, information on disease status among family members of an affected individual can be used to derive a genetic risk ratio. It can provide a rationale for performing genetic studies to identify the susceptibility alleles and has been used extensively in the mapping of complex diseases. The recurrence risk ratio, λ_R, is the ratio of disease manifestation in other family members to the affected individual compared with the disease prevalence in the general population.

The sibling recurrence risk ratio is commonly used, where the numerator would represent the risk of manifesting the disease given that one's sibling is affected:

$$\lambda S = \frac{\Pr(D \text{ in a sibling/ affected case})}{K}$$

where K is the prevalence of the disease in the general population.

Cross-References

▶ Allele
▶ Gene

References and Further Reading

Risch, N. (1990a). Linkage strategies for genetically complex traits. I. Multilocus models. *American Journal of Human Genetics, 46*, 222–228.
Risch, N. (1990b). Linkage strategies for genetically complex traits. II. The power of affected relative pairs. *American Journal of Human Genetics, 46*, 229–241.

Regression Analysis

J. Rick Turner
Campbell University College of Pharmacy and Health Sciences, Buies Creek, NC, USA

Synonyms

Linear regression; Multiple regression; Regression modeling

Definition

In regression analysis it is assumed that a change in variable x will lead to a change in variable y. It is often the case that the researcher wishes to predict the value of y for a given value of x (Campbell et al. 2007).

Consider the case of linear regression and the plotting of a fitted regression line. In cases where linear regression is appropriate there is only one independent variable. Conventionally, the dependent variable is plotted on the vertical axis (y-axis) and the independent variable is plotted on the horizontal axis (x-axis). The equation $y = \alpha + \beta x$ is defined as the linear regression equation. Alpha (α) is the intercept, and Beta (β) is the regression coefficient (Greek letters are used to clarify that these are population parameters). The regression equation is a model that is used to describe or model the relationship between y and x. When the graph is plotted, alpha is the value of the equation when $x = 0$, and beta is the slope of the line drawn (plotted). An increase of x of one unit will be associated with a change in y of beta units.

A set of data is used to create the plot, and then to draw the regression line. Imagine a set of data describing hemoglobin levels and age in a set of 20 women. The individual subjects' data can be represented as a set of 20 paired observations, and these points can be plotted on the graph. The best fitting linear regression line is then drawn. This line enables the determination of alpha and beta. Then, for any value of x, the appropriate value of y as given by this model can be calculated.

Since outcomes in behavioral medicine research are often influenced by more than one independent variable, the linear regression model can easily be extended to the technique of multiple regression. Multiple regression can address various questions of interest, including examination of the relationship between continuous variables while allowing for a third variable, and adjusting for differences in confounding factors between experimental groups (Machin et al. 2007). Examples are provided in the "References and Readings" section of this entry.

Cross-References

▶ Data
▶ Experimental Group
▶ Multivariate Analysis
▶ Univariate Analysis

References and Further Reading

Campbell, M. J., Machin, D., & Walters, S. J. (2007). *Medical statistics: A textbook for the health sciences* (4th ed.). Chichester: Wiley.
Naicker, N., Richter, L., Mathee, A., Becker, P., & Norris, S. A. (2011). Environmental lead exposure and sociobehavioral adjustment in the early teens: The birth to twenty cohort. *Science of the Total Environment, 414*, 120–125.
Smith, K. J., Blizzard, L., McNaughton, S. A., Gall, S. L., Dwyer, T., & Venn, A. J. (2011). Takeaway food consumption and cardio-metabolic risk factors in young adults. *European Journal of Clinical Nutrition*. (Epub ahead of print).
Soureti, A., Hurling, R., van Mechelen, W., Cobain, M., & Chinapaw, M. (2011). Moderators of the mediated effect of intentions, planning, and saturated-fat intake in obese individuals. *Health Psychology*. (Epub ahead of print).

Regression Modeling

▶ Regression Analysis

Regulation of Expression

▶ Gene Expression

Rehabilitation

Bengt H. Sjölund
University of Southern Denmark, Odense, DK, Denmark

Synonyms

Habilitation

Definition

According to the World Report on Disability, rehabilitation is "a set of measures that assist individuals who experience, or are likely to experience, disability to achieve and maintain optimal functioning in interaction with their environments" (World Health Organization [WHO] 2011).

Description

Rehabilitation literally means "redressing" (*Latin habitat – dress*). While there are many definitions of this concept, the world health organization (WHO) has defined rehabilitation as "a process aimed at enabling disabled persons to reach and maintain their optimal physical, sensory, intellectual, psychological and social functional levels. Rehabilitation provides disabled people with the tools they need to attain independence and self-determination." Thus, the aim of rehabilitation has traditionally been seen as facilitating the normalization of human functioning after injury, disease, or due to congenital defects. It is usually said to comprise a number of coordinated measures of medical, psychological, social, educational and vocational nature. The Convention of the Rights of Persons with Disabilities, in its article 26 calls for "appropriate measures ... to enable persons with disabilities to attain and maintain their maximum independence, full physical, mental, social and vocational ability, and full inclusion and participation in all aspects of life" (United Nations 2006).

Background. Modern rehabilitation originated in British experiences of people with spinal cord injuries during the Second World War, where the neurosurgeon Dr. Ludwig Guttmann at Stoke-Mandeville pioneered the development of reliable rehabilitation programs for those with paraplegia and tetraplegia. Apart from crisis intervention, these programs placed strong emphasis on conservative treatment of the spinal fractures and on preventive measures, such as prophylactic bed positioning to avoid pressure sores, to empty the urinary bladder at regular intervals, and to train adequate techniques for breathing and coughing in high injuries. Effective techniques for independently taking care of personal hygiene as well as transferring were also developed, e.g., between a bed, a chair, and a wheelchair, including the effective handling of transport vehicles. After post-acute rehabilitation, a lifelong follow-up ensued. The result was that the remaining number of life years increased from 1 to 2 years after the injury (even in young people), to today's normal life span for a paraplegic person, usually at an independent level, and a moderately reduced life span for the tetraplegic person, as a rule partly dependent.

In the mid-twentieth century, Physical and Rehabilitation Medicine (PRM) was established as an independent specialty in Western health care. It currently defines itself as "concerned with the promotion of physical and cognitive functioning, behavior, quality of life (activities and participation) and with the prevention, diagnosis, treatment and rehabilitation management of people with disabling medical conditions and co-morbidity across all ages" (Gutenbrunner et al. 2007).

Rehabilitation services have gradually been expanded to include people disabled by stroke, neurological disease, traumatic brain injury, chronic pain, cardiac and pulmonary insufficiency, cancer, mental disorders, and other disabling conditions. Generally speaking, rehabilitation can be considered a re-adaptive process, where the disabled person adapts his/her set of values to a different, more restricted life situation. Originally, rehabilitation was based on a biomedical model, where problems in functioning of an individual were seen as due to a deviation from "normal" organ function. In the 1970s, the social model of disability was launched by disabled people's organizations, where problems in functioning were instead viewed as society's exclusion (by its design and organization) of such persons. These models have more recently been replaced by the biopsychosocial model of disability, recognizing biological as well as social factors (ICF, WHO 2001). This model is now acknowledged among both organizations of people with disabilities and among professional organizations.

The Interdisciplinary Team

It was recognized that many different health professions apart from physicians and nurses were necessary in the daily work to fulfill the multiple needs of people receiving rehabilitation services. This led to the development of *rehabilitation teams*, supervised by the rehabilitation physician. Today, these teams ideally contain psychologists (with cognitive-behavioral or neuropsychological background), physiotherapists, occupational therapists, social workers, nurses and sometimes vocational specialists, speech therapists, and recreational therapists. The expected norm in such *interdisciplinary* teams is group decision making, both in assessment, rehabilitation planning, and treatment. In the team, the disabled person is considered the most important member, both in planning and in decision making.

Rehabilitation Strategies

Common rehabilitation strategies are used, where the various team professionals contribute important components. The team members share responsibility for the rehabilitation given. The team conference, led by anyone of the team members, is the important forum for lateral communication and for decision making. A comprehensive rehabilitation plan is formulated, where time frames, types of intervention, and responsible therapists are given, all communicated to and agreed with the disabled person. This concept allows a free exchange of ideas, may benefit from group synergies in problem solving, and facilitates the use of common strategies and coordination. However, it can be time consuming and the team members need training in the team process.

Disability Assessment, Rehabilitation and the ICF

An important part of the work is disability assessment, usually with a team approach, and greatly helped by the development of the International Classification of Functioning, Disability and Health (ICF) (WHO 2001). Special rating instruments provide supplementary information in this task. The ICF is based on the biopsychosocial model and is a *components of health* classification. It has advanced the understanding and assessment of disability in that it classifies both problems in human functioning (health conditions) and the context in which people with different levels of functioning live and act. The problems are characterized in three interconnected areas:

- *Impairments* are problems in body function or structure such as a significant deviation or loss.
- *Activity limitations* are difficulties an individual may have in executing activities.
- *Participation restrictions* are problems an individual may experience in involvement in life situations.

It is the *interaction* between a health condition and contextual factors, both environmental and personal that may be experienced as a *disability*. *Environmental factors* make up the physical, social, and attitudinal environment in which people live and conduct their lives, whereas *personal factors* are the particular background of an individual's life and living, and may include gender, race, age, other health conditions, fitness, lifestyle, habits, upbringing, coping styles, social background, education, profession, past and current experience, overall behavior pattern and character style, individual psychological assets, and other characteristics.

Disability and Rehabilitation. Defining disability as an interaction means that disability is no longer the attribute of the person (World Report on Disability; WHO and World Bank 2011). The prevalence of disability in different countries varies greatly, not only due to differences in definitions but also in context, including cultural values. The current definition of rehabilitation (supra), "a set of measures that assist individuals who experience, or are likely to experience, disability to achieve and maintain optimal functioning in interaction with their environments," emphasizes firstly that disability is something experienced, i.e., subjective, and secondly that changing an individual's environment, e.g., by housing adaptation or by educating the family to change attitudes, is also part of rehabilitation. Consequently, rehabilitation is cross-sectional and often carried out by health professionals in cooperation with specialists on education, social welfare and employment. The fact that disability is seen as a subjective experience may also explain the core role of cognitive therapy as an important component in many rehabilitation programs, where modifications of thought patterns along with influencing the links between the individual's thoughts, emotions, and behaviors is vital.

ICF and Rehabilitation. It is obvious with the evolution of the ICF as a conceptual model and the disability concept that rehabilitation should be defined in relation to these notions. An attempt to do so was elaborated in cooperation with several professional rehabilitation organizations by Stucki et al. (2007) and importantly, further developed by integrating the perspective of the disabled person to describe rehabilitation as a health strategy (Meyer et al. 2011) (Table 1).

Community-Based Rehabilitation

If there are few health professional resources such as in developing countries, *community-based rehabilitation* (CBR) performed locally by community groups, health assistants, families, and friends may be an alternative (Chatterjee et al. 2003; Gona et al. 2010; Dalal et al. 2010). CBR

Rehabilitation, Table 1 ICF-based conceptual description of rehabilitation strategy, modified version (ICF terms are marked in bold; from Meyer et al. 2011 with permission)

Rehabilitation is the health strategy which, based on WHO's **integrative model** of **functioning, disability and health** applies and integrates
Approaches to assess **functioning** in light of **health conditions**
Approaches to optimize a **person's capacity**
Approaches that build on and strengthen the resources of the **person**
Approaches that provide a **facilitating environment**
Approaches that develop a **person's performance**
Approaches that enhance a person's health-related quality of life in partnership between person and provider and in appreciation of the person's perception of his or her position in life over the course of a **health condition** and in all age groups; along and across the continuum of care, including hospitals, rehabilitation facilities and the community, and across sectors, including health, education, labor and social affairs; with the goal to enable persons with **health conditions** experiencing or likely to experience **disability** to achieve and maintain optimal **functioning**

started in Europe as rehabilitation in the home or in the work place in the 1970s as a cheaper alternative to institution-based rehabilitation and has spread rapidly in low-income countries, often advocated and performed by human rights activists and non-health professionals working with development with the additional goal to transform and strengthen local communities in third world countries.

The Effectiveness of Rehabilitation

The evidence base for the effectiveness of modern rehabilitation is now considerable, e.g., for traumatic brain injury and stroke (Cicerone et al. 2011), spinal cord injury (Martin Ginis et al. 2010), chronic musculoskeletal pain (Norlund et al. 2009; Schonstein et al. 2003), cardiac insufficiency (Dalal et al. 2010), breast cancer (Duijts et al. 2011), and some mental diseases (Twamley et al. 2003).

In summary, rehabilitation as the health strategy of functioning represents a unique health service delivery system that contributes markedly to restoring and maintaining health for people with disabilities in most developed countries, but has insufficient resources in others. It is often substituted by voluntary community-based services in developing countries. Since many of the functional disturbances treated emanates from the nervous system, the rapidly expanding new neurobiology, having demonstrated plasticity, regeneration, and adult-born neural stem cells in adult man, will provide fascinating new therapeutical possibilities for the rehabilitation of persons with disabilities in the years to come.

Cross-References

▶ Occupational Therapy
▶ Physiotherapy

References and Readings

Chatterjee, S., Patel, V., Chatterjee, A., & Weiss, H. A. (2003). Evaluation of a community-based rehabilitation model for chronic schizophrenia in rural India. *The British Journal of Psychiatry, 182*, 57–62.

Cicerone, K. D., Langenbahn, D. M., Braden, C., Malec, J. F., Kalmar, K., Fraas, M., Felicetti, T., et al. (2011). Evidence-based cognitive rehabilitation: Updated review of the literature from 2003 through. *Archives of Physical Medicine and Rehabilitation, 92*, 519–530.

Dalal, H. M., Zawada, A., Jolly, K., Moxham, T., & Taylor, R. S. (2010). Home based versus centre based cardiac rehabilitation: Cochrane systematic review and meta-analysis. *British Medical Journal, 340*, b5631. Review. Erratum in: BMJ. 2010;340:c1133.

Duijts, S. F., Faber, M. M., Oldenburg, H. S., van Beurden, M., & Aaronson, N. K. (2011). Effectiveness of behavioral techniques and physical exercise on psychosocial functioning and health-related quality of life in breast cancer patients and survivors – a meta-analysis. *Psycho-Oncology, 20*, 115–126.

Gona, J. K., Xiong, T., Muhit, M. A., Newton, C. R., & Hartley, S. (2010). Identification of people with disabilities using participatory rural appraisal and key informants: A pragmatic approach with action potential promoting validity and low cost. *Disability and Rehabilitation, 32*(1), 79–85.

Gutenbrunner, C., Ward, A. B., & Chamberlain, M. A. (Eds.). (2007). White book on physical and rehabilitation medicine in Europe. *Journal of Rehabilitation Medicine, 39*(Suppl. 45), 1–48.

Martin Ginis, K. A., Jetha, A., Mack, D. E., & Hetz, S. (2010). Physical activity and subjective well-being among people with spinal cord injury: A meta-analysis. *Spinal Cord, 48*, 65–72.

Meyer, T., Gutenbrunner, C., Bickenbach, J., Cieza, A., Melvin, J., & Stucki, G. (2011). Towards a conceptual description of rehabilitation as a health strategy. *Journal of Rehabilitation Medicine, 43*, 765–769.

Norlund, A., Ropponen, A., & Alexanderson, K. (2009). Multidisciplinary interventions: Review of studies of return to work after rehabilitation for low back pain. *Journal of Rehabilitation Medicine, 41*, 115–121.

Schonstein, E., Kenny, D. T., Keating, J., & Koes, B. W. (2003). Work conditioning, work hardening and functional restoration for workers with back and neck pain. *Cochrane Database of Systematic Reviews, 1*, CD001822.

Stucki, G., Cieza, A., & Melvin, J. (2007). The international classification of functioning, disability and health: A unifying model for the conceptual description of the rehabilitation strategy. *Journal of Rehabilitation Medicine, 39*, 279–285.

Twamley, E. W., Jeste, D. V., & Lehman, A. F. (2003). Vocational rehabilitation in schizophrenia and other psychotic disorders: A literature review and meta-analysis of randomized controlled trials. *The Journal of Nervous and Mental Disease, 191*, 515–523.

United Nations. (2006). *Convention on the rights of people with disabilities*. New York: Author. Retrieved November 14, 2006, from http://www.un.org/disabilities/convention/conventionfull.

World Health Organization (WHO). (2001). *ICF: International classification of functioning, disability and health*. Geneva: Author. September 3, 2011, Also available online, http://www.who.int/classifications/icf/en/.

World Health Organization (WHO), World Bank. (2011). *World report on disability*. Geneva: Author. Retrieved November 14, 2011, from http://www.who.int/disabilities/world_report/2011/en/.

Rehabilitation Psychology

▶ Psychosocial Adjustment

Relapse, Relapse Prevention

M. Kathleen B. Lustyk and Gabriana Navarrete
Department of Behavioral and Social Sciences, Embry–Riddle Aeronautical University, Prescott, AZ, USA

Synonyms

Remission and remission prevention

Definition

Relapse, as a clinical term, is the loss of ground gained towards positive behavior change or the return of problem behavior following a period of cessation. Not unlike a lapse, which is an initial setback or a single occurrence of the problem behavior, relapse is often associated with feelings of guilt and shame, and accompanied by self-degrading thoughts. Relapse prevention is an approach to therapy or education that helps one identify and anticipate triggers or precipitators of relapse. Relapse prevention also teaches behavioral coping strategies for managing high-risk situations in which triggers are present as well as coping strategies for urges, cravings, and negative emotional states that often precipitate relapse.

Description

With substance use disorders, relapse is the return to problematic substance use following a period of abstinence. Relapse is a major roadblock to treatment efficacy for substance use disorders because the majority of those trying to change addictive behaviors or attempt abstinence will relapse. Given what we know about the neurobiology of addiction, the high occurrence of relapse is not surprising. With substance use disorders, the brain's pleasure circuit is usurped such that what was once perceived as a pleasurable experience (e.g., drug use) becomes necessary to prevent a painful experience (i.e., withdrawal). The habit circuits involved in the addictive behaviors become entrained. For example, with habitual drug use, a trigger can produce a small amount of activity in the pleasure circuit and this pleasure "appetizer" can increase the desire or craving for the abused substance as well as the motivation to seek out and use the abused substance. Thus, triggers can tap the habit circuitry, which may ultimately result in relapse.

Triggers or high-risk precipitators of relapse often arise in interpersonal situations where people or the environment can serve as powerful reminders of the pleasure and behaviors that once sustained the addiction. For example, an abstinent alcoholic may find the pub they used to frequent a powerful cue for drinking. Stress and other negative emotional states may also serve as triggers, especially if the habitual behavior served as a coping strategy to reduce stress or improve negative affect. The powerful role that even a deleterious coping strategy can have on stress and affect has motivated the continued study and application of Harm Reduction methods for managed use for substance use disorders.

Harm Reduction Therapy takes on a much different approach in comparison to 12-step or other abstinence-based therapies. While abstinence may be the only approach that provides full protection from the adverse effects of substance use disorders, harm reduction strategies can help suffers manage problem behaviors such as substance use before abstinence is achieved or in its stead. Harm reduction focuses on changing behaviors and use in order to minimize the health, social, and economic impacts associated with problematic substance use. However, therapeutic progress takes on a different definition with Harm Reduction as managed use constitutes progress. Thus, unlike abstinence, those who suffer from addiction in harm reduction therapy continue with their usage but at a decreased and managed level. The thought is that a decreased consumption or usage will reduce the risks and subsequently result in a higher rate of success in the treatment for substance use disorders.

In the presence of a trigger, relapse is not inevitable but is more likely without therapy. The way in which a person with a substance use disorder approaches the trigger can have profound effects on the outcome. If, for example, a person with a substance use disorder find themselves in high-risk situations whereby triggers result in a lapse, they may respond by removing themselves from that situation and chalk it up to a learning experience such that they will need to face similar situations differently in the future. Conversely, one could suffer an abstinence violation effect whereby the person berates himself or herself for failing to remain abstinent. As such, an abstinence violation effect may compound the impact of negative affect on relapse if, for example, the suffer convinces themselves that they will never be successful in managing their addiction and give in to full relapse.

A primary goal of relapse prevention therapy is the identification and prevention of high-risk situations that may lead to the return of problematic behavior. Prevention may be achieved through the implementation of coping strategies that facilitate positive behavior changes aimed at enhancing self-efficacy, managing lapses, and restructuring thought processes (prolapse). In the case of substance use disorders, replace prevention reduces the return of substance misuse. One such strategy that has become a popular relapse prevention therapy for substance use disorders incorporates mindfulness. Mindfulness teaches one how to cultivate nonjudgmental, nonreactive present moment awareness. This type of awareness can allow for a kind of "space" between a person's sensations or feelings and their ultimate reaction to them. This space may ultimately break the habit cycle. Mindfulness-based relapse prevention therapy incorporates cognitive-behavioral Relapse Prevention skills with mindfulness training to increase awareness and skillful action in high-risk situations. Mindfulness-based relapse prevention therapy is an effective aftercare treatment for substance use disorders, reducing relapse and substance-related problems. As an example, mindfulness-based relapse prevention therapy exerts salutary effects on negative affect and feelings of craving. Among other high-risk conditions associated with relapse, stress or psychological distress, and stressors or stressful life events, are among the most frequently endorsed reasons for relapse in those with substance use disorders. Mindfulness-based relapse prevention therapy is associated with reduced stress reactivity in the face of a stressor suggesting enhanced self-regulation in a high-risk or stress inducing situation (Fig. 1).

Readers interested in learning more about mindfulness-based relapse prevention therapy

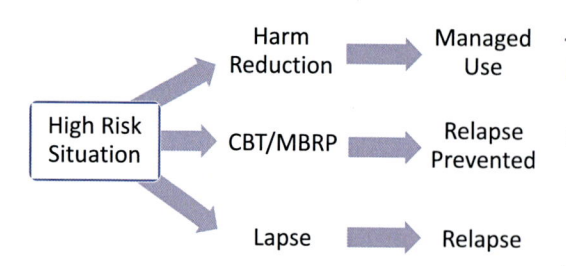

Relapse, Relapse Prevention, Fig. 1 In the presence of high-risk situations, various processes can be engaged with differing outcomes. (**a**) harm reduction therapy allows for use in moderation which regulates problem behavior by keeping it managed within limits, (**b**) cognitive-behavioral therapy (CBT) and/or mindfulness-based relapse prevention therapy utilize skills to prevent relapse such as meditation (**c**), in the absence of therapy, a lapse is likely to lead to relapse

are referred to the Bowen et al. (2011) reference listed below.

Cross-References

▶ Addiction
▶ Mindfulness

References and Further Reading

Bowen, S., Chawla, N., & Marlatt, A. G. (2011). *Mindfulness-based relapse prevention for addictive behaviors: A clinician's guide.* New York: Guilford Press.
Logan, D. E., & Marlatt, A. G. (2010). Harm reduction therapy: A practice-friendly review of research. *Journal of Clinical Psychology, 66*(2), 201–214.
Lustyk, M. K. B., Chawla, M., Nolan, R., & Marlatt, G. A. (2009). Mindfulness meditation research: Issues of participant screening, safety procedures, and researcher training. *Advances in Mind-Body Medicine, 24*(1), 20–30.
Marlatt, G. A., & Donovan, D. M. (2005). *Relapse prevention* (2nd ed.). New York: Guilford Press.

Relational Distress

▶ Social Conflict

Relationship Conflict

▶ Social Conflict

Relationship Processes

▶ Interpersonal Processes

Relationship Stress

▶ Family Stress

Relative Risk

J. Rick Turner
Campbell University College of Pharmacy and Health Sciences, Buies Creek, NC, USA

Definition

Relative risk is best defined in conjunction with absolute risk. For this example, we can define risk as the likelihood of an adverse consequence in two behavioral medicine interventions, Treatment A and Treatment B. Imagine that the risk is 1 in 10 for Treatment A and 2 in 10 for Treatment B. In this case, a relative risk statement can be made, saying that the probability of the event occurring following Treatment B is twice the probability of the event occurring following Treatment A. However, the same relative risk statement can be made for probabilities of 1 in 1,000,000 and 2 in 1,000,000. However, the absolute risks are vastly different: 1 and 2 in 10; and 1 and 2 in a million.

Description

Relative risk is often captured by a relative risk ratio. Consider a hypothetical trial in which the interventional treatment group receives a stress-reduction program intended to become an add-on treatment for patients with a serious disease that leads to heart attacks. This group of subjects is already receiving certain medication that is the "standard of care" for this condition. Subjects in the control group do not receive the stress-reduction intervention, but they too are receiving the standard of care medication. The trial is designed to investigate whether the standard of care medication plus the add-on intervention leads to fewer heart attacks than the standard of care medication alone.

The number of heart attacks is determined for each treatment group, and a relative risk ratio is calculated by considering the number of heart attacks in the treatment group as the numerator and the number of heart attacks in the control group as the denominator. If the number of events in each treatment group were to be precisely the same (the likelihood of which is vanishingly small), the value of the risk ratio will be unity, represented here as 1.00. If the number of events in the treatment group is less than that for the control treatment group, the value will be less than 1.00. Conversely, if the number of events in the treatment group is greater than that for the control treatment group, the value will be greater than 1.00.

Imagine that the value of the relative risk ratio is 0.80. This value conveys that, in this single trial, the addition of the stress-reduction program to the standard of care medication led to a 20% reduction in risk of heart attack. To estimate the true but unknown relative risk for the general patient population, confidence intervals (CIs) are placed around this value of 0.80, which in this context is called the relative risk point estimate. Let us calculate a two-sided 95% CI, which can be defined as a range of values that we are 95% confident that will cover the true but unknown population risk ratio. Imagine that the lower and upper limits of the 95% CI are 0.70 and 0.92, respectively. (The calculation of a ratio means that these limits do not fall symmetrically around the point estimate.) The confidence interval provides insight into the likely occurrence of heart attacks in the general population receiving the stress-reduction program. The following statement can now be made:

- The data obtained from this single trial are compatible with as little as an 8% decrease and as much as a 30% decrease in the risk of a heart attack in the general population, and our best estimate is a decrease of 20%.

Consider now a scenario in which the relative risk point estimate is 1.50, and the lower and upper bounds of a two-sided 95% CI placed around this point estimate are 1.35 and 1.68, respectively. Such data would show that adding the stress-reduction intervention to the standard of care medication actually *increased* the risk of heart attack. The interpretation of such results is as follows:

- The data obtained from this single trial are compatible with as little as a 35% increase and as much as a 68% increase in risk of heart attack in the general population, and our best estimate is an increase in risk of 50%.

Cross-References

▶ Absolute Risk

Relaxation

▶ Psychophysiologic Recovery

Relaxation Techniques

▶ Stress Management

Relaxation Techniques/Therapy

Hiroe Kikuchi
Department of Psychosomatic Medicine, Center Hospital, National Center for Global Health and Medicine, Tokyo, Japan

Definition

Relaxation techniques/therapy are techniques for reducing stress and inducing relaxation.

Description

Relaxation techniques/therapy increase parasympathetic nervous system activity, thereby decreasing the opposing sympathetic nervous system activity such as the fight or flight phenomenon and decreasing arousal. There are a variety of techniques for inducing relaxation. Probably, the most common are variants of Jacobson's progressive muscle relaxation training. Other methods include autogenic training, use of relaxation imagery, biofeedback, and practices derived from meditation and yoga techniques (Jorm et al. 2008).

With regard to psychiatric illnesses, relaxation techniques/therapy are often used as a competing stimulus during systematic desensitization and as part of a comprehensive intervention strategy for the reduction of anxiety. They are more effective at reducing self-rated depressive symptoms than no or minimal treatment, while data on clinician-rated depressive symptoms are less conclusive. However, they are not as effective as psychological treatment (Jorm et al. 2008). In addition, progressive muscle relaxation training has significant therapeutic efficiency in chronic insomnia in adult patients (Taylor and Roane 2010).

With regard to physical symptoms or diseases, relaxation techniques/therapy have positive effects on pain reduction (Palermo et al. 2010). In addition, they have a mild to moderate effect on reducing hot flushes in women with a history of breast cancer (Rada et al. 2010). Although many studies tried to investigate the effect of relaxation techniques/therapy on primary hypertension, the evidence in favor of causal association between relaxation and blood pressure reduction is weak due to the poor quality of the studies (Dickinson et al. 2008). Therefore, further research is required to investigate the possibility of relaxation on physical symptoms or diseases.

Cross-References

▶ Biofeedback
▶ Meditation
▶ Yoga

References and Further Readings

Dickinson, H. O., Campbell, F., Beyer, F. R., Nicolson, D. J., Cook, J. V., Ford, G. A., et al. (2008). Relaxation therapies for the management of primary hypertension in adults. *Cochrane Database of Systematic Reviews, 23*, CD004935.

Jorm, A. F., Morgan, A. J., & Hetrick, S. E. (2008). Relaxation for depression. *Cochrane Database of Systematic Reviews, 8*, CD007142.

Palermo, T. M., Eccleston, C., Lewandowski, A. S., Williams, A. C., & Morley, S. (2010). Randomized controlled trials of psychological therapies for management of chronic pain in children and adolescents: An updated meta-analytic review. *Pain, 148*, 387–397.

Rada, G., Capurro, D., Pantoja, T., Corbalán, J., Moreno, G., Letelier, L. M., et al. (2010). Non-hormonal interventions for hot flushes in women with a history of breast cancer. *Cochrane Database of Systematic Reviews, 8*, CD004923.

Taylor, D. J., & Roane, B. M. (2010). Treatment of insomnia in adults and children: A practice-friendly review of research. *Journal of Clinical Psychology, 66*, 1137–1147.

Reliability and Validity

Yori Gidron
SCALab, Lille 3 University and Siric Oncollile, Lille, France

Definition

These two concepts are the basis for assessment in most scientific work in medical and social sciences. Reliability refers to the degree of consistency in measurement and to the lack of error. There are several types of indices of reliability. Internal reliability (measured by Cronbach's alpha) is a measure of repeatability of a measure. In psychometrics, a questionnaire of, for example, ten items is said to be reliable if its internal reliability coefficient is at least 0.70. This reflects approximately the mean correlation between each score on each item, with all remaining item scores, repeated across all items. Methodologically, this reflects a measure of repeatability, a basic premise of science. Another type of reliability is inter-rater reliability, which refers to the degree of agreement between two or more observers, evaluating a patient's behavior, for example. Thus, in the original type A behavior interview, which currently places more emphasis on hostility, researchers provide a measure of inter-rater reliability, reflecting their agreement on an observed behavior. Finally, test-retest reliability refers to stability of a measure over time, for example, over 2 weeks, 1 month, or 4 years. For example, hostility has a strong test-retest reliability over 1 year of $r = 0.85$, $p < 0.0001$ (Barefoot et al. 1983). This reliability can indicate stability of a measure and of the psychological phenomenon being assessed.

Validity of instruments refers to the degree to which instruments assess the construct they aim to measure. To test this, researchers have developed several types of validity indices. Face validity reflects the degree to which items of a scale "appear" to assess the construct they claim to, based on the meaning of items. This can be judged by participants or experts rating the relevance of each item to the construct being investigated. Construct validity is a higher and more theoretical level of validity and refers to the degree to which scores on a scale correlate with scores on other measures of other constructs, with which they should be theoretically correlated. For example, a scale of anxiety would be expected to correlate with life events in one's past, the latter being a possible trigger of current anxiety levels. Concurrent validity refers to correlations between scores of two different measures of the same construct, for example, between two anxiety scales. Criterion validity occurs when scores on an instrument predict or correlate with an accepted criterion, for example, anxiety being associated with observed behavioral responses to a stressor. Alternatively, criterion validity can be measured by showing that anxiety scores of a group of patients with clinically high anxiety levels (e.g., post-traumatic stress disorder) are higher than those of a healthy control group, also referred to as discriminant validity. Finally, predictive validity reflects the degree to which scores on an instrument predict in time the outcome of people in the future. For example, an anxiety scale has predictive validity if it predicts health-care utilization over the next 12 months.

Another type of validity, a very important one, is internal validity. This reflects the confidence a researcher may have in his or her inferences from a study. This can be achieved by choosing an adequate study design, sampling, and methodological and statistical control over confounders. However, it also results from close consideration and measurement of all possible variables in a study, from sampling, to reliability and validity of tests, to control over confounders, etc. To the extent that these are achieved, the attribution of observed results to the effects of an independent variable or a predictor variable may be internally valid. Internal validity is perhaps the outmost important issue in scientific investigation, and a study can be scientifically valid if its internal validity is maintained. The extent to which these two issues have been carefully regarded can be seen as questionable when viewing a recent crucial study published in *Science*, in which very few previously statistically significant results observed in 100 different past studies were subsequently replicated (Aarts et al. 2015). Reliability and validity should thus be seen as at least important and give prior importance before "statistical significance."

Cross-References

▶ Psychometric Properties
▶ Psychometrics

References and Further Readings

Aarts, A. A., Anderson, J. E., Anderson, C. J., Attridge, P. R., Attwood, A., Axt, J., Babel, M., Bahník, S., Baranski, E., Barnett-Cowan, M., Bartmess, E., Beer, J., Bell, R., Bentley, H., Beyan, L., Binion, G., Borsboom, D., Bosch, A., Bosco, F. A., Bowman, S. D., Brandt, M. J., Braswell, E., Brohmer, H., Brown, B. T., Brown, K., Brüning, J., Calhoun-Sauls, A., Callahan, S. P., Chagnon, E., Chandler, J., Chartier, C. R., Cheung, F., Christopherson, C. D., Cillessen, L., Clay, R., Cleary, H., Cloud, M. D., Cohn, M., Cohoon, J., Columbus, S., Cordes, A., Costantini, G., Cramblet Alvarez, L. D., Cremata, E., Crusius, J., DeCoster, J., DeGaetano, M. A., Della Penna, N., den Bezemer, B., Deserno, M. K., Devitt, O., Dewitte, L., Dobolyi, D. G., Dodson, G. T., Donnellan, M., Donohue, R., Dore, R. A., Dorrough, A., Dreber, A., Dugas, M., Dunn, E. W., Easey, K., Eboigbe, S., Eggleston, C., Embley, J., Epskamp, S., Errington, T. M., Estel, V., Farach, F. J., Feather, J., Fedor, A., Fernández-Castilla, B., Fiedler, S., Field, J. G., Fitneva, S. A., Flagan, T., Forest, A. L., Forsell, E., Foster, J. D., Frank, M. C., Frazier, R. S., Fuchs, H., Gable, P., Galak, J., Galliani, E. M., Gampa, A., Garcia, S., Gazarian, D., Gilbert, E., Giner-Sorolla, R., Glöckner, A., Goellner, L., Goh, J. X., Goldberg, R., Goodbourn, P. T., Gordon-McKeon, S., Gorges, B., Gorges, J., Goss, J., Graham, J., Grange, J. A., Gray, J., Hartgerink, C., Hartshorne, J., Hasselman, F., Hayes, T., Heikensten, E., Henninger, F., Hodsoll, J., Holubar, T., Hoogendoorn, G., Humphries, D. J., Hung, C. O., Immelman, N., Irsik, V. C., Jahn, G., Jäkel, F., Jekel, M., Johannesson, M., Johnson, L. G., Johnson, D. J., Johnson, K. M., Johnston, W. J., Jonas, K., Joy-Gaba, J. A., Kappes, H. B., Kelso, K., Kidwell, M. C., Kim, S. K., Kirkhart, M., Kleinberg, B., Knežević, G., Kolorz, F. M., Kossakowski, J. J., Krause, R. W., Krijnen, J., Kuhlmann, T., Kunkels, Y. K., Kyc, M. M., Lai, C. K., Laique, A., Lakens, D., Lane, K. A., Lassetter, B., Lazarević, L. B., LeBel, E. P., Lee, K. J., Lee, M., Lemm, K., Levitan, C. A., Lewis, M., Lin, L., Lin, S., Lippold, M., Loureiro, D., Luteijn, I., Mackinnon, S., Mainard, H. N., Marigold, D. C., Martin, D. P., Martinez, T., Masicampo, E. J., Matacotta, J., Mathur, M., May, M., Mechin, N., Mehta, P., Meixner, J., Melinger, A., Miller, J. K., Miller, M., Moore, K., Möschl, M., Motyl, M., Müller, S. M., Munafo, M., Neijenhuijs, K. I., Nervi, T., Nicolas, G., Nilsonne, G., Nosek, B. A., Nuijten, M. B., Olsson, C., Osborne, C., Ostkamp, L., Pavel, M., Penton-Voak, I. S., Perna, O., Pernet, C., Perugini, M., Pipitone, R. N., Pitts, M., Plessow, F., Prenoveau, J. M., Rahal, R. M., Ratliff, K. A., Reinhard, D., Renkewitz, F., Ricker, A. A., Rigney, A., Rivers, A. M., Roebke, M., Rutchick, A. M., Ryan, R. S., Sahin, O., Saide, A., Sandstrom, G. M., Santos, D., Saxe, R., Schlegelmilch, R., Schmidt, K., Scholz, S., Seibel, L., Selterman, D. F., Shaki, S., Simpson, W. B., Sinclair, H. C., Skorinko, J. L., Slowik, A., Snyder, J. S., Soderberg, C., Sonnleitner, C., Spencer, N., Spies, J. R., Steegen, S., Stieger, S., Strohminger, N., Sullivan, G. B., Talhelm, T., Tapia, M., te Dorsthorst, A., Thomae, M., Thomas, S. L., Tio, P., Traets, F., Tsang, S., Tuerlinckx, F., Turchan, P., Valášek, M., van't Veer, A. E., Van Aert, R., van Assen, M., van Bork, R., van de Ven, M., van den Bergh, D., van der Hulst, M., van Dooren, R., van Doorn, J., van Renswoude, D. R., van Rijn, H., Vanpaemel, W., Vásquez Echeverría, A., Vazquez, M., Velez, N., Vermue, M., Verschoor, M., Vianello, M., Voracek, M., Vuu, G., Wagenmakers, E. J., Weerdmeester, J., Welsh, A., Westgate, E. C., Wissink, J., Wood, M., Woods, A., Wright, E., Wu, S., Zeelenberg, M., & Zuni, K. (2015). PSYCHOLOGY. Estimating the reproducibility of psychological science. *Science, 349*, 1–8.

Barefoot, J. C., Dahlstrom, W. G., & Williams, R. B., Jr. (1983). Hostility, CHD incidence, and total mortality: A 25-year follow-up study of 255 physicians. *Psychosomatic Medicine, 45*, 59–63.

Del Greco, L., Walop, W., & McCarthy, R. H. (1987). Questionnaire development: 2. Validity and reliability. *CMAJ, 136*, 699–700.

Religion

▶ Religiousness/Religiosity
▶ Spirituality

Religion/Spirituality

Stephen Gallagher and Warren Tierney
Department of Psychology, Faculty of Education and Health Sciences, University of Limerick, Castletroy, Limerick, Ireland

Synonyms

Religiosity; Religiousness; Spiritual; Spirituality

Definition

Even though there is much dispute among researchers regarding accurate definitions of spirituality and religion, it is generally accepted that spirituality concerns the exploration for the sacred, celestial, or transcendent side of life, while religion can be defined as a perception, influence, and behavior which emerges from a consciousness of, or alleged contact with, metaphysical entities which are deemed to perform an essential role in human life. Moreover, in contemporary society, the formation of a dichotomy is being witnessed: with spirituality representing the personal, subjective, inner-directed, unsystematic, liberating expression and religion signifying a formal, authoritarian, institutionalized inhibiting expression. Yet the concept of religion may further be separated into two categories: intrinsic and extrinsic religion. Intrinsic religion is an internalized faith which becomes an innate outlook on life. Extrinsic is focused more on individual practices driven by external motives, such as improved social standing or acceptance. Although religion and spirituality at times appear to be polarized concepts, for the moment, at least, it is impossible to completely segregate the two concepts as the search for the sacred occurs within various faith traditions, and most researchers agree that they are in fact overlapping constructs.

Description

Associations Between Spirituality, Religion, and Health

Historically, it was argued that the study of the natural and explicable phenomena belonged to science, whereas the relatively unexplained belonged to religion. This was very pertinent to the field of medicine. Nowadays, however, there is a strong realization that health involves the interaction of mind, body, and more. In fact, health is far more than a physical matter. Much of this realization has been attributed to a substantial body of literature which has accumulated over the last number of decades connecting spirituality, religion, and communal religious involvement to a variety of health outcomes (Hill and Pargament 2003; Koenig 2009; McCullough and Willoughby 2009; Powell et al. 2003). The links between spirituality and health are discussed elsewhere in this encyclopedia (see ▶ "Spirituality"). Even though the vast majority of studies report a beneficial effect of religion on health, this research has been the subject of considerable controversy. For example, religious involvement is strongly correlated with health-related factors, such as functional status, lifestyle, and social support, which may confound associations between religious observance, beliefs, and health (Sloan et al. 1999). Further, longitudinal studies have found differential stress-buffering effects: protective against multiple events but not discrete events (Schnittker 2001). It could be that religious coping is used as a last resort when individuals feel overwhelmed when dealing with multiple stressful episodes, especially when their personal coping resources fail or prove to be inadequate (Gallagher et al. 2015). However, what adds to this controversy is that the precise mechanisms behind the links between religion and health are not yet clear and are the subject of much research (Powell et al. 2003; Seeman et al. 2003).

A number of possible psychological, social, and physiological mediators have been proposed to account for this connection. For example, it could be that prayer may help people deal with unpleasant situations or that faith promotes a positive disposition which facilitates coping. It is also becoming increasingly evident that religious/spiritual coping strategies can be divided into positive (e.g., seeking support from clergy, forgiveness, reappraisal) and negative (e.g., spiritual discontent, pleading for direct intercession, punishing God reappraisal) forms; positive forms typically relate to more positive outcomes, whereas negative religious coping strategies are generally related to more negative outcomes (Hill and Pargament 2003). Moreover, religious affiliations are associated with the practice of healthy lifestyles, and the social aspect of attending religious rituals, i.e., church, promotes social integration, all of which are linked to better health (Sloan and Ramakrishnan 2006). Further, religious attendance has been found to be inversely related to inflammatory cytokine high interleukin-6 levels (>5 pg/ml), providing supportive evidence of a direct link between religious observance and health (Koenig et al. 1997); this observed association was somewhat attenuated after controlling for age, sex, race, education, chronic illnesses, and physical functioning, implying that other factors may be driving the observed effects. In addition, the proponents of these links between religion and health would argue that the strongest evidence comes from intervention studies, demonstrating the positive effect of intercessory prayer on cardiovascular health (Townsend et al. 2002). However, in a very recent Cochrane Review, it was found that this particular evidence was rather weak and that trials of this type of intervention should not be undertaken, stating that they "would prefer to see any resources available for such a trial used to investigate other questions in health care" (Roberts et al. 2009). Another issue that needs to be addressed is the differential effects of intrinsic and extrinsic religion on psychological distress. Studies have indicated that intrinsic religious individuals who attend religious services demonstrate reduced anxiety, whereas extrinsically motivated individuals who attend services tend to portray anxiety (Koenig 2009). How these different religious concepts relate to physical health outcomes is still unclear, but the link between psychological distress and ill health is well established (Roberts et al. 2009; Rugulies 2002).

How to Measure Spirituality and Religion

Measuring spirituality and religion has proven to be a very difficult task due to the researcher's inability to completely differentiate between religion and spirituality. This inadequacy has unlocked Pandora's box, due to the paradoxical question: is one measuring or has one measured spirituality or religion? Or are these religious measurements tapping into other constructs such as social support? Nonetheless, there are a number of measures available for measuring spirituality (see entry on ▶ "Spirituality") and religion: the Religious Involvement Scale (Piedmont et al. 2009) is a useful scale to test how involved individuals are in religious activities; the Multi-Religion Identity Measure (Abu-Rayya et al. 2009) is a scale which can be used accurately in order to distinguish between members of different religions; and the Religious Coping Scale (RCOPE) (Pargament et al. 2000) can be used to assess religious coping. If one wants to measure both spirituality and religion, the Assessment of Spirituality and Religious Sentiments (ASPIRES) (Piedmont 2004) scale can be used, which has proved to have reliability and discriminant validity. Finally, and more recently, an Implicit Christian Humanist Implicit Association Test (Ventis et al. 2010) has been developed to measure both religion and spirituality which may have stronger behavioral correlates.

Cross-References

▶ Religiousness/Religiosity
▶ Spirituality

References and Further Readings

Abu-Rayya, H., Abu-Rayya, M., & Khalil, M. (2009). The multi-religion identity measure: A new scale for use with diverse religions. *Journal of Muslim Mental Health, 4,* 124–138.

Allport, G. W., & Ross, J. M. (1967). Personal religious orientation and prejudice. *Journal of Personality and Social Psychology, 5*, 432–443.

Gallagher, S., Phillips, A. C., Lee, H. A. N., & Carroll, D. (2015). The association between spirituality and depression in parents caring for children with developmental disabilities: Social support and/or last resort. *Journal of Religion and Health, 54*(1), 358–370.

Hill, P. C., & Pargament, K. I. (2003). Advances in the conceptualization and measurement of religion and spirituality: Implications for physical and mental health research. *American Psychologist, 58*, 64–74.

Koenig, H. G. (2009). Research on religion, spirituality, and mental health: A review. *Canadian Journal of Psychiatry, 54*, 283–291.

Koenig, H. G., Cohen, H. J., George, L. K., Hays, J. C., Larson, D. B., & Blazer, D. G. (1997). Attendance at religious services, interleukin-6, and other biological parameters of immune function in older adults. *International Journal of Psychiatry in Medicine, 27*, 233–350.

Koenig, H. G., McCullough, M. E., & Larson, D. B. (Eds.). (2001). *Handbook of religion and health*. New York: Oxford University Press.

McCullough, M. E., & Willoughby, B. B. (2009). Religion, self-regulation, and self-control: Associations, explanations, and implications. *Psychological Bulletin, 135*, 69–93.

Pargament, K. I., Koenig, H. G., & Perez, L. M. (2000). The many methods of religious coping: Development and initial validation of the RCOPE. *Journal of Clinical Psychology, 56*, 519–543.

Piedmont, R. L. (2004). *Assessment of Spirituality and Religious Sentiments (ASPIRES) technical manual*. Columbia: Author.

Piedmont, R. L., Ciarrochi, J. W., Dy-Liacco, G. S., & Williams, J. G. (2009). The empirical and conceptual value of the spiritual transcendence and religious involvement scales for personality research. *Psychology of Religion and Spirituality, 1*(3), 162–179.

Powell, L. H., Shahabi, L., & Thoresen, C. E. (2003). Religion and spirituality: Linkages to physical health. *American Psychologist, 58*, 36–52.

Roberts, L., Ahmed, I., Halls, S., & Davison, A. (2009). Intercessory prayer for the alleviation of ill health. *Cochrane Database Systematic Review, 2*, CD000368. https://doi.org/10.1002/14651858.CD000368.pub3.

Rugulies, R. (2002). Depression as a predictor for coronary heart disease a review and meta-analysis. *American Journal of Preventive Medicine, 23*, 51–61.

Schnittker, J. (2001). When is faith enough? The effects of religious involvement on depression. *Journal for the Scientific Study of Religion, 40*, 393–411.

Seeman, T. E., Dubin, L. F., & Seeman, M. (2003). Religiosity/spirituality and health: A critical review of the evidence for biological pathways. *American Psychologist, 58*, 53–63.

Sloan, R. P., & Ramakrishnan, R. (2006). Science, medicine, and intercessory prayer. *Perspectives in Biological Medicine, 49*, 504–514.

Sloan, R. P., Bagiella, E., & Powell, T. (1999). Religion, spirituality, and medicine. *Lancet, 353*, 664–667.

Townsend, M., Kladder, V., Ayele, H., Mulligan, T., et al. (2002). Systematic review of clinical trials examining the effects of religion on health. *Southern Medical Journal, 95*, 1429–1434.

Ventis, W., Ball, C. T., & Viggiano, C. (2010). A Christian humanist implicit association test: Validity and test – retest reliability. *Psychology of Religion and Spirituality, 2*, 181–189.

Religiosity

▶ Religion/Spirituality
▶ Spirituality

Religious Beliefs

▶ Spiritual Beliefs

Religious Ceremony

▶ Religious Ritual

Religious Coping

Jennifer Wortmann
Mental Health and Chaplaincy, VA Mid-Atlantic MIRECC, Durham, NC, USA

Synonyms

Negative religious coping; Religious struggle; Spiritual coping; Spiritual struggle

Definition

Religious coping is religiously framed cognitive, emotional, or behavioral responses to stress, encompassing multiple methods and purposes as well as positive and negative dimensions.

Description

Religion and spirituality translate into coping responses to stress insofar as they serve as available and compelling orienting systems and especially when stressors test "the limits of personal powers" (Pargament 1997, p. 310). Religion can provide a framework for understanding emotional and physical suffering and can facilitate perseverance or acceptance in the face of stressors. Religious coping encompasses religiously framed cognitive, emotional, or behavioral responses to stress. It may serve many purposes, including achieving meaning in life, closeness to God, hope, peace, connection to others, self-development, and personal restraint (Pargament 1997). Who uses religious coping depends on individual (e.g., degree of personal religious commitment), situational (e.g., stressfulness of the event), and cultural factors (Harrison et al. 2001). The outcomes of religious coping depend in part on the appropriateness of the coping method to the stressor (Pargament 1997; e.g., Park et al. 2012).

Early measures of coping very briefly assessed a limited array of religious coping strategies (Carver et al. 1989; Lazarus and Folkman 1984). The RCOPE religious coping scale by Pargament and colleagues expanded measurement of religious coping to include methods to find meaning, gain control, gain comfort and closeness to God, and achieve a life transformation (Pargament et al. 2000), and a brief version has shown good psychometric properties (Pargament et al. 2011). Additional measures have been developed to capture the related but somewhat broader domains of spiritual struggles (e.g., Exline et al. 2014; Wood et al. 2010). Measurement of diverse methods of religious coping permits researchers and clinicians to assess specific beliefs, experiences, or practices that differentially relate to health.

Religious coping may be active or passive in nature. An actively collaborative religious coping style in which a person considers him or herself partners with God in resolving a problem has been found to be more common and more effective than either a self-directing or passive style (Pargament 1997). Religious coping methods that have been shown to have a generally positive relationship with psychological adjustment to stress (Ano and Vasconcelles 2005), hence positive religious coping, include the collaborative style, benevolent reappraisal of the stressor, and seeking spiritual support from God, clergy, or members of one's religious group. Religious coping is increasingly being researched in the contexts of multiple illnesses, and suspected mechanisms through which religious coping can influence health include relaxation, sense of control, and the promotion of healthy behaviors. Positive religious coping may alleviate the negative physical impacts of stress, yet more research is needed to isolate the specific strategies and mechanisms (Krause 2011). Although research has failed to show consistent relations between positive religious coping methods and physical health, future research may incorporate sophisticated design and proposed psychosocial (e.g., meaning, social support, meditation) and physiological mediation pathways (Park 2007; Seybold 2007). Moderation analyses may also help identify which individuals benefit under in particular circumstances (e.g., Pirutinsky et al. 2012).

Research has demonstrated consistent relations between negative religious coping methods and poorer mental and physical health (Ano and Vasconcelles 2005; Powell et al. 2003), including poorer health in the context of physical disease, such as increased risk of suicidal ideation in advanced cancer patients (Trevino et al. 2014) and depressive symptoms and poor quality of life in individuals with HIV/AIDS (Lee et al. 2014). Negative religious coping, also known as spiritual struggle, encompasses interpersonal, intrapersonal, and divine categories, including conflict with religious others, questioning, guilt, and perceived distance from or negative views of a higher power (Pargament 2007). Religious coping may also be a negative force in health if it interferes with receipt of necessary treatments (e.g., passive religious deferral).

Although generally less common than positive coping in response to stress (Abu-Raiya and Pargament 2015), negative religious coping is common in people facing serious or life-threatening illness. As such, researchers have recommended incorporating assessment of positive and negative religious coping in clinical practice to identify those at risk for the negative impacts of spiritual struggles and have begun to develop recommendations regarding interventions targeted at spiritual struggles (Pargament 2007).

Cross-References

▶ Coping
▶ Religion/Spirituality
▶ Religiousness/Religiosity
▶ Spirituality and Health
▶ Spirituality, Measurement of

References and Further Readings

Abu-Raiya, H., & Pargament, K. I. (2015). Religious coping among diverse religions: Commonalities and divergences. *Psychology of Religion and Spirituality, 7*, 24–33. https://doi.org/10.1037/a0037652.

Ano, G. G., & Vasconcelles, E. B. (2005). Religious coping and psychological adjustment to stress: A meta-analysis. *Journal of Clinical Psychology, 61*, 461–480.

Carver, C. S., Scheier, M. F., & Weintraub, J. K. (1989). Assessing coping strategies: A theoretically based approach. *Journal of Personality and Social Psychology, 56*, 267–283.

Exline, J. J., & Rose, E. D. (2013). Religious and spiritual struggles. In R. F. Paloutzian & C. L. Park (Eds.), *Handbook of the psychology of religion and spirituality* (2nd ed., pp. 380–398). New York: Guilford Press.

Exline, J. J., Pargament, K. I., Grubbs, J. B., & Yali, A. M. (2014). The religious and spiritual struggles scale: Development and initial validation. *Psychology of Religion and Spirituality, 6*, 208–222. https://doi.org/10.1037/a0036465.

Harrison, M. O., Koenig, H. G., Hays, J. C., Eme-Akwari, A., & Pargament, K. I. (2001). The epidemiology of religious coping: A review of recent literature. *International Review of Psychiatry, 13*, 86–93.

Krause, N. (2011). Stress, religious-based coping, and physical health. Toward a sociological theory of religion and health. In A. J. Blasi (Ed.), *Toward a sociological theory of religion and health* (pp. 207–238). Leiden: Koninklijke Brill NV.

Lazarus, R. S., & Folkman, S. (1984). *Stress, appraisal, and coping*. New York: Springer.

Lee, M., Nezu, A. M., & Nezu, C. M. (2014). Positive and negative religious coping, depressive symptoms, and quality of life in people with HIV. *Journal of Behavioral Medicine, 37*, 921–930. https://doi.org/10.1007/s10865-014-9552-y.

Pargament, K. I. (1997). *The psychology of religion and coping: Theory, research, practice*. New York: Guilford Press.

Pargament, K. I. (2007). *Spiritually integrated psychotherapy: Understanding and addressing the sacred*. New York: Guilford Press.

Pargament, K. I., Koenig, H. G., & Perez, L. M. (2000). The many methods of religious coping: Development and initial validation of the RCOPE. *Journal of Clinical Psychology, 56*, 519–543.

Pargament, K. I., Ano, G. G., & Wachholtz, A. B. (2005). The religious dimension of coping: Advances in theory, research, and practice. In R. F. Paloutzian & C. L. Park (Eds.), *Handbook of the psychology of religion and spirituality* (pp. 479–495). New York: Guilford Press.

Pargament, K., Feuille, M., & Burdzy, D. (2011). The Brief RCOPE: Current psychometric status of a short measure of religious coping. *Religions, 2*, 51–76.

Park, C. L. (2007). Religiousness/spirituality and health: A meaning systems perspective. *Journal of Behavioral Medicine, 30*, 319–328.

Park, C. L., Sacco, S. J., & Edmondson, D. (2012). Expanding coping goodness-of-fit: Religious coping, health locus of control, and depressed affect in heart failure patients. *Anxiety, Stress & Coping: An International Journal, 25*, 137–153. https://doi.org/10.1080/10615806.2011.586030.

Pirutinsky, S., Rosmarin, D. H., & Holt, C. L. (2012). Religious coping moderates the relationship between emotional functioning and obesity. *Health Psychology, 31*, 394–397. https://doi.org/10.1037/a0026665.

Powell, L. H., Shahabi, L., & Thoresen, C. E. (2003). Religion and spirituality: Linkages to physical health. *American Psychologist, 58*, 36–52.

Seybold, K. (2007). Physiological mechanisms involved in religiosity/spirituality and health. *Journal of Behavioral Medicine, 30*, 303–309.

Trevino, K. M., Balboni, M., Zollfrank, A., Balboni, T., & Prigerson, H. G. (2014). Negative religious coping as a correlate of suicidal ideation in patients with advanced cancer. *Psycho-Oncology, 23*, 936–945. https://doi.org/10.1002/pon.3505.

Wood, B. T., Worthington, E. J., Exline, J. J., Yali, A. M., Aten, J. D., & McMinn, M. R. (2010). Development, refinement, and psychometric properties of the Attitudes Toward God Scale (ATGS-9). *Psychology of Religion and Spirituality, 2*, 148–167. https://doi.org/10.1037/a0018753.

Religious Practice

▶ Religious Ritual

Religious Ritual

Login S. George and Crystal L. Park
Department of Psychology, University of
Connecticut, Storrs, CT, USA

Synonyms

Church attendance; Prayer; Religious ceremony; Religious practice; Religious service; Service attendance

Definition

A religious ritual is any repetitive and patterned behavior that is prescribed by or tied to a religious institution, belief, or custom, often with the intention of communicating with a deity or supernatural power. Rituals may be performed individually or collectively during predetermined times (e.g., praying at specific times of day), elicited by events (e.g., mourning rituals performed after a death), or performed sporadically (e.g., praying at various times throughout the day).

Description

Rituals are an important aspect of religion because they allow believers to express and reaffirm their belief systems. One of the primary purposes of rituals is communication. Rituals communicate or are intended to communicate to self, others, or deities. They convey information regarding the commitments, beliefs, and values of the individuals performing the ritual and link them to the larger religious tradition. They reaffirm the religious frameworks individuals use to conceptualize and understand life and, thus, endow a sense of meaning. Religious rituals also serve other psychosocial functions such as emotional control, social support, and community cohesion. By structuring and prescribing behavior, rituals may ease anxiety and uncertainty and promote stability and understanding in social interactions. It is thought that religious rituals may affect physical and mental health through the psychosocial functions that they serve.

In the context of health, prayer is one of the most common religious rituals examined. Studies of relationships between prayer and health have produced contradictory findings. Some have demonstrated favorable links between the two. For example, a longitudinal study of healthy elderly adults found that prayer was related to reduced mortality rates even after many potential confounds such as demographics, health practices, and social support were controlled for (Helm et al. 2000). In contrast, cross-sectional studies have found unfavorable relationships between prayer and health such that higher levels of prayer are related to more disability and pain. A possible explanation for this negative relationship is that those who are ill and suffering may turn to prayer as a way to deal with their distress. Prayer may become particularly relied upon when individuals are facing stress or illness in that prayer can be an important coping resource. The contradictory findings regarding prayer and health may also be due to the failure of many studies to examine factors such as frequency and content of prayer. Prayer can be categorized into different types based on its content, and evidence suggests that different types of prayer may have differing relationships with health and well-being. As of now, it seems that the relationship between prayer and health is a complex one and one that is yet to be fully explored or understood.

Numerous studies have also looked at relationships between frequency of service attendance and health. Ample evidence points to a strong positive relationship between the two. For example, a review of the literature concluded that there was a 25% reduction in mortality rates among those who attended religious services even after confounds and risk factors (such as demographics, healthy lifestyle, social support, and depression) were taken into account (Powell et al. 2003). A meta-analysis that included data from over 125,000 participants found a similar 25% reduction in mortality rates even after potential confounding variables were taken into account (McCullough et al. 2000). Many pathways through which service attendance affects health have been proposed; service attendance may affect health by generating strong positive emotions, encouraging healthy behaviors, and providing access to resources and social support.

Other forms of religious rituals exist besides religious service and prayer, and such forms of rituals may be related to health as well. For example, religious mourning rituals have been postulated to play a role in constructively dealing with grief. Mourning rituals may provide a sense of mastery and control during a highly stressful and uncertain time by prescribing to individuals what ought to be done. Other collective rituals such as participation in religious festivals or ceremonies may foster social bonding and yield a sense of community and social support. Although it can be reasoned that such forms of rituals may affect health as it is related to many salutary psychosocial functions such as social support and a sense of control, currently there is very little empirical literature linking them to health.

In conclusion, although scholars have theorized that religious rituals serve a wide array of functions such as social cohesion, sense of meaning, emotional control, and personal control, all of which have been shown to be related to better health, very little research has examined the full linkages. With the exception of participation in formal worship services as strongly linked to better health, few solid conclusions regarding links between religious rituals and physical health can be drawn at this point. These questions await further empirical attention.

Cross-References

▶ Beliefs
▶ Coping
▶ Emotional Control
▶ Grieving
▶ Prayer
▶ Religion/Spirituality
▶ Social Support

References and Readings

Helm, H. M., Hays, J. C., Flint, E. P., Koenig, H. G., & Blazer, D. G. (2000). Does private religious activity prolong survival? A six-year follow-up study. *Journals of Gerontology A: Biological and Medical Science, 55*, 400–405.

Lee, B. Y., & Newberg, A. B. (2005). Religion and health: A review and critical analysis. *Zygon, 40*, 443–468.

Masters, K. S., & Spielmans, G. I. (2007). Prayer and health: Review, meta-analysis, and research agenda. *Journal of Behavioral Medicine, 30*, 329–338.

McCullough, M. E., Hoyt, W. T., Larson, D. B., Koenig, H. G., & Thoresen, C. (2000). Religious involvement and mortality: A meta-analytic review. *Health Psychology, 19*, 211–222.

Powell, L. H., Shahabi, L., & Thoresen, C. E. (2003). Religion and spirituality: Linkages to physical health. *American Psychologist, 58*, 36–52.

Pruyser, P. (1968). *A dynamic psychology of religion*. New York: Harper & Row.

Rappaport, R. (1999). *Ritual and religion in the making of humanity*. Cambridge, England: Cambridge University Press.

Spilka, B. (2005). Religious practice, ritual, and prayer. In R. F. Paloutzian & C. L. Park (Eds.), *Handbook of the psychology of religion and spirituality* (pp. 435–459). New York: Guilford.

Religious Service

▶ Religious Ritual

Religious Social Support

Chad Barrett
Department of Psychology, University of Colorado, Denver, CO, USA

Synonyms

Church-based support

Definition

Religious social support can be described as the social support individuals receive as a result of their religious beliefs and participation in religious activities. Social support refers to the size of one's social network and the perception of belonging to one or more groups. It also includes perceptions of received, provided, and expected emotional and tangible support from one's social network (Cohen et al. 2000). Thus, religious social support refers to the emotional and tangible support that one receives, provides, and expects from one's religious community. It may also refer to the size of one's social network as a result of participation in religious and spiritual activities (Debnam et al. 2011; Krause et al. 2001). Religious support is a multidimensional construct that has sometimes been operationalized differently across various studies. Most definitions of religious social support include the amount of religious involvement (usually indicated by frequency of attending religious services and related activities). Religious involvement is intended as a proxy measure of the social interaction and supportive relationships that one may form with fellow members of a religious community. Religious social support can be further specified according to type (emotional or spiritual) and source (clergy or laity members) of the support (Debnam et al. 2011). Occasionally, religious support includes a person's perception of emotional and tangible support received from supernatural entities as a result of religious or spiritual beliefs and activities. A four-dimensional model of religious social support has been described in the Brief Multidimensional Measure of Religiousness/Spirituality for Use in Health Research (NIA working group/Fetzer Institute 1999). The four dimensions are emotional support provided, emotional support received, negative interaction, and anticipated support.

Description

There is a broad literature linking religiosity and spirituality to mental and physical health (George et al. 2002; Koenig 2009; Koenig et al. 2001; Oman and Thoresen 2005). In general, though not always, the large number of studies examining the relationship between religiosity and spirituality and mental and physical health suggest that religious and spiritual activities have a salutary influence on a variety of variables related to mental and physical health. Numerous studies involving participants in a variety of settings, from different ethnic backgrounds, in different age groups, and in different countries, some of which used longitudinal designs or random controlled trials, have found evidence that religious and spiritual activities are mostly related to better coping with stress and less depression, suicide, anxiety, and substance abuse (Koenig 2009). The positive influence of religion and spirituality goes beyond the mere absence of psychopathology to include greater general happiness, satisfaction with life, and sense of meaning and purpose (Miller and Kelley 2005). They are also related to better physical health, better health behaviors, and longer survival (George et al. 2002; Oman and Thoresen 2005; McCullough et al. 2000; Powell et al. 2003). People who attend religious services and activities once a week or more tend to have fewer illnesses, recover more quickly from illness, and live longer than those who attend less frequently (George et al. 2002). There is also evidence that they have lower blood pressure and reduced risk of hypertension. Many religious communities encourage health-promoting behaviors. Individuals who attend religious activities tend to engage in more exercise and less smoking and heavy drinking, and they tend to wear their seat belts more often. Further, they are more likely to seek preventative medical care and comply with medical treatment. At least one longitudinal study of over 2500 community participants spanning 30 years found that people who attended religious services more often were also more likely to adopt and maintain healthy behaviors, such as exercising and avoiding smoking and abusing alcohol (Oman and Thoresen 2005). At least two reviews found evidence from several large-scale studies that religious involvement is related to lower mortality rates (McCullough et al. 2000; Powell et al. 2003). In both studies, on average, increased religious activity reduced mortality rates by about 25%.

It is likely that the influence religion and spirituality have on mental and physical health is partially mediated by religious social support. Social support in general, (i.e., social support that is not specific to religiously based social support) has often been related to better physical and mental health (Taylor 2011). Involvement in religious and spiritual communities seems to provide individuals with opportunities to develop greater social support. Individuals who participate in religious and spiritual communities may have additional, and/or unique, opportunities to benefit from social support. People who regularly attend religious and spiritual activities, compared to those who attend less frequently, typically have larger social networks and engage in more activities in which they provide or receive social support (Ellison et al. 2010; Oman and Thoresen 2005). Increased participation in religious community activities is associated with larger and more stable social networks and with more perceived social, and emotional, support (George et al. 2002; Strawbridge et al. 2001). Further, the quality of religious social support may be better. Members of religious and spiritual communities tend to share similar beliefs, worldviews, values, backgrounds, and experiences. They may also have more opportunities to share intimate moments, significant life experiences, and develop long-term friendships and bonds. They may feel more closely connected as a result of participating in common worship, prayer, services, or social groups and activities. In addition, religious and spiritual teachings that promote prosocial values can encourage and facilitate providing and receiving emotional and tangible support, especially during times of stress (Ellison and George 1994).

Religious social support may help individuals cope with stress by encouraging healthy coping strategies and may help them construct a sense of meaning and purpose. Religious social support can also provide individuals wcith a sense of shared burden and comfort. Another way religious social support may influence physically and mentally is by encouraging healthy behaviors. Most religious and spiritual communities encourage their members to abstain from harmful behaviors such as drug and alcohol abuse, smoking, and unsafe sex. Dimensions of religious social support have been related to better eating and exercising habits (Debnam et al. 2011; Oman and Thoresen 2005; McCullough et al. 2000; Powell et al. 2003). However, the evidence for the mediating role of religious social support is mixed with some studies finding evidence for the mediating role of religious social support and some not finding this (George et al. 2002).

It is also important to note that increased involvement in religious and spiritual communities can sometimes have negative consequences. Religious and spiritual participation can sometimes be a source of stress rather than comfort. Interactions may be more negative than positive. For example, in religious communities where certain things such as divorce or homosexuality are strongly condemned, individuals and families experiencing these issues may encounter a variety of negative interactions with community members. In some cases, religious communities may reinforce unhealthy beliefs and behaviors. They can promote perfectionism, negative self-views, and exacerbate feelings of guilt, worry, and anxiety. They can perpetuate mental illness by interpreting pathological symptoms in religious and moralistic terms. Further, some religious communities may discourage members from seeking and adhering to medical treatment for physical and mental health issues (Exline and Rose 2005; Miller and Kelley 2005). Quite often, the negative reality of religious and spiritual activity exists alongside the positive benefits. Thus, religious social support includes both positive and negative elements.

Elements of religious and spiritual activities likely to influence health and mental health include public participation (e.g., attendance at religious services and related activities), religious affiliation (i.e., belonging to religious groups or denominations), private religious practices (e.g., prayer, meditation, reading religious literature), and religious coping (relying on religion to help cope with stressful situations) (George et al. 2002).

Cross-References

▶ Religion/Spirituality
▶ Religious Coping
▶ Social Support

References and Readings

Cohen, S., Underwood, L., & Gottlieb, B. H. (2000). *Social support measurement and intervention: A guide for health and social scientists*. New York: Oxford University Press.

Debnam, K., Holt, C. L., Clark, E. M., Roth, D. L., & Southward, P. (2011). Relationship between religious social support and general social support with health behaviours in a national sample of African Americans. *Journal of Behavioural Medicine*. Retrieved December 1, 2011, from http://0-www.springerlink.com.skyline.ucdenver.edu/content/243t686161407262/

Ellison, C. G., & George, L. K. (1994). Religious involvement, social ties, and social support in a southeastern community. *Journal for the Scientific Study of Religion, 33*, 46–61.

Ellison, C., Hummer, R., Burdette, A., & Benjamins, M. (2010). Race, religious involvement, and health: The case of African Americans. In C. G. Ellison & R. A. Hummer (Eds.), *Religion, families, and health: Population-based research in the United States* (pp. 321–348). New Brunswick: Rutgers University Press.

Exline, J. J., & Rose, E. (2005). Religious and spiritual struggles. In R. F. Paloutzian & C. L. Park (Eds.), *Handbook of the psychology of religion and spirituality* (pp. 435–459). New York: Guilford.

Fetzer Institute, National Institute on Aging Working Group. (1999). *Multidimensional measurement of religiousness/spirituality for use in health research*. Kalamazoo: John E. Fetzer Institute.

George, L. K., Ellison, C. G., & Larson, D. B. (2002). Explaining the relationships between religious involvement and health. *Psychological Inquiry, 13*, 190–200.

Koenig, H. G. (2009). Research on religion, spirituality, and mental health: A review. *Canadian Journal of Psychiatry, 54*, 283–291.

Koenig, H. G., McCullough, M. E., & Larson, D. B. (2001). *Handbook of religion and health*. New York: Oxford University Press.

Krause, N., Ellison, C., Shaw, B. A., Marcum, J. P., & Boardman, J. D. (2001). Church-based social support and religious coping. *Journal for the Scientific Study of Religion, 40*, 637–656.

McCullough, M. E., Hoyt, W. T., Larson, D. B., Koenig, H. G., & Thoresen, C. (2000). Religious involvement and mortality: A meta-analytic review. *Health Psychology, 19*, 211–222.

Miller, L., & Kelley, B. S. (2005). Relationships of religiosity and spirituality with mental health and psychopathology. In R. F. Paloutzian & C. L. Park (Eds.), *Handbook of the psychology of religion and spirituality* (pp. 435–459). New York: Guilford.

Oman, D., & Thoresen, C. E. (2005). Do religion and spirituality influence health? In R. F. Paloutzian & C. L. Park (Eds.), *Handbook of the psychology of religion and spirituality* (pp. 435–459). New York: Guilford.

Powell, L. H., Shahabi, L., & Thorensen, C. E. (2003). Religion and spirituality: Linkages to physical health. *American Psychologist, 58*, 36–52.

Strawbridge, W. J., Shema, S. J., Cohen, R. D., & Kaplan, G. A. (2001). Religious attendance increases survival by improving and maintaining good health practices, mental health, and stable marriages. *Annals of Behavioral Medicine, 23*, 68–74.

Taylor, S. E. (2011). Social support: A Review. In M. S. Friedman (Ed.), *The handbook of health psychology* (pp. 189–214). New York: Oxford University Press.

Religious Struggle

▶ Religious Coping

Religiousness

▶ Religion/Spirituality
▶ Spirituality

Religiousness and Health

▶ Spirituality and Health

Religiousness/Religiosity

Stephen Gallagher and Warren Tierney
Department of Psychology, Faculty of Education and Health Sciences, University of Limerick, Castletroy, Limerick, Ireland

Synonyms

Religion; Spirituality

Definition

The terms religiousness and religiosity are used interchangeably but often defined as an individual's conviction, devotion, and veneration toward a divinity. However, in its most comprehensive use, religiosity can encapsulate all dimensions of religion, yet the concept can also be used in a narrow sense to denote an extreme view and overdedication to religious rituals and traditions. This rigid form of religiosity in essence is often viewed as a negative side of the religious experience; it can be typified by an overinvolvement in religious practices which are deemed to be beyond the social norms of one's faith.

Description

Religiousness/Religiosity and Health

As the use of the concept religiosity has a certain ambiguity in its definition, the lack of clarification can lead to much confusion among researchers. Further, adding to this complexity is the fact that research has found both negative and positive relationships between religiosity and a variety of health outcomes (Miller and Kelley 2005). Thus, future researchers may need to investigate not only linear patterns but to test for nonlinear associations between these particular constructs and need to appreciate that religiosity can often be used to represent an extreme view and overdedication to religious rituals and traditions that are positioned outside social norms. Indeed, such obsessive behaviors are frequently viewed as pathological, and perhaps it is these excessive practices that underlie the negative ill-health associations that have been observed. Moreover, some researchers have proposed a bidirectional and interaction model to explain these complex relationships (Erwin-Cox et al. 2007).

Measuring Religiosity/Religiousness

When one is measuring religiosity and religiousness, they are in fact measuring how religious an individual is. The Faith Maturity Scale (Benson et al. 1993) is an 11-item self-report questionnaire which is segregated into two subscales: horizontal and vertical faith maturity. The vertical scale assesses closeness to God, while the horizontal subscale reviews the existent to which faith has motivated an individual to assist another person. The Centrality of Religiosity Scale (CRS) measures the general intensities of five theoretical defined core dimensions of religiosity: the public practice, private practice, religious experience, ideology, and intellectual dimensions (Huber and Huber 2012). Also, religiousness can be measured using a number of scales such as the Religiosity Index (Piedmont 2001) and the Religion Schema Scale (Streib et al. 2010). While the Mature Religiosity Scale (de Vries-Schot et al. 2012) measures a combination of healthy religiosity and salutary faith and is primarily concerned with their protective roles in mental health. However, as researchers neglect to consider that religiousness may also denote religiosity, one must analyze specific questions from the scales in order to assess the religiosity of an individual. Similarly, it is not yet clear whether these scales allow for assessment of the more extreme aspects of religiosity which have been associated with ill health.

Cross-References

▶ Religion
▶ Spirituality

References and Further Readings

Benson, P. L., Donahue, M. J., & Erikson, J. A. (1993). The faith maturity scale: Conceptualization, measurement, and empirical validation. *Research in the Social Scientific Study of Religion, 5*, 1–26.

de Vries-Schot, M. R., Pieper, J. Z. T., & van Uden, M. H. F. (2012). Mature religiosity scale: Validity of a new questionnaire. *European Journal of Mental Health, 7*(2012), 57–71.

Erwin-Cox, B., Hoffman, L., Grimes, C. S. M., & Fehl, S. (2007). Spirituality, health, and mental health: A holistic model. In K. Rockefeller (Ed.), *Psychology, spirituality and healthcare*. Westport: Praiger Books.

Huber, S., & Huber, O. W. (2012). The centrality of religiosity scale (CRS). *Religions, 3*, 710–724.

Miller, L., & Kelley, B. (2005). Relationships of religiosity and spirituality with mental health and psychopathology. In R. F. Paloutzian & C. L. Park (Eds.), *Handbook of the psychology of religion and spirituality*. New York: Guilford Press.

Piedmont, R. L. (2001). Spiritual transcendence and the scientific study of spirituality. *Journal of Rehabilitation, 67*, 4–14.

Streib, H., Hood, R. R., & Klein, C. (2010). The religious schema scale: Construction and initial validation of a quantitative measure for religious styles. *The International Journal for the Psychology of Religion, 20*, 151–172.

REM Sleep

Salvatore Insana
Western Psychiatric Institute and Clinic, Pittsburgh, PA, USA

Synonyms

Active sleep; Paradoxal sleep; Phasic REM; Tonic REM

Definition

Rapid eye movement (REM) sleep is a behavioral classification of sleep that is characteristic to rapid jerky eye movements and is associated with increased incidence of dream activity. REM is present in humans from birth throughout the life span and is expressed by all terrestrial mammals as well as birds.

Description

Rapid eye movement (REM) sleep is widely known by its shortened acronym "REM" sleep – when pronounced, REM rhymes with "gem." Sleep can be measured with polysomnography (PSG). Polysomnographically measured sleep can be classified into distinct categories that include N1, N2, N3, and REM – the focus of this entry. REM can be classified as defined by the 2007 American Academy of Sleep Medicine sleep scoring manual (Iber et al. 2007) and is similarly classified according to the Rechtschaffen and Kales "classic criteria" (Rechtschaffen and Kales 1968). REM sleep was given its name due to the rapid and jerky eye movements that occur during this behavioral state. Another common term used to describe REM sleep is "paradoxal sleep" because brain activity during REM sleep has a striking resemblance to that observed during wakefulness, hence the paradox. The term "paradoxal sleep" was coined in the late 1950s by Michel Jouvet, M.D.

REM sleep was discovered and first reported in the early 1950s by Eugene Aserinsky, Ph.D. and his mentor Nithaniel Kleitman, Ph.D. The discovery was made through Aserinsky's doctoral dissertation study, serendipitously, when Aserinsky observed rapid eye movements among his sleeping participants (Aserinsky and Kleitman 1953). During the late 1950s and early 1960s, William C. Dement, M.D., Ph.D. began researching REM sleep in greater detail (e.g., Dement and Kleitman 1957), which initiated his to-be legendary career in sleep science, and provided a platform for sleep science to advance. During the 1950s and 1960s era, the groundbreaking discovery of REM sleep lead to the acknowledgment of brain activity during sleep, which countered the conventional wisdom that the brain was inactive during this behavioral state. In sum, the discovery of REM sleep propagated the investigations that built the foundation for the development of modern sleep medicine as it stands today (Dement 2005).

A characteristic component of REM sleep is an unstructured pattern of low amplitude (4–7 Hz) mixed frequency neurological activity, as measured by electroencephalography. The neurological activity during REM sleep displays sawtooth wave forms or trains of sharp triangular waves that occur at 2–6 Hz. Behavioral and physiological changes occur during REM sleep, including rapid eye movements, poikilothermia, atonia (i.e., low or absent muscle tone), fast bursts of transient muscle activity, shallow irregular breathing, increased heart rate and blood pressure, increased genital blood flow, and increased neurological oxygen and glucose metabolism. Poikilothermia is the loss of thermoregulatory control, resulting in the body temperature gravitating toward the ambient environmental temperature; sweating and shivering also cease. Atonia is when the skeletal musculature essentially enters a state of paralysis, which likely functions to avoid acting out the dreams that typically occur during REM sleep. Transient increases in heart rate, blood pressure, and irregular breathing typically occur during dream content and co-occur with rapid eye movements. Increased genital blood flow leads to erections that are unrelated to dream content for men and increased vaginal blood flow for women. Dreams typically occur during REM sleep (Dement and Kleitman 1957); brain activity associated with dreams increases, which propagates increased neurological oxygen and glucose metabolism. Due to the multiple physiological and behavioral expressions during REM sleep, REM sleep can be further subdescribed as phasic or tonic. Phasic is the occurrence of rapid eye movements and muscle twitches, whereas tonic is the more constant state of REM between the phasic events.

Typically, sleep transitions from wake into N1, followed by N2, followed by N3, and then followed by REM – this progressive series is termed a "sleep cycle." Sleep cycles typically occur throughout sleep at approximately 50-min intervals among infants and approximately 90–110-min intervals among adults. Several sleep cycles occur throughout the night, and the time spent in the different sleep stages changes within each sleep cycle. During the first sleep cycle, REM may only last several minutes; REM episodes within each subsequent sleep cycle become progressively longer throughout the night. Thus, typically, the first portion of the night primarily consists of non-REM sleep (i.e., N1, N2, and N3), and the second portion of the night primarily consists of REM sleep.

Although the true function of sleep, and particularly REM sleep, is unknown, to date several functions of REM sleep have been delineated (e.g., Rector et al. 2009; Siegel 2009). Dreams typically occur during REM sleep; although, the purpose of dreaming remains unknown. REM sleep may stimulate the brain during sleep through dreaming. REM sleep appears central to memory formation, where REM sleep and non-REM sleep (N1, N2, N3) complement each other to process and consolidate various memory forms (Diekelmann and Born 2010; Stickgold and Walker 2007). REM sleep also appears to be central to emotion regulation (Walker and van der Helm 2009). Despite the unknown purpose of REM sleep, it appears necessary to obtain. For example, total sleep deprivation, as well as experimentally induced REM sleep deprivation, leads to a compensatory increase in time spent in REM sleep during the following sleep episode, a phenomenon known as REM rebound. Furthermore, REM sleep has been observed among all terrestrial mammals and birds, but not reptiles.

Entering directly into REM sleep from wake, instead of into N1 first, is associated with a sleep disorder called narcolepsy. Several parasomnias are particularly linked to REM sleep, including nightmares, isolated sleep paralysis, and REM sleep behavior disorder. REM sleep disturbances are implicated in and are associated with numerous psychiatric disorders, including depression, schizophrenia, bipolar disorder, and posttraumatic stress disorder.

Human Development: From birth to approximately 6 months post-term, infant sleep patterns are classified into either REM or NREM; during the birth–6-month postterm period, these classifications are also referred to as active sleep and quiet sleep, respectively. Following 6 months post-term, infant NREM sleep patterns become more complex and can be categorized into N1, N2, and N3 sleep stages – in addition to REM sleep. During the first few postterm months, infants spend approximately 50% of time in both REM and NREM sleep. During childhood, the percentage of time spent in REM sleep drops off, levels out to approximately 25% of the entire sleep time, and then gradually decreases across the life span. Across the life span, generally, the percentages of N1 and N2 sleep increase, whereas N3 and REM sleep decrease (Ohayon et al. 2004).

Cross-References

▶ Non-REM Sleep
▶ Polysomnography
▶ Sleep
▶ Sleep Architecture

References and Readings

Aserinsky, E., & Kleitman, N. (1953). Regularly occurring periods of eye motility, and concomitant phenomena, during sleep. *Science, 118*, 273–274.
Dement, W. C. (2005). History of sleep medicine. *Neurologic Clinics, 23*, 945–965.
Dement, W., & Kleitman, N. (1957). Cyclic variations in EEG during sleep and their relation to eye movements, body motility, and dreaming. *Electroencephalography and Clinical Neurophysiology, 9*, 673–690.
Diekelmann, S., & Born, J. (2010). The memory function of sleep. *Nature Reviews. Neuroscience, 11*, 114–126.
Iber, C., Ancoli-Israel, S., Chesson, A., Quan, S. F., & for the American Academy of Sleep Medicine. (2007). *The AASM manual for the scoring of sleep and associated events: Rules, terminology and technical specifications* (1st ed.). Westchester: American Academy of Sleep Medicine.
Ohayon, M. M., Carskadon, M. A., Guilleminault, C., & Vitiello, M. V. (2004). Meta-analysis of quantitative sleep parameters from childhood to old age in healthy individuals: Developing normative sleep values across the human lifespan. *Sleep, 27*, 1255–1273.
Rechtschaffen, A., & Kales, A. (1968). *A manual of standardized, techniques and scoring system for sleep stages in human subjects.* Washington, DC: NIH Publication No. 204, US Government Printing Office.
Rector, D. M., Schei, J. L., Van Dongen, H. P., Belenky, G., & Krueger, J. M. (2009). Physiological markers of local sleep. *The European Journal of Neuroscience, 29*, 1771–1778.
Siegel, J. M. (2009). Sleep viewed as a state of adaptive inactivity. *Nature Reviews. Neuroscience, 10*, 747–753.
Stickgold, R., & Walker, M. P. (2007). Sleep-dependent memory consolidation and reconsolidation. *Sleep Medicine, 8*, 331–343.
Walker, M. P., & van der Helm, E. (2009). Overnight therapy? The role of sleep in emotional brain processing. *Psychological Bulletin, 135*, 731–748.

Remission and Remission Prevention

▶ Relapse, Relapse Prevention

Renin

George J. Trachte
Academic Health Center, School of Medicine-Duluth Campus, University of Minnesota, Duluth, MN, USA

General Background

Renin is an aspartyl protease that raises blood pressure, retains sodium, and alters gene transcription to adversely affect the kidney and heart. Renin cleaves a decapeptide, angiotensin I, from a large hepatic protein, angiotensinogen. Angiotensin-converting enzyme activates angiotensin I to the octapeptide, angiotensin II, by removal of two amino acids from the carboxyl terminus. Angiotensin II interacts with AT1 receptors to mediate most renin effects. The system is involved with the pathology of the following: congestive heart failure, myocardial infarction, hypertension, and diabetes mellitus (renal damage). Inhibitors of the system are beneficial in treating these pathologies and include direct renin inhibitors, angiotensin-converting enzyme inhibitors, and angiotensin receptor antagonists.

Physiological Relevance

The renin-angiotensin system is thought to be important in adaptations to low-salt diets and normal development of the kidneys in utero.

Control of Renin Release

Renin is secreted from the kidney in response to the following: lower renal artery blood pressure, reduced dietary sodium intake, sympathetic nerve activation, and prostaglandins. Renin release is inhibited by elevated renal artery pressure, increased sodium consumption, ß-receptor antagonists, and atrial natriuretic peptide.

Renin Tissue Localization and Molecular Biology

In addition to the kidney, renin (REN) mRNA is found in multiple organs, including the brain. The REN gene codes for a large 406 amino acid protein (pre-pro-renin). The removal of 23 amino acids from the carboxyl terminal results in the formation of prorenin. The final activation step removes 43 amino acids from the amino terminal to form the 340 amino acid active protein known as renin. Both renin and prorenin are secreted into the circulation. Prorenin can be activated by binding to its receptor even in the absence of conversion to renin. The enzyme converting prorenin to renin has not been identified but is believed to be specific to the kidney because nephrectomized patients or animals contain no renin in their circulation but prorenin is present. Inhibitors of the prorenin receptor have been shown to be beneficial in diabetic nephropathy and hypertension.

Behavioral Actions of Renin

Renin and other components of the renin-angiotensin system are present in the brain and are believed to impact memory negatively and to exacerbate Alzheimer's disease and other neurodegenerative disorders, potentially because the prorenin receptor tends to promote the formation of reactive oxidative products. Prorenin receptors are present on substantia nigra neurons where they augment toxicity in dopaminergic neurons, potentially worsening Parkinson's disease. Renin secretion polymorphisms also are one of five pathway-wide associations for schizophrenia. Results with the prorenin receptor and prorenin-processing enzyme are absolutely specific for the renin pathway and should assist in determining relevant behavioral effects of the system in the future. In contrast, angiotensin-converting enzyme inhibitors or polymorphisms have multiple behavioral effects, but these could be unrelated to the renin-angiotensin system because of the nonspecific nature of the angiotensin-converting enzyme. Alterations in angiotensin-converting enzyme activity have been associated with the following: greater physical activity, improved cognition, panic disorder, depression, suicide, autism, physical aggression, schizophrenia, and Alzheimer's disease.

Repeated Measures Design

▶ Crossover Design

Repetitive Thinking

▶ Perseverative Cognition
▶ Worry

Repression

▶ Defensiveness

Repressive Coping

▶ Defensiveness

Reproductive Health

Ulrike Ehlert[1] and Simona Fischbacher[2]
[1]Department of Psychology, University of Zurich, Zurich, Switzerland
[2]Klinische Psychologie und Psychotherapie, Universität Zürich, Zürich, Switzerland

Definition

As a part of general health and development, reproductive health, which refers to the reproductive processes and functions, is essential in adolescence and adulthood and also affects one's well-being beyond the reproductive years. Healthy development of the reproductive system in the fetus and during early childhood is required to achieve reproductive capacity. Reproductive maturity is usually reached after puberty, a phase characterized by biologically based growth and change processes modulated by psychosocial factors. In adulthood, when reproductive capacity is completely developed, a healthy menstrual cycle and male reproductive functioning are biological requirements for reproduction. Furthermore, individual reproductive goals need to be developed and pursued. For women, the fertile phase ends rapidly with menopause, whereas men usually experience a gradual decrease in fertility with increase in age.

Description

A Biopsychological Approach to Reproductive Health

From a biopsychological perspective, the association between psycho-endocrinological or psycho-immunological factors and reproductive processes is of interest. Deviations from the healthy sex hormone secretion are associated with the development and maintenance of various chronic diseases and modulate neurotransmitter systems associated with psychiatric disorders. On the other hand, infertility and diseases of the reproductive system affect one's psychological well-being and may lead to impairments in social life, work productivity, interpersonal relationships, and sexuality (Stanton et al. 2002).

Stress is one of the most potent factors affecting reproductive health and is related to several reproductive disorders, such as cycle length disorders, infertility, premenstrual syndrome, or erectile dysfunction. The bidirectional interaction between the hypothalamic-pituitary-adrenal (HPA) axis, as the most prominent stress-associated hormone system, and the hypothalamic-pituitary-gonadal (HPG) axis is well documented. The HPA axis exerts an inhibitory effect on the HPG axis, due to the inhibiting action of corticotropin-releasing hormone (CRH), arginine-vasopressin (AVP), and CRH-induced beta-endorphin release. In addition, cortisol suppresses secretion of the gonadotropin-releasing hormone (GnRH) and the luteinizing hormone (LH), and inhibits ovarian sex steroids (estrogen and progesterone) and testosterone. Sex steroids, on the other hand, have a modulating effect on the HPA axis (Creatsas et al. 2006).

Women's Reproductive Health

Women's reproductive health includes not only reproductive processes, a healthy reproductive system, and reproductive functioning, but also psychological well-being and a safe and satisfying sexual life. The biological basis of women's reproductive health is a healthy and ovulatory menstrual cycle. This entry will give a brief overview on the endocrinological processes of a healthy menstrual cycle.

Endocrinology of female reproduction and the menstrual cycle: The most important physiological function of the hypothalamic-pituitary-ovarian (HPO) axis is the control of reproduction. This hormonal system includes the hypothalamic GnRH, which is controlled by the GnRH-pulse generator, the pituitary gonadotropes, and sex-hormones produced by the ovaries. The menstrual cycle can be divided into three successive phases: the follicular phase, the ovulatory phase, and the luteal phase. Menstrual bleeding marks the first day of the follicular phase and occurs after the decrease in levels of progesterone and estrogen at the end of the previous cycle. At the beginning of the follicular phase, the follicle-stimulating hormone (FSH) stimulates the development of several follicles, resulting in a slow increase in a woman's estrogen level. As the estradiol level increases, its negative feedback on the pituitary inhibits secretion of FSH; consequently, the FSH level decreases. Shortly before ovulation occurs, maturation of the dominant follicle and the corresponding peak in estrogen level lead to a positive feedback on LH, generating a preovulatory LH surge. This surge causes the follicle to swell and rupture. Ovulation usually occurs after the LH surge. The following luteal phase is characterized by the formation of the corpus luteum and its production of progesterone and estrogen, which help to prepare the endometrium for implantation and maintenance of pregnancy. High progesterone level exerts negative feedback on the GnRH pulse frequency, and consequently, FSH and LH secretions decrease. Lacking stimulation by FSH and LH, the corpus luteum regresses after approximately 14 days. The following decline in estrogen and progesterone levels remove the negative feedback control on FSH, and its level increases again to initiate the next menstrual cycle.

The first day of menstrual bleeding is counted as the beginning of the menstrual cycle, which lasts until the day before the next onset of menses. Between the ages of 20 and 40 years, the average cycle length ranges from 27 to 30 days. Whereas the follicular phase can vary in length (13–15 days), the luteal phase lasts approximately 14 days, correlating with the life span of the corpus luteum. Menstrual cycle lengths vary most after menarche and before menopause, mainly because of anovulatory cycles (Rees et al. 2005).

Women's Reproductive Disorders

Reproductive health is influenced by a number of different factors, such as age, genetics, lifestyle, and exposure to environmental toxins. Thus, women's reproductive health not only includes the healthy aspects of reproduction but also diseases and conditions that negatively affect the female reproductive system. Reproductive disorders, defined as abnormalities in the reproductive system, reduce reproduction and often affect overall health, psychological well-being, and sex life. This section will provide a brief outline of selected menstrual cycle–related reproductive disorders from the perspective of behavioral medicine.

Menstrual Cycle–Related Disorders

Cycle Length Disorders and Bleeding Disorders: Cycle length disorders and bleeding disorders are deviations from normative patterns of menstrual functioning in terms of menstruation frequency or bleeding pattern. Cycle length disorders and bleeding disorders are often associated with anovulatory cycles and infertility. The most common are oligomenorrhea, amenorrhea, menorrhagia, and spotting or breakthrough bleeding. Oligomenorrhea is defined as infrequent menstruation, with 5–9 periods within 1 year; amenorrhea is the absence of a menstrual period. Primary amenorrhea (or the absence of a menstrual period until the age of 16) is a relatively rare disorder, whereas secondary amenorrhea (i.e., the absence of a menstrual period for 3 or more months) affects about 3% of women during the reproductive years (Rees et al. 2005). Menorrhagia is defined as prolonged and/or abnormally heavy periods, with a blood loss of more than 80 ml/period. Spotting or breakthrough bleeding usually affects young or perimenopausal women. Cycle length disorders or bleeding disorders can have organic, endocrine, or psychosocial causes. Exposure to chronic stress or traumatic events seems to influence the hypothalamic pulse generator, leading to a disturbance of reproductive function. Behavioral factors like restraint eating or excessive exercise may contribute to the development of menstrual disorders. In addition, there is a close association between eating disorders, such as anorexia nervosa or obesity, and cycle length disorders (Creatsas et al. 2006).

Dysmenorrhea: Dysmenorrhea is defined as pelvic pain associated with the bleeding phase of the menstrual cycle and can be classified as either primary or secondary, depending on the absence or presence of an identifiable pelvic pathology. Painful cramping is felt in the lower abdomen or back area and is often accompanied by somatic or psychological symptoms, for example, headache, nausea, vomiting, dizziness, restlessness, fatigue, and depressed mood. Dysmenorrhea often interferes with daily activities and may result in absenteeism from school or work (Stanton et al. 2002). The cause of dysmenorrhea can be either organic (e.g., endometriosis) or functional (associated with excessive production of prostaglandines). Studies have shown that affected women show a learning history of enhanced body vigilance and anticipated pain-avoidance behavior. The widely used therapy options for dysmenorrhea are nonsteroidal anti-inflammatory drugs (NSAIDs) to inhibit prostaglandin production and oral contraceptives to suppress ovulation. Pain relief can also be achieved by behavioral therapy methods, such as relaxation techniques or an increase in (physical) activity.

Premenstrual Syndrome and Premenstrual Dysphoric Disorder: Up to 90% of women of reproductive age experience some degree of premenstrual symptoms. A smaller group of women report symptoms meeting criteria of premenstrual syndrome (PMS), and less than 10% of women are classified as having premenstrual dysphoric disorder (PMDD). According to the *Diagnostic and Statistical Manual of Mental Health Disorders* 5th edition (in development process; www.dsm5.org), indications of PMDD include depressive symptoms (decreased interest in usual activities, depressed mood, self-deprecating thoughts, difficulty concentrating, hopelessness, affective lability, and change in sleep and appetite), anxiety symptoms (feeling of tension or anxiety, irritability or anger, and feeling overwhelmed), and physical symptoms (bloating, breast tenderness, and joint or muscle pain). Symptoms begin in the late luteal phase and remit after the onset of the follicular phase. Women suffering from PMDD often experience impairment of work productivity and interpersonal relationships and increased healthcare utilization. Although the etiology of PMS/PMDD has not been definitely established, studies suggest that the cause of PMS/PMDD is allopregnanolone and $GABA_A$ receptor dysfunction, serotonin abnormalities, and a special sensitivity to the withdrawal or fluctuation of estrogen and progesterone (Freeman 2003). Depending on the predominant symptoms, different treatment options seem to be effective: oral contraceptives, stress management training, exercise, dietary regulation, vitamins, herbal preparations, cognitive behavioral therapy (CBT), and selective serotonin reuptake inhibitors (SSRIs) (Rapkin 2003).

Endometriosis: Endometriosis is a common gynecological condition that affects women of reproductive age. It is a condition in which extrauterine, glandular, and stromal endometrial-like tissue grows in physiologically abnormal locations, often within the fallopian tubes, on the outside of the tubes and ovaries, or on the surface of the uterus and intestines. These cells are influenced by monthly hormonal changes; they build up during the menstrual cycle and are shed as levels of sex steroids decrease. Endometriosis is associated with several symptoms, including chronic pelvic pain, dysmenorrhea, menstrual disorders, infertility, dyspareunia (painful intercourse), and dysuria (painful or difficult urination). The exact cause of endometriosis remains unknown; several factors have been suggested, for example, the presence of estrogen, retrograde menstruation, hereditary factors, immune system function, and environmental influence. In addition, discrepancies between the reported location of pain and endoscopic findings make it difficult for women and their gynecologists to handle the symptoms. Affected women present greater susceptibility to mood disturbances, and depressive or anxiety symptoms may play a role in the maintenance of pelvic pain (Gao et al. 2006).

Polycystic Ovary Syndrome: Polycystic ovary syndrome (PCOS) is one of the most common endocrine disorders, affecting about 5–10% of women of childbearing age. Symptoms are heterogeneous and include oligo- or anovulation, biochemical or clinical hyperandrogenism (hirsutism, acne, and alopecia), polycystic ovaries, hyperinsulinemia, infertility, and obesity. The exact etiology has not yet been clarified, but considerable knowledge of the underlying pathophysiologic mechanism and management has been gained. Various lines of evidence suggest a genetic component, but the candidate genes have yet to be identified. Several hypotheses have been proposed to explain the pathogenesis of PCOS:

(a) An alteration in LH pulse frequency and amplitude, resulting from an increased frequency of GnRH pulses and leading to increased androgen synthesis in the theca cells within the ovary
(b) Hyperinsulinemia, resulting from insulin resistance and acting synergistically with LH to stimulate ovarian testosterone production and decrease serum sex hormone–binding globulin (SHBG) concentrations
(c) A primary defect of sex steroid synthesis, leading to increased androgen production and anovulation

The treatment of PCOS depends on the predominant symptoms and the women's stage of life (Jones et al. 2008). The management (e.g., lifestyle management and exercise) of PCOS is directed toward improving the woman's health-related quality of life. A growing body of evidence suggests that affected women are at increased risk for cardiovascular disease, type II diabetes mellitus, dyslipidemia, metabolic syndrome, and affective disorders (Azziz 2007).

Reproductive Health Issues Not Related to the Menstrual Cycle
The following disorders are not related to the endocrinological processes of the menstrual cycle but to female sexual health.

Vulvodynia: Vulvodynia is defined as vulvar discomfort (burning, irritation, or sharp pain) often accompanied by sexual dysfunction and affective distress in the absence of anatomic or neurologic findings. Many factors have been proposed to be possible causes (e.g., genetic, immune, or hormonal factors), yet the etiology remains unknown. Comorbidity with psychosomatic disorders, such as irritable bowel syndrome or fibromyalgia, points to a potential psychosomatic cause. Vulvar discomfort affects one's psychological well-being, relationship quality, and sexuality; however, only a few randomized controlled studies have been conducted to study vulvodynia. Apart from numerous medical treatment options (including topical, oral, and injectable medications), biofeedback and relaxation techniques are helpful, especially when vaginismus is concomitant. There is growing evidence that CBT for pain management reduces pain severity and improves sexual functioning in women suffering from vulvodynia.

Pruritus Vulva: Pruritus vulva is characterized by severe itching of the external female genitalia. It can be caused by infections, systemic diseases, or mechanical stimulation. Scratching, which relieves the physical discomfort, may eventually lead to chronic painful sensations in the vulva area. Therapeutic interventions, such as psychoeducation, diverting attention, and development of new coping skills, seem to be promising approaches.

Other Common Reproductive Diseases/Disorders
- Ovarian cancer
- Cervical cancer
- Neoplasia and dysplasia of the cervix
- Uterine cancer
- Sexually transmitted diseases
- Pelvic inflammatory disease/pelvic pain
- Ovarian cysts
- Benign/malignant breast ailments
- Medical complications during gestation
- Low birth weight
- Reduced fertility/infertility

Male Reproductive Health
The endocrinology of male reproduction and a healthy reproductive system are biological requirements for successful reproduction and an important part of overall health in men. The following section will describe the endocrinology of male reproduction and the healthy male reproductive system.

Endocrinology of Male Reproduction and the Male Reproductive System: The male morphologic reproductive system includes the hypothalamic-pituitary-testicular (HPT) axis, penis, scrotum, epididymis, vas deferens, accessory glands, seminal vesicles, prostate, and urethra. The testes have two important functions: production of sperm and synthesis of androgen (testosterone). Both functions are regulated by an endocrine feedback mechanism of the hypothalamus and the pituitary. The pulsatile hypothalamic release of GnRH causes the secretion of FSH and LH. Whereas FSH primarily acts on Sertoli cells to facilitate spermatogenesis, LH acts on Leydig cells in the testicular interstitium to stimulate steroidogenesis, particularly of testosterone. Testosterone is necessary for spermatogenesis, and together with inhibin (which is secreted by the Sertoli cells), it downregulates LH and FSH release via a negative feedback loop (Nieschlag and Behre 2001).

Male Reproductive Disorders

The above-mentioned endocrinological functioning of male reproduction describes healthy male reproduction. However, male reproduction can be diminished by a variety of diseases and conditions. In the following section, selected male reproductive disorders will be discussed.

Hypogonadism: Primary or secondary hypogonadism is a defect of the testes, resulting in inadequate production of androgen (causing androgen deficiency) and germ cells. Primary hypogonadism is caused by abnormal testicular function. Reasons for primary hypogonadism include genetic disorders (e.g., Klinefelter's syndrome), viral orchitis, and the influence of toxins, among others. Secondary hypogonadism results from a malfunction in the hypothalamus or pituitary gland, which inhibits secretion of pituitary hormones. Symptoms of hypogonadism can be observed in the developing fetus (e.g., improperly formed external genitals), during puberty (e.g., absence of testicular growth and secondary sexual characteristics), and adulthood (e.g., decreased fertility). Hypogonadism is associated with loss of libido, erectile dysfunction, concentration problems, decreased interest in activities, depression, irritability, sleep disorders, loss of muscle strength, and loss of bone density. The most commonly used therapy for hypogonadism is testosterone replacement therapy (Nieschlag and Behre 2001).

Erectile Dysfunction: Erectile dysfunction is defined as the "consistent inability to achieve or maintain an erection sufficient for satisfactory sexual performance." The prevalence rate ranges from 7% for men aged between 18 and 29 years to 18% for men aged between 50 and 59 years. The cause of erectile dysfunction can be organic or psychogenic. Several risk factors have been detected, including cardiovascular disease, hypertension, smoking, stress, and alcohol or drug abuse. Psychosocial distress, relationship problems, depression, and performance anxiety seem to be potential psychosocial causes. The management of erectile dysfunction includes lifestyle modification, medication (sildenafil citrate), psychotherapy, and surgery. There is evidence that psychotherapy improves erectile functioning, interpersonal assertiveness, and relationship satisfaction and reduces anxiety in men suffering from erectile dysfunction (Nieschlag and Behre 2001).

Chronic Prostatitis/Chronic Pelvic Pain Syndrome: Chronic prostatitis/chronic pelvic pain syndrome (CP/CPPS) is characterized by pain in the pelvis or perineum, which may be accompanied by ejaculatory disturbances, dysuria, fatigue, low libido, and erectile dysfunction. Chronic prostatitis/chronic pelvic pain syndrome can result either from a bacterial infection (5–10% of all cases) or may not be associated with an identifiable cause, which is the most common type of CP/CPPS. Several different causes have been suggested (including immunological, neurological, endocrine, and psychological causes), yet the actual cause remains unknown. Recently published studies have shown that several traditionally used medications (antimicrobials, anti-inflammatories, and alpha-blockers) do not significantly ameliorate symptoms of CP/CPPS (Tripp et al. 2004). Affected men often report helplessness, catastrophic thinking about pain, pain-contingent resting for coping with pain, and a low perceived control over pain. There is primary evidence that psychotherapy, which focuses on decreasing negative thoughts and emotional responses related to pain while building up self-management skills, is predictive of positive treatment outcomes for patients with CP/CPPS (Nickel et al. 2007).

Other Common Reproductive Diseases/Disorders
- Infertility
- Sexually transmissible diseases
- Testicular cancer

Reproductive Health in Middle-Aged and Elderly Men

Whereas women show an unavoidable clear cessation of reproductive capacity, men usually maintain fertility through old age. Similar to women, men may also experience physical and psychological symptoms due to changing concentrations of steroid hormones from midlife onward. Age-related decline in insulin, growth hormone, thyroid hormones, aldosterone, melatonin, and progesterone has been demonstrated. Cortisol, on the other hand, increases with advancing age. Testosterone and bioavailable testosterone show a decline of 35–50% between the ages of 20 and 80 years, whereas the LH level increases slightly with age. In addition to age-related variations in hormone concentrations, loss of circadian rhythm of LH and testosterone levels has been demonstrated. Furthermore, sex hormone–binding globulin (SHBG) increases with age, leading to reduced bioavailable testosterone (Hermann et al. 2000).

Partial Androgen Deficiency in Aging Men: If decline in testosterone levels is associated with symptoms of androgen deficiency, the condition is called andropause, androgen deficiency in aging men, or partial androgen deficiency in aging men. The incidence and prevalence of androgen deficiency (or unequivocally low serum testosterone levels) in middle-aged men and elderly men are difficult to determine, particularly because of controversial diagnostic criteria and because some of the symptoms are also experienced by normal aging men. Androgen deficiency is associated with symptoms similar to those experienced by menopausal women or men suffering from hypogonadism. Several studies have indicated that testosterone replacement therapy can improve many of these parameters in middle-aged and elderly men. However, the risks of testosterone replacement therapy (e.g., cardiovascular disease) have not been fully assessed.

Other Age-Associated Disorders: Several age-associated histomorphological alterations of the testes have been observed. Age seems to have a negative impact on spermiogenesis, and there is an association between chromosomal abnormalities in spermatozoa and age. One of the most common age-associated morbid changes is prostate hyperplasia (benign enlargement of the prostate); it is sometimes accompanied by erectile dysfunction, which affects quality of life and can cause mood disorders and relationship problems. The major risk factor for erectile dysfunction is age, with an incidence rate of 5–15% for complete impotence and a prevalence of 52% (of erectile dysfunction of any grade) in men between the ages of 40 and 70 years.

Summary

As a part of general health, reproductive health, which refers to the processes and functions of the reproductive system, is essential across the life span. From a biopsychological perspective, a close association between the endocrinology of the reproductive system and psychosocial well-being is of interest. Normal and healthy functioning of the reproductive system and processes is one of the biological fundaments of psychosocial well-being. Nevertheless, reproductive health includes the diseases, disorders, and conditions that affect the functioning of the male and female reproductive system, their sexual life, and mental health.

Cross-References

▶ Androgen
▶ Breast Cancer
▶ Endometriosis
▶ Erectile Dysfunction
▶ Estrogen
▶ Family Planning
▶ Gestation
▶ Menopause
▶ Puberty
▶ Sex Hormones
▶ Sexual Functioning
▶ Women's Health

References and Readings

Azziz, R. (Ed.). (2007). *The polycystic ovary syndrome. Current concepts on pathogenesis, and clinical care*. New York: Springer.

Creatsas, G., Mastorakos, G., & Chrousos, G. P. (Eds.). (2006). *Women's health and disease. Gynecologic, endocrine, and reproductive issues*. Boston: Blackwell.

Freeman, E. W. (2003). Premenstrual syndrome and premenstrual dysphoric disorder: Definitions and diagnosis. *Psychoneuroendocrinology, 28*, 25–37.

Gao, X., Yeh, Y. C., Outley, J., Simon, J., Botteman, M., & Spalding, J. (2006). Health-related quality of life burden of women with endometriosis: A literature review. *Current Medical Research and Opinion, 22*(9), 1787–1797.

Hermann, M., Untergasser, G., Rumpold, H., & Berger, P. (2000). Aging of the male reproductive system. *Experimental Gerontology, 35*, 1267–1279.

Jones, G. L., Hall, J. M., Balen, A. H., & Ledger, W. L. (2008). Health-related quality of life measurement in women with polycystic ovary syndrome: A systematic review. *Human Reproduction Update, 14*, 15–25.

Nickel, J. C., Mullins, C., & Tripp, D. A. (2007). Development of an evidence-based cognitive behavioral treatment program for men with chronic prostatitis/chronic pelvic pain syndrome. *World Journal of Urology, 26*, 167–172.

Nieschlag, E., & Behre, H. M. (Eds.). (2001). *Andrology. Male reproductive health and dysfunction*. Berlin: Springer.

Rapkin, A. (2003). A review of treatment of premenstrual syndrome and premenstrual dysphoric disorder. *Psychoneuroendocrinology, 28*, 39–53.

Rees, M., Hope, S., & Ravnikar, V. (Eds.). (2005). *The abnormal menstrual cycle*. Oxfordshire: Taylor & Francis Group.

Stanton, A. L., Lobel, M., Sears, S., & Stein De Luca, R. (2002). Psychosocial aspects of selected issues in women's reproductive health: Current status and future directions. *Journal of Consulting and Clinical Psychology, 70*(3), 751–770.

Tripp, D. A., Nickel, J. C., Landis, J. R., Wang, Y. L., & Knauss, J. S. (2004). Predictors of quality of life and pain in chronic prostatitis/chronic pelvic pain syndrome: Findings from the National Institutes of Health Chronic Prostatitis Cohort Study. *British Journal of Urology International, 94*, 1279–1282.

Research Benefits

▶ Research Participation, Risks and Benefits of

Research Ethics Committee

▶ Ethics Committee
▶ Human Subjects Committee
▶ Institutional Review Board (IRB)

Research Methodology

J. Rick Turner
Campbell University College of Pharmacy and Health Sciences, Buies Creek, NC, USA

Synonyms

Study methodology

Definition

Research methodology falls in between study design (including the design of a clinical trial) and data management and analysis. It is concerned with the acquisition of optimum quality data.

Three factors are of central importance in determining the attainment of statistical significance:

1. Variation *between* the two sets of data (one receiving the behavioral intervention of interest, the test treatment group, and one receiving a control treatment, the control treatment group). This is between-groups variation.
2. Variation *within* the two sets of data, or within-groups variation.
3. The total number of subjects participating in the study (the sum of subjects in each treatment group), sometimes expressed as the size of the trial.

The following statements can then be made for each of these factors, assuming in each case that the other two factors remain constant:

- The greater the between-groups variation (operationalized as the greater the difference between the group means, i.e., the greater the treatment effect), the more likely it is that the difference will attain statistical significance.
- The greater the within-groups variation, the less likely it is that the difference will attain statistical significance.
- The greater the number of subjects participating in the trial, the more likely it is that the difference will attain statistical significance.

Notice that two of these three factors address variation. Consider the first statement, which is intuitively the most straightforward. The larger the treatment effect, the more likely it is to attain statistical significance. That is, all other factors being constant, the greater the treatment's efficacy the more likely it is that compelling evidence for the use of the new treatment is provided.

The influence of the treatment can be considered a systematic influence. It is the signal in which we are interested. In contrast, in the present context, the within-groups variation can be regarded as nonsystematic variation, or the noise against which we desire to detect the signal. This noise has two components: biological variation and random error. Since we all have unique biological systems, including those pertinent to a treatment's influence on the body (a statement that is true for identical twins and other identical births given the gene-environment interactions they experience), biological variation is inevitable and perfectly normal.

In contrast, random error can be addressed. Indeed, minimizing random error is a key focus of research methodology. There are multiple instances where such error can occur, with the following being just a few examples:

- Administering the wrong behavioral treatment to a subject on one or more occasions during the trial.
- Employing measurement equipment that is substandard (e.g., blood pressure monitors).
- Conducting blood pressure measurements in an inconsistent manner (e.g., using the dominant arm sometimes and the nondominant arm at others).
- Recording a measurement incorrectly.
- Misplacing data.

Optimum quality research methodology contributes to optimum quality data. All researchers must strive to the greatest extent possible to execute their role in a study flawlessly to reduce random error, thus allowing the trial the best opportunity of accurately assessing the test treatment's characteristics.

Cross-References

▶ Efficacy

Research Participation, Risks and Benefits of

Marianne Shaughnessy
School of Nursing, University of Maryland, Baltimore, MD, USA

Synonyms

Research benefits; Research risks

Definition

Voluntary decision to engage in a process of *organized scientific inquiry (research)*.

Description

The conduct of human subjects research relies on the voluntary participation of persons in research studies. The design of a particular study and definition of the population of interest will define which person or populations will be sought for recruitment into a research study. The decision to participate in a research study begins with a process known as informed consent. Informed consent is referred to as a process because continued review and education must be offered throughout every stage of participation in a study, and consent to continue participation is ongoing. Through this process, participants are continually informed about the requirements of their participation, any known risks associated with participation, and any potential benefits (to themselves or to a larger community) that may result from their participation. Prior to the start of research projects, an institutional review board will review the risks and benefits of proposed research from a scientific and human subject's perspective. However, before actually enrolling in a research study, every participant (or legally authorized representative, in the event the participant cannot consent on his/her own behalf) should understand the potential risks and benefits to the individual associated with participation in the research. The risks and benefits of participation must be explained completely to all potential participants and, ideally, the participant communicates a thorough understanding of the research procedures, risks, and benefits prior to providing initial consent. In some cases, not all the risks of participation may be known. It is not uncommon for researchers to include a statement in the consent form advising potential participants that there may be unknown risks to participation.

Examples of some of the risks involved in research participation may include physical injury, as may occur when testing the safety of a new drug or medical device, or psychological injury, such as the diagnosis of a mental health problem during testing or data collection. There may also be a financial cost associated with research participation, such as treatment of research related illnesses or injuries not covered by the research study or the participant's medical insurance. However, generally speaking, the most common risk encountered is the breach of confidential information collected during the course of participation in human subjects research. The Health Insurance Portability and Accountability Act of 1996 (HIPAA) has had a significant impact on the way all protected health information (PHI) is collected and stored in both clinical and research arenas; therefore, researchers are required to make provisions to safeguard an individual's health information collected as part of their research participation (U.S. Department of Health and Human Services [DHHS] 2011).

Examples of some of the benefits of research participation may include direct physical benefit, such as relief from disease symptoms from the use of an experimental drug or other intervention. Psychological benefits may evolve through a targeted mental health intervention. Often, subjects will agree to participate in research with the knowledge that there may be no direct benefit to self but that they are making a contribution to science and therefore the greater good of society. Some research studies offer direct financial compensation for participation, but this practice causes concern regarding the potential for payment to unduly influence participation and thus obscure risks, impair judgment, or encourage misrepresentation (Grady 2005). The research application and consent form should state how any risks will be minimized, and the institutional review board or regulatory body overseeing research should carefully evaluate the research study protocol to ensure that overall, benefits outweigh the risks.

Cross-References

▶ Confidentiality
▶ Protection of Human Subjects

References and Readings

Grady, C. (2005). Payment of clinical research subjects. *Journal of Clinical Investigation, 115*(7), 1681–1687.
U.S. Department of Health and Human Services. (2011). Health information privacy. Accessed May 2, 2011, from http://www.hhs.gov/ocr/privacy/

Research Risks

▶ Research Participation, Risks and Benefits of

Research to Practice Translation

Bonnie Spring[1], Angela Fidler Pfammatter[2], Sara A. Hoffman[3] and Jennifer L. Warnick[4]
[1]Department of Preventive Medicine, Feinberg School of Medicine, Northwestern University, Chicago, IL, USA
[2]Feinberg School of Medicine, Northwestern University, Chicago, IL, USA
[3]Feinberg School of Medicine, Northwestern University, Evanston, IL, USA
[4]University of Florida, Gainesville, FL, USA

Synonyms

Dissemination and implementation; Knowledge translation; Translational research

Definition

Research to practice translation is the process of adapting principles and findings from scientific investigation in order to apply them in real-world practice (Sung et al. 2003; Woolf 2008). The translational process typically proceeds through a series of phases: T1 (translation of fundamental research findings to develop new practical applications), T2 (adaptation of efficacious treatments into a form that is effective in usual practice settings), and T3 (dissemination and implementation of research-tested interventions so that they are taken up widely by care systems and become usual practice). Although T1, T2, and T3 are all part of research to practice translation, the phrase connotes an emphasis on the later stages, particularly T3. The problem addressed is the slow and incomplete uptake of scientific discoveries into clinical and public health practice. Barriers that impede translation include lack of resources for practitioner training, resistance to change, competing institutional priorities, and lack of infrastructure to support new practices.

Description

Background

A bifurcation between basic and applied research has characterized US science policy since the mid-1940s. In the wake of World War II, Vannevar Bush, Science Advisor to President Franklin D. Roosevelt, wrote an advisory entitled "Science: The Endless Frontier." In it, he advocated for major federal investment in basic science research as the engine that would drive the postwar economy. Bush drew a distinction between basic research, motivated fundamentally by curiosity and a quest for understanding, versus applied research, motivated by the need to solve practical problems. He contended that new insights from basic research are the prime mover of technological and medical progress. Because major advances result from discoveries in remote, unexpected scientific domains, it is virtually impossible to predict which basic scientific inquiries will produce major advances. Consequently, Bush aimed to protect unfettered, curiosity-driven pursuit of scientific understanding from being constrained by worries about whether the knowledge to be gained had any practical use. Arguing that industrial and medical progress would stagnate if basic research were neglected, he succeeded in prompting major federal investment in basic research, including creation of what was to become the National Science Foundation.

Over the next half century, it gradually became apparent that the insights emerging from basic science research were not being translated into practical applications. An analysis by Balas and Boren (2000) indicated that, even after 17 years, only 14% of research knowledge is adopted into practice. By 2001, the Institute of Medicine (IOM) used the term "chasm" to describe the gap between scientific knowledge and actual clinical practice. There was also growing realization that Vannevar Bush's contention that "applied research invariably drives out pure" drew too sharp a dichotomy. In a 1996 book entitled, *Pasteur's Quadrant*, Donald Stokes presented a fourfold table, whereby research could be either low or high on both quest for fundamental understanding and considerations about use. Stokes argued that the most generative, valuable research falls into *Pasteur's Quadrant*, inspired simultaneously *both* by the need to solve a practical problem *and* by curiosity to understand how nature works. A consequence of these realizations has been some realignment of budget allocations at the National Institutes of Health (NIH) to support greater investment in translational and applied research. In fiscal year 1998, the NIH allocated 31% of its budget to applied research and 57% to basic science (Institute of Medicine [IOM] 1998). By fiscal year 2007, the amount allocated to applied research was 41%, increasing to 48% by fiscal year 2016 (National Science Board 2004; NIH 2016).

New Research Approaches to Facilitate Translation

In 2003, the Institute of Medicine's Clinical Round Table presented a schema to conceptualize blockades within the translational pipeline (Sung et al. 2003). The identified obstacles are shown in Fig. 1 (adapted from Sung et al. 2003).

Although T1 translation remains a concern, attention has focused increasingly on blockages later in the pipeline. There has been major federal investment in comparative effectiveness research to address a T2 blockage: determining which treatments work best in usual practice, as contrasted with research settings. Moreover, a further translational phase (T3 – implementation) has been recognized, acknowledging the need to overcome system-level obstacles that impede uptake of best research-tested practices into institutions and health-care systems (Westfall et al. 2007) (see also entry on ▶ "Translational Behavioral Medicine"). Practice-based research and community-based participatory research (CBPR) are two research approaches now being applied to learn how to overcome implementation barriers (Woolf 2008).

An insight that is driving attention toward later phase translation is the desire to scale evidence-based interventions to bring their benefits to more of the population. A highly efficacious treatment available to very few will have less public health impact than a less effective treatment available to many (Glasgow et al. 2006). Stated differently, population-level impact is the product of efficacy and reach (Abrams et al. 1996).

Comparative Effectiveness Research

The US Agency for Health Research and Quality (AHRQ) defines comparative effectiveness research (CER) as the conduct and synthesis of research that compares the benefits and harms of

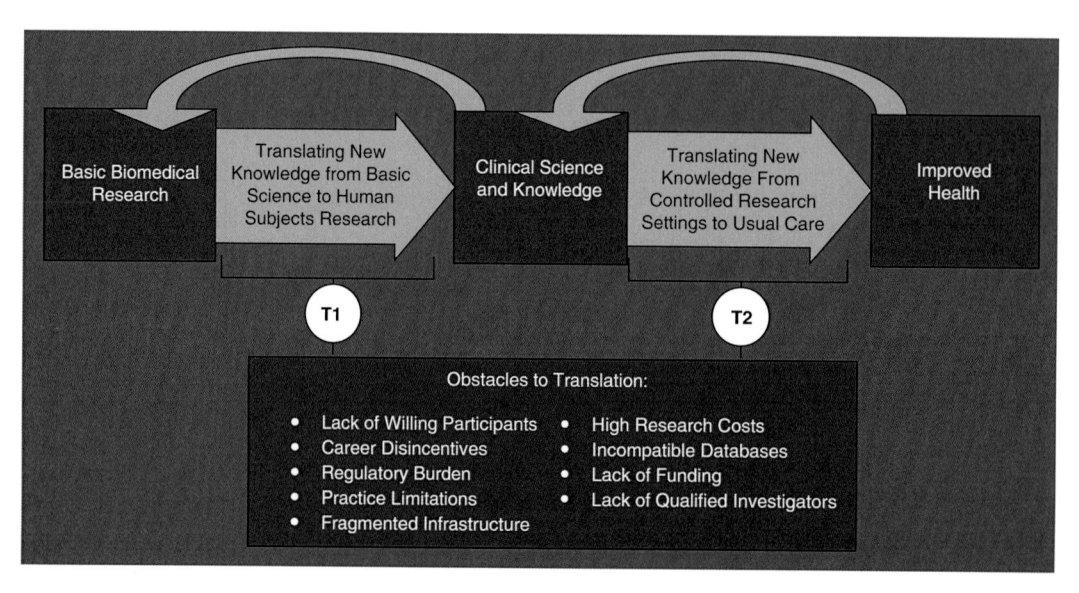

Research to Practice Translation, Fig. 1 Translating basic biomedical research into clinical practice and improved health outcomes (Adapted from Sung et al. 2003)

different strategies to prevent, diagnose, treat, and monitor health conditions in "real-world" settings. CER is a T2 research strategy that addresses practitioners' need to know the relative merits of treatment options available to them. CER takes two main forms: (1) systematic evidence reviews that evaluate benefits and harms of treatment options for different groups of people on the basis of preexisting research and (2) new studies that generate evidence about the effectiveness of health-care practices in usual practice. The most common CER methodologies have been randomized controlled trials (RCTs) (60% of total CER), followed by systematic reviews (14%), and retrospective observational studies (6%). The most common CER interventions have been pharmacological (34% of total CER), delivery system (20%), and behavioral (16%) (Department of Health and Human Services [DHHS] and Federal Coordinating Council for Comparative Effectiveness Research 2009).

Implementation Research

The aim of T3 or implementation research (IR) is to learn how to overcome barriers that limit the uptake of evidence-based practices into usual care. A core insight is that "if we want more evidence-based practice, we need more practice-based evidence" (Green and Kreuter 2005). Few practitioners or health-care system administrators appreciate being admonished by academic researchers for not following scientific practices. Many respond that the research evidence they are being asked to follow is rarefied: derived from patients, clinicians, and settings different from those in the contexts where they work. They advocate making translational processes more bidirectional, so that an understanding of the practice context informs the genesis of relevant research.

Practice-Based Research

Because primary care is the gateway by which most of the population accesses health care, it offers a major channel to deliver evidence-based care to the public. In 1999, Congress enabled the Agency for Health Research and Quality (AHRQ) to establish practice-based research networks (PBRNs) that engage groups of experienced, practicing clinicians in framing research questions whose answers could improve the practice of primary care (Green and Hickner 2006). By helping practices collaborate to address quality improvement questions with rigorous research methods, AHRQ hopes that PBRNs can produce research findings that are more immediately relevant to clinicians and therefore readily assimilated into everyday practice.

Patient-Centered Outcomes Research Institute (PCORI)

Despite a voluminous body of medical research, too often the evidence doesn't answer questions that patients, clinicians, and insurers face routinely. To address this challenge, Congress authorized the Patient-Centered Outcomes Research Institute (PCORI) as part of the Patient Protection and Affordable Care Act of 2010. PCORI is charged to identify critical unanswered questions about health care, fund comparative effective research (CER), and disseminate the results in ways that end users will find most valuable. This means engaging patients as partners in the research endeavor by learning which approaches to care are most responsive to patients' concerns, circumstances, and preferences. The resultant patient-centered research reconfigures the direction of the translational pipeline that has historically flowed from researcher to practitioner to patient. By engaging patients, providers, insurers, and payers together as stakeholders in the research process, PCORI facilitates collective engagement in the process of expanding evidence-based practice and health-care quality (Selby et al. 2015).

Community-Based Participatory Research

Whereas both patient-centered research and community-based participatory research (CBPR) engage end users in the production of research, CBPR goes a step further by integrating social action into the research motivation. CBPR aims explicitly to reduce health disparities, overcome social injustice, and improve community well-being. In contrast, social action is not a required part of the research funded by PCORI. Guided by a core set of values, CBPR builds on community strengths and resources; facilitates collaboration, co-learning, and capacity building; and balances investment in knowledge generation with a long-term commitment to action that supports equity and benefits the community (Israel et al. 2008). A guiding principle of community-based participatory research is that culture, religious values, and economic factors specific to a community are integral to any decision about best practices. Consequently, multiple community stakeholders, rather than just a core research team, need to participate in all aspects of the research enterprise so that the resulting findings are relevant, responsive to stakeholder concerns, and therefore implemented. An underlying premise of this approach is that an equitable standing and distribution of power between researchers and the community is most likely to empower the community to implement emergent evidence-based practices as part of a long-lasting community commitment to health-care improvement (Muhammad et al. 2015).

Educating Researchers and Practitioners About Translation

Research to practice translation is still an evolving field with the overarching goal of improving healthcare practice. Several training resources are available about research to practice translation. First, the NIH Office of Behavioral and Social Science Research (OBSSR) offers a residential summer training institute on Dissemination and Implementation Research in Health (https://obssr-archive.od.nih.gov/scientific_areas/translation/dissemination_and_implementation/index.aspx). Another OBSSR-funded resource that can be accessed remotely and free of charge is the Evidence-Based Behavioral Practice (EBBP) site available at www.ebbp.org. Among the interactive online learning modules available at ebbp.org are several dedicated to (a) shared decision-making with individuals, (b) collaborative decision-making with communities, (b) stakeholder perspectives about research and evidence-based practice, and (c) implementation. Finally, a third set of resources involve several new scholarly journals: *The Journal of Translational Medicine* (2003), *Science: Translational Medicine* (2009), and *Translational Behavioral Medicine* (2011).

Cross-References

▶ Evidence-Based Behavioral Medicine (EBBM)
▶ Translational Behavioral Medicine

References and Further Reading

Abrams, D. B., Orleans, C. T., Niaura, R., Goldstein, M. G., Prochaska, J. O., & Velicer, W. (1996). Integrating individual and public health perspectives for treatment of tobacco dependence under managed care: A combined stepped care and matching model. *Annals of Behavioral Medicine, 18*, 290–304.

Balas, E. A., & Boren, S. A. (2000). Managing clinical knowledge for health care improvement. In J. Bemmel & A. T. McCray (Eds.), *Yearbook of medical informatics* (pp. 65–70). Stuttgart: Schattauer Publishing Company.

Bush, V. (1945). *Science, the endless frontier: A report to the president by Vannevar Bush, director of the office of scientific research and development*. Washington, DC: United States Government Printing Office.

Department of Health and Human Services & Federal Coordinating Council for Comparative Effectiveness Research. (2009). *Report to the president and the congress* [Internet]. Washington, DC: HHS; [cited 2011 Jan 11]. Available from http://www.hhs.gov/recovery/programs/cer/cerannualrpt.pdf

Glasgow, R. E., Klesges, L. M., Dzewaltowski, D. A., Estabrooks, P. A., & Vogt, T. M. (2006). Evaluating the impact of health promotion programs: Using the RE-AIM framework to form summary measures for decision making involving complex issues. *Health Education Research, 21*(3), 688–694.

Green, L. A., & Hickner, J. (2006). A short history of primary care practice-based research networks: From concept to essential research laboratories. *The Journal of the American Board of Family Medicine, 19*(1), 1–10.

Green, L. W., & Kreuter, M. W. (2005). *Health program planning: An educational and ecological approach* (4th ed.). Boston: McGraw Hill.

Institute of Medicine Committee on the NIH Research Priority-Setting Process. (1998). *Scientific opportunities and public needs: Improving priority setting and public input at the national institutes of health*. Washington, DC: National Academies Press.

Israel, B. A., Schulz, A. J., Parker, E. A., & Becker, A. B. (2008). Review of community-based research: Assessing partnership approaches to improve public health. *Annual Review of Public Health, 19*, 173–202.

Muhammad, M., Wallerstein, N., Sussman, A. L., Avila, M., Belone, L., & Duran, B. (2015). Reflections on researcher identity and power: The impact of positionality on community based participatory research (CBPR) processes and outcomes. *Critical Sociology, 41*(7–8), 1045–1063.

National Institutes of Health. (2016). *FY 2012 – FY 2017 distribution of budget authority percentage for basic and applied research*. [Internet] from: https://officeofbudget.od.nih.gov/pdfs/FY16/Basic%20and%20Applied%20FY%202002%20-%20FY%202017%20R2%20-%20V.pdf. Retrieved 7/2/2016.

National Science Board. (2004). *Science and engineering indicators 2004 (NSB 04–01)*. Arlington: National Science Foundation, Division of Science Resources Statistics.

Selby, J. V., Forsythe, L., & Sox, H. C. (2015). Stakeholder-driven comparative effectiveness research: An update from PCORI. *JAMA, 314*(21), 2235–2236.

Stokes, D. (1997). *Pasteur's quadrant: Basic science and technological innovation*. Washington, DC: Brookings Institute.

Sung, N. S., Crowley, W. F., Jr., Genel, M., Salber, P., Sandy, L., Sherwood, L. M., et al. (2003). Central challenges facing the national clinical research enterprise. *Journal of the American Medical Association, 289*, 1278–1287.

Westfall, J. M., Mold, J., & Fagnan, L. (2007). Practice-based research-"blue highways" on the NIH roadmap. *Journal of the American Medical Association, 297*(4), 403–406.

Woolf, S. H. (2008). The meaning of translational research and why it matters. *Journal of the American Medical Association, 299*(2), 211–213.

Residential Treatment

▶ Substance Abuse: Treatment

Resilience

▶ Resilience: Measurement
▶ Salutogenesis
▶ Williams LifeSkills Program

Resilience to Adversity

Melissa Julian[1], Chelsea Romney[2], Nicole E. Mahrer[3] and Christine Dunkel Schetter[4]
[1]George Washington University, Washington, DC, USA
[2]University of California, Los Angeles (UCLA), Los Angeles, CA, USA
[3]Department of Psychology, University of La Verne, La Verne, CA, USA
[4]Department of Psychology, University of California, Los Angeles (UCLA), Los Angeles, CA, USA

Definition

Resilience is the capacity of a system to adapt successfully to challenges that threaten system functioning, survival, or development.

Description

Resilience refers to the process of withstanding or overcoming stress with minimal disturbance to one's functioning, physical and mental health, and well-being (Rutter 1999) and is primarily studied within the context of trauma and severe stress. Early research focused on children who did remarkably well over time despite experiencing early adversity. More recent research has focused on recovery following traumatic events or disasters, such as the September 11th terrorist attack in New York City or Hurricane Katrina in New Orleans. With the growing focus on positive psychology in the past few decades, resilience in the context of stress and coping has become a bourgeoning area of research across many types of stressors, contexts, and groups of people.

Resilience may be conceptualized in three ways – as responses to major stressors, as outcomes of the coping process, or as factors that facilitate adaptive responses. The last approach conceptualizes resilience as a set of protective factors or resources, either socioenvironmental or innate, that enable an individual to adaptively respond to stressors (Dunkel Schetter and Dolbier 2011). All of these approaches fit under the umbrella of resilience as an overarching concept (Luthar et al. 2000; Zautra et al. 2010). Once thought to be an extraordinary phenomenon, we now know that resilience, even following major adversity, is fairly common (Masten 2014). Resilience can also be viewed from an evolutionary perspective. Humans innately have capacities to manage and overcome stress; some people may even grow or thrive in the aftermath of adversity (Bonanno 2004).

Current approaches define resilience within a systems framework as the capacity of a system to adapt successfully to challenges that threaten system function, survival, or development (Masten 2018). Resilience operates at multiple levels and is embedded in systems that span from the community level to the psychological and biological systems within a single individual. For example, a community can be resilient by having disaster preparedness plans in place, holding emergency drills, and generally preparing individuals to respond safely and calmly. Just as communities differ in their resilience capacity, so do individuals.

An individual's resilience capacity is not stable, but rather changes over time and differs across contexts (Rutter 2006). For example, a person may seem to be resilient in the context of chronic stressors such as neighborhood-related adversity or academic stress, but not in the context of relationship conflict. Resilience can also change across the lifespan, such that a person might become more or less resilient over certain developmental periods. Resilience has been studied in early childhood, adolescence, and through older adulthood, and there is evidence that all age ranges have the ability to enhance their resilience capacity. However, children tend to be particularly resilient and are especially skilled at building resilience if given the opportunity (Masten 2014).

Resilience is a multicomponent and dynamic phenomenon with many possible contributors. Given a systems perspective, a person can be resilient in certain areas more than others and across biological, social, or psychological levels.

The factors that contribute to a person's resilience capacity can be referred to as *resilience resources*. Dunkel Schetter and Dolbier (2011) developed a taxonomy of six categories of resilience resources.

Personality or dispositional resources include relatively stable traits such as being an optimistic person by nature (dispositional optimism) and personality factors from the Big Five personality cluster, such as conscientiousness and agreeableness. *Self and ego-related resources* include a person's self-efficacy, mastery, and self-esteem. Having a positive view of the self and of one's ability is important in being able to overcome adversities and the challenges they pose (Marmot 2003). Extensive research indicates that both *personality* and *self and ego-related resources* contribute to favorable outcomes following stress.

Interpersonal and social factors include perceived available support and having a strong social network. Perceiving that others are available as a source of support is a powerful resource that has been linked with several health benefits (Uchino 2004). However, in times of adversity, actual received emotional, tangible, or instrumental support from family and close friends is critical in increasing one's resilience capacity.

World views and culturally based beliefs and values include resources such as spirituality and religious beliefs or practices, which have a multitude of positive implications for dealing with hardships throughout life (Cheadle and Schetter 2017). Factors such as believing that there is a higher power and believing that the higher power has a beneficial role in one's life can be helpful in one's ability to cope in the face of difficulties. Cultural factors such as familism in Latinos, or collectivism in Asian cultures, can also be protective.

Behavioral and cognitive skills include resources such as emotion regulation skills and active coping which enable a person to manage stress. For example, mindfulness and relaxation techniques that promote calmness in the face of stress are adaptive ways to cope with many types of adversity (Brown et al. 2007).

The final category, *endowed or acquired resources*, includes resources such as high socioeconomic status, a genetic predisposition to good health, and strong cognitive abilities. For example, research indicates that both education and income generally enhance health and well-being and are valuable resources in the context of stress as well.

While some resilience resources are fairly stable and inflexible, other resilience resources can be learned and practiced. For example, coping and emotion regulation skills or building a greater social support network are factors that can be fostered, but changing one's socioeconomic status is much more difficult. Counselors can help individuals process specific or ongoing events, learn how to reframe thoughts, and provide tools for emotional coping. Although personal growth in the face of adversity can often be difficult, a focus on fostering these more malleable resilience resources may enhance individuals' ability to adapt to stressors with minimal disturbance to functioning or well-being.

Currently, researchers use various measures to assess resilience. Two established measures are the Connor-Davidson Resilience Scale (CD-RISC; Connor and Davidson 2003) and the Brief Resilience Scale (BRS; Smith et al. 2008). Recently, our group has developed a brief resilience measure for young adults in higher education settings. The Resilience Resources Scale (RRS) is a 12-item instrument that assesses several of the specific personal and social factors that contribute to one's resilience capacity.

In conclusion, resilience refers to a system's capacity to adaptively respond to and withstand challenges, whether they are traumatic events or chronic stressors. Resilience research can help advance our understanding of the processes affecting at-risk individuals. An individual's capacity to be resilient will change throughout the lifespan and vary across situations. Resilience resources contribute to a person's resilience capacity, and further study of them may be particularly useful in the development of interventions to promote resilience for people of all ages.

References and Further Reading

Bonanno, G. A. (2004). Loss, trauma, and human resilience: Have we underestimated the human capacity to thrive after extremely aversive events? *American Psychologist, 59*(1), 20–28. https://doi.org/10.1037/0003-066X.59.1.20.

Brown, K. W., Ryan, R. M., & Creswell, J. D. (2007). Mindfulness: Theoretical foundations and evidence for its salutary effects. *Psychological Inquiry, 18*(4), 211–237. https://doi.org/10.1080/10478400701598298.

Cheadle, A. C. D., & Schetter, C. D. (2017). Untangling the mechanisms underlying the links between religiousness, spirituality, and better health. *Social and Personality Psychology Compass, 11*(2), 1–10. https://doi.org/10.1111/spc3.12299.

Connor, K. M., & Davidson, J. R. T. (2003). Development of a new resilience scale: The Connor-Davidson Resilience Scale (CD-RISC). *Depression and Anxiety, 18*(2), 76–82. https://doi.org/10.1002/da.10113.

Dunkel Schetter, C., & Dolbier, C. (2011). Resilience in the context of chronic stress and health in adults. *Social and Personality Psychology Compass, 5*(9), 634–652. https://doi.org/10.1111/j.1751-9004.2011.00379.x.

Luthar, S. S., Cicchetti, D., & Becker, B. (2000). The construct of resilience: A critical evaluation and guidelines for future work. *Child Development, 71*(3), 543–562. https://doi.org/10.1111/1467-8624.00164.

Marmot, M. (2003). Self esteem and health. *British Medical Journal, 327*(7415), 574–575. https://doi.org/10.1136/bmj.327.7415.574.

Masten, A. S. (2014). *Ordinary magic: Resilience in development*. New York: The Guilford Press.

Masten, A. S. (2018). Resilience theory and research on children and families: Past, present, and promise. *Journal of Family Theory and Review, 10*(1), 12–31. https://doi.org/10.1111/jftr.12255.

Rutter, M. (1999). Resilience concepts and findings: Implications for family therapy. *Journal of Family Therapy, 21*, 119–144. https://doi.org/10.1111/1467-6427.00108.

Rutter, M. (2006). Implications of resilience concepts for scientific understanding. *Annals of the New York Academy of Sciences, 1094*(1), 1–12. https://doi.org/10.1196/annals.1376.002.

Smith, B. W., Dalen, J., Wiggins, K., Tooley, E., Christopher, P., & Bernard, J. (2008). The brief resilience scale: Assessing the ability to bounce back. *International Journal of Behavioral Medicine, 15*(3), 194–200. https://doi.org/10.1080/10705500802222972.

Uchino, B. N. (2004). *Social support and physical health: Understanding the health consequences of relationships*. New Haven/London: Yale University Press.

Zautra, A. J., Hall, J. S., & Murray, K. E. (2010). Resilience: A new definition of health for people and communities. In J. R. Reich, A. J. Zautra, & J. S. Hall (Eds.), *Handbook of adult resilience* (pp. 3–30). New York: Guilford.

Resilience Training

▶ Williams LifeSkills Program

Resilience: Measurement

Hannah Süss and Susanne Fischer
Clinical Psychology and Psychotherapy, Institute of Psychology, University of Zurich, Zurich, Switzerland

Synonyms

Hardiness; Resilience; Sense of coherence – measurement

Definition

Resilience is a relatively stable trajectory of healthy functioning after a potentially stressful event, which is characterized by transient symptoms and minimal impairment.

Description

The above definition of resilience implies the occurrence of a *potential stressor* as well as the presence of certain *resilience factors*, which contribute to a *beneficial* rather than a pathological *outcome* (Bonanno 2004; Bonanno and Diminich, 2013; Bonanno et al. 2011). Despite general consensus on the conceptualization of resilience, there are ambiguities in how its components are operationalized.

Regarding *potential stressors*, operationalization depends on the individual research question and on the population of interest. In studies on children and adolescents, the focus is usually on adverse early life events, such as childhood trauma, or on socioeconomic deprivation as a variant of chronic stress. In adults, trauma occurring during the adult life span, critical life events, and various forms of chronic stress have been the subject of most research. In terms of chronic stress, important topics have been resilience in the face of chronic diseases (e.g., Deshields et al. 2016; Goubert and Trompetter 2017; Tan-Kristanto and Kiropoulos, 2015) and minority stress (e.g., Babatunde-Sowole et al. 2016; Woodward et al. 2017). Most studies adopt self-reported measurement approaches, such as structured interviews or checklists and questionnaires to retrospectively assess potential stressors. Such measures are sometimes complemented by biological parameters, such as brain activity, autonomic, endocrine, or immune parameters, which may serve as indicators of long-lasting physiological changes in response to severe or long-lasting stress.

In order to measure *beneficial outcomes* after previous exposure to stressors, composite indices across multiple behavioral domains of functioning (e.g., school or recreational activities) are often created in children and adolescents. Also, achievement of developmental milestones can be used as an indicator of successful adaptation. Such measurements commonly rely on evaluations and ratings provided by parents or teachers. In contrast, studies investigating adults are mostly designed within clinical contexts. As a consequence, beneficial outcomes equal the absence of somatic symptoms, physical diseases, psychological distress, or mental disorders. The assessment of physical and mental well-being usually relies on self-reported measures, but again, structured interviews may be used to determine the absence or presence of particular illnesses.

There are two types of *resilience factors*: psychological and biological. In order to assess psychological resilience factors, several questionnaires have been developed over the past decades (Ahern et al. 2006; Pangallo et al. 2015; Windle et al. 2011). Some refer to global resilience constructs, such as sense of coherence (Antonovsky 1979), hardiness (Kobasa 1979), or ego-resiliency (Block and Block 1980). Further global resilience scales are the Resilience Scale (RS; Wagnild and Young 1993), the Connor-Davidson Resilience Scale (CD-RISC; Connor and Davidson 2003), and the Resilience Scale for Adults (RSA; Friborg et al. 2003). The RS was developed based on interviews with community-dwelling older women after experience of critical life events. Principal component analysis of the 25 items revealed two factors labeled "personal competence" and "acceptance of self and life." The scale has been employed in population based as well as clinical contexts. The CD-RISC, by contrast, predominantly consists of questions addressing coping behavior. A preliminary validation study conducted by the authors yielded a structure of five factors based on the 25 items of the test. Application of the instrument has so far mostly been limited to clinical trials. Finally, the RSA also incorporates items on external resilience factors, such as social support. Overall, five dimensions were empirically found to adequately describe the resilience concept as suggested by the authors, namely, personal competence, social competence, family coherence, social support, and personal structure. The scale has been used in studies in both healthy participants and patient samples. Moreover, a number of scales to measure resilience with regard to specific chronic diseases are now available. One example for this is the Resilience Scale Specific to Cancer (RS-SC; Ye et al. 2018). Finally, a number of more specific traits have commonly been associated with resilience, and for all of these, questionnaires are available. These include self-efficacy (Sherer et al. 1982), positive affectivity (Watson et al. 1988), optimism (Scheier et al. 1994), self-esteem (Rosenberg 1965), active coping (Folkman and Lazarus 1988), and social support (Sarason et al. 1983).

While resilience factors have traditionally been examined psychometrically, more recent research has sought to identify biological underpinnings of resilience (Charney, 2004; Feder et al. 2009; Russo et al. 2012). Studies in this area of research usually utilize experimental designs directed at exploring the biological processes involved in beneficial outcomes in the aftermath of a stressor. Concerning neuronal processes, researchers have demonstrated that various brain structures and pathways, such as the medial prefrontal cortex, the hippocampal pathway and the mesolimbic pathway are involved in resilience (Han and Nestler 2017; Liu et al. 2018). In addition, according to Walker et al. (2017), the following markers are particularly promising in serving as biological resilience factors: noradrenaline, corticotropin-releasing hormone (CRH), neuropeptide Y (NPY), the acoustic startle response, cardiovascular stress reactivity (response amplitude), heart rate variability (HRV), cortisol, dehydroepiandrosterone (DHEA), glucocorticoid sensitivity, and pro-inflammatory cytokines. The authors postulate that resilient individuals are characterized by lower concentrations of noradrenaline, CRH and pro-inflammatory cytokines, a decreased acoustic startle response, lower cardiovascular stress reactivity, higher concentrations of NPY and DHEA, and a higher HRV. Notably, with regard to cortisol and glucocorticoid sensitivity, depending on the outcome measure, (i.e., absence or presence of a particular illness), lower or higher concentrations may favor resilience. For instance, hyperactivity of the hypothalamic-pituitary-adrenal (HPA) axis has been found in melancholic depression, alcohol use disorder, and eating disorders (Chrousos 2009). In contrast, posttraumatic stress disorder or somatic symptom disorders seem to be associated with diminished HPA activity. Finally, research into genetic factors fostering resilient trajectories has recently gained momentum. Accumulating evidence shows that polymorphisms within various genes that code for components of the HPA axis, such as *NR3C1* and *FKBP5*, seem to play an important role in facilitating beneficial outcomes after the occurrence of a potential stressor (Zannas and West 2014).

Cross-References

▶ Active Coping
▶ Chronic Disease or Illness
▶ Coping
▶ Hardiness
▶ Life Events
▶ Minority Subgroups
▶ Optimism and Pessimism: Measurement
▶ Positive Affectivity
▶ Resilience
▶ Self-Efficacy
▶ Self-Esteem
▶ Sense of Coherence
▶ Social Support
▶ Stress
▶ Stress, Early Life
▶ Stress, Posttraumatic

References and Further Reading

Ahern, N. R., Kiehl, E. M., Lou Sole, M., & Byers, J. (2006). A review of instruments measuring resilience. *Issues in Comprehensive Pediatric Nursing, 29*, 103–125.

Antonovsky, A. (1979). *Health, stress, and coping: New perspectives on mental and physical well-being*. San Francisco: Jossey-Bass.

Babatunde-Sowole, O., Power, T., Jackson, D., Davidson, P. M., & DiGiacomo, M. (2016). Resilience of African migrants: An integrative review. *Health Care for Women International, 37*, 946–963.

Block, J. H., & Block, J. (1980). The role of ego-control and ego-resiliency in the organization of behavior. In W. A. Collins (Ed.), *Development of cognition, affect, and social relations: The Minnesota Symposia on child psychology*. Hillsdale: Erlbaum.

Bonanno, G. A. (2004). Loss, trauma, and human resilience: Have we underestimated the human capacity to thrive after extremely aversive events? *American Psychologist, 59*, 20–28.

Bonanno, G. A., & Diminich, E. D. (2013). Annual research review: Positive adjustment to adversity–trajectories of minimal–impact resilience and emergent resilience. *Journal of Child Psychology and Psychiatry, 54*, 378–401.

Bonanno, G. A., Westphal, M., & Mancini, A. D. (2011). Resilience to loss and potential trauma. *Annual Review of Clinical Psychology, 7*, 511–535.

Charney, D. S. (2004). Psychobiological mechanisms of resilience and vulnerability: Implications for successful adaptation to extreme stress. *The American Journal of Psychiatry, 161*, 195–216.

Chrousos, G. P. (2009). Stress and disorders of the stress system. *Nature Reviews Endocrinology, 5*, 374–381.

Connor, K. M., & Davidson, J. R. (2003). Development of a new resilience scale: The Connor-Davidson resilience scale (CD-RISC). *Depression and Anxiety, 18*, 76–82.

Deshields, T. L., Heiland, M. F., Kracen, A. C., & Dua, P. (2016). Resilience in adults with cancer: Development of a conceptual model. *Psycho-Oncology, 25*, 11–18.

Feder, A., Nestler, E. J., & Charney, D. S. (2009). Psychobiology and molecular genetics of resilience. *Nature Reviews Neuroscience, 10*, 446–457.

Folkman, S., & Lazarus, R. S. (1988). *Manual for the ways of coping questionnaire*. Palo Alto: Consulting Psychological Press.

Friborg, O., Hjemdal, O., Rosenvinge, J. H., & Martinussen, M. (2003). A new rating scale for adult resilience: What are the central protective resources behind healthy adjustment? *International Journal of Methods in Psychiatric Research, 12*, 65–76.

Goubert, L., & Trompetter, H. (2017). Towards a science and practice of resilience in the face of pain. *European Journal of Pain, 21*, 1301–1315.

Han, M. H., & Nestler, E. J. (2017). Neural substrates of depression and resilience. *Neurotherapeutics, 14*, 677–686.

Kobasa, S. C. (1979). Stressful life events, personality, and health: An inquiry into hardiness. *Journal of Personality and Social Psychology, 37*, 1–11.

Liu, H., Zhang, C., Ji, Y., & Yang, L. (2018). Biological and psychological perspectives of resilience: Is it possible to improve stress resistance? *Frontiers in Human Neuroscience, 12*, 1–12.

Martin, M. M., & Rubin, R. B. (1995). A new measure of cognitive flexibility. *Psychological Reports, 76*, 623–626.

Pangallo, A., Zibarras, L., Lewis, R., & Flaxman, P. (2015). Resilience through the lens of interactionism: A systematic review. *Psychological Assessment, 27*, 1–20.

Rosenberg, M. (1965). *Society and the adolescent self-image*. Princeton: Princeton University Press.

Russo, S. J., Murrough, J. W., Han, M. H., Charney, D. S., & Nestler, E. J. (2012). Neurobiology of resilience. *Nature Neuroscience, 15*, 1475–1484.

Sarason, I. G., Levine, H. M., Basham, R. B., & Sarason, B. R. (1983). Assessing social support: The social support questionnaire. *Journal of Personality and Social Psychology, 44*, 127–139.

Scheier, M. F., Carver, C. S., & Bridges, M. W. (1994). Distinguishing optimism from neuroticism (and trait anxiety, self-mastery, and self-esteem): A reevaluation of the life orientation test. *Journal of Personality and Social Psychology, 67*, 1063–1078.

Sherer, M., Maddux, J. E., Mercandante, B., Prentice-Dunn, S., Jacobs, B., & Rogers, R. W. (1982). The self-efficacy scale: Construction and validation. *Psychological Reports, 51*, 663–671.

Tan-Kristanto, S., & Kiropoulos, L. A. (2015). Resilience, self-efficacy, coping styles and depressive and anxiety symptoms in those newly diagnosed with multiple sclerosis. *Psychology, Health & Medicine, 20*, 635–645.

Wagnild, G. M., & Young, H. M. (1993). Development and psychometric evaluation of the resilience scale. *Journal of Nursing Measurement, 1*, 165–178.

Walker, F. R., Pfingst, K., Carnevali, L., Sgoifo, A., & Nalivaiko, E. (2017). In the search for integrative biomarker of resilience to psychological stress. *Neuroscience & Biobehavioral Reviews, 74*, 310–320.

Watson, D., Clark, L. A., & Tellegen, A. (1988). Development and validation of brief measures of positive and negative affect: The PANAS scales. *Journal of Personality and Social Psychology, 54*, 1063–1070.

Windle, G., Bennett, K. M., & Noyes, J. (2011). A methodological review of resilience measurement scales. *Health and Quality of Life Outcomes, 9*, 1–18.

Woodward, E. N., Banks, R. J., Marks, A. K., & Pantalone, D. W. (2017). Identifying resilience resources for HIV prevention among sexual minority men: A systematic review. *AIDS and Behavior, 21*, 2860–2873.

Ye, Z. J., Liang, M. Z., Li, P. F., Sun, Z., Chen, P., Hu, G. Y., Yu, Y. L., Wang, S. N., & Qiu, H. Z. (2018). New resilience instrument for patients with cancer. *Quality of Life Research, 27*, 355–365.

Zannas, A. S., & West, A. E. (2014). Epigenetics and the regulation of stress vulnerability and resilience. *Neuroscience, 264*, 157–170.

Resilient Aging

▶ Positive Aging

Resistance Training

Roland Thomeé
Department of Rehabilitation Medicine,
Sahlgrenska University Hospital, Göteborg,
Sweden

Definition

Resistance training has an impact on many-body systems such as the muscular, respiratory, skeletal, and neural, but also the immune, endocrine, and metabolic (Deschenes and Kraemer 2002).

Description

Resistance training has been used for a very long time. There is documentation from 700 B.C. of the very strong Bybon in Greece lifting a 140 kg rock over his head with only one hand. The legendary Milon from Italy lifted a new born calf every day until the calf was a full-grown bull. This is the first documentation of progressive resistance training (Fry and Newton 2002). Among the pioneers in research on resistance training Thomas L. De Lorme needs to be mentioned. In 1946 he presented a method for resistance training using the one repetition maximum (1RM) (De Lorme 1946). This concept is still widely used today describing the intensity used in resistance training programs.

In order to achieve the desired response on the body it is important to understand the basic principles of resistance training. Resistance training can, according to the American Sports Medicine Institute (http://www.asmi.org/), be defined as a gradual overload of the musculoskeletal system resulting in improved capacity. In general resistant training is often synonymous with strength training. Depending on the design the resistance training program can result in improved muscle strength, muscle volume, muscle power, or muscle endurance. Motor control can improve with better balance, coordination, and technique. Also tendons, ligaments, articular cartilage, and bones can improve their capacity as a result of resistance training (Deschenes and Kraemer 2002).

There are several methods available and various effects of the resistance training program are achieved depending on the frequency, intensity, and volume of the training (Wernbom et al. 2007). The program needs to specify the number of weeks of training, the number of training sessions performed per week, the number of exercises used for each muscle group, the number of sets and repetitions used for each exercise, and how long time of rest is given in between sets and exercises. For general strength training it can be recommended that the program consists of two session per week, two exercises per major muscle group, two to three sets of 8–12 repetitions per exercise with 30 s of rest in between sets and exercises (Haskell et al. 2007). In order to improve muscle power, i.e., the ability to produce a high force rapidly, a moderate load moved as fast as possible is recommended. For muscular endurance the number of repetitions should exceed 20 and the rest between sets and exercises decreased to a minimum (Wernbom et al. 2007).

One mode of strength training can be classified as dynamic external resistance, including free weights and weight machines, where the resistance is moved through the range of motion of the joint. Another mode can be classified as accommodating resistance, for example, isokinetic (the speed of movement is constant and the resistance offered by the machine accommodates to the applied force through the whole range of motion). A third mode can be classified as isometric resistance where no movement occurs during muscle force development. For the first two modes one usually differs concentric from eccentric muscle action. In a concentric muscle action the muscle shortens while developing force and in the eccentric muscle action the muscle lengthens while developing force. There is no evidence as of now for the superiority of any mode and/or type of muscle action over other modes and types (Wernbom et al. 2007). Given sufficient frequency, intensity, and volume of work, all three types of muscle actions can induce significant increased muscle volume at an impressive rate.

Cross-References

▶ Isometric/Isotonic Exercise

References and Readings

De Lorme, T. L. (1946). Heavy resistance exercises. *Archives of Physical Medicine and Rehabilitation, 27*, 607–630.
Deschenes, M. R., & Kraemer, W. J. (2002). Performance and physiologic adaptations to resistance training. *American Journal of Physical Medicine & Rehabilitation, 81*(11 Suppl), S3–S16. https://doi.org/10.1097/01.PHM.0000029722.06777.E9.
Fry, A. C., & Newton, R. U. (2002). A brief history of strength training and basic principles and concepts. In W. Kraemer & K. Häkkinen (Eds.), *Strength training for sport* (pp. 1–19). Oxford: Blackwell Scientific.
Haskell, W. L., Lee, I. M., Pate, R. R., Powell, K. E., Blair, S. N., Franklin, B. A., & Bauman, A. (2007). Physical activity and public health: Updated recommendation for adults from the American College of Sports Medicine and the American Heart Association. *Medicine and Science in Sports and Exercise, 39*(8), 1423–1434. https://doi.org/10.1249/mss.0b013e3180616b27.00005768-200708000-00027 [pii].
Wernbom, M., Augustsson, J., & Thomee, R. (2007). The influence of frequency, intensity, volume and mode of strength training on whole muscle cross-sectional area in humans. *Sports Medicine, 37*(3), 225–264. 3734 [pii].

Resource Management

▶ Multiphase Optimization Strategy (MOST)

Respect

Catharina Vogt[1] and Nadine Skoluda[2]
[1]RespectResearchGroup, University of Hamburg, Hamburg, Germany
[2]Faculty of Psychology, University of Vienna, Vienna, Austria

Synonyms

Appreciation; Civility; Recognition (means of acknowledgment); Responsiveness

Antonyms

Disrespect; Rudeness

Definition

Having its nomological roots in the Latin verb *respicere* meaning to "look around," "show consideration," and "pay attention to someone," the term respect was coined by philosophers (e.g., Darwall 1977; Dillon 1992), with Immanuel Kant (1785) being the most prominent. With the aim of sharpening the concept of respect, researchers argued for a differentiation from connotatively related concepts such as acceptance, care, courtesy, status, tolerance, trust, dignity, affirmation, or even justice (e.g., Rogers and Ashforth 2017; van Quaquebeke et al. 2007) leading to the definition by Van Quaquebeke and Eckloff (2010, p. 344): "A person who respects another person acts in such a manner that it in return engenders a feeling in the other person of being appreciated in his/her importance and worth as a person." Accordingly, the setting of respect requires a social interaction, with one person (sender) who is paying attention and is responsive to another person (recipient) who is perceiving these actions as such, resulting in feelings of belongingness and/or being recognized and valued (De Cremer and Tyler 2005). Thus the concept of respect in an interaction is only justified if the intended recipient has also perceived the sent respect as such. However, the concept of respect is often used inconsistently; its meaning is shaped by the situational context; and so respect research is faced with the challenge of investigating the various meanings and integrating the results into an overall picture (Rogers and Ashforth 2017). Due to the criticism of semantically ambiguous definitions of respect (Frei and Shaver 2002; van Quaquebeke et al. 2007), and its ambiguous use in everyday language, researchers have proposed a division of the term into two parts: horizontal (general/recognition) respect and vertical (particular/appraisal) respect (Darwall 1977; Decker and Van Quaquebeke 2015; Grover 2014; Rogers and Ashforth 2017; van Quaquebeke et al. 2007). By means of both horizontal and vertical respect, those who show respect communicate how they relate to those to whom the respect was targeted at. Of note, horizontal respect and vertical respect are intertwined and can be simultaneously present in the same social situation.

The central component of horizontal respect is the recognition and unconditional consideration of a person as an equal counterpart, regardless of his/her qualities and achievements, on the basis of his/her human dignity (Lalljee et al. 2007; Renger and Simon 2011). Correspondingly, potentially every human being can be respected horizontally. At the core of horizontal respect is the equality of both, the sender and the recipient of respect. This facilitates the formation of a "We" unit between the sender and recipient (Rogers and Ashforth 2017). Horizontal respect is typically dichotomous, communicating respect or disrespect (van Quaquebeke et al. 2007).

Vertical respect refers to the recognition of a person's expertise or abilities. This emphasizes the "Me" (Rogers and Ashforth 2017), as it focuses on the inequality between the sender and the recipient based on the evaluation of the recipient in terms of their achievements, qualities, and behaviors in comparison to the respect sending person.

By virtue of their characteristics, respect recipients stand out positively from those who show respect to them. Through vertical respect, senders signal that they are open to the influence of the respect recipient (van Quaquebeke et al. 2007). Vertical respect can be seen as a dimensional continuum.

Within the respect research, the construct of respect varies broadly: it is operationalized as an attitude (e.g., Lalljee et al. 2007), behavior (e.g., Voigt et al. 2017), expectation (e.g., Van Quaquebeke and Eckloff 2010), need (Tay and Diener 2011), perception (De Cremer and Tyler 2005; Greguras and Ford 2006; perception of received and sent respect, respectively), stressor (Semmer et al. 2007), and value (Ng and Diener 2014).

Description

Social Interaction/Context

Due to its interactional nature, respect plays a role in all domains of society. Within the occupational context, organizational respect (e.g., Grover 2014), respectful leadership (e.g., Van Quaquebeke and Eckloff 2010), respectful inquiry (Van Quaquebeke and Felps 2018), respect as a motivator (e.g., Renger and Simon 2011), and lack of respect as a job stressor (e.g., Semmer et al. 2007) have been investigated in various contexts of leader-follower teams in corporations, as well as in prisons (e.g., Rogers and Ashforth 2017), schools (Mertz et al. 2015), public service (e.g., police) (e.g., Warren 2011), politics (e.g., Molders and Van Quaquebeke 2017), professional sports (Prestwich and Lalljee 2009), and primary healthcare settings such as medical or therapeutic contexts (e.g., Koskenniemi et al. 2018; Murante et al. 2017) and nurse-physician collaborations (Wang et al. 2018). Within the private domain, respect is suggested to play an important role in close relationships between friends, family members, and intimate partners (e.g., Frei and Shaver 2002; Selcuk and Ong 2013).

Functions and Findings

Even though mutual respect is the basis for successful cooperation and is believed to be one of the most important ethical values of our time (Ng and Diener 2014), the term and its practical implications have only been the focus of research since the 2000s. Regarding the function of respect, horizontal and vertical respect address the needs and values of social belongingness and social reputation/self-esteem (De Cremer and Mulder 2007). Further, respect is thought to act as a "social lubricant and glue" (p. 197; van Quaquebeke et al. 2007) and can thus contribute to how individuals evaluate the quality of social interactions or interpersonal relationships. For example, respect plays a pivotal role in conflict resolution (De Cremer 2003). Beyond its social functions, perceived respect is believed to contribute to individual's well-being (e.g., Tay and Diener 2011). According to the effort-reward imbalance model (ERI; Siegrist et al. 2004), a model of occupational gratification crisis, respect can be understood as a form of (social) reward and can even act as a motivating factor for behavior.

Whereas disrespect has detrimental effects on perceived stress (e.g., see also "stress-as-offense-to-self," Semmer et al. 2007), sleep quality (Pereira et al. 2014), performance capability, and functioning in interpersonal relationships (Lind et al. 1998; Miller 2001), a high degree of perceived respect is associated with individuals' vitality (Selcuk and Ong 2013), self-esteem (De Cremer and Tyler 2005), general health (Vinberg 2008), relationship quality (Frei and Shaver 2002), job performance (Rogers et al. 2017), self-determination and job satisfaction (Decker and Van Quaquebeke 2015), commitment to ones' in-group (Erez et al. 2009), organizational participation (Stürmer et al. 2008), creativity (Carmeli et al. 2015), autonomy (Renger and Simon 2011), pride (Boezeman and Ellemers 2008), and positive affect and mood (Strahler et al. 2019).

Cross-References

▶ Interpersonal Relationships
▶ Job Performance
▶ Job Satisfaction/Dissatisfaction
▶ Self-esteem
▶ Sleep
▶ Stress
▶ Well-being

References and Readings

Boezeman, E. J., & Ellemers, N. (2008). Pride and respect in volunteers' organizational commitment. *European Journal of Social Psychology, 38*, 159–172.

Carmeli, A., Dutton, J. E., & Hardin, A. E. (2015). Respect as an engine for new ideas: Linking respectful engagement, relational information processing and creativity among employees and teams. *Human Relations, 68*(6), 1021–1047.

Darwall, S. L. (1977). Two kinds of respect. *Ethics, 88*(1), 36–49.

De Cremer, D. (2003). Noneconomic motives predicting cooperation in public good dilemmas: The effect of received respect on contributions. *Social Justice Research 16*(4), 367–377.

De Cremer, D., & Mulder, L. B. (2007). A passion for respect: On understanding the role of human needs and morality. *Gruppendynamik und Organisationsberatung, 38*(4), 439–449.

De Cremer, D., & Tyler, T. R. (2005). Am I respected or not? Inclusion and reputation as issues in group membership. *Social Justice Research, 18*, 121–153.

Decker, C., & Van Quaquebeke, N. (2015). Getting respect from a boss you respect: How different types of respect interact to explain subordinates' job satisfaction as mediated by self-determination. *Journal of Business Ethics, 131*(3), 543–556.

Dillon, R. S. (1992). Respect and care – toward moral integration. *Canadian Journal of Philosophy, 22*(1), 105–131.

Erez, A., Sleebos, E., Mikulincer, M., Van Ijzendoorn, M. H., Ellemers, N., & Kroonenberg, P. M. (2009). Attachment anxiety, intra-group (dis)respect, actual efforts, and group donation. *European Journal of Social Psychology, 39*(5), 734–746.

Frei, J. R., & Shaver, P. R. (2002). Respect in close relationships: Prototype definition, self-report assessment, and initial correlates. *Personal Relationships, 9*(2), 121–139.

Greguras, G. J., & Ford, J. M. (2006). An examination of the multidimensionality of supervisor and subordinate perceptions of leader-member exchange. *Journal of Occupational and Organizational Psychology, 79*, 433–465.

Grover, S. L. (2014). Unraveling respect in organization studies. *Human Relations, 67*(1), 27–51.

Kant, I. (1785). *Groundwork of the metaphysics of morals*. Cambridge, UK: Cambridge University Press.

Koskenniemi, J., Leino-Kilpi, H., Puukka, P., Stolt, M., & Suhonen, R. (2018). Being respected by nurses: Measuring older patients' perceptions. *International Journal of Older People Nursing, 13*(3), e12127.

Lalljee, M., Laham, M., & Tam, T. (2007). Unconditional respect for persons: A social psychological analysis. *Gruppendynamik und Organisationsberatung, 38*, 451–464.

Lind, E. A., Kray, L., & Thompson, L. (1998). The social construction of injustice: Fairness judgments in response to own and others unfair treatment by authorities. *Organizational Behavior and Human Decision Processes, 75*(1), 1–22.

Mertz, C., Eckloff, T., Johannsen, J., & Van Quaquebeke, N. (2015). Respected students equal better students: Investigating the links between respect and performance in schools. *Journal of Educational and Developmental Psychology, 5*, 74–86.

Miller, D. T. (2001). Disrespect and the experience of injustice. *Annual Review of Psychology, 52*, 527–553.

Molders, C., & Van Quaquebeke, N. (2017). When and how politicians' disrespect affects voters' trust in the political system: The roles of social judgments and category prototypicality. *Journal of Applied Social Psychology, 47*(9), 515–527.

Murante, A. M., Seghieri, C., Vainieri, M., & Schafer, W. L. A. (2017). Patient-perceived responsiveness of primary care systems across Europe and the relationship with the health expenditure and remuneration systems of primary care doctors. *Social Science & Medicine, 186*, 139–147.

Ng, W., & Diener, E. (2014). What matters to the rich and the poor? Subjective well-being, financial satisfaction, and postmaterialist needs across the world. *Journal of Personality and Social Psychology, 107*(2), 326–338.

Pereira, D., Semmer, N. K., & Elfering, A. (2014). Illegitimate tasks and sleep quality: An ambulatory study. *Stress and Health, 30*(3), 209–221.

Prestwich, A., & Lalljee, M. (2009). The determinants and consequences of intragroup respect: An examination within a sporting context. *Journal of Applied Social Psychology, 39*(5), 1229–1253.

Renger, D., & Simon, B. (2011). Social recognition as an equal: The role of equality-based respect in group life. *European Journal of Social Psychology, 41*(4), 501–507.

Rogers, K. M., & Ashforth, B. E. (2017). Respect in organizations: Feeling valued as "we" and "me". *Journal of Management, 43*(5), 1578–1608.

Rogers, K. M., Corley, K. G., & Ashforth, B. E. (2017). Seeing more than orange: Organizational respect and positive identity transformation in a prison context. *Administrative Science Quarterly, 62*(2), 219–269.

Selcuk, E., & Ong, A. D. (2013). Perceived partner responsiveness moderates the association between received emotional support and all-cause mortality. *Health Psychology, 32*(2), 231–235.

Semmer, N. K., Jacobshagen, N., Meier, L. L., & Elfering, A. (2007). Occupational stress research: The "stress-as-offense-to-self" perspective. In J. Houdmont & S. McIntyre (Eds.), *Occupational health psychology: European perspectives on research, education and practice* (Vol. 2, pp. 43–60). Castelo da Maia: ISMAI Publishers.

Siegrist, J., Starke, S., Chandola, T., Godin, I., Marmot, M., Niedhammer, I., et al. (2004). The measurement of effort-reward imbalance at work: European comparisons. *Social Science & Medicine, 58*(8), 1483–1499.

Strahler, J., Nater, U. M., & Skoluda, N. (2019). Associations between health behaviors and factors on markers of healthy psychological and physiological functioning: A daily diary study. *Annals of Behavioral Medicine*, kaz018. https://academic.oup.com/abm/advance-article-abstract/doi/10.1093/abm/kaz018/5498794?redirectedFrom=fulltext.

Stürmer, S., Simon, B., & Loewy, M. I. (2008). Intraorganizational respect and organizational participation: The mediating role of collective identity. *Group Processes & Intergroup Relations, 11*(1), 5–20.

Tay, L., & Diener, E. (2011). Needs and subjective well-being around the world. *Journal of Personality and Social Psychology, 101*(2), 354–365.

Van Quaquebeke, N., & Eckloff, T. (2010). Defining respectful leadership: What it is, how it can be measured, and another glimpse at what it is related to. *Journal of Business Ethics, 91*, 343–358.

Van Quaquebeke, N., & Felps, W. (2018). Respectful inquiry: A motivational account of leading through asking questions and listening. *Academy of Management Review, 43*(1), 5–27.

van Quaquebeke, N., Henrich, D. C., & Eckloff, T. (2007). "It's not tolerance I'm asking for, it's respect"! A conceptual framework to differentiate between tolerance, acceptance and (two types of) respect. *Gruppendynamik und Organisationsberatung, 38*(2), 185–200.

Vinberg, S. (2008). Workplace health interventions in small enterprises: A Swedish longitudinal study. *Work – A Journal of Prevention Assessment & Rehabilitation, 30*(4), 473–482.

Voigt, R., Camp, N. P., Prabhakaran, V., Hamilton, W. L., Hetey, R. C., Griffiths, C. M., et al. (2017). Language from police body camera footage shows racial disparities in officer respect. *Proceedings of the National Academy of Sciences of the United States of America, 114*(25), 6521–6526.

Wang, Y. Y., Wan, Q. Q., Guo, J., Jin, X. Y., Zhou, W. J., Feng, X. L., et al. (2018). The influence of effective communication, perceived respect and willingness to collaborate on nurses' perceptions of nurse-physician collaboration in China. *Applied Nursing Research, 41*, 73–79.

Warren, P. Y. (2011). Perceptions of police disrespect during vehicle stops: A race-based analysis. *Crime & Delinquency, 57*(3), 356–376.

Respiratory Sinus Arrhythmia

Randall Steven Jorgensen
Department of Psychology, Syracuse University, Syracuse, USA

Synonyms

Heart rate variability (HRV)

Definition

In mammals, heart rate (HR) ordinarily accelerates during inspiration and decelerates during expiration, and the tenth cranial nerve (i.e., vagus nerve) exerts a profound influence on this heart rate variability (HRV). This oscillation of R-wave (the sharp upward spike of the QRS complex associated with the contraction of the heart) to R-wave intervals (RRI) is a cardiorespiratory phenomenon called respiratory sinus arrhythmia (RSA); since RRI, which are inversely related to moment-to-moment HR, reflect vagal stimulation, noninvasive measures of RSA are commonly used to estimate autonomic cardiovascular control (Grossman and Taylor 2007). The "peak to valley" time-domain estimate, usually quantified in milliseconds (ms), corresponds to the inspiratory-expiratory difference in RRI. For estimates based on spectral analysis and other frequency-domain approaches, RRI variation is estimated within the respiratory frequency range (.15–.4 Hz); to reflect statistical units of variance, ms^2 is commonly used. For steady-state conditions (viz., respiratory parameters, momentary physical activity, metabolic activity, and autonomic tone remain nearly constant), these estimates are almost perfectly correlated (Grossman and Taylor). These noninvasive measures' covariation with cardiac vagal tone, however, can be confounded by such factors as respiratory rate and volume, changes in physical and metabolic activity, body weight, age, and sympathetic nervous system tone; this confounding is more pronounced in between-group designs (e.g., high blood pressure vs. normal blood pressure groups) than within-subject designs (e.g., examining within-person changes in RSA following atropine administration) (Grossman and Taylor 2007).

The vagus has been posited to be a key factor in emotional regulation and health (Thayer and Lane 2009). Researchers, therefore, have used noninvasive measures of HRV and RSA to predict health and psychological well-being. These ostensible markers of cardiac vagal tone are reported to covary with cardiovascular disease, anxiety, depression, and childhood behavior disorders (Berntson et al. 2007; Thayer and Lane 2007). Even when the predicted associations are revealed, the (a) correlational designs; (b) paucity of multivariate/multilevel studies cutting across anatomical, physiological, and behavioral domains; and (c) inadequate controls of confounds (e.g., bodily motion and respiration rate) make interpretation of underlying causal and multiply determined pathways ambiguous (Berntson et al. 2007). At minimum, it is important to take into account and address the confounding variables discussed earlier (for guidelines, see Grossman and Taylor 2007).

Cross-References

▶ Heart Rate Variability
▶ Parasympathetic

References and Readings

Berntson, G. G., Cacioppo, J. T., & Grossman, P. (2007). Whither vagal tone. *Biological Psychology, 74*, 297–300. https://doi.org/10.1016/j.biopsycho.2006.08.006.

Grossman, P., & Taylor, E. W. (2007). Toward understanding respiratory arrhythmia: Relations to cardiac vagal tone, evolution, and biobehavioral functions. *Biological Psychology, 74*, 263–285. https://doi.org/10.1016/j.biopsycho.2005.11.014.

Thayer, J. F., & Lane, R. D. (2007). The role of vagal function in the risk for cardiovascular disease and mortality. *Biological Psychology, 74*, 224–242. https://doi.org/10.1016/j.biopsycho.2005.11.013.

Thayer, J. F., & Lane, R. D. (2009). Claude Bernard and the heart-brain connection: Further elaboration of a model of neurovisceral integration. *Neuroscience and Biobehavoioral Reviews, 33*, 81–88. https://doi.org/10.1016/j.neubiorev.2008.08.004.

Response Inhibition

▶ Behavioral Inhibition

Response to Disability

▶ Psychosocial Adjustment

Responses to Stress

▶ General Adaptation Syndrome

Responsibility

▶ Self-Blame

Responsiveness

▶ Respect

Rest Pain

▶ Peripheral Arterial Disease (PAD)/Vascular Disease

Retrospective Study

Jane Monaco
Department of Biostatistics, The University of North Carolina at Chapel Hill, Chapel Hill, NC, USA

Definition

A study in which the outcome of interest has already occurred when the study initiated is commonly referred to as retrospective study.

Some investigators have used the terms retrospective and case-control interchangeably. This usage is misleading since study designs other than case-control studies can be retrospective. For example, in a retrospective cohort study (Okasha et al. 2002) examining the relationship between body mass index (BMI) during early adulthood and cancer death, both the exposure and the outcome had occurred at the initiation of the study. University students' weight and height information was obtained from annual physical records at the University of Glasgow health service from 1948 to 1968. Cancer mortality was determined based on a central registry in Scotland that identifies the cause of death (National Health Service Central Register). Subjects with BMI in the highest quartile were found to be at higher risk of cancer death than individuals in the lowest BMI quartile.

In a retrospective study, data may be collected based on clinical records, employment records, or memory. These retrospective data can be more prone to bias, such as recall bias, than prospective designs studying the same association.

Some investigators may also use the term "retrospective" in a different way, referring to the timing of the measurements of the exposure and outcome; studies in which the exposure is measured after the outcome is measured can be referred to as retrospective (Rothman and Greenland 1998, pp. 74–75).

Cross-References

▶ Case-Control Studies
▶ Cohort Study

References and Further Reading

Kleinbaum, D. G., Sullivan, K. M., & Barker, N. D. (2007). *A pocket guide to epidemiology*. New York: Springer.
Okasha, M., McCarron, P., McEwen, J., & Davey Smith, G. (2002). Body mass index in young adulthood and cancer mortality: A retrospective cohort study. *Journal of Epidemiology and Community Health, 56*, 780–784.
Rothman, K. J., & Greenland, S. (1998). *Modern epidemiology*. Philadelphia: Lippencott-Raven.

Return to Baseline

▶ Psychophysiologic Recovery

Return to Work

Beth Grunfeld
Department of Psychological Sciences, Birkbeck College, University of London, London, UK

Synonyms

Occupational rehabilitation; Sickness absence; Vocational rehabilitation

Definition

Return-to-work (RTW) status is regarded as a return to normal work-related activity following illness or return to suitable employment that takes account of post-illness ability and priorities.

Description

Scope
Mental illness and musculoskeletal diseases are the most common causes of long-term sickness, although other chronic conditions such as heart disease and cancer make a significant contribution to recorded sickness absence. It is estimated that each UK employee loses an estimated 30.4 days of productivity annually as a consequence of sick days or underperformance resulting from ill-health. This is estimated to cost employers between 2 and 16% of annual salary costs due to lost productivity and as a consequence of implementing sickness management systems. In Australia, lost productivity through absenteeism is estimated to cost $33 billion, with a total of 92 million working days being lost each year. While in the USA, illness-related lost productivity costs an estimated $530 billion per year with around 893 million days lost due to illness. These figures include all cause illnesses and any duration of illness. Return to work is specifically concerned with returning to the work place following longer periods of absence, which is important as it is known that the longer a person is absent from the workplace, the greater the risk of non-return.

Costs of Being Out of Work
Employment is important not only for individual financial reasons but also because being out of work is thought to contribute to, and aggravate, adverse health outcomes. A 10% reduction in health-related quality of life (in absolute terms) has been observed as a consequence of unemployment, and the largest impact is observed in the domains of anxiety and depression (Norström et al. 2019), a finding that has endured over the past two decades. Not working is associated with reduced self-esteem, lowered self-efficacy, and decreased belief in one's ability to return to the workplace (Creed et al. 2001). The relationship between unemployment and negative health outcomes is thought to be mediated by factors such as lower socioeconomic status, financial anxiety, and a chronic stress pathway involving temporary lowered immunity whereby lower natural killer cell cytotoxicity (NKCC) associated with unemployment reflects differences in the cytotoxic capacity of the cell.

Factors Influencing Return to Work
Many patients do well following treatment; however, some experience ongoing negative outcomes from the disease or treatment (including pain, fatigue, and low mood) that may impact everyday functioning, including work. For example, over a quarter of cancer survivors report high symptom burden 1-year post-diagnosis, even after treatment termination (Shi et al. 2011). Furthermore, return-to-work rates have been shown to vary across cancer types (Cooper et al. 2013), and longer return-to-work times have been

reported among patients undergoing certain treatments (surgery/chemotherapy) or experiencing fatigue.

In addition to disease- and treatment-related factors, non-modifiable demographic factors, such as higher education and socioeconomic status, are associated with successful return to work. More recently, psychological factors have been shown to impact on effective return to work including self-efficacy, lower levels of fear avoidance, positive expectations of recovery, and illness cognitions (Cooper et al. 2013). Such psychological factors may be modifiable through psychoeducational strategies presenting the opportunity for intervention to improve return to work.

Conversely, poorer return-to-work outcomes are associated with older age, being female, greater reported pain and depression, work requiring high physical demands, and greater disability or work limitations. In addition, among employees with mental health conditions, multiple short sickness absences, or a period of 8 days or more of sickness absence per year are associated with high risk for subsequent long-term sickness absence (Sumanen et al. 2017). Furthermore, although some illnesses (including specific cancer types) have a high return-to-work rate, we know that a significant proportion of patients return to work too early, or in an inappropriate manner, which results in them taking additional sick leave or leaving the workplace.

Interventions to Support Return to Work

Several interventions to support working have been developed across illness groups, including musculoskeletal disorders, back pain, cancer, heart disease, and multiple sclerosis. These interventions have tended to focus on ergonomic adaptation within the workplace with the aim of minimizing the risk of physical injuries, likely to be experienced by these patient groups. Interventions targeted at patients with cancer include a 12-week occupational physician-led intervention focused on increasing physical activity to support return to work (Groeneveld et al. 2012), a case management approach involving signposting/referring patients to services (e.g., physiotherapy, occupational, or psychological therapy) to support return to work (Hubbard et al. 2013), and a tool that cancer survivors use to guide discussions about working (Munir et al. 2013). However, this tool focused on interactions with employers and health-care professionals and not on patients' beliefs and barriers that impact workability (one's perception of one's ability to work) and influence work behavior. Furthermore, a Cochrane review reported low-quality evidence for return-to-work rates for psychoeducational interventions (interventions that encompass a broad range of activities that combine educational and other activities such as counseling and supportive care); however, this was based on only two studies: one that focused on teaching self-care behaviors to manage fatigue and one comprising lectures focused on side effects, stress, and coping. The review concluded that there was a need for more high-quality randomized controlled trials (de Boer et al. 2015). Furthermore, a meta-synthesis of qualitative research studies highlighted the need for vocational interventions with patients to be person centered and for such interventions to acknowledge the role of social, clinical, and work-related factors (Wells et al. 2013).

Methodological Considerations

Studies of the incidence of sickness absence often utilize employer or national data registries. These provide reliable and comprehensive data about absence but lack wider data about participants and their health-related background, including important diagnostic information. Furthermore, studies have tended to examine return to work within discrete groups, for example, a particular illness, but few have examined factors influencing return to work across illnesses or among participants with comorbidities. Such an approach could help identify modifiable factors that could inform more generic, cost-effective intervention packages to support return to work following illness.

Cross-References

▶ Cancer Survivorship
▶ Health-Related Quality of Life
▶ Vocational Rehabilitation
▶ Work

References and Further Reading

Cooper, A. F., Hankins, M., Rixon, L., Eaton, E., & Grunfeld, E. A. (2013). Distinct work-related, clinical and psychological factors predict return to work following treatment in four different cancer types. *Psychooncology, 22*(3), 659–667.

Creed, P. A., Bloxsome, T. D., & Johnston, K. (2001). Self-esteem and self-efficacy outcomes for unemployed individuals attending occupational skills training programs. *Community, Work & Family, 4*, 285–303.

de Boer, A. G., Taskila, T. K., Tamminga, S. J., et al. (2015). Interventions to enhance return-to-work for cancer patients. *Cochrane Database of Systematic Reviews*, https://doi.org/10.1002/14651858. CD007569.

Groeneveld, I. F., de Boer, A. G., & Frings-Dresen, M. H. (2012). A multidisciplinary intervention to facilitate return to work in cancer patients: Intervention protocol and design of a feasibility study. *BMJ Open, 2*, e001321.

Hubbard, G., Gray, N. M., Ayansina, D., et al. (2013). Case management vocational rehabilitation for women with breast cancer after surgery: A feasibility study incorporating a pilot randomised controlled trial. *Trials, 14*, 175.

Munir, F., Kalawsky, K., Wallis, D. J., et al. (2013). Using intervention mapping to develop a work-related guidance tool for those affected by cancer. *BMC Public Health, 13*, 6.

Norström, F., Waenerlund, A. K., Lindholm, L., Nygren, R., Sahlén, K. G., & Brydsten, A. (2019). Does unemployment contribute to poorer health-related quality of life among Swedish adults? *BMC Public Health, 19*(1), 457.

Shi, Q., Smith, T. G., Michonski, J. D., Stein, K. D., Kaw, C., & Cleeland, C. S. (2011). Symptom burden in cancer survivors 1 year after diagnosis: A report from the American Cancer Society's studies of cancer survivors. *Cancer, 117*(12), 2779–2790.

Sumanen, H., Pietilainen, O., Lahelma, E., & Rahkonen, O. (2017). Short sickness absence and subsequent sickness absence due to mental disorders – A follow-up study among municipal employees. *BMC Public Health, 17*, 15.

Wells, M., Williams, B., Firnigl, D., et al. (2013). Supporting 'work-related goals' rather than 'return to work' after cancer? A systematic review and meta-synthesis of 25 qualitative studies. *Psychooncology, 22*, 1208–1219.

Revised Life Orientation Test (LOT-R)

▶ Optimism and Pessimism: Measurement

Rheumatoid Arthritis: Psychosocial Aspects

Toshihide Hashimoto
Division of Rehabilitation, Joumou Hospital, Maebashi, Japan

Synonyms

RA

Definition

Rheumatoid arthritis is a chronic, systemic, and progressive inflammatory disease that is characterized by swelling, pain, and deformity of the joints. It affects not only synovial joints but also many tissues and organs of the body.

Description

Rheumatoid Arthritis (RA)

RA affects about 0.5–1.0% of the general population worldwide. Women are afflicted two to three times more often than men. Individuals between 40 and 60 years of age are more prone to RA, but people can be affected at any age. Although the cause of RA has not been fully elucidated, genetics, infection, hormones, and the environment play a major role in the onset and progression of RA.

The initial symptoms of RA generally occur in the smaller joints (e.g., finger or wrist joints) and gradually spread symmetrically to the larger joints (e.g., elbow or knee joints). In affected joints, inflammation first occurs in the synovial membrane. Abnormal synovium, called "pannus," multiplies gradually and results in cartilage damage and bone erosion and ultimately leading to destruction of the joints. Consequently, RA patients suffer from joint symptoms, such as pain, swelling, stiffness, deformity, and restriction of motion.

In addition, inflammation involved in RA may affect various organs, including the lung, heart and blood vessels, kidneys, bone, and skin. RA patients also experience some general symptoms due to chronic inflammation, such as anemia, fatigue, low-grade fever, sleep disorder, and lack of appetite.

These symptoms can cause physical disability and various psychosocial problems in RA patients. Consequently, many RA patients experience loss of income, reduction/loss of recreational and social activities, and disability in doing housework and taking care of children. These physical and social disabilities are likely to disturb their interpersonal relationships and lead to psychological disorders. Depression and anxiety have also been known to cause increased pain and other RA-related symptoms (Erickson et al. 2016; Firestein 2016; McInnes and Schett 2011).

Psychological Distress of RA Patients

Depression is significantly more common among RA patients than healthy individuals. Recent meta-analyses have revealed the prevalence of major depressive disorder to be 16.8% based upon standard clinical interviews and depressive symptoms to be between 14.8% and 38.8% based upon screening tools. These figures are presumed to be higher than that of the general population and similar to or higher than those of other chronic conditions.

Many factors have been associated with depression of RA patients. In terms of RA-related symptoms, increases in self-reported pain, fatigue, and physical disability are likely to lead to a more depressive state. The causal relationship between pain, fatigue, disability, and depression is complex and is considered multidirectional. On the other hand, the association between depression and indices of inflammation (i.e., C-reactive protein (CRP), erythrocyte sedimentation rate (ESR), swollen joint count, grip strength, and radiological status) remains contradictory.

Recently, psychosocial factors have been emphasized as important variables that are associated with depression. In general, increased depression among RA patients is related to being female, of a younger age, with a lower income, less employment, greater work disability, more social stress, less social support, dysfunctional familial background, maladaptive coping strategy, and distorted cognition.

In clinical practice, objective clinical variables (CRP, ESR, or joint count) and subjective patient-reported physical symptoms are considered as important indices of treatment effectiveness. However, clinicians do not tend to pay close attention to the mood state of RA patients. Depressed RA patients may not verbally express their emotions, because they judge that their emotional and physical conditions are a part of their RA symptoms, and often hesitate to admit their mental distress. Accordingly, depression in RA patients is most likely underestimated by clinicians. Thus, all health-care professionals should attempt to observe whether RA patients exhibit latent depression (Bruce 2008; Matcham et al. 2013; Sheehy et al. 2006).

Relationship Between RA-Related Symptoms and Psychosocial Factors

Pain, fatigue, and physical disability are RA-related symptoms that need to be addressed by all health-care professionals. Pain is the most common and basic symptom among RA patients. Fatigue is also common and the most burdensome symptom. The prevalence of fatigue ranges greatly, from 40% to 80%, most likely because the definitions and methods of measurement are not uniform. Fatigue is perceived as a frustrating or exhausting state, which impacts every situation of life, and persists for a long time. Pain, fatigue, and physical disability influence the psychological well-being and social participation among RA patients. Moreover, psychosocial factors, i.e., perception of symptoms, self-efficacy, coping strategy, social stress, and social support, play important roles in modifying the process and outcome of RA-related symptoms and psychological distress.

The perception of symptoms remains an individual belief, in how RA will influence oneself, how long RA will last, whether RA can be controlled, and what the outcomes of RA are. RA patients with negative beliefs, such as "catastrophizing" (the tendency to focus on symptoms and predict extremely negative outcomes) or "helplessness" (the belief that nothing can be done by oneself to deal with symptoms), may manifest increased symptoms and poor psychological well-being. On the other hand, self-efficacy (the confidence in one's ability to accomplish sufficiently a desired outcome) and an adaptive coping strategy (the suitable and effective process to deal with stresses and difficulties of life) are considered to improve symptoms and psychological distress.

All health-care professionals should make efforts to inform RA patients of the cause, treatment, clinical course, and result of RA at the early stage of their disease, before they have poor perception of symptoms and acquire maladaptive coping strategies. There are indications that cognitive behavioral therapy (CBT) and mindfulness are effective for the treatment of pain and depression in RA patients, particularly when administered at the early stage of the disease. These interventions would help patients to manage RA-related symptoms and comorbidities, by learning coping strategies to manage pain, other physical symptoms, and emotional consequences, that would prevent the development of psychological difficulties associated with RA (Backman 2006; Bruce 2008; Repping-Wuts et al. 2009; Sharpe 2016; Sheehy et al. 2006).

Relevance to Clinical Practice

During the past second decade, drug treatment for RA has improved significantly. Conventional synthetic disease-modifying antirheumatic drugs (csDMARDs) and biological DMARDs (drugs that block or modify the effect of factors of the immune system, such as cytokines and cells) have been introduced to RA patients in the early stage. These new medications effectively reduce the inflammation of RA and prevent the advancement of joint erosion and deformities. These drug therapies have the potential to reduce not only RA-related symptoms but also comorbidities. Consequently, the clinical course of RA could change significantly, leading to a decrease in the number of patients who suffer from pain, fatigue, disability, and psychosocial distress.

However, such medications have several problems, including potential side effects (e.g., lung or liver dysfunction, infection, or malignancy), ineffectiveness for some patients, and the high cost of treatment. While many, but not all, patients are expected to benefit from these medical advancements in RA, they will likely experience new psychosocial problems. Therefore, health-care professionals must further examine psychosocial factors that accompany new therapies to evaluate both the positive and negative influences on patients (Humphreys et al. 2016; O'Dell 2016; Singh et al. 2016).

Cross-References

▶ Psychosocial Characteristics
▶ Psychosocial Factors

References and Further Reading

American College of Rheumatology (ACR). Retrieved from http://www.rheumatology.org

Backman, C. L. (2006). Arthritis and pain. Psychosocial aspects in the management of arthritis pain. *Arthritis Research & Therapy, 8*, 221–227.

Bruce, T. O. (2008). Comorbid depression in rheumatoid arthritis: Pathophysiology and clinical implications. *Current Psychiatry Reports, 10*, 258–264.

Erickson, A. R., et al. (2016). Chapter 70: Clinical features of rheumatoid arthritis. In G. S. Firestein, R. C. Budd, S. E. Gabriel, I. B. McInnes, & J. R. O'Dell (Eds.), *Kelley & Firestein's textbook of rheumatology* (10th ed.). Philadelphia: Saunders.

Firestein, G. S. (2016). Chapter 69: Etiology and pathogenesis of rheumatoid arthritis. In G. S. Firestein, R. C. Budd, S. E. Gabriel, I. B. McInnes, & J. R. O'Dell (Eds.), *Kelley & Firestein's textbook of rheumatology* (10th ed.). Philadelphia: Saunders.

Humphreys, J., Hyrich, K., & Symmons, D. (2016). What is the impact of biologic therapies on common co-morbidity in patients with rheumatoid arthritis? *Arthritis Research & Therapy, 18*, 282.

Matcham, F., Rayner, L., Steer, S., & Hotopf, M. (2013). The prevalence of depression in rheumatoid arthritis: A systematic review and meta-analysis. *Rheumatology, 52*, 2136–2148.

McInnes, I. B., & Schett, G. (2011). The pathogenesis of rheumatoid arthritis. *The New England Journal of Medicine, 365*, 2205–2219.

O'Dell, J. R. (2016). Chapter 71: Treatment of rheumatoid arthritis. In G. S. Firestein, R. C. Budd, S. E. Gabriel, I. B. McInnes, & J. R. O'Dell (Eds.), *Kelley & Firestein's textbook of rheumatology* (10th ed.). Philadelphia: Saunders.

Repping-Wuts, H., van Riel, P., & van Achterberg, T. (2009). Fatigue in patients with rheumatoid arthritis: What is known and what is needed. *Rheumatology, 48*, 207–209.

Sharpe, L. (2016). Psychosocial management of chronic pain in patient with rheumatoid arthritis: Challenge and solutions. *Journal of Pain Research, 9*, 137–146.

Sheehy, C., Murphy, E., & Barry, M. (2006). Depression in rheumatoid arthritis – Underscoring the problem. *Rheumatology, 45*, 1325–1327.

Singh, J. A., Saag, K. G., Bridgers, S. L., Jr., Akl, E. A., Bannuru, R. R., Sullivan, M. C., et al. (2016). 2015 American College of Rheumatology Guideline for the treatment of rheumatoid arthritis. *Arthritis and Rheumatism, 68*, 1–26.

The European League Against Rheumatism (EULAR). Retrieved from http://www.eular.org

Ribosomal RNA

▶ RNA

Rief, Winfried

Alexandra Martin
Friedrich-Alexander University Erlangen-Nürnberg, University Hospital, Erlangen, Erlangen, Germany

Biographical Information

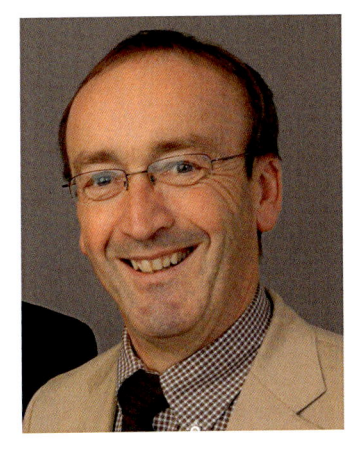

Winfried Rief was born in Ellwangen, Germany, on May 12, 1959. He is married to Sabine and has a son. Rief studied physics at the University of Karlsruhe, Germany (1978–1979), and psychology at the University of Trier, Germany (1979–1984), receiving a Diploma in psychology in 1984. His doctoral thesis presented EEG-based research about "Visual Information Processing in Chronic Schizophrenics" and led to the awarding of the Ph.D. degree at the University of Konstanz in 1987.

Rief completed postgraduate training in cognitive-behavioral therapy (1988) and is a licensed Psychological Psychotherapist. He gained excellent clinical experiences and was Head of the psychology department at the Roseneck Hospital in Prien (1989–2000), a behavioral medicine center specialized in the inpatient treatment of eating disorders, anxiety, somatoform disorders, and other conditions, which is affiliated with the Medical Faculty of the University of Munich. He accomplished the "Habilitation" – the regular German academic qualification for professorship – at the University of Salzburg, Austria in 1994.

Rief was appointed as Professor of Clinical Psychology and Psychotherapy at the University of Marburg, Germany, in 2001 and since then has chaired the division for clinical psychology. He is also Head of the Outpatient Clinic for Psychological Interventions and Head of the postgraduate training program in cognitive-behavior therapy. He has been an invited guest professor for research visits at the University of Auckland Medical School, New Zealand (2002), Harvard Medical School Institute of Psychiatry (2004), and at the University of California, San Diego, Department of Psychiatry (2009).

Rief is an active participant in many professional organizations. He was President of the German Society of Behavioral Medicine and Behavior Modification (DGVM; 2001–2005). He served as Member and as Chair of the speaker group of the section for "Clinical Psychology and Psychotherapy" in the German Psychological Society (Fachgruppe Klinische Psychologie und Psychotherapie in der Deutschen Gesellschaft für Psychologie DGPs; 1996–1998; 2005–2008). He was one of the founding members of the German Society of Biofeedback, and later served as

President in this organization (DGBFB 2000–2004). He organized many national and international scientific meetings, for example, the "International Symposium on Somatoform Disorders" (co-sponsored by the Division of Mental Health of the World Health Organization; Prien, 1997), the Congress of the German Society of Behavioral Medicine (Prien, 1999, co-organized with Prof. Dr. Manfred Fichter), the International Congress "Somatoform Disorders" (Marburg 2002), the International Congress of Behavioral Medicine (Mainz 2004, co-organized with Prof. Dr. Wolfgang Hiller), and the Annual Meetings of the German Society of Biofeedback (2001, 2007). Rief is recipient of the Biofeedback Foundation of Europe Award for Excellent Scientific Contribution (2004).

Rief has been appointed as reviewer for several research funding organizations, including the Deutsche Forschungsgemeinschaft (DFG) (German Research Foundation), Swiss National Fonds (SNF), NIHR Biomedical Research Center for Mental Health, and the Institute of Psychiatry/King's College London. In 2011, he was elected as coordinator for DFG grants in the field of clinical and health psychology in Germany. He currently serves or has served as an editorial board member in several scientific journals (*Behavioural and Cognitive Psychotherapy; British Journal of Health Psychology; Cognitive Behaviour Therapy; Current Opinion in Psychiatry; Psychology and Health; Psychotherapie in Psychiatrie, Psychosomatik und Klinischer Psychologie; Verhaltenstherapie; Zeitschrift für Psychiatrie, Psychologie und Psychotherapie ZPPP*).

Major Accomplishments

Rief is a world-leading scientist in the field of *somatoform disorders*. For more than 20 years, his research has considerably advanced the knowledge about epidemiology, etiology, and effective treatments of somatoform disorders. He has shown that medically unexplained symptoms are not only prevalent in medical settings, but also common in the general population. With the Screening for Somatoform Symptoms (SOMS) he and Professor Wolfgang Hiller provided a reliable and valid instrument to assess somatoform syndromes that are associated with considerable distress, disability, and health care utilization. One of his most recent research projects (funded by a DFG grant) aimed to investigate course and classification of medically unexplained physical complaints in the general population. Against the background of current proposals to improve the classification of somatoform disorders and related syndromes in the Diagnostic and Statistical Manual of Mental Disorders DSM-5 and the International Classification of Diseases ICD-11, Rief and colleagues were the first who tested the most prominent classification proposals (such as the Complex Somatic Symptom Disorder). Their results showed that classification criteria that include positive psychological features (such as somatic illness attribution and illness behavior) are advantageous in identifying people with health care needs and disability as compared to approaches that focus simply on symptom count and the absence of sufficient medical explicability (Rief et al. 2011c). Based on his expertise in the classification of somatoform disorders Rief was appointed as an ICD-11 representative of the International Association for the Study of Pain IASP to coordinate revision proposals for pain diagnoses, and he was Member of the Expert Conference on Somatic Presentations of Mental Disorders (Task: Preparation of classification criteria for ICD-11 and DSM-V) under the auspices of the American Psychiatric Association (APA), the National Institute of Health (NIH), and the World Health Organization (WHO) 2006).

Rief has always been interested in processes that contribute to etiology and maintenance of somatoform disorders. He demonstrated the roles of cognitive processes such as symptom interpretation and memory biases (Rief et al. 2006b), of illness behaviors, and especially of neurobiological and psychoneuroimmunological processes in somatoform disorders (Rief and Barsky 2005; Rief and Broadbent 2007).

Rief and his colleagues conducted a number of randomized clinical trials to evaluate the effects of different intervention strategies in somatoform syndromes (all funded by research grants from the DFG, the Federal Ministry of Education, Research BMBF Germany, and others). These studies demonstrated, for example, that a cognitive-behavior group -based inpatient treatment is effective in somatoform disorders, and that even a minimal intervention program designed for subjects in primary care results in symptom improvement. The evaluation of a special training program for general practitioners to improve management of patients with unexplained physical symptoms showed a reduction in health care utilization, but appeared not to be sufficient to improve disability in patients. Rief will continue to develop psychological treatments further to enhance their clinical effects in somatoform disorders.

Placebo effects and placebo and nocebo mechanisms are one of Rief's most recent research fields (Rief et al. 2006a). He has published meta-analytical results showing that close to 70% of positive effects of antidepressants are already reported for the placebo group. In line with his interest in the development of somatic symptoms, he was able to show that expectation of side effects results in higher side effect rates in clinical trials. Consequently, many subjects discontinuing drug intake because of side effects were shown to be in the placebo group. He is the spokesperson of a German Research Unit "Expectation and conditioning as basic mechanisms of placebo and nocebo effects," which covers eigth subprojects on placebo and nocebo mechanisms (total budget about 2.7 Mio. EUR; local budget for Rief's work is 640,000,- EUR). Together with colleagues of this research unit, he has published new proposals for study design in clinical trials (Rief et al. 2011b).

Rief's breadth of research interests in the field of behavioral medicine is demonstrated by additional studies he has conducted in obesity (e.g., BMBF grants' "Counseling of obese patients including genetic findings" and "Psychosocial, legal, and ethical aspects of genetic and molecular obesity research"), cancer (Rief et al. 2011a), tinnitus (e.g., DFG grant "Psychophysiological aspects and treatment of chronic tinnitus" (Weise et al. 2008), chronic pain, CBT in schizophrenia, side effect assessment in clinical trials, and public health issues. In international projects, he has collaborated with distinguished members of Harvard Medical School (A. Barsky), UCSD (J. Dimsdale), Auckland Medical School (K. Petrie), and many others. His current publication record includes more than 300 publications in peer-reviewed journals, 15 books and co-edited books, and numerous book sections.

Cross-References

▶ Biofeedback
▶ International Society of Behavioral Medicine
▶ Nocebo and Nocebo Effect
▶ Placebo and Placebo Effect
▶ Psychophysiology: Theory and Methods
▶ Somatoform Disorders

References and Readings

Rief, W., & Barsky, A. J. (2005). A psychobiological perspective on somatoform disorders. *Psychoneuroendocrinology, 30*, 996–1002.

Rief, W., & Broadbent, E. (2007). Explaining medically unexplained symptoms-models and mechanisms. *Clinical Psychology Review, 27*, 821–841.

Rief, W., Avorn, J., & Barsky, A. J. (2006a). Medication-attributed adverse effects in placebo groups. Implications for assessment of adverse effects. *Archives of Internal Medicine, 166*(2), 155–160.

Rief, W., Heitmüller, A. M., Reisberg, K., & Rüddel, H. (2006b). Why reassurance fails in patients with unexplained symptoms-an experimental investigation of remembered probabilities. *PLoS Medicine, 3*(8), e269. https://doi.org/10.1371/journal.pmed.0030269.

Rief, W., Bardwell, W. A., Dimsdale, J. E., Natarajan, L., Flatt, S. W., Pierce, J. P. for the Women's Healthy Eating and Living (WHEL) Study Group. (2011a). Long-term course of pain in breast cancer survivors:

A four year longitudinal study. *Breast Cancer Research and Treatment, 130*, 579–586.

Rief, W., Bingel, U., Schedlowski, M., & Enck, P. (2011b). Mechanisms involved in placebo and nocebo responses and implications for drug trials. *Clinical Pharmacology and Therapeutics, 90*, 722–726.

Rief, W., Mewes, R., Martin, A., Glaesmer, H., & Braehler, E. (2011c). Evaluating new proposals for the psychiatric classification of patients with multiple somatic symptoms. *Psychosomatic Medicine, 73*, 760–768.

Weise, C., Heinecke, K., & Rief, W. (2008). Biofeedback-based behavioural treatment for chronic tinnitus-results of a randomised controlled trial. *Journal of Consulting and Clinical Psychology, 76*, 1046–1057.

Ringing in the Ears

▶ Tinnitus

Risk Aversion

▶ Risk Perception

Risk Factors

▶ Diathesis-Stress Model

Risk Factors and Their Management

Bernt Lindahl
Occupational and Environmental Medicine, Department of Public Health and Clinical Medicine, Umeå University, Umeå, Sweden

Definition

The term "risk factor" describes factors that are associated with an increased risk of developing a disease but that are not sufficient to cause the disease. In this topic, risk factors for our most important noncommunicable diseases, such as cardiovascular disease (CVD), type 2 diabetes, and certain forms of cancer, are discussed. Special emphasis is on explaining the link between an individual's choice of lifestyle (behaviors) and these diseases. This link is called "the metabolic syndrome" and can be described as a group of risk factors that occur together, are modifiable by lifestyle change, and increase the risk for CVD and diabetes. Some implications of this lifestyle metabolic syndrome association may also be drawn to other diseases, such as dementia and depression. Management of these cardio-metabolic risk factors is primarily behavior modification or long-term lifestyle change. Often, the lifestyle treatment needs to be complimented by pharmacologic treatment for some specific risk factors, such as LDL-cholesterol and high blood pressure.

Description

Risk Factors

During the last four decades, it has been said that three risk factors, often called the traditional risk factors, could explain 50% of the risk of getting an acute heart attack or an acute myocardial infarction (AMI). The three risk factors were smoking, serum cholesterol, and blood pressure. In 2004, the Interheart study was published, and this worldwide case–control study found nine modifiable risk factors to explain 90% of the risk of getting AMI (Yusuf et al. 2004). The study compared 15,000 cases of AMI with the same number of controls without having AMI. They found that smoking and lipid disorder, mainly high total and LDL-cholesterol, were the most powerful of these nine risk factors. The others were blood pressure, diabetes, abdominal obesity, psychosocial factors, physical activity, fruit and vegetables, and alcohol consumption. The last three of these risk factors were in reality protecting factors, since a higher level of physical activity, fruit and vegetables, and alcohol were associated with a lower rate of AMI. The strength of this worldwide study is that the risk factor pattern for AMI was the same among men and women, between different geographical regions of the world and also between different racial or ethnic groups (Yusuf et al. 2004).

Smoking

Smoking is perhaps the most important risk factor for cardiovascular disease (CVD), and if one was to be confronted with a patient with CVD and several other risk factors, who still was a smoker, the foremost advice would be to discuss how to stop smoking (Burell and Lindahl 2008). The consequences of smoking and how to work with tobacco and smoking cessation will be dealt with elsewhere.

Lipids

Disturbances in blood lipids are strong risk factors for atherosclerosis and cardiovascular disease, such as coronary heart disease, stroke, and peripheral artery disease. There are two main forms of lipids in the blood: cholesterol and triglycerides. Total cholesterol can be subdivided into low density lipoprotein (LDL)-cholesterol, sometimes called bad cholesterol since it increases the risk of cardiovascular disease, and high density lipoprotein (HDL)-cholesterol, sometimes called good cholesterol since it reduces the risk of cardiovascular disease (Faergeman 2008). As a rule of thumb, in order to avoid atherosclerosis and risk of CVD, an individual's total cholesterol should be below 5 mmol/L, LDL-cholesterol below 3 mmol/L, triglycerides below 2 mmol/L, and HDL-cholesterol above 1 mmol/L. For some individuals, the lipid goals need to be even more advanced. In secondary prevention, for instance, when you already have had one heart attack and you want to prevent another one, the aim for the LDL-cholesterol level may be below 2.5 mmol/L or 2.0 mmol/L. All patients with cardiovascular disease, diabetes, and familial high cholesterol belong to this group of individuals (Faergeman 2008).

Obesity, Insulin Resistance, and the Metabolic Syndrome

Obesity has long been the main modifiable risk factor for type 2 diabetes, and during the last decade, a nearly explosive growth over the world of both obesity and diabetes has been demonstrated. This development has mostly been attributed to developed countries, but has also increasingly been found in many developing countries (Barnett and Kumar 2004; Björntorp 2001). Obesity is often defined as a condition of excessive fat accumulation in adipose tissue to the extent that health may be impaired and is the result of an imbalance between energy intake and expenditure (Björntorp 2001). If an individual consumes more energy than he/she spends, fat tissue will accumulate, and obesity may follow. According to the World Health Organization (WHO), obesity is defined as a body mass index (BMI) of 30 kg/m^2 or more. Although obesity per se is a strong risk factor for diabetes and CVD, it was discovered already in the beginning of the 1950s that the male form of obesity having most of the fat deposit localized around the waist, i.e., abdominal obesity, was an even stronger risk factor (Barnett and Kumar 2004; Björntorp 2001). A waist circumference of 94 cm (37 in.) in men and 80 cm (32 in.) in women has been shown to increase the risk of getting diabetes and CVD, and this risk is further increased with a waist of 102 cm (40 in.) or above in men and 88 cm (35 in.) or above in women. The first level could be seen as an alerting zone, i.e., an obligation to inform the individual about the increased risk and discuss possible solutions. The second level is often called "an action level," implying that these individuals really ought to be offered inclusion in a lifestyle program (Björntorp 2001).

Portal-Visceral Hypothesis and Insulin Resistance

Several of the nine modifiable risk factors from the Interheart study are highly correlated to each other, i.e., they are more often than by chance found together in the same individual. As shown in Fig. 1, low physical activity in combination with high energy intake and sustained psychosocial stress will increase the risk of developing obesity and especially abdominal obesity. A large amount of abdominal fat, which is more metabolically active than subcutaneous fat, will release large amounts of fatty acids to the blood circulation. Large amounts of free fatty acids at muscular level will reduce the uptake of glucose

Risk Factors and Their Management, Fig. 1 The metabolic syndrome: the link between lifestyle, type 2 diabetes, and cardiovascular disease

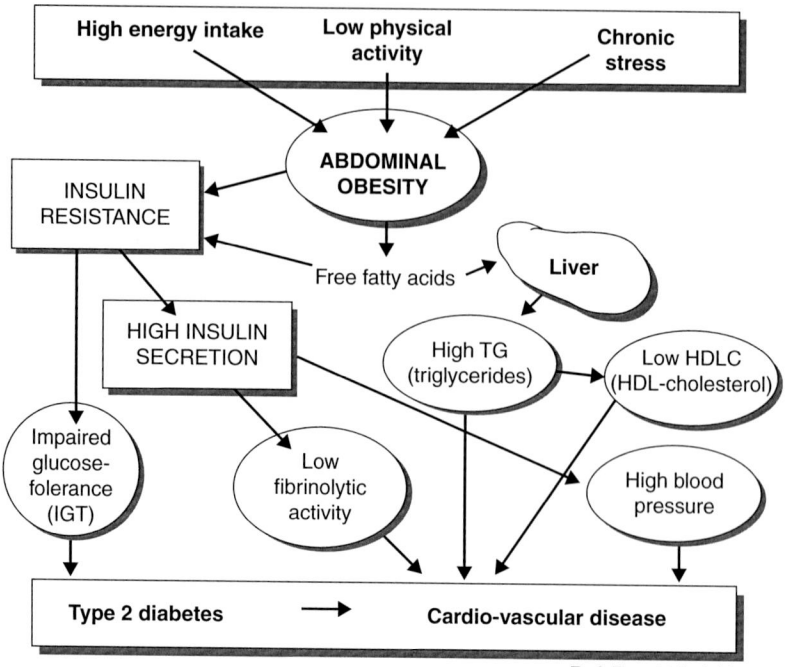

Ref. Bernt Lindahl

due to a subnormal insulin action. A state of insulin resistance will follow, which may be defined as a state in which a given concentration of insulin produces a less than expected biological effect. The small increase in glucose concentration in the circulation that will follow will in turn increase the secretion of insulin from the beta cells in the pancreas. Glucose uptake at muscular level will be restored, despite that insulin resistance still exists. However, the price to pay is a larger than normal insulin secretion. This could go on for years with increasing body weight, waist circumference, insulin resistance, and high beta cell activity. The long-term problem is that the beta cells get exhausted and lose their ability to produce insulin (Kumar and O'Rahilly 2005).

In the beginning of such a development, the amount of insulin secreted is not high enough to take care of the carbohydrates after a meal and plasma glucose often rises to levels beyond the normal. This is called a state of impaired glucose tolerance (IGT), and without a lifestyle change, this state will worsen to type 2 diabetes in about 50% of the cases within a 10-year period. IGT is a reversible state, and much attention in primary prevention of type 2 diabetes has been devoted to find and to treat this group of high-risk individuals. Impaired glucose tolerance (IGT) as well as impaired fasting glucose (IFG), i.e., having a higher than normal plasma glucose in the fasting state but not after a meal, may be called prediabetic states (Ganz 2005; Kumar and O'Rahilly 2005).

Other effects of insulin resistance and high insulin secretion are the appearance of risk factors such as high blood pressure and a specific lipid disturbance, characterized by high levels of triglycerides and low levels of HDL-cholesterol. This lipid combination is relatively common and considered to be a strong risk factor for CVD. The combination of these multiple risk factors for diabetes and cardiovascular disease is called "the metabolic syndrome" (Fig. 1). Other names for this risk state are syndrome X, the deadly quartet, or the insulin resistance syndrome. The description above is based upon the portal-visceral hypothesis for the mechanism of developing insulin resistance. However, other mechanisms have also been discussed (Kumar and O'Rahilly 2005).

Adipose Tissue as an Endocrine Organ

During the last 15 years, our knowledge of fat tissue has changed tremendously, from being just a reservoir for energy to being the largest endocrine organ in the body. The handling of energy intake and expenditure and of hunger and satiety as well as effects on blood pressure and inflammatory systems are regulated, at least in part, by hormones or hormone-like substances (adipokines) produced and secreted from fat cells in adipose tissue (Kumar and O'Rahilly 2005).

Ectopic Fat Accumulation

A third possible mechanism for the development of insulin resistance and increased risk for diabetes is "ectopic fat" accumulation. The definition of ectopic fat is that it is accumulation of fat cells in other tissues than adipose tissue. It has been shown that ectopic fat in liver and muscle tissues is associated with central (liver) and peripheral (muscles) insulin resistance, and accumulation of fat droplets in the neighborhood of the beta cells in the pancreas has been associated with a disturbance in insulin secretion (Kumar and O'Rahilly 2005).

Type 2 Diabetes and Cardiovascular Disease

From population studies, using different metabolic syndrome definitions, as much as 20–25% of the adult population has been found to have a metabolic syndrome. Besides having the risk of developing diabetes, the risk of getting CVD is two- to threefold higher among those with the metabolic syndrome. Today, type 2 diabetes, due to its strong correlation with CVD (macrovascular complications of diabetes), is by many considered to be in its essence a cardiovascular disease, and among diabetes patients, there is a three- to fourfold increased risk for CVD. Importantly, much points to the fact that the CVD risk already starts to rise when the individuals start to accumulate body fat and is clearly increased in the state of the metabolic syndrome, and even more so in impaired glucose tolerance. In other words, the risks of developing type 2 diabetes and cardiovascular disease should be seen as parallel phenomena, and not as a simple case of diabetes being followed by CVD (the "common soil" hypothesis). This has of course large implications on when in this process of development it is optimal to start the prevention or treatment of these risk states or diseases (Ganz 2005; Kumar and O'Rahilly 2005).

The strong association between diabetes and CVD could also be demonstrated from another point of view. In a recent Swedish study on acute myocardial infarction patients submitted to hospital care and followed up 3 months later with among other things an oral glucose tolerance test, it was demonstrated that only 35% of the AMI patients had normal glucose concentrations. A majority of the cases (65%) had either unknown diabetes or prediabetes (Norhammar et al. 2002).

Other Related Diseases

The same kind of reasoning as above, using the same risk factor pattern, has also given rise to implications for other types of diseases (outcomes), such as certain types of cancers (mainly breast, colon, and prostate), dementia, and depression. However, our knowledge is much more limited in this area of research.

Management of Risk Factors

Behavior Modification and Long-Term Lifestyle Change

As discussed above, in reality, many of our most important risk factors for noncommunicable diseases, such as type 2 diabetes and cardiovascular disease as well as certain forms of cancer, dementia, and depression, are the same and are also associated with each other in a complex pattern of interrelationships, such as in the metabolic syndrome (Fig. 1). An individual's choice of lifestyle will have great impact on these relationships, and the metabolic syndrome may be seen as the link between the lifestyle of an individual and the risk to develop type 2 diabetes and cardiovascular disease for that individual. Of course, heredity also influences many of these interrelationships, but this is a risk factor that, at least today, is unmodifiable. Behavior modification inducing long-term lifestyle change with increased physical activity and a lowered energy intake, often based upon a low-fat high-fiber diet, and sometimes also the inclusion of stress management techniques in the lifestyle change, has been the standard for an intensive lifestyle change program. Studies using this approach often achieve a weight loss of 5–10% of the initial body weight (Barnett and Kumar 2004; Burell and Lindahl 2008; Ganz 2005). Although, this is a relatively modest weight loss for someone having obesity, it has been shown to generate large beneficial effects on the metabolism. However, it seems crucial that the weight loss is achieved by a lifestyle change. An intensive lifestyle program induces a multitude of effects that protect against both cardiovascular disease and type 2 diabetes. In the Finnish Diabetes Prevention Study (DPS), a weight loss difference between the intensive lifestyle group and the control group of 2.7 kg after 2 years resulted in a reduction of diabetes development of 58% at the 3-year follow-up (Tuomilehto et al. 2001).

Effects of Physical Activity

There is a strong inverse relationship between physical activity, type 2 diabetes, and cardiovascular disease, and the evidence for this relationship must be considered as solid (Burell and Lindahl 2008). Furthermore, a large body of evidence examining the effects of physical activity on cardiovascular risk factors has also documented beneficial effects, mainly a lowering of blood pressure and a less atherogenic lipid profile. A paradigm shift concerning physical activity was launched in 1995, proclaiming that even less intensive and shorter bouts of physical activity may have health promoting effects (Pate et al. 1995). It was shown that a dose corresponding to an energy expenditure of 1000 kcal per week significantly lowered all-cause mortality by 20–30%, and CVD mortality possibly even more. This level of energy expenditure corresponds to about 30 min of moderately intensive physical activity each day, i.e., brisk walks, bicycling, and swimming. An updated version of this physical activity statement was published in 2007 (Haskell et al. 2007).

Effects of a Healthy Diet

In the last decade, our understanding of how nutrients and foods promote cardiac health or increase the risk for diabetes and cardiovascular disease has grown substantially, but the search for an optimal composition of food intake is far from over. Diets that are higher in monounsaturated fatty acids, fiber, and low glycemic foods (slow carbohydrates) appear to improve insulin resistance, blood glucose, and blood lipids. Additionally, three food intake strategies to prevent cardiovascular disease have been suggested. First, to increase intake of unsaturated fats and decrease intake of saturated and trans-fats, second, to increase intake of omega-3 fatty acids, and last, to increase consumption of fruits, vegetables, nuts, and whole grains (Hu and Willett 2002).

Adherence to a Long-Term Lifestyle Change

Two key features of such an intensive lifestyle program in order to achieve adherence are goal-setting and self-monitoring. The goals should be realistic, measurable, concrete, and engaging, and there should be both short- and long-term goals. Simple ways of self-monitoring key behaviors, such as food intake and physical activity, should also be included in such a lifestyle program (Burell and Lindahl 2008; Ganz 2005).

Management of Specific Risk Factors: High LDL-Cholesterol and High Blood Pressure

In addition to a comprehensive lifestyle program, some specific risk factors need to be treated with medications, either because the lifestyle program is insufficient to handle the risk factor in an optimal way or because healthy lifestyle change does not impact enough on the risk factor in question. In order to lower LDL-cholesterol, lipid-modifying drugs, especially use of statins, are the standard treatment in cases with familial high cholesterol levels and in patients with cardiovascular disease and type 2 diabetes (Faergeman 2008). In order to control high blood pressure, a lifestyle change is often not enough, and the use of antihypertensive drugs is customary.

Cross-References

▶ Behavior Change

References and Further Reading

Barnett, A. H., & Kumar, S. (Eds.). (2004). *Obesity & diabetes*. Chichester: Wiley.
Björntorp, P. (Ed.). (2001). *International textbook of obesity*. Chichester: Wiley.
Burell, G., & Lindahl, B. (2008). Management of specific behavioural risk factors – Exercise, obesity and smoking. In I. M. Graham & R. B. D'Agostino (Eds.), *Therapeutic strategies in cardiovascular risk* (pp. 201–211). Oxford: Clinical Publishing.
Faergeman, O. (2008). Management of specific risk factors – Lipids. In I. M. Graham & R. B. D'Agostino (Eds.), *Therapeutic strategies in cardiovascular risk* (pp. 213–232). Oxford: Clinical Publishing.
Ganz, M. (Ed.). (2005). *Prevention of type 2 diabetes*. Chichester: Wiley.
Haskell, W. L., Lee, I.-M., Pate, R. R., Powell, K. E., Blair, S. N., Franklin, B. A., et al. (2007). Physical activity and public health. Updated recommendation for adults from the American College of Sports Medicine and the American Heart Association. *Circulation, 116*, 1081–1093.
Hu, F. B., & Willett, W. C. (2002). Optimal diets for prevention of coronary heart disease. *Journal of the American Medical Association, 288*, 2569–2578.
Kumar, S., & O'Rahilly, S. (Eds.). (2005). *Insulin resistance*. Chichester: Wiley.
Norhammar, A., Tenerz, Å., Nilsson, G., Hamsten, A., Efendic, S., & Rydén, L. (2002). Glucose metabolism in patients with acute myocardial infarction and no previous diagnosis of diabetes mellitus: A prospective study. *Lancet, 359*, 2140–2144.
Pate, R. R., Pratt, M., Blair, S. N., Haskell, W. L., Macera, C. A., Bouchard, C., et al. (1995). Physical activity and public health. A recommendation from the Centers for Disease Control and Prevention and the American College of Sports Medicine. *Journal of the American Medical Association, 273*, 402–407.
Tuomilehto, J., Lindström, J., Eriksson, J. G., Valle, T. T., Hämäläinen, H., Lanne-Parikka, P., et al. (2001). Prevention of type 2 diabetes mellitus by changes in lifestyle among subjects with impaired glucose tolerance. *New England Journal of Medicine, 344*, 1343–1350.
Yusuf, S., Hawken, S., Ounpuu, S., Dans, T., Avezum, A., Lanas, F., et al. (2004). Effect of potentially modifiable risk factors associated with myocardial infarction in 52 countries (the INTERHEART study): Case–control study. *Lancet, 364*, 937–952.

Risk Perception

Catherine Darker[1] and Anna C. Whittaker[2]
[1]Public Health and Primary Care, Institute of Population Health, School of Medicine, Trinity College Dublin, The University of Dublin, Dublin, Ireland
[2]School of Sport, Faculty of Health Science and Sport, University of Stirling, Stirling, UK

Synonyms

Risk aversion; Risk-taking

Definition

Risk perceptions are beliefs about potential harm or the possibility of a loss. It is a subjective judgment that people make about the characteristics and severity of a risk.

Description

The degree of risk associated with a given behavior is generally considered to represent the likelihood and, given its occurrence, the consequences of harmful effects that result from that behavior. To perceive risk includes evaluations of the probability as well as the consequences of an uncertain outcome. There are three dimensions of perceived risk – perceived likelihood (the probability that one will be harmed by the hazard), perceived susceptibility (an individual's constitutional vulnerability to a hazard), and perceived severity (the extent of harm a hazard would cause). Risk perceptions are central to many health behavior theories. For example, models that have been developed specifically to predict health behavior such as the health belief model (Rosenstock 1966), the protection motivation theory (Rogers 1975), and the self-regulation model (Leventhal et al. 1980) all contain constructs that explicitly focus on risk perceptions. In addition, other models such as the theory of reasoned action (Fishbein and Ajzen 1975), the theory of planned behavior (Ajzen 1985), and the social cognitive theory (Bandura 1977) also include perceptions of risk indirectly via other constructs.

Biases and Heuristics in Risk Assessment

The estimation of risk tends to be a complex process that depends on factors such as the context in which the risk information is presented and the way the risk is being described and also on personal and cultural characteristics. Tversky and Kahneman (1973) proposed that when faced with the difficult task of judging risk, people use a limited number of strategies, called heuristics, to simplify these judgments. These heuristics can be useful shortcuts for thinking for most of us most of the time, but they may lead to inaccurate judgments in some situations in which case they become cognitive biases. There are three broad biases that can affect risk perceptions, and these are the availability heuristic, the representativeness heuristic, and the anchoring and adjustment heuristic.

Availability heuristic is a phenomenon in which people predict the frequency or likelihood of an event, or a proportion within a population, based on how easily an example can be brought to mind (Tversky and Kahneman 1973). We make decisions based on the knowledge that is readily available in our minds rather than examining all the alternatives. Most of the time, our brains use the availability heuristic without us even realizing it. Often this gives our brains the quick shortcut to the answer we need, and in many cases the judgments are accurate. However, as with any shortcut, sometimes the availability heuristic can lead us to make mistakes. Some events are easier to recall than others, not because they are more common but because they stand out in our minds.

Representativeness heuristic is an occurrence in which individuals assess the frequency of a particular event based solely on the generalization of a previous similar event (Gilovich et al. 2002). Naturally, relying on past experiences can be beneficial and allow for quick conclusions to be reached, but the cost of being able to make quick decisions is oftentimes accuracy. The fact that a mental representation, which can be compared to a new situation, exists in your memory does not have any bearing on how likely that representation is to occur in reality.

Anchoring and adjustment heuristic is a phenomenon in which people start with one piece of known information, known as an anchor, and then adjust said information to create an estimate of an unknown risk (Epley and Gilovich 2006). The adjustment, however, is usually conservative, and hence, the final judgment is usually biased toward the anchor.

Psychometric Paradigm of Risk Assessment

The "psychometric paradigm" developed by Slovic, Fischhoff, and Lichtenstein was a landmark in research about public attitudes toward risks (Fischhoff et al. 1978, 1983; Slovic et al. 1980, 1982, 1985). These studies demonstrated that the public is not irrational. Ordinary people simply use a broader definition of "risks" than experts when making their judgments about which ones are of most concern to them. "Experts" base their risk ratings on the expected number of fatalities. "Lay people," in contrast, have a richer definition of risk. This incorporates a number of more qualitative characteristics such as "voluntariness" (whether people have a choice about whether they face the risk), "immediacy of effect" (the extent to which the effect is immediate or might occur at some later time), and "catastrophic potential" (whether many people would be killed at once). Slovic et al. (1985) identified and analyzed 18 characteristics of this kind using factor analysis and found that they could be resolved into three factors broadly defined as "dread," "unknown," and "exposure." Further, high perceived risk, and hence a desire for societal regulation, was associated. Psychometric paradigm assumes that with appropriate design of survey instruments, many of these factors can be quantified (Slovic 1992).

Research within the psychometric paradigm turned to focus on the roles of affect, emotion, and stigma in influencing risk perception. Psychometric research identified a broad domain of characteristics that may be condensed into three high-order factors: (1) the degree to which a risk is understood, (2) the degree to which it evokes a feeling of dread, and (3) the number of people exposed to the risk. A dread risk elicits visceral feelings of terror, uncontrollability, catastrophe, and inequality. An unknown risk is new and unknown to science. The more a person dreads an activity, the higher its perceived risk and the more that person wants the risk reduced (Slovic et al. 1982).

Cross-References

▶ Cancer Risk Perceptions
▶ Cognitive Appraisal
▶ Perceived Benefits
▶ Perceived Risk
▶ Risky Behavior

References and Further Reading

Ajzen, I. (1985). From intentions to actions: A theory of planned behavior. In J. Kuhl & J. Beckman (Eds.), *Action-control: From cognition to behavior* (pp. 11–39). Heidelberg: Springer.
Bandura, A. (1977). Self-efficacy: Toward a unifying theory of behavior change. *Psychological Review, 84*, 191–215.
Epley, N., & Gilovich, T. (2006). The anchoring-and-adjustment heuristic: Why the adjustments are insufficient. *Psychological Science, 17*, 311–318.
Fischhoff, B., Slovic, P., Lichtenstein, S., Read, S., & Combs, B. (1978). How safe is safe enough? A psychometric study of attitudes towards technological risks and benefits. *Policy Studies, 9*, 127–152.
Fischhoff, B., Slovic, P., & Lichtenstein, S. (1983). The public vs. 'the experts'. In V. T. Covello, W. G. Flamm, J. V. Rodricks, & R. G. Tardiff (Eds.), *The analysis of actual vs. perceived risks* (pp. 235–249). New York: Plenum.
Fishbein, M., & Ajzen, I. (1975). *Belief, attitude and intention and behavior: An introduction to theory and research*. Reading: Addison-Wesley.
Gilovich, T., Griffin, D., & Kahneman, D. (2002). *Heuristics and biases -the psychology of intuitive judgment*. New York: Cambridge University Press.
Kahneman, D., & Tversky, A. (1973). On the psychology of prediction. *Psychological Review, 80*, 237–251.
Leventhal, H., Meyer, D., & Nerenz, D. (1980). The common sense representation of illness danger. *Medical Psychology, 2*, 7–30.
Plous, S. (1993). *The psychology of judgment and decision making*. New York: McGraw-Hill.
Rogers, R. W. (1975). A protection motivation theory of fear appeals and attitude change. *Journal of Psychology, 91*, 93–114.
Rosenstock, I. M. (1966). Why people use health services. *The Milbank Memorial Fund Quarterly, 44*, 94–127.
Slovic, P. (1992). Perception of risk: Reflections on the psychometric paradigm. In S. Krimsky & D. Golding (Eds.), *Social theories of risk* (pp. 117–152). Westport: Praeger.
Slovic, P. (2000). *The perception of risk*. Sterling: Earthscan.
Slovic, P., Fischhoff, B., & Lichtenstein, S. (1980). Facts and fears: Understanding perceived risk. In R. C. Schwing & W. A. Albers (Eds.), *Societal risk assessment: How safe is safe enough?* (pp. 181–216). New York: Plenum Press.
Slovic, P., Fischhoff, B., & Lichtenstein, S. (1982). Why study risk perception? *Risk Analysis, 2*, 83–93.
Slovic, P., Fischhoff, B., & Lichtenstein, S. (1985). Characterizing perceived risk. In R. W. Kates, C. Hohenemser, & J. X. Kasperson (Eds.), *Perilous progress: Managing the hazards of technology*. Boulder: Westview Press.
Tversky, A., & Kahneman, D. (1973). Availability: A heuristic for judging frequency and probability. *Cognitive Psychology, 5*, 207–232.
Tversky, A., & Kahneman, D. (1974). Judgments under uncertainty: Heuristics and biases. *Science, 185*, 1124–1131.
Wildavsky, A., & Dake, K. (1990). Theories of risk perception: Who fears what and why? *American Academy of Arts and Sciences (Daedalus), 119*, 41–60.

Risk Pooling

▶ Health Insurance: Comparisons

Risk Reduction

▶ Harm Reduction

Risk Taking

▶ Risky Behavior

Risk-Benefit Assessment

▶ Benefit-Risk Estimation

Risk-Benefit Ratio

▶ Benefit-Risk Estimation

Risk-Taking

▶ Risk Perception

Risky Behavior

Tereza Killianova
Free University of Brussels (VUB), Jette, Belgium

Synonyms

Risk taking

Definition

Risky behavior or risk-taking behavior is defined according to Trimpop (1994) as "any consciously, or non-consciously controlled behavior with a perceived uncertainty about its outcome, and/or about its possible benefits, or costs for the physical, economic or psycho-social well-being of oneself or others." In addition to this broad definition, there are other definitions of risky behavior depending on the field of research. While in the economic view, risk is defined in terms of the variability of possible monetary outcomes, in the clinical literature, the risk is generally defined as exposure to possible loss or harm (Schonberg et al. 2011). Turner et al. (2004) described risk-taking behavior further as either a socially unacceptable volitional behavior with a potentially negative outcome in which precautions are not taken, such as speeding, drinking and driving, drugs abuse, unprotected sex, ..., or a socially accepted behavior in which the danger is recognized (climbing, competitive sports,...). This description is important when looking at the relation between risk-taking behavior and injuries. It has been shown that risk-taking behavior is associated with an increased chance of sustaining an injury. However, this relation was not shown in the case of high-skilled, risk-taking sports (Turner et al. 2004). Risky behavior can be a direct consequence and manifestation of a risk-taking personality or of sensation-seeking personality. These can be reliably assessed by various existing questionnaires. In behavior medicine, risk behavior is an important factor to consider, since it is a predictor of various adverse health outcomes. In the domain of driving, risky behaviors, such as excessive speeding or driving under the influence of alcohol, are known predictors of traffic accidents (Jonah 1997), one of the 10 leading causes of mortality worldwide. In infectious diseases, risky behavior in the form of unprotected sex or having multiple partners often co-occurs (Biglan et al. 1990) and can increase the risk of HIV/AIDS, a leading cause of death in Africa. Thus, identifying people likely to perform risky behaviors and developing and testing interventions to prevent risky behaviors are crucial for contributing to prevention of diseases and adverse health outcomes at the individual and social levels.

Cross-References

▶ Risk Perception

References and Readings

Biglan, A., Metzler, C. W., Wirt, R., Ary, D., Noell, J., Ochs, L., et al. (1990). Social and behavioral factors associated with high-risk sexual behavior among adolescents. *Journal of Behavioral Medicine, 13*, 245–261.

Jonah, B. A. (1997). Sensation seeking and risky driving: A review and synthesis of the literature. *Accident Analysis and Prevention, 29*, 651–665.

Schonberg, T., Fox, C. R., & Poldrack, R. A. (2011). Mind the gap: Bridging economic and naturalistic risk-taking with cognitive neuroscience. *Trends in Cognitive Sciences, 15*(1), 11–19.

Trimpop, R. (1994). *The psychology of risk taking behavior*. Amsterdam: Elsevier Science.

Turner, C., McClure, R., & Pirozzo, S. (2004). Injury and risk-taking behavior-a systematic review. *Accident Analysis and Prevention, 36*, 93–101.

Risky Drinking Episode

▶ Binge Drinking

RNA

Jana Strahler
Clinical Biopsychology, Department of Psychology, University of Marburg, Marburg, Germany

Synonyms

Coding RNA; Messenger RNA; mRNA; Noncoding RNA; Ribosomal RNA; rRNA; Transfer RNA; tRNA

Definition

Ribonucleic acid (RNA) is a chain of multiple nucleotides (a polynucleotide) consisting of a molecule of sugar (ribose), a molecule of phosphoric acid, and a nucleic base (uracil, cytosine, guanine, or adenine). In contrast to DNA, RNA is normally single-stranded. Its main function within the cell is the conversion of the genetic information into proteins, i.e., gene expression. There are different RNA molecules exerting different functions, the so-called coding and noncoding RNA. Coding RNA, also called messenger RNA (*mRNA*), copies information from the DNA and carries this information to the ribosome, the cell organelle where protein synthesis takes place. There are different forms of noncoding RNA with transfer RNA and ribosomal RNA being the most important. Transfer RNA (*tRNA*) molecules take amino acids and transport them to the ribosome. Ribosomal RNA (*rRNA*) is the fundamental part of the ribosome and catalyzes protein synthesis.

Research has demonstrated that various types of stressors modulate RNA. For instance, social isolation, chronic stress, and low socioeconomic status are associated with immunological impairment mediated via alterations in immune-related RNA expression. In contrast, there is also evidence for an RNA-regulating effect of positive psychological states.

Cross-References

▶ DNA
▶ Gene Expression

References and Readings

Cole, S. W., Hawkley, L. C., Arevalo, J. M., Sung, C. Y., Rose, R. M., & Cacioppo, J. T. (2007). Social regulation of gene expression in human leukocytes. *Genome Biology, 8*(9), R189.

Sloan, E. K., Capitanio, J. P., Tarara, R. P., Mendoza, S. P., Mason, W. A., & Cole, S. W. (2007). Social stress enhances sympathetic innervation of primate lymph nodes: Mechanisms and implications for viral pathogenesis. *Journal of Neuroscience, 27*(33), 8857–8865.

Robert Wood Johnson Foundation

Stephanie Ann Hooker
Department of Psychology, University of Colorado Denver, Denver, CO, USA

Basic Information

The Robert Wood Johnson Foundation (RWJF) is one of the world's largest private philanthropic foundations, with a mission of improving public health in the United States. Upon his death, Robert Wood Johnson II (of Johnson & Johnson Services Inc.) dedicated virtually all of his fortune to establish this foundation.

The RWJF funds projects that are "innovative" and have "measurable impact" in seven different program areas. These program areas include childhood obesity, coverage (health care), human capital (preparation of health professionals), pioneer (innovative health-related technologies), public health, quality/equality (health care), and vulnerable populations. Within these seven program areas, the RWJF funds a variety of different types of projects including service demonstrations, gathering and monitoring of health-related statistics, public education, training and fellowship programs, policy analysis, health services research, technical assistance, communications activities, and evaluations. In 2009, the RWJF funded $350 million in grants, and approximately 20% of the funding was dedicated to research-related projects.

Major Impact on the Field

The RWJF seeks to better society and the lives of Americans through its philanthropic contributions. Some notable past efforts include the creation of the 911 emergency response system across the United States; the introduction of new methods for the research, prevention, and treatment of tobacco use; and the establishment of the field of end-of-life/palliative care.

Each year, the RWJF publishes a book entitled *To Improve Health and Health Care: The Robert Wood Johnson Foundation Anthology*. The book focuses on approximately 10 different topics every year and describes why the foundation funded certain topics, what the program activities were, what was accomplished, how the program fits with RWJF, and what lessons were learned. The most recent volume (XIV) focused on health and health care of vulnerable populations. This anthology is one way the foundation examines its impact on public health, and it is available on the foundation's website.

Cross-References

▶ Palliative Care
▶ Public Health

References and Further Reading

Isaacs, S. L., & Dolby, D. C. (Eds.). (2011). *To improve health and health care: The Robert Wood Johnson Foundation anthology* (Vol. XIV). San Francisco: Jossey-Bass.

Robert Wood Johnson Foundation. (2011). Retrieved July 15, 2011 from http://www.rwjf.org

rRNA

▶ RNA

Rumination

Yori Gidron
SCALab, Lille 3 University and Siric Oncollile, Lille, France

Definition

Rumination is both a state and trait tendency to focus on negative events, emotions, and symptoms and their occurrence, causes, and consequences (Nolen-Hoeksema 1991; Rydstedt et al. 2011). Multiple conceptualizations of rumination exist, each having its own measure, and tested in different contexts. The majority of research has tested and shown rumination to play a key role in the onset and maintenance of depression. However, some research also shows that it causes and maintains distress in physically ill patients (see review by Soo et al. 2009). Rumination is a marker of poor adaptation, since it is thought to prolong one's psychophysiological response to a stressor even long after it has ended. In a review of this domain, Brosschot (2010) views rumination as part of perseverative cognitions, where people have a sustained cognitive representation of past stressors, beyond their mere existence. Brosschot also contends that much of the effects of rumination could also be unconscious, even impacting one's well-being during sleep. Furthermore, rumination is thought to mediate the association between stress and one's psychophysiological responses. Rumination, which amplifies one's failure to achieve goals, can be contrasted with more constructive self-reflection which is more distant and less immersed in one's experiences. Supporting this, among people moderately high on rumination, promotion failure predicted depressive symptoms. In contrast, among people high on self-reflection, promotion failure was not predictive of severe increases in depressive symptoms (Jones et al. 2009). Looking at physiological indices of stress, Rydstedt et al. (2011) found that rumination interacted synergistically with job ambiguity (a known stressor) in relation to morning cortisol in British workers. As such, rumination amplified the effects of job ambiguity on a physiological marker of stress, namely, morning cortisol. Thus, rumination amplifies and worsens the impact of negative events, both in terms of their "duration" and in terms of their possible psychophysiological consequences. A study conducted by Klein et al. (2012) assessed implicit job-stress associations using the implicit association test. This could reflect to some extent an unconscious measure of rumination about work. Only this implicit measure significantly and positively correlated with waking cortisol, while an explicit measure of job intrusions did not (Klein et al. 2012). This result supports the contention of Brosschot (2010) that even implicit rumination may exert long-term psychophysiological consequences. Some research shows that meditation can reduce levels of rumination. A relevant study by Hanstede et al. (2008) found that meditation led to greater reductions in obsessive-compulsive symptoms, related to rumination, compared to a wait-list control condition. The health consequences, mechanisms, and the ability to reduce rumination with meditation all require further research.

Cross-References

▶ Coping Strategies
▶ Negative Thoughts
▶ Neuroticism
▶ Perseverative Cognition
▶ Psychophysiologic Reactivity
▶ Worry

References and Further Readings

Brosschot, J. F. (2010). Markers of chronic stress: Prolonged physiological activation and (un)conscious perseverative cognition. *Neuroscience and Biobehavioral Reviews, 35*, 46–50.

Hanstede, M., Gidron, Y., & Nyklíček, I. (2008). The effects of a mindfulness intervention on obsessive-compulsive symptoms in a non-clinical student population. *Journal of Nervous and Mental Diseases, 196*, 776–779.

Jones, N. P., Papadakis, A. A., Hogan, C. M., & Strauman, T. J. (2009). Over and over again: Rumination, reflection, and promotion goal failure and their interactive effects on depressive symptoms. *Behaviour Research and Therapy, 47*, 254–259.

Klein, M., Weksler, N., Gidron, Y., Heldman, E., Gurski, E., Smith, O. R., & Gurman, G. M. (2012). Do waking salivary cortisol levels correlate with anesthesiologist's job involvement? *Journal of Clinical Monitoring and Computing, 26*, 407–413.

Nolen-Hoeksema, S. (1991). Responses to depression and their effects on the duration of depressive episodes. *Journal of Abnormal Psychology, 100*(4), 569–582.

Rydstedt, L. W., Cropley, M., & Devereux, J. (2011). Long-term impact of role stress and cognitive rumination upon morning and evening saliva cortisol secretion. *Ergonomics, 54*, 430–435.

Soo, H., Burney, S., & Basten, C. (2009). The role of rumination in affective distress in people with a chronic physical illness: A review of the literature and theoretical formulation. *Journal of Health Psychology, 14*, 956–966.

S

Saccharide

▶ Carbohydrates

Saliva

▶ Salivary Biomarkers

Salivary Biomarkers

Douglas A. Granger[1] and Sara B. Johnson[2]
[1]Center for Interdisciplinary Salivary Bioscience Research, School of Nursing, Bloomberg School of Public Health, and School of Medicine The Johns Hopkins University, Baltimore, MD, USA
[2]School of Medicine and Bloomberg School of Public Health, Johns Hopkins School of Medicine, Baltimore, MD, USA

Synonyms

Analytes; Biomarkers; Saliva

In the interest of full disclosure, DAG is founder and Chief Strategy and Scientific Advisor at Salimetrics LLC (State College, PA). DAG's relationship with Salimetrics LLC is managed by the policies of the Conflict of Interest Committee at the Johns Hopkins University School of Medicine.

© Springer Nature Switzerland AG 2020
M. D. Gellman (ed.), *Encyclopedia of Behavioral Medicine*,
https://doi.org/10.1007/978-3-030-39903-0

Definition

Behavioral medicine research is increasingly being influenced by theoretical models that explain individual differences in behavior and disease risk as a function of interrelated biological, behavioral, social, and contextual forces. This multi-level theoretical approach follows technical innovations that have made measuring the activity of many biological systems straightforward, portable, and cost efficient. Saliva, in particular, has received attention as a biospecimen; sample collection is perceived as feasible, cost-efficient, and safe, and salivary assays as reliable and accurate (see Table 1). A single oral fluid specimen can provide information about a range of physiologic systems, chemical exposures, and genetic variability relevant to basic biological function, health, and disease. The purpose of this review is to provide a road map for investigators interested in integrating this unique biospecimen into the next generation of studies in behavioral medicine.

Description

Oral fluid as a biospecimen: "Saliva" is a composite of oral fluids secreted from many different glands. The source glands are located in the upper posterior area of the oral cavity (*parotid gland* area), lower area of the mouth between the cheek and jaw (*submandibular gland* area), and under the tongue (*sublingual gland* area). There are also

Salivary Biomarkers, Table 1 Perceived advantages of oral fluids as a research specimen compared to serum

"Minimally invasive"	Considered "acceptable and noninvasive" by research participants and patients
	Collection is quick, non-painful, uncomplicated
"Safety"	Reduces transmission of infectious disease by eliminating the potential for accidental needle sticks
	CDC does not consider saliva a class II biohazard unless visibly contaminated with blood
"Self-collection"	Allows for community- and home-based collection
	Enables specimen collection in special populations
"Economics"	Eliminates the need for a health care intermediary (e.g., phlebotomist, nurse)
	Resources for collection and processing samples are of low cost and available
"Accuracy"	Salivary levels of many analytes represent the "free unbound fraction" or biological active fraction in the general circulation

Source: US Department of Health and Human Services (2000)

many minor secretory glands in the lip, cheek, tongue, and palate. A small fraction of oral fluid (i.e., crevicular fluid) comes from serum leakage, either from the cleft area between teeth and gums, or from mucosal injury or inflammation. In the presence of significant mucosal or epithelial inflammation, however, serum constituents may contribute substantially to oral fluids. Each secretory gland produces a fluid that differs in volume, composition, and constituents. Oral fluid is water-like in composition and has a pH (acidity) between 6 and 9; it has minimal buffering capacity, so substances placed in the mouth can change salivary acidity very quickly.

An understanding of how a given analyte makes its way into oral fluid is key to interpreting individual differences in that analyte, as well as its association with outcomes of interest. Many of the salivary analytes of interest in biobehavioral research are serum constituents (e.g., steroid hormones). Serum constituent analytes are transported into saliva either by *filtration* between the tight spaces between acinus or duct cells in the salivary glands, or by *diffusion* through acinus or duct cell membranes. In contrast, some analytes found in oral fluids are synthesized, stored, and released from the granules within the secretory cells of the salivary glands (i.e., enzymes, mucins, cystatins, histatins). Still others are components of humoral immunity (antibodies, complement) or compounds (cytokines) secreted by immune cells (neutrophils, macrophages, lymphocytes). In addition to these analytes, saliva contains sufficient cellular material to obtain high quantity and quality DNA (Zimmerman et al. 2007).

The *rate* of saliva secretion can significantly influence levels of salivary analytes produced locally in the mouth (e.g., alpha-amylase (sAA), secretory IgA) as well as those that migrate into saliva from blood by filtration (e.g., dehydroepiandrosterone-sulfate and other conjugated steroids) (Malamud and Tabak 1993). Oral fluid secretion is influenced by many factors, including the day-night cycle, chewing movement of the mandibles, taste and smell, medications that cause dry mouth, as well as medical conditions and treatments that affect salivary gland function (e.g., radiation therapy, Sjögren's syndrome). It is important to note, therefore, that for analytes influenced by flow rate, the measured concentration or activity of the analyte (e.g., U/mL, pg/mL) must be multiplied by the flow rate (mL/min). The resulting measure is expressed as *output as a function of time* (e.g., U/min, pg/min).

Sample Collection: Even under normative-healthy conditions, more than 250 species of bacteria are present in oral fluids (Paster et al. 2001). During upper respiratory infections, oral fluids are highly likely to contain agents of disease. Oral fluid specimens should, therefore, be handled with *universal precautions* when used in research and diagnostic applications.

Saliva collection devices have historically involved cotton-based absorbent materials. Placed in the mouth for 2–3 min, oral fluids rapidly saturate the cotton; fluids are subsequently recovered by centrifugation or compression. Most of the time, this approach is convenient, simple, and time-efficient. However, when the sample volume is small, the specimen can be diffusely distributed in the cotton fibers, making sample recovery problematic (Harmon et al. 2007). The process of absorbing oral fluid with cotton and other materials also interferes with several salivary immunoassays (Groschl and Rauh 2006). Further, where in the mouth oral swabs are placed may affect the measured levels or activity of some salivary analytes (e.g., Beltzer et al. 2010). Standardizing swab placement instructions and monitoring compliance can minimize this threat to measurement validity.

In early studies, saliva flow was often stimulated using techniques that involved chewing or tasting various substances (e.g., gums, waxes, sugar crystals, powdered drink mixes). When not used minimally and/or consistently, some of these methods may change immunoassay performance (Granger et al. 2007). Indirectly, stimulants also influence levels of salivary analytes that depend on saliva flow rate (SIgA; dehydroepiandrosterone-sulfate (DHEA-S); Neuropeptide Y (NPY); Vasoactive Intestinal Peptide, (VIP)). Researchers are advised to avoid these techniques.

Collecting *whole saliva* by "passive drool" (Granger et al. 2007) is an alternative collection approach that minimizes many of the threats to validity described above. Briefly, participants imagine they are chewing their favorite food, slowly moving their jaws in a chewing motion, and allowing oral fluid to pool in their mouth. Next, they gently force the specimen through a short plastic drinking straw into a vial. The advantages of this procedure include the following: (1) A large sample volume may be collected relatively quickly (3–5 min). (2) Target collection volume may be confirmed by visual inspection in the field. (3) The fluid collected is a pooled specimen mixture of the output from all salivary glands. (4) The procedure does not introduce interference related to stimulating or absorbing saliva. (5) Collection materials are of very low cost. (6) Samples can be aliquoted and archived for future assays.

Blood Leakage into Oral Fluid: Blood poses a threat to the validity of salivary analyte measurements because most analytes are present in serum in much higher levels (10–100-fold) than in saliva. Specifically, to meaningfully index *systemic* (vs oral) biological activity, analyte levels in saliva must be highly correlated with levels measured in serum. This serum-saliva association depends, in part, on circulating molecules being appropriately and consistently transported into oral fluids (Malamud and Tabak 1993). When the integrity of diffusion or filtration is compromised (e.g., through blood leakage directly into salivary fluid), the level of the serological marker in saliva will be affected. Blood leakage into oral fluid is more common among individuals with poor oral health (i.e., open sores, periodontal disease, gingivitis), certain infectious diseases (e.g., HIV), and tobacco users. Samples visibly contaminated with blood present varying degrees of yellow-brownish hue. Kivlighan et al. (2004) have proposed a five-point Blood Contamination in Saliva Scale (BCSS) that rates contamination from one (no visible color) to five (deep, rich, dark yellow or brown). Under healthy conditions, BCSS ratings ($N = 42$) averaged 1.33 ($SE = .08$); after microinjury caused by vigorous tooth brushing, ratings averaged 2.42 ($SE = .19$).

Particulate Matter and Interfering Substances: As noted above, items placed in the mouth can influence the integrity of oral fluid samples. Food residue in the oral cavity may introduce particulate matter in samples, change salivary pH or composition, and/or contain substances (e.g., bovine hormones, active ingredients in medications, enzymes) that cross-react with assays. Accordingly, research participants should not eat or drink for 20 min prior to sample donation. In the event that they do eat in this time window, participants should rinse their mouths with water. Importantly, however, they must wait at least 10 min after rinsing before a specimen is collected to avoid artificially lowering estimates of salivary analytes. Access to food and drink should be carefully planned and scheduled when study designs involve repeated sample collections over long time periods.

Sample Handling, Transport, and Storage: Typically, once specimens are collected, they should be kept cold or frozen. Refrigeration prevents degradation of some salivary analytes and restricts the activity of protolytic enzymes and growth of bacteria. Conservatively, it is recommended that samples be kept frozen. At minimum, samples should be kept cold (on ice or refrigerated) and frozen later on the day of collection. Repeated freeze-thaw cycles should be avoided. DHEA, estradiol, and progesterone are very sensitive to freeze-thaw, whereas DNA, cortisol, testosterone, and sAA are robust (up to at least three cycles). Freeze-thaw cycles should be considered in the context of plans to aliquot and archive frozen samples for future assays. It should also be noted that some salivary analytes (e.g., neuropeptides) may require specimens be collected into pre-chilled storage vials (Carter et al. 2007) or treated with neuropeptidase inhibitors (e.g., EDTA, aprotinin) to minimize degradation (Dawidson et al. 1997). For large-scale national surveys, investigators working in remote areas, or patients collecting samples at home, freezing and shipping these frozen samples can be logistically complex and cost-prohibitive. In such circumstances, the impact of the handling and storage conditions should be documented by pilot work, or alternative biospecimens should be considered.

Medications: As noted above, many medications can indirectly affect some analytes by reducing salivary flow (e.g., diuretics, hypotensives, antipsychotics, antihistamines, barbiturates, hallucinogens, cannabis, and alcohol). Further, the condition for which the medication is prescribed or taken may itself directly influence analyte levels or activity (Granger et al. 2009). Few behaviorally oriented studies involving salivary analytes comprehensively document medication usage. Further, a lack of normative data coupled with wide individual variation in salivary analyte levels makes it impractical to identify improbable values due to medication use (unless the value is not physiologically plausible).

Medications that are applied intranasally, inhaled, or applied as oral topicals (e.g., teething gels) are of particular concern. Residue in the oral cavity left by these substances may change saliva composition and/or interfere with antibody-antigen binding in immunoassays. The name, dosage, and schedule of all medications taken (prescription and nonprescription) within 48 h should be recorded and used to statistically evaluate the possibility that medication use is driving analyte-outcome relationships.

Assays for Salivary Analytes: Immunoassays are the main laboratory techniques employed to assess levels and activity of salivary analytes. Most immunoassays share two basic steps. Antibodies prepared against a specific salivary analyte are coated to the bottom of a microtiter plate well; these antibodies are used to capture the target molecules. Conversely, antigens may be coated to the wells to capture antibodies present in the sample. Most modern assays employ a labeling design known as enzyme immunoassay (EIA), which uses enzymes coupled to antigens or antibodies (i.e., the enzyme conjugate). To measure salivary cortisol, for instance, antibodies to cortisol are fixed to the plastic surface of a microtiter well. The specimen and a cortisol-enzyme conjugate are added into the well and incubated. During the incubation, cortisol from the sample and the cortisol-enzyme conjugate compete for available antibody-binding sites. The well is then rinsed to remove unbound materials. Next, a substrate is added that reacts with the enzyme conjugate to produce a color. The degree of color in each reaction well is measured in units of optical density (OD). The more cortisol in the sample, the lower the amount of cortisol-conjugate that is bound to the plate, and the lower the OD in that reaction well. To determine concentrations of cortisol in the unknown samples, samples with known concentrations of cortisol (standards) are analyzed as part of each assay. Results from the standards are used to establish a calibration curve from which concentration/volume units can be interpolated from OD.

Operationalizing Individual Differences: A "basal level" is the level or activity of an analyte that represents the "stable state" of the host during a resting period. One approach to assessing "basal" levels is to sample early in the morning before the events of the day are able to contribute variation. However, day-to-day variability differs across salivary analytes depending on a number of factors including inherent variation in the production/release of the analytes, rate of their metabolism/degradation, and their sensitivity to environmental influences. Therefore, a single time-point measure of salivary analytes (other than invariant genetic polymorphisms) is unlikely to yield meaningful insight into an individual's true "basal level." The reliability of "basal" estimates of salivary analytes can be enhanced by sampling at the same time of day across a number of days, then aggregating (by averaging assay results or physically pooling specimens) across days.

Most salivary biomarker/analyte studies have involved a reactivity/regulation paradigm; this approach uses repeated samples to evaluate time-dependent changes in analytes (i.e., cortisol, sAA) in response to (or in anticipation of) a discrete event. The number of samples collected depends on the research question and logistical and practical issues (e.g., participant's tolerance for sampling burden). The optimal design for the measurement of salivary cortisol and sAA reactivity and regulation involves a pre-pre-[task]-post-post-post sampling scheme with samples collected on arrival to the lab (after consent) immediately before the task, then again immediately, 10-, 20- and 40-min post-challenge. Although some studies have yielded consistent mean-level differences in the patterns of cortisol response following a stressful or novel event, there are more often significant individual differences in stress-reactivity. Some individuals exhibit unexpected patterns of change (or no change), as well as continuously increasing or decreasing analyte levels over time.

An important component of variability in salivary analyte levels, both within and between individuals, is the diurnal rhythm. Most salivary hormone levels (e.g., cortisol) are high in the morning, decline before noon, and then decline more slowly in the afternoon and evening hours (Nelson 2005). By contrast, levels of sAA show the opposite pattern with low levels in the morning and higher levels in the afternoon (Nater et al. 2007). The nonlinear nature of these patterns requires multiple sampling time points to create adequate statistical models. A typical sampling design for salivary cortisol would involve sampling immediately upon waking, 30-min post-waking, midday (around noon), in the late afternoon, and immediately prior to bed.

Many analytical techniques have been used to model individual differences in diurnal rhythm including mean levels, evaluating the awakening response, and calculating summary measures of analytes over time (e.g., area under the curve, Pruessner et al. 2003). Another approach, growth curve modeling (McArdle and Bell 2000), has recently gained popularity for a number of reasons. Briefly, growth models allow the level and slope of the diurnal rhythm to be examined in the same model and their distinct effects on predictors can be evaluated; they minimize the impact of error or noise in measured values; and the presence of individual differences in the diurnal rhythm can be statistically tested (e.g., McArdle and Bell 2000).

Another analytical approach, hierarchical linear modeling (HLM) allows investigators to estimate values across the day for an individual, based on several samples (Bryk and Raudenbush 1992). Then, deviations from these expected values can be predicted from momentary states and feelings (e.g., mood states) about activities reported at that time of day. Documenting everyday events and emotions that help explain changes in analyte levels or activity across a time period of interest may strengthen causal inference when paired with samples across multiple days. For example, in studies focusing on cortisol, samples are collected approximately 20 min after a diary entry. Computerized handheld devices have made self-assessments quite feasible.

Analytes in Saliva of Interest to Behavioral Medicine: To date, most biobehavioral research has focused on a small number of salivary analytes, that is, cortisol, testosterone, DHEA, and sAA. In fact, however, the salivary proteome has recently been characterized, and includes more than 1,000 analytes (Hu et al. 2007). These analytes provide information about the following: (1) systemic body processes, (2) local oral biology, (3) surrogate markers of physiological activity, (4) antibodies, (4) medications and environmental exposures, and (5) genetic factors. Each category of analyte is briefly discussed below and summarized in Table 2.

The first group of analytes is present in saliva because oral fluid represents an ultra-filtrate of analytes found in the bloodstream (i.e., serum constituents). Because of high serum-saliva correlations, measuring these analytes in saliva enables investigators to make interferences about systemic physiological states. Adrenal and gonadal hormones are exemplars of this category of salivary markers (e.g., see Table 2).

Most analytes in oral fluid are produced locally in the oral cavity and are secreted from salivary glands. While individual differences in these salivary analytes may reflect systemic processes, a major contributor is local oral biology (e.g., local inflammatory processes, oral health and disease). Many salivary immune and inflammatory markers such as neopterin, beta-2-microglobulin, cytokines, and C-reactive protein (see Table 2) fall into this category. Markers in this group may be less interesting to investigators outside the fields of oral biology and oral health.

A third group of salivary analytes is produced locally by salivary glands, but the levels vary predictably with systemic physiological activation. For example, sympathetic nervous system activation affects the release of catecholamines from nerve

Salivary Biomarkers, Table 2 Salivary analytes of potential interest to biobehavioral research

Endocrine		
Aldosterone	Estradiol, Estriol, Esterone	
Androstenedione	Progesterone; 17-OH Progesterone	
Cortisol	Testosterone	
Dehydroepiandrosterone, and –sulfate	Melatonin	
Adiponectin, leptin, ghrelin	Oxytocin, Vassopressin	
Immune/inflammation		
Secretory immunoglobulin A (SIgA)	Beta-2-microglobulin (B_2M)	
Neopterin	Cytokines	
Soluble tumor necrosis factor receptors	C-reactive protein (CRP)	
Autonomic nervous system		
Alpha-amylase (sAA)	Neuropeptide Y (NPY)	
Vasoactive intestinal peptide (VIP)	Chromogranin A	
Nucleic acids		
Human genomic	mRNA	
Mitochondrial	Microbial	
Bacterial	Viral	
Antibodies specific for antigens		
Measles	Hepatitis A	Herpes simplex
Mumps	Hepatitis B	Epstein-Barr
Rubella	Hepatitis C	HIV
Pharmaceuticals/environmental chemicals		
Cotinine	Alcohol	Pesticides
Meth-, amphetamine	Lithium	Metals
Methadone	Cocaine	Opiods
Marijuana (THC)	Caffeine	Phenytoin
Bisphenol-A (BPA)	Barbituates	

Sources: Cone and Huestis (2007), Malamud and Tabak (1993), Tabak (2007), and US Department of Health and Human Services (2000)

endings, and these compounds' action on adrenergic receptors influences the activity of the salivary glands. For instance, salivary alpha-amylase is considered a *surrogate marker* of ANS activation, as are salivary measures of neuropeptide Y and vasoactive intestinal peptide.

Antibodies to specific antigens (e.g., HIV antibodies) comprise another group of salivary analytes. Table 2 offers several additional examples. Antibodies in oral fluids reflect an individual's immunological history and pathogen/microbe exposure. Further, depending on the specific antibody measured, they may reflect local and/or systemic immune activity. To date, relatively few biobehavioral studies have taken advantage of the information provided by salivary antibodies.

A variety of pharmaceuticals, abused substances, and environmental contaminants can be quantitatively monitored in oral fluids (see Table 2). One example is bisphenol-A (BPA) – a constituent of polycarbonate plastic and epoxy resins used in water bottles, baby bottles, and food containers that may leach into food and drink. Daily BPA exposures below the US Human Exposure limit (50 ug/kg/day) have been linked to permanent changes in genitalia, early puberty, and reversal of sex differences in brain structure (Maffini et al. 2006).

A final group of analytes has been made possible by recent technical advances allowing high quantity and quality DNA to be extracted from whole saliva (Zimmerman et al. 2007). Saliva samples collected to assess individual differences in salivary analytes, and biomarkers can yield reliable and valid information about genetic polymorphism.

Conclusion and Future Directions: As the gateway to the body, the mouth senses and responds to the external world, and reflects what is happening inside the body. Oral fluids provide insight into environmental exposures and contaminants, and serve as an early warning system for disease and infection. Genetic analyses using oral fluids can help explain individual differences, predict outcomes of medical treatments, and identify polymorphisms that affect disease risk and resilience. As the number of substances that can be reliably measured in saliva increases, oral fluid may become an increasingly attractive alternative to collecting blood. The wealth of information provided by salivary analytes has the potential to greatly enrich behavioral medicine research.

Cross-References

- Adrenal Glands
- Adrenergic Activation
- Antibodies
- Autonomic Nervous System (ANS)
- Behavioral Immunology
- Biobehavioral Mechanisms
- Central Nervous System
- Chronobiology
- Circadian Rhythm
- Cortisol
- Genetics
- Public Health
- Stress

References and Readings

Adam, E. (2006). Transactions among adolescent trait and state emotion and diurnal and momentary cortisol activity in naturalistic settings. *Psychoneuroendocrinology, 31*, 664–679.

Arendorf, T. M., Bredekamp, B., Cloete, C. A., & Sauer, G. (1998). Oral manifestations of HIV infection in 600 South African patients. *Journal of Oral Pathology & Medicine, 27*, 176–179.

Beall, C. M., Worthman, C. M., Stallings, J., Strohl, K. P., Brittenham, G. M., & Barragan, M. (1992). Salivary testosterone concentration of Aymara men native to 3,600 m. *Annals of Human Biology, 19*, 67–78.

Beltzer, E. K., Fortunato, C. K., Guaderrama, M. M., Peckins, M. K., Garramone, B. M., & Granger, D. A. (2010). Salivary flow on alpha-amylase: Collection technique, duration, and oral fluid type. *Physiology and Behavior, 101*, 289–296.

Booth, A., Johnson, D. R., Granger, D. A., Crouter, A. C., & McHale, S. (2003). Testosterone and child and adolescent adjustment: The moderating role of parent-child relationships. *Developmental Psychology, 39*, 85–98.

Brandtzaeg, P. (2007). Do salivary antibodies reliably reflect both mucosal and systemic immunity? *Annals of the New York Academy of Science, 1098*, 288–311.

Bryk, A. S., & Raudenbush, S. W. (1992). *Hierarchical linear models*. Newbury Park: Sage.

Carter, C. S., Pournajafi-Nazarloo, H., Kramer, K. M., Ziegler, T. E., White-Traut, R., Bello, D., & Schwertz, D. (2007). Oxytocin: Behavioral associations and potential as a salivary biomarker. *Annals of the New York Academy of Science, 1098*, 312–322.

Chard, T. (1990). *An introduction to radioimmunoassay and related techniques* (4th ed.). Amsterdam, NY: Elsevier.

Cone, E. J., & Huestis, M. A. (2007). Interpretation of oral fluid tests for drugs of abuse. *Annals of the New York Academy of Science, 1098*, 51–103.

Dabbs, J. M., Jr. (1991). Salivary testosterone measurements: Collecting, storing, and mailing saliva samples. *Physiology and Behavior, 49*, 815–817.

Dawidson, I., Blom, M., Lundeberg, T., Theodorsson, E., & Angmar-Mansson, B. (1997). Neuropeptides in the saliva of healthy subjects. *Life Sciences, 60*, 269–278.

Flinn, M. V., & England, B. G. (1995). Childhood stress and family environment. *Current Anthropology, 36*, 854–866.

Granger, D. A., Kivlighan, K. T., Fortunato, C., Harmon, A. G., Hibel, L. C., Schwartz, E. B., & Whembolua, G.-L. (2007). Integration of salivary biomarkers into developmental and behaviorally-oriented research: Problems and solutions for collecting specimens. *Physiology and Behavior, 92*, 583–590.

Granger, D. A., Hibel, L. C., Fortunato, C. K., & Kapelewski, C. H. (2009). Medication effects on salivary cortisol: Tactics and strategy to minimize impact in behavioral and developmental science. *Psychoneuroendocrinology, 34*, 1437–1448.

Groschl, M., & Rauh, M. (2006). Influence of commercial collection devices for saliva on the reliability of salivary steroids analysis. *Steroids, 71*, 1097–1100.

Gunnar, M. R., & Vasquez, D. (2001). Low cortisol and a flattening of the expected daytime rhythm: Potential indices of risk in human development. *Development and Psychopathology, 13*, 515–538.

Gunnar, M., Mangelsdorf, S., Larson, M., & Hertsgaard, L. (1989). Attachment, temperament, and adrenocortical activity in infancy: A study of psychoendocrine regulation. *Developmental Psychology, 3*, 355–363.

Haeckel, R., & Bucklitsch, I. (1987). Procedures for saliva sampling. *Journal of Clinical Chemistry and Biochemistry, 25*, 199–204.

Harmon, A. G., Hibel, L. C., Rumyansteva, O., & Granger, D. A. (2007). Measuring salivary cortisol in studies of child development: Watch out–what goes in may not come out of saliva collection devices. *Developmental Psychobiology, 49*, 495–500.

Harmon, A. G., Towe, N. R., Fortunato, C. K., & Granger, D. A. (2008). Differences in saliva collection location and disparities in baseline and diurnal rhythms of alpha-amylase: A preliminary note of caution. *Hormones and Behavior, 54*, 592–596.

Hellhammer, J., Fries, E., Schweusthal, O. W., Schlotz, W., Stone, A. A., & Hagemann, D. (2007). Several daily measurements are necessary to reliably assess the cortisol rise after awakening: State- and trait components. *Psychoneuroendocrinology, 32*, 80–86.

Horvat-Gordon, M., Granger, D. A., Schwartz, E. B., Nelson, V., & Kivlighan, K. T. (2005). Oxytocin is not a valid biomarker when measured in saliva by immunoassay. *Physiology and Behavior, 16*, 445–448.

Hu, S., Loo, J. A., & Wong, D. T. (2007). Human saliva proteome analysis. *Annals of the New York Academy of Science, 1098*, 323–329.

Kivlighan, K. T., Granger, D. A., Schwartz, E. B., Nelson, V., Curran, M., & Shirtcliff, E. A. (2004). Quantifying blood leakage into the oral mucosa and its effects on the measurement of cortisol, dehydroepiandrosterone, and testosterone in saliva. *Hormones and Behavior, 46*, 39–46.

Kugler, J., Hess, M., & Haake, D. (1992). Secretion of salivary immunoglobulin A in relation to age, saliva flow, mood states, secretion of albumin, cortisol, and catecholamines in saliva. *Journal of Clinical Immunology, 12*, 45–49.

Maffini, M. V., Rubin, B. S., Sonnenschein, C., & Soto, A. M. (2006). Endocrine disruptors and reproductive health: The case of bisphenol-A. *Molecular and Cellular Endocrinology, 254*, 179–186.

Malamud, D., & Tabak, L. (1993). Saliva as a diagnostic fluid. *Annals of the New York Academy of Sciences, 694*, 216–233.

McArdle, J. J., & Bell, R. Q. (2000). An introduction to latent growth models for developmental data analysis. In T. D. Little, K. U. Schnabel, & J. Baumert (Eds.), *Modeling longitudinal and multiple-group data: Practical issues, applied approaches, and specific examples* (pp. 69–107). Hillsdale: Lawrence Erlbaum Associates.

McArdle, J. J., & Nesselroade, J. (1994). Using multivariate data to structure developmental change. In S. H. Cohen & H. W. Reese (Eds.), *Life-span developmental psychology* (pp. 223–267). Hillsdale: Lawrence Erlbaum Associates.

Melnick, R., Lucier, G., Wolfe, M., Hall, R., Stancel, G., Prins, G., Gallo, M., Reuhl, K., Ho, S. M., Brown, T., Moore, J., Leakey, J., Haseman, J., & Kohn, M. (2002). Summary of the national toxicology program's report of the endocrine disruptors low-dose peer review. *Environmental Health Perspectives, 110*, 427–431.

Nater, U. M., Rohleder, N., Schlotz, W., Ehlert, U., & Kirschbaum, C. (2007). Determinants of the diurnal course of salivary alpha-amylase. *Psychoneuroendocrinology, 32*, 392–401.

Nelson, R. J. (2005). *An introduction to behavioral endocrinology.* Sunderland: Sinauer Associates.

Nemoda, Z., Horvat-Gordon, M., Fortunato, C. K., Beltzer, E. K., Scholl, J. L., & Granger, D. A. (2011). Assessing genetic polymorphisms using DNA extracted from cells present in saliva samples. *BMC Medical Research Methodology, 11*, 170.

Nieuw Amerongen, A. V., Ligtenberg, A. J. M., & Veerman, E. C. I. (2007). Implications for diagnostics in the biochemistry and physiology of saliva. *Annals of the New York Academy of Science, 1098*, 1–6.

Paster, B. J., Boches, S. K., Galvin, J. L., Ericson, R. E., Lau, C. N., Levanos, V. A., Sahasrabudhe, A., & Dewhirst, F. E. (2001). Bacterial diversity in human subgingival plaque. *Journal of Bacteriology, 183*, 3770–3783.

Pruessner, J., Kirschbaum, C., Meinlschmid, G., & Hellhammer, D. H. (2003). Two formulas for computation of the area under the curve represent measures of total hormone concentration versus time-dependent change. *Psychoneuroendocrinology, 28*, 916–931.

Raff, H., Homar, P. J., & Skoner, D. P. (2003). New enzyme immunoassay for salivary cortisol. *Clinical Chemistry, 49*, 203–204.

Rees, T. D. (1992). Oral effects of drug abuse. *Critical Reviews in Oral Biology and Medicine, 3*, 163–184.

Reibel, J. (2003). Tobacco and oral diseases. Update on the evidence, with recommendations. *Medical Principles and Practice, 12*(Suppl. 1), 22–32.

Santavirta, N., Konttinen, Y. T., Tornwall, J., Segerberg, M., Santavirta, S., Matucci-Cerinic, M., & Bjorvell, H. (1997). Neuropeptides of the autonomic nervous system in Sjogren's syndrome. *Annals of Rheumatoid Disease, 56*, 737–740.

Scannapieco, F. A., Papandonatos, G. D., & Dunford, R. G. (1998). Associations between oral conditions and respiratory disease in a national sample survey population. *Annals of Periodontology, 3*, 251–256.

Schwartz, E. B., Granger, D. A., Susman, E. J., Gunnar, M. R., & Laird, B. (1998). Assessing salivary cortisol in studies of child development. *Child Development, 69*, 1503–1513.

Shirtcliff, E. A., Granger, D. A., Schwartz, E. B., & Curran, M. J. (2001). Use of salivary biomarkers in biobehavioral research: Cotton based sample collection methods can interfere with salivary immunoassay results. *Psychoneuroendocrinology, 26*, 165–173.

Smyth, J. M., Ockenfels, M. C., Gorin, A. A., Cately, D., Porter, L. S., Kirschbaum, C., Hellhammer, D. H., & Stone, A. A. (1997). Individual differences in the diurnal cycle of cortisol. *Psychoneuroendocrinology, 22*, 89–105.

Sreebny, L. M., & Schwartz, S. S. (1997). A reference guide to drugs and dry mouth – 2nd edition. *Gerodontology, 14*, 33–47.

Stone, A. A., Broderick, J. E., Schwartz, J. E., Shiffman, S., Litcher-Kelly, L., & Calvanese, P. (2003). Intensive momentary reporting of pain with an electronic diary: Reactivity, compliance, and patient satisfaction. *Pain, 104*, 343–351.

Tabak, L. A. (2007). Point-of-care diagnostics enter the mouth. *Annals of the New York Academy of Science, 1098*, 7–14.

U.S. Department of Health and Human Services. (2000). *Oral health in America: A report of the surgeon general*. Rockville: U.S. Department of Health and Human Services, National Institute of Dental and Craniofacial Research, National Institutes of Health.

Veerman, E. C. I., Van Den Keijbus, P. A. M., Vissink, A., & Nieuw Amerongen, A. V. (1996). Human glandular saliva: Their separate collection and analysis. *European Journal of Oral Science, 104*, 346–352.

Zimmerman, B. G., Park, N. J., & Wong, D. T. (2007). Genomic targets in saliva. *Annals of the New York Academy of Science, 1098*, 184–191.

Salt, Intake

Kelly Doran
University of Maryland, Baltimore School of Nursing, Baltimore, MD, USA

Synonyms

Sodium; Sodium chloride

Definition

Salt is a dietary element made up of sodium and chlorine (U.S. National Library of Medicine and National Institutes of Health 2011a).

Description

A majority (90%) of sodium consumed comes from salt (Centers for Disease Control & Prevention 2011). The body needs a small amount of sodium for fluid regulation, nerve impulse transmission, and muscle function. The kidneys are responsible for retaining sodium (if body stores are low) or excreting sodium through urine (if body stores are too high). However, if the kidneys do not excrete enough sodium, the excess sodium will accumulate in the blood. This can lead to high blood pressure, from an increase in fluid volume in the arteries, ultimately putting additional stress on the heart (Mayo Clinic 2011a; U.S. National Library of Medicine and National Institutes of Health 2011a).

Recommendations

For children ages 1–3, 4–8, and 9–13, the recommended daily sodium intake is 1,500 mg, ≤1,900 mg, and ≤2,200 mg, respectively. Those ages 14 and older are recommended to consume ≤2,300 mg a day (U.S. Department of Agriculture and U.S. Department of Health and Human

Services 2015). However, the American Heart Association recommends the general public to reduce their sodium intake to no more than 1,500 mg per day (American Heart Association Presidential Advisory 2011). In addition, those with certain diseases (e.g., cirrhosis and congestive heart failure) may be recommended lower sodium intake levels by their primary care providers (U.S. National Library of Medicine and National Institutes of Health 2011b).

A half of a teaspoon of salt is approximately 1,200 mg of sodium, and one teaspoon of salt is approximately 2,300 mg of sodium (American Heart Association 2011). More than 85% of Americans consume 2,300 mg of sodium or more a day; the average intake of sodium for Americans over 2 years of age is 3,400 mg per day (Centers for Disease Control & Prevention 2011; U.S. Department of Agriculture and U.S. Department of Health and Human Services 2010). Diets high in sodium have been associated with an increased risk for high blood pressure, heart disease, and stroke (American Heart Association 2011). Generally, when salt intake is reduced, it only takes a few weeks for blood pressure to decrease (Centers for Disease Control & Prevention 2011).

Identifying Sources of Sodium

Most foods naturally contain sodium (U.S. National Library of Medicine and National Institutes of Health 2011b); however, this form of sodium only accounts for about 12% of daily sodium intake. An additional 11% of sodium intake comes from cooking at home and adding salt while eating. A majority (77%) of the sodium Americans consume comes from processed foods, foods bought at stores, packaged foods, and foods cooked at restaurants (Centers for Disease Control & Prevention 2010). Sodium is added to foods to act as a preservative, cure meat, retain moisture, and enhance color and flavor (American Heart Association 2011; U.S. Department of Agriculture and U.S. Department of Health and Human Services 2010). When food and beverages were grouped in 96 categories, the top six categories that contributed the most sodium to Americans' diets included yeast breads, chicken and chicken mixed dishes, pizza, pasta and pasta dishes, cold cuts, and condiments (National Cancer Institute 2010).

Reading food labels is important for determining sodium intake because milligrams of sodium in food can vary even for the same type of food. For instance, a slice of frozen pizza can range from 450 to 1,200 mg of sodium (Centers for Disease Control & Prevention 2011). However, caution should be used reading the %DV (daily value) on the food label because the percentage is based on 2,400 mg, which is 100 or 900 mg higher than the recommended daily sodium intake depending on recommended group (U.S. Department of Agriculture and U.S. Department of Health and Human Services 2015; U.S. Food and Drug Administration 2011; American Heart Association Presidential Advisory 2011). Food packaging messages can be confusing (Centers for Disease Control & Prevention 2011). For example, a package message titled unsalted or no salt added simply means no salt was added while processing the food; yet, reading the label is important because some of the ingredients may contain sodium (Mayo Clinic 2011b). Additionally, looking at the ingredients list can help determine if sodium was added. Sodium is sometimes called different names; some examples include baking soda, monosodium glutamate, and sodium nitrite (U.S. National Library of Medicine and National Institutes of Health 2011b; Mayo Clinic 2011b).

Methods for Reducing Sodium

Some methods for reducing the amount of sodium consumed can include (Mayo Clinic 2011b; National Heart, Lung and Blood Institute n.d.; National Library of Medicine and National Institutes of Health 2010; U.S. Department of Agriculture and U.S. Department of Health and Human Services 2010; American Heart Association 2011):

- Following specific heart-healthy diets (e.g., dietary approaches to stop hypertension, which is also called the DASH diet)
- Eating fresh foods
- Using food labels to purchase items low in sodium
- Ordering lower sodium items when eating out
- Using healthy salt substitutes to replace salt

Cross-References

▶ Hypertension

References and Further Readings

American Heart Association. (2011). Sodium (salt or sodium chloride). Retrieved 15 Apr 2011, from http://www.heart.org/HEARTORG/GettingHealthy/NutritionCenter/HealthyDietGoals/Sodium-Salt-or-Sodium-Chloride_UCM_303290_Article.jsp

American Heart Association Presidential Advisory. (2011). Population-wide reduction in salt consumption recommended. Retrieved 15 Apr 2011, from http://www.newsroom.heart.org/index.php?s=43%26item=1237

Centers for Disease Control & Prevention. (2010). Sodium and food sources. Retrieved 15 Apr 2011, from http://www.cdc.gov/salt/food.htm

Centers for Disease Control & Prevention. (2011). Sodium fact sheet. Retrieved 15 Apr 2011, from http://www.cdc.gov/dhdsp/data_statistics/fact_sheets/fs_sodium.htm

Mayo Clinic. (2011a). Sodium: How to tame your salt habit now. Retrieved 15 Apr 2011, from http://www.mayoclinic.com/health/sodium/NU00284

Mayo Clinic. (2011b). Sodium: How to tame your salt habit now (continued). Retrieved 15 Apr 2011, from http://www.mayoclinic.com/health/sodium/NU00284/NSECTIONGROUP=2

National Cancer Institute. (2010). Sources of sodium among the US population, 2005–06. Risk factor monitoring and methods branch website. *Applied Research Program*. Retrieved 22 Mar 2012, from http://riskfactor.cancer.gov/diet/foodsources/sodium/

National Library of Medicine, & National Institutes of Health. (2010). Tasty stand-ins for salt. *NIH Medline Plus, 5*, 15.

National Heart, Lung and Blood Institute. (2003). Your guide to lowering high blood pressure: Healthy eating. Retrieved 15 Apr 2011, from http://www.nhlbi.nih.gov/hbp/prevent/h_eating/h_eating.htm

U.S. Department of Health and Human Services, & U.S. Department of Agriculture. (2010). Available at http://health.gov/dietaryguidelines/dga2010/dietaryguidelines2010.pdf

U.S. Department of Health and Human Services, & U.S. Department of Agriculture. (2015–2020). *Dietary guidelines for Americans* (8th ed.). Dec 2015. Available at http://health.gov/dietaryguidelines/2015/guidelines/

U.S. Food and Drug Administration (2011). How to understand and use the nutrition facts label. Retrieved 15 Apr 2011, from http://www.fda.gov/food/labelingnutrition/consumerinformation/ucm078889.htm

U.S. National Library of Medicine, & National Institutes of Health (2011a). Dietary sodium. Retrieved 15 Apr 2011, from http://www.nlm.nih.gov/medlineplus/dietarysodium.html

U.S. National Library of Medicine, & National Institutes of Health (2011b). Sodium in diet. Retrieved 15 Apr 2011, from http://www.nlm.nih.gov/medlineplus/ency/article/002415.htm

Salutogenesis

Sefik Tagay
Department of Psychosomatic Medicine and Psychotherapy, University of Duisburg-Essen, Essen, North Rhine-Westphalia, Germany

Synonyms

Hardiness; Resilience; Self-efficacy; Sense of coherence

Definition

The medical sociologist Aaron Antonovsky (1923–1994) introduced the term "salutogenesis" which derives from the Latin "salus = health" and the Greek "genesis = origin." Antonovsky was mainly interested in the question of what creates and what sustains health rather than explaining the causes of disease in the pathogenic direction (Antonovsky 1979, 1987, 1993). In his salutogenetic model, he described health as a continuum between total ease (health) and total disease rather than a health-disease dichotomy. Therefore, his most important research question was: What causes health (salutogenesis)? (rather than what are the reasons for disease (pathogenesis)). The core concepts of salutogenesis show great conceptual overlap with the theory of "hardy personality" (Kobasa 1979, 1982), the theory of "self-efficacy" (Bandura 1977), and with the theory of "resilience" (Werner and Smith 1982).

The central terms of the salutogenetic theory are sense of coherence (SOC) and general resistance resources (GRRs). Antonovsky postulates that the status of health and well-being depends on these personal and environmental resources (Antonovsky 1979, 1987).

Description

Sense of Coherence (SOC)

Sense of coherence explains why humans in stressful situations stay well and are even able to improve their physical, mental, and social well-being. Antonovsky (1993) suggested that SOC depicts a stable and long-lasting way of looking at the world. He postulated that SOC is mainly formed in the first three decades of life and then becomes relatively stable.

Antonovsky defined SOC as a:

> Global orientation that expresses the extent to which one has a pervasive, enduring though dynamic feeling of confidence that (1) the stimuli, deriving from one's internal and external environments in the course of living are structured, predictable, and explicable; (2) the resources are available to one to meet the demands posed by these stimuli; and (3) these demands are challenges, worthy of investment and engagement. (Antonovsky 1987, p. 19)

The SOC consists of three dimensions (Antonovsky 1987) as follows:

1. *Comprehensibility (cognitive component)*: The internal and external environments are interpreted as understandable, consistent, structured, and predictable.
2. *Manageability (behavioral component)*: Individuals consider resources to be personally available to help them cope adequately with demands or problems.
3. *Meaningfulness (motivational component)*: This dimension refers to the extent to which a person feels that life makes sense, and that problems and demands are worth investing energy in. Additionally, it determines whether a situation is appraised as challenging, and whether it is worth making commitments and investments in order to cope with it.

According to Antonovsky (1987) the third component is the most important aspect of SOC.

General Resistance Resources (GRRs)

The general resistance resources (GRRs) are biological and psychosocial factors that make it easier for people to perceive their lives as predictable, controllable, and understandable. Typical GRRs are money, intelligence, social support, self-esteem, ego-strength, healthy behavior, traditions, and culture. These types of resources can help the person to deal in a better way with the challenges of life. In general, the GRRs lead to life experiences that promote a better SOC (Antonovsky 1987).

Measuring Sense of Coherence

With the Sense of Coherence (SOC) Scale, there is only one instrument that measures sense of coherence worldwide. Antonovsky (1987) developed the SOC as a self-report questionnaire with Likert-type items; higher scores indicate a better SOC. This instrument exists in a long form (SOC-29) and in a short form (SOC-13). In the long form, 11 items refer to "comprehensibility," 8 items refer to "meaningfulness," and 10 items refer to "manageability." The SOC scale is a reliable, valid, and cross-culturally applicable instrument. SOC seems to be a multidimensional concept rather than a unidimensional one (Eriksson and Lindström 2005). By 2007, the SOC questionnaire has been used in at least 44 languages all over the world (Singer and Brähler 2007).

Sense of Coherence and Health (Empirical Evidence)

Empirical evidence shows a strong association between SOC and mental health. A large number of studies consistently reveal a negative relationship of SOC with depression, anxiety, and post-traumatic symptoms (Antonovsky 1993; Eriksson and Lindström 2007; Tagay et al. 2006, 2009). In a recent review, Eriksson and Lindström (2007) synthesized empirical findings on SOC and examined its capacity to explain health and its dimensions. SOC was strongly related to perceived health. The stronger the SOC, the better the perceived health in general. This relation was manifested in study populations regardless of age, sex, ethnicity, nationality, and study design. Therefore, numerous authors assert that there is substantial empirical support for the idea that SOC promotes health. A strong SOC is associated with successful coping with the inevitable stressors that individuals encounter in the course of their daily lives, and therefore, with better outcomes (Antonovsky 1993; Eriksson and Lindström 2007). All in all, SOC seems to have a main, moderating, or mediating role in the explanation of health, and it seems to be able to predict health (Schnyder et al. 1999; Tagay et al. 2011).

Cross-References

▶ Coping
▶ Health
▶ Optimism
▶ Self-Esteem
▶ Stress
▶ Well-Being

References and Readings

Antonovsky, A. (1979). *Health, stress, and coping*. San Francisco/Washington/London: Jossey-Bass.
Antonovsky, A. (1987). *Unraveling the mystery of health*. San Francisco/London: Jossey-Bass.
Antonovsky, A. (1993). The structure and properties of the sense of coherence scale. *Social Science & Medicine, 36*, 725–733.
Bandura, A. (1977). Self-efficacy: Toward a unifying theory of behavioral change. *Psychological Review, 84*, 191–215.
Eriksson, M., & Lindström, B. (2005). Validity of Antonovsky's sense of coherence scale. *Journal of Epidemiology and Community Health, 59*, 460–466.
Eriksson, M., & Lindström, B. (2007). Antonovsky's sense of coherence scale and it's relation with quality of life – a systematic review. *Journal of Epidemiology and Community Health, 61*, 938–944.
Kobasa, S. C. (1979). Stressful life events, personality, and health. *Journal of Personality and Social Psychology, 37*, 1–11.
Kobasa, S. C. (1982). The hardy personality: Toward a social psychology of stress and health. In G. S. Sanders & J. Suls (Eds.), *Social psychology of health and illness* (pp. 3–32). Hillsdale: Erlbaum.
Schnyder, U., Büchi, S., Mörgeli, H., Senky, T., & Klaghofer, R. (1999). Sense of coherence-a mediator between disability and handicap? *Psychotherapy and Psychosomatics, 68*, 102–110.
Singer, S., & Brähler, E. (2007). *Die "Sense of coherence scale". Testhandbuch zur deutschen Version*. Göttingen: Vandenhoeck & Ruprecht.
Tagay, S., Erim, Y., Brähler, E., & Senf, W. (2006). Religiosity and sense of coherence – protective factors of mental health and well-being? *Zeitschrift für Medizinische Psychologie, 4*, 165–171.
Tagay, S., Mewes, R., Brähler, E., & Senf, W. (2009). Sense of coherence in female patients with bulimia nervosa: A protective factor of mental health? *Psychiatrische Praxis, 36*, 30–34.
Tagay, S., Düllmann, S., Schlegl, S., Nater-Mewes, R., Repic, N., Hampke, C., Brähler, E., Gerlach, G., & Senf, W. (2011). Effects of inpatient treatment on eating disorder symptoms, health-related quality of life and personal resources in anorexia and bulimia nervosa. *Psychotherapie, Psychosomatik, Medizinische Psychologie, 61*(7), 319–327.
Werner, E., & Smith, R. (1982). *Vulnerable but invincible. A longitudinal study of resilient children and youth*. New York: McGraw Hill.

Sample Size Estimation

J. Rick Turner
Campbell University College of Pharmacy and Health Sciences, Buies Creek, NC, USA

Synonyms

Sample-size calculation; Sample-size determination; Study size

Definition

Sample-size estimation is the process by which a researcher decides how many subjects to include in a given clinical trial. Sample-size estimation is a critical part of the design of clinical trials, and, like all design issues, this must be addressed in the study protocol before the trial commences.

Description

Many sources use the terms sample-size determination or sample-size calculation when discussing this issue. The term sample-size estimation emphasizes that deciding on the sample size that will be employed in a clinical trial is a process of estimation that involves both statistical and clinical informed judgment and not a process of simply calculating the "right" answer. It is true that mathematical calculations are made in this process, and, for a given set of values that are placed into the appropriate formula in any given circumstance, a precise answer will be given. However, the values that are placed into the formula are chosen by the researcher.

Some of the values that need to be entered into the formula are typically chosen from a standard set of possibilities, with the researcher deciding which of several generally acceptable values is best suited for the intentions of a given trial. Other values are estimates based on data that may be available in existing literature or may have been collected in an earlier trial. These include the estimated treatment effect and the variability associated with the estimated treatment effect.

The likelihood of a successful outcome (at least from the point of view that "success" means obtaining a statistically significant result) can be increased by increasing the sample size. When designing a study, the researcher wants to ensure that a large enough sample size is chosen to be able to detect an important difference that does in fact exist. It is certainly possible that a trial can fail to demonstrate such a difference simply because the sample size chosen was too small. Therefore, it might appear reasonable to think that a very big sample size is a good idea. However, increasing the sample size increases the expenses, difficulties and overall length of a trial. Somewhere, for each researcher and each study, an acceptable sample size needs to be chosen that balances the likelihood of a statistically significant result with the cost and time involved in conducting the clinical trial.

Several variables need to be considered in the process of sample-size estimation. The values of these variables in any given case can be chosen by the researcher based on several considerations. Relevant terms include:

- Type I errors and Type II errors. A Type I error occurs when a significant result is "found" when it does not really exist, and a Type II error occurs when one fails to find a significant difference that actually exists.
- The probability of making a Type I error, α. This is also the level of statistical significance chosen, typically 0.05, but it is possible to choose 0.01 or even more conservative values.
- The probability of making a Type II error, β. A probability value must be between 0 and 1: therefore, β will be between 0 and 1.
- Power, calculated as $1 - \beta$. Since the probability represented by β will be between 0 and 1, power will also be between 0 and 1 since it is defined as $1 - \beta$. The power of a statistical test is the probability that the null hypothesis is rejected when it is indeed false. Since rejecting the null hypothesis when it is false is extremely desirable, it is generally regarded that the power of a study should be as great as practically feasible.

Sample-size estimation can be performed for any study design. In each case, the respective formula will be used to estimate the sample size required. For the formula used in the type of study design discussed in some entries in the Methodology section (i.e., a comparison of a new behavioral medicine treatment or intervention with an existing one), each of the variables we have discussed will have certain influences on the sample size, N, that will be given by the formula. These influences, i.e., their relationships with N given that all of the others remain the same, can be summarized as follows:

- The smaller the chosen value of α, the larger the value of N that will be given.

- The smaller the chosen value of β, the larger the value of N that will be given. This is because power is defined as 1 − β. As β decreases, power increases; as power increases, the larger the value of N that will be given.
- The larger the standardized effect size, the smaller the value of N that will be given. The standardized treatment effect is the estimated treatment effect divided by the variability associated with it.

Cross-References

▶ False-Negative Error
▶ False-Positive Error
▶ Probability
▶ Study Protocol

Sample-Size Calculation

▶ Sample Size Estimation

Sample-Size Determination

▶ Sample Size Estimation

Sarcopenia

Oliver J. Wilson[1] and Anton J. M. Wagenmakers[2]
[1]Institute for Sport, Physical Activity and Leisure, Leeds Beckett University, Leeds, UK
[2]Research Institute for Sport and Exercise Sciences, Liverpool John Moores University, Liverpool, UK

Synonyms

Anabolic resistance; Disuse atrophy; Skeletal muscle atrophy

Definition

Sarcopenia is a syndrome characterized by a progressive generalized loss of skeletal muscle mass and strength with a risk of adverse outcomes such as physical disability, poor quality of life, and death. Sarcopenia is derived from Greek "sarx" for flesh and "penia" for loss.

Description

The global population aged 60 years or older is expected to more than double from 901 million in the year 2015 to 2.1 billion by 2050 (www.un.org). A common result of the aging process is the loss of skeletal muscle mass. This is associated with metabolic disease such as type 2 diabetes (Park et al. 2009), impaired physical performance (e.g., walking and rising from a chair), self-reported disability (Janssen et al. 2002), and the increased risk of accidental falls (Szulc et al. 2005) and fractures (Fiatarone Singh et al. 2009). Hip fractures are among the most common site of fracture in elderly individuals (Johnell and Kanis 2006), and elderly hip fracture patients have a threefold higher all-cause age- and sex-standardized risk of mortality than the general population (Panula et al. 2011). Consequently, maintaining muscle mass will be very important for lowering the socioeconomic burden of an aging population.

The age-related loss of skeletal muscle mass and physical function was termed sarcopenia by Rosenberg (1989). The European Working Group on Sarcopenia in Older People (EWGSOP) now defines sarcopenia as "a syndrome characterized by progressive and generalized loss of skeletal muscle mass and strength with a risk of adverse outcomes such as physical disability, poor quality of life and death" (Cruz-Jentoft et al. 2010). The EWGSOP suggests three stages of severity for sarcopenia that depends on the cutoff points appropriate to the measurement technique used to measure muscle mass, strength, and physical performance. The "presarcopenia" stage is present in individuals who combine a low muscle mass without impact on skeletal muscle strength or physical performance. "Sarcopenia" is the stage in which individuals combine a low muscle mass with either a low muscle strength or low physical performance. Finally, "severe sarcopenia" is present in individuals who combine a low muscle mass with a low muscle strength and low physical performance. In a systematic review, the estimated prevalence of sarcopenia using EWGSOP criteria was 1–29% in community-dwelling individuals and 14–33% of those receiving long-term care (Cruz-Jentoft et al. 2014). Using other diagnostic criteria, Baumgartner et al. (1998) observed the prevalence of sarcopenia in >50% of males and females aged >80 years.

Sarcopenia can be masked by weight stability in the presence of a concomitant increase in fat mass. However, the prolonged accumulation of fat mass can lead to obesity, resulting in "sarcopenic obesity." This presents further complications as excess fat mass which, in association with chronic low-level pro-inflammatory cytokines, can result in the development of insulin resistance in a variety of tissues such as the endothelium of the microvasculature and within skeletal muscle fibers. This leads to periods of hyperglycemia, hyperinsulinemia, and hyperlipidemia and the development of type 2 diabetes and cardiovascular disease (Wagenmakers et al. 2006, 2016).

The genesis of sarcopenia can be attributable to physical inactivity and inadequate nutrition among other factors (Table 1).

Effect of Age on Skeletal Muscle

Skeletal muscle mass peaks between 20 and 30 years of age and the loss of muscle mass begins in the fourth decade (Janssen et al. 2000). The loss of muscle mass is more notable in lower than upper limbs (Janssen et al. 2000) with leg skeletal muscle mass lost at an average rate of approximately 1% per year for males and females during their eighth decade (Goodpaster et al. 2006). Most individuals aged over 70 years will possess about 80% of the muscle mass of those aged 20–30 years.

Sarcopenia, Table 1 Summary of the potential mechanisms underpinning sarcopenia

Whole body
Reduced physical activity and muscle disuse
Loss of motor neurons
Reduced growth hormone and insulin-like growth factor-I production
Chronic pro-inflammatory state
Increased glucocorticoid production and receptor activity
Malnutrition
Muscular
Reduced number and proliferative capacity of skeletal muscle satellite cells
Mitochondrial DNA mutations and apoptosis
Increased intracellular production of glucocorticoids
Impaired insulin-mediated increase in microvascular perfusion
Blunting of the effects of amino acids on muscle protein synthesis
Blunting of the effects of insulin on muscle protein breakdown
Impaired transcriptional responses of muscle to exercise and nutrition

Leg strength can be lost at an average rate of approximately 2.8% and 3.8% per year for females and males aged >70 years over a 3-year period (Goodpaster et al. 2006). This exceeds the annual loss of muscle mass and suggests a reduction in muscle quality (force per unit area of tissue) with age. Muscle power also declines with age, and low muscle power is associated with a two- to threefold greater risk of impaired physical performance than low muscle strength (Bean et al. 2003). The effect of age on muscle strength and power has been termed dynapenia (Manini and Clark 2012). The loss of skeletal muscle mass and strength is evident even in those who engage in regular aerobic or resistance exercise.

Sarcopenia and dynapenia have been linked to the age-related loss of spinal motor neurons (Aagaard et al. 2010). This leads to a reduction in the number and size of muscle fibers and results in impaired muscle mechanical performance (Aagaard et al. 2010). Some of the denervated muscle fibers are reinnervated by surviving motor units, leading to the formation of very large motor units and the appearance of fiber-type grouping (Andersen 2003). Of the remaining muscle fibers, atrophy is more notable in type II fibers. In people aged 88 years, type II fibers had atrophied in size to about 43% of a matched group of 25-year-olds, but type I fibers had atrophied in size to about 75% of their younger counterparts (Andersen 2003). These effects, in combination with an age-related decline in neuromuscular function, lead to impaired muscle mechanical performance and a reduced ability to complete normal daily living tasks such as walking and rising from a chair (Aagaard et al. 2010). Further age-related changes include the infiltration of fat and connective tissue within the muscle and a reduction in type II fiber satellite cell content (Koopman and van Loon 2009). A reduction in the oxidative capacity of skeletal muscle is also observed with age and is likely attributable to a reduction in mitochondrial content and/or function. This results in poor endurance and increased fatigability, compromising the ability to live an independent lifestyle. Poor oxidative capacity is also mechanistically linked to the development of insulin resistance and type 2 diabetes (Wagenmakers et al. 2006, 2016).

Protein Metabolism in the Elderly

Contemporary evidence suggests basal rates of muscle protein synthesis (MPS) and muscle protein breakdown (MPB) in the elderly equal that of younger individuals and does not explain the age-related loss of muscle mass (Wall et al. 2014). Instead, sarcopenia might be attributable to anabolic resistance, the reduced ability to mount a youthful response of MPS to protein ingestion, and/or muscle loading (Witard et al. 2016). The mechanisms underlying anabolic resistance remain to be elucidated, but impairments may exist at the cellular level (e.g., protein/amino acid digestion, absorption, and transport) and molecular level (e.g., Akt-mTOR-p70S6K signaling pathway) (Wall et al. 2014; Witard et al. 2016). These may impede the availability of amino acids for MPS and blunt the sensing and transduction of amino acid- and/or insulin-dependent signaling, thereby limiting the stimulation of MPS and the inhibitory effects of insulin on MPB. As exercise increases the sensitivity of the muscle to the anabolic effects of protein intake, increasing the physical activity rates of the elderly may help counteract anabolic resistance (Wall et al. 2014).

Muscle loss and anabolic resistance may also develop through periods of reduced physical activity and muscle disuse. An accelerated loss of muscle mass and blunting of postprandial MPS in elderly individuals after 2 weeks of reduced daily physical activity have been reported (Breen et al. 2013). Suggestions have also been made that an accelerated loss of muscle mass during periods of illness leading to bed rest (<10 days) is irreversible and will lead to stepwise reductions in muscle mass (Wall et al. 2013).

The age-associated decline in daily physical activity and total energy expenditure also leads to a gradual reduction of both the calorie and protein intake, if the dietary protein content is kept constant. Consequently, sedentary and frail elders may fail to consume the current recommended daily allowance (RDA) for protein intake (0.8 g/kg body mass). An increase of the protein intake of the diet from ±15 to ≥ 20 En% is enough to prevent this deficit (Houston et al. 2008). In addition, such an increase will be more effective in maximally stimulating (post-exercise) MPS and, therefore, attenuating the loss of muscle mass (Houston et al. 2008; Wall et al. 2014; Witard et al. 2016).

Resistance Training in the Elderly

Resistance exercise training is a potent stimulator of MPS, leading to increased muscle mass (mostly attributable to type II fiber hypertrophy) and strength in the young, elderly, frail elderly, and older individuals presenting with comorbidities. Resistance training therefore offers an effective strategy to counteract sarcopenia and improve functional muscle capacity. The American College of Sports Medicine (Chodzko-Zajko et al. 2009) recommends progressive resistance training at least 2 days per week using 8–10 exercises involving the major muscle groups over 8–12 repetitions. Gains in muscular endurance of up to 200% have also been reported after completing moderate- to high-intensity resistance training (Chodzko-Zajko et al. 2009). An increase in mitochondrial protein content and oral glucose tolerance has also been reported in the elderly after resistance training (Frank et al. 2016).

Conclusion

Sarcopenia contributes to the increased risk of falls, fractures, and functional impairment and increased dependency. The loss of muscle mass is also associated with type 2 diabetes. Anabolic resistance to protein and exercise may contribute to the development of sarcopenia, and this may be further exacerbated through periods of reduced physical activity or bed rest. The accelerated loss of muscle mass during these periods may be irreversible. However, resistance exercise is a potent stimulator of MPS, and progressive resistance training results in improved muscle mass and strength and will give older individuals the confidence to continue to engage in aerobic exercise such as walking. The combination of resistance and aerobic exercise is optimal to maintain metabolic health until a very high age.

Cross-References

▶ Atrophy
▶ Cytokines
▶ Glucocorticoids
▶ Insulin
▶ Physical Inactivity

References and Further Readings

Aagaard, P., Suetta, C., Caserotti, P., Magnusson, S. P., & Kjaer, M. (2010). Role of the nervous system in sarcopenia and muscle atrophy with aging: Strength training as a countermeasure. *Scandinavian Journal of Medicine & Science in Sports, 20*, 49–64.

Andersen, J. L. (2003). Muscle fibre type adaptation in the elderly human muscle. *Scandinavian Journal of Medicine & Science in Sports, 13*, 40–47.

Baumgartner, R. N., Koehler, K. M., Gallagher, D., Romero, L., Heymstleld, S. B., Ross, R. R., Garry, P. G., & Lindeman, R. D. (1998). Epidemiology of sarcopenia among the elderly in New Mexico. *American Journal of Epidemiology, 147*(8), 755–763.

Bean, J. F., Leveille, S. G., Kiely, D. K., Bandinelli, S., Guralnik, J. M., & Ferrucci, L. (2003). A comparison of leg power and leg strength within the InCHIANTI study: Which influences mobility more? *Journals of Gerontology. Series A, Biological Sciences and Medical Sciences, 58*(8), 728–733.

Breen, L., Stokes, K. A., Churchward-Venne, T. A., Moore, D. R., Baker, S. K., Smith, K., Atherton, P. J., & Phillips, S. M. (2013). Two weeks of reduced activity decreases leg lean mass and induces "anabolic resistance" of myofibrillar protein synthesis in healthy elderly. *Journal of Clinical Endocrinology and Metabolism, 98*(6), 2604–2612.

Chodzko-Zajko, W. J., Proctor, D. N., Fiatarone Singh, M. A., Minson, C. T., Nigg, C. R., & Salem, G. J. (2009). Exercise and physical activity for older adults. *Medicine & Science in Sports & Exercise, 41*, 1510–1530.

Cruz-Jentoff, A. J., Baeyens, J. P., Bauer, J. M., Boirie, J. M., Cederholm, T., Landi, F., Martin, F. C., Michel, J. P., Rolland, Y., Schneider, S. M., Topinkova, E., Vandewoude, M., & Zamboni, M. (2010). Sarcopenia: European consensus on definition and diagnosis: Report of the European working group on sarcopenia in older people. *Age and Ageing, 39*(4), 412–423.

Cruz-Jentoft, A. J., Landi, F., Schneider, S. M., Zúñiga, C., Arai, H., Boirie, Y., Chen, L. K., Fielding, R. A., Martin, F. C., Michel, J. P., Sieber, C., Stout, J. R., Studenski, S. A., Vellas, B., Woo, J., Zamboni, M., & Cederholm, T. (2014). Prevalence of and interventions for sarcopenia in ageing adults: A systematic review. Report of the International Sarcopenia Initiative (EWGSOP and IWGS). *Age and Ageing, 43*(6), 748–759.

Fiatarone Singh, M. A., Singh, N. A., Hansen, R. D., Finnegan, T. P., Allen, B. J., Diamond, T. H., Diwan, A. D., Lloyd, B. D., Williamson, D. A., Smith, E. U., Grady, J. N., Stavrinos, T. M., & Thompson, M. W. (2009). Methodology and baseline characteristics for the sarcopenia and hip fracture study: A 5-year prospective study. *Journal of Gerontolgical Advances in Biological Sciences and Medical Sciences, 64A*(5), 568–574.

Frank, P., Andersson, E., Pontén, M., Ekblom, B., Ekblom, M., & Sahlin, K. (2016). Strength training improves muscle aerobic capacity and glucose tolerance in elderly. *Scandinavian Journal of Medicine & Science in Sports, 26*(7), 764–773.

Goodpaster, B. H., Park, S. W., Harris, T. B., Kritchevsky, S. B., Nevitt, M., Schwartz, A. V., Simonsick, E. M., Tylavsky, F. A., Visser, M., & Newman, A. B. (2006).

The loss of skeletal muscle strength, mass, and quality in older adults: The health, aging and body composition study. *The Journals of Gerontology. Series A, Biological Sciences and Medical Sciences, 61*(10), 1059–1064.

Houston, D. K., Nicklas, B. J., Ding, J., Harris, T. B., Tylavsky, F. A., Newman, A. B., Lee, J. S., Sahyoun, N. R., Visser, M., Kritchevsky, S. B., & Health ABC Study. (2008). Dietary protein intake is associated with lean mass change in older, community-dwelling adults: The Health, Aging, and Body Composition (Health ABC) Study. *American Journal of Clinical Nutrition, 87*(1), 150–155.

Janssen, I., Heymsfield, S. B., Wang, Z., & Ross, R. (2000). Skeletal muscle mass and distribution in 468 men and women aged 18–88 yr. *Journal of Applied Physiology, 89*(1), 81–88.

Janssen, I., Heymsfield, S. B., & Ross, R. (2002). Low relative skeletal muscle mass (sarcopenia) in older persons is associated with functional impairment and physical disability. *Journal of the American Geriatrics Society, 50*(5), 889–896.

Johnell, O., & Kanis. (2006). An estimate of the worldwide prevalence and disability associated with osteoporotic fractures. *Osteoporosis International, 17*, 1726–1733.

Koopman, R., & van Loon, L. J. (2009). Aging, exercise, and muscle protein metabolism. *Journal of Applied Physiology, 106*, 2040–2048.

Manini, T. M., & Clark, B. C. (2012). Dynapenia and aging: An update. *Journals of Gerontology. Series A, Biological Sciences and Medical Sciences, 67*(1), 28–40.

Panula, J., Pihlajamäki, H., Mattila, V. M., Jaatinen, P., Vahlberg, T., Aarnio, P., & Kivela, S. L. (2011). Mortality and cause of death in hip fracture patients aged 65 or older – A population-based study. *BMC Musculoskeletal Disorders, 12*(105), 1–6.

Park, S. W., Goodpaster, B. H., Lee, J. S., Kuller, L. H., Boudreau, R., de Rekeneire, N., Harris, T. B., Kritchevsky, S., Tylavsky, F. A., Nevitt, M., Cho, Y. W., & Newman, A. B. (2009). Excessive loss of skeletal muscle mass in older people with type 2 diabetes. *Diabetes Care, 32*, 1993–1997.

Rosenberg, I. (1989). Summary comments: Epidemiological and methodological problems in determining nutritional status of older persons. *American Journal of Clinical Nutrition, 50*, 1231–1233.

Szulc, P., Beck, T. J., Marchand, F., & Delmas, P. D. (2005). Low skeletal muscle mass is associated with poor structural parameters of bone and impaired balance in elderly men – The MINOS study. *Journal of Bone and Mineral Research, 20*(5), 721–729.

Wagenmakers, A. J., vanRiel, N. A., Frenneaux, M. P., & Stewart, P. M. (2006). Integration of the metabolic and cardiovascular effects of exercise. *Essays in Biochemistry, 42*, 193–210.

Wagenmakers, A. J., Strauss, J. A., Shepherd, S. O., Keske, M. A., & Cocks, M. (2016). Increased muscle blood supply and transendothelial nutrient and insulin transport induced by food intake and exercise: Effect of obesity and ageing. *Journal of Physiology, 594*, 2207–2222.

Wall, B. T., Dirks, M. L., & van Loon, L. J. C. (2013). Skeletal muscle atrophy during short-term disuse: Implications for age-related sarcopenia. *Ageing Research Reviews, 12*, 898–906.

Wall, B. T., Cermak, N. M., & van Loon, L. J. C. (2014). Dietary protein considerations to support active ageing. *Sports Medicine, 44*(2), S185–S194.

Witard, O. C., McGlory, C., Hamilton, D. L., & Phillips, S. M. (2016). Growing older with health and vitality: A nexus of physical activity, exercise and nutrition. *Biogerontology, 17*, 529–546.

www.un.org United Nations, Department of Economic and Social Affairs: Population Division. (2015). *World population prospects: The 2015 revision, key findings and advance tables.* Accessed 25 Aug 2016.

Saturated Fats

▶ Fat, Dietary Intake

Saturated Fatty Acids

▶ Fat: Saturated, Unsaturated

SBM

▶ Society of Behavioral Medicine

Scale Development

Yori Gidron
SCALab, Lille 3 University and Siric Oncollile, Lille, France

Synonyms

Questionnaire development

Definition

Scale development is an essential stage in the assessment of constructs and variables in behavior medicine and in any social and health science. Scales are used for assessment of self-reported variables including mood, daily disability, various types of symptoms, adherence to recommended diet, etc. Though there is no explicit "rule" for the stages of scale development, certain steps need to be included for claiming that a scale is reliable and valid. The reliability of a scale is very important and refers to its repeatability and lack of measurement error. This is tested by internal reliability tests (Cronbach's α) and by a test-retest reliability of scores over time. Validity is an essential aspect of a scale and refers to the extent to which it measures what it claims to measure. This is tested by several manners including "face validity," concurrent validity, construct validity, and criterion validity. When developing a scale, it is essential to have a clear definition of the concept it refers to. Thus, for example, an anxiety scale should not have items assessing depression since these are not the same construct. After choosing an acceptable definition for the construct, a group of "experts" on the construct meets to provide items or even topics related to the construct, from which the researcher creates items. The chosen items will reflect the most common topics or items suggested by the expert panel. The panel can be experts from the field (psychologists, physicians, etc.) and patients who experienced the issue under investigation, thus reflecting experienced "experts." Then, the investigator can ask another group of experts or patients to rate the relevance of each item to the construct, reflecting face validity. The items with a mean relevance above a chosen criterion will be selected for the preliminary scale. Next, the researcher administers the scale to a larger sample, with theoretically relevant additional tests. This will enable to test the internal reliability, concurrent validity against another scale assessing the same construct, and the construct validity against scales assessing theoretically related constructs. Finally, an acceptable criterion (e.g., ill vs. healthy sample) will enable to test the scale's criterion validity. Predictive validity can also be tested by examining whether the scale's scores predict a certain event or outcome in the future, beyond the effects of known confounders. For example, Barefoot et al. (1989) tested the predictive validity of a shorter hostility scale derived from the original Ho scale in the Minnesota Multiphasic Personality Inventory. They found that the brief scale which included cynicism, hostile affect, and aggressive responding predicted death better than the original full Ho scale, supporting the brief scale's predictive validity. These steps are needed for scale development, to verify a scale's reliability and validity, for use in research and clinical evaluations.

Cross-References

▶ Reliability and Validity

References and Further Readings

Barefoot, J. C., Dodge, K. A., Peterson, B. L., Dahlstrom, W. G., & Williams, R. B., Jr. (1989). The Cook-Medley hostility scale: Item content and ability to predict survival. *Psychosomatic Medicine, 51*, 46–57.

Clark, L. A., & Watson, D. (1995). Constructing validity: Basic issues in objective scale development. *Psychological Assessment, 3*, 309–319.

Scatter

▶ Dispersion

Scenario Design

▶ Scenario-Based Design

Scenario-Based Design

Colleen Stiles-Shields
Loyola University, Chicago, IL, USA
Northwestern University, The University of Chicago, Chicago, IL, USA

Synonyms

Scenario design; Scenario-based design; User-centered design approaches

Definition

Scenario-based design is a validated and user-centered design approach, used early in the design process of a technology or product, which relies upon "scenarios" or stories to capture the elements of interaction between a person and a future product.

Description

Scenario-based design (SBD) refers to a family of validated user-centered design approaches that use "scenarios," or stories, to inform the design of a technology or product. These scenarios are narratives, which may be in the form of text, storyboards, videos, etc. The scenarios are created and utilized to concretely define a user's experience of an interaction with a technology, what happens during that interaction, and how it happens. Indeed, given that scenarios are like stories, they have characters, character goals and actions, and a plot within a larger setting. Through the use of scenarios, the use of the product becomes contextualized and more explicit, thereby informing ultimate design decisions (Carroll 1985; Rosson and Carroll 2002).

Use in the Design of Behavioral Intervention Technologies

SBD is increasingly being utilized in the field of behavioral medicine, primarily in designing behavioral intervention technologies (BITs). As BITs tend to be designed by interdisciplinary teams, ranging from engineers to psychologists (Schueller et al. 2014), SBD lends well to the design process across disciplines. Indeed, SBD's use of scenarios to contextualize a BIT interaction is similar to the use of case vignettes to establish clinical practice techniques (a training practice common in medical and clinical fields), while also being a design approach familiar to technologists, usability experts, and engineers. Further, the use of SBD provides a common framework and language for the interdisciplinary team to utilize throughout the design process (Carroll 2000). Recent examples of the use of SBD include BITs targeting well-being and mental health in youth (Blythe and Wright 2006; Bødker 2000; Orlowski et al. 2015) and apps targeting symptoms of depression and anxiety in adults (Mohr et al. 2017; Stiles-Shields et al. 2016). Additionally, in examining the impact of the use of SBD in the design of medication alerts for prescribers, system usability improved, errors were reduced, and the prescribers reported a decrease in perceived work load (Russ et al. 2014). For the purposes of direct application of SBD to the design process of BITs, the remainder of the description of SBD will utilize the design of a mobile treatment app for adults with depression as an example.

Framework

The framework of SBD involves three primary phases: Analysis, Design, and Prototype and Evaluation (Rosson and Carroll 2002). The first phase of the framework is *Analysis*, in which claims about current practices and possible stakeholders are identified through the use of *Problem Scenarios*. Problem Scenarios depict the story of a user in a current practice. To represent the user, personas are often created to elucidate the benefits and challenges that may be incorporated and/or addressed through the design process. For the example of the design of an app for depression, the persona demographics could be informed by samples of adults interested in treatments delivered through technology, treatment-seeking patients in traditional community or clinic settings, and/or national prevalence rates of adults with depression. These personas would be individualized (e.g., "Sara," a 21-year-old Latina with moderate depression who moved to a new city within the last year), and then used in Problem Scenarios designed to highlight benefits and challenges associated with seeking depression treatment through current practices (e.g., face-to-face therapy, medication, and/or self-help resources). A *Claims Analysis* would follow, with the intention to reveal positive and negative features about current practice. For example, a design team might consider varying positive (e.g., a therapist can directly address "Sara's" concerns as they are brought up in the moment) and negative (e.g., "Sara" might need to wait several weeks for an initial therapy session, possibly impacting her motivation and symptomology) features of a face-to-face therapy session (e.g., a "current practice" for depression treatment). A stakeholder analysis would also follow. *Stakeholders* include anyone who might be impacted by the product. Stakeholders might have conflicting interests from other stakeholders, and may be Primary (use the product), Secondary (provide input or receive output from the product), or Tertiary (no direct involvement but effected by successes or failures). For example, in the design of an app for adults with depression, stakeholders might include: patients with depression (Primary); researchers and clinical providers (Secondary); and users of future iterations of the app, the immediate social network of the patient, referral sources, developers and technologists, and other mHealth researchers (Tertiary). Through the Analysis process of SBD, designers elucidate the positive and negative elements of current practices for stakeholders, while identifying how a new product will maintain, enhance, or alter current practice (Carroll 1985; Rosson and Carroll 2002).

The second phase of the SBD framework is *Design*, in which multiple iterations of designs are completed through analyses of Design Claims informed by *Activity Scenarios, Information Design Scenarios, and Interaction Design Scenarios*. Activity Scenarios are persona interactions with the new technology, and therefore serve as initial depictions of the transformation from the current practice to the new design features. The intended output of Activity Scenarios is *Design Claims*, which detail new features and their purposes. For example, an Activity Scenario for the design of an app for depression may depict "Sara" locating the app on an app store and learning about the functionality through pop up notifications at app launch; a Design Claim from this scenario would include brief, informative notifications at initial launch. Information Design Scenarios add nuance to the Activity Scenarios, such that they make perceptual details more explicit. The ultimate aim of this process is to identify how a user might perceive or interpret the product and/or information provided. For example, an Information Design Scenario would describe specifically what the launch notification reads to "Sara" and how she might interpret that information. Finally, Interaction Design Scenarios extend the design process initiated by the previous scenarios by explicitly detailing the actions a user might take, and how the system would respond. For example, these scenarios would provide step-by-step information about "Sara's" launch of the app, what is presented, how she proceeds, etc. Throughout the Design phase of the SBD framework, multiple iterations are completed across personas to inform and enrich the design (Carroll 1985; Rosson and Carroll 2002).

The final phase of the SBD framework is *Prototype and Evaluation*. Resulting from the multiple iterations of scenarios created during the Analysis and Design phases, *Prototypes* may be created as preliminary models of aspects of the designed product. Prototypes may range from simple (e.g., paper drawings, tending to be less costly and time intensive) to complex/realistic (e.g., an initial version of a mobile app, tending to have greater validity). The purpose of creating prototypes in the SBD process is to engage in usability evaluations of the designs. These evaluations may be formative (i.e., occurring during the design and development) or summative (i.e., occurring at the end of the development stage; Tullis and Albert 2008; Please see "Usability Testing" entry for more information). This evaluative process enables teams to finalize their designs and prepare for the ultimate creation of a new product.

Benefits

Multiple benefits of SBD have been highlighted in the literature. First, scenarios evoke careful attention and reflection for design teams through their use of depictions of persona experiences with the product. This process often highlights how well design ideas align with ultimate user and designer goals. Second, scenarios allow for flexibility, in that they are easily revised, but can also promote concrete solutions to identified problems. Third, scenarios can be created from multiple perspectives and levels, and for varying purposes. They can anchor design discussions in specific work products, across multiple disciplines, and design team members. Finally, scenarios are easily abstracted and categorized, promoting the recognition, use, and reuse of generalizations or patterns that emerge in interactions with the designed product (Carroll 1985, 2000; Rosson and Carroll 2002). SBD therefore stands as a promising and accessible means for interdisciplinary teams to design BITs, or other products which may promote behavioral health.

Cross-References

▶ Usability Testing

References and Further Reading

Blythe, M. A., & Wright, P. C. (2006). Pastiche scenarios: Fiction as a resource for user centred design. *Interacting with Computers, 18*(5), 1139–1164. https://doi.org/10.1016/j.intcom.2006.02.001.

Bødker, S. (2000). Scenarios in user-centred design—Setting the stage for reflection and action. *Interacting with Computers, 13*(1), 61–75. https://doi.org/10.1016/S0953-5438(00)00024-2.

Carroll, J. M. (1985). *Scenario-based design: Envisioning work and technology in system development*. New York: Wiley.

Carroll, J. M. (2000). Five reasons for scenario-based design. *Interacting with Computers, 13*(1), 43–60. https://doi.org/10.1016/S0953-5438(00)00023-0.

Mohr, D. C., Tomasino, K. N., Lattie, E. G., Palac, H. L., Kwasny, M. J., Weingardt, K., et al. (2017). IntelliCare: An eclectic, skills-based app suite for the treatment of depression and anxiety. *Journal of Medical Internet Research, 19*(1). https://doi.org/10.2196/jmir.6645.

Orlowski, S. K., Lawn, S., Venning, A., Winsall, M., Jones, G. M., Wyld, K., et al. (2015). Participatory research as one piece of the puzzle: A systematic review of consumer involvement in design of technology-based youth mental health and well-being interventions. *JMIR Human Factors, 2*(2). https://doi.org/10.2196/humanfactors.4361.

Rosson, M. B., & Carroll, J. M. (2002). *Usability engineering: Scenario-based development of human-computer interaction*. San Francisco: Morgan Kaufmann.

Russ, A. L., Zillich, A. J., Melton, B. L., Russell, S. A., Chen, S., Spina, J. R., et al. (2014). Applying human factors principles to alert design increases efficiency and reduces prescribing errors in a scenario-based simulation. *Journal of the American Medical Informatics Association, 21*(e2), e287–e296. https://doi.org/10.1136/amiajnl-2013-002045.

Schueller, S. M., Begale, M., Penedo, F. J., & Mohr, D. C. (2014). Purple: A modular system for developing and deploying behavioral intervention technologies. *Journal of Medical Internet Research, 16*(7). https://doi.org/10.2196/jmir.3376.

Stiles-Shields, C., Montague, E., & Mohr, D. C. (2016). *The use of scenario-based design for the development of behavioral intervention technologies*. International Society for Research on Internet Interventions (ISRII) 8th scientific meeting, Washington, DC.

Tullis, T., & Albert, B. (2008). *Measuring the user experience: Collecting, analyzing, and presenting usability metrics*. Burlington: Morgan Kaufmann Publishers.

Schneiderman, Neil

Neil Schneiderman
Department of Psychology, Behavioral Medicine Research Center, University of Miami, Coral Gables, FL, USA

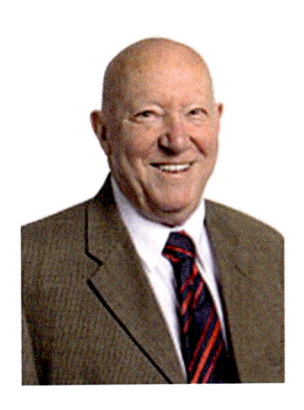

Neil Schneiderman was born in Brooklyn, New York, on February 24, 1937. He has been married to his wife Eleanor since 1960 and is the father of three children and grandfather of five. Schneiderman received his A.B.. degree from Brooklyn College, spent 2 years in the US Army, earned his Ph.D. degree in Psychology from Indiana University, and received postdoctoral training in Neurophysiology and Neuropharmacology in the Physiological Institute of the University of Basel, Switzerland. Schneiderman was appointed as assistant professor at the University of Miami, Coral Gables, Florida, in 1965, rising through the ranks to become professor in 1974. He subsequently received secondary appointments as professor of Medicine, Public Health Sciences, Psychiatry and Behavioral Sciences, and Biomedical Engineering. In 1989, he was awarded an endowed chair as the James L. Knight Professor of Health Psychology. Since 1986, he has served as the director of the Division of Health Psychology in the Department of Psychology and as director of the University of Miami Behavioral Medicine Research Center. He also served extensively as chair of the NIH-funded University of Miami General Clinical Research Center Advisory Committee. Schneiderman has directed pre- and postdoctoral NIH training grants involving cardiovascular disease from the National Heart, Lung, and Blood Institute (NHLBI) since 1979 and HIV/AIDS from the National Institute of Mental Health (NIMH) from 1993 to 2017.

Schneiderman was the second editor in chief of the journal *Health Psychology* before becoming founding editor in chief of the *International Journal of Behavioral Medicine*. Within the NIH, he served as a member of the Biopsychology Study Section, NHLBI Research Training Review Committee, and NIMH Health Behavior and Prevention Review Committee. In the American Psychological Association (APA), he was chair of the Board of Scientific Affairs and is a fellow in the Divisions of Experimental Psychology (3), Behavioral Neuroscience and Comparative Psychology (6), and Health Psychology (38) as well as a former president of Division 38. A founding fellow of the Academy of Behavioral Medicine Research, Schneiderman later served as president of that organization. Schneiderman also served as president of the International Society of Behavioral Medicine (ISBM). He is a fellow of the Society of Behavioral Medicine and of the American College of Clinical Pharmacology. He is also the recipient of the APA Distinguished Scientific Contribution Award (1994), Society of Behavioral Medicine Distinguished Scientist Award (1997), ISBM Outstanding Scientific Achievement Award (2004), and American Psychosomatic Society Distinguished Scientist Award (2014).

Major Accomplishments

Schneiderman's first two empirical research articles were published in *Science* in 1962. Written with his academic mentor, Isidore Gormezano, the papers described animal models of eyelid and nictitating membrane Pavlovian conditioning in rabbits. These preparations were suitable for concomitantly studying behavioral and neurophysiological processes in conscious, minimally restrained animals. Subsequently, Schneiderman added heart rate conditioning to the repertoire of animal models, and for the next several decades, he and his colleagues traced neuronal pathways involved in Pavlovian conditioning of cardiovascular responses in rabbits. This began with identifying the cells of origin of vagal cardioinhibitory motoneurons in the rabbit medulla, using histochemistry, microstimulation, and single neuron extracellular electrophysiological recordings, and continued with mapping the central nervous system pathways that mediated conditioned and unconditioned cardiovascular adjustments. Key collaborators included James Schwaber, Marc Kaufman, Howard Ellenberger, and Michael Spyer. The study of central nervous system pathways mediating differentiated patterns of cardiovascular adjustments also led Schneiderman and his colleagues including Marc Gellman, Barry Hurwitz, Maria Llabre, and Pat Saab to conduct an important series of psychophysiological studies in humans. They described differentiated patterns of neurohormonal and cardiovascular responses to separate behavioral stressors as a function of race, gender, and hypertensive status. These responses were also shown to be influenced by such psychosocial factors as harassment and hostility. Subsequently, Schneiderman collaborated with Philip McCabe, Armando Mendez, and other Miami scientists in documenting the psychosocial prevention of atherosclerosis progression in a rabbit model of coronary artery disease.

Because of Schneiderman's interest in relationships among biological regulation, psychosocial factors, and disease processes, it was not surprising that he also joined with colleagues including MaryAnn Fletcher, Gail Ironson, and Nancy Klimas relatively early in the HIV/AIDS epidemic to study relationships between psychosocial variables and endocrine-immune regulation in HIV-infected patients, when AIDS was beginning to ravage the Miami community. This, in turn, led Schneiderman, Michael Antoni, and their collaborators to begin to use group-based cognitive behavior therapy and relaxation training in randomized controlled trials to influence psychosocial, endocrine, and immune factors and even to reduce HIV viral load to undetectable levels in patients who were failing their regimen of highly active antiretroviral drugs.

Schneiderman's broad research experience, including intervention studies with clinical patients, prepared him to serve as principal investigator of the Miami Field Center for the NIH/NHLBI "Enhancing Recovery in Coronary Heart Disease Patients (ENRICHD)" randomized trial. The trial compared cognitive behavior therapy and usual care in post-myocardial infarction patients. Although that trial produced null results in terms of morbidity and mortality, Schneiderman and colleagues conducted a secondary analysis that suggested that the trial appeared to decrease morbidity and mortality in White men, but not in women or minority patients. Based on the supposition that the null result in the ENRICHD trial was due to the protocol not being sufficiently tailored to women, Schneiderman joined with Kristina Orth-Gomér and other Swedish colleagues to conduct the "Stockholm Women's Intervention Trial for Coronary Heart Disease (SWITCHD)." This trial, which used group-based cognitive behavior therapy and relaxation training in women previously hospitalized for myocardial infarction or coronary revascularization, showed a significant decrease in mortality rate for the intervention compared with a usual care group. Similar results have now also been reported by others.

In addition to Schneiderman's contributions in basic science and in clinical trials research, he has been actively involved in population-based observational studies such as those with Ronald Goldberg and Jay Skyler. As the principal investigator of the Miami Field Center of the NIH/NHLBI multicenter Hispanic Community Health Study/Study of Latinos, Schneiderman and his colleagues in Miami, including Frank Penedo, David Lee, and Marc Gellman, as well as investigators in the Bronx, Chicago, and San Diego are characterizing the health status and disease burden of Hispanic adults living in the United States, describing the positive and negative consequences of immigration and acculturation in relation to lifestyle and access to health care and assessing likely causal factors of disease in this diverse population. This study, sponsored by the NIH, was initiated in 2006 and is funded until 2024. Between 2008 and 2011, 16,415 women and men 18–74 years of age, who self-identified as being Hispanic or Latino, completed a 6.5 h baseline clinical exam. Participants were recruited from a stratified random sample of households in defined committees in the Bronx, Chicago, Miami, and San Diego, thus including a wide range of ancestral backgrounds. The study assessed risk factors and prevalence of heart, lung, blood, and sleep disorders, liver and kidney dysfunction, diabetes, cognitive impairment, dental problems, and hearing disorder. A second clinic exam was conducted on 80% of the original cohort between 2014 and 2017, and a third exam is being conducted between 2019 and 2023. The emphasis of clinic exams 2 and 3 is on long-term follow-up and disease incidence. In summary, Schneiderman's contributions have been in terms of basic science, population-based observational studies, and randomized clinical trials.

Cross-References

▶ International Society of Behavioral Medicine

References and Further Readings

Ironson, G. H., Gellman, M. D., Spitzer, S. B., Llabre, M. M., Pasin, R. D., Weidler, D. J., et al. (1989). Predicting home and work blood pressure measurements from resting baselines and laboratory reactivity in black and white Americans. *Psychophysiology, 26*, 174–184.

Orth-Gomér, K., Schneiderman, N., Wang, H., Walldin, C., Blom, M., & Jernberg, T. (2009). Stress reduction prolongs life in women with coronary disease: The Stockholm women's intervention trial for coronary heart disease (SWITCHD). *Circulation. Cardiovascular Quality and Outcomes, 2*, 25–32. https://doi.org/10.1161/CIRCOUTCOMES.108.812859.

Schneiderman, N., Fuentes, I., & Gormezano, I. (1962). Acquisition and extinction of the classically conditioned eyelid responses in the albino rabbit. *Science, 136*, 650–652.

Schneiderman, N., Saab, P. G., Catellier, D. J., Powell, L. H., DeBusk, R. F., Williams, R. B., et al. (2004). Psychosocial treatment within sex by ethnicity subgroups in the enhancing recovery in coronary heart disease (ENRICHD) clinical trial. *Psychosomatic Medicine, 66*, 475–483.

Schwaber, J., & Schneiderman, N. (1975). Aortic nerve activated cardioinhibitory neurons and interneurons. *American Journal of Physiology, 229*, 783–789.

Scientific Psychology

▶ Psychological Science

Screen Time

Sally A. M. Fenton
School of Sport, Exercise and Rehabilitation Sciences, University of Birmingham, Birmingham, UK

Synonyms

Computer use; Screen-based behaviors; Sedentary behavior; TV viewing

Definition

The time spent engaged in screen-based behaviors. *These behaviors can be performed while being sedentary or physically active.*

Screen time refers to the time spent engaged in "screen-based" behaviors, such as watching television (TV) and using a smartphone, tablet, or computer (Tremblay et al. 2017). Screen time is the most studied component sedentary behavior (i.e., waking behavior ≤1.5 metabolic equivalents, while in a sitting, reclining, or lying posture), with researchers typically examining the link between screen-based sedentary behaviors and several health indicators – such as adiposity and cardio-metabolic (including diabetes and metabolic syndrome) and a cardiovascular outcome (van Ekris et al. 2017).

Much of the existing research in this domain includes observational studies investigating the adverse health consequences of TV viewing time among children and adults. Overall, results of both cross-sectional and prospective studies are suggestive of a positive (adverse) relationship between TV viewing and adiposity indicators among youth, such as overweight/obesity, body-mass-index, and body fat (%) (Biddle et al. 2017, 2018). In addition, prospective studies in adults suggest higher levels of TV viewing are linked to increased risk of cardiovascular, cancer, and all-cause mortality (Dunstan et al. 2010). However, authors consistently emphasize that the associations observed between TV viewing with studied health outcomes may be bi-directional in nature (i.e., we cannot rule out reverse causality) and might be mediated or moderated by coexisting behaviors, such as physical activity (Biddle et al. 2018). These considerations are not exclusive to studies examining the health implications of TV viewing, but extend to other screen-based behavior, such as using a computer, smartphones, tablet, or screen-based entertainment systems.

With this in mind, future research that considers the mediating roles of concomitant health behaviors in the associations between screen time and various health outcomes is critical, particularly when we consider how advances in modern technology have changed the manner in which people access and engage in screen-based behaviors. For example, increased use of smartphones and tablets – not of which will be engaged in through sitting – have contributed to overall declines in TV viewing (Ofcom 2018). Consequently, screen-based behaviors can be engaged when being sedentary (e.g., at home, watching TV) or while being active (e.g., using a phone while walking, exergames), across many contexts (e.g., home, school, work, travel) and for many different purposes (e.g., work/study, recreation). The changing technological landscape that is facilitating access to screen-based behaviors is therefore essential to consider when studying the role of "screen time" – and the diverse behaviors this may encompass – for health indicators in different populations.

In their recent "Terminology Consensus Project," the Sedentary Behaviour Research Network highlight caveats to the definition of screen time, emphasizing the importance of describing whether screen-based behaviors are undertaken while sitting, stationary, or being physically active, as well the context (and type) of screen time. Specific definitions include:

- **Sedentary screen time:** Time spent using a screen-based device (e.g., smartphone, tablet, computer, television) while being sedentary in any context (e.g., school, work, recreational). ****Currently, the most commonly researched definition of screen time.**
- **Active screen time:** Time spent using a screen-based device (e.g., smartphone, tablet, computer, television) while not being stationary in any context (e.g., school, work, recreational). Examples of active screen time include playing active video games and running on a treadmill while watching television.
- **Stationary screen time:** Time spent using a screen-based device (e.g., smartphone, tablet, computer, television) while being stationary in any context (e.g., school, work, recreational).
- **Recreational screen time:** Time spent in screen-based behaviors that are not related to school or work.

In conducting future research centered on the health consequences of screen time, the development of new measures aligned with these nuanced definitions will be essential. Such measures should serve to assess the specific type of screen-based behavior, as well as the behavioral and environmental context in which it occurs.

Cross-References

▶ Lifestyle, Sedentary
▶ Sedentary Behaviors
▶ Sedentary Time

References and Further Readings

Biddle, S. J. H., Garcia Bengoechea, E., Pedisic, Z., Bennie, J., Vergeer, I., & Wiesner, G. (2017). Screen time, other sedentary behaviours, and obesity risk in adults: A review of reviews. *Current Obesity Reports, 6*(2), 134–147. https://doi.org/10.1007/s13679-017-0256-9.

Biddle, S. J. H., Pearson, N., & Salmon, J. (2018). Sedentary behaviors and adiposity in young people: Causality and conceptual model. *Exercise and Sport Sciences Reviews, 46*(1), 18–25. https://doi.org/10.1249/JES.0000000000000135.

Dunstan, D. W., Barr, E. L., Healy, G. N., Salmon, J., Shaw, J. E., Balkau, B., et al. (2010). Television viewing time and mortality: The Australian diabetes, obesity and lifestyle study (AusDiab). *Circulation, 121*(3), 384–391. https://doi.org/10.1161/CIRCULATIONAHA.109.894824.

Ofcom. (2018). *Media nations: UK 2018*. Retrieved from https://www.ofcom.org.uk/__data/assets/pdf_file/0014/116006/media-nations-2018-uk.pdf.

Tremblay, M. S., Aubert, S., Barnes, J. D., Saunders, T. J., Carson, V., Latimer-Cheung, A. E., et al. (2017). Sedentary Behavior Research Network (SBRN) – Terminology Consensus Project process and outcome. *The International Journal of Behavioral Nutrition and Physical Activity, 14*(1), 75. https://doi.org/10.1186/s12966-017-0525-8.

van Ekris, E., Altenburg, T. M., Singh, A. S., Proper, K. I., Heymans, M. W., & Chinapaw, M. J. M. (2017). An evidence-update on the prospective relationship between childhood sedentary behaviour and biomedical health indicators: A systematic review and meta-analysis. *Obesity Reviews, 18*(6), 712–714. https://doi.org/10.1111/obr.12526.

Screen-Based Behaviors

▶ Screen Time

Screening

Yori Gidron
SCALab, Lille 3 University and Siric Oncollile, Lille, France

Synonyms

Early detection

Definition

Screening refers to the process of surveying a population or sample of a population, in the attempt to identify people at risk for or with a given health condition. Screening is a crucial part of epidemiology, as it informs about the prevalence and risk factors of various health conditions in a population. Furthermore, screening is crucial for preventive medicine, since it enables to identify people who may benefit from primary, secondary, or tertiary interventions. Screening for primary prevention reflects identifying people without a risk factor (e.g., hypertension, depression), to prevent the risk factor and subsequent illnesses. Screening for secondary prevention could be among people with a risk factor, to prevent an illness. And screening for tertiary prevention would be done to prevent relapse or mortality in people already ill (e.g., after a first myocardial infarction). Screening could be in relation to psychosocial factors such as hostility or anxiety, to behavioral risk factors of disease such as smoking or excessive alcohol drinking, and to genetic profiles. For implementing screening tests in clinical use to reliably predict disease risk or prognosis, it is crucial to know the relative risk for a disease in people high and low on a screening risk factor as well as the correct value of "false positives" (Wald and Morris 2011). It is of utmost importance to identify the criteria or cutoffs for screening in clear, precise, and operational manners (e.g., smoking more than ten cigarettes/day, depression score above 10 on the Center for Epidemiological Studies Depression Scale). Screening then enables either to study specific subpopulations at risk for health conditions or for treating them. One important criterion for screening tests is their accuracy. A test is thought to be 95% accurate if in 95% of the times it predicts correctly who has a disease (sensitivity) and if 95% of the time it predicts correctly who does not have a disease (specificity). Screening also enables to increase one's therapeutic and statistical effects, since by excluding people below a certain cutoff, researchers can prevent a "floor effect" of therapeutic effectiveness. Regretfully, such exclusion is often not practiced in psychological intervention trials. In clinical practice, the cutoffs used to screen are a function of previously defined cutoffs from research or clinical studies, a function of how severe a risk the researchers aim to identify, and the available therapeutic resources that can be allocated for treating the "screened in" subpopulation later. Furthermore, in randomized controlled trials (RCT), the more strict screening criteria are, the longer could be the trial's duration as the sought patient profile becomes more scarce. Thus, the screening criteria are a function of the research question and available resources for such screening and subsequent treatment, and this is a vital part of clinical epidemiology and research and of therapeutic preventative interventions.

Cross-References

▶ Cancer Prevention
▶ Epidemiology
▶ Population-Based Study
▶ Population Health

References and Further Readings

Wald, N. J., & Morris, J. K. (2011). Assessing risk factors as potential screening tests. A simple assessment tool. *Archives of Internal Medicine, 171*, 286–291.

Screening, Cognitive

Richard Hoffman
Academic Health Center, School of Medicine-Duluth Campus University of Minnesota, Duluth, MN, USA

Synonyms

Cognitive impairment tests; Cognitive status tests; Dementia screening tests; Mental status examination

Definition

Cognitive screening is a brief, performance-based assessment of one or more domains of neurobehavioral or cognitive functioning. These assessments typically are completed using standardized cognitive screening tests that can be completed at bedside or in the clinic in 20–30 min or less, often accompanied by interview information elicited from family members or other informants who know the examinee well and can comment on their observations about the examinee's behaviors or changes in their behaviors.

Description

Cognitive screening tests are very commonly used in behavioral medicine, neuropsychology, neuropsychiatry, and primary care medicine. Surveys indicate that cognitive screening instruments are used by over 50% of practitioners in neuropsychiatry and such tests have become a mainstay in the practice of medicine over the course of the last 35 years. Because cognitive screening tests are brief and require a minimum of specialized testing equipment, they can in most cases be administered at bedside, in a busy clinic, or in the emergency department and serve to identify those patients who might benefit from more extensive workups, including neuroimaging, metabolic assays and blood work, or more extensive neuropsychological testing. Cognitive screening tests are used as one central component in the initial differential diagnosis of delirium versus dementia and are perhaps most frequently used in the initial screening for dementias and mild cognitive impairment (MCI), both of which are underdiagnosed in their earliest stages in primary care practice due to the subtlety of their initial presenting symptoms.

Changes in cognitive functioning are frequently seen as a consequence of a number of neurological and general medical diseases, including dementias and degenerative diseases of the cerebral cortex and subcortical regions of the brain. In addition to central nervous system diseases, cognition may also be affected by other systemic diseases, including respiratory, cardiovascular, and renal diseases as well as some infectious diseases, diseases of the liver and pancreas, nutritional deficiencies, metabolic diseases and diabetes, adverse effects of medications, and exposure to toxic substances. Judicious use of cognitive screening instruments can provide evidence to suggest an underlying medical disorder heretofore undiagnosed and may help guide the use of medications and medication dosages, as well as provide information that may prompt the treatment of reversible conditions, such as reversible dementias and pseudodementias.

Cognitive screening tests can help detect deficits associated with disorders that are commonly missed in a standard psychiatric intake interview, especially in emergency room settings, including patients who present with mild disorientation or evidence of possible substance abuse. In addition, many primary psychiatric disorders have significant effects on cognition, such as affective disorders and schizophrenia, and some focal neurological disorders such as focal strokes, neoplasias, and seizure disorders may have combined cognitive and affective sequelae.

Among the most commonly used and well-researched brief cognitive screening tests are the

Mini-Mental State Examination (MMSE), the Cognitive Capacities Screening Examination (CCSE), and the Short Portable Mental Status Questionnaire (SPMSQ), but there are numerous cognitive screening tests available to practitioners at the present time, and these are listed in Table 1. Although there is considerable variability in the component sections of the cognitive screening tests listed in Table 1, in general each contains some assessment of orientation (does the patient know who they are, where they are, and know the day and date), attention and concentration, language skills, memory and immediate recall of verbal information, and visuospatial or drawing/copying skills. Most cognitive screening tests are designed to be completed within 10 min or less. The BIMC, the ACE-R, the CASI, the Cognistat, the RBANS, the HSCS, and the CAMCOG-R contain more extensive subtests and may require up to 30 min to complete. The Mattis Dementia Rating Scale requires 20–45 min to complete and provides assessment of attention, initiation perseveration, visuospatial construction, reasoning, and memory.

Since 1988, there have been several cognitive screening tests designed to be administered by phone or telehealth link, often used in epidemiological studies as more extensive follow-up instruments after an initial administration face-to-face of a brief screening instrument such as the MMSE or the SASSI. Six such instruments are listed in Table 1.

Also listed in Table 1 are five-guided interview or informant-based cognitive screening instruments which are designed to document information from family members or caregivers of patients regarding observed cognitive decline, changes in behavior, or – in the case of the Deterioration Cognitive Observee (DECO) instrument – changes in activity level, long-term memory, short-term memory, visuospatial processing, and new skill learning. Although these can be used as stand-alone measures, they are perhaps best used to complement the findings from cognitive screening tests directly administered to the patient in question.

There is now considerable interest in the development of cognitive screening tests for specific at-risk populations, and recent examples include a

Screening, Cognitive, Table 1 Cognitive screening tests

Brief cognitive screening tests
AB Cognitive Screen (ABCS)
Abbreviated Mental Test Score (AMTS)
Addenbrooke's Cognitive Examination III (ACE-III)
Animal Fluency Test
Blessed Information-Memory-Concentration Test (BIMC)
Blessed Orientation-Memory-Concentration Test (OMC)
Brief Alzheimer Screen (BAS)
Brief Cognitive Assessment Tool (BCAT)
Brief Cognitive Rating Scale (BCRS)
Brief Interview for Mental Status (BIMS)
Brief Memory and Executive Test (BMET)
Bowles-Langley Technology/Ashford Memory Test
Cambridge Cognitive Examination-Revised (CAMCOG-R)
Clock Drawing Test (CDT)
Cognitive Abilities Screening Instrument (CASI)
Cognitive Assessment Screening Test (CAST)
Cognistat (also known as the Neurobehavioral Cognitive Status Examination or NCSE)
Cognitive Capacity Screening Examination (CCSE)
Cognitive Disorders Examination (Codex)
Cognitive Failures Questionnaire (CFQ)
Cognitive Performance Scale (CPS)
Cognitive Screening Battery for Dementia in the Elderly
Community Screening Interview for Dementia (CSI'D')
Computer-Administered Neuropsychological Screen for Mild Cognitive Impairment (CANS-MCI)
Continuous Recognition Test
Dementia Questionnaire (DQ)
DemTect
Double Memory Test
Eurotest
Fototest
Free and Cued Selective Reminding Test/Five Words Test
Fuld Object Memory Evaluation
Galveston Orientation and Amnesia Test (GOAT)
General Practitioner Assessment of Cognition (GPCOG)
Geriatric Evaluation of Mental Status (GEMS)
Hasegawa Dementia Scale-Revised (HDS-R)
High Sensitivity Cognitive Screen (HSCS)
Hopkins Verbal Learning Test (HVLT)
Imon Cognitive Impairment Screening Test (ICIS)
Isaacs' Set Test of Verbal Fluency
Kingston Standardized Cognitive Assessment
Kokmen Short Test of Mental Status (STMS)
Mattis Dementia Rating Scale (DRS)

(continued)

Screening, Cognitive, Table 1 (continued)

Memory and Executive Screening (MES)
Memory Impairment Screen (MIS)
Memory Orientation Screening Test (MOST)
Mental Alteration Test (MAT)
Mental Status Questionnaire (MSQ)
Middlesex Elderly Assessment of Mental State (MEAMS)
Mini-Addenbrooke's Cognitive Examination (M-ACE)
Mini-Cog
Mini-Mental Status Examination (MMSE)
Mini-Severe Impairment Battery (Mini-SIB)
Modified Mini-Mental Status Examination (3MS)
Modified WORLD Test (WORLD)
Montpellier Screen (Mont)
Montreal Cognitive Assessment (MoCA)
Neurobehavioral Cognitive Status Examination (NCSE)
Philadelphia Brief Assessment of Cognition
Poppelreuter Overlapping Figure
Queen Square Screening Test for Cognitive Deficits
Quick Mild Cognitive Impairment Screen (Qmci)
Quick Test for Cognitive Speed (AQT)
Rapid Dementia Screening Test (RDST)
Repeatable Battery for the Assessment of Neuropsychological Status (RBANS)
Revised Mattis Dementia Rating Scale (DRS-2)
Rowland Universal Dementia Assessment Scale (RUDAS)
Saint Louis University Mental Status Examination (SLUMS)
Severe Impairment Battery (SIB)
Seven-Minute Screen (7MS)
Severe MMSE
Short and Sweet Screening Instrument (SASSI)
Short Blessed Test (SBT)
Short Cognitive Battery (B2C)
Short Cognitive Evaluation Battery (SCEB)
Short Memory Questionnaire (SMQ)
Short Portable Mental Status Questionnaire (SPMSQ)
Short Test of Mental Status (STMS)
Six-item Cognitive Impairment Test (6CIT)
Six-Item Screener (SIS)
Sweet 16
Takeda Three Colors Combination Test
TE4D-Cog
Test for the Early Detection of Dementia from Depression (TE4D-Cog)
Test Your Memory Test (TYM)
Three Word Recall (3WR)
Time and Change Test (T&C)
Trail Making Test (TMT)
(continued)

Screening, Cognitive, Table 1 (continued)

Tree Drawing Test (TDT; Koch's Baum Test)
Verbal Fluency Categories (VFC)
Verbal Fluency Animals (VFA)
Visual Association Test
Cognitive screening tests for specialized patient populations
High Sensitivity Cognitive Screen
HIV Dementia Scale
Immediate Post-Concussion Assessment and Cognitive Testing (ImPACT)
Mini-Mental Parkinson (MMP)
Informant- or proxy-rated screening instruments
The Alzheimer Disease 8 (AD8)
Blessed Dementia Rating Scale (BDRS)
Deterioration Cognitive Observee (DECO)
Informant Questionnaire for Cognitive Decline in the Elderly (IQCODE)
Quick Dementia Rating Scale (QDRS)
Telephone and mail screening instruments
Dementia Questionnaire
Five-Minute Telephone Version of the Short Blessed Test (SBT)
Minnesota Cognitive Acuity Screen
Structured Telephone Interview for Dementia Assessment (STIDA)
Telephone Interview for Cognitive Status (TICS)
Telephone MMSE (TMMSE)

cognitive screening test designed to assess changes in cognition in Parkinson patients (MMP), two cognitive screening tests designed to detect the early signs of AIDS-related dementia in AIDS patients (the High Sensitivity Cognitive Screen test and the HIV Dementia Scale), and a recently developed test to screen for post-concussion cognitive changes, the Immediate Post-Concussion Assessment and Cognitive Testing (ImPACT).

With the aging of the population have come an increased interest in cognitive screening in geriatric populations and the increased need to identify early signs of dementia and early signs of mild cognitive impairment, especially as new treatments are developed that are capable of modifying the progression of dementias. In primary care medicine, the standard of practice in the very near future may well include cognitive screening of all patients over the age of 75 in addition to screening of all younger patients when there is a reason to suspect cognitive impairment.

Cross-References

▶ Neuropsychology

References and Further Reading

Cullen, B., O'Neill, B., Evans, J. J., Coen, R. F., & Lawlor, B. A. (2007). A review of screening tests for cognitive impairment. *Journal of Neurology, Neurosurgery, and Psychiatry, 78*, 790–799.

Demakis, G. J., Mercury, M. G., & Sweet, J. J. (2000). Screening for cognitive impairments in primary care settings. In M. E. Maruish (Ed.), *Handbook of psychological assessment in primary care settings* (pp. 555–582). London: Lawrence Erlbaum.

Larner, A. (Ed.). (2017). *Cognitive screening instruments: A practical approach.* New York: Springer.

Lonie, J. A., Tierney, K. M., & Ebmeier, K. P. (2009). Screening for mild cognitive impairment: A systematic review. *International Journal of Geriatric Psychiatry, 24*, 902–915.

Malloy, P. F., Cummings, J. L., Coffey, C. E., Duffy, J., Fink, M., Lauterbach, E. C., et al. (1997). Cognitive screening instruments in neuropsychiatry: A report of the Committee on Research of the American Neuropsychiatric Association. *Journal of Neuropsychiatry and Clinical Neurosciences, 9*, 189–197.

Mitchell, A. J., & Malladi, S. (2010). Screening and case finding tools for the detection of dementia. Part I: Evidence-based meta-analysis of multidomain tests. *American Journal of Geriatric Psychiatry, 18*, 759–782.

Mitrushina, M. (2009). Cognitive screening methods. In I. Grant & K. M. Adams (Eds.), *Neuropsychological assessment of neuropsychiatric and neuromedical disorders* (pp. 101–126). New York: Oxford University Press.

Tombaugh, T. N., & McIntyre, N. J. (1992). The mini-mental state examination: A comprehensive review. *Journal of the American Geriatrics Society, 40*, 922–935.

Seasonal Affective Disorder

Kathryn A. Roecklein and Patricia M. Wong
Department of Psychology, University of Pittsburgh, Pittsburgh, PA, USA

Synonyms

Bipolar disorder, with seasonal pattern; Major depressive disorder, with seasonal pattern

Definition

The most common presentation of seasonal affective disorder (SAD) is recurrent depressive episodes in winter followed by spring remission (Rosenthal et al. 1984). SAD is diagnosed according to the American Psychiatric Association not as a separate disorder, but rather as a course specifier to describe the pattern of depressive episodes in patients meeting criteria for major depressive disorder, or bipolar I or II disorder (American Psychiatric Association [DSM-IV-TR] 2000). Criteria for the seasonal specifier include (1) recurrence of major depressive episodes at a specific time of year; (2) full remission (or change to mania/hypomania) from depression also recurring at a specific time of year; (3) at least two major depressive episodes meeting criteria 1 and 2 within the last 2 years, with no occurrence of nonseasonal depression within the same period; and (4) experiencing a greater number of major depressive episodes meeting SAD criteria than that of nonseasonal depression throughout the individual's lifetime (American Psychiatric Association [DSM-IV-TR] 2000).

Description

Epidemiology. SAD is characterized by depressed mood, anhedonia, and fatigue, as well as higher rates of appetite increase, weight gain, and hypersomnia compared to nonseasonal major depression (Magnusson and Partonen 2005). Ten to twenty percent of patients with depression seeking outpatient treatment have a seasonal pattern of recurrences, and SAD accounts for 10–22% of all unipolar and bipolar mood disorders (Roecklein et al. 2010). A notable characteristic of sleep in SAD is that, in contrast with the predominance of insomnia in nonseasonal depression, a majority of individuals with SAD experience hypersomnia (68–80%; e.g., Rosenthal et al. 1985). Given that seasonality, the tendency to vary in mood and behavior across the seasons (Kasper et al. 1989; Rosen et al. 1990), is normally distributed, a range of mild to severe seasonal changes are likely to occur in behavioral medicine research and practice.

Etiology. Etiological models propose that seasonal changes in the environment, being light levels or other conditioned cues, trigger onset in fall or winter (Rohan et al. 2009; Sohn and Lam 2005). Lewy et al. (1987) proposed that winter changes in day length lead to a delay in internal circadian rhythms relative to clock time or other rhythms like sleep and wake. Wehr et al. (2001) proposed that winter changes in day length are encoded by nocturnal melatonin release duration as a "circadian signal of change of season," leading to behavioral and physiological changes in humans similar to those of seasonally breeding mammals. Transforming environmental light levels to neural signals is mediated by a retinal pathway to the central clock, and this pathway could be differentially sensitive across individuals, leading some to be vulnerable to insufficient input in winter (Hebert et al. 2002). These circadian and retinal hypotheses may interact with one another, as well as with the monoamine hypothesis (i.e., serotonin and dopamine) and cognitive behavioral mechanisms (Rohan et al. 2009).

Treatment. The recommended first-line treatment for SAD is light therapy, while antidepressants are also commonly used (Lam and Levitt 1999). Light therapy typically requires daily exposure to 10,000-lux of white or full-spectrum fluorescent light for at least 30 min, although efforts to refine the wavelength and reduce duration are being tested clinically. Among antidepressants, Bupropion XL is the first FDA-approved drug for the treatment of winter depression. A double-blind, placebo-controlled, multisite trial testing Bupropion XL on adults with a history of SAD demonstrated that the overall proportion of depression recurrences following treatment was lower for those taking Bupropion (16%) than for those using a placebo (28%; Modell et al. 2005), although the low rate of recurrence indicates a significant placebo response. In addition, cognitive behavioral therapy is as effective as light therapy for acute treatment during a depressive episode, and has prophylactic effects 1 year later in reducing the risk of a subsequent episode (Rohan et al. 2004). Given that multiple empirically validated treatments are available, detecting seasonal patterns in clinical settings can improve patient outcomes.

Implications for behavioral medicine. Seasonal variations in mood and behavior are relevant to Behavioral Medicine research and clinical practice. Such implications can be divided into specific biopsychosocial components including biological characteristics (e.g., genetic risk for seasonality, neurotransmitter and neurohormonal seasonal fluctuations), behaviors (e.g., seasonal changes in physical activity, sleep, substance use, and eating behavior), and social factors (e.g., seasonal changes in social activity rhythms). Candidate behavioral mechanisms in SAD include behavioral disengagement (i.e., lack of response-contingent positive reinforcement) as well as emotional and psychophysiological reactivity to light and seasonal visual stimuli. Several biological mechanisms in SAD have also been proposed (Rohan et al. 2009). The circadian phase shift hypothesis suggests that in the fall and winter months, the timing of different circadian rhythms (e.g., melatonin release, sleep-wake cycle) is out of phase, or desynchronized from other rhythms and/or environmental factors (e.g., dusk/dawn cycle). Another hypothesis is that individuals with SAD have retinas that are less sensitive to light; low environmental light levels in the winter then lead to subthreshold levels of light information transmitted to the brain. The photoperiodic hypothesis proposes that some individuals with SAD maintain biological mechanisms to track changes in photoperiod, a circadian signal of change between seasons, evidenced by individuals with SAD who demonstrate a longer duration of nocturnal melatonin release in the winter months. Rohan et al. (2009) proposed that behavioral and cognitive mechanisms contribute to a psychological vulnerability that, when integrated with biological vulnerabilities, may explain the onset, maintenance, or remission of SAD. Although these separate mechanisms have been shown to play a role in SAD, it is not yet clear if these factors are mechanistic in the cause or maintenance of the disease.

Cross-References

▶ Circadian Rhythm
▶ Depression: Symptoms
▶ Psychiatric Diagnosis
▶ Unipolar Depression

References and Further Readings

American Psychiatric Association. (2000). *Diagnostic and statistical manual of mental disorders* (4th). Washington, DC: Author.

Hebert, M., Dumont, M., & Lachapelle, P. (2002). Electrophysiological evidence suggesting a seasonal modulation of retinal sensitivity in subsyndromal winter depression. *Journal of Affective Disorders, 68*(2–3), 191–202.

Kasper, S., Wehr, T. A., Bartko, J. J., Gaist, P. A., & Rosenthal, N. E. (1989). Epidemiological findings of seasonal changes in mood and behavior. A telephone survey of Montgomery County, Maryland. *Archives of General Psychiatry, 46*(9), 823–833.

Lam, R. W., & Levitt, A. J. (Eds.). (1999). *Clinical guidelines for the treatment of seasonal affective disorder.* Vancouver: Clinical & Academic.

Lewy, A. J., Sack, R. L., Miller, L. S., & Hoban, T. M. (1987). Antidepressant and circadian phase-shifting effects of light. *Science, 235*(4786), 352–354.

Magnusson, A., & Partonen, T. (2005). The diagnosis, symptomatology, and epidemiology of seasonal affective disorder. *CNS Spectrums, 10*(8), 625–634.

Modell, J. G., Rosenthal, N. E., Harriett, A. E., Krishen, A., Asgharian, A., Foster, V. J., et al. (2005). Seasonal affective disorder and its prevention by anticipatory treatment with bupropion XL. *Biological Psychiatry, 58*(8), 658–667.

Roecklein, K. A., Rohan, K. J., & Postolache, T. T. (2010). SAD: Is seasonal affective disorder a bipolar variant? *Current Psychiatry, 9*(2), 42–54.

Rohan, K. J., Roecklein, K. A., & Haaga, D. A. F. (2009). Biological and psychological mechanisms of seasonal affective disorder: A review and integration. *Current Psychiatry Reviews, 5*(1), 37–47.

Rohan, K. J., Tierney Lindsey, K., Roecklein, K. A., & Lacy, T. J. (2004). Cognitive-behavioral therapy, light therapy, and their combination in treating seasonal affective disorder. *Journal of Affective Disorders, 80*, 273–283.

Rosen, L. N., Targum, S., Terman, M., Bryant, M., Hoffman, H., Kasper, S., et al. (1990). Prevalence of seasonal affective disorder at four latitudes. *Psychiatry Research, 31*(2), 131–144.

Rosenthal, N. E., Sack, D. A., Gillin, J. C., Lewy, A. J., Goodwin, F. K., & Davenport, Y. (1984). Seasonal affective disorder. A description of the syndrome and preliminary findings with light therapy. *Archives of General Psychiatry, 41*(1), 72–80.

Rosenthal, N. E., Sack, D., James, S., Parry, B., Mendelson, W., Tamarkin, L., et al. (1985). Seasonal affective disorder and phototherapy. *Annals of the New York Academy of Sciences, 453*, 260–269.

Sohn, C. H., & Lam, R. W. (2005). Update on the biology of seasonal affective disorder. *CNS Spectrums, 10*(8), 635–646.

Wehr, T. A., Duncan, W. C., Jr., Sher, L., Aeschbach, D., Schwartz, P. J., Turner, E. H., et al. (2001). A circadian signal of change of season in patients with seasonal affective disorder. *Archives of General Psychiatry, 58*(12), 1108–1114.

Secondary Care

▶ Clinical Settings

Secondary Gain

▶ Symptom Magnification Syndrome

Secondary Parkinsonism

▶ Parkinson's Disease: Psychosocial Aspects

Secondary Prevention Programs

▶ Cardiac Rehabilitation

Secondhand Smoke

Susan J. Bondy
Dalla Lana School of Public Health, University of Toronto, Toronto, ON, Canada

Synonyms

Environmental tobacco smoke; Involuntary exposure to tobacco smoke; Passive smoking

Definition

The exposure to, and effects of, inhalation of cigarette smoke by an individual other than the active smoker. The term is also applied, more specifically, to smoke exhaled by an active smoker that remains in the environment.

Description

Secondhand smoke includes sidestream smoke from the end of a lit cigarette and exhaled smoke (United States Department of Health and Human Services 2006, 2010; World Health Organization International Agency for Research on Cancer 2004). Harmful components identified specifically in cigarette smoke measured in the air include gases (e.g., carbon monoxide), droplets, and respirable particles which result from the release, combustion, and partial combustion of the tobacco leaves and cigarette paper, as well as flavorants, additives, and other chemicals introduced at agricultural, manufacturing, or packaging stages (California Environmental Protection Agency 2005a). Secondhand smoke, has been shown to contain elevated levels of a large number of known and probable human carcinogens as well as many other toxins with proven causal links to human health conditions (California Environmental Protection Agency 2005b; Institute of Medicine 2010; United States Department of Health and Human Services 2010; United States Environmental Protection Agency, Office of Research and Development, Office of Health and Environmental Assessment & U.S. EPA 1992; World Health Organization International Agency for Research on Cancer 2004). It has been estimated that, in 2004, one third of all children and nonsmoking adults worldwide were exposed to secondhand smoke, and that this avoidable exposure was responsible for over 600,000 premature deaths or 1% of all deaths (Oberg et al. 2010). As with active smoking, there is no confirmed risk-free level of exposure to secondhand cigarette smoke (United States Department of Health and Human Services 2006, 2010).

Concentrations of secondhand smoke (and resulting levels of toxic exposure) vary widely and are influenced by: the number of cigarettes and rate of active smoking; the time elapsed since cigarettes were lit and extinguished; the volume of the affected air space; ventilation, air exchange rates, and direction of air flow; and the duration of exposure (California Environmental Protection Agency 2005a). Air concentrations in occupational and private settings, where smoking is permitted, often exceed occupational safety standards for specific agents, and biomarker levels in heavily exposed nonsmokers can overlap levels observed in active smokers (California Environmental Protection Agency 2005b; United States Department of Health and Human Services 2006). Exposure levels in outdoor settings can vary from negligible to concentrations similar to indoor levels if the passive smoker is exposed to the stream of smoke (Institute of Medicine 2010).

Measuring exposure for research, surveillance, and program evaluation may be achieved through air sampling or use of markers of human exposure in biological samples. Air monitoring assesses for concentrations for one or more specific component of tobacco smoke or respirable particulates of specific sizes (Institute of Medicine 2010; United States Department of Health and Human Services 2006). The most widely used biomarkers include exhaled carbon monoxide, and cotinine (a metabolite of nicotine) in saliva, urine, or blood samples. Other biomarkers used in research include, metabolites other than cotinine and concentrations of known carcinogens, as well as through use of other biological media (e.g., testing for accumulated cotinine and nicotine in hair samples from exposed individuals, even newborns as an indication of late prenatal exposure).

Over 40 years of evidence exists on the adverse health effects caused by passive smoke exposure. This evidence has been summarized in prominent reports by international health agencies including International Agency for Research on Cancer (IARC) (International Agency for Research on Cancer 2004, 2009), the Office of the United States Surgeon General (United States

Department of Health and Human Services 2006, 2010), and others (California Environmental Protection Agency 2005b; Institute of Medicine 2010). The major classes of health effects linked to passive smoking include cancers, respiratory disorders, cardiovascular diseases, reproductive effects, and adverse effects on pre-and postnatal growth and development.

Carcinogenic effects of passive smoking can be expected to be consistent with those for active smoking (International Agency for Research on Cancer 2004), and for both, the increased risk is dose-dependent. Secondhand smoke has a confirmed causal role in the development of lung cancer in exposed nonsmokers (California Environmental Protection Agency 2005b; International Agency for Research on Cancer 2004; United States Department of Health and Human Services 2006) and is suggested to increase the risks of nasal and nasopharyngeal cancers in adults (California Environmental Protection Agency 2005b; United States Department of Health and Human Services 2006). There is also evidence to suggest secondhand smoke increases the risk of all childhood cancers, studied collectively, as well as specific childhood cancers (California Environmental Protection Agency 2005b; United States Department of Health and Human Services 2006). For several cancers with definitive evidence linking them to active smoking (including various digestive, kidney, and bladder cancers), there is not sufficient quantitative data to show a causal association with secondhand smoke exposure in humans (International Agency for Research on Cancer 2009). The role of secondhand smoke in breast cancer remains more controversial with The California EPA (California Environmental Protection Agency 2005b) being the first health agency to draw the conclusion of a causal association, while other agencies have not concluded that there is a strong link between active or passive cigarette smoke exposure and breast cancer (International Agency for Research on Cancer 2009; United States Department of Health and Human Services 2010).

Conclusive evidence of noncancer respiratory effects of passive smoking include lower respiratory tract illness in children and adults, prevalence of asthma in children, and severity of asthma in children and adults (United States Department of Health and Human Services 2006). Secondhand smoke also causes recurrent otitis media and middle ear effusion in children (United States Department of Health and Human Services). Passive smoke exposure has also been found to cause adverse and lasting effects on lung function and lung development in children associated with prenatal passive smoking and secondhand exposure in childhood (United States Department of Health and Human Services). Secondhand smoke has been identified as a risk factor for sudden infant death syndrome, with sufficient evidence to suggest a causal association, and associated with a small reduction in birth weight when nonsmoking mothers are exposed while pregnant (United States Department of Health and Human Services).

In terms of cardiovascular diseases, secondhand smoke exposure is accepted as a cause of coronary heart disease morbidity and mortality in adult women and men as well as acute cardiac events (Institute of Medicine 2010; United States Department of Health and Human Services 2006). Even brief exposure to environmental cigarette smoke can lead to vascular function changes and arrhythmic effects associated with acute cardiovascular events in susceptible individuals (Institute of Medicine 2010; United States Department of Health and Human Services 2010).

The World Health Organization Framework Convention on Tobacco Control (FCTC) requires that all signatory nations adopt and enforce measures to protect their populations from exposure to tobacco smoke (World Health Organization 2003, 2011). Protecting the population from secondhand smoke is identified as a key, evidence-based, measure to reduce death, disease, and disability caused by tobacco (World Health Organization 2003). FCTC guidelines (and others International Agency for Research on Cancer 2009; United States Department of Health and Human Services 2006, 2010) recommend that this be achieved through making all environments 100% smoke free as opposed to reliance on ventilation or creation of designated smoking spaces, which have proven ineffective. Legislation and other measures should apply equally to outdoor spaces wherever there is evidence of exposure (United States Department of Health and Human Services 2006, 2010; World Health Organization 2011).

A number of educational, legislative, occupational, and clinical interventions to eliminate exposure to tobacco smoke have been implemented and evaluated. Evidence from several countries has shown that legislated bans in a variety of settings including workplaces, bars, and restaurants have been effective in terms of: achievement of compliance, improved air quality, reduced human biomarker levels of exposure, and a corollary effect of reducing smoking prevalence among individuals exposed to the restrictions (Institute of Medicine 2010; International Agency for Research on Cancer 2009; United States Department of Health and Human Services 2006). There is also growing evidence that event rates for acute cardiac events have been reduced successfully by legislative and other interventions to eliminate smoking in workplaces and other settings and reduce secondhand smoke exposure (Institute of Medicine 2010; United States Department of Health and Human Services 2010).

Cross-References

▶ Cancer and Smoking
▶ Heart Disease and Smoking
▶ Institute of Medicine
▶ Smoking and Health
▶ Smoking Behavior
▶ Smoking Cessation
▶ Tobacco Control
▶ Tobacco Use
▶ World Health Organization (WHO)

References and Readings

California Environmental Protection Agency. (2005a). *Proposed identification of environmental tobacco smoke as a toxic air contaminant. Part A: Exposure assessment*. Sacramento: California Environmental Protection Agency, Office of Environmental Health Hazard Assessment.

California Environmental Protection Agency. (2005b). *Proposed identification of environmental tobacco smoke as a toxic air contaminant. Part B: Health effects*. Sacramento: California Environmental Protection Agency, Office of Environmental Health Hazard Assessment.

Institute of Medicine. (2010). *Secondhand smoke exposure and cardiovascular effects: Making sense of the evidence*. Washington, DC: Committee on Secondhand Smoke Exposure and Acute Coronary Events, Board on Population Health and Public Health Practice, Institute of Medicine of the National Academies.

International Agency for Research on Cancer. (2004). *IARC monographs on the evaluation of carcinogenic risks to humans* (volume 83: Tobacco smoke and involuntary smoking). Lyon: International Agency for Research on Cancer.

International Agency for Research on Cancer. (2009). *IARC handbook of cancer prevention. volume 13: Evaluating the effectiveness of smoke-free policies*. Lyon: International Agency for Research on Cancer, World Health Organization.

Oberg, M., Jaakkola, M. S., Woodward, A., Peruga, A., & Pruss-Ustun, A. (2010). Worldwide burden of disease from exposure to second-hand smoke: A retrospective analysis of data from 192 countries. *Lancet, 377*(9760), 139–146.

United States Department of Health and Human Services. (2006). *The health consequences of involuntary exposure to tobacco smoke: A report of the Surgeon General*. Rockville: United States Department of Health and Human Services, Public Health Service, Office of the Surgeon General.

United States Department of Health and Human Services. (2010). *How tobacco smoke causes disease: The biology and behavioral basis for smoking-attributable diseases. A report of the Surgeon General*. Rockville: United States Department of Health and Human Services, Public Health Service, Office of the Surgeon General.

United States Environmental Protection Agency, Office of Research and Development, Office of Health and Environmental Assessment & U.S. EPA. (1992). *Respiratory health effects of passive smoking (also known as exposure to secondhand smoke or environmental tobacco smoke ETS)*. EPA/600/6-90/006F. Washington, DC: United States Environmental Protection Agency (US EPA).

World Health Organization. (2003). *WHO framework convention on tobacco control*. Geneva: Author.

World Health Organization. (2011). *WHO framework convention on tobacco control: Guidelines for implementation Article 5.3; Article 8; Articles 9 and 10; Article 11; Article 12; Article 13; Article 14–2011 edition*. Geneva: Author.

World Health Organization International Agency for Research on Cancer. (2004). *IARC monographs on the evaluation of carcinogenic risks to humans. volume 83: Tobacco smoke and involuntary smoking*. Lyon: International Agency for Research on Cancer.

Sedentary Activity

▶ Lifestyle, Sedentary

Sedentary Behavior

▶ Screen Time

Sedentary Behaviors

Yori Gidron
SCALab, Lille 3 University and Siric Oncollile, Lille, France

Synonyms

Physical inactivity

Definition

Sedentary behaviors are an increasingly common problem worldwide, with important health consequences. These behaviors include long durations of sitting in front of the TV or the computer, playing computer or TV games, and a general lack of peripheral limb movements. These behaviors have risen due to a multitude of reasons including technological advancements, greater dependence on transportation, urbanization and hence smaller distances to work or schools spent walking, the omnipresence of TV and computers, and our dependence on such means for information, work, leisure, and communication. Various measures and scales exist to assess sedentary behaviors, and these depend on the type of behaviors assessed, the time frame the questions refer to (days, weeks, etc.), and the response format (e.g., a Likert scale or hours). This variability in assessment and use of different cutoffs could of course impact on the prevalence of sedentary behaviors identified in various samples. The prevalence of sedentary behaviors was found to be 58% in a nationally representative sample of Americans aged between 20 and 59 years. When looking just at sitting, one in four Americans spends 70% of their waking time sitting. Furthermore, people in developed countries may spend 4 h a day watching TV and 1 h a day in their vehicle. Importantly, the metabolic and health consequences of sedentary behaviors are distinct from the effects of lack of physical exercise (Owen et al. 2010). In a 21-year follow-up study, the number of hours riding in a car, alone or in combination with hours in front of a TV, significantly predicted cardiovascular disease mortality, independent of confounders (Warren et al. 2010). In contrast, taking daily breaks from sedentary behaviors is related to reduced waist circumference and to improved metabolic outcomes, independent of total amount of sedentary behaviors and of physical exercise (Healy et al. 2008). Mental health problems such as anxiety and depression are also associated with more sedentary behaviors, independent of general physical activity level (de Wit et al. 2011). Finally, an important study examined prospectively over 25 years the relationship between sedentary behavior (TV viewing >3 h/day) and long-term cognitive functions using various measures of processing speed and executive functioning. Indeed, sedentary behavior significantly predicted longer processing speed and poorer executing functioning (inhibition), independent of multiple confounders such as education, age, sex, and hypertension (Hoang et al. 2016). Thus, sedentary behaviors are an important topic for research and intervention in behavior medicine.

Cross-References

▶ Cardiovascular Risk Factors
▶ Lifestyle, Sedentary
▶ Obesity: Causes and Consequences
▶ Physical Activity and Health

References and Further Readings

de Wit, L., van Straten, A., Lamers, F., Cuijpers, P., & Penninx, B. (2011). Are sedentary television watching and computer use behaviors associated with anxiety and depressive disorders? *Psychiatry Research, 186,* 239–243.

Healy, G. N., Dunstan, D. W., Salmon, J., Cerin, E., Shaw, J. E., Zimmet, P. Z., et al. (2008). Breaks in sedentary time: Beneficial associations with metabolic risk. *Diabetes Care, 31,* 661–666.

Hoang, T. D., Reis, J., Zhu, N., Jacobs, D. R., Jr., Launer, L. J., Whitmer, R. A., Sidney, S., & Yaffe, K. (2016). Effect of early adult patterns of physical activity and television viewing on midlife cognitive function. *Journal of the American Medical Association – Psychiatry, 73,* 73–79.

Owen, N., Healy, G. N., Matthews, C. E., & Dunstan, D. W. (2010). Too much sitting: The population health science of sedentary behavior. *Exercise and Sport Sciences Reviews, 38,* 105–113.

Warren, T. Y., Barry, V., Hooker, S. P., Sui, X., Church, T. S., & Blair, S. N. (2010). Sedentary behaviors increase risk of cardiovascular disease mortality in men. *Medicine and Science in Sports and Exercise, 42,* 879–885.

Sedentary Time

Ciara M. O'Brien[1], Joan L. Duda[1], George D. Kitas[2] and Sally A. M. Fenton[1]
[1]School of Sport, Exercise and Rehabilitation Sciences, University of Birmingham, Birmingham, UK
[2]Russells Hall Hospital, The Dudley Group NHS Foundation Trust, Dudley, UK

Definition

Sedentary Time (vs. Sedentary Behavior)

Sedentary behavior has been defined as "any waking behavior characterized by an energy expenditure ≤ 1.5 metabolic equivalents (METs), while in a sitting, reclining or lying posture" (Tremblay et al. 2017). Common sedentary behaviors include watching television, reading a book, working at a computer, and driving motorized transport.

Sedentary time refers to the sum of all sedentary behaviors that are undertaken throughout the course of a day. For example, time spent traveling to work by car, sitting working at an office desk, and watching television during leisure time all represent different sedentary behaviors but accumulate to contribute toward "total sedentary time." However, within the field of sedentary behavior research, the terms sedentary time and sedentary behavior are often used interchangeably, and incorrectly.

Description

Measurement of Sedentary Time

Methods employed to assess sedentary time include both self-report measures and objective devices. Until recently, self-report measures were more frequently used in large-scale studies or epidemiological research due to their ease of application and relatively low-cost. Examples include diaries and questionnaires, such as the Bouchard Physical Activity Record and the International Physical Activity Questionnaire, respectively. However, the validity of the data collected using these measures is somewhat limited, due to social desirability bias and errors in participant recall. Moreover, most self-report measures largely focus on assessing specific sedentary behaviors (e.g., screen-based behaviors such as television viewing) rather than overall time spent sedentary.

Objective devices, such as accelerometers and posture sensors, are being more readily employed for the measurement of sedentary time due to their superior validity and reliability relative to self-report measures. Accelerometers (e.g., the ActiGraph) assess sedentary time on the basis of accelerations recorded over prespecified time periods (epochs). These accelerations are subsequently converted to accelerometer "counts," which are interpreted against validated "count thresholds" or "cut points," to determine the frequency and duration of sedentary time. Numerous cut points have been developed for this purpose, for example, Troiano et al. (2008) defines adults' sedentary time as ≤ 99 counts per minute (cpm), and Freedson et al. (2005) have proposed cut points of ≤ 149 cpm to classify sedentary time in children. Such cut points have been derived by establishing the upper limit of accelerometer counts recorded while undertaking activities requiring ≤ 1.5 METs (measured with indirect calorimetry). Consequently, accelerometers enable measurement of sedentary time on the basis of energy expenditure, but they typically do not afford the ability to determine the posture at which the behavior was undertaken. This may lead to misclassification of low energy, non-sitting behaviors (e.g., standing) as contributors toward sedentary time. Similarly, posture sensors (e.g., the activPAL) are not able to quantify the energy cost of sitting/lying behaviors they measure and therefore may misclassify seated active behaviors (e.g., cycling) as sedentary time. Bearing these limitations in mind, devices that have the ability to combine both accelerometry and posture classification should provide the most comprehensive and accurate assessment of sedentary time.

Sedentary Time and Health

The problem of sedentariness is receiving increased attention due to the high prevalence of this behavior among youth, adults, and older adults, coupled with growing evidence for the role of sedentary time in the development of poor health (Biswas et al. 2015; Hoare et al. 2016). For example, epidemiological research indicates that adolescents accumulate 6 h/day of accelerometer-assessed sedentary time, and sedentary time estimates increase with age (Collings et al. 2014). For adults, the National Health and Nutrition Examination Survey (Healy et al. 2011) indicated that sedentary time represents around 50–60% of waking hours when measured with accelerometry. Still, older adults represent the most sedentary age group, with sedentary time estimates of almost 10 h per day (Harvey et al. 2015).

The adverse health consequences of high sedentary time include increased risk of developing cardiovascular disease, type 2 diabetes, metabolic syndrome, and compromised mental health (Biswas et al. 2015; Hoare et al. 2016). Furthermore, a review of recent epidemiological studies indicated a probable causal positive association between sedentary time and all-cause mortality (Biddle et al. 2016). Importantly, the deleterious health consequences of sedentary time are observed to be independent of participation in moderate-vigorous physical activity (i.e., activity ≥ 3 METs).

Still, despite growing evidence for negative health consequences of sedentary time, studies are yet to determine exactly "how much" sedentary time is bad for us. As a result, current guidelines can only recommend reducing overall sedentary time. Research examining the dose-response association between sedentary time and poor health is therefore necessary to refine sedentary time guidelines.

Cross-References

▶ Cardiovascular Risk Factors
▶ Lifestyle, Sedentary
▶ Sedentary Behaviors
▶ Type 2 Diabetes

References and Further Reading

Biddle, S. J., Bennie, J. A., Bauman, A. E., Chau, J. Y., Dunstan, D., Owen, N., et al. (2016). Too much sitting and all-cause mortality: Is there a causal link? *BMC Public Health, 16*, 635.

Biswas, A., Oh, P. I., Faulkner, G. E., Bajaj, R. R., Silver, M. A., Mitchell, M. S., et al. (2015). Sedentary time and its association with risk for disease incidence, mortality, and hospitalization in adults: A systematic review and meta-analysis. *Annals of Internal Medicine, 162*(2), 123–132.

Collings, P. J., Wijndaele, K., Corder, K., Westgate, K., Ridgway, C. L., Dunn, V., et al. (2014). Levels and patterns of objectively-measured physical activity volume and intensity distribution in UK adolescents: The ROOTS study. *International Journal of Behavioral Nutrition and Physical Activity, 11*(23), 1–12.

Freedson, P. S., Pober, D., & Janz, K. F. (2005). Calibration of accelerometer output for children. *Medicine and Science in Sports and Exercise, 37*(11 Suppl), S523–S530.

Harvey, J. A., Chastin, S. F., & Skelton, D. A. (2015). How sedentary are older people? A systematic review of the amount of sedentary behaviour. *Journal of Aging and Physical Activity, 23*(3), 471–487.

Healy, G. N., Matthews, C. E., Dunstan, D. W., Winkler, E. A., & Owen, N. (2011). Sedentary time and cardiometabolic biomarkers in US adults: NHANES 2003-06. *European Heart Journal, 32*(5), 590–597.

Hoare, E., Milton, K., Foster, C., & Allender, S. (2016). The associations between sedentary behaviour and mental health among adolescents: A systematic review. *International Journal of Behavioral Nutrition and Physical Activity, 13*(1), 108.

Tremblay, M. S., Aubert, S., Barnes, J. D., Saunders, T. J., Carson, V., Latimer-Cheung, A. E., et al. (2017). Sedentary behaviour research network (SBRN) – Terminology consensus project process and outcome. *International Journal of Behavioral Nutrition and Physical Activity, 14*(75), 1–17.

Troiano, R. P., Berrigan, D., Dodd, K. W., Mâsse, L. C., Tilert, T., & McDowell, M. (2008). Physical activity in the United States measured by accelerometer. *Medicine and Science in Sports and Exercise, 40*(1), 181–188.

Seek Feedback

▶ Self-Monitoring

Selection Bias

▶ Bias

Selective Serotonin Reuptake Inhibitors (SSRIs)

Michael Kotlyar[1] and John P. Vuchetich[2]
[1]Department of Experimental and Clinical Pharmacology, College of Pharmacy, University of Minnesota, Minneapolis, MN, USA
[2]Department of Psychiatry, University of Minnesota School of Medicine, Minneapolis, MN, USA

Synonyms

Celexa®; Citalopram; Escitalopram; Fluoxetine; Fluvoxamine; Lexapro®; Luvox®; Paroxetine; Paxil®; Prozac®; Sertraline; Zoloft®

Definition

The SSRIs are a family of medications that act primarily (but not exclusively) by inhibiting serotonin reuptake pumps (Finley 2009; Sussman 2009). These medications are used to treat a variety of psychiatric disorders including depression, generalized anxiety disorder, obsessive-compulsive disorder (OCD), panic disorder, premenstrual dysphoric disorder, bulimia nervosa, social phobia, and posttraumatic stress disorder (Sussman). Clinicians should consult the product labeling for each individual medication to determine the indications that each drug is currently approved to treat, since not all of the SSRIs are indicated in the treatment of all of these disorders (although in some cases there is data in the literature suggesting efficacy for a given agent for the treatment of conditions for which it does not have an indication). In the treatment of most types of depression, the SSRIs have similar efficacy to older classes of medications such as the tricyclic antidepressants. However better tolerability at therapeutic doses and lower toxicity in overdose has led to an increased use of SSRIs and decreased use of these older agents over the past several decades (American Psychiatric Association [APA] 2010; Baldessarini 2006; Finley 2009). As with all antidepressants, full therapeutic effects are not observed for as long as 8 weeks in the treatment of depression or longer in the treatment of other disorders (such as OCD), however some symptoms may start to improve sooner (APA 2010; Finley 2009; Kirkwood et al. 2008). In the treatment of depression, all of the SSRIs are thought to be approximately equally effective and therefore initial choice of therapy is often based on factors such as patient preference, prior response to the medication, cost, side effect profile of the individual agents, and the probability that a drug interaction will occur between the antidepressant being chosen and the other medications that the patient is on (APA 2010; Finley 2009). Although the mechanism of action of the SSRIs is similar, lack of efficacy following treatment with one of the drugs in this class does not necessarily predict lack of efficacy by another medication in this class (APA 2010).

There are currently six medications classified as SSRIs that are approved for marketing in the United States (i.e., fluoxetine, paroxetine, sertraline, citalopram, escitalopram, and fluvoxamine) (APA 2010). The SSRIs are similar in many respects; however, important differences between agents are present. Some of these differences are in the side effect profiles of the various drugs and in the likelihood of each drug contributing to a drug-drug interaction with other medications that a patient is taking.

All of the SSRIs have been commonly associated with side effects such as gastrointestinal complaints (e.g., nausea and diarrhea), disturbances in sleep and headache (APA 2010; Finley 2009). Although an individual patient could have any of the sides effects listed, fluoxetine is generally considered the most likely to cause insomnia while paroxetine is often considered to be the most sedating. In many patients, these side effects decrease after the first week of therapy. Additionally, all of the SSRIs have been associated with sexual dysfunction (in both men and women) with the most common symptom reported being delayed orgasm, although decreased interest in sex or erectile dysfunction can also occur (APA 2010; Finley 2009). Since many patients may not spontaneously report sexual side effects, clinicians should inform patients that these may occur and determine if these have been problematic. Serotonin syndrome which includes neurobehavioral (e.g., lethargy and mental status changes), autonomic (e.g., sweating, blood pressure, and heart rate changes), and neuromuscular (e.g., rigidity and tremor) signs and symptoms has been rarely reported with the use of an SSRI as mono-therapy (Chyka 2008). However, the risk of serotonin syndrome increases when SSRIs are used in combination with other serotonergic agents, particularly with monoamine oxidase inhibitors (MAOIs) (APA 2010; Chyka 2008). SSRIs have also been associated with increased bleeding risk, likely due to the presence of serotonin transporters on blood platelets (Sussman 2009). Other side effects such as increased sweating, osteoporosis, bruxism, akathisia, and hyponatremia have been reported occasionally as have a wide range of other side effects (APA 2010; Finley 2009). As with all antidepressants, the SSRIs carry a warning regarding increased suicidality, particularly in children, adolescents, and young adults (under age 24) during the initial stages of therapy (Sussman 2009).

Substantial differences between the SSRIs are present in the pharmacokinetic properties of the agents and in the likelihood that the drug can contribute to drug-drug interactions. For example, fluoxetine is notable for its long half-life (i.e., 4–6 days) and that of its active metabolite norfluoxetine (4–16 days) (Teter et al. 2008). A longer half-life means that any side effects will persist for a longer period of time after discontinuation of the medication. Discontinuation of SSRIs has been associated with withdrawal symptoms characterized by headache, anxiety, flu-like symptoms, and paresthesias (APA 2010). Therefore, it is advisable to taper the medication when possible. The likelihood of a withdrawal syndrome is less likely in SSRIs with longer half-lives (such as fluoxetine) since the decline in the concentration of medications occurs more gradually.

Many of the SSRIs have been found to interact with other medications, some of which may be commonly co-administered with the SSRIs. The cytochrome P450 (CYP450) superfamily of enzymes is responsible for the metabolism of a large number of medications. There are numerous specific isoenzymes within the CYP450 superfamily of enzymes and the degree to which each is affected by an individual SSRI varies considerably. For example, paroxetine and fluoxetine are both strong inhibitors of CYP2D6 (with fluoxetine being a moderate inhibitor of several other CYP450 isoenzymes) (APA 2010; Finley 2009). Since antidepressants are frequently co-administered with other medications, care should be taken to identify and manage any potential drug-drug interactions. It is important to consider the impact of drug interactions both when initiating an enzyme inhibitor (since concentrations of affected medications can increase) and when discontinuing an enzyme inhibitor (since concentrations of affected medication can decrease).

Cross-References

▶ Anxiety Disorder
▶ Depression: Symptoms

References and Readings

American Psychiatric Association. (2010). *Practice guideline for the treatment of patients with major depressive disorder* (3rd ed.). Washington, DC: Author. *The American Journal of Psychiatry, 167*(Suppl. 10), 1–124.

Baldessarini, R. J. (2006). Drug therapy of depression and anxiety disorders. In L. S. Goodman, A. Gilman, L. L. Brunton, J. S. Lazo, & K. L. Parker (Eds.), *Goodman & Gilman's the pharmacological basis of therapeutics* (11th ed.). New York: McGraw-Hill, Medical.

Chyka, P. A. (2008). Clinical toxicology. In J. T. DiPiro, R. L. Talbert, G. C. Yee, G. R. Matzke, B. G. Wells, & L. M. Posey (Eds.), *Pharmacotherapy: A pathophysiologic approach* (7th ed.). New York: McGraw-Hill Medical.

Finley, P. R. (2009). Mood disorders: Major depressive disorders. In M. A. Koda-Kimble, L. Y. Young, B. K. Alldredge, R. L. Corelli, B. J. Gugielmo, W. A. Kradjan, & B. R. Williams (Eds.), *Applied therapeutics: The clinical use of drugs* (9th ed.). Philadelphia: Wolters Kluwer Health/Lippincott Williams & Wilkins.

Kirkwood, C. K., Makela, E. H., & Wells, B. G. (2008). Anxiety disorders: Posttraumatic stress disorder and obsessive-compulsive disorder. In J. T. DiPiro, R. L. Talbert, G. C. Yee, G. R. Matzke, B. G. Wells, & L. M. Posey (Eds.), *Pharmacotherapy: A pathophysiologic approach* (7th ed.). New York: McGraw-Hill Medical.

Sussman, N. (2009). Selective serotonin reuptake inhibitors. In B. J. Sadock, V. A. Sadock, P. Ruiz, & H. I. Kaplan (Eds.), *Kaplan & Sadock's comprehensive textbook of psychiatry* (9th ed.). Philadelphia: Wolters Kluwer Health/Lippincott Williams & Wilkins.

Teter, C. J., Kando, J. C., Wells, B. G., & Hayes, P. E. (2008). Depressive disorders. In J. T. DiPiro, R. L. Talbert, G. C. Yee, G. R. Matzke, B. G. Wells, & L. M. Posey (Eds.), *Pharmacotherapy: A pathophysiologic approach* (7th ed.). New York: McGraw-Hill Medical.

Self, The

▶ Self-Identity

Self-Assessment

▶ Self-examination

Self-Attitude

▶ Self-Concept
▶ Self-image

Self-Blame

Stephanie Ann Hooker
Department of Psychology, University of Colorado Denver, Denver, CO, USA

Synonyms

Responsibility

Definition

Self-blame is the attribution that the consequences one experiences are a direct result of one's actions or character. In the context of behavioral medicine, this may be either beneficial or harmful depending on if it leads to positive behavior change or increased negative affectivity and lack of behavior change.

Description

Self-blame is indirectly related to perceived control, where individuals who self-blame more often also are more likely to believe they have greater control over their lives. Because enhancements in perceived self-control are adaptive to psychological well-being, one may assume that self-blame may also be adaptive. However, this is not always the case.

Janoff-Bulman (1979) proposed two types of self-blame: (1) an adaptive, control-oriented response where the focus is on the individual's behavior and (2) a maladaptive, esteem-oriented response where the focus is on the individual's character. Self-blame is adaptive when individuals recognize that they had some control over the situation but failed to act appropriately. Thus, these individuals can modify their behavior for future events. On the other hand, self-blame is maladaptive when individuals blame their character flaws for the outcome; this is referred to as characterological self-blame. These flaws are generally seen as stable, so these individuals make no efforts to change. This can lead to recurrence of the same problems and feelings of helplessness and depression.

Although Janoff-Bulman's (1979) theory of self-blame seems plausible, there is little support for these notions in the literature. Two studies did not support the theory that behavioral self-blame is adaptive in breast cancer patients; rather, behavioral self-blame was positively associated with symptoms of anxiety and depression (Bennett et al. 2005; Glinder and Compas 1999). Moreover, Bennett et al. found that both forms of self-blame were unrelated to perceptions of control, which directly contradicts the theory of self-blame.

However, one study of head and neck cancer patients supported Janoff-Bulman's (1979) theory. Low behavioral self-blame (smoking specific) was related to greater likelihood of continued smoking after the cancer diagnosis (Christensen et al. 1999). The relationship held for those patients with high and low perceived control over cancer recurrence, although those with low perceived control had almost a three times greater probability of continued smoking after a cancer diagnosis than those with higher perceived control over cancer recurrence. Furthermore, in this study, it appeared that specific behavior self-blame was more predictive of behavior than a general behavioral self-blame. The authors suggest this may be because of the patients' knowledge of how specific behaviors related to the likelihood of having cancer and that patients do not attribute their behavior in general as the cause of cancer. This study illustrates the importance of understanding how patients' attributions of self-blame, perceived control, and knowledge of their condition may interact in predicting behavior change following a cancer diagnosis.

In the literature self-blame may be used interchangeably with responsibility. However, there are important differences between self-blame and responsibility that should be recognized. Self-blame differs from responsibility in that self-blame suggests that one intentionally brings about negative consequences, whereas responsibility is related more to perceived control over the event (Voth and Sirois 2009). Indeed, Voth and Sirois demonstrated in their study of patients with inflammatory bowel disease that self-blame is related to poor psychological adjustment, whereas responsibility is related to better psychological adjustment. Self-blame was associated with increased use of avoidant coping strategies, whereas responsibility was associated with decreased use of avoidant coping strategies. Avoidant coping was related to poorer psychological adjustment.

Theories of self-blame in behavioral medicine suggest that self-blame has maladaptive and adaptive qualities. Self-blame can be adaptive when individuals recognize their past actions caused their negative consequences, and they also recognize that their behavior is modifiable. Thus, individuals can make positive behavior changes in these cases, which can improve health. However, self-blame is maladaptive when it is primarily characterological in nature. This may lead individuals to feel helpless and to have poorer psychological adjustment to disease. Thus, it is imperative for researchers to properly define the self-blame construct for their research in order to further understand self-blame's role in behavioral medicine.

References and Further Reading

Bennett, K. K., Compas, B. E., Beckjord, E., & Glinder, J. G. (2005). Self-blame and distress among women with newly diagnosed breast cancer. *Journal of Behavioral Medicine, 28*, 313–323.

Christensen, A. J., Moran, P. J., Ehlers, S. L., Raichle, K., Karnell, L., & Funk, G. (1999). Smoking and drinking behavior in patients with head and neck cancer: Effects of behavioral self-blame and perceived control. *Journal of Behavioral Medicine, 22*, 407–418.

Glinder, J. G., & Compas, B. E. (1999). Self-blame attributions in women with newly diagnosed breast cancer: A prospective study of psychological adjustment. *Health Psychology, 18*, 475–481.

Janoff-Bulman, R. (1979). Characterological versus behavioral self-blame: Inquiries into depression and rape. *Journal of Personality and Social Psychology, 37*, 1798–1809.

Voth, J., & Sirois, F. M. (2009). The role of self-blame and responsibility in adjustment to inflammatory bowel disease. *Rehabilitation Psychology, 54*, 99–108.

Self-Care

Linda C. Baumann[1] and Alyssa Ylinen[2]
[1]School of Nursing, University of Wisconsin-Madison, Madison, WI, USA
[2]Allina Health System, St. Paul, MN, USA

Synonyms

Self-management

Definition

Self-care as described by Orem (1995) is "action of persons who have developed or developing capabilities to use appropriate, reliable and valid measures to regulate their own functioning and development in stable or changing environments" (p. 43). Self-care is both caring "for" oneself and "by" oneself. Self-care promotes well-being and is a perceived condition of personal existence characterized by experiences of contentment, pleasure, and happiness. It is associated with health and with sufficiency of resources. This definition is consistent with Diener's (2009) concept of subjective well-being as an individual's global judgment of values and standards that are significant to life satisfaction.

A paradigm that is emerging in health-care delivery for people with chronic conditions is that they are their own principal caregivers; health-care professionals act as consultants and advisors in supporting them in self-care and self-management of their condition. This paradigm of collaborative care and self-management education involves shared decision making between providers and patients. Self-management education includes providing patients with information, problem-solving skills, and behavioral strategies to enhance their lives.

Diabetes is an excellent example of a health condition that requires self-management skills to maintain optimal control through healthy eating, being active, taking medications, monitoring, problem solving, reducing risks, and healthy coping. http://www.diabeteseducator.org/DiabetesEducation/Patient_Resources/AADE7_PatientHandouts.html Self-management education can occur in group settings where peers can provide emotional support and practical information for problem solving. In addition to knowledge and skills, self-care behaviors are determined by attitudes and beliefs, social and environmental influences, and self-efficacy expectations.

Description

Self-care is the thoughts and actions a person takes to achieve or maintain health and well-being.

Cross-References

▶ Self-Management

References and Further Readings

Bodenheimer, T., Lorig, K., Holman, H., & Grumbach, K. (2002). Patient self-management of chronic disease in primary care. *Journal of the American Medical Association, 288*, 2469–2475.

Diener, E. (2009). *The science of well-being*, (Social indicators book series, Vol. 37). New York: Springer.

Orem, D. E. (1995). *Nursing: Concepts and practice* (6th ed.). St. Louis: Mosby.

Self-Concept

Tara McMullen
Doctoral Program in Gerontology, University of Maryland Baltimore and Baltimore County, Baltimore, MD, USA

Synonyms

Self-attitude; Self-identity; Self-image

Definition

Self-concept can be defined as one's beliefs about oneself.

Description

Self-concept is a difficult yet important terms to define as self-concept attempts to explain human behavior (micro). Defining self-concept is difficult as a large number of terms use the term 'self' to define some sort of individualistic behavior (Burns 1980). However, in its simplest form, self-concept can be defined as one's beliefs about oneself. Carl Rogers (1951) suggested that oneself, or the "self," plays a role in the development of personality and behavior.

Self-concept can be seen as what an individual understands him or herself to be, cultivated by the appraisal of oneself (Epstein 1973). Self-concept is an organized system of learned beliefs, perceptions, and feelings that aid in the understanding of oneself. Simply, self-concept is the perception an individual has of one's personal characteristics, formed and shaped by society and attitudes. The understanding of oneself is established by one's character, personality, traits, and appearance. Self-concept is developed from an individual's "I," "me," and/or "mine" experience (Burns 1980).

As individuals age, their self-concept is organized and reorganized by their social and nonsocial experiences (Burns 1980). Characteristics in an individual's social environment structure understanding of who the individual is (Epstein 1973). The self-concept or the "who am I" assessed by the individual can be defined and then redefined as the individual encounters many life experiences. In this sense, self-concept can be designated as a multifaceted phenomenon that is dynamic and can change due to experiences, environments, and social affiliations (Markus and Wurf 1987). Thus, self-concept is not fixed and is based individual on the context or situation. Moreover, Burns (1980) suggests that individuals may have many overlapping self-concepts that have been shaped and developed by various beliefs, experiences, and events. Therefore, self-concept can be seen as a multifaceted and individualized process.

An individual can develop a positive or negative self-concept based entirely on the evaluations of oneself. Bailey (2003) states that self-concept is associated with individualistic qualities that can be assessed rather than measured. "Nonmeasurable" aspects to one's self can be seen as physical attributes, religious preferences, and/or personality traits (Bailey 2003). Thus, self-concept is a learned trait. Rogers (1951) suggests that the self, through self-concept, must be maintained in order to avoid anxiety and stress. This ability to maintain one's self-concept can be achieved through the maintenance of self-esteem (Rosenberg 1979). It has been suggested that self-concept consists of one's self-image and one's self-esteem (Burns 1980). Self-image can be defined as the perception individuals have of themselves physically, psychologically, philosophically, and politically, developed through the agency of their societal experiences and development (Fisher 1986; Statt 1990). Self-esteem is operationally defined as an individual's orientation toward oneself (Rosenberg 1965); self-worth, motivations, and perceptions encompass the conceptualization of an individual's understanding of who they are (Rosenberg 1965). Thus, the process in which individuals view themselves constructed by the perceptions they have of their self-worth aids in the development of self-concept.

Self-concept can be measured in children and adults by means of various psychometric scales such as the Tennessee Self Concept Scale (Fitts 1991) and the Piers-Harris Children's Self-Concept Scale (Piers 1984).

Cross-References

▶ Self-Blame
▶ Self-esteem
▶ Self-examination
▶ Self-Identity
▶ Self-image

References and Readings

Bailey, J. A. (2003). Self-image, self-concept, and self-identity revisited. *Journal of the National Medical Association, 95*, 383–386.
Burns, R. B. (1980). *Psychology for the health professions*. Lancaster: MTP Press.
Epstein, S. (1973). The self-concept revisited – Or a theory of a theory. *The American Psychologist, 28*, 404–416.
Fisher, S. (1986). *Development and structure of the body image* (Vol. 1). Hillsdale: Erlbaum.
Fitts, W. H. (1991). *Tennessee self-concept scale manual*. Los Angeles: Western Psychological Services.
Harriman, P. L. (1947). *The new dictionary of psychology*. New York: The Philosophical Library.
Markus, H., & Nurius, P. (1986). Possible selves. *The American Psychologist, 41*, 954–969.
Markus, H., & Wurf, E. (1987). The dynamic self-concept: A social psychological perspective. *Annual Review of Psychology, 38*, 299–337.
Piers, E. V. (1984). *Revised manual for the Piers-Harris children's self-concept scale*. Los Angeles: Western Psychological Services.
Piers, E. V. (1986). *The Piers-Harris children's self-concept scale, revised manual*. Los Angeles: Western Psychological Services.
Rogers, C. R. (1951). *Client-centered counselling*. Boston: Houghton-Mifflin.
Rosenberg, M. (1965). *Society and the adolescent self-image*. Princeton: Princeton University Press.
Rosenberg, M. (1979). *Conceiving the self*. New York: Basic Books.
Rosenberg, M. (1986). *Conceiving the self*. Malabar: Krieger.
Rosenberg, M. (1989). *Society and the adolescent self-image*. Middeltown: Wesleyan University Press.
Statt, D. (1990). *The concise dictionary of psychology*. New York: Routledge.

Self-Conception

▶ Self-image

Self-Consciousness

▶ Self-image

Self-Construal

▶ Self-Identity

Self-Control

▶ Behavioral Inhibition
▶ Self-Regulation Model

Self-Control Capacity

▶ Self-Regulatory Capacity

Self-Control Failure

▶ Self-Regulatory Fatigue

Self-Determination Theory

Lauren Law, Dawn Wilson and Hannah G. Lawman
Department of Psychology, University of South Carolina, Columbia, SC, USA

Synonyms

Cognitive evaluation theory

Definition

Self-determination theory is a theory of human motivation that describes two distinct types of motivation: autonomous (regulated through natural and internal processes such as inherent enjoyment or satisfaction) and controlled (regulated through externally held demands and social expectations). Autonomous motivation can be elicited and sustained through social–environmental factors including high autonomy, competence, and relatedness and may contribute to long-term maintenance of a behavior change.

Description

Self-determination theory (SDT) is a theory of human motivation that describes motivation in two distinct types: autonomous and controlled (Deci and Ryan 2008). Autonomous motivation, which includes intrinsic and well-internalized extrinsic motivation, is regulated through natural and internal processes such as inherent satisfaction and can be thought of as an individual's innate desire to engage in healthy behaviors independent of external influences. Autonomous motivation can be elicited and sustained through social contextual conditions including social support from significant others that facilitates intrinsic motivation (e.g., autonomy, competence, and relatedness) in contrast to conditions that undermine one's innate propensity for it such as authoritarian or highly controlled interpersonal interactions (Ryan and Deci 2000). An intrinsically motivated individual may engage in healthy eating because it aligns with his/her self-concept and is enjoyable. Controlled (extrinsic) motivation is regulated through externally held demands and expectations that are contingent on rewards or punishments. An extrinsically motivated individual may engage in healthy eating for approval from peers or to avoid health consequences rather than inherent enjoyment or self-satisfaction. While both types of motivation represent an individual's intention to act, health behavior outcomes resulting from autonomous versus controlled motivation may be qualitatively different. A growing evidence base shows that autonomous motivation may more likely contribute to the maintenance of health behaviors compared to controlled motivation (Ng et al. 2012).

SDT provides a framework for understanding motivational influences on health behaviors, such as healthy diet, physical activity, safe sex practices, and substance use. The conceptualization of motivation on a continuum allows for distinctions to be made in the type and quality of motivation that may contribute to different outcomes. SDT makes distinctions between autonomous and controlled motivation with autonomous motivation being more inherently enjoyable, long-lasting, and internally regulated, while controlled motivation consists of motivation that is primarily driven by externally held demands, social pressures, and reinforcers (Deci and Ryan 2008). For example, controlled motivation based on social pressures has been shown to be negatively related to fruit and vegetable intake compared to autonomous motivation which positively predicted this health behavior (McSpadden et al. 2016).

SDT originally conceptualized the motivation continuum as ranging from amotivation to extrinsic to intrinsic motivation. Amotivation is conceptualized as having no intention to act and has been associated with a lack of outcome value, as well as a lack of beliefs about the link between behavior and desired outcome, or competence in performing the behavior. On the one end of the continuum, motivation is hypothesized to be regulated extrinsically and controlled by rewards and punishments or other externally regulated processes. Extrinsic motivation may be broken down into subcategories based on increasing levels of intrinsic regulation: extrinsic, introjected (i.e., somewhat external regulation or internal rewards and/or punishments), and identified (somewhat internal regulation and holds personal importance; Deci and Ryan 1985; Ryan and Deci 2000). At the other end of the continuum, intrinsic motivation is regulated or controlled by an individual's inherent satisfaction, novelty, and drive. Previous research has supported beneficial effects of intrinsic motivation compared to extrinsic motivation in substance abuse treatment outcomes (Zeldman et al. 2004) and in predicting mental health and job outcomes in the workplace (Vansteenkiste et al. 2007). However, some researchers have combined extrinsic and introjected into controlled-type motivation and combined identified and intrinsic into autonomous-type motivation (Deci and Ryan 2008). This has resulted in a shift of the primary motivation differentiation moving toward autonomous and controlled in conceptualizing intrinsic and extrinsic in a more dynamic fashion.

SDT emphasizes the role of social context in understanding health behavior motivation and suggests its influence on behavior is through affecting social contextual conditions that may help to elicit and sustain intrinsic motivation. These conditions are described as psychological needs that are inherent to being human and consist of the needs for competence, autonomy, and relatedness. Social relationships (e.g., social support), environmental characteristics (e.g., built environment, resources), and cultural practices and norms (e.g., gender roles) can influence these psychological needs and in turn facilitate or undermine one's sense of intrinsic motivation for engaging in healthy behaviors (Deci and Ryan 1985, 2008; Ryan and Deci 2000). An intervention to increase physical activity, the Active by Choice Today trial, focused on increasing social support (relatedness), teaching behavioral skills (competence), and encouraging choice (autonomy) to provide conditions that facilitate the development of autonomous motivation to be physically active for a lifetime (Wilson et al. 2008). This trial showed a significant intervention effect on increasing accelerometry estimates of physical activity in youth during the afterschool program as compared to a general health education program (Wilson et al. 2011). Similarly, researchers and clinicians interested in reducing substance use have utilized autonomy-supportive strategies for resisting peer pressure (competence) for substance use while preserving positive peer relationships (relatedness) and increasing their choices for alternative activities (autonomy; Williams et al. 2000).

Application of SDT to interventions with other behavioral change theories, such as Social Cognitive Theory (SCT) or Family Systems Theory (FST), has also been implemented in recent trials. For example, the Families Improving Together for Weight Loss trial combined essential elements from SCT including self-monitoring and goal setting and FST including family communication skills and social support with SDT strategies that promoted parental autonomy-supportive communication to enhance motivation for health behavior change in overweight African American adolescents (Wilson et al. 2015). Integrating evidenced-based theoretical frameworks will allow researchers to design comprehensive interventions that are relevant and effective in improving long-term health behaviors.

There is growing evidence that interventions that address cognitive and social factors related to health behavior change may also have ripple effects, such as impacting additional physical, mental, and social health outcomes that were not the intended targeted outcomes (Wilson 2015). This suggests that these health behavior interventions may have far-reaching benefits and impact population health more broadly. Mata et al. (2009) found that increased motivation for exercise behavior also had positive effects on eating self-regulation in a weight control intervention, suggesting that utilizing SDT in health behavior interventions may support multiple health behavior change. Further, a recent meta-analysis of studies utilizing SDT in health interventions showed positive relationships between supportive health climates that emphasized autonomous motivation and mental and physical health, suggesting that positive health climate-based interventions may be a cost-effective strategy to improve a variety of health outcomes (Ng et al. 2012). In addition, a recent study found that applying SDT to financial incentives was a cost-effective strategy for increasing adherence to existing treatments (Kullgren et al. 2016). However, it is important to utilize theories of motivation, such as SDT, in behavioral economics studies to better understand which types of incentive structures may yield consistent positive changes across different settings (Haff et al. 2015).

In conclusion, SDT has been shown to be a promising theory for individual health behavior change that emphasizes the importance of a positive social context in fostering motivation over time and across health behaviors. Applications of SDT, especially when coupled with other evidenced-based theoretical frameworks of behavior change, show strong promise for future interventions that could be important for improving population level health outcomes.

Cross-References

▶ Health Behaviors
▶ Motivational Interviewing

References and Further Reading

Deci, E. L., & Ryan, R. M. (1985). *Intrinsic motivation and self-determination in human behavior*. New York: Plenum Press.

Deci, E. L., & Ryan, R. M. (2008). Facilitating optimal motivation and psychological well-being across life's domains. *Canadian Psychology, 49*(1), 14–23.

Haff, N., Patel, M. S., Lim, R., Zhu, J., Troxel, A. B., Asch, D. A., & Volpp, K. G. (2015). The role of behavioral economic incentive design and demographic characteristics in financial incentive-based approaches to changing health behaviors: A meta-analysis. *American Journal of Health Promotion, 29*(5), 314–323.

Kullgren, J. T., Williams, G. C., Resnicow, K., An, L. C., Rothberg, A., Volpp, K. G., & Heisler, M. (2016). The promise of tailoring incentives for healthy behaviors. *International Journal of Workplace Health Management, 9*(1), 2–16.

Mata, J., Silva, M. N., Vieira, P. N., Carraça, E. V., Andrade, A. M., Coutinho, S. R., . . ., & Teixeira, P. J. (2009). Motivational "spill-over" during weight control: Increased self-determination and exercise intrinsic motivation predict eating self-regulation. *Health Psychology, 28*(6), 709.

McSpadden, K. E., Patrick, H., Oh, A. Y., Yaroch, A. L., Dwyer, L. A., & Nebeling, L. C. (2016). The association between motivation and fruit and vegetable intake: The moderating role of social support. *Appetite, 96*, 87–94.

Ng, J. Y., Ntoumanis, N., Thøgersen-Ntoumani, C., Deci, E. L., Ryan, R. M., Duda, J. L., & Williams, G. C. (2012). Self-determination theory applied to health contexts a meta-analysis. *Perspectives on Psychological Science, 7*(4), 325–340.

Ryan, R. M., & Deci, E. L. (2000). Self-determination theory and the facilitation of intrinsic motivation, social development, and well-being. *American Psychologist, 55*(1), 68–78.

Vansteenkiste, M., Neyrinck, B., Niemiec, C. P., Soenens, B., Witte, H., & Broeck, A. (2007). On the relations among work value orientations, psychological need satisfaction and job outcomes: A self-determination theory approach. *Journal of Occupational and Organizational Psychology, 80*(2), 251–277.

Wilson, D. K. (2015). Behavior matters: The relevance, impact, and reach of behavioral medicine. *Annals of Behavioral Medicine, 49*(1), 40–48.

Williams, G. C., Cox, E. M., Hedberg, V. A., & Deci, E. L. (2000). Extrinsic life goals and health-risk behaviors in adolescents. *Journal of Applied Social Psychology, 30*(8), 1756-1771.

Wilson, D. K., Kitzman-Ulrich, H., Williams, J. E., Saunders, R., Griffin, S., Pate, R., et al. (2008). An overview of "The Active by Choice Today" (ACT) trial for increasing physical activity. *Contemporary Clinical Trials, 29*(1), 21–31.

Wilson, D. K., Van Horn, M. L., Kitzman-Ulrich, H., Saunders, R., Pate, R., Lawman, H. G. . . ., & Mansard, L. (2011). Results of the "Active by Choice Today" (ACT) randomized trial for increasing physical activity in low-income and minority adolescents. *Health Psychology, 30*(4), 463–471.

Wilson, D. K., Kitzman-Ulrich, H., Resnicow, K., Van Horn, M. L., George, S. M. S., Siceloff, E. R., . . ., & Coulon, S. (2015). An overview of the Families Improving Together (FIT) for weight loss randomized controlled trial in African American families. *Contemporary Clinical Trials, 42*, 145–157.

Zeldman, A., Ryan, R. M., & Fiscella, K. (2004). Motivation, autonomy support, and entity beliefs: Their role in methadone maintenance treatment. *Journal of Social and Clinical Psychology, 23*(5), 675–696.

Self-Directed Violence

▶ Suicide

Self-Efficacy

Jorie Butler
Department of Psychology, University of Utah, Salt Lake City, UT, USA

Definition

Self-efficacy: Self-efficacy is the belief in personal ability to successfully perform challenging life tasks. Self-efficacy plays an important role in a person's emotions, cognitions, motivational activities, and behaviors across a variety of activities.

Description

Self-efficacy is rooted within Social Cognitive Theory (Bandura 1986) in which people are characterized as active agents of control within their own lives – dynamically influencing their personal environments by organizing responses to opportunities, reflecting on past performances, and self-regulating behavior. Self-efficacy influences response organization, develops in part from reflection, and contributes to self-regulation, particularly, by fostering approach-oriented behavior and persistence in the face of obstacles. Attribution Theory (Weiner 1992), which includes the properties of locus, stability, controllability, also provides a framework for understanding self-efficacy. Locus reflects the cause of a situation as internal or external to a person. Stability reflects how changeable the situation is perceived to be. Controllability is an indicator of whether the person can willfully change a situation. A negative situation such as reaching an unhealthy weight could be interpreted as internal (*Being this heavy is my fault*), stable (*I've always been too heavy*), and uncontrollable (*It doesn't matter what I eat, I just get heavier*), resulting in poor self-efficacy for weight control in the future. In contrast, reaching an unhealthy weight could be interpreted as external (*Weight gain is common with age*), unstable (*This weight came on, it can come off!*), and controllable (*Now that I realize I'm eating too much and moving too little, I can change that behavior*), producing opportunities for improvements in future self-efficacy.

Social Learning Theory (Bandura 1977b) explains development of self-efficacy via four principle pathways: mastery experiences, modeling, social persuasion, and physiology. Past experiences are most predictive of future experiences. People engage in tasks and actions, interpret the outcome, and develop perceptions of their competence within the task domain. Mastery experiences result from multiple successes and promote self-efficacy. Failures are detrimental to developing self-efficacy, although the negative impact of failures is diminished when failures occur attempting a task that has been successfully completed on multiple occasions. The primacy of mastery experiences in self-efficacy development speaks to the titration between efficacy development and actual performance. Self-efficacy develops in domains in which skills are acquired often through the combination of effortful practice and natural talent. Self-efficacy development can be fostered by modeling, particularly when successful completion of activities is modeled by someone viewed as admirable and possessing desired capabilities of the observer. Conversely, a model who fails to perform a desired activity can weaken an observer's sense of competence for performing the activity. Social persuasions involve effective encouragement (not empty praise) that can be instrumental in fostering self-efficacy when the tasks are achievable or nearly achievable. Negative social persuasion deflates self-efficacy. Social persuasion is an important pathway by which parents, teachers, coaches, employment supervisors, and others can facilitate or damage developing self-efficacy. Physiological responses during task attempts influence self-efficacy development. Emotional states indicative of negative arousal such as stress and fear are indicators that the task is difficult and may indicate anticipated failure. In contrast, excitement, anticipation of fun, happiness, or a sense of work "flow" indicate positively developing efficacy. Individuals experiencing negative adjustment periods – such as depressive states or grief – will have difficulty developing self-efficacy. Self-efficacy can develop more freely when negative emotional states are resolved.

Self-efficacy influences behavior across many domains, including the choices of activities to become involved in effortful work to complete activities, persistence in the face of setbacks or failures, and resilience following adversity (Schunk and Pajares 2005). Individuals tend to avoid activities for which they anticipate poor performance and approach tasks for which they anticipate success. Thus, individuals with low self-efficacy in a given domain may avoid it all together, thus contributing to narrowing of life skills. High self-efficacy contributes to task engagement. High self-efficacy is also associated with effortful engagement in tasks – particularly when intrinsic motivation to engage in the task is also present. Persistence in the face of setbacks is more likely when individuals have high self-efficacy for the task. With the expectation for eventual failure (a component of low self-efficacy), persistence is unlikely. In addition, when failures or enduring obstacles are encountered, low self-efficacy may contribute to a sense of failure and withdrawal from the situation whereas high self-efficacy may contribute to resilience.

Self-efficacy is an integral component of a number of models designed to explain health behavior – primarily because self-efficacy contributes to the willingness to try to change undesirable health behavior, successful implementation of health behavior change, and persistently maintaining health behavior change over time. The Theory of Reasoned Action was extended to form the Theory of Planned Behavior. The extension incorporated self-efficacy as a key factor in changing health behavior along with personal attitudes toward change and the attitudes of significant others toward the change (Ajzen 1991). Self-efficacy was also incorporated into the Health Belief Model during the 1980s – reflecting understanding of the importance of the construct in promoting health (Rosenstock et al. 1988). The Health Behavior Change Model (Prochaska and Velicer 1997) incorporates self-efficacy as a contributor to stages of change. Self-efficacy can influence a person's thoughts about needing change (in the contemplation stage).

A person high in self-efficacy will anticipate success and may progress more quickly to the active preparation stage – involving active planning for change behaviors. In addition, self-efficacy will influence effective active change (action stage) as persons high in self-efficacy may more effectively respond to setbacks with persistence and resilience. This quality of those high in self-efficacy also contributes to effective sustainment of the changed behavior (maintenance stage).

Self-efficacy is generally best understood in specific domains and the concept is well supported across multiple domains including school performance, athletic achievement, occupational arenas, and in health behaviors including health maintenance (such as diet and exercise), recovery from acute events such as surgery, and coping with chronic illness or dangerous diagnoses. There is some evidence for a generalized self-efficacy as individuals expect better competence for activities when they have demonstrated aptitude in other activities in the past (Smith 1989). Self-efficacy contributes a theoretically grounded explanation for the myriad ways in which people shape their own environments by seeking out opportunities for success, persisting in the face of hard work and adversity, learning from past experiences, and responding with resilience to failure.

Cross-References

▶ Efficacy
▶ Efficacy Cognitions
▶ Hopelessness
▶ Locus of Control
▶ Salutogenesis
▶ Self-Concept
▶ Self-Image
▶ Theory of Reasoned Action

References and Further Readings

Ajzen, I. (1991). The theory of planned behavior. *Organizational Behavior and Human Decision Processes, 50*, 179–211.
Ajzen, I., & Fishbein, M. (1980). *Understanding attitudes and predicting social behavior*. Englewood Cliffs: Prentice-Hall.

Bandura, A. (1977a). Self-efficacy: Toward a unifying theory of behavioral change. *Psychological Review, 84*, 191–215.

Bandura, A. (1977b). *Social learning theory.* Englewood Cliffs: Prentice-Hall.

Bandura, A. (1986). *Social foundations of thought and actions: A social cognitive theory.* Englewood Cliffs: Prenctice-Hall.

Fishbein, M., & Ajzen, I. (1975). *Belief, attitude, intention, and behavior: An introduction to theory and research.* Reading: Addison-Wesley.

Prochaska, J. O., & Velicer, W. F. (1997). The transtheoretical model of health behavior change. *American Journal of Health Promotion, 12*, 38–48.

Rosenstock, I. M., Strecher, V. J., & Becker, M. H. (1988). Social learning theory and the health belief model. *Health Education Quarterly, 15*, 175–183.

Schunk, D. H., & Pajares, F. (2005). Competence perceptions and academic functioning. In A. J. Elliot & C. S. Dweck (Eds.), *Handbook of competence and motivation* (pp. 84–104). New York: Guilford Press.

Smith, R. E. (1989). Effects of coping skills training on generalized self-efficacy and locus of control. *Journal of Personality and Social Psychology, 56*, 228–233.

Walker, J. (2001). *Control and the psychology of health: Theory, measurement and applications.* Buckingham: Open University Press.

Weiner, B. (1986). *An attributional theory of motivation and emotion.* New York: Springer.

Weiner, B. (1992). *Human motivation: Metaphors, theories, and research.* Newbury Park: Sage.

Self-esteem

Shin-ichi Suzuki[1] and Koseki Shunsuke[2]
[1]Faculty of Human Sciences, Graduate School of Human Sciences, Waseda University, Tokorozawa-shi, Saitama, Japan
[2]Faculty of Psychology and Education, J. F. Oberlin University, Machida-shi, Tokyo, Japan

Synonyms

Pride; Self-respect

Definition

Self-esteem can be defined as a positive self-evaluation or a concept broader than confidence. It refers to an individual's cognitive appraisal that is constant over time. A positive self-appraisal indicates higher self-esteem, and a negative self-appraisal indicates lower self-esteem. Self-esteem is not perceived anytime, but it essentially influences one's actions, consciousness, or attitude. One who is perceived to have high self-esteem pursues goals aggressively and actively. Further, they are perceived to be amiable by themselves or by others. In this sense, self-esteem becomes indispensable to mental health or social adaptation.

In the previous study concerning self-esteem, an individual's self-esteem was considered in terms of not only his or her tendency and degrees of appraisal, which could be positive or negative, but also its relationship with the individual's cognitive faculty. James (1890) propounded that "self-esteem is successes divided by desire." This formula suggests that just thinking that one could succeed in the desired field increases self-satisfaction. This formula is similar to the theory on the gap between ideal self and real self (Rogers et al. 1951).

An individual's self-esteem strongly correlates with the affection, unconditional acceptance, and nurturing attitude that the parents display. Self-esteem can be measured in various ways, the most representative being Rosenberg's (1965) questionnaire and Coopersmith's (1967) scales. Because each scale may be different in terms of its dimensionalities or factors, it is necessary to consider the characteristics of the scales used or interpreted on a case-by-case basis.

Cross-References

▶ Attitudes
▶ Cognitive Appraisal
▶ Self-Concept

References and Further Reading

Coopersmith, S. (1967). *The antecedents of self-esteem.* San Francisco: WH Freeman.

James, W. (1890). *The principles of psychology.* New York: Holt.

Rogers, C. R., Dorfman, E., Gordon, T., & Hobbs, N. (1951). *Client-centered therapy: Its current practice, implications, and theory.* Boston: Houghton Mifflin.

Rosenberg, M. (1965). *Society and adolescent self-image.* Princeton: Princeton University Press.

Self-Evaluate

▶ Self-Monitoring

Self-Evaluation

▶ Self-examination

Self-examination

Tara McMullen
Doctoral Program in Gerontology, University of Maryland Baltimore and Baltimore County, Baltimore, MD, USA

Synonyms

Self-assessment; Self-evaluation; Self-monitoring; Self-rating

Definition

Self-examination can be seen as a process of evaluation or appraisal of one's qualities, traits, and characteristics.

Description

Self-examination can be seen as a process of evaluation or appraisal of one's qualities, traits, and characteristics. The evaluation of one's qualities, traits, and characteristics helps develop one's self-image and aids in the development of one's self-awareness or self-concept. Self-examination may result in a positive or negative self-feeling, which may enhance or decrease individuals' ideas about themselves. The evaluation of oneself can be seen as the attempt to understand one's motivations and behaviors. In addition, the examination of oneself is likely to affect self-esteem, which may affect self-image. Individuals who deem themselves as worthy may have a greater self-esteem, which may maintain one's "self." Rogers (1951) suggests that the self must be maintained in order to avoid anxiety and stress. Further, theorists often define self-examination as the evaluation or rating of oneself. This evaluation or rating is often defined as the degree to which an individual is self-aware and may result in a negative or positive self-actualization. This formed self-awareness helps develop the basis of individual self-regulation or the ability of one to control one's behaviors and actions (Hull 2002). Therefore, an individual defines one's self-concept from the degree to which the individual self-examines their personal traits, motivations, behaviors.

The act of self-examination may result in individuals self-monitoring themselves. Self-monitoring can be seen as the degree to which an individual manages or controls the image presented to others in social circumstances (Rawn et al. 2007). An individual who is a "high self-monitor" may be adept at self-monitoring and motivated to alter individual behavior in order to impact the responses of peers in social situations (Rawn et al. 2007). An individual who is a "low self-monitor" remains constant in individual behavior and will not alter individual behavior in social situations (Rawn et al. 2007). Further, the act of self-examination may result in self-criticism, or the awareness that individual traits and/or characteristics do not compare to the ideal self-image one may have for oneself. This self-criticism may be a result of the self-examination of one's strengths and weaknesses and may increase the evaluation of one's image. One may examine and reexamine individual strengths and weaknesses in order to measure self-actualization, or the fulfillment of one's potential (Maslow 1943, 1976). Therefore, the greater the self-actualization, the more defined one's self-concept may be, and possibly the greater the self-acceptance an individual may have for oneself. Self-acceptance is defined as the attitude toward one's self and ones individual qualities (English und English 1958).

Research that explores how self-evaluation impacts everyday situations has become common. For example, Judge, Locke, and Durham (1997), in a study exploring workplace job satisfaction, found that individuals with greater self-evaluations were more likely to have a higher self-esteem, self-efficacy, personal control, and emotional stability and were motivated to perform well in the workplace. Judge et al. (1997) conceptually define self-esteem, self-efficacy, locus of control, and "neuroticism-stability" as core self-evaluations. Judge et al. suggest that core self-evaluations are the "fundamental, subconscious conclusions individuals reach about themselves, other people, and the world" (Judge et al. 1998).

Cross-References

▶ Self-blame
▶ Self-concept
▶ Self-esteem
▶ Self-identity
▶ Self-image

References and Readings

English, H. B., & English, A. C. (1958). *A comprehensive dictionary of psychology and psychoanalytic terms*. New York: Longmans, Green.

Hull, J. G. (2002). Modeling the structure of self-knowledge and the dynamics of self-regulation. In A. Tesser, D. A. Stapel, & J. V. Wood (Eds.), *Self and Motivation: Emerging Psychological Perspectives* (pp. 173–206). Washington, DC: American Psychological Association.

Judge, T. A., Locke, E. A., & Durham, C. C. (1997). The dispositional causes of job satisfaction: A core evaluations approach. *Research in Organizational Behavior, 19*, 151–188.

Judge, T. A., Locke, E. A., Durham, C. C., & Kluger, A. N. (1998). Dispositional effects on job and life satisfaction: The role of core evaluations. *Journal of Applied Psychology, 83*, 17–34.

Maslow, A. H. (1943). A theory of human motivation. *Psychological Review, 50*, 37.

Maslow, A. H. (1976). Self-actualization psychology. In J. Fadiman & R. Frager (Eds.), *Personality and personal growth*. New York: Harper Collins.

Rawn, C. D., Mead, N., Kerkhof, P., & Vohs, K. D. (2007). The influence of self-esteem and ego threat on decision making. In K. D. Vohs, R. F. Baumeister, & G. Loewenstein (Eds.), *Do Emotions Help or Hurt Decision Making? A Hedgefoxian Perspective* (pp. 157–182). New York: Russell Sage Foundation Press.

Rogers, C. (1951a). Perceptual reorganization in client-centered therapy. In R. R. Blake & G. V. Ramsey (Eds.), *Perception: An approach to personality*. New York: Ronald Press.

Rogers, C. (1951b). *Client-centered therapy (pp. 13–71)*. Boston: Houghton Mifflin Company.

Self-Experimentation

▶ Quantified Self

Self-Identity

Katherine T. Fortenberry[1], Kate L. Jansen[2] and Molly S. Clark[3]
[1]Department of Family and Preventative Medicine, The University of Utah, Salt Lake City, UT, USA
[2]Behavioral Health, Midwestern University, Glendale, AZ, USA
[3]Midwestern University College of Health Sciences, Clinical Psychology, Glendale, AZ, USA

Synonyms

Self-concept; Self-construal; Self-perspective; Self-schema; Self-system; Self, The; Sense of self

Definition

Self-identity can be conceptualized as a dynamic, contextually based system (Baumeister 1998). It is a complex structure centered in memory and cognition that helps define who we are, how we relate to others, and our place in the world (Swann and Bosson 2008). It is also considered a key motivating force that influences personality and behavior. Self-identity is thought to drive our interactions with others (Andersen and Chen 2002), goals and future roles (Markus and Wurf 1987), and experience of emotions (Higgins 1989). Self-identity is also believed to regulate and motivate behavior by providing key self-regulation through a feedback system (Carver and Scheier 2002).

Description

A person's self-views are considered fundamental to how he or she interprets events, experiences emotion, and behaves. Individuals have distinct identities in different social roles, and differentiation into multiple role-related selves (e.g., self as a student, self as an athlete) is a process of normal development that begins in adolescence or earlier (Oosterwegel and Oppenheimer 2002). Self-identity differs in content and structure across individuals, and likely varies as a function of culture or gender (Cross and Madson 1997).

Research has examined the importance of the organization of positive and negative attributes within self-identity, namely, compartmentalization (i.e., negative attributes enclosed within a single role) and integration (i.e., negative attributes spread across multiple roles; see Showers and Zeigler-Hill 2007). The structure of self-identity is considered contextual and fluctuates between situations as different aspects of the self-structure are activated, strongly relating to mood and self-esteem. A person with a compartmentalized self-structure would experience more positive moods when a role containing predominantly positive attributes is activated frequently, but experience negative moods when a role containing negative attributes is activated. In contrast, both positive and negative attributes are frequently activated in an integrated self-structure, moderating the adverse emotional consequences of activating negative beliefs.

Self-identity is also conceptualized as dynamic. Andersen and Chen (2002) take an interpersonal developmental approach to understanding self-identity in different situations. In their theory of the relational self, they suggest that self-identity develops through interactions with significant others, who set *exemplars*, or cognitive templates stored in long-term memory. These exemplars are set in motion by environmental cues, so that behavior with different individuals varies based upon the active exemplar. Therefore, *who we are now* may differ when with different people.

In addition to describing *who we are now*, views of self-identity also describe *who we may become*. Higgins (1987) suggests that a driving force in self-identity is comparison of the *actual* self to the *ideal* self and *ought* self. A discrepancy between the selves is thought to cause negative psychological states, which initiate behavior that is designed to reduce the discrepancy. Similarly, Carver and Scheier (1998) describe that all individuals strive toward goals, which organize and motivate behavior. Comparisons between future goals and current behavior create emotions that drive future behavior. Positive emotions are experienced and behavior is reinforced when an action is judged to move us closer to a goal; negative emotions are experienced and behavior may change when an action is inconsistent with attaining a goal. Therefore, self-identity is part of a regulatory system that not only reflects, but also drives, who we are and who we will become.

Markus and Nurius (1986) suggest that current self-identity is strongly influenced by *possible selves*, or who we either want to become, or fear becoming, in the future. In this view, self-identity is fluid, continuously developing as possible selves are achieved, modified, or relinquished. Possible selves are thought to directly influence current behavior by providing movement toward or away from possible selves (i.e., approaching hoped-for selves or avoiding feared selves). Exposure to possible selves has been shown to influence exercise behavior (Ouellette et al. 2005) and school involvement in adolescents (Oyserman et al. 2002) over time. Possible selves are thus considered to play key roles in self-regulatory processes of motivation and behavior (Hoyle and Sherrill 2006). By comparing current self-identity with future selves, possible selves provide a framework in which to interpret and contextualize *who we are now*.

Self-identity is important for Behavioral Medicine because one's self-conceptions can influence how one responds to chronic illness, and can be altered by the experience of chronic illness. As views of the future are highly impacted by circumstances, major life events are likely to lead to changes in these views and, likewise, to changes in self-identity (Tesser et al. 2002). The diagnosis of a chronic illness is an example of this type of event. Adverse outcomes are likely if an illness contains attributes that reflect negatively onto an individual's self-identity. For example, individuals with lung cancer are more likely than individuals with prostate or breast cancer to associate stigma and self-blame with their illness, leading to negative psychological outcomes (Else-Quest et al. 2009). However, a growing body of literature suggests that positive outcomes such as perceptions of personal growth, improvements in life priorities and important relationships, and positive changes in personality (i.e., increased patience, tolerance, and empathy) can also occur as a result of dealing with adverse circumstances such as a chronic illness (Pakenham 2005; Tedeschi and Calhoun 2004).

Self-identity is also relevant to health promotion and illness prevention behaviors. Self-identity plays key roles in self-regulatory processes of motivation and behavior (Hoyle and Sherrill 2006), with the potential to influence health behavior in both positive and negative ways. For example, contemplating an image of a future possible self as an exerciser or non-exerciser influenced exercise behavior at four-week follow-up (Ouellette et al. 2005). Additionally, individuals' self-identity related to both smoking and quitting smoking independently predicted future attempts to quit. In contrast, sexually active teens who viewed STD's as more stigmatized were significantly less likely to have received STD screening over the last year (Cunningham et al. 2009). Goals that individuals wish to achieve, and views of who they are as they achieve these goals, are thought to be continuously present in the self-concept, providing a feedback loop that regulates these behaviors.

Cross-References

▶ Benefit Finding
▶ Chronic Disease Management
▶ Posttraumatic Growth
▶ Self-Concept
▶ Self-Image
▶ Self-Regulation
▶ Stigma

References and Further Readings

Andersen, S. M., & Chen, S. (2002). The relational self: An interpersonal social-cognitive theory. *Psychological Review, 109*, 619–645.

Baumeister, R. R. (1998). The self. In D. T. Gilbert, S. T. Fiske, & G. Lindzey (Eds.), *The handbook of social psychology* (Vol. 1, 4th ed., pp. 680–740). New York: McGraw-Hill.

Carver, C. S., & Scheier, M. F. (1998). *On the self-regulation of behavior*. New York: Cambridge University Press.

Carver, C. S., & Scheier, M. F. (2002). Coping processes and adjustment to chronic illness. In A. J. Christensen & M. H. Antoni (Eds.), *Chronic physical disorders: Behavioral medicine's perspective* (pp. 47–68). Malden: Blackwell.

Cross, S. E., & Madson, L. (1997). Models of the self: Self-construals and gender. *Psychological Bulletin, 122*, 5–37.

Cunningham, S. D., Kerrigan, D. L., Jennings, J. M., & Ellen, J. M. (2009). Relationships between perceived STD-related stigma, STD-related shame and STD screening among a household sample of adolescents. *Perspectives on Sexual and Reproductive Health, 41*, 225–230.

Else-Quest, N. M., LoConte, N. K., Schiller, J. H., & Hyde, J. S. (2009). Perceived stigma, self-blame, and adjustment among lung, breast, and prostate cancer patients. *Psychology and Health, 24*, 949–964.

Higgins, E. T. (1987). Self-discrepancy: A theory related self and affect. *Psychological Review, 94*, 319–340.

Higgins, E. (1989). Continuities in self-regulatory and self-evaluative processes: A developmental theory relating self and affect. *Journal of Personality, 57*, 407–444.

Hoyle, R. H., & Sherrill, M. R. (2006). Future orientation in the self-system: Possible selves, self-regulation, and behavior. *Journal of Personality, 74*(6), 1674–1696.

Markus, H., & Nurius, P. (1986). Possible selves. *American Psychologist, 41*, 954–969.

Markus, H., & Wurf, E. (1987). The dynamic self-concept: A social psychological perspective. *Annual Review of Psychology, 38*, 299–337.

Oosterwegel, A., & Oppenheimer, L. (2002). Jumping to awareness of conflict between self-representations and its relation to psychological wellbeing. *International Journal of Behavioral Development, 26*, 548–555.

Ouellette, J. A., Hessling, R., Gibbons, F. X., Reis-Bergan, M., & Gerrard, M. (2005). Using images to increase exercise behavior: Prototypes versus possible selves. *Personality and Social Psychology Bulletin, 31*, 610–620.

Oyserman, D., Terry, K., & Bybee, D. (2002). A possible selves intervention to enhance school involvement. *Journal of Adolescence, 25*, 313–326.

Pakenham, K. I. (2005). Benefit finding in multiple sclerosis and associations with positive and negative outcomes. *Health Psychology, 24*, 123–132.

Showers, C. J., & Zeigler-Hill, V. (2007). Compartmentalization and integration: The evaluative organization of contextualized selves. *Journal of Personality, 75*(6), 1181–1204.

Swann, W. B., & Bosson, J. K. (2008). Identity negotiation: A theory of self and social interaction. In R. W. Robins & L. A. Pervin (Eds.), *Handbook of personality psychology: Theory and research* (3rd ed., pp. 448–471). New York: Guilford Press.

Tedeschi, R. G., & Calhoun, L. G. (2004). Posttraumatic growth: Conceptual foundations and empirical evidence. *Psychological Inquiry, 15*, 1–18.

Tesser, A., Crepaz, N., Collins, J. C., Cornell, D., & Beach, S. R. H. (2002). Confluence of self-esteem regulation mechanisms: On integrating the self-zoo. *Personality and Social Psychology Bulletin, 26*, 1476–1489.

Self-image

Tara McMullen
Doctoral Program in Gerontology, University of Maryland Baltimore and Baltimore County, Baltimore, MD, USA

Synonyms

Self-attitude; Self-concept; Self-conception; Self-consciousness; Self-identity

Definition

Self-image is how an individual thinks they should be (English and English 1958). An individual's self-image is comprised of many attitudes, opinions, and ideals.

Description

Like self-concept, self-image is conceptually a difficult term to define due to the large number of varied terms using "self" as a phrase to define some sort of behavior (Burns 1980). However, self-image is important as it delineates how a self-aware individual views themselves or their image, which further establishes one's self-concept (Harriman 1947). Self-image is how an individual thinks they should be (English and English 1958). An individual's self-image is comprised of many attitudes, opinions, and ideals. Self-image develops at a young age and is a process which develops throughout the lifespan. Beginning at a young age, self-image can be seen as a physical process (Statt 1990). However, self-image is developed not only from body image and physical aspects but also from concepts shaped by society and attitudes.

Self-image is a measurable assessment of one's characteristics. Measurable aspects belonging to an individual build and maintain an individual's self-image. Measurable aspects can be identified as achievements and appearance (Bailey 2003). Self-image is how an individual perceives him/herself based on measurable traits developed at an early age (Bailey 2003). Like self-concept, an individual's self-image may be a learned trait structured from an individual's attitude toward a group, idea, object, and so forth (Rosenberg 1989). Thus, defined behavior may emerge from self-image; however, this behavior is not seen as fixed as it may deviate with the occurrence of different experiences and roles (Burns 1980). In addition, self-image may be affected by an individual's self-esteem. Self-esteem is defined as an individual's orientation toward oneself

(Rosenberg 1965). Rosenberg (1989) suggested that the more uncertain an individual is in regard to who they perceive he/she is, the more likely the individual will have a lowered self-esteem. A lower degree of self-esteem may render a negative self-image, diverging from the ideal self-image individuals may hold for themselves (Burns 1980). The ideal self can be defined as who an individual aspires to be. The ideal self is one part of self-concept and helps individuals better evaluate who they are (Burns 1980).

How individuals perceive who they are may depend on the individual's social environment and/or culture. Self-image can further be characterized as the perception an individual has of who he/she is physically, psychologically, philosophically, and politically, developed through the agency of individual societal experiences and development (Fisher 1986; Statt 1990). Individuals may develop a self-image that is associated with societal roles and norms (Markus and Kitayama 1991). Individuals in collectivist or individualistic cultures may establish who they are based on the culture in which they were raised. A collectivist culture accentuates individual's social roles and responsibilities within the context of social groups, while an individualistic culture accentuates individual identity and achievements (Nevid 2009). Thus, experiences and culture aid in the development of one's self-image. In defining individual roles, culture imparts a strong effect on the individual self-image.

Self-image has been measured in many populations by means of various psychometric scales such as the Rosenberg Self-Esteem Scale (Rosenberg 1989). Further, theory, such as the Social Identity Theory (Tajfel and Turner 1979) and the Objective Self-Awareness Theory (Duval and Wicklund 1972) have emerged from interpretations of self-image and self-consciousness.

Cross-References

▶ Body Image and Appearance-Altering Conditions
▶ Self-Concept

References and Readings

Bailey, J. A. (2003). Self-image, self-concept, and self-identity revisited. *Journal of the National Medical Association, 95*, 383–386.

Burns, R. B. (1980). *Psychology for the health professions*. Lancaster: MTP Press.

Duval, T. S., & Wicklund, R. A. (1972). *A theory of objective self-awareness*. New York: Academic Press.

English, H. B., & English, A. C. (1958). *A comprehensive dictionary of psychology and psychoanalytic terms*. New York: Longmans, Green.

Fisher, S. (1986). *Development and structure of the body image* (Vol. 1). Hillsdale: Erlbaum.

Fitts, W. H. (1991). *Tennessee self concept scale, manual*. Los Angeles: Western Psychological Services.

Harriman, P. L. (1947). *The new dictionary of psychology*. New York: The Philosophical Library.

Markus, H., & Kitayama, S. (1991). Culture and the self: Implication for cognition, emotion, and motivation. *Psychology Review, 98*, 224–253.

Markus, H., & Nurius, P. (1986). Possible selves. *The American Psychologist, 41*, 954–969.

Markus, H., & Wurf, E. (1987). The dynamic self-concept: A social psychological perspective. *Annual Review of Psychology, 38*, 299–337.

Nevid, J. S. (1990). *Essentials of psychology: Concepts and applications* (2nd ed.). Boston: Houghton Mifflin Company.

Nevid, J. S. (2009). *Psychology: Concepts and applications* (3rd ed.). Belmont: Cengage.

Rogers, C. (1951a). Perceptual reorganization in client-centered therapy. In R. R. Blake & G. V. Ramsey (Eds.), *Perception: An approach to personality*. New York: Ronald Press.

Rogers, C. (1951b). *Client-centered therapy* (pp. 13–71). Boston: Houghton Mifflin Company.

Rosenberg, M. (1965). *Society and the adolescent self-image*. Princeton: Princeton University Press.

Rosenberg, M. (1979). *Conceiving the self*. New York: Basic Books.

Rosenberg, M. (1986). *Conceiving the self*. Malabar: Krieger.

Rosenberg, M. (1989). *Society and the adolescent self-image*. Middletown: Wesleyan University Press.

Statt, D. (1990). *The concise dictionary of psychology*. New York: Routledge.

Tajfel, H., & Turner, J. C. (1979). An integrative theory of intergroup conflict. In W. G. Austin & S. Worchel (Eds.), *The social psychology of intergroup relations* (pp. 33–47). Monterey: Brooks/Cole.

Self-Inflicted Injurious Behavior

▶ Suicide

Self-Management

Andrea Wallace
College of Nursing, University of Iowa, Iowa City, IA, USA

Synonyms

Self-care

Definition

The process of actively engaging in activities aimed at controlling the negative effects of an illness, particularly a chronic illness, on one's health.

Description

Self-management concerns the acquisition of knowledge, as well as application of skills, necessary to engage in a complex set of health-promoting behaviors in the context of daily living. This process of integrating a number of complex behaviors in an effort to maintain wellness often involves problem-solving, decision-making, resource utilization, and communicating with multiple health-care providers. The ability to adapt health behaviors based on physiological or psychological information is a key element of self-management. The importance of self-management is undergirded by its role in health outcomes: It has been demonstrated that those who successfully engage in self-management activities experience better health-related outcomes for a number of chronic conditions.

Based on early studies of those living with chronic conditions, it has been proposed that the tasks related to self-management generally fall within three primary categories addressing: (1) medical management, which includes activities such as taking medications or adhering to a special diet; (2) role management, which includes actions allowing one to adopt roles that accommodate for ones condition; and (3) emotional management, which includes actions aimed at coping with emotions associated with an illness, such as uncertainty, depression, and fear (Corbin and Strauss 1988). It follows, then, that a wide array of psychosocial factors play a role in one's ability to successfully engage in self-management including, but not limited to, social support, motivation, confidence (self-efficacy), and depression. In addition, the ability to read and understand written information (literacy), understand and manipulate numerical information (numeracy), verbal memory, planning, and motor speed have all been associated with disease self-management behavior.

Although disease-specific self-management education is widely accepted as beneficial, its effect on health outcomes has been difficult to establish, primarily due to variability in the nature of the programs and populations tested. Because of the complexity associated with self-management, education and support aiming to train patients to manage their chronic disease attempt to address the many factors and tasks associated with self-management as well as tailor training to the individual needs of patients. However, some common elements among self-management education programs include general information about an illness (e.g., physiology), establishing and personalizing a treatment or self-care "plan" that addresses the behaviors necessary for improved disease outcomes and strategies to facilitate health-related behavior change and maintenance (Funnell et al. 2009; Lorig and Holman 2003). Many programs are guided by a specific theoretical framework and plan training to target variables believed to be important facilitators and barriers to self-management such as means of promoting patients' perceived self-efficacy (confidence) in engaging in health-promoting activities (Bandura 1997). A recent focus has been on the feasibility and broad dissemination of programs facilitating self-management and behavior change.

Driven by rising prevalence, costs, and poor outcomes associated with chronic illnesses, health-care settings have recently begun to focus on models of service delivery that best support patients' self-management needs. Although these efforts have been given a number of names, some common elements include easy access to health-care providers, providing disease-specific education, incorporating interdisciplinary teams of health-care providers (e.g., physicians, social workers, physical therapists), proactive reminders to both clinicians and patients about health maintenance needs (e.g., routine blood tests), and strategies for supporting the adoption and maintenance of health-promoting behaviors, such as behavioral goal setting between health-care providers and patients (Bodenheimer et al. 2002a, b; Patient-Centered Primary Care Collaborative 2010; The MacColl Institute for Healthcare Innovation 2010).

Cross-References

▶ Behavior Change
▶ Chronic Disease Management
▶ Disease Management
▶ Fatigue
▶ Health Behaviors
▶ Health Promotion
▶ Self-Care
▶ Self-efficacy

References and Readings

Bandura, A. (1997). *Self-efficacy: The exercise of control.* New York: Freeman.
Bodenheimer, T., Wagner, E. H., & Grumbach, K. (2002a). Improving primary care for patients with chronic illness. *Journal of the American Medical Association, 288*(14), 1775–1779.
Bodenheimer, T., Wagner, E. H., & Grumbach, K. (2002b). Improving primary care for patients with chronic illness: The chronic care model, Part 2. *Journal of the American Medical Association, 288*(15), 1909–1914.
Corbin, J., & Strauss, A. (1988). *Unending work and care: Managing chronic illness at home.* San Francisco: Jossey-Bass.
Funnell, M. M., Brown, T. L., Childs, B. P., Haas, L. B., Hosey, G. M., & Jensen, B. (2009). National standards for diabetes self-management education. *Diabetes Care, 32*(Suppl. 1), S87–S94.

Lorig, K. R., & Holman, H. (2003). Self-management education: History, definition, outcomes, and mechanisms. *Annals of Behavioral Medicine, 26*(1), 1–7.
Patient-Centered Primary Care Collaborative. (2010). *Patient-centered medical Home.* Retrieved 24 Jan-2010, from http://www.pcpcc.net/patient-centered-medical-home
The MacColl Institute for Healthcare Innovation. (2010). *The chronic care model.* Retrieved 24 Jan-2010, from http://www.improvingchroniccare.org/index.php?p=The_Chronic_Care_Model%26s=2

Self-Management Education

▶ Diabetes Education

Self-medication

Nicole Brandt
School of Pharmacy, University of Maryland, Baltimore, MD, USA

Synonyms

Self-treatment

Definition

Self-medication is the use of medications, treatments, and/or substances by an individual without a medical prescription. Self-medication is the most popular form of self-care, which is defined as the personal preservation of health through prevention and self-treatment of ailments (Ryan et al. 2009). In regards to self-care, substances used to self-medicate include but are not limited to over-the-counter (OTC) medications, nutritional supplements, and other nonprescription medications. The number of OTC medications has increased significantly, allowing more individuals to practice self-medication. These nonprescription medications can be purchased at various locations such as pharmacies, supermarkets, and retail superstores (Wazaify et al. 2005).

This increase in self-medicating practices entails both advantages and disadvantages. The benefits of self-medication include increased access to treatment, increased patient involvement in their own health care, economical choices, and evidence of cost-effectiveness compared to prescription treatments in some situations. The drawbacks of self-treatment are the threat of misuse and abuse of medications, incorrect self-diagnosis, a delay in appropriate treatment, and an increased risk of drug-drug interactions (Hughes et al. 2001). Due to the many risks listed above, safety is a major concern with self-medication. To ensure safety with self-treatment, patient education about the medication is a necessity (Bradley and Blenkinsopp 1996). Pharmacists are in a pivotal position to help ensure appropriate and safe use of various medications by patients that are obtained without a prescription.

Cross-References

▶ Nutritional Supplements
▶ Self-care
▶ Self-management

References and Readings

Bradley, C., & Blenkinsopp, A. (1996). Over the counter drugs: The future for self medication. *British Medical Journal, 312*, 835–837.
Hughes, C. M., McElnay, J. C., & Fleming, G. F. (2001). Benefits and risks of self medication. *Drug Safety, 24*(14), 1027–1037.
Ryan, A., Wilson, S., Taylor, A., & Greenfield, S. (2009). Factors associated with self-care activities among adults in the United Kingdom: A systematic review. *BMC Public Health, 9*, 96.
Wazaify, M., Shields, E., Hughes, C. M., & McElnay, J. C. (2005). Societal perspectives on over-the-counter (OTC) medicines. *Family Practice, 22*, 170–176.

Self-Monitor

▶ Self-Monitoring

Self-Monitoring

David Cameron[1] and Thomas L. Webb[2]
[1]Information School, The University of Sheffield, Sheffield, UK
[2]Department of Psychology, The University of Sheffield, Sheffield, UK

Synonyms

Seek feedback; Self-evaluate; Self-monitor

Definition

Self-monitoring can refer to (1) self-monitoring expressive behavior and self-presentation (the extent to which people observe and control their expressive behavior and self-presentation) and (2) self-monitoring goal progress (periodically noting current state and comparing these perceptions with whichever goals are currently relevant).

Description

Self-Monitoring Expressive Behavior and Self-Presentation

People differ in the extent to which they self-monitor (observe and control) their expressive behavior and self-presentation. High self-monitors think about how they appear to others and take care to portray themselves in a socially appropriate manner. Thus, high self-monitors are likely to monitor their facial expression, content of speech, tone of voice, expressed emotionality, and so on. In contrast, low self-monitors do not monitor these things, either because they lack the ability to do so or because they are not motivated to do so.

A number of studies have examined differences between high and low self-monitors. For example, low self-monitors tend to behave in ways that are more consistent with their attitudes and are better able to imagine how their own behavior relates to particular traits (e.g., the extent to which they are sociable). In contrast, individuals who score high on self-monitoring scales are particularly sensitive to social cues and are better able to imagine the prototypic type of person that would be described as holding a particular trait (e.g., a sociable person), perhaps because they are keen to be able to tailor their own behavior so as to demonstrate certain traits (e.g., to appear sociable). High self-monitors are even more likely to choose friends who facilitate the construction of their own situationally appropriate appearances and romantic partners with an attractive physical appearance. The idea that people self-monitor their expressive behavior has been hugely influential, and these studies just only hint at the wealth of differences.

The self-monitoring scale was developed to measure these individual differences. There are 25 items including "I guess I put on a show to impress or entertain people"; "in different situations and with different people, I often act like very different persons"; and "even if I am not enjoying myself, I often pretend to be having a good time." The scale was revised by Lennox and Wolfe who proposed a shorter 13-item scale with 6 items measuring sensitivity to the expressive behavior of others (e.g., "I am often able to read people's true emotions correctly through their eyes") and 7 items measuring the ability to modify self-presentation (e.g., "once I know what the situation calls for, it's easy for me to regulate my actions accordingly"). Lennox and Wolfe also proposed a separate 20-item "Concern for Appropriateness" scale measuring cross-situational variability (e.g., "different people tend to have different impressions about the type of person I am") and attention to social comparison information (e.g., "I usually keep up with clothing style changes by watching what others wear"). Despite this revision (and others), there remains a debate over exactly what the self-monitoring scale measures.

Self-Monitoring Goal Progress

A separate, but potentially overlapping, literature has examined whether and how people monitor their current standing in relation to their personal goals, for example, whether and how people assess if they are on track to maintain a healthy weight. While monitoring goal progress can involve feedback from external sources, people can, and do, self-monitor. Self-monitoring in this sense involves periodically noting one's current state and comparing these perceptions with whichever goals are currently relevant. For example, a person with the goal to reach a particular weight for their health might monitor caloric intake and physical activity. Monitoring goal progress, therefore, involves a series of processes from deciding to seek information (e.g., I need to monitor the suitability of the food I consume), becoming aware of and directing attention toward relevant information (e.g., looking at nutritional information), interpreting the information (e.g., this indicates a high-/low-fat/sugar content), and so on. Relevant goals provide both a comparative standard and also a schema for making sense of the information available. The person can monitor behavior (e.g., food chosen) or the outcomes of behavior (e.g., at routine health checkups). Monitoring may also vary on a temporal dimension (e.g., hourly, daily, weekly, or monthly) and can occur with respect to goals represented at different levels of specificity, for example, monitoring progress toward relatively high-level values comprising principles (or "be" goals, e.g., to be healthy), specific behavioral goals (or "do" goals, e.g., to take more exercise), or even the performance of motor programs (e.g., "one last rep").

Monitoring goal progress is central to a number of models of goal striving and self-regulation (e.g., control theory), but only a few studies have examined the effect of manipulating the likelihood that people would or could self-monitor. Polivy et al. (1986) investigated the effect of being able to monitor consumption on unhealthy eating. Participants were asked to taste some chocolates and to "eat as many as necessary to ensure accurate ratings." Unbeknown to participants, the researchers manipulated how easy it was for participants to monitor their consumption; some participants were asked to leave their chocolate wrappers on the table, others to place them in a wastebasket that was already half full of wrappers. The main finding was that participants asked to leave their wrappers on the table (and so, presumably, found it easy to monitor how many chocolates they had eaten) ate less than those asked to put the wrappers in the wastebasket. Quinn et al. (2010) found that self-monitoring helped people to break bad habits. Across two studies, prompting participants to use vigilant monitoring (thinking "don't do it" and watching carefully for mistakes) proved more effective in helping participants to avoid habitual responses (e.g., staying up too late, eating too much) than prompting stimulus control (removing oneself from the situation or removing the opportunity to perform the behavior). Prompting or facilitating behavioral monitoring has also proven an influential technique for promoting goal attainment. In summary, people who self-monitor their current standing in relation to their goals tend to be better able to achieve their goals and make changes to their behavior than people who do not.

Cross-References

▶ Behavior Change
▶ Self-examination
▶ Self-Regulation

References and Further Reading

Abraham, C., & Michie, S. (2008). A taxonomy of behavior change techniques used in interventions. *Health Psychology, 27*, 379–387.
Ajzen, I., Timko, C., & White, J. B. (1982). Self-monitoring and the attitude behavior relation. *Journal of Personality and Social Psychology, 42*, 426–435.
Ashford, S. J., & Cummings, L. L. (1983). Feedback as an individual resource: Personal strategies of creating information. *Organizational Behavior and Human Performance, 32*, 370–398.
Carver, C. S., & Scheier, M. F. (1982). Control theory: A useful conceptual framework for personality, social, clinical, and health psychology. *Psychological Bulletin, 92*, 111–135.
Carver, C. S., & Scheier, M. F. (1990). Origins and functions of positive and negative affect: A control process view. *Psychological Review, 97*, 19–35.
Gangestad, S. W., & Snyder, M. (2000). Self-monitoring: Appraisal and reappraisal. *Psychological Bulletin, 126*, 530–555.
Kluger, A. N., & DeNisi, A. (1996). The effects of feedback interventions on performance: A historical review, a meta-analysis, and a preliminary feedback intervention theory. *Psychological Bulletin, 119*, 254–284.
Lennox, R. D., & Wolfe, R. N. (1984). Revision of the self-monitoring scale. *Journal of Personality and Social Psychology, 46*, 1349–1364.
Polivy, J., Herman, C. P., Hackett, R., & Kuleshnyk, I. (1986). The effects of self-attention and public attention on eating in restrained and unrestrained subjects. *Journal of Personality and Social Psychology, 50*, 1253–1260.
Quinn, J. M., Pascoe, A., Wood, W., & Neal, D. T. (2010). Can't help yourself? Monitor those bad habits. *Personality and Social Psychology Bulletin, 36*, 499–511.
Snyder, M. (1974). Self-monitoring expressive behavior. *Journal of Personality and Social Psychology, 30*, 526–537.
Snyder, M. (1979). Self-monitoring processes. *Advances in Experimental Social Psychology, 12*, 85–128.
Snyder, M., & Cantor, N. (1980). Thinking about ourselves and others: Self-monitoring and social knowledge. *Journal of Personality and Social Psychology, 39*, 222–234.
Snyder, M., Gangestad, S., & Simpson, J. A. (1983). Choosing friends as activity partners: The role of self-monitoring. *Journal of Personality and Social Psychology, 45*, 1061–1072.
Snyder, M., Berscheid, E., & Glick, P. (1985). Focusing on the exterior and the interior: Two investigations of the initiation of personal relationships. *Journal of Personality and Social Psychology, 48*, 1427–1439.

Self-Monitoring of Blood Glucose

▶ Glucose Meters and Strips

Self-Murder

▶ Suicide

Self-Perspective

▶ Self-Identity

Self-Rating

▶ Self-examination

Self-Regulation

▶ Self-Regulation Model

Self-Regulation Model

Pablo A. Mora[1] and Gozde Ozakinci[2]
[1]Department of Psychology, The University of Texas at Arlington, Arlington, TX, USA
[2]Health Psychology, School of Medicine, University of St Andrews, St Andrews, UK

Synonyms

Model of self-regulation; Self-control; Self-Regulation

Definition

Self-regulation is a dynamic and systematic process that involves efforts to modify and modulate thoughts, emotions, and actions in order to attain goals.

Description

Self-regulation refers to the dynamic cognitive, affective, and behavioral processes that underlie goal attainment. It is important to note that not all types of situations involving goal attainment or problem solving constitute self-regulation. What makes self-regulation unique is that the target of problem solving is set by or focuses on the individual (i.e., self), its "machinery" (e.g., physical problems such as symptoms), and subjective feelings or affect.

Models of self-regulation are based on the idea of cybernetic control and propose that actions are regulated by a TOTE (Test, Operate, Test, Exit) feedback control loop. Central to the idea of feedback loop is the corrective actions that result from the detection and evaluation of discrepancies between input (internal or external) and a reference value. In the context of health, "feeling good" (i.e., not having any symptoms) can be considered a reference value or goal. Thus, when a person experiences a headache (i.e., discrepancy between current state and feeling good), he or she will engage in corrective actions to rid himself or herself of the headache such as taking a pain reliever or resting. If the headache subsides (i.e., test has determined that the discrepancy was eliminated), then the loop ends (i.e., exit). If not, then a new loop will begin.

These self-regulation principles have been widely applied to the study and explanation of multiple psychological phenomena. Psychological models of self-regulation diverge in terms of their foci of interest and emphases; however, they do share core features. Common features of psychological self-regulation models are: (1) goal setting, (2) developing and enacting strategies to achieve these goals, (3) developing criteria to determine proximity to the goal, and (4) determining, based on goal proximity, whether corrective actions are needed or whether the goal needs to be revised. Self-regulation is an iterative process that may require constant evaluation to ensure that the distance between the person's status and the goal is the desired one. One additional commonality shared by behavioral models is the importance they ascribe to affective experiences as integral to self-regulation. Affect, as a core component of the motivational system, can be the reference value that triggers self-regulatory behaviors, be the product of progress toward a goal or lack thereof (i.e., negative affect resulting from not attaining a goal), and/or influence cognitions and behaviors involved in self-regulatory activities (e.g., symptom perception). Models that integrate affective experiences with self-regulation propose that problem-focused and emotion-focused goals and the behavioral processes used by individuals to attain such goals operate in a parallel yet interrelated fashion (see commonsense model of self-regulation, stress-behavior model advanced by Lazarus and Folkman, or work on self-regulation of affect conducted by Carver and Scheier).

Hierarchical Structure of Goals

Goals are usually differentiated and hierarchically organized in terms of their level of abstraction (Carver and Scheier 1990a). At the highest level of abstraction, one can find goals related to self-concepts (e.g., ideal self and undesired self), self-assessments (e.g., self-rated health), and general affect (e.g., depressed or happy mood). Specific, concrete actions such as daily activities performed by an individual (e.g., buying low fat food) are at the lower level of the hierarchy. Attaining higher-order goals requires that lower-level goals are accomplished; that is, lower-level goals constitute routes to higher-order ones (e.g., buying and consuming low fat food in order to achieve better health). Abstract goals also provide internal consistency and coherence to lower-level goals and to the actions performed to achieve specific higher-order goals. The relationship between goals of different levels of abstraction is quite dynamic. Thus, while a single abstract goal can be attained by pursuing multiple lower-level, concrete goals, it is also possible to simultaneously attain multiple, distinct higher-order goals by setting and pursuing the same lower-level, concrete goals. For instance, a person can get closer to their ideal, healthy self and farther from their undesired, decrepit self by engaging in similar lower-level self-regulatory activities (e.g., engaging in regular exercises and eating a healthful diet).

Feedback Loops and Behavioral Strategies Involved in Goal Attainment

In self-regulation, goals provide the reference values for feedback loops and motivate and guide actions. Individuals may engage in two types of overall feedback loops depending on whether the reference value (i.e., goal) represents a desired state (i.e., approach) or whether it represents an undesired one (i.e., avoidance, Carver 2006). Behavior directed toward desired goals is regulated by a negative feedback loop. In this case, a reduction of the discrepancy between the current state (i.e., input) and the goal (i.e., reference value) dominates the individual's actions. Behaviors involved in the avoidance of reference value, on the other hand, are controlled by a positive feedback loop. Thus, efforts are deployed to maintain or enlarge a discrepancy between the input and the reference value. Many times avoiding an undesired state may require that individuals set desired goals. For example, infirmity (undesired goal) can be avoided by establishing a regime of regular exercise and a healthy diet (desired goals). One can argue that positive feedback loops are part of larger negative feedback loops that motivate individuals to reduce discrepancy between their current status and the reference value. In the case discussed above, an individual for whom avoiding infirmity is critical will need to develop achievable, concrete goals in order to appraise progress. Thus, the reference value for "avoiding infirmity" can take the form of "being symptom-free," a goal that is regulated by a negative feedback loop.

The two strategies discussed above assume that goals set by an individual are attainable; however, there are situations in which, regardless of effort, goal attainment can become difficult or impossible. In such situations, abandoning activities directed at the pursuit of the goal will result in better adjustment than maintaining goal-directed efforts. Research has shown that goal disengagement can result in improved well-being if goal-directed efforts are focused on alternative goals when available. If alternative goals are unavailable, inability to disengage from goal pursuit can result in frustration, negative affect, and increased stress (Miller and Wrosch 2007). For older adults, goal disengagement and goal reengagement may be a key strategy for adjustment to physical changes and for successful aging.

Goal attainment and affect. As indicated above, affect can be an indicator of progress toward the attainment of a goal. Carver and Scheier (1990b) have proposed a second feedback process that monitors whether a person's efforts are being successful in attaining a goal. Success in closing the gap between one's status and a given goal results in positive affect. Slow progress or failure to attain a goal, on the other hand, results in negative affect. Individuals differ in terms of the reference values they use to determine what constitutes acceptable or unacceptable progress. Accordingly, similar rates of discrepancy reduction can result in two very different responses if the individuals use different criteria to appraise the effectiveness of their actions.

Research on self-discrepancies provides an interesting example of how proximity to a goal can elicit positive or negative moods (Mora et al. in press). These data have shown that individuals who felt they were farther from being at their worst (i.e., undesired self) reported less anxiety and depression and more happiness than their counterparts who felt closer to their feared self. These affective experiences can, in turn, influence subsequent evaluations of progress and actions. Negative mood arisen from perceptions that progress toward a goal is slow can result in maladaptive behaviors especially if new actions are focused on reducing negative feelings. Depressive feelings may alter perceptions of control over their environment and future outcomes, and lead individuals to give up on their efforts to attain a goal. Despite its critical and multifaceted role in self-regulation, there is a dearth of research examining the multiple interactive ways in which cognitive/behavioral and affective self-regulation operates.

Organization of Goals and Actions: Goal Cognitions

Germane to the relationships among goals of different levels of abstraction are goal cognitions (Karoly 1993) and action plans (Leventhal 1970). Goal cognitions are mental models or schemas that organize domain-specific goals and actions or procedures to attain those goals (in health literature, goal cognitions are referred as illness representations). For instance, a schema for an abstract, higher-order goal of "being healthy" would involve several less abstract concrete goals such as engaging in exercise, eating healthful food, and improving coping skills. These goals, in turn, would be connected in the mental schema to more concrete, lower-level goals such as setting days to go the gym, eating more complex carbohydrates, and learning how to meditate to reduce stress. Action plans translate aspects of goal pursuit (e.g., beliefs, attitudes, evaluation criteria) into actual, concrete behaviors. These behaviors help link goals at different levels of abstraction and provide continuity to the pursuit of abstract goals. In the current example, being healthy requires the person to set and attain multiple concrete goals. Goal cognitions will specify the action plans required to attain the concrete goals in route to reach the higher-order, abstract goal. Thus, to attain the various goals on route to being healthy, the person will need to engage in actions such as joining a gym, building a routine of going to the gym, and choosing the specific workout routine (e.g., cardio and/or weightlifting).

Conscious and Nonconscious Aspects of Self-Regulation

Although the terms "goal setting" and "self-regulation" suggest conscious volition, processes involved in self-regulation are the result of both automatic and intentional behaviors. Awareness of every single process involved in self-regulation would unnecessarily tax the organism and result in maladaptation. Action plans required for the attainment of a goal can become automated behaviors if goal pursuit is an ongoing activity. For instance, the management of a chronic condition such as hypertension requires that people take medications every day. To ensure that doses are not missed, a person may decide to put pills in a case and place this case on top of the counter next to the coffee maker. By doing this, taking the pill can become an automated behavior that imposes a minimal burden on the cognitive system of the individual. It is in consciousness, however, where automatic and intentional processes are integrated. Ensuring that doses have not been missed, the person needs to engage in a conscious decision-making process (e.g., pick up the pill case and count the remaining pills).

Recently, investigators interested in the volitional aspects of self-regulation have been devoting increased attention to the idea of self-control. Although sometimes self-control and self-regulation are used interchangeably, self-control refers to the capacity to consciously and effortfully regulate one's affect, cognitions, and behaviors (Hagger et al. 2010). In attempting to explain the reasons individuals engage in maladaptive behaviors (e.g., smoking), researchers have argued that self-control is a limited resource (Ego Strength model: Baumeister et al. 2007). The Ego Strength model argues that self-control works as "a muscle" that can become tired after repeated use (i.e., ego depletion). In other words, a person's capacity to engage in self-control becomes reduced following previous acts of self-control. Although the idea of ego depletion has received support from experimental studies, a recent meta-analysis suggests that the strength model does not fully explain the mechanisms underlying self-control and additional theoretical perspectives need to be integrated into the strength model (Hagger et al. 2010). The results from the meta-analysis suggest that motivation, fatigue, self-efficacy, and affect are involved in self-control and ego-depletion processes. Further research in this area is needed to better understand how self-control and ego depletion operate in real world contexts in which long-term and unplanned attempts at self-control occur frequently.

Moderators of Self-Regulation

Self-regulation occurs within particular settings and is, thus, influenced by individual, social, and cultural factors. Personality, an individual factor, has been implicated in various processes of self-regulation such as appraisal, coping, and behaviors (Cervone et al. 2006). For instance, research has shown that individuals high in neuroticism (one of the big five personality traits) consistently and reliably perceive and report more physical symptoms than their low neuroticism counterparts (Watson and Pennebaker 1989). Because physical symptoms are a departure from normal functioning, increases in symptomatology may trigger prompt self-regulatory actions (e.g., care seeking) if symptoms are perceived to be indicators of imminent threat. Research on coping has revealed that individual differences such as optimism and pessimism influence goal pursuit. Specifically, individuals who have positive views about the future tend to engage in problem-focused coping, whereas individuals who perceive the future as uncertain tend to either engage in emotion-focused coping or else disengage from goal pursuit (Rasmussen et al. 2006). Personality can also have an impact on the selection of specific behaviors used by individuals to deal with threat. There is evidence that individuals high in optimism and conscientiousness who face stressful situations select coping procedures that improve well-being and adjustment (O'Connor et al. 2009).

Social factors and culture can also influence the various stages of self-regulation from goal setting to selection and performance of corrective actions through multiple pathways. Social comparisons can help individuals to determine the origin of their physical symptoms (e.g., food poisoning if everybody at dinner has the same symptoms or stomach flu if symptoms are unique to one person) and, thereby, select the necessary corrective actions to deal with such symptoms (Leventhal et al. 1997). Research has also demonstrated that social relations (i.e., social network size) can influence long-term self-regulatory activities such as participation in cardiac rehabilitation among patients with acute coronary syndrome (Molloy et al. 2008).

Culture has been shown to influence the type of stimuli that trigger self-regulation, the content of goals, the specific corrective actions, and the appraisal criteria involved in goal attainment. Anthropological research has shown that the interpretation and attribution of bodily symptoms varies across culture. This body of evidence suggests that culturally determined illness models are powerful determinants of the ways people experience illness conditions. For example, work on depression has shown that among certain ethnic groups (e.g., Chinese), depression is usually experienced as a somatic disorder (Kleinman 1977). This difference in experience can shape what actions are taken to remediate the problem (e.g., seeing a primary care physician instead of a mental health specialist) and the criteria to determine the success of the remedial actions (e.g., improvement in physical versus affective well-being). The impact of culture on the construction and development of the self has led some authors to question the idea that self-regulation is set by and focuses on the individual. In collectivistic cultures where the self is construed as closely interrelated to others, goal setting can be motivated by a need to please the person's social network (Trommsdorff 2009). Future research needs to determine whether the mechanisms of self-regulation guided by interrelatedness are different from those underlying self-regulation of intraindividual processes.

Self-Regulation and Health

Although most models of self-regulation have originated outside the domain of behavioral medicine (see the Commonsense Model of Self-regulation for an exception), the use of self-regulatory principles and ideas to understand health-related behaviors has been relatively widespread. Models such as the Health Beliefs Model, Theory of Reasoned Action, and Social Cognitive Theory which focus on specific aspects of self-regulation such as social (e.g., norms) and psychological (e.g., self-efficacy) determinants have been utilized to understand self-regulation of health behaviors. In general, the use of these models has focused more on the description of predictors of goals rather than on the underlying mechanisms that explain self-regulatory behaviors. In addition, goal pursuit is usually examined by these models as a single-event rather than a continuous process (Maes and Karoly 2005). Recent efforts, however, have been directed at the understanding and examination of self-regulation as a process by investigating how goal-directed behaviors in health domains are initiated and maintained. Evidence has provided convincing support that the various phases of self-regulation are controlled by different processes. Studies examining health behaviors such as smoking cessation and engagement in exercise activities have revealed that factors such as self-efficacy and attitudes toward the specific behavior are important determinants of initiation. Maintenance of health behaviors, on the other hand, is influenced by factors such as satisfaction with behavioral change. A recent study examining data from participants in a smoking cessation program provided further evidence of the complexity of self-regulation processes (Baldwin et al. 2009). In this study, the authors found that maintenance of health-related behaviors was a heterogeneous process and that the factors that influenced satisfaction with behavioral maintenance varied according to whether they had quit smoking recently or not.

Final Remarks

Literature and research on self-regulation has grown rapidly over the past 20 years. New research has expanded the understanding of self-regulation mechanisms but more research is needed. Some of the research questions that remained underexplored include changes in self-regulation over time, factors that contribute to long-term self-regulatory behaviors (e.g., adherence to medical treatment for chronic conditions), and the multiple and simultaneous pathways through which cognitive and affective self-regulation interact.

New opportunities provided by advances in technology, especially in brain imaging, are opening exciting areas of inquiry (e.g., cognitive neuroscience of self-regulation). Similarly, increased understanding of the psychophysiology of stress offers an invaluable opportunity to understand how self-regulatory processes get under the skin.

Cross-References

▶ Active Coping
▶ Behavioral Intervention
▶ Common-Sense Model of Self-regulation
▶ Optimism
▶ Self-Efficacy
▶ Self-Regulatory Capacity
▶ Self-Regulatory Fatigue

References and Further Readings

Baldwin, A. S., Rothman, A. J., & Jeffery, R. W. (2009). Satisfaction with weight loss: Examining the longitudinal covariation between people's weight-loss-related outcomes and experiences and their satisfaction. *Annals of Behavioral Medicine, 38*, 213–224.

Baumeister, R. F., & Vohs, K. D. (2004). *Handbook of self-regulation: research, theory, and applications*. New York: Guilford Press.

Baumeister, R. F., Vohs, K. D., & Tice, D. M. (2007). The strength model of self-control. *Current Directions in Psychological Science, 16*(6), 351–355. https://doi.org/10.1111/j.1467-8721.2007.00534.x.

Boekaerts, M., Zeidner, M., & Pintrich, P. R. (1999). *Handbook of self-regulation*. San Diego\London: Academic Press.

Carver, C. (2006). Approach, avoidance, and the self-regulation of affect and action. *Motivation and Emotion, 30*(2), 105–110. https://doi.org/10.1007/s11031-006-9044-7.

Carver, C. S., & Scheier, M. (1990a). Principles of self-regulation: Action and emotion. In E. T. Higgins, R. M. Sorrentino, et al. (Eds.), *Handbook of motivation and cognition: Foundations of social behavior* (Vol. 2, pp. 3–52). New York: Guilford Press.

Carver, C. S., & Scheier, M. F. (1990b). Origins and functions of positive and negative affect: A control-process view. *Psychological Review, 97*(1), 19–35.

Carver, C. S., & Scheier, M. F. (1998). *On the self-regulation of behavior*. New York: Cambridge University Press.

Cervone, D., Shadel, W. G., Smith, R. E., & Fiori, M. (2006). Self-regulation: Reminders and suggestions from personality science. *Applied Psychology: An International Review, 55*(3), 333–385. https://doi.org/10.1111/j.1464-0597.2006.00261.x.

Folkman, S., & Lazarus, R. S. (1988). The relationship between coping and emotion: Implications for theory and research. *Social Science & Medicine, 26*(3), 309–317.

Hagger, M. S., Wood, C., Stiff, C., & Chatzisarantis, N. L. D. (2010). Ego depletion and the strength model of self-control: A meta-analysis. *Psychological Bulletin, 136*(4), 495–525. https://doi.org/10.1037/a0019486.

Karoly, P. (1993). Mechanisms of self-regulation: A systems view. *Annual Review of Psychology, 44*, 23–52.

Kleinman, A. M. (1977). Depression, somatization and the "new cross-cultural psychiatry". [Case reports comparative study]. *Social Science and Medicine, 11*(1), 3–10.

Leventhal, H. (1970). Findings and theory in the study of fear communications. In L. Berkowitz (Ed.), *Advances in experimental social psychology* (Vol. 5, pp. 120–186). New York: Academic.

Leventhal, H. (1983). Behavioral medicine: Psychology in health care. In D. Mechanic (Ed.), *Handbook of health, health care, and the health professions* (pp. 709–743). New York: The Free Press.

Leventhal, H., Hudson, S., & Robitaille, C. (1997). Social comparison and health: A process model. In B. P. Buunk & F. X. Gibbons (Eds.), *Health, coping, and well-being: Perspectives from social comparison theory* (pp. 411–432). Mahwah: Lawrence Erlbaum Associates.

Maes, S., & Karoly, P. (2005). Self-regulation assessment and intervention in physical health and illness: A review. *Applied Psychology, 54*(2), 267–299. https://doi.org/10.1111/j.1464-0597.2005.00210.x.

Miller, G. E., & Wrosch, C. (2007). You've gotta know when to fold'em. *Psychological Science, 18*(9), 773–777. https://doi.org/10.1111/j.1467-9280.2007.01977.x.

Molloy, G. J., Perkins-Porras, L., Strike, P. C., & Steptoe, A. (2008). Social networks and partner stress as predictors of adherence to medication, rehabilitation attendance, and quality of life following acute coronary syndrome. *Health Psychology, 27*(1), 52–58. https://doi.org/10.1037/0278-6133.27.1.52.

Mora, P. A., Musumeci-Szabo, T. J., Popan, J., Beamon, T., & Leventhal, H. (in press). Me at my worst: Exploring the relationship between the undesired self, health, and mood among older adults. *Journal of Applied Social Psychology*.

O'Connor, D., Conner, M., Jones, F., McMillan, B., & Ferguson, E. (2009). Exploring the benefits of conscientiousness: An investigation of the role of daily stressors and health behaviors. *Annals of Behavioral Medicine, 37*(2), 184–196. https://doi.org/10.1007/s12160-009-9087-6.

Rasmussen, H. N., Wrosch, C., Scheier, M. F., & Carver, C. S. (2006). Self-regulation processes and health: The importance of optimism and goal adjustment. *Journal of Personality, 74*(6), 1721–1747. https://doi.org/10.1111/j.1467-6494.2006.00426.x.

Schunk, D. H., & Zimmerman, B. J. (1994). *Self-regulation of learning and performance: issues and educational applications*. Hillsdale, NJ: Lawrence Erlbaum Associates.

Trommsdorff, G. (2009). Culture and development of self-regulation. *Social and Personality Psychology Compass, 3*(5), 687–701. https://doi.org/10.1111/j.1751-9004.2009.00209.x.

Watson, D., & Pennebaker, J. W. (1989). Health complaints, stress, and distress: Exploring the central role of negative affectivity. *Psychological Review, 96*(2), 234–254.

Self-Regulatory Ability

▶ Self-Regulatory Capacity

Self-Regulatory Capacity

David Cameron[1] and Thomas L. Webb[2]
[1]Information School, The University of Sheffield, Sheffield, UK
[2]Department of Psychology, The University of Sheffield, Sheffield, UK

Synonyms

Self-control capacity; Self-regulatory ability; Strength model of self-control

Definition

Self-regulatory capacity refers to people's ability to exert control over their thoughts, feelings, and actions, for example, the capacity to inhibit prejudice, make oneself feel better, or select healthy food. However, self-regulatory capacity is thought to be a limited resource that (i) is temporarily depleted by exertions of self-control (an effect termed "ego-depletion") and (ii) differs in strength from person to person.

Description

Limited Self-Regulatory Capacity

Self-regulatory capacity refers to an individual's ability to exert control over their behavior, thoughts, and feelings. The capacity for self-regulation differs between individuals and can differ intraindividually dependent on situational factors, such as the experience of self-regulatory fatigue. Self-regulation is closely related to goal-driven behavior and is characterized by the process of attempting to work toward a desired held goal. For example, in terms of health behavior, an individual may regulate their diet to reach a specific weight or resist a personal temptation such as cigarettes to reach their goal of overcoming a smoking addiction. Self-regulatory capacity would influence how successfully an individual pursues such goals, alongside other factors such as the prepotency of the action that needs to be overcome. The modal model of self-regulatory capacity (strength model) poses that persistence with self-regulation can lead to a temporary state of self-regulatory fatigue and lapses of self-regulation can occur. In terms of the prior examples, this could include short-term gratifications such as deviations from a planned diet or the resumption of smoking.

Self-regulatory capacity can be measured using a wide variety of cognitive or behavioral tests. Examples include persistence at impossible (e.g., completing unsolvable anagrams) or aversive (e.g., consuming unpleasant drinks, squeezing a handgrip, cold pressor) tasks; response time or errors made in inhibition tasks (Stroop task, stop signal); resisting temptation (limiting alcohol consumption); and suppression of emotional expression. The key criterion for a task measuring self-regulatory capacity is the requirement for the person to override an otherwise dominant response (e.g., the desire to give up, to read the words in the Stroop task). Tasks that are simply difficult (e.g., complex math puzzles) or stressful (e.g., watching an emotional video) are unlikely to reflect the same ability. The strength model argues that self-regulation draws from a universal pool – that exerted effort at one self-regulation task impairs ability at performing a subsequent, seemingly distinct, task. Presenting these tasks in sequence is a commonly used method to examine self-regulatory capacity.

Self-regulatory capacity has an important relation to health behavior. Many behaviors which are considered to have long-term benefits, such as eating a healthy diet or maintaining an exercise regimen, are notably absent from people's routines, while behaviors that are demonstrably harmful in the long term such as smoking, unhealthy diets, unprotected sexual intercourse, or substance abuse are common in society. The contrast between these behaviors can be seen in the temporal distance between the costs and benefits: behaviors associated with improved health typically only show a beneficial change over the longer term, while the costs (such as the self-regulatory effort in changing behavior) are high in the short term, whereas behaviors that show a high cost of being harmful to health in the long term offer immediate benefits (such as the satiation of an immediate desire or need). In the context of temporal self-regulation theory, self-regulatory capacity acts as a moderator of the link between an individual's intentions for health behavior, which are shaped by the temporal differences between perceived costs and benefits for an action, and the individual's actual observed behavior. A greater capacity for self-regulation is predicted to be associated with the ability to overcome prepotent responses, such as habitual smoking, and follow intentions for behavior, such as intention to quit smoking. Limited capacity for regulation is predicted to be associated with lapses in self-control and the resumption of prepotent responses; so despite the intention to quit smoking, this would not translate into actionable behavior.

Nature of Self-Regulatory Capacity

The precise nature of self-regulatory capacity remains elusive – since the development of the strength model in 1994, a multitude of studies using the two-task paradigm indicate a limited self-regulatory capacity; a meta-analysis of these suggests a reliable effect. However, more recent research challenges the size and reliability of effects previously observed.

Self-regulatory capacity has been linked to the biological substrate of blood glucose levels – Gailliot and colleagues (2007) identify that depletion of self-regulatory capacity was correlated with blood glucose levels and that performance on self-regulatory tasks could be restored with blood glucose supplements (namely, lemonade). The strength model has since been updated to situate a central monitor of available, or potentially available, glucose as a candidate for momentary self-regulatory capacity.

Self-regulatory capacity's apparent dependence on glucose availability suggests a similarity with executive functions known to be affected by available glucose levels (e.g., the attentional system). Self-regulation is considered to exist alongside this diverse array of higher cognitive processes and may work in concert with others, particularly that of planning and error detection. Self-regulation can be considered as a goal-driven process because it is used by an individual who seeks to override one state of behavior, thoughts, or feelings with another goal state. As such, an individual is required to recruit multiple executive processes to reach goal states: representations of one's current state and goal state must be held alongside a plan for how to achieve the goal state, detection of discrepancy (or error) between these two states must occur, and self-regulation to change the current experienced state toward the goal is required. Apparent failures in the wider system of self-regulation may not be restricted to a depleted self-regulatory capacity; related systems such as that of error detection may impair self-regulation if there is an incorrect perception of error between the current state and desired state.

Like other aspects of executive function, self-regulatory capacity is associated with the frontal lobes. Both neuroimaging and lesion studies indicate that self-regulatory actions such as the control of behavioral and emotional output is closely associated with the ventromedial prefrontal cortex. In addition, the ventromedial-orbitofrontal cortex has been particularly associated with the self-regulatory process of suppressing previously rewarding responses. Damage to this area often results in a diminished or absent ability to inhibit immediately rewarding actions, even though the semantic knowledge of an action's inappropriateness may still be intact. These regions associated with self-regulatory capacity show high connectivity will executive areas related to the processes involved in self-monitoring, which support the process of self-regulation. The anterior cingulate cortex is associated with the degree and nature of conflict between competing responses to situations such as the short-term desire to satiate an immediate need against the longer-term goal for a healthier lifestyle. The dorsolateral prefrontal cortex has been associated with the resolution of detected response conflict alongside attentional and planning behavior. These regions working in cohort are considered to form the neural circuitry underpinning self-regulation.

Individual Differences in Self-Regulatory Capacity

In addition to situational demands on self-regulatory capacity, there is also a body of research suggesting that there may be stable individual differences in self-regulatory capacity. Some people simply seem better than others at, for example, selecting healthy food, cheering themselves up, and acting in an egalitarian manner. In support of this idea, Hofmann et al. (2008) found that individual differences in working memory capacity moderated participants' ability to self-regulate their sexual interest, consumption of tempting food, and anger expression. In a similar vein, a number of authors have proposed measures of self-regulatory capacity such as the Self-Control Behavior Inventory, the Self-Control Questionnaire, and the Brief Self-Control Scale (BSCS). In each case, differences have been found between people that reliably map onto various self-control outcomes such as task performance, impulse control, interpersonal relations, and so on.

Building Self-Regulatory Capacity

Much like with general executive function training, there is a significant interest in the possibility that self-regulatory capacity can be improved in individuals through practice. Meta-analysis of training studies indicates that training can have a positive effect on some elements of self-regulatory capacity, particularly when measured using the two-task paradigm.

Cross-References

▶ Cold Pressor Task
▶ Ego-Depletion
▶ Emotion
▶ Limited Resource
▶ Prejudice
▶ Self-Control
▶ Self-Report Inventory
▶ Stroop Color-Word Test
▶ Working Memory

References and Further Reading

Baumeister, R. F., & Vohs, K. D. (2018). Strength model of self-regulation as limited resource: Assessment, controversies, update. In *Self-regulation and self-control* (pp. 78–128). New York: Routledge.

Brandon, J. E., Oescher, J., & Loftin, J. M. (1990). The self-control questionnaire: An assessment. *Health Values, 14*, 3–9.

Carter, E. C., & McCullough, M. E. (2014). Publication bias and the limited strength model of self-control: Has the evidence for ego depletion been overestimated? *Frontiers in Psychology, 5*, 823.

Fagen, S. A., Long, N. J., & Stevens, D. J. (1975). *Teaching children self-control: Preventing emotional and learning problems in the elementary school.* Columbus: Charles E. Merrill.

Friese, M., Frankenbach, J., Job, V., & Loschelder, D. D. (2017). Does self-control training improve self-control? A meta-analysis. *Perspectives on Psychological Science, 12*(6), 1077–1099.

Gailliot, M. T., Baumeister, R. F., DeWall, C. N., Maner, J. K., Plant, E. A., Tice, D. M., Brewer, L. E., & Schmeichel, B. J. (2007). Self-control relies on glucose as a limited energy source: Willpower is more than a metaphor. *Journal of Personality and Social Psychology, 92*, 325–336.

Hagger, M. S., Wood, C., Stiff, C., & Chatzisarantis, N. L. D. (2010). Ego depletion and the strength model of self-control: A meta-analysis. *Psychological Bulletin, 136*, 495–525.

Hagger, M. S., Chatzisarantis, N. L., Alberts, H., Anggono, C. O., Batailler, C., Birt, A. R., ..., Calvillo, D. P. (2016). A multilab preregistered replication of the ego-depletion effect. *Perspectives on Psychological Science, 11*(4), 546–573.

Hall, P. A., & Fong, G. T. (2013). Temporal self-regulation theory: Integrating biological, psychological, and ecological determinants of health behavior performance. In *Social neuroscience and public health* (pp. 35–53). New York: Springer.

Hofmann, W., Friese, M., Gschwendner, T., Wiers, R. W., & Schmit, M. (2008). Working memory capacity and self-regulatory behavior: Toward an individual differences perspective on behavior determination by automatic versus controlled processes. *Journal of Personality and Social Psychology, 95*, 962–977.

Tangney, J. P., Baumeister, R. F., & Boone, A. L. (2004). High self-control predicts good adjustment, less pathology, better grades, and interpersonal success. *Journal of Personality, 72*, 271–324.

Self-Regulatory Fatigue

David Cameron[1] and Thomas L. Webb[2]
[1]Information School, The University of Sheffield, Sheffield, UK
[2]Department of Psychology, The University of Sheffield, Sheffield, UK

Synonyms

Ego-depletion; Limited resource; Self-control failure

Definition

Self-regulatory fatigue refers to the temporary depletion of individuals' capacity for self-control. In a state of self-regulatory fatigue, individuals find it harder to resist making impulsive purchases, inhibit prejudice, or regulate their own emotions (an effect often termed "ego-depletion"). Self-regulatory fatigue arises from the extended use of self-regulation, which is thought to be a limited resource.

Description

Limited Self-Regulatory Capacity
Self-regulatory fatigue describes the temporary impairment in self-control performance after prior exertions of self-control (an effect also referred to as "ego-depletion"). The strength model of self-regulation draws the analogy between muscular fatigue and self-regulatory fatigue. Muscular fatigue occurs after repeated or prolonged acts of physical exertion, where longer or more effortful exertions lead to a greater experience of fatigue. Similarly, persistent acts of self-regulation, such as the overriding of impulses, result in a mental fatigue, limiting the effectiveness of further regulatory efforts. Again, longer or more effortful exertions of self-regulation lead to a greater experience of self-regulatory fatigue. Like muscular fatigue, rest and recuperation are hypothesized to restore the temporary depletion in self-regulatory strength.

It is important to distinguish between subjective and actual self-regulatory fatigue, although the two can coincide. Self-regulatory persistence and ego-depletion is associated with the physiological indications and subjective feelings of fatigue such as somnolence and decreased attention. Subjective fatigue is thought to mediate between exertions of self-regulation and subsequent decrements in self-regulatory ability. However, subjective fatigue – or the belief that one is fatigued – can have effects that are independent of actual fatigue. Despite experiencing prior effortful self-regulation, individuals perceiving themselves to be low in fatigue can engage in subsequent regulation more effectively than those perceiving themselves to be high in fatigue. A second contributing factor to the state of self-regulatory fatigue is motivation. Individuals may cease persistence at self-regulation if they believe that the effort exerted during self-regulation costs more than the outcome of self-regulation is worth. Self-regulatory fatigue is, therefore, not merely a state of exhaustion in which the individual is willing to engage a task and yet unable to persist but can also lead to acquiescence – the person willfully consents to relax self-control because they are not motivated to do otherwise.

Measuring Self-Regulatory Fatigue
The strength model poses that exertions of self-regulation draw from a limited self-regulatory capacity. However, this hypothesis of capacity has proven difficult to objectively measure. A range of cognitive or behavioral tests have been implemented to measure self-regulatory fatigue. Common examples include persistence at impossible (e.g., unsolvable puzzles) or unpleasant (e.g., consuming unpleasant drinks, cold pressor) tasks; response time or errors made in inhibition tasks (modified Stroop task, go/no-go); resisting temptation (limiting alcohol consumption); and regulating facial expression. In such cases, the primary means for measuring self-regulatory fatigue is a comparison of

performance at a self-regulatory task between individuals in a depleted state (those having exerted prior self-regulation) against individuals in a non-depleted state (those having completed a difficult task such as complex math problems that does not require self-regulation). As a result, self-regulatory fatigue and the presence of a limited resource are only measured indirectly; thus the relationship between subjective fatigue, motivation, and self-regulatory fatigue remains unclear.

Attempts at more direct and biological measures of self-regulatory fatigue have been made. Blood glucose levels have been reported to show a correlation with self-regulatory fatigue, suggesting a positive link between available caloric energy to the brain and available mental resource. However, glucose supply itself is not thought to be a causal link to self-regulatory fatigue, as glucose dynamics are too small to account for differences between depleted and non-depleted states. The strength model for self-regulatory fatigue has more recently been revised to incorporate a monitor of potentially available (rather than direct levels of) glucose as a possible driver of self-regulatory fatigue. Alternative physiological measures, such as glycogen store levels and heart rate variability, have also been suggested as means of measuring resource availability and self-regulatory fatigue.

Overcoming Self-Regulatory Fatigue

While the primary means to counteract self-regulatory fatigue are rest and recuperation, the effects of self-regulatory fatigue may be moderated or counteracted by a number of other means. The induction of a positive mood by others, including humor and laughter, observation of others undergoing successful self-regulation, salient social goals, primed ideas of success, a broadened mindset through self-affirmation, external attribution of the causes of depletion, perception of a low state of fatigue, simultaneous tensing or firming of muscles, and monetary incentives all serve to encourage individuals to persist at self-regulation. However, in many cases, this increased persistence is considered to deprioritize conservation of remaining resources rather than a reduction in fatigue. Poor performance in an unannounced third self-regulatory task after the standard two-task design often indicates that depleted participants have persisted beyond their typical point of self-regulatory fatigue rather than overcoming fatigue. Further interventions, such as the prior practice of self-regulation tasks or the formulation of implementation intentions ("if... then...") plans), serve to encourage persistence at self-regulation through moderating the effort required to expend during successful self-regulation.

Wider Implications of Self-Regulatory Fatigue

Self-regulatory fatigue has been implicated in a number of problems for both the individual and society. While warnings about substance abuse, risky sexual practice, and unhealthy diets are extensively promoted, there equally exists a widespread failure of individuals to adhere to these guidelines or rules. Experimental studies such as those examining alcohol or unhealthy food consumption demonstrate that these behaviors are affected by both self-regulatory fatigue and individuals' chronic tendencies. A chronic tendency that is typically suppressed, such as a high temptation to drink alcohol, becomes more likely to shape behavior when an individual is depleted. In contrast, an individual with low trait temptation to drink alcohol might show no change in alcohol consumption when depleted because it is not necessary to engage in self-regulation. Further examples of behaviors affected by self-regulatory fatigue include impulsive or overspending, emotional regulation such as anger management, interpersonal interaction, self-presentation or impression formation, and stereotype suppression.

Cross-References

▶ Ego-Depletion
▶ Fatigue
▶ Limited Resource
▶ Self-Control
▶ Self-Report Inventory
▶ Working Memory

References and Further Reading

Baddeley, A. (2007). *Chapter 13: Working memory, thought and action*. New York: Oxford University Press.

Baumeister, R. F., & Vohs, K. D. (2018). Strength model of self-regulation as limited resource: Assessment, controversies, update. In *Self-regulation and self-control* (pp. 78–128). New York: Routledge.

Baumeister, R. F., Heatherton, T., & Tice, D. M. (1994). *Losing control: How and why people fail at self-regulation*. London: Academic.

Baumeister, R. F., Gailliot, M., DeWall, N., & Oaten, M. (2006). Self-regulation and personality: How interventions increase regulatory success, and how depletion moderates the effects of traits on behavior. *Journal of Personality, 74*, 1773–1802.

Baumeister, R. F., Tice, D. M., & Vohs, K. D. (2018). The strength model of self-regulation: Conclusions from the second decade of willpower research. *Perspectives on Psychological Science, 13*(2), 141–145.

Beedie, C. J., & Lane, A. M. (2012). The role of glucose in self-control: Another look at the evidence and an alternative conceptualization. *Personality and Social Psychology Review, 16*(2), 143–153.

Gailliot, M. (2008). Unlocking the energy dynamics of executive functioning: Linking executive functioning to brain glycogen. *Perspectives on Psychological Science, 3*, 245–263.

Self-Report

Jane Upton
Department of Psychology, William James College, Newton, MA, USA

Synonyms

Self-report inventory

Definition

Self-report includes an individual's reports about what they are feeling, what they are doing, and what they recall happening in the past (Stone et al. 2009).

These are captured by validated self-report questionnaires, of which there are many. Indeed, one of the challenges facing behavioral medicine is the bewildering variety of measurement instruments (Dekker 2009). Although validated, the limitations of self-report questionnaires are that the researcher is dependent on the research participant to be completely truthful and unbiased and to be able to accurately remember details.

References and Further Reading

Dekker, J. (2009). Measurement instruments in behavioral medicine. *International Journal of Behavioural Medicine, 16*, 89–90. https://doi.org/10.1007/s12529-009-9049-1.

Stone, A., Turkkan, J., Bachrach, C., Jobe, J., Kuftzman, H., Cain, V., et al. (2009). *The science of self-report*. Taylor & Francis e-library. Retrieved from http://books.google.co.uk/books

Self-Report Inventory

► Self-Report

Self-Reported Patient Outcome Measure

► Health Assessment Questionnaire

Self-Respect

► Self-esteem

Self-Schema

► Self-Identity

Self-System

► Self-Identity

Self-Tracking

▶ Quantified Self

Self-Treatment

▶ Self-medication

Seligman, Martin

Stephanie Ann Hooker
Department of Psychology, University of Colorado Denver, Denver, CO, USA

Biographical Information

Dr. Martin Seligman

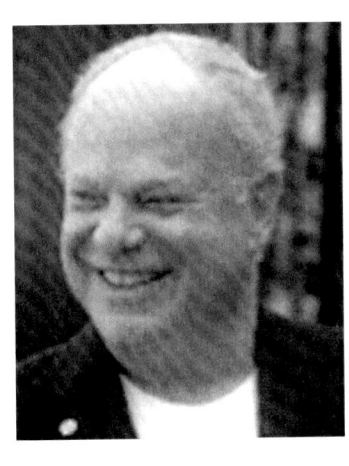

Martin E. P. Seligman was born August 12, 1942, in Albany, NY. He received his A.B.. from Princeton University in 1964 and his Ph.D. in Psychology from the University of Pennsylvania in 1967 (Shah n.d.). After receiving his doctorate, he began his career as an assistant professor at Cornell University in Ithaca, NY. He soon returned to the University of Pennsylvania where he was promoted to associate professor and to professor of Psychology and then to director of the Clinical Training Program. He is currently the Zellerbach Family Professor of Psychology in the Department of Psychology at the University of Pennsylvania and the director of the Positive Psychology Center (University of Pennsylvania 2007). Early in his career, Seligman studied depression and defined the theory of learned helplessness and pessimism. His worked progressed from a focus on pessimism to optimism, and hence from depression to happiness. He believed that psychology focused too much on mental illness and not enough on health and flourishing; thus, he pioneered the field of positive psychology in 2000 (Seligman and Csikzentmihalyi 2000).

Major Accomplishments

In 1996, Seligman was elected president of the American Psychological Association (APA) by the largest vote in history. As president, he chose the theme of positive psychology and called for an integration of human flourishing, strengths, and virtues into the science and practice of psychology. He noted that psychology and psychiatry had focused primarily on mental illness (e.g., depression, suffering, victimization, anger, anxiety), but had forgotten positive forms of mental health (e.g., positive emotion, engagement, positive relationships, purpose, accomplishment) (Seligman 2008). His mission in the APA paralleled his personal mission to promote positive psychology.

In 2008, he began his next mission: to promote a new movement in psychology, positive health (Seligman 2008). He argued that people desire more than just the absence of suffering and pain; they desire well-being and flourishing that in itself can be protective against mental illness and disease. Thus, he defined positive health as the subjective, biological, and functional realms that can predict positive aspects of mental health, e.g., longevity, positive emotion, prognosis, and suggested areas for which positive health could be incorporated into studies of well-being and illness.

Seligman has published 20 books and over 200 articles on motivation and personality, including best sellers such as *Learned Optimism*, *Authentic Happiness*, and *The Optimistic Child*

(Shah n.d.). He is one of the most often-cited psychologists and the thirteenth most likely name to appear in a general psychology textbook (TED Conferences LLC 2008). Seligman also created the Masters of Applied Positive Psychology program at the University of Pennsylvania. Many institutions, including the National Institute on Aging, the National Science Foundation, and the National Institute of Mental Health, have supported his research. He has received numerous awards, including two Distinguished Scientific Contribution awards from the APA, the William James Fellow Award, and the James McKeen Cattell Fellow Award from the Association for Psychological Science, the MERIT Award from the National Institute of Mental Health, the Laurel Award of the American Association for Applied Psychology and Prevention, and the Lifetime Achievement Award of the Society for Research in Psychopathology.

Cross-References

▶ Learned Helplessness
▶ Optimism
▶ Positive Psychology

References and Readings

Seligman, M. E. P. (1975). *Helplessness: On depression, development, and death.* San Francisco: W. H. Freeman.
Seligman, M. E. P. (1990). *Learned optimism.* New York: Knopf.
Seligman, M. E. P. (1993). *What you can change and what you can't: The complete guide to successful self-improvement.* New York: Knopf.
Seligman, M. E. P. (1996). *The optimistic child: Proven program to safeguard children from depression and build lifelong resilience.* New York: Houghton Mifflin.
Seligman, M. E. P. (2002). *Authentic happiness: Using the new positive psychology to realize your potential for lasting fulfillment.* New York: Free Press.
Seligman, M. (2008). Positive health. *Applied Psychology. An International Review, 57,* 3–18.
Seligman, M., & Csikzentmihalyi, M. (2000). Positive psychology: An introduction. *American Psychologist, 55,* 5–14.
Shah, N. (n.d.). *Seligman, Martin E. P.* Retrieved 15 July 2011 from http://www.pabook.libraries.psu.edu/palitmap/bios/Seligman_Martin.html

TED Conferences, LLC. (2008). *Speakers: Martin Seligman: Psychologist.* Retrieved 15 July 2011 from http://www.ted.com/index.php/speakers/martin_seligman.html
The Trustees of the University of Pennsylvania. (2006). *Authentic happiness.* http://www.authentichappiennes.sas.upenn.edu/seligman.aspx
University of Pennsylvania. (2007). *Positive psychology center: Seligman bio.* Retrieved 15 July 2011 from http://www.ppc.sas.upenn.edu/bio.htm

Selye, Hans

Adrienne Stauder
Institute of Behavioural Sciences, Semmelweis University Budapest, Budapest, Hungary

Biographical Information

Dr. Hans Selye 1973

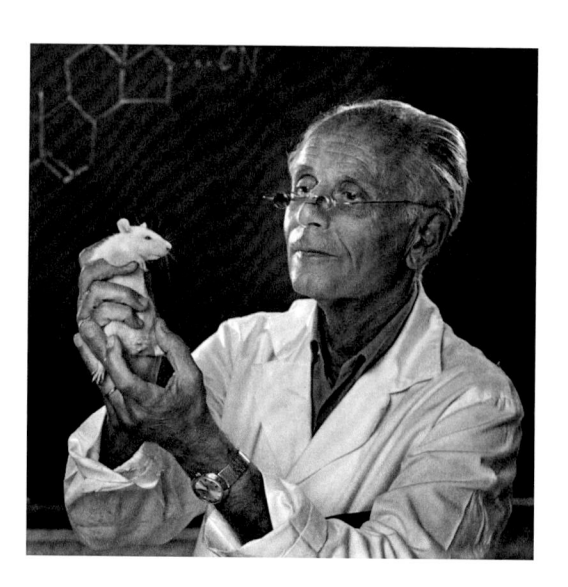

Photo by Yousuf Karsh

Hans Selye was born on January 26, 1907, in Vienna, Austria. His mother Maria Felicitas Langbank was an Austrian, his father Hugo Selye was a Hungarian military surgeon, and his grandfather and great grandfather were family doctors. Selye completed his elementary and secondary school education in Komarno (Slovakia). Since 1924 he studied medicine in Prague, Rome, and Paris, and obtained his diploma at the German University of Prague in 1929. He started his research at the Institute of Experimental Pathology in Prague, and got his doctorate in biochemistry in 1931.

A Rockefeller Research Fellowship allowed Selye to continue his scientific career at the Department of Biochemical Hygiene of the Johns Hopkins University in Baltimore in 1931, and then from 1932 at the Department of Biochemistry of the McGill University in Montreal. He became lecturer then associate professor in biochemistry, and also in histology. He received Canadian citizenship in 1939, and became Doctor of Sciences in 1942. From 1945 to 1976 he directed the Institute of Experimental Medicine and Surgery (IMCE) at the University of Montreal, which gained international reputation under his leadership. After his retirement he remained active as founding president of the International Institute of Stress in Montreal (1976), and as co-founder of the Hans Selye Foundation (1979) until his death on October 15, 1982.

Selye held honorary doctorates from 18 universities, was a member of the Academy of Science of the Royal Society of Canada and 43 scientific societies, was an honorary citizen of many cities and countries, and received numerous high-ranking awards and distinctions. He was nominated for the Nobel Prize in physiology or medicine for 10 consecutive years (first in 1949), but he never received it. In 2006 he was inducted as a member of the Canadian Medical Hall of Fame.

Major Accomplishments

Selye is one of the most well-known, most productive scientists of the twentieth century. He wrote his name in the history of science by introducing the concept of stress. As a result of his work the word "stress" previously used in other contexts gained a physiological meaning and has been adopted in all languages. His research work had great impact in the field of endocrinology, physiology, biochemistry, epidemiology of chronic diseases, and behavioral medicine, not only on scientific thinking but also among lay people all around the world. Selye authored or coauthored 39 books and over 1,600 scientific articles, and his work has been estimated to have been cited in more than 300,000 scientific papers, although Somorjai (2007) could compile a list of only 800 of all his publications.

Selye's most important finding, the discovery of the stress syndrome, was accidental during his attempts to isolate a special female hormone from the placenta (Selye 1964, 1967b). The originality of his thinking was that he started to research the significance of the nonspecific reactions that he observed. His first short note describing "the nonspecific response to nocuous agents" was published in Nature in 1936, followed in the same year by a longer article in The British Journal of Experimental Pathology describing the General Adaptation Syndrome. In the following years, he systematically developed his comprehensive theory on stress (Selye 1950) and envisaged the existence of diseases of adaptation (Selye 1946).

His researches on steroids turned his interest to the inflammatory process (Selye 1943, 1949, 1965), then to the phenomena of calciphylaxis (Selye 1962) and of thrombohemorrhagy (Selye 1967a). Through these experiments he confirmed his hypothesis that diseases such as heart disease, rheumatoid arthritis, anaphylaxis, depression, autoimmune diseases, and Alzheimer disease are in fact all diseases of adaptation. Although his experiments were always on animals, over the years Selye became more and more interested in how his research results could be applied to medicine and to society. While his original definition of stress – "nonspecific response of the living organism to any stimuli, for example, effort, focused attention, pain, illness, failure, joy, success, that cause changes," – implied that the stressor can be either pleasant or unpleasant, since similar physiological/biochemical changes are produced, he later made the distinction between good stress (eustress) and bad stress (distress) (Selye 1974).

Selye expanded his model to include Perception, Conditioning Factors, and Coping Mechanisms. This so-called *Selye – Smith Conceptual Model of Stress Variables* served as theoretical basis to the comprehensive course "Stress Management for Optimal Health" offered by Selye's Institute first to health professionals and then to the lay public (Smith and Selye 1979). Selye proposed that stress education and stress management should be important elements of preventive medicine.

Research was a passion for Selye. He was very much interested in great discoveries, the history and psychology of science, and in personal characteristics of scientists. These topics appeared in his lectures, books, and also in his every day discussions. He emphasized that original ideas were the most important elements in research that must be tested and proved by well-designed experiments. He also gave special attention to research methodology. On one hand, he was reluctant to adapt complicated technological methods, and he emphasized in all forums that one always should try to view the entire organism in its complexity and not to get lost with tiny little details without considering how they relate to the whole organism (Selye 1967b). On the other hand he introduced new methods in experimental surgery (Selye et al. 1960). He also carefully selected his laboratory assistants based on their skillfulness.

Effective information processing was another key element of Selye's exceptional productivity. He systematically developed his library that became world famous. He worked out his own "Symbolic Shorthand System for Medicine and Physiology" (SSS) that was subsequently published and used until the start of the computer era (Selye and Mishra 1957). He also followed a very structured daily schedule at his Institute as well as in his private life (Selye 1964). Selye was also a charismatic teacher. He shared his knowledge and his devotion to science with his fellow workers and students, exerting a deep influence on their lives and careers. He invited talented young researchers from all over the world to work in his Institute. He also invited many world renowned professors (the so-called Claude Bernard Professors). Thus, young researchers had the opportunity to meet famous personalities. They not only delivered one or two lectures, but participated in daily routine of the Institute and at informal dinners and discussions at Selye's house. Selye also traveled over the world and very often he obtained the recognition of his audience not only by his research results and presentation style, but also by giving his lecture in the language of the respective country. He not only shared his experiences with the scientific community, but could transmit his knowledge about stress, the process of scientific research, and related subjects to the general lay population by writing several popular books such as The Stress of Life (1956), From Dream to Discovery (1964), In Vivo: The Case for Supramolecular Biology (1967b), and Stress without Distress (1974) that have been translated into many languages.

Selye's scientific heritage is formally maintained by the Hans Selye Foundation, Montreal, Canada, www.stresscanada.org.

Cross-References

▶ Coping
▶ Stress
▶ Stress: Appraisal and Coping

References and Readings

Berczi, I. Stress and disease: The contribution of Hans Selye to: Neuroimmune Biology. A personal reminiscence. Retrieved March 30, 2012 from http://home.cc.umanitoba.ca/~berczii/page2.htm

Selye, H. (1936a). A syndrome produced by diverse nocuous agents. *Nature, 138*, 32.

Selye, H. (1936b). Thymus and adrenals in the response of the organism to injuries and intoxications. *British Journal of Experimental Pathology, 17*, 234–248.

Selye, H. (1943). Morphological changes in the fowl following chronic overdosage with various steroids. *Journal of Morphology, 73*, 401.

Selye, H. (1946). The general adaptation syndrome and the diseases of adaptation. *Journal of Clinical Endocrinology, 6*, 117–230.

Selye, H. (1949). Effect of ACTH and cortisone upon an anaphylactoid reaction. *Canadian Medical Association Journal, 61*, 553–556.

Selye, H. (1950). *Stress*. Montreal: Acta.

Selye, H. (1956). *The stress of life*. New York: McGraw Hill.

Selye, H. (1962). *Calciphylaxis*. Chicago: University of Chicago Press.

Selye, H. (1964). *From dream to discovery*. New York: McGraw Hill.

Selye, H. (1965). *The mast cells.* Washington, DC: Butterworths.

Selye, H. (1967a). Experimental thrombohemorrhagic phenomena. *The American Journal of Cardiology, 20*(2), 153–160.

Selye, H. (1967b). *In vivo: The case for supramolecular biology.* New York: Livesight.

Selye, H. (1974). *Stress without distress* (p. 364). Philadelphia: Lippincott.

Selye, H. (1979). *The stress of my life: A scientist's memory.* New York: Van Nostrand Reinhold.

Selye, H., & Mishra, R. K. (1957). Symbolic shorthand system for medicine and physiology. *Federation Proceedings, 16*(3), 704–706.

Selye, H., Bajusz, E., Grasso, S., & Mendell, P. (1960). Simple techniques for the surgical occlusion of coronary vessels in the rat. *Angiology, 11*, 398–407.

Smith, M. J. T., & Selye, H. (1979). Stress: Reducing the negative effects of stress. *The American Journal of Nursing, 11*, 1953–1955.

Somorjai, N. (2007). Bibliography Hans Selye. Retrieved March 30, 2012 from http://www.selyesociety.hu/pdf/Selye_bibliography_2011.pdf.

Stauder, A., & Kovács, P. B. (Eds.). (2007). *Stress. A memorial book on the birth centenary of Hans Selye.* Budapest: Downtown Artists' Society.

The American Institute of Stress: Hans Selye and The Birth of Stress. Retrieved March 30, 2012 from http://www.stress.org/hans.htm.

Université de Montréal: Hans Selye: Une vie en images. Retrieved March 30, 2012 from http://www.archiv.umontreal.ca/exposition/Hans_Selye/index.html

SEM

▶ Structural Equation Modeling (SEM)

Semenogelase

▶ Prostate-Specific Antigen (PSA)

Seminin

▶ Prostate-Specific Antigen (PSA)

Seminoma

▶ Cancer, Testicular

Senescence

▶ Immunosenescence

Senior

▶ Elderly

Sense of Coherence

▶ Salutogenesis

Sense of Coherence – Measurement

▶ Resilience: Measurement

Sense of Self

▶ Self-Identity

Separation

▶ Divorce and Health

SEPs

▶ Needle Exchange Programs

Sera

▶ Serum

Serious Games

▶ Health Gaming

Serostatus: Seronegative and Seropositive

Angela White
Department of Psychology, University of Connecticut, Storrs, CT, USA

Synonyms

HIV status

Definition

Serostatus refers to the extent to which HIV antibodies can be detected in an individual's serum. This detection is an indicator of HIV infection.

Description

An individual is considered to be seronegative when the amount of HIV antibodies are not sufficient enough to be detected using an antibody test, although indication of HIV infection can be determined through the use of more sensitive culture, antigen, and viral gene detection techniques (Fultz 1989; Kaslow and Francis 1989; O'Malley 1988). Individuals who are seronegative may not produce HIV antibodies for months or year after HIV infection, or they may stop producing these antibodies after some unknown time interval. There is a long incubation period associated with being seronegative; individuals may not show physical symptoms associated with HIV/AIDS for several months or years after the initial HIV infection. As such, it is difficult to determine the ability of seronegative individuals to spread HIV (Kaslow and Francis 1989).

An individual is considered to be seropositive when HIV antibodies are detected on a HIV antibody test (Fultz 1989; O'Malley 1988). Individuals who have detectable HIV antibodies are considered to be "HIV-positive." The period of time between HIV infection and seroconversion (the presence of detectable antibodies in the serum) may range from 2 weeks to 3 months; this period of time is referred to as the "window period" (Stine 2003).

Some individuals who are seropositive, or "HIV-positive," exhibit symptoms associated with an acute mononucleosis-like syndrome immediately after being infected with HIV. This syndrome has been known as acute HIV syndrome or acute retroviral syndrome; its symptoms include sweats, lethargy, headaches, muscle aches, fever, and sore throat (Fultz 1989; Stine 2003). Not all seropositive individuals experience this syndrome. Other seropositive individuals remain asymptomatic for several weeks. All seropositive individuals, whether symptomatic or asymptomatic, are infected with HIV and can infect others through blood and genital secretions and by transmission from mother to fetus (Fultz 1989; O'Malley 1988). In 2001, the Center for Disease Control and Prevention proposed the Serostatus Approach to Fighting the HIV Epidemic (SAFE) program to encourage awareness that individuals may be HIV-positive even if they appear to be outwardly healthy. This program attempted to reduce the spread of HIV by extending prevention services and improving treatment adherence for individuals with a seropositive status and by providing training to individuals who give these services (Normand et al. 1995; Stine 2003).

Being notified of a seropositive status is associated with behavioral and psychological changes. For instance, individuals who receive a positive test result may reduce their high-risk sexual activity. However, they also may experience increased stress and depression. Also, these individuals may feel compelled to disclose their HIV status to family, friends, and potential sexual parents. Some barriers associated with the disclosing HIV status include the disclosure of a stigmatized identity (such as being gay or an intravenous drug user), the fear of losing health insurance or employment, and the concern of being stigmatized by family and friends (Stall et al. 1989).

References and Readings

Black, P. H., & Levy, E. M. (1988). The HIV seropositive state and progression to AIDS: An overview of factors promoting progression. In P. O'Malley (Ed.), *The AIDS epidemic: Private rights and the public interest* (pp. 97–107). Boston: Beacon.

Fultz, P. (1989). The biology of human immunodeficiency viruses. In R. A. Kaslow & D. P. Francis (Eds.), *The epidemiology of AIDS: Expression, occurrence, and control of human immunodeficiency virus type 1 infection* (pp. 3–17). New York: Oxford University Press.

Kaslow, R. A., & Francis, D. P. (1989). Epidemiology: General considerations. In R. A. Kaslow & D. P. Francis (Eds.), *The epidemiology of AIDS: Expression, occurrence, and control of human immunodeficiency virus type 1 infection* (pp. 117–135). New York: Oxford University Press.

Normand, J., Vlahov, D., & Moses, L. E. (1995). *Preventing HIV transmission: The role of sterile needles and bleach*. Washington, DC: National Academy Press.

O'Malley, P. (1988). *The AIDS epidemic: Private rights and the public interest*. Boston: Beacon.

Stall, R., Coates, T. J., Mandel, J. S., Morales, E. S., & Sorensen, J. L. (1989). Behavioral factors and intervention. In R. A. Kaslow & D. P. Francis (Eds.), *The epidemiology of AIDS: Expression, occurrence, and control of human immunodeficiency virus type 1 infection* (pp. 266–281). New York: Oxford University Press.

Stine, G. J. (2003). *AIDS update 2003: An annual overview of acquired immune deficiency syndrome*. Upper Saddle River: Prentice Hall.

Serotonin

Marc D. Gellman
Behavioral Medicine Research Center,
Department of Psychology, University of Miami,
Miami, FL, USA

Definition

Serotonin (5-hydroxytryptamine or 5-HT) is a neurotransmitter that is particularly important in central nervous system modulation.

Description

Serotonin (5-hydroxytryptamine or 5-HT) is synthesized from the amino acid tryptophan. It is a major neurotransmitter, considered an indolamine monoamine, that is particularly important in central nervous system modulation, especially in the brain. Serotonin is also found in peripheral sites and regarded as a neuromodulator. In the periphery, serotonin is found in enteric neurons, part of the autonomic nervous system that governs the functions of the gastrointestinal tract. Serotonin is also found in blood platelets and cells of the gut.

In the brain serotonin plays an important neuromodulatory role involved in the regulation of mood, appetite, and sleep and in the cognitive functions of learning and memory.

Serotonin plays an important role in mental processes and has been implicated in many psychiatric disorders. Modulation of serotonin at synapses is thought to be a major action of several classes of pharmacological antidepressants, including selective serotonin reuptake inhibitors (SSRIs). It is uncertain whether low serotonin levels contribute to depression or if depression causes a fall in serotonin levels.

Cross-References

▶ Antidepressant Medications
▶ Central Nervous System
▶ Depression: Treatment
▶ Sleep

References and Further Reading

Pilowsky, P. (Ed.). (2019). *Serotonin: The mediator that spans evolution.* London: Academic. https://doi.org/10.1016/C2013-0-14440-6.

Serotonin Transporter Gene

Anett Mueller[1] and Turhan Canli[2]
[1]Department of Psychology, State University of New York at Stony Brook, Stony Brook, NY, USA
[2]Department of Psychology, Stony Brook University Psychology B-214, Stony Brook, NY, USA

Synonyms

SERT; SLC6A4 (solute carrier family 6, member 4)

Definition

In humans, the gene that encodes for the serotonin transporter is called the serotonin transporter gene which is modulated by the functional serotonin-transporter-linked polymorphism (5-HTTLPR), a variable number of tandem repeats in the 5′ promoter region.

Description

The neurotransmitter *serotonin* (5-hydroxytryptamine, 5-HT) is probably best known for its modulation of neural activity and the modulation of various neuropsychological processes such as mood, perception, emotion, and cognition. Serotonin is also implicated in the pathogenesis of many psychiatric and neurological disorders and furthermore, it is involved in brain development and plasticity of brain areas related to cognitive and emotional processes (Berger et al. 2009; Trevor et al. 2010). Additionally, the serotonin transporter is considered to be the initial site of action of broadly used antidepressant drugs, such as selective serotonin uptake inhibitors (SSRIs), and several potentially neurotoxic compounds.

Following neuronal stimulation, serotonin is transmitted into the synaptic cleft and then binds to receptors on the membrane of the postsynaptic neuron. Serotonin is then removed from the synaptic cleft via special proteins, called *transporters*. Serotonin transporters are located in the serotonin neuron; they transport serotonin from the synaptic cleft back into the presynaptic neuron in both the brain and many peripheral tissues terminals. In humans, the gene that codes for the serotonin transporter contains a number of common variants (polymorphisms), including the serotonin-transporter-linked promoter region (*5-HTTLPR*) of the serotonin transporter gene (SLC6A4). This polymorphism is located upstream of the transcription start site on the long arm of the 17th chromosome (17q11.1-q12). The majority of alleles are composed of either fourteen ("short" or "*S*" allele) or sixteen repeated ("long" or "*L*" for allele) units, which differentially modulate on the expression and function of 5-HTT. The short form of *5-HTTLPR* has been associated with a reduced transcription of the 5-HTT gene, which leads to a decreased 5-HTT expression and availability and also a reduced 5-HT uptake (Lesch et al. 1996). In addition to the *S* and *L* alleles, there is an A > G single nucleotide polymorphism (SNP), a single nucleotide variation in a genetic sequence, upstream of the repetitive region that comprises the *5-HTTLPR*. The derived L_G allele has been associated with decreased 5-HTT transcription relative to the L_A allele. The frequency of *5-HTTLPR* alleles can vary substantially across ethnic groups, thus, showing population stratification.

The short allele variant of *5-HTTLPR* was first reported to be associated with personality traits such as neuroticism and harm avoidance (Lesch et al.,). Subsequent work has reported *5-HTTLPR* allelic variation to a wide range of phenotypes including aggression, anxiety, and affective disorders. Most studies have implied that *5-HTTLPR* has only a moderate impact on these behavioral predispositions of 3–4% or less of the total variance. The less active *S* allele has been associated, either by itself or in interaction with adverse life events, with abnormal levels of anxiety, fear, and depression. Despite the association between presence of the *S* allele and psychopathology, studies of patient responsiveness to SSRIs suggest no strong link between *5-HTTLPR* genotype and drug effectiveness.

However, if the *S* allele produced only deleterious consequences, evolutionary pressures should have led to its removal from the gene pool. Thus, more recent studies have begun to accrue evidence for favorable phenotypes associated with the *S* allele. For example, studies revealed an improved performance in (social) cognition in individuals with the *S* allele (Homberg and Lesch 2010). On the other hand, the *L* allele, originally viewed as the protective allele, also has negative associations with at-risk phenotypes, such as cardiovascular health (e.g., increased cardiovascular reactivity and greater probability of myocardial infarction) (Fumeron et al. 2002; Williams et al. 2001) or certain psychiatric diseases (e.g., psychosis or posttraumatic stress disorder, PTSD) (Goldberg et al. 2009; Grabe et al. 2009). In addition to allelic association on observed phenotypes, there is growing evidence for gene-by-environment (G x E) interactions, suggesting that individuals possessing the *S* allele are predisposed to an increased risk for major depression or suicidal ideation as a function of early life stress. The first evidence for this G x E interaction in humans was presented by Caspi et al. (2003) who investigated more than 800 individuals over 23 years and found that life stress and depression was moderated by the *5-HTTLPR* genotype. Individuals with the *S* allele showed a higher probability of depressive symptoms, diagnosis of depression and suicidal attempts when exposed to stressful life events. However, replication studies have shown somewhat inconsistent results and thus, these findings are still a matter of debate. In addition to behavioral studies, non-invasive functional MRI (fMRI) studies have also shown that structural and functional characteristics of neural circuits involved in emotion and cognition can be moderated by the interaction of life stress and 5-HTTLPR genotype.

Most recently, investigators have come to recognize the potential gene regulatory role of epigenetic mechanisms in mediating environmental effects on brain function and on behavior (Rutter et al. 2006). For example, it has been argued that environmental influences bear the potential to persistently modify neuronal units during early development by epigenetic programming of emotionality (Weaver et al. 2004; Weaver 2007). This has first been shown with respect to the glucocorticoid receptor gene and individual differences in rodents' stress reactivity: variations in maternal care have been shown to modify the expression of genes that regulate behavioral and endocrine responses to stress and hippocampus synaptic development. Thus, alterations of particular genomic regions within the 5-HTT in response to varying environmental conditions might serve well as a major source of variation in biological and behavioral phenotypes. Indeed, there is now emerging evidence linking *5-HTTLPR* genotype to individual differences in epigenetic methylation (Philibert et al. 2007, 2008).

Studies that use biological endophenotypes, such as stress-induced HPA activation, might be more strongly associated with a specific polymorphism than a psychiatric disorder (Uher and McGuffin 2010). However, given the fact that brain serotonin and more specifically *5-HTTLPR* shows pleiotropic behavioral effects, we need to learn and understand more about the biological function and how *5-HTTLPR* becomes associated with various different phenotypes. The modulation of these multiple behavioral processes might very likely be regulated by multiple serotonin receptors that are expressed in multiple brain regions. In summary, *5-HTTLPR* seems to play an important, though not yet fully understood, role in behavioral medicine. We will likely gain new serotonergic drugs and disease treatments as well as a more thorough understanding of complexity of human biology from this research.

Cross-References

▶ Depression
▶ Gene-Environment Interaction
▶ Serotonin

References and Readings

Berger, M., Gray, J. A., & Roth, B. L. (2009). The expanded biology of serotonin. *Annual Review of Medicine, 60*, 355–366.

Caspi, A., Sugden, K., Moffitt, T. E., Taylor, A., Craig, I. W., Harrington, H., et al. (2003). Influence of life stress on depression: moderation by a polymorphism in the 5-HTT gene. *Science, 301*(5631), 386–389.

Fumeron, F., Betoulle, D., Nicaud, V., Evans, A., Kee, F., Ruidavets, J. B., et al. (2002). Serotonin transporter gene polymorphism and myocardial infarction: Etude Cas-Temoins de l'Infarctus du Myocarde (ECTIM). *Circulation, 105*(25), 2943–2945.

Goldberg, T. E., Kotov, R., Lee, A. T., Gregersen, P. K., Lencz, T., Bromet, E., et al. (2009). The serotonin transporter gene and disease modification in psychosis: Evidence for systematic differences in allelic directionality at the 5-HTTLPR locus. *Schizophrenia Research, 111*(1–3), 103–108.

Grabe, H. J., Spitzer, C., Schwahn, C., Marcinek, A., Frahnow, A., Barnow, S., et al. (2009). Serotonin transporter gene (SLC6A4) promoter polymorphisms and the susceptibility to posttraumatic stress disorder in the general population. *The American Journal of Psychiatry, 166*(8), 926–933.

Homberg, J. R., & Lesch, K. P. (2010). Looking on the bright side of serotonin transporter gene variation. *Biological Psychiatry, 69*, 513–519.

Lesch, K. P., Bengel, D., Heils, A., Sabol, S. Z., Greenberg, B. D., Petri, S., et al. (1996). Association of anxiety-related traits with a polymorphism in the serotonin transporter gene regulatory region. *Science, 274*(5292), 1527–1531.

Philibert, R., Madan, A., Andersen, A., Cadoret, R., Packer, H., & Sandhu, H. (2007). Serotonin transporter mRNA levels are associated with the methylation of an upstream CpG island. *American Journal of Medical Genetics. Part B, Neuropsychiatric Genetics, 144B*(1), 101–105.

Philibert, R. A., Sandhu, H., Hollenbeck, N., Gunter, T., Adams, W., & Madan, A. (2008). The relationship of 5HTT (SLC6A4) methylation and genotype on mRNA expression and liability to major depression and alcohol dependence in subjects from the Iowa Adoption Studies. *American Journal of Medical Genetics. Part B, Neuropsychiatric Genetics, 147B*(5), 543–549.

Rutter, M., Moffitt, T. E., & Caspi, A. (2006). Gene-environment interplay and psychopathology: Multiple varieties but real effects. *Journal of Child Psychology and Psychiatry, 47*(3–4), 226–261.

Trevor, A. J., Katzung, B. G., & Masters, S. B. (2010). *Katzung and Trevor's pharmacology examination and board review* (9th ed.). New York: McGraw-Hill Medical.

Uher, R., & McGuffin, P. (2010). The moderation by the serotonin transporter gene of environmental adversity in the etiology of depression: 2009 update. *Molecular Psychiatry, 15*(1), 18–22.

Weaver, I. C. (2007). Epigenetic programming by maternal behavior and pharmacological intervention. Nature versus nurture: Let's call the whole thing off. *Epigenetics, 2*(1), 22–28.

Weaver, I. C., Cervoni, N., Champagne, F. A., D'Alessio, A. C., Sharma, S., Seckl, J. R., et al. (2004). Epigenetic programming by maternal behavior. *Nature Neuroscience, 7*(8), 847–854.

Williams, R. B., Marchuk, D. A., Gadde, K. M., Barefoot, J. C., Grichnik, K., Helms, M. J., et al. (2001). Central nervous system serotonin function and cardiovascular responses to stress. *Psychosomatic Medicine, 63*(2), 300–305.

SERT

▶ Serotonin Transporter Gene

Sertraline

▶ Selective Serotonin Reuptake Inhibitors (SSRIs)

Serum

Briain O. Hartaigh
School of Sport and Exercise Sciences,
The University of Birmingham, Edgbaston,
Birmingham, UK

Synonyms

Antiserum; Sera

Definition

Serum is blood plasma with the coagulatory proteins removed. It is a clear, pale-yellow, thin, and sticky fluid that moistens the surface of serous membranes or that is secreted by such membranes when they become inflamed. In blood, serum is obtained after coagulation, upon separating whole blood into its solid and liquid components. This is achieved whereby blood is drawn from the subject and is allowed to naturally form a blood clot. After blood is allowed to clot and stand, a centrifuge is used to extract the red blood cells and the blood clot, which contains platelets and fibrinogens. In practice, blood serum is used in numerous diagnostic tests as well as blood typing.

Cross-References

▶ Antibodies
▶ Antigens

References and Further Reading

Abbas, A. K., & Lichtman, A. H. (2004). *Basic immunology: Functions and disorders of the immune system* (2nd ed.). Philadelphia: Saunders.

Service Attendance

▶ Religious Ritual

Sex

▶ Sexual Behavior

Sex Hormones

▶ Estrogen

Sexual Activity

▶ Sexual Behavior

Sexual Behavior

Jennifer L. Brown
Department of Behavioral Sciences and Health Education, Emory University School of Public Health, Atlanta, GA, USA

Synonyms

Sex; Sexual activity

Definition

There is a diverse array of activities that can be classified as sexual behavior: masturbation, oral-genital stimulation (oral sex), penile-vaginal intercourse (vaginal sex), and anal stimulation or anal intercourse. Sexual behaviors may also include activities to arouse the sexual interest of others or attract partners. Individuals engage in sexual behaviors for a variety of reasons, differ in their acceptability based on societal norms, and change across the lifespan.

Description

What is Sexual Behavior: Types of Sexual Behaviors

Sexual behavior includes a wide variety of activities individuals engage in to express their sexuality (Crooks and Baur 2008). Abstinence and celibacy are terms used for individuals who do not engage in certain or any sexual behaviors. Kissing and touching are sexual behaviors that stimulate the erogenous zones of one's partner. Masturbation is a sexual behavior referring to stimulation of one's genitals to create sexual pleasure. Individuals may also engage in oral stimulation of a partner's genitals; terms used to describe oral-genital stimulation include: oral sex (referring broadly to oral-genital stimulation), cunnilingus (oral stimulation of the vulva), and fellatio (oral stimulation of the penis). Anal stimulation includes either touching around the anus or penile insertion in the anus (often referred to as anal sex). Penile-vaginal intercourse involves insertion of the penis into a female's vagina; this behavior too has a variety of other synonymous terms (e.g., vaginal sex, coitus). The frequency that these and other sexual behaviors are engaged in has enormous individual variability and may differ based upon many factors (e.g., social acceptability, age).

Sexual Behavior: The Role of Societal Norms

Societal norms for acceptable sexual behaviors differ across cultures. Paraphilia refers to less common sexual behaviors within a given society or culture; an example of such behavior is a fetish. In some cultures, the nature of the relationship affects which behaviors are deemed acceptable. For instance, sexual behavior may be deemed appropriate only within the context of marriage. Similarly, societal perspectives on sexual orientation may influence whether sexual behaviors are viewed as socially acceptable.

Reasons for Sexual Behavior Engagement

Individuals engage in sexual behaviors for a multitude of reasons. Sexual behavior may be engaged in to experience sexual pleasure, sexual arousal, or orgasm. Procreation or a desire for children may motivate sexual behavior. Sexual behaviors may also be used to earn money or acquire other goods or services; prostitution refers to the exchange of a sexual behavior for monetary or other compensation. Additionally, pornography may motivate engagement in sexual behaviors. Unfortunately, sexual behaviors also occur in nonconsensual or coerced contexts (e.g., rape) and in the form of abuse (e.g., child sexual abuse) or sexual exploitation (e.g., pedophilia). Sexual behavior engagement may also have unintended consequences (e.g., unplanned pregnancy) or pose health risks associated with the acquisition of sexually transmitted diseases, including human immunodeficiency virus (HIV).

Developmental Perspectives on Sexual Behavior Engagement

Engagement in sexual activity changes across one's lifespan, and there is considerable variation in sexual development (Crooks and Baur 2008). During childhood, sexual behaviors may include self-stimulation of the genitals or engagement in play that may be viewed as sexual in nature (e.g., "playing doctor" with a peer). Puberty typically occurs during adolescence and results in dramatic physical changes including the development of secondary sex characteristics. Adolescence is typically linked to increases in sexual activity, both self-stimulation behaviors and sexual behavior with partners. During adulthood, and as people age, there is considerable individual variation of sexual behavior engagement.

Cross-References

▶ Condom Use
▶ HIV Infection
▶ HIV Prevention
▶ Sexual Functioning
▶ Sexual Hookup
▶ Sexual Risk Behavior

References and Readings

Crooks, R., & Baur, K. (2008). *Our sexuality* (10th ed.). Pacific Grove: Thomson.

Sexual Dysfunction

▶ Sexual Functioning

Sexual Functioning

Robyn Fielder
Center for Health and Behavior, Syracuse University, Syracuse, NY, USA

Synonyms

Sexual dysfunction

Definition

Sexual functioning is characterized by absence of difficulty moving through the stages of sexual desire, arousal, and orgasm, as well as subjective satisfaction with the frequency and outcome of individual and partnered sexual behavior.

Description

Sexual functioning is an important aspect of quality of life. Our understanding of sexual functioning is influenced by not only the current state of medical knowledge but also the social values upheld in our culture. Healthy sexual functioning is characterized by a lack of pain or discomfort during sexual activity and a lack of physiological difficulty moving through the three-phase sexual response cycle of desire, arousal, and orgasm. In addition, sexual functioning is indicated by subjective feelings of satisfaction with the frequency of sexual desire and sexual behavior, as well as subjective pleasure during individual and partnered sexual activity.

Kaplan's three-phase model is the basis for current models of healthy sexual response. The desire phase consists of sexual fantasies and desire to engage in sexual behavior. The arousal phase involves subjective feelings of pleasure along with physiological changes conducive to sexual intercourse. Males experience penile tumescence and erection, and females experience pelvic vasocongestion and vaginal lubrication. The orgasm phase consists of peak feelings of sexual pleasure and a release of sexual tension. Males ejaculate semen, whereas females experience contractions of the outer vaginal wall; additionally, in both males and females, the anal sphincter contracts. Individuals may experience physiological and/or psychological difficulties at any or all of the three phases of sexual response. A resolution period, characterized by relaxation and, for males, a refractory period, follows orgasm.

Etiology of Sexual Dysfunction

The etiology of sexual problems is often a complex combination of biological/medical, psychological, and social factors. For example, the sexual dysfunction may be secondary to a chronic health condition or psychotropic medication. In other cases, performance anxiety, low mood, or previous traumatic experiences may impair sexual functioning. Moreover, conflicts within a relationship as well as within the larger sociocultural context may affect an individual's sexual functioning. Due to the variety of potential predisposing, precipitating, and maintaining factors, clinicians are encouraged to take a biopsychosocial approach to assessment and treatment of problems in sexual functioning.

Sexual Dysfunction Disorders

Consistent with the medical model of disease, most research and scholarship focuses on sexual dysfunction rather than healthy sexual functioning. The American Psychiatric Association's Diagnostic and Statistical Manual of Mental Disorders (2000) describes nine main disorders of sexual dysfunction, which are grouped into four categories: desire, arousal, orgasm, and pain. All nine disorders share some common diagnostic criteria: the dysfunction is persistent and recurrent; the dysfunction is not substance-induced, due to a general medical condition, or part of another Axis I mental disorder; and the dysfunction causes clinically significant distress or interpersonal difficulty. Sexual dysfunctions are also classified according to their onset (lifelong or acquired), context (generalized or situational), and etiology (due to psychological factors or due to combined psychological and medical factors). Additional diagnostic options include sexual dysfunction due to a general medical condition, substance-induced sexual dysfunction, and sexual dysfunction not otherwise specified.

Desire disorders are characterized by lack of interest in sex, absence of sexual fantasies and sexual behavior, or fear of sexual contact. In hypoactive sexual desire disorder, there is a low level of sexual fantasy and desire for sex. In sexual aversion disorder, genital sexual contact is feared and actively avoided.

Arousal disorders are characterized by difficulty attaining or maintaining sexual arousal. Male erectile disorder is the most researched type of sexual dysfunction and receives the most media attention, particularly since the advent of Sildenafil (Viagra) in 1998. Erectile dysfunction is the inability to maintain an erection adequate for sexual penetration until completion of sexual activity. Female sexual arousal disorder is the inability to attain or maintain vaginal lubrication until completion of sexual activity.

Orgasm disorders are characterized by delay in or absence of orgasm on one extreme, or, on the other extreme, by occurrence of orgasm before the individual wants. In female orgasmic disorder and male orgasmic disorder, orgasm is delayed or absent despite normal sexual arousal and sufficient sexual stimulation. Premature ejaculation describes the occurrence of ejaculation with minimal stimulation before, upon, or soon after penetration and before the individual wants to orgasm.

Sexual pain disorders are characterized by genital pain that is not due to a general medical condition. In dyspareunia, which affects both males and females, genital pain occurs during sex. In vaginismus, involuntary muscle spasms of the vagina prevent penetration or may cause pain if it is attempted.

Prevalence of Sexual Dysfunction

Epidemiological surveys suggest problems with sexual functioning are common among the general population. For example, prevalence rates of premature ejaculation, erectile dysfunction, and female orgasmic disorder are 5%, 5%, and 10%, respectively, among community samples (Wincze and Carey 2001). Symptoms that do not meet full diagnostic criteria for a sexual dysfunction disorder are likely much more common. Patients struggling with sexual health problems may be reluctant to seek medical consultation due to embarrassment or privacy concerns. Many health care providers are also uncomfortable discussing sexuality, so patients' sex-related questions and concerns may be neglected in clinical settings.

Assessment of Sexual Functioning

Clinicians are advised to employ multimethod assessment of sexual functioning by including medical, psychosocial, and psychophysiological components. All three perspectives provide valuable information that aids in diagnosing sexual dysfunction, hypothesizing the etiology of the problem, and developing an appropriate treatment plan.

A medical evaluation is an essential piece of the sexual functioning assessment. A general physical examination allows for biological causes (e.g., general medical conditions, such as diabetes or cancer, as well as other vascular, neurologic, or hormonal conditions) to be ruled out. A gynecological or urological exam ensures no anatomical complications. Physical symptoms, such as bleeding or pain, can also be addressed. Medical providers should attend to any notable medical history (e.g., surgeries) as well as any prescription medications or substance use that may affect sexual functioning.

For the psychosocial evaluation, an interview is essential to learn about the onset, frequency, intensity, and duration of the presenting complaint(s). In addition, clinicians should assess pertinent areas including family history, adolescence, significant relationships in adulthood, sexual history, and sexual abuse or trauma. Although an individual patient may present with sexual complaints, difficulties with sexual functioning are often better understood in the context of the individual's sexual relationship. In many cases (e.g., when working with a patient who is married or in a committed relationship), involving the patient's sexual partner in the psychosocial evaluation (with the patient's permission) facilitates a better resolution. It is often advisable to interview the patient's sexual partner separately to find out more about the presenting complaint. A joint interview with the patient and his or her partner also provides additional insight into the couple's interaction style, relationship quality, and non-sex-related problems that may cause interpersonal tension. For some patients, self-administered questionnaires may be used to supplement the psychosocial interview. Questionnaires may provide an easier method whereby to disclose sensitive information compared to a face-to-face interview.

The third potential component of the evaluation is psychophysiological assessment. Depending on the presenting complaint, psychophysiological measures can be quite helpful in differential diagnosis. For example, nocturnal penile tumescence is the gold standard for differential diagnosis for male patients with erectile dysfunction. Inability to obtain erections during sleep indicates a medical cause, whereas ability to maintain erections during sleep suggests a psychosocial cause.

Treatment of Sexual Dysfunction

Often the first therapeutic intervention occurs during the comprehensive assessment. During the psychosocial and medical evaluations, clinicians normalize the patient's problem, provide information, and correct misunderstandings. Formal treatment plans will depend on the presumed cause of the sexual dysfunction. Medical treatments include options such as pharmacotherapy (e.g., Viagra for erectile dysfunction), gels and creams (e.g., lubricating gels to compensate for problems with female arousal), hormone replacement therapy (e.g., testosterone to increase sexual desire), and surgery (e.g., penile implants to treat organic erectile dysfunction). Psychological treatments include psychoeducation about healthy sexual functioning, behaviorally focused sex therapy with the patient or the patient and his or her partner (e.g., using the stop-start technique to treat premature ejaculation), interpersonally focused couples therapy with the patient and his or her partner (e.g., working on trust or communication), or more traditional individual therapy with the patient (e.g., treating mood, anxiety, or trauma symptoms).

Cross-References

▶ Sexual Behavior

References and Readings

American Psychiatric Association. (2000). *Diagnostic and statistical manual of mental disorders* (4th ed., text revision). Washington, DC: Author.

Balon, R., & Segraves, R. T. (Eds.). (2005). *Handbook of sexual dysfunction* (Medical psychiatry series, Vol. 30). Boca Raton: Taylor & Francis.

Balon, R., & Segraves, R. T. (Eds.). (2009). *Clinical manual of sexual disorders*. Arlington: American Psychiatric Publishing.

Carey, M. P., & Gordon, C. M. (1995). Sexual dysfunction among heterosexual adults: Description, epidemiology, assessment, and treatment. In L. Diamant & R. McAnulty (Eds.), *The psychology of sexual orientation, behavior, and identity: A handbook* (pp. 165–196). Westport: Greenwood.

Fagan, P. J. (2004). *Sexual disorders: Perspectives on diagnosis and treatment*. Baltimore: The Johns Hopkins University Press.

IsHak, W. W. (Ed.). (2008). *The guidebook of sexual medicine*. Beverly Hills: A & W Publishing.

Maurice, W. L. (1999). *Sexual medicine in primary care*. St. Louis: Mosby.

Nusbaum, M., & Rosenfeld, J. A. (2005). *Sexual health across the lifecycle: A practical guide for clinicians*. Cambridge: Cambridge University Press.

Rowland, D. L., & Incrocci, L. (Eds.). (2008). *Handbook of sexual and gender identity disorders*. Hoboken: Wiley.

Wincze, J. P., & Carey, M. P. (2001). *Sexual dysfunction: Guide for assessment and treatment* (2nd ed.). New York: Guilford.

Sexual Hookup

Robyn Fielder
Center for Health and Behavior, Syracuse University, Syracuse, NY, USA

Synonyms

Casual sex; Hooking up

Definition

A sexual hookup is a sexual interaction between partners who are not dating or in a committed romantic relationship. There is no universal definition of sexual hookups, but qualitative research has begun to converge on the most common interpretation of hookup, which has three main components. First, hookups may involve a range of sexual behaviors, from kissing to sex. Kissing and sexual touching occur more frequently, but oral and vaginal sex occur during a significant minority of hookups. Anal sex during a hookup is rare. The variety of sexual behaviors that can occur during hookups causes ambiguity. From a research or public health perspective, behavioral specificity is needed to distinguish among different levels of sexual risk behavior. Condom use is rare during oral sex hookups, suggesting a potential risk for sexually transmitted diseases.

Second, hookup partners are not dating or in a committed romantic relationship. They may be friends, acquaintances, or strangers, or they may have been in a romantic relationship in the past. The most common connection between partners is friendship. Third, hookups do not signify an impending romantic commitment, so partners typically do not expect a relationship to result from the encounter. Instead, hookups are expected to serve a utilitarian function of sexual pleasure. However, individuals may desire a relationship with their hookup partner, and some engage in hookups with the hope that a relationship will eventually develop. Besides these three main criteria, hookups are also understood in terms of what they lack (emotional attachment and commitment). Emerging adults' descriptions of typical hookups are highly consistent, even between those who have and have not hooked up.

Several biomedical, sociocultural, and college environment changes occurring over the past 50 years have contributed to emergence of the hookup culture. Notably, emerging adults increasingly choose to postpone serious committed relationships to focus on self-development. Hookups offer a convenient way to obtain sexual intimacy without the commitment or time investment required by a relationship. Accordingly, hooking up has become very common among adolescents and emerging adults. A minority of middle and high school students and the majority of college students report hookup experience. Hooking up has replaced traditional dating as the main way to explore relationships and sexual behavior on college campuses. Hookup behavior among similarly aged noncollege attending youth is rarely studied.

Research has investigated several characteristics of sexual hookups. Hookups frequently co-occur with alcohol use, and alcohol use is a strong predictor of hookup behavior. Hookups are often spontaneous, but some individuals plan to hook up (either with a particular partner or with anyone). A variety of sexual, emotional, and social motives may lead individuals to hook up, such as sexual desire, intoxication, excitement, and desire to feel attractive. Some hookup partners interact only once, but some hook up multiple times, which is sometimes known as "friends with benefits." Hookups are also related to casual sex, as both lack emotional attachment. The main differences are the greater variety of sexual behaviors and partner types involved in hookups compared to casual sex and the extent to which hooking up has become a normative experience for youth.

Cross-References

▶ Condom Use
▶ Sexual Behavior
▶ Sexual Risk Behavior

References and Readings

Bogle, K. A. (2008). *Hooking up: Sex, dating, and relationships on campus.* New York: New York University Press.

Owen, J. J., Rhoades, G. K., Stanley, S. M., & Fincham, F. D. (2010). "Hooking up" among college students: Demographic and psychosocial correlates. *Archives of Sexual Behavior, 39,* 653–663.

Stinson, R. D. (2010). Hooking up in young adulthood: A review of factors influencing the sexual behavior of college students. *Journal of College Student Psychotherapy, 24,* 98–115.

Sexual Maturation

▶ Puberty

Sexual Orientation

Jason W. Mitchell
Center for AIDS Intervention Research, Medical College of Wisconsin, Milwaukee, WI, USA

Definition

Sexual orientation is the sexual attraction, emotional, and/or romantic state that a person endures toward women, men, or both sexes. Sexual orientation also pertains to a person's sense of identity that is tied to these attractions, behaviors, and membership into a community with similar individuals (American Psychological Association [APA] 2011). Therefore, sexual orientation is the compilation of a person's sexual behavior and sense of sexual identity.

These two core components of sexual orientation are developed across a person's life span, yet many believe it to be an innate and fixed state (APA 2011). Nonetheless, an individual's sexual orientation is often characterized with a label, such as heterosexuality, homosexuality, or bisexuality. Sometimes asexuality is also considered as a separate entity of sexual orientation. Those labels normally, but not always, incorporate and include the individuals' sexual identity and sexual behavior of her or his sexual orientation. Because sexuality may be viewed as a fluid construct, an individual's sexual behavior may change over time while maintaining the same sexual identity. An example of this phenomenon would be when a heterosexual male experiments sexually with another male. Another exception to this generalization is when a self-identified lesbian woman has sex with a male. As such, these categories exist on a continuum of sexuality.

Scientists and psychologists have created measures of sexual orientation to better assess an individuals' sexuality. Typically, these measures will include a range of "solely heterosexual" to "solely homosexual" with "bisexuality" falling somewhere in between these two categories and "asexuality" not being included. A variety of measurements exist to assess sexual orientation. However, an individual's sexual orientation may change over time, and as such, measuring this construct at a single point in time (i.e., cross-sectional study) does have its limitations. Nonetheless, more studies are including a variety of measures that assess the sexual behavior and identity dimensions of sexual orientation.

The most well-recognized measurement of sexual orientation for males and females is the Kinsey scale (Kinsey et al. 1948, 1953). The scale ranges from 0 for "exclusively heterosexual with no homosexual" to 6 for "exclusively homosexual." The original scale does not include an "asexual" rating or category nor does it take into account any changes of sexual orientation over a period of time. Since then, other measurements of sexual orientation have been created and reviewed. For more information and references, please refer to the further readings section.

Cross-References

▶ Sexual Behavior

References and Readings

American Psychological Association. (2011). *Sexual orientation and homosexuality.* Retrieved 4 Feb 2011 from http://www.apa.org/topics/sexuality/orientation.aspx

Chung, Y. B., & Katayama, M. (1996). Assessment of sexual orientation in lesbian/gay/bisexual studies. *Journal of Homosexuality, 30*(4), 49–62.

Kinsey, A., Pomeroy, W., & Martin, C. (1948). *Sexual behavior in the human male.* Philadelphia: Saunders. ISBN 978-0253334121.

Kinsey, A., Pomeroy, W., Martin, C., & Gebhard, P. (1953). *Sexual behavior in the human female.* Philadelphia: Saunders. ISBN 978-0253334114.

Sell, R. L. (1996). The sell assessment of sexual orientation: Background and scoring. *Journal of Gay, Lesbian, and Bisexual Identity, 1*(4), 295–310.

Sexual Risk

▶ Sexual Risk Behavior

Sexual Risk Behavior

Theresa Senn
Center for Health and Behavior, Syracuse University, Syracuse, NY, USA

Synonyms

Sexual risk; Unprotected sex

Definition

Sexual risk behavior is any sexual behavior (typically condom-unprotected oral, vaginal, or anal intercourse) that puts one at risk for an adverse health outcome. Adverse health outcomes may include an unwanted pregnancy or contracting a sexually transmitted disease (STD), including human immunodeficiency virus (HIV).

Vaginal intercourse is the only sexual behavior that puts an individual at risk for unwanted pregnancy. There are many methods for reducing the risk of unwanted pregnancy, including hormonal contraceptives, correct and consistent condom use, surgical methods such as a vasectomy or tubal ligation, and other methods such as an intrauterine device or a diaphragm.

Sexual behavior falls on a continuum from no risk to low risk to high risk for contracting an STD. The risk level of the sexual behavior depends on the STD under consideration. For example, with respect to HIV, masturbation incurs virtually no risk, oral sex is low risk, and vaginal and anal intercourse are high-risk behaviors. However, oral sex is a high-risk behavior for contracting some STDs such as gonorrhea.

The risk level of a particular sexual behavior also depends on with whom the behavior occurs. Any sexual behavior that occurs when an individual is alone is generally no risk because the individual is not at risk of contracting an STD from him- or herself. In addition, any sexual behavior that occurs within the context of a mutually monogamous relationship, in which both individuals are not infected with any STDs (especially when confirmed by testing), confers no risk of contracting an STD for either individual. Sexual behavior puts an individual at risk for contracting an STD only when his or her sexual partner is infected with an STD.

The risk of a particular sexual behavior also depends on the individual's sexual network. Sexual risk increases with an increasing number of sexual partners, and/or an increasing number of a sex partner's partners, because there is an increasing likelihood that one of these individuals is infected with an STD. In other words, the larger the sexual network, the greater the sexual risk.

STDs can have serious consequences, including epididymitis in men, pelvic inflammatory disease and pregnancy complications in women, infertility, and cancer (Centers for Disease Control and Prevention 2010d). In addition, the presence of another STD facilitates the transmission of HIV through sexual exposure (Centers for Disease Control and Prevention 2007). HIV weakens the immune system, ultimately leading to death when the immune system is so weakened it is unable to fight off infections or cancers (Centers for Disease Control and Prevention 2010a). STDs can also have negative relationship and social consequences due to the stigma surrounding some STDs.

The majority of STDs are either bacterial or viral (Holmes et al. 2008). In general, bacterial STDs can be cured with antibiotics, although some STDs are becoming resistant to antibiotics that had previously successfully treated the disease (Centers for Disease Control and Prevention 2010b). Viral STDs have no cure, although there are medications that can help to manage outbreaks or viral load. STDs may sometimes be cleared from the body with no treatment (Centers for Disease Control and Prevention 2010c).

Condoms are an effective way to reduce the risk of contracting an STD when they are used consistently and correctly. Although the value of condoms for the prevention of some STDs that can be transmitted through genital-to-genital contact, such as human papillomavirus and herpes simplex virus, has been debated, recent evidence suggests that condoms reduce the risk of STD infection from these pathogens as well (Holmes et al. 2008).

Numerous factors influence sexual risk behavior. These factors can be broadly categorized into individual-level factors, partner- or relationship-level factors, and social or structural factors. Researchers have typically focused on only one level of influence at a time, although the integration of individual-level, partner or relationship-level, and social or structural factors has recently been attempted in the Network-Individual-Resource Model for HIV prevention (Johnson et al. 2010).

The relation between individual-level factors and sexual risk behavior has been extensively researched. Numerous health behavior theories, including the health belief model, social-cognitive theory, the theory of planned behavior, and the information-motivation-behavioral skills model, have been used to explain why individuals engage in sexual risk behavior (Fisher and Fisher 2000). Constructs from these models such as perceived risk, benefits of and barriers to risk reduction, self-efficacy, social norms, attitudes, intentions, and skills have been associated with sexual risk behavior (Fisher and Fisher 2000).

Because sexual risk behavior usually occurs within a dyad, researchers have begun to consider partnership-level influences on sexual behavior. At the partnership level, variables such as intimate partner violence and the balance of power in a relationship may influence sexual risk behavior. There are few existing theories that incorporate partner influences on sexual risk behavior; one exception is a framework recently proposed by Karney et al. (2010), which posits that sexual risk behavior is influenced by the ability to communicate about and coordinate sexual behavior, which, in turn, is influenced by the individual beliefs and motivations of each partner as well as by the nature of the relationship.

Although it is commonly accepted that social and structural factors influence sexual risk behavior, because of the complexity and breadth of these factors, it is difficult to develop a general model that predicts how these factors influence sexual risk behavior. Several broad frameworks have been suggested that specify different levels of structural influence (Gupta et al. 2008). Structural factors that influence sexual risk behavior vary depending on the social, cultural, and economic conditions faced by the population under study. Some structural factors associated with sexual risk behavior include gender inequality and poverty (Gupta et al. 2008). In the United States, one factor that has received considerable recent attention is the male-to-female ratio. Social and structural factors such as the high mortality rate among African American males due to disease and violence, high rate of incarceration among African American males, and high rates of poverty and unemployment among African American males (making them less desirable as potential husbands) have led to an unbalanced ratio of available African American men to women. This shortage of men relative to women may reduce women's power in relationships and their ability to insist on monogamy, ultimately leading to high rates of partner concurrency (Adimora and Schoenbach 2002).

Behavioral medicine researchers and practitioners have played an important role in the design and evaluation of interventions to reduce sexual risk behavior. Numerous interventions have been developed to target the individual-level determinants of sexual risk behavior. These interventions, particularly those that include motivational and skills elements, are effective in reducing sexual risk behavior (Crepaz et al. 2007, 2009; Johnson et al. 2006). Few interventions have been developed to target the partnership-level determinants of sexual risk behavior (Karney et al. 2010); this is an important area for future research. Although there are challenges to implementing and evaluating structural interventions, some programs, such as microcredit programs for women and policies requiring condoms be used for sex work, have successfully reduced sexual risk behavior in some settings (Gupta et al. 2008).

Additional research on structural-level sexual risk reduction interventions is needed, as is research on interventions that target multiple levels of influence.

References and Readings

Adimora, A. A., & Schoenbach, V. J. (2002). Contextual factors and the black–white disparity in heterosexual HIV transmission. *Epidemiology, 13*, 707–712.

Centers for Disease Control and Prevention. (2007). *CDC fact sheet: The role of STD prevention and treatment in HIV prevention*. Retrieved 6 Jan 2011 from http://cdc.gov/std/HIV/stds-and-hiv-fact-sheet.pdf

Centers for Disease Control and Prevention. (2010a). *Basic information about HIV and AIDS*. Retrieved 6 Jan 2011 from http://www.cdc.gov/hiv/topics/basic/index.htm

Centers for Disease Control and Prevention. (2010b). *CDC fact sheet: Basic information about antibiotic-resistant gonorrhea (ARG)*. Retrieved 6 Jan 2011 from http://cdc.gov/std/Gonorrhea/arg/basic.htm

Centers for Disease Control and Prevention. (2010c). *CDC fact sheet: Genital HPV*. Retrieved 6 Jan 2011 from http://cdc.gov/std/hpv/hpv-fact-sheet-press.pdf

Centers for Disease Control and Prevention. (2010d). *CDC fact sheets: Sexually transmitted diseases*. Retrieved 6 Jan 2011 from http://cdc.gov/std/healthcomm/fact_sheets.htm

Crepaz, N., Horn, A. K., Rama, S. M., Griffin, T., Deluca, J. B., Mullins, M. M., et al. (2007). The efficacy of behavioral interventions in reducing HIV risk sex behaviors and incident sexually transmitted disease in Black and Hispanic sexually transmitted disease clinic patients in the United States: A meta-analytic review. *Sexually Transmitted Diseases, 34*, 319–332.

Crepaz, N., Marshall, K. J., Aupont, L. W., Jacobs, E. D., Mizuno, Y., Kay, L. S., et al. (2009). The efficacy of HIV/STI behavioral interventions for African American females in the United States: A meta-analysis. *American Journal of Public Health, 99*, 2069–2078.

Fisher, J. D., & Fisher, W. A. (2000). Theoretical approaches to individual-level change in HIV risk behavior. In J. L. Peterson & R. J. DiClemente (Eds.), *Handbook of HIV prevention* (pp. 3–55). New York: Kluwer Academic/Plenum.

Gupta, G. R., Parkhurst, J. O., Ogden, J. A., Aggleton, P., & Mahal, A. (2008). Structural approaches to HIV prevention. *The Lancet, 372*, 764–775.

Holmes, K. K., Sparling, P. F., Stamm, W. E., Piot, P., Wasserheit, J. N., et al. (2008). Introduction and overview. In K. K. Holmes, P. F. Sparling, W. E. Stamm, P. Piot, J. N. Wasserheit, L. Corey, et al. (Eds.), *Sexually transmitted diseases* (4th ed., pp. xvii–xxv). New York: McGraw Hill.

Johnson, B. T., Carey, M. P., Chaudoir, S. R., & Reid, A. E. (2006). Sexual risk reduction for persons living with HIV: Research synthesis of randomized controlled trials, 1993 to 2004. *Journal of Acquired Immune Deficiency Syndromes, 41*, 642–650.

Johnson, B. T., Redding, C. A., DiClemente, R. J., Mustanski, B. S., Dodge, B., Sheeran, P., et al. (2010). A network-individual-resource model for HIV prevention. *AIDS and Behavior, 14*, S204–S221.

Karney, B. R., Hops, H., Redding, C. A., Reis, H. T., Rothman, A. J., & Simpson, J. A. (2010). A framework for incorporating dyads in models of HIV-prevention. *AIDS and Behavior, 14*, S189–S203.

Sexuality and Stress

Hanna M. Mües[1] and Urs M. Nater[2]
[1]Department of Clinical and Health Psychology, Faculty of Psychology, University of Vienna, Vienna, Austria
[2]Department of Psychology, University of Vienna, Vienna, Austria

Introduction

According to many therapy manuals and self-help guides on sexuality, stress is the number one factor inhibiting sexual desire. However, no sufficient empirical evidence can be found to support this claim. Since both sexuality and stress are important factors of everyday life and contribute substantially to health (e.g., McEwen 1998; World Health Organization [WHO] 2006), this entry attempts to provide a summary of the current state of knowledge regarding how sexuality and stress might be intertwined.

Sexuality

Human sexuality plays a central role throughout life (WHO 2006) and "encompasses sex, gender identities and roles, sexual orientation, eroticism, pleasure, intimacy and reproduction" (WHO 2006, p. 5). There are three key components of sexual experience and behavior, based on the sexual response cycle (Masters and Johnson 1966), modified by Kaplan (1979), and repeatedly reported in the scientific literature: sexual desire, sexual arousal, and orgasm. According to Bancroft, sexual desire and arousal are "two 'windows' into the complexity of sexual arousal [...], one focusing on the incentive motivation component (desire) and the other on the arousal component (excitement)" (2009, p. 65). An orgasm, often seen as the goal of sexual activity, is associated with pleasure and reduced tension (Bancroft 2009). The importance of these factors is also evident in the division of sexual dysfunctions presented in the Diagnostic and Statistical Manual of Mental Disorders (DSM-5; American Psychiatric Association 2013).

Among other factors, sexuality is influenced by psychological, social, and biological factors (WHO 2006) such as reproductive hormones, which play an essential role in human sexual development, sexual function, and sexual experience and behavior (Bancroft 2009). The main reproductive hormones include steroid (e.g., testosterone, estradiol) and peptide hormones (e.g., vasopressin, oxytocin). Androgens, such as testosterone, and estrogens, such as estradiol, are produced by the testes as well as the ovaries and play an important role for sexuality in both men and women. Testosterone seems to be especially relevant for sexual desire and arousal in both men and women (Bancroft 2009).

Given that sexuality plays such an essential role throughout life, maintaining sexual health is highly important. Sexual health can be defined as "a state of physical, emotional, mental and social well-being in relation to sexuality; it is not merely the absence of disease, dysfunction or infirmity" (WHO 2006, p. 5). It "requires a positive and respectful approach to sexuality and sexual relationships, as well as the possibility of having pleasurable and safe sexual experiences, free of coercion, discrimination and violence" (WHO 2006, p. 5).

A sexual dysfunction, by contrast, is characterized as a sexual problem that occurs recurrently or in the majority of sexual contacts, leads to significant distress, lasts for at least half a year and cannot directly be explained by another mental disorder, severe relationship distress, or other significant stressors, a disease, or substance or medication intake (American Psychiatric Association 2013). The most common sexual dysfunctions have been found to involve lack of sexual desire (prevalence rates between 10% and 61.5%) and lack of sexual arousal (prevalence rates between 12% and 49%) in women, and premature ejaculation (prevalence rates between 1% and 10%) and erectile dysfunction (prevalence rates between 1% and 10% for individuals younger than 40 years old) in men (McCabe et al. 2016).

Stress

Acute stress can be caused by potential stressors such as major life events or situations necessitating a "fight or flight" response, while chronic stress can be caused by potential stressors such as daily hassles. Whether an individual perceives a potential stressor as a stressor is determined by the individual's perception of the situation as well as the individual's general health (McEwen 1998). Specifically, according to the transactional model of stress and coping, in a step called "primary appraisal", a situation is evaluated as irrelevant, positive, or, as in the case of a stressor, dangerous (Lazarus and Folkman 1984). In a concomitant step called "secondary appraisal", available resources and coping strategies are analyzed. Depending on "primary appraisal" and "secondary appraisal", a stressful situation can be categorized as harm or loss, a threat or a challenge by an individual and can thus differ between individuals (Lazarus and Folkman 1984). Acute and chronic stress can both have negative long-term consequences (McEwen 1998).

The Association between Sexuality and Stress

Sexual experience and behavior seems to be negatively associated with stress (e.g., Abedi et al. 2015), although there is some contrasting evidence regarding sexual desire, which can be seen as a component of sexual experience and behavior (Morokoff and Gillilland 1993; Raisanen et al. 2018).

Results from cross-sectional studies: Specifically, stress has been negatively associated with the frequency of sexual intercourse in women (Abedi et al. 2015). Furthermore, while one study reported that stress was negatively associated with sexual desire in women (Abedi et al. 2015), another study found a positive association between stress and sexual desire in both women and men (Morokoff and Gillilland 1993). In women, in the study by Abedi et al. (2015), sexual arousal and lubrication were negatively associated with stress, while Hamilton and Meston (2013) also found a negative association between genital arousal and levels of stress as well as cortisol levels, but did not find a significant association between psychological arousal and stress. Moreover, the study by Abedi et al. (2015) also reported a negative association between stress and satisfaction as well as stress and orgasm, and a positive association between stress and sexual pain in women.

Results from experiments inducing stress: One of the few experimental studies to have investigated the association of sexual experience and behavior with stress found that receiving a sexual reward in the form of viewing mildly erotic images compared to viewing neutral images before participating in the Trier Social Stress Test (TSST) positively affected stress in men: Participants in the reward condition showed significantly lower cortisol reactivity during the TSST compared to participants in the neutral condition (Creswell et al. 2013).

Results from longitudinal studies: In addition, some studies have examined the link between sexual experience and behavior and stress longitudinally. Specifically, stress was negatively associated with sexual desire for partnered sexual activity in women but positively associated with sexual desire for partnered sexual activity in men, and not associated with sexual desire for non-partnered sexual activity in men or women (Raisanen et al. 2018). Furthermore, the authors found that testosterone was negatively associated with sexual desire for partnered sexual activity in women and with sexual desire for non-partnered sexual activity in women with lower levels of stress, but positively associated with sexual desire for non-partnered sexual activity in women with high levels of stress. In men, testosterone was not associated with sexual desire for partnered sexual activity, but positively associated with sexual desire for non-partnered sexual activity. Stress moderated the association between testosterone and sexual desire for non-partnered sexual activity but not between testosterone and sexual desire for partnered sexual activity (Raisanen et al. 2018). In addition, research has shown a negative association of same-day stress with occurrence of sexual intercourse, genital stimulation, and orgasm with and without the partner in women (Burleson et al. 2007). Stress was also negatively associated with frequency of sexual activity, satisfaction, and relationship satisfaction in women (Bodenmann et al. 2010). Contrasting these findings, Hall, Kusunoki, Gatny, and Barber found that women with moderate to severe stress symptoms showed a significantly higher frequency of sexual intercourse (2014). Furthermore, in line with these results, intimacy, including sexual intercourse, was significantly associated with lower levels of daily salivary cortisol (Ditzen et al. 2008). Also, sexual intercourse led to better blood pressure reactions under stress compared to engagement in other or no sexual activities (Brody 2006). In another study, experiencing a stressful day increased the probability of engaging in sexual intercourse the next day, although this probability was higher for men than for women (Ein-Dor and Hirschberger 2012). Furthermore, sexual intercourse on 1 day led to lower levels of stress the next day for both genders. While this link between stress and sexual intercourse was unaffected by relationship satisfaction for women, men with lower relationship satisfaction showed a higher stress relief following sexual intercourse (Ein-Dor and Hirschberger 2012). In addition, physical affection on 1 day predicted lower stress on the following day in women (Burleson et al. 2007). Similarly, genital stimulation and orgasm with a partner predicted lower stress the next day, but only for women with a shorter relationship duration; no such effect was found for women with longer relationship duration. Stress, however, did not significantly affect any of the variables on the following day in this study in women (Burleson et al. 2007).

Outlook

So far, study findings on the link between sexual experience and behavior and stress are not straightforward. Few studies have investigated this link bidirectionally or longitudinally. Moreover, there is little research investigating this relationship in daily life, thus limiting the ecological validity of previous studies. Additionally, studies comparing the sex-stress link between men and women are scarce. Hence, future research will need to focus on investigating the bidirectional link between sexual experience and behavior and stress in both men and women, ideally in a setting characterized by high ecological validity. Furthermore, while the assessment of stress requires a multidimensional measurement approach (Nater 2018), previous analyses have rarely sampled and included biological stress parameters such as cortisol or alpha-amylase, even though it is widely known that these parameters not only represent the human stress reaction biologically but have also been associated with negative health consequences (e.g., Kudielka and Kirschbaum 2014). Similarly, testosterone has been linked to both sexual desire and arousal (e.g., Bancroft 2009). Thus, future studies should incorporate a comprehensive measurement of biological parameters (e.g., cortisol, alpha-amylase, and testosterone) and thus fulfill the requirements of a multidimensional measurement approach. Finally, to date, no studies have investigated the sex-stress link in the everyday life of patients diagnosed with a sexual dysfunction, even though acquiring knowledge in this area might inform further valuable treatment options. Hence, future research should investigate the association between sexual experience and behavior and stress in individuals with diagnosed sexual dysfunctions such as female sexual interest/arousal disorder, as this is one of the most frequently occurring sexual dysfunctions.

Cross-References

▶ Daily Stress
▶ Immune Responses to Stress
▶ Mental Stress
▶ Perceived Stress
▶ Perceptions of Stress
▶ Psychological Stress
▶ Sexual Behavior
▶ Sexual Functioning
▶ Stress
▶ Stress Reactivity
▶ Stress Responses
▶ Stress, Emotional
▶ Stress: Appraisal and Coping
▶ Stress-Related Disorders
▶ Trier Social Stress Test

References and Further Reading

Abedi, P., Afrazeh, M., Javadifar, N., & Saki, A. (2015). The relation between stress and sexual function and satisfaction in reproductive-age women in Iran: A cross-sectional study. *Journal of Sex & Marital Therapy, 41*(3), 384–390. https://doi.org/10.1080/0092623X.2014.915906.

American Psychiatric Association. (2013). *Diagnostic and statistical manual of mental disorders: DSM-5* (5th ed.). Washington, DC: American Psychiatric Publishing.

Bancroft, J. (2009). *Human sexuality and its problems* (3rd ed.). Edinburgh: Churchill Livingstone.

Bodenmann, G., Atkins, D. C., Schär, M., & Poffet, V. (2010). The association between daily stress and sexual activity. *Journal of Family Psychology, 24*(3), 271–279. https://doi.org/10.1037/a0019365.

Brody, S. (2006). Blood pressure reactivity to stress is better for people who recently had penile-vaginal intercourse than for people who had other or no sexual activity. *Biological Psychology, 71*, 214–222. https://doi.org/10.1016/j.biopsycho.2005.03.005.

Burleson, M. H., Trevathan, W. R., & Todd, M. (2007). In the mood for love or vice versa? Exploring the relations among sexual activity, physical affection, affect, and stress in the daily lives of mid-aged women. *Archives of Sexual Behavior, 36*(3), 357–368. https://doi.org/10.1007/s10508-006-9071-1.

Creswell, J. D., Pacilio, L. E., Denson, T. F., & Satyshur, M. (2013). The effect of a primary sexual reward manipulation of cortisol responses to psychosocial stress in men. *Psychosomatic Medicine, 75*(4), 397–403. https://doi.org/10.1097/PSY.0b013e31828c4524.

Ditzen, B., Hoppmann, C., & Klumb, P. (2008). Positive couple interactions and daily cortisol: On the stress-protecting role of intimacy. *Psychosomatic Medicine, 70*(8), 883–889. https://doi.org/10.1097/PSY.0b013e318185c4fc.

Ein-Dor, T., & Hirschberger, G. (2012). Sexual healing: Daily diary evidence that sex relieves stress for men and women in satisfying relationships. *Journal of Social and Personal Relationships, 29*(1), 126–139. https://doi.org/10.1177/0265407511431185.

Hall, K. S., Kusunoki, Y., Gatny, H., & Barber, J. (2014). Stress symptoms and the frequency of sexual intercourse among young women. *Journal of Sexual Medicine, 11*(8), 1982–1990. https://doi.org/10.1111/jsm.12607.

Hamilton, L. D., & Meston, C. M. (2013). Chronic stress and sexual function in women. *Journal of Sexual Medicine, 10*(10), 2443–3454. https://doi.org/10.1111/jsm.12249.

Kaplan, H. S. (1979). *Disorders of sexual desire and other new concepts and techniques in sex therapy*. New York: Brunner/Mazel.

Kudielka, B. M., & Kirschbaum, C. (2014). Sex differences in HPA axis responses to stress: A review. *Biological Psychology, 69*, 113–132. https://doi.org/10.1016/j.biopsycho.2004.11.009.

Lazarus, R. S., & Folkman, S. (1984). *Stress, appraisal, and coping*. Berlin: Springer.

Masters, W. H., & Johnson, V. E. (1966). *Human sexual response*. Boston: Little, Brown.

McCabe, M. P., Sharlip, I. D., Lewis, R., Atalla, E., Balon, R., Fisher, A. D., et al. (2016). Incidence and prevalence of sexual dysfunction in women and men: A consensus statement from the fourth international consultation on sexual medicine 2015. *The Journal of Sexual Medicine, 13*(2), 144–152. https://doi.org/10.1016/j.jsxm.2015.12.034.

McEwen, B. S. (1998). Protective and damaging effects of stress mediators. *New England Journal of Medicine, 338*(3), 171–179. https://doi.org/10.1056/NEJM199801153380307.

Morokoff, P. J., & Gillilland, R. (1993). Stress, sexual functioning, and marital satisfaction. *The Journal of Sex Research, 30*(1), 43–53. https://doi.org/10.1080/00224499309551677.

Nater, U. M. (2018). The multidimensionality of stress and its assessment. *Brain, Behavior, and Immunity, 73*, 159–160. https://doi.org/10.1016/j.bbi.2018.07.018.

Raisanen, J. C., Chadwick, S. B., Michalak, N., & van Anders, S. M. (2018). Average associations between sexual desire, testosterone, and stress in women and men over time. *Archives of Sexual Behavior, 47*(6), 1613–1631. https://doi.org/10.1007/s10508-018-1231-6.

Stoléru, S., Fonteille, V., Cornélis, C., Joyal, C., & Moulier, V. (2012). Functional neuroimaging studies of sexual arousal and orgasm in healthy men and women: A review and meta-analysis. *Neuroscience & Biobehavioral Reviews, 36*(6), 1481–1509. https://doi.org/10.1016/j.neubiorev.2012.03.006.

World Health Organization (WHO). (2006). *Defining sexual health: Report of a technical consultation of sexual health, 28–31 January 2002*. Sexual Health Document Series. Geneva. Retrieved from http://www.who.int/reproductivehealth/publications/sexual_health/defining_sexual_health.pdf

Sexually Transmitted Disease/Infection (STD/STI)

▶ AIDS: Acquired Immunodeficiency Syndrome
▶ HIV Infection

Sexually Transmitted Diseases (STDs)

Theresa Senn
Center for Health and Behavior, Syracuse University, Syracuse, NY, USA

Synonyms

Sexually transmitted infections; Venereal diseases

Definition

A sexually transmitted disease is a disease that is transmitted through sexual contact (World Health Organization).

Our knowledge of sexually transmitted diseases (STDs) is still evolving. Currently, at least 35 pathogens that can be transmitted sexually have been identified (Holmes et al. 2008). Although some sexually transmissible pathogens can be transmitted through other routes besides sexual contact, generally a disease is classified as an STD when the primary method of transmission in a population is sexual contact (Holmes et al.).

There are five different types of pathogens that can be transmitted sexually: (a) bacteria, such as gonorrhea or chlamydia; (b) viruses, such as human immunodeficiency virus (HIV), herpes simplex virus, or human papillomavirus (HPV); (c) protozoa, such as trichomoniasis; (d) fungi, such as *Candida albicans* (although the primary mode of transmission for this pathogen is not sexual); and (e) ectoparasites, such as pubic lice (Holmes et al. 2008). Depending on the pathogen, STDs can be transmitted through bodily fluids (e.g., blood, semen, cervicovaginal fluid), feces, or skin-to-skin contact. Thus, the transmission of an STD usually involves vaginal or anal intercourse, oral sex (including oral-genital contact and oral-anal contact), or genital-to-genital contact.

STD symptoms vary depending on the pathogen involved, as well as the sex of the infected person and the site of infection. Symptoms associated with some of the more common STDs include blisters or ulcers, pain or burning during urination, discharge, abdominal pain, and pain during intercourse. However, many individuals who are infected with an STD do not have any symptoms (Centers for Disease Control and Prevention 2010d). Such "asymptomatic" individuals may unknowingly infect a sexual partner with the STD.

Testing for STDs is generally conducted in medical facilities (although community- and home-based testing protocols are now available). Depending on the STD, testing may involve urethral or cervical swabs, swabs taken from the site of an ulcer, urine testing, blood testing, and clinical examination (Centers for Disease Control and Prevention 2010d). In the United States, some STDs must be reported (by health-care providers) to county, state, or federal health authorities; for example, positive test results for chlamydia, gonorrhea, and syphilis must be reported to the Centers for Disease Control and Prevention for disease surveillance and monitoring (Centers for Disease Control and Prevention 2009).

STDs can have serious consequences, including epididymitis in men, pelvic inflammatory disease and pregnancy complications in women, infertility, and cancer (Centers for Disease Control and Prevention 2010d). In addition, individuals who are co-infected with HIV and another STD are more likely to transmit HIV through sexual exposure, and individuals who are infected with an STD are more likely to acquire HIV through sexual exposure from an HIV-positive partner (Centers for Disease Control and Prevention 2007). HIV weakens the immune system, ultimately leading to death when the immune system is so weakened it is unable to fight off infections and cancers (Centers for Disease Control and Prevention 2010a). STDs can also have negative interpersonal and social consequences due to the stigma surrounding some STDs.

The majority of STDs are either bacterial or viral (Holmes et al. 2008). In general, bacterial STDs can be cured with antibiotics, although some STDs are becoming resistant to many classes of antibiotics that had previously successfully treated the disease (Centers for Disease Control and Prevention 2010b). Viral STDs have no cure, although there are medications that can help to manage outbreaks or viral load. STDs such as HPV may sometimes be cleared from the body with no treatment (Centers for Disease Control and Prevention 2010c).

An individual's likelihood of acquiring an STD is based on his or her sexual behavior and the risk of transmission per sexual act with an infected partner. Sexual behaviors that affect the likelihood of acquiring an STD include the number of sexual partners, the number of unprotected sexual acts, and the types of unprotected sexual acts. The risk of transmission per sexual act depends in part on the pathogen as well as the individual's biology. Different pathogens are associated with different risks of transmission per sexual act. Biological factors associated with transmission risk include the individual's immune response and the mucosal surface area exposed during the sexual act; women, for example, are more likely than men to be infected with an STD through vaginal intercourse because women have a larger mucosal surface area that is exposed during vaginal intercourse, and young women are more likely to acquire an STD because they have an immature cervix. STD risk is also affected by the STD prevalence in an individual's sexual network, which is influenced by the rate of sexual partner change, partner concurrency (i.e., multiple, overlapping sexual partnerships), and degree of disassortative mixing (i.e., sexual partners who are dissimilar in certain characteristics, such as age or sexual activity Garnett 2008).

To date, some types of HPV and some types of hepatitis are the only STDs that can be prevented through vaccination. Other medical strategies are currently being developed for STD prevention, such as vaginal microbicides and preexposure prophylaxis. STDs can also be prevented through behavioral change. Abstaining from sexual contact is the only certain way to prevent most STDs. However, other behavioral strategies including correct and consistent condom use, engaging in sexual activity only with one partner who is not infected with any STD and who has no other sexual partners, and having fewer sexual partners will reduce the likelihood of acquiring an STD.

Behavioral medicine can play a large role in STD prevention. Behavioral interventions can promote sexual risk reduction behavior, by encouraging individuals to use condoms consistently and correctly for all sexual activity, be in a mutually monogamous sexual relationship with an uninfected partner, or adopt other strategies that will reduce the risk of contracting an STD. Behavioral interventions have been shown to be effective in reducing sexual risk behavior and STDs in a variety of populations (Crepaz et al. 2007, 2009; Johnson et al. 2006). Behavioral medicine can also play a role in encouraging the adoption of biomedical strategies. For example, behavioral medicine strategies could be used to encourage STD and HIV testing, vaccine acceptance, the completion of medications for curable STDs and adherence to medications for viral STDs, and male circumcision, which may reduce the spread of STDs and HIV.

Cross-References

▶ Sexual Risk Behavior

References and Readings

Centers for Disease Control and Prevention. (2007). *CDC fact sheet: The role of STD prevention and treatment in HIV prevention*. Retrieved 6 Jan 2011 from http://cdc.gov/std/HIV/stds-and-hiv-fact-sheet.pdf

Centers for Disease Control and Prevention. (2009). *Sexually transmitted disease surveillance, 2008*. Atlanta: U.S. Department of Health and Human Services, Centers for Disease Control and Prevention, National Center for HIV/AIDS, Viral Hepatitis, STD, and TB Prevention, Division of STD Prevention.

Centers for Disease Control and Prevention. (2010a). *Basic information about HIV and AIDS*. Retrieved 6 Jan 2011 from http://www.cdc.gov/hiv/topics/basic/index.html

Centers for Disease Control and Prevention. (2010b). *CDC fact sheet: Basic information about antibiotic-resistant gonorrhea (ARG)*. Retrieved 6 Jan 2011 from http://cdc.gov/std/Gonorrhea/arg/basic.htm

Centers for Disease Control and Prevention. (2010c). *CDC fact sheet: Genital HPV*. Retrieved 6 Jan 2011 from http://cdc.gov/std/hpv/hpv-fact-sheet-press.pdf

Centers for Disease Control and Prevention. (2010d). *CDC fact sheets: Sexually transmitted diseases*. Retrieved 6 Jan 2011 from http://cdc.gov/std/healthcomm/fact_sheets.htm

Crepaz, N., Horn, A. K., Rama, S. M., Griffin, T., Deluca, J. B., Mullins, M. M., et al. (2007). The efficacy of behavioral interventions in reducing HIV risk sex behaviors and incident sexually transmitted disease in Black and Hispanic sexually transmitted disease clinic patients in the United States: A meta-analytic review. *Sexually Transmitted Diseases, 34*, 319–332.

Crepaz, N., Marshall, K. J., Aupont, L. W., Jacobs, E. D., Mizuno, Y., Kay, L. S., et al. (2009). The efficacy of HIV/STI behavioral interventions for African American females in the United States: A meta-analysis. *American Journal of Public Health, 99*, 2069–2078.

Garnett, G. P. (2008). The transmission dynamics of sexually transmitted infections. In K. K. Holmes, P. F. Sparling, W. E. Stamm, P. Piot, J. N. Wasserheit, L. Corey, et al. (Eds.), *Sexually transmitted diseases* (4th ed., pp. 27–40). New York: McGraw Hill.

Holmes, K. K., Sparling, P. F., Stamm, W. E., Piot, P., Wasserheit, J. N., et al. (2008). Introduction and overview. In K. K. Holmes, P. F. Sparling, W. E. Stamm, P. Piot, J. N. Wasserheit, L. Corey, et al. (Eds.), *Sexually transmitted diseases* (4th ed., pp. xvii–xxv). New York: McGraw Hill.

Johnson, B. T., Carey, M. P., Chaudoir, S. R., & Reid, A. E. (2006). Sexual risk reduction for persons living with HIV: Research synthesis of randomized controlled trials, 1993 to 2004. *Journal of Acquired Immune Deficiency Syndromes, 41*, 642–650.

World Health Organization. *Health topics: Sexually transmitted infections*. Retrieved 6 Jan 2011 from http://www.who.int/topics/sexually_transmitted_infections/en/

Sexually Transmitted Infections

▶ Sexually Transmitted Diseases (STDs)

SF-36

Stephanie Ann Hooker
Department of Psychology, University of Colorado Denver, Denver, CO, USA

Synonyms

Short form 36

Definition

The SF-36 is a 36-item self-report measure of health-related quality of life. It has eight subscales measuring different domains of health-related quality of life: physical functioning (PF), role-physical (RP), bodily pain (BP), general health (GH), vitality (VT), social functioning (SF), role-emotional (RE), and mental health (MH). Two component scores are derived from the eight subscales: a physical health component score and a mental health component score. The SF-36 also includes a single item that assesses perceived change in health status over the past year. Higher scores on all subscales represent better health and functioning. From its development to 2011, more than 16,000 articles were published using the SF-36. SF-36 is also known as the Short Form 36 Health Survey Questionnaire.

Description

Development

Ware and colleagues (Stewart and Ware 1992; Ware 1988, 1990) developed the SF-36 from the Medical Outcomes Study, a study of the health, well-being, and functioning of randomly selected patients seen by randomly selected physicians and other medical providers in three large metropolitan areas. Items were chosen for the SF-36 because they were items commonly used in other health surveys and the domains were ones that seemed to be commonly affected by differing health and disease states. After 10 years of use, the SF-36 was revised to address wording and response choice categories. The SF-36 version 2 (SF-36v2) is the current version (Ware et al. 2007).

Health Domain Scales

Physical Functioning (PF). The PF scale is a 10-item measure of physical limitation in a range of activities from vigorous exercise to performing self-care activities.

Role-Physical (RP). The RP scale contains four items and measures limitations in various roles, including work and daily activities.

Bodily Pain (BP). The BP scale has two items that measure body pain intensity and the extent to which pain interferes with daily activities.

General Health (GH). The five-item GH scale measures overall self-rated health.

Vitality (VT). The VT scale has four items that measure vitality, energy level, and fatigue and is meant to be a measure of subjective well-being.

Social Functioning (SF). The SF scale includes two items that measure the impact of physical and mental health on social functioning.

Role-Emotional (RE). The RE scale measures role limitations due to mental health difficulties with three items, including amount of time spent on work or other activities, amount of work accomplished, and the care with which work is performed.

Mental Health (MH). The MH scale has five items that measure anxiety, depression, loss of behavioral/emotional control, and psychological well-being.

Component Summary Scales

Component summaries were developed to reduce the number of scores derived from this measure from 8 to 2. They also have the advantages of having smaller confidence intervals than the health domain scales and limiting floor and ceiling effects. The Physical Component Summary (PCS) combines items from the PF, RP, BP, and GH scales, and the Mental Health Component Summary (MCS) combines items from the VT, SF, RE, and MH scales. Each provides one score to assess physical and mental health, respectively.

Reliability

Estimates for internal consistency reliability are very good for all subscales. The two component summary scores show evidence for very high internal consistency ($\alpha = .95$ and $\alpha = .93$ for the PCS and MCS, respectively). Internal consistency estimates for the health domain scales are also high, ranging from $\alpha = .83$ (GH) to $\alpha = .95$ (RP) (Ware et al. 2007). Evidence suggests that test-retest reliability for the SF-36 over a 3-week interval is very good, with estimates of .94 and .81 for the PCS and MCS scales, respectively (Ware et al. 1995).

Validity

The SF-36 has been widely used in health research, and the user manual (Ware et al. 2007) provides a comprehensive list of studies offering evidence for the scales' construct validity. The content of the SF-36 survey was compared with other well-known health surveys to establish content validity (cf., Ware et al. 1994, for a list of references).

Options

Along with the 36-item SF-36, the shorter 12-item (SF-12) and 8-item (SF-8) versions of the SF are also available. Both shorter versions offer scores on all eight health domains and the two component summary scores. Versions 1 and 2 of both the SF-36 and the SF-12 are available for use (there is only one version of the SF-8). All forms are available in the standard 4-week recall and the acute 1-week recall versions. Additionally, the SF-8 is available in a 24-h recall version.

Administration

The survey is designed for adults 18 and over and can be given in a self-report paper/pencil format or in an interview format. The SF-36 and its other forms are available for licensure from QualityMetric Incorporated (www.qualitymetric.com).

Cross-References

▶ Health-Related Quality of Life

References and Readings

Quality Metric Incorporated. (2011). http://www.qualitymetric.com/

Stewart, A. L., & Ware, J. E., Jr. (Eds.). (1992). *Measuring functioning and well-being: The medical outcomes study approach*. Durham: Duke University Press.

Ware, J. E., Jr. (1988). *How to score the revised MOS short-form health scales*. Boston: Institute for the Improvement of Medical Care and Health, New England Medical Center.

Ware, J. E., Jr. (1990). Measuring patient function and well-being: Some lessons from the medical outcomes study. In K. A. Heitgoff & K. N. Lohr (Eds.), *Effectiveness and outcomes in health care: Proceedings of an invitational conference by the Institute of Medicine Division of Health Care Services* (pp. 107–119). Washington, DC: National Academy Press.

Ware, J. E., Jr., Kosinski, M., DeBrota, D. J., Andrejasich, C. M., & Bradt, E. W. (1995, October). *Comparison of patient responses to SF-36 Health Surveys that are self-administered, interview administered by telephone, and computer-administered by telephone*. Paper presented at the Eastern Regional Meeting of the American Federation for Clinical Research, New York, NY.

Ware, J. E., Jr., Gandek, B., & The IQOLA Project Group. (1994). The SF-36 health survey: Development and use in mental health research and the IQOLA project. *International Journal of Mental Health, 23*, 49–73.

Ware, J. E., Jr., Kosinski, M., Bjorner, J. B., Turner-Bowker, D. M., Gandek, B., & Meruish, M. E. (2007). *User's manual for the SF-36v2 health survey* (2nd ed.). Lincoln: Quality Metric Incorporated.

Short Form 36

▶ SF-36

Shortness of Breath

▶ Dyspnea

Sick Headache

▶ Migraine Headache

Sickness Absence

▶ Return to Work

Sickness Behavior

Aric A. Prather
Center for Health and Community, University of California, San Francisco, CA, USA

Synonyms

Cytokine-induced depression; Inflammation-associated depression

Definition

Sickness behavior is a coordinated set of adaptive behavioral changes that occur in physically ill animals and humans during the course of infection. These behaviors include lethargy, depressed mood, reduced social exploration, loss of appetite, sleepiness, hyperalgesia, and, at times, confusion. This set of behaviors often accompanies fever and is considered a motivational state responsible for reorganizing an ill individual's perceptions and actions to enable better coping with infection (Dantzer et al. 2008).

Description

Sickness behavior is a normal response to infection and is characterized by endocrine, autonomic, and behavioral changes triggered by soluble proteins produced at the site of infection. Activated immune cells, such as macrophages and dendritic cells, release biochemical mediators called pro-inflammatory cytokines, such as interleukin (IL)-1, IL-6, and tumor necrosis factor (TNF)-alpha, which coordinate the local and systemic inflammatory response during active infection. These inflammatory mediators, in turn, act on the brain facilitating behavioral changes associated with sickness.

Much of the evidence supporting a link between pro-inflammatory cytokines and sickness behaviors comes from experimental studies in animals and humans. Peripheral and central administration of IL-1 and TNF-alpha in healthy laboratory animals induces fever and behavioral symptoms of sickness, including depressed activity, decreased food intake, and a curled posture. Sexual behavior is similarly reduced, particularly among females. IL-1 receptor antagonist (IL-1RA) blocks the biological effects of IL-1 when co-administered at 100- to 1000-fold excess dose with IL-1. Treatment with IL-1RA abrogates the depressing effect on social behavior but not food-motivated behavior, suggesting that IL-1 is a key mechanism in social function (Bluthe et al. 1992). Similar effects are seen when IL-1RA is injected directly into the brain. Time course studies of the behavioral effects of IL-1 in animals show changes in social exploration gradually develop within 2 h of peripheral administration whereas changes in food-motivated behavior reach a maximum by 1 h following treatment. Interestingly, IL-6 administered systemically or centrally has no behavioral effects despite inducing a fever response. That said, IL-6 does have the capacity to potentiate the effects of subthreshold dose of IL-1 administration suggesting that IL-6 may be behaviorally active only in the context of other pro-inflammatory mediators.

In humans, administration of endotoxin, a component of the outer membrane of Gram-negative bacteria, leads to systemic elevations in pro-inflammatory cytokines. This stimulus has been shown to cause participants to experience flu-like symptoms (e.g., fever, chills) as well as fatigue and depressed affect (reviewed in DellaGioia and Hannestad 2010). Moreover, a recent study demonstrated that subjects exposed experimentally to endotoxin led to increased self-reported levels of depressed mood and reduced activity in the ventral striatum in response to reward cues (Eisenberger et al. 2010), which is consistent with anhedonia.

There is substantial overlap between the behavioral components of sickness behavior and major depression in humans. As such, pro-inflammatory cytokines are proposed to participate in the pathophysiology of depression and potentially account for the high prevalence of depression among the medically ill (Smith 1991; Raison et al. 2006; Dantzer et al. 2008). Patients treated with immune-activating medications, such as IFN-a therapy prescribed for patients suffering with Hepatitis C or certain cancers, show elevated rates of depression compared to patients undergoing alternative therapies (Raison et al. 2006). Indeed, patients undergoing IFN-a therapy tend to experience depressive symptoms coupled with anxiety and irritability over a background of neurovegetative sickness–like symptoms, including sleep disorders, fatigue, and decreased appetite. While the mood disturbances generally occur between 4 and 12 weeks of treatment, the neurovegetative symptoms occur more rapidly, within the first 2 weeks of treatment.

Significant research efforts have focused on the neurochemical effects of inflammation that underlie sickness behavior and related depressive symptoms. Experimental animal data demonstrates that pro-inflammatory cytokines enhance indoleamine 2,3 dioxygenase (IDO) that peaks 24-h after endotoxin administration. This increase in IDO leads to a decrease in tryptophan (TRP), an essential amino acid that is actively transported into the brain for the synthesis of serotonin. IDO also leads to a decrease in kynurenine (KYN) and other tryptophan-related metabolites. Animals pretreated with a potent anti-inflammatory agent that blocks pro-inflammatory cytokines in the periphery and in the brain show significant reductions in both sickness and depressive behaviors. In contrast, animals treated with an inhibitor of IDO show a reduction in depressive behaviors but not neurovegetative symptoms, providing important evidence for the role of tryptophan metabolism in cytokine-induced depression (Dantzer et al. 2008). It is anticipated that this research will have important implications for effective treatment of inflammation-related depression in humans.

Cross-References

▶ Depression: Symptoms
▶ Illness Behavior
▶ Inflammation
▶ Psychoneuroimmunology

References and Further Readings

Bluthe, R. M., Dantzer, R., & Kelley, K. W. (1992). Effects of interleukin-1 receptor antagonist on the behavioral effects of lipopolysaccharide in rat. *Brain Research, 573*, 318–320.

Dantzer, R., Bluthe, R. M., Castanon, N., Kelley, K. W., Konsman, J. P., Laye, S., et al. (2007). Cytokines, sickness behavior, and depression. In R. Ader (Ed.), *Psychoneuroimmunology* (4th ed., pp. 281–318). New York: Academic Press.

Dantzer, R., O'Connor, J. C., Freund, G. G., Johnson, R. W., & Kelley, K. W. (2008). From inflammation to sickness and depression: When the immune system subjugates the brain. *Nature Neuroscience Reviews, 9*, 46–56.

DellaGioia, N., & Hannestad, J. (2010). A critical review of human endotoxin administration as an experimental paradigm of depression. *Neuroscience and Biobehavioral Reviews, 34*, 130–143.

Eisenberger, N. I., Berkman, E. T., Inagaki, T. K., Rameson, L. T., Mashal, N. M., & Irwin, M. R. (2010). Inflammation-induced anhedonia: Endotoxin reduces ventral striatum responses to reward. *Biological Psychiatry, 15*, 748–754.

Miller, A. H., Maletic, V., & Raison, C. L. (2009). Inflammation and its discontents: The role of cytokines in the pathophysiology of major depression. *Biological Psychiatry, 65*, 732–741.

Raison, C. L., Capuron, L., & Miller, A. H. (2006). Cytokines sing the blues: Inflammation and pathogenesis of depression. *Trends in Immunology, 27*, 24–31.

Smith, R. S. (1991). The macrophage theory of depression. *Medical Hypotheses, 35*, 298–306.

Siegrist, Johannes

Johannes Siegrist
Work Stress Research, Centre for Health and Society Faculty of Medicine, University of Düsseldorf, Life Science Center, Düsseldorf, Germany

Johannes Siegrist was born in Zofingen, Switzerland, on August 6, 1943. His nationality is Swiss, and he is married to Karin and has two daughters. Siegrist studied Sociology, Social Psychology, Philosophy, and History at the Universities of Basel (Switzerland) and Freiburg i.Br. (Germany). He received his M.A. (1967) and his Ph.D. (1969) in Sociology at the University of Freiburg. After postdoctoral training at the Universities of Ulm and Freiburg, he accomplished his habilitation in Sociology at the University of Freiburg (1973). In 1973, he was appointed as Professor of Medical Sociology at the Faculty of Medicine, University of Marburg (Germany), where he served until 1992, interrupted by Visiting Professorships at the Institute for Advanced Studies in Vienna (Austria) and at the Johns Hopkins Bloomberg School of Public Health in Baltimore, USA. In 1992, Siegrist was appointed as Professor of Medical Sociology and Director of the Department of Medical Sociology at the Faculty of Medicine, Heinrich Heine University of Dusseldorf, Germany, and as Director of the Postgraduate Training Program of Public Health at the same university. After his retirement in 2012, he was granted a Senior Professorship at this university to continue his research activities (Fig. 1).

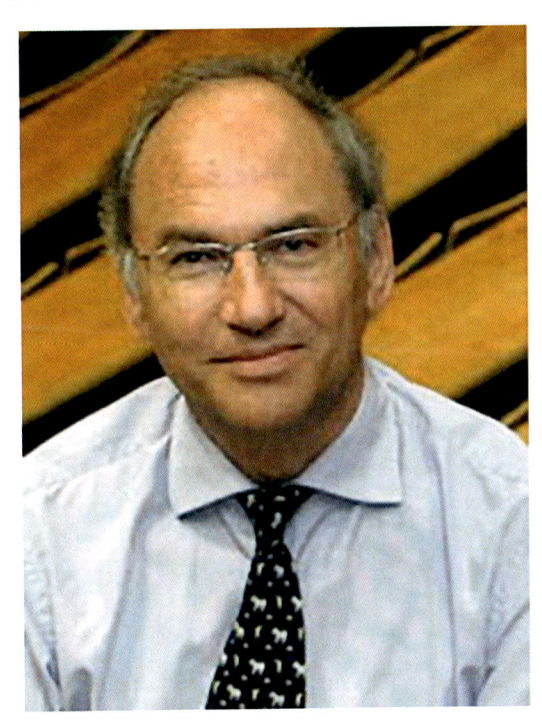

Siegrist, Johannes, Fig. 1 Johannes Siegrist

Siegrist has been President of the International Society of Behavioral Medicine (ISBM; 1996–1998), President of the European Society of Health and Medical Sociology (1990–1992), and Director of the European Science Foundation Program on Social Variations in Health Expectancy in Europe (1999–2003). He was Chair of the Section "Behavioral Sciences" of Academia Europaea (2004–2012), member of the Expert Panel of the German Research Foundation (2006–2010), and member of a Scientific Committee and two working groups of the German Academy of Sciences Leopoldina (since 2011).

He has been a Task Group Leader to the Marmot Review (Strategic Review of Health Inequalities in England post-2010) for the British Government, with a focus on work and health. In this same function, he has coordinated and edited a report on employment and working conditions in the context of the "Review of Social Determinants of Health and the Health Divide in the WHO European Region," commissioned by the WHO European Office in 2011. Since 2015, he is a member of the Advisory Board of OECD on guidelines for measuring the quality of working environments and a lead author of the report on social progress prepared by the International Panel for Social Progress (IPSP).

Siegrist served as Associate Editor or Advisory Board Member of several international journals (e.g., *International Journal of Behavioral Medicine*, *Social Science & Medicine*, *Social Psychiatry and Psychiatric Epidemiology*, *Work & Stress*, *European Journal of Public Health*, *Scandinavian Journal of Work, Environment and Health*).

The awards he received include Honorary Member of the European Society of Health and Medical Sociology where he also received the Research Award, Member of Academia Europaea (London), and Corresponding Member of the Heidelberg Academy of Sciences. He received the Salomon Neumann Award of the German Society of Social Medicine and Prevention, the Hans Roemer Award of the German College of Psychosomatic Medicine, and the Belle van Zuylen Chair at the University of Utrecht, the Netherlands.

Major Accomplishments

Siegrist's major contribution to scientific research concerns the development and test of a theoretical model of an adverse psychosocial work environment, with the aim of explaining stress-related disorders, termed "effort-reward imbalance" (ERI). The model posits that failed reciprocity of effort spent and rewards received at work ("high cost-low gain") elicits strong negative emotions and psychobiological stress responses with adverse long-term effects on health. Starting from cross-sectional and longitudinal epidemiological research in the late 1970s and early 1980s, together with collaborators Ingbert Weber, Karin Siegrist, Richard Peter, and others at Marburg University, he systematically elaborated and expanded research on the ERI model in a network of national and international scientific collaboration. The questionnaire measuring the model has been incorporated in a number of epidemiological studies (e.g., Whitehall II, GAZEL, CONSTANCES, German Socioeconomic Panel, German National Cohort Study) and was successfully applied in other sociocultural contexts (e.g., Japan) and in rapidly developing societies (e.g., China, Brazil).

Evidence from prospective cohort studies indicates that continued experience of failed reciprocity in terms of the ERI model is associated with significantly elevated odds of stress-related disorders. Most robust results are available on depression and coronary heart disease. Additionally, findings point to elevated risks of alcohol dependence, type 2 diabetes, reduced health functioning, sickness absence, and disability. This epidemiological evidence was supplemented by experiments and "naturalistic" studies (e.g., ambulatory blood pressure and heart rate monitoring), where reduced immune function, enhanced autonomic activity, and altered release patterns of stress hormones were linked to ERI, often in a dose-response relationship. Siegrist was also involved in some intervention studies where measures of reducing ERI at work were followed by improvements of well-being and mental health.

Siegrist applied the ERI model to other types of contractual social exchange, e.g., voluntary work, marital, or parent-child relations. Available results support the notion that failed reciprocity in core social roles exerts negative effects on health and well-being, suggesting a basic link between perceived injustice of effortful exchange and the development of stress-related disorders in humans. Siegrist has expanded this research with a focus on retirement, volunteering, and healthy aging, together with Morten Wahrendorf and other colleagues, in the frame of the Survey of Health, Ageing and Retirement in Europe (SHARE) and additional longitudinal investigations on aging populations. As a crosscutting topic of his long-lasting research career, Siegrist has put special emphasis on explaining and reducing avoidable social inequalities in health, both as a scientist and as an advocate for different stakeholders where he has proposed evidence-based policy recommendations for improving quality of work and employment and for reducing the burden of stress-related disease.

Cross-References

▶ International Society of Behavioral Medicine
▶ Occupational Health

References and Further Reading

Siegrist, J., & Marmot, M. (Eds.). (2006). *Social inequalities in health: New evidence and policy implications.* Oxford: Oxford University Press.

Siegrist, J., & Wahrendorf, M. (Eds.). (2016). *Work stress and health in a globalized economy: The model of effort-reward imbalance.* Dordrecht: Springer.

Siegrist, J., Starke, D., Chandola, T., Godin, I., Marmot, M., Niedhammer, I., & Peter, R. (2004). The measurement of effort-reward imbalance at work. European comparisons. *Social Science & Medicine, 58*, 1483–1499.

Simulation Games

▶ Health Gaming

Singing and Health

Genevieve A. Dingle[1] and Stephen Clift[2]
[1]The University of Queensland, Brisbane, QLD, Australia
[2]Sidney de Haan Research Centre for Arts and Health, Canterbury Christ Church University, Canterbury, UK

Synonyms

Choir; Choral singing; Group singing; Vocal group

Definition

Singing in health contexts typically involves participants with one or more health condition(s) gathering to sing together at weekly rehearsals and sometimes performing within a hospital or health service or in the community. Sessions commonly include a series of warm-up exercises, learning new songs as a group, and singing songs already in the singers' repertoire. Singing groups may be led by musicians, music educators, music therapists, or community musicians. Typically one or more health professionals are in attendance to support participants who require it. Some health choirs are for patients only while others feature patients and staff, or patients and carers, singing together.

Description

Examples of single condition choirs include the "Sing to Live" choir for people affected by breast cancer in Illinois; the "Brainwaves" and "Stroke a Chord" choirs in Australia for adults who have experienced a stroke; "Sing Your Lungs Out" choir in New Zealand and "Singing for Better Breathing" choirs in the UK for people who have chronic obstructive pulmonary disease; and "Remini-Sing" choir in Australia and "Singing for the Brain" in the UK for people with dementia and their carers. Other choirs include singers with a variety of diagnoses, for instance, the "Choir of Hard Knocks" in Australia comprises adults who are socially marginalized as a result of their mental illness, addiction, neurological condition, disability, or other ongoing health condition.

The purpose of health choirs is to improve the health and wellbeing of participants, rather than merely to keep patients occupied or, at the other extreme, to achieve an elite level of musical performance. These health aims may be met through the physical demands of standing, moving, and controlling the breath during regular singing rehearsals (e.g., Skingley et al. 2018) and the cognitive demands of listening, producing the correct sounds with the correct timing, learning and recalling lyrics and melodies, and coordinating movements such as swaying, tapping, and clicking while singing. The wellbeing aims may be met through the social bonding effects of group singing (e.g., Pearce et al. 2015) as well as the uplifting effect group singing has on emotions (e.g., Dingle et al. 2017). The social and emotional effects of choir singing may be particularly important for individuals affected by chronic health conditions whose ability to socialize may be adversely affected as a consequence of their health condition and its treatment. Indeed, a cross-national survey study of 1779 choristers revealed that singers perceived the following health benefits: social connection, physical and physiological benefits (specifically respiratory health), cognitive stimulation, mental health, enjoyment, and transcendence (Moss et al. 2018).

Emerging research shows that group singing is related to improved health and wellbeing among adults affected by cancers. For instance, one study examined the impact of singing on mood, stress, and immune response in three populations affected by cancer: carers ($n = 72$), bereaved carers ($n = 66$), and patients ($n = 55$). Assessments taken before and after 1 h of singing showed that singing was associated with significant reductions in negative emotions and increases in positive emotions, accompanied by significant increases in a majority of measured cytokines (substances secreted by cells as part of an immune response). Furthermore, singing was associated with reductions in cortisol, beta-endorphin, and oxytocin levels. These positive effects of singing were found in all three groups (Fancourt et al. 2016). In a Welsh study with 816 participants, a sub-sample of 203 completed initial, 3-month and 6-month questionnaires. Over time, measures of vitality and overall mental health improved, while levels of anxiety reduced significantly in both patients and non-patients (Reagon et al. 2017).

In the area of respiratory health, a review of six studies reported that singing has the potential to improve health-related quality of life, particularly related to physical health, and levels of anxiety without causing significant side effects. Qualitative data indicate that singing is an enjoyable experience for patients, who consistently report that it helps them to cope with their condition better (Lewis et al. 2016).

In relation to cognitive health, choir singing has been found to improve measures of cognitive functioning and wellbeing among healthy older adults (e.g., Coulton et al. 2015; Dingle et al. 2018). Much research is currently focusing on the potential benefits of choir singing for people with dementias. For instance, a Finnish study recruited 89 dyads (people with early dementia and their caregivers) and randomized them to a 10-week singing coaching group, a 10-week music listening coaching group, or a usual care control group (Särkämö et al. 2013). Compared with usual care, both weekly singing and music listening improved mood, orientation, and remote episodic memory and to a lesser extent, also attention and executive function and general cognition. Singing also enhanced short-term and working memory and caregiver wellbeing, whereas music listening had a positive effect on quality of life.

Turning to mental health, a systematic review of studies of choir singing for adults experiencing mental health conditions found that the results of seven longitudinal studies showed that while people with mental health conditions participated in choir singing, their mental health and wellbeing significantly improved with moderate to large effect sizes (Williams et al. 2018). Often physical health conditions were also featured in these samples, although changes in physical health measures were less frequently reported. Moreover, six qualitative studies based on interviews with choir participants yielded converging themes, indicating that group singing can provide enjoyment, improve emotional states, develop a sense of belonging, and enhance self-confidence in participants.

Taken together, this body of research on choir singing shows that it is associated with improvements in biological measures such as improved immune functioning and decreased stress hormone levels; improved lung functioning among people with respiratory conditions; improved cognitive performance in older adults; and improved self-reported mood, mental health, and wellbeing. Often these benefits extend to family members and carers who are also affected by the health condition and its treatment.

Cross-References

▶ Music and Health

References and Further Reading

Coulton, S., Clift, S., Skingley, A., & Rodriguez, J. (2015). Effectiveness and cost-effectiveness of community singing on mental health-related quality of life of older people: Randomised controlled trial. *The British Journal of Psychiatry, 207*(3), 250–255. https://doi.org/10.1192/bjp.bp.113.129908.

Dingle, G. A., Williams, E., Jetten, J., & Welch, J. (2017). Choir singing and creative writing enhance emotion regulation in adults with chronic mental health conditions. *British Journal of Clinical Psychology, 56*(4), 443–457. https://doi.org/10.1111/bjc.12149.

Dingle, G., Ellem, R., Davidson, R., Haslam, C., Clift, S., Humby, M., Stathis, A., & Williams, E. (2018). *Live wires music program connects and aids cognitive performance of older adults.* Paper presented at the Australian Association for cognitive behaviour therapy national conference, Brisbane, 25–27 Oct 2018.

Fancourt, D., Williamon, A., Carvalho, L. A., Steptoe, A., Dow, R., & Lewis, I. (2016). Singing modulates mood, stress, cortisol, cytokine and neuropeptide activity in cancer patients and carers. *eCancer, 10*, 631. https://doi.org/10.3332/ecancer.2016.631.

Lewis, A., Cave, P., Stern, M., Welch, L., Taylor, K., Russell, J., Doyle, A., Russell, A., McKee, H., Clift, S., Bott, J., & Hopkinson, N. S. (2016). Singing for lung health – A systematic review of the literature and consensus statement. *NPJ Primary Care Respiratory Medicine, 26*, 16080. https://doi.org/10.1038/npjpcrm.2016.80.

Moss, H., Lynch, J., & O'Donoghue, J. (2018). Exploring the perceived health benefits of singing in a choir: An international cross-sectional mixed-methods study. *Perspectives in Public Health, 138*(3), 160–168. https://doi.org/10.1177/1757913917739652.

Pearce, E., Launay, J., & Dunbar, R. I. M. (2015). The icebreaker effect: Singing mediates fast social bonding. *Royal Society Open Science, 2*, 150221. https://doi.org/10.1098/rsos.150221.

Reagon, C., Gale, N., Dow, R., Lewis, I., & van Duersen, R. (2017). Choir singing and health status in people affected by cancer. *European Journal of Cancer Care, 26*, e12568. https://doi.org/10.1111/ecc.12568.

Särkämö, T., Tervaniemi, M., Laitinen, S., Numminen, A., Kurki, M., Johnson, J. K., & Rantanen, P. (2013). Cognitive, emotional, and social benefits of regular musical activities in early dementia: Randomized controlled study. *The Gerontologist, 54*(4), 634–650. https://doi.org/10.1093/geront/gnt100.

Skingley, A., Clift, S., Hurley, S., Price, S., et al. (2018). Community singing groups for people with chronic obstructive pulmonary disease: Participant perspectives. *Perspectives in Public Health, 133*(1), 66–75. https://doi.org/10.1177/1757913917740930.

Williams, E., Dingle, G., & Clift, S. (2018). A systematic review of mental health and wellbeing outcomes of group singing for adults with a mental health condition. *European Journal of Public Health*. https://doi.org/10.1093/eurpub/cky115. Accepted 26 May 2018.

Single Nucleotide Polymorphism (SNP)

J. Rick Turner
Campbell University College of Pharmacy and Health Sciences, Buies Creek, NC, USA

Synonyms

SNP (pronounced "snip")

Definition

The term "single nucleotide polymorphism" contains two defining criteria. First, it refers to a single nucleotide, i.e., an individual base pair, that can differ between individuals. Second, the word polymorphism indicates that a particular nucleotide change of interest is shared by at least 1% of the population.

SNPs occur when one base pair replaces another base pair in a point mutation (see DNA entry for discussion of bases). For example, an A-T pairing may be replaced by a G-C pairing. Such a mutation does not typically harm the organism.

Cross-References

▶ DNA
▶ Polymorphism

References and Further Reading

Britannica. (2009). *The Britannica guide to genetics (Introduction by Steve Jones)*. Philadelphia: Running Press.

Single Subject

▶ Outcome for the Single Case: Random Control Index, Single Subject Experimental Design, and Goal Attainment Scale

Single-Case Experimental, or N of 1 Clinical Trials

▶ Outcome for the Single Case: Random Control Index, Single Subject Experimental Design, and Goal Attainment Scale

Situational Responsiveness

▶ Job Performance

Skeletal Muscle Atrophy

▶ Sarcopenia

Skin Cancer Prevention: Sun Protection, Sun Safety, Sunscreen Use

Karen Glanz
Schools of Medicine and Nursing, University of Pennsylvania, Philadelphia, PA, USA

Definition

Skin cancer is the most commonly diagnosed cancer in the United States, with more than one million Americans diagnosed with skin cancer each year. The incidence of skin cancer has increased dramatically worldwide in the last decade. Both main types of skin cancer – malignant melanoma and non-melanoma skin cancer (NMSC) – are now significant public health concerns. While skin cancer rates are increasing, it is considered one of the most preventable types of cancer.

The greatest risk factor for skin cancer is exposure to ultraviolet radiation, or UV radiation, which comes mainly from the sun. Behavioral recommendations for primary prevention of skin cancer include: limit time spent in the sun, avoid the sun during peak hours (10 a.m. to 4 p.m.), use sunscreen with a sun protection factor (SPF) of 15 or higher when outside, wear protective clothing (hats, shirts, pants) and sunglasses, seek shade when outdoors, and avoid sunburn. These behaviors, if consistently practiced, can help prevent all forms of skin cancer. There is some concern that using sunscreen will lead people who are trying to get a suntan to stay in the sun for a longer time, so another recommendation for prevention is not to intentionally bake in the sun or seek a tan.

Additional, important recommendations for behaviors to prevent skin cancer and related morbidity and mortality include performing regular skin self-examination and seeking professional evaluation of suspicious skin changes. Further, avoidance of indoor tanning and the use of tanning salons and tanning beds (also called "solaria") are strongly recommended.

An understanding of patterns of behavior can help to guide efforts to prevent skin cancer. More people take precautions at the beach or on vacation than when taking outdoor recreation. Parents are more likely to protect their children than themselves. Children are more often protected from UV radiation if their parents also protect themselves. Adolescents seem especially resistant to advice about skin cancer prevention and minimizing sun exposure.

Most skin cancer prevention interventions reported in the literature are directed at the general population through school-based curricula, multicomponent community programs, or media campaigns, and some recent trials have targeted people with high sun exposure at work or during outdoor recreation. Children, adolescents, and adults at high risk are important audiences for skin cancer prevention.

This chapter provides an overview of skin cancer prevention for the general population and groups at increased risk due to genetic or environmental exposures. The reference sources include evidence reviews, key research articles reporting on well-designed studies, and works addressing issues in measurement and methodology for skin cancer prevention research and evaluation.

Description

Evidence Reviews

An extensive evidence review of strategies to prevent skin cancer was undertaken by the Task Force on Community Preventive Services, and the results and recommendations were published in Saraiya et al. (2004). This report presents the results of systematic reviews of the effectiveness of interventions to prevent skin cancer by reducing exposure to ultraviolet radiation (UVR). The Task Force on Community Preventive Services found that education and policy approaches were effective when implemented in primary schools and in recreational or tourism settings but found insufficient evidence to determine effectiveness in other settings. This evidence review is currently being updated to reflect the continuing growth of the scientific literature on behavioral interventions to prevent skin cancer during the past decade.

Comprehensive Community Programs Including Mass Media

There is a long history of comprehensive, multi-component community skin cancer prevention programs, especially in Australia, where skin cancer is highly prevalent. These programs include mass media and communication campaigns as an integral part of these community programs.

Two related sun protection programs have been conducted in Australia for more than 20 years: Slip! Slop! Slap! from 1980 to 1988 and SunSmart from 1988 to the present (Montague et al. 2001). These programs have played an important role in changing the whole society's approach to the sun and have resulted in marked reductions in sun exposure. An examination of trends in behavioral risk factors for skin cancer over 15 years was examined in an Australian population exposed to the SunSmart program including SunSmart television advertising. Higher exposure to SunSmart advertising in the weeks before the interview increased preferences for not tanning, hat and sunscreen use, and greater clothing protection. These results indicate that sustained multicomponent programs with media campaigns can both prompt and reinforce skin cancer preventive behaviors.

Interventions in Schools

The most often studied settings for skin cancer prevention programs are schools, and there is good evidence that educational and policy interventions can be effective in primary schools (Saraiya et al. 2004). Of the many reported studies, a few are particularly well designed, carefully described, have long follow-up periods, and/or use objective outcome measures. The Kidskin intervention trial in Western Australia is particularly noteworthy and had a 6-year follow-up period. The "Kidskin" study involved three groups: control, "moderate," and "high" intervention. Results showed that children in the intervention groups – especially the "high" group – reported less sun exposure and spent less time outdoors in the middle of the day. There was little difference between groups in the wearing of hats or sunscreen (Milne et al. 2001). Children in the intervention groups – especially the high group – were less tanned at the end of the summer; this effect was greater for the back than for the forearms. There was also a smaller increase in the number of nevi (or moles) on the backs of children in the intervention groups (English et al. 2005). Further, the program had a positive effect on hat wearing on the playground, especially in the "high" intervention groups, but did not change children's use of shade at lunchtime (Giles-Corti et al. 2004).

Outdoor Workers

Outdoor workers are at high risk for skin cancer because they receive regular and significant solar UVR exposure. In a well-designed study to reduce UVR exposure among ski instructors, greater program implementation was associated with less sunburn. In an intervention for US Postal Service workers, regular sunscreen and hat use were higher among the intervention group than among the control group after 3 months and at 3-year follow-up (Mayer et al. 2007, 2009).

Recreation Settings

Intense and prolonged sun exposure often occurs during outdoor recreation activities. High UVR exposure, often with minimal clothing, tends to occur at beach and swimming pool settings. Other outdoor recreation settings include camps, zoos, and parks. Large and well-designed studies of skin cancer prevention in these locations have been reported. Effective skin cancer prevention programs for children have been evaluated in swimming pool settings (Glanz et al. 2002; Glanz et al. 2005) and for beachgoers at Northeastern (Weinstock et al. 2002) and Midwestern (Pagoto et al. 2003) beaches as well as at zoos (Mayer et al. 2001).

High-Risk Groups

Targeting skin cancer prevention to people at high risk may result in greater effects of preventive strategies and an efficient public health strategy. Risk factors for skin cancer include age, sun-sensitive phenotypes, excess sun exposure, family history, personal history of skin cancer or precancerous lesions, and some other medical conditions. There is a need to develop low-cost, effective interventions to improve skin cancer prevention and early detection behaviors among a broader population of persons at moderate and high risk. (Geller et al. 2006) and Glanz, Schoenfeld, and Steffen (2010) describe studies of effective tailored interventions that specifically target individuals at high risk, either siblings of melanoma patients or adults determined to be at moderate or high risk for skin cancer. These studies focused on both prevention and skin examinations. A study of a group of people who have tested positive in genetic testing for skin cancer-related mutations and found that positive genetic test results led to greater intentions to obtain total body skin examinations and adhere to skin self-examination recommendations (Aspinwall et al. 2008).

Screening and Early Detection

Screening for skin cancer through health-care-provider skin exams and skin self-examination has the potential to help detect skin cancers at an earlier stage (i.e., when they are thinner) so that they are more curable and less serious. Although there has not been a large randomized trial of skin screening in the United States, an Australian trial reported by Aitken et al. (2006) provides promising evidence of the impact of skin screening and how it can be successfully implemented. A randomized trial was conducted to determine whether a multicomponent intervention can increase total skin self-examination (TSSE) performance. Participants received instructional materials, a video, and a brief counseling session and a brief follow-up phone call and tailored feedback letters. Results showed that the intervention group increased TSSE performance in the intervention group compared to the control group (Weinstock et al. 2007). A follow-up article aimed to identify the most important Check-It-Out intervention components for promoting TSSE. Results showed that watching the video, using the hand mirror, shower card, American Cancer Society brochure, sample photographs, and finding the health educator helpful were associated with performing TSSE at 2 months, 12 months, or both. The studies of high-risk groups reported by Geller et al. (2006) and Glanz et al. (2010) also targeted behavioral outcomes of skin self-examination and thorough examination of all moles.

Measurement and Methodology

Advances in skin cancer prevention depend on good quality research and ideally different intervention studies that can be compared to understand the impact of various strategies. Most skin cancer prevention studies uses verbal reports, or self-report, to measure habitual sun exposure and solar protection behaviors. Despite the well-known limitations of verbal reports of behavior, these measures are the most practical for use in both population surveillance and descriptive and intervention research (Glanz and Mayer 2005). Therefore, the comparability of assessments across population-based surveys and outcome measures used in intervention research is important, and a core set of measures was recently published by a diverse group of investigators in the field (Glanz et al. 2008). In addition, because it is important to continue to build a research tool kit for measures other than surveys, including objective biological measures and observational measures, recent research to validate self-reports of sunscreen use (Glanz et al. 2009) and other behaviors is of particular importance to the field.

Conclusion

Skin cancer prevention interventions have demonstrated modest success, with the majority of programs being conducted in school settings. It is believed that the ideal intervention strategies for reducing exposure to ultraviolet radiation (UVR) exposure are coordinated, sustained, community-wide approaches that combine education, mass media, and environmental and structural changes. Interventions within specific organizational settings such as schools, health care, recreation programs, and workplaces provide useful ways to reach important audiences like children and are suitable venues for structural supports such as environmental and policy change that complement educational efforts. It is generally agreed that environmental and structural changes also need to be part of successful skin cancer prevention efforts. Advances in measurement and methods in skin cancer prevention research will contribute to future efforts to address this important and widespread health and behavior problem.

Cross-References

▶ Cancer Prevention

References and Readings

Aitken, J. F., Janda, M., Elwood, M., Youl, P. H., Ring, I. T., & Lowe, J. B. (2006). Clinical outcomes from skin screening clinics within a community-based melanoma screening program. *Journal of the American Academy of Dermatology, 54*, 105–114.

Aspinwall, L. G., Leaf, S. L., Dola, E. R., Kohlmann, W., & Leachman, S. A. (2008). CDKN2A/p16 genetic test reporting improves early detection intentions and practices in high-risk melanoma families. *Cancer Epidemiology, Biomarkers & Prevention, 17*, 1510–1519.

English, D. R., Milne, E., Jacoby, P., Giles-Corti, B., Cross, D., & Johnston, R. (2005). The effect of a school-based sun protection intervention on the development of melanocytic nevi in children: 6-year follow-up. *Cancer Epidemiology, Biomarkers & Prevention, 14*, 977–980.

Geller, A. C., Emmons, K. M., Brooks, D. R., Powers, C., Zhang, Z., Koh, H. K., Heeren, T., Sober, A. J., Li, F., & Gilchrest, B. A. (2006). A randomized trial to improve early detection and prevention practices among siblings of melanoma patients. *Cancer, 107*, 806–814.

Giles-Corti, B., English, D., Costa, C., Milne, E., Cross, D., & Johnston, R. (2004). Creating SunSmart schools. *Health Education Research, 19*, 98–109.

Glanz, K., & Mayer, J. A. (2005). Reducing UVR exposure to prevent skin cancer: Methodology and measurement. *American Journal of Preventive Medicine, 29*, 131–142.

Glanz, K., Geller, A. C., Shigaki, D., Maddock, J., & Isnec, M. R. (2002). A randomized trial of skin cancer prevention in aquatic settings: The Pool Cool program. *Health Psychology, 21*, 579–587.

Glanz, K., Steffen, A., Elliott, T., & O'Riordan, D. (2005). Diffusion of an effective skin cancer prevention program: Design, theoretical foundations, and first-year implementation. *Health Psychology, 24*, 477–487.

Glanz, K., Yaroch, A. L., Dancel, M., Saraiya, M., Crane, L. A., Buller, D. B., et al. (2008). Measures of sun exposure and sun protection practices for behavioral and epidemiologic research. *Archives of Dermatology, 144*, 217–222.

Glanz, K., McCarty, F., Nehl, E. J., O'Riordan, D. L., Gies, P., Bundy, L., et al. (2009). Validity of self-reported sunscreen use by parents, children and lifeguards. *American Journal of Preventive Medicine, 36*, 63–69.

Glanz, K., Schoenfeld, E. R., & Steffen, A. (2010). Randomized trial of tailored skin cancer prevention messages for adults: Project SCAPE. *American Journal of Public Health, 100*, 735–741.

Mayer, J. A., Lewis, E. C., Eckhardt, L., Slymen, D., Belch, G., Elder, J., et al. (2001). Promoting sun safety among zoo visitors. *Preventive Medicine, 33*, 162–169.

Mayer, J. A., Slymen, D. J., Clapp, E. J., Pichon, L. C., Eckhardt, L., Eichenfield, L. F., et al. (2007). Promoting sun safety among US postal service letter carriers: Impact of a 2-year intervention. *American Journal of Public Health, 97*, 559–565.

Mayer, J. A., Slymen, D. J., Clapp, E. J., Pichon, L. C., Elder, J. P., Sallis, J. F., et al. (2009). Long-term maintenance of a successful occupational sun safety intervention. *Archives of Dermatology, 145*, 88–89.

Milne, E., English, D. R., Johnston, R., Cross, D., Borland, R., Giles-Corti, B., et al. (2001). Reduced sun exposure and tanning in children after 2 years of a school-based intervention (Australia). *Cancer Causes and Control, 12*, 387–393.

Montague, M., Borland, R., & Sinclair, C. (2001). Slip! Slop! Slap! and SunSmart, 1980-2000: Skin cancer control and 20 years of population-based campaigning. *Health Education & Behavior, 28*, 290–305.

Pagoto, S., McChargue, D., & Fuqua, R. (2003). Effects of a multicomponent intervention on motivation and sun protection behaviors among midwestern beachgoers. *Health Psychology, 22*, 429–433.

Saraiya, M., Glanz, K., Briss, P. A., Nichols, P., White, C., Das, D., et al. (2004). Interventions to prevent skin cancer by reducing exposure to ultraviolet radiation – a systematic review. *American Journal of Preventive Medicine, 27*, 422–466.

Weinstock, M. A., Rossi, J. S., Redding, C. A., & Maddock, J. E. (2002). Randomized controlled community trial of the efficacy of a multicomponent stage-matched intervention to increase sun protection among beachgoers. *Preventive Medicine, 35*, 584–592.

Weinstock, M. A., Risica, P. M., Martin, R. A., Rakowski, W., Dubé, C., Berwick, M., et al. (2007). Melanoma early detection with thorough skin self-examination: The "check it out" randomized trial. *American Journal of Preventive Medicine, 32*, 517–524.

SLC6A4 (Solute Carrier Family 6, Member 4)

▶ Serotonin Transporter Gene

Sleep

Martica H. Hall
Department of Psychiatry, University of Pittsburgh, Pittsburgh, PA, USA

Definition

Sleep is a complex reversible neurobiological state characterized by closed eyes, behavioral quiescence, and perceptual disengagement from one's surroundings.

Description

Healthy adults cycle between two types of sleep during the typical nocturnal sleep period: non-rapid eye movement (NREM) sleep and rapid eye movement (REM) sleep. When healthy adults fall asleep, they enter NREM sleep and usually move from lighter stages of sleep (e.g., Stages N1 and N2) to deeper sleep (e.g., Stage N3) before entering their first REM sleep period. The terms "light" and "deep" sleep refer to the ease with which one can be awakened from sleep and become fully oriented to one's surroundings. The descent from light into deep NREM sleep is characterized by decreasing inputs from external stimuli, a slowing of catabolic processes, and an increase in parasympathetic nervous system activity. In contrast, REM sleep is characterized by autonomic instability and active mental activity. In healthy adults, individual NREM-REM cycles generally last approximately 90 min, although the duration of sleep cycles varies across individuals. During the first third of the night, NREM sleep is more prevalent, whereas REM sleep becomes more prevalent during the last third of the night.

Sleep can be characterized along multiple dimensions. Here we focus on four dimensions of sleep that have been most widely evaluated in relation to health and functioning; these include sleep *duration*, *continuity*, *architecture*, and *quality*. It is important to recognize that each of these dimensions of sleep changes across the life span, from infancy through old age and may, additionally, be moderated by sex, race/ethnicity, and mental and physical health conditions (Carrier et al. 2001; Carskadon and Dement 2005; Hall et al. 2009; Ohayon et al. 2004).

Sleep Duration

The two most commonly assessed indices of sleep duration include "time in bed" and "total sleep time." Operationally, time in bed (TIB) may be defined as total hours elapsed between getting into bed to go to sleep at night ("good night time") and waking up in the morning ("good morning time"). Total sleep time (TST) may be operationalized as time in bed minus the amount of time needed to fall asleep ("sleep latency") and amount of time spent awake during the night ("wakefulness after sleep onset").

Sleep duration is one of the most widely studied dimensions of sleep in relation to health and functioning (see entry on ▶ "Sleep Duration, ▶ Sleep and Health"). For the most part, this literature has documented robust associations among sleep duration extremes (generally, <6 h or >8 h) and indices of morbidity and mortality. One meta-analysis of 23 studies reported pooled relative risk (RR) values of 1.10 (95% CI = 1.06–1.15) and 1.23 (95% CI = 1.17–1.30) for all-cause mortality and short and long sleep duration, respectively (Gallicchio and Kalesan 2009).

It must be noted, however, that studies using objective measures (actigraphy, PSG) of sleep duration and health outcomes are lacking. This issue is especially important given discrepancies between self-reported and objective indices of sleep duration, which may be confounded by other risk factors for morbidity and mortality such as age, sex, race, BMI, and comorbidities. Nor do measures of sleep duration differentiate between individuals with or without primary sleep disorders such as sleep apnea and insomnia, which have been widely linked to health and functioning (Boivin 2000; Somers 2005).

Sleep Continuity

Measures of sleep continuity focus on one's ability to initiate and maintain sleep (see ▶ "Sleep Continuity, ▶ Sleep Fragmentation" entries). *Sleep latency* refers to the amount of time it takes to fall asleep (e.g., minutes from "good night time" to onset of sleep), whereas *wakefulness after sleep onset* (WASO) refers to the total amount of wakefulness during the sleep period (e.g., minutes of wakefulness between sleep onset and "good morning time"). *Sleep efficiency* is a proportional sleep continuity measure which refers to the percentage of time in bed spent asleep. Although operational definitions may differ across laboratories, sleep efficiency is commonly calculated as follows: (time spent asleep/ time in bed) × 100.

Compared to sleep duration, fewer population-based studies have evaluated relationships among sleep continuity and indices of health and functioning. Several studies have linked self-reported sleep continuity disturbances with incident Type2 diabetes and cardiovascular disease (as reviewed by Mezick et al. under review). Although few in number, other studies have reported significant cross-sectional associations between objectively assessed sleep continuity disturbances and health outcomes including obesity, increased blood pressure, increased inflammation, decreased circulating natural killer cell numbers, and the metabolic syndrome (Hall et al. 1998; Knutson et al. 2009; Mills et al. 2007). In their longitudinal study of sleep and all-cause mortality in healthy older adults, Dew and colleagues reported that participants with PSG-assessed sleep latencies of greater than 30 min were at 2.14 times greater risk of death (95% CI = 1.25–3.6) compared to those who fell asleep in less than 30 min, after adjusting for age, medical burden, and other relevant covariates (Dew et al. 2003).

Emerging evidence based on experimental models of sleep fragmentation suggests that endocrine, immune, metabolic, and autonomic mechanisms may be important pathways through which sleep continuity disturbances influence health and functioning (Bonnet and Arand 2003; Janackova and Sforza 2008; Redwine et al. 2003; Tartar et al. 2009). In terms of its relevance to behavioral medicine and health, sleep continuity appears to be exquisitely sensitive to psychological and social factors such as stress, loneliness, relationship quality, and socioeconomic status Akerstedt et al. 2002; Cacioppo et al. 2002; Cartwright and Wood 1991; Friedman et al. 2005; Hall et al. 2008).

Sleep Architecture

Sleep architecture refers to the pattern or distribution of visually scored NREM and REM sleep stages as well as quantitative measures derived from power spectral analysis of the EEG (see "▶ Sleep Architecture" entry). Within NREM sleep, measures of sleep architecture include stages N1-N3. Lighter stages of sleep are characterized by low-amplitude, fast-frequency EEG activity whereas deeper stages of sleep are characterized by high-amplitude, low-frequency EEG activity generated by rhythmic oscillations of thalamic and cortical neurons (see Jones 2005).

Patients with medical disorders including cardiovascular and kidney disease, diabetes, and cancer exhibit lighter sleep architecture profiles compared to healthy individuals (e.g., Jauch-Chara et al. 2008; Ranjbaran et al. 2007). Yet, these studies do not indicate whether sleep architecture profiles were a contributing cause or consequence of disease. Both possibilities are plausible given experimental evidence of bidirectional relationships among components of sleep architecture and physiological processes important to health and functioning including metabolic, endocrine, autonomic, and immune mechanisms (e.g., Hall et al. 2004; Opp 2006; Rasch et al. 2007). The longitudinal study of sleep and mortality by Dew et al. (2003) is the only published study, to date, that has evaluated relationships among measures of sleep architecture and indices of morbidity or mortality. In this study, risk for mortality was significantly higher in individuals with extreme amounts of REM sleep (upper and lower 15th percentile of the sample distribution); the visually scored slow-wave sleep percentage was also modestly associated with survival time.

Experimental manipulation of sleep architecture, although technically complex, may be an especially promising approach to disentangling cause and effect and evaluating cellular and molecular mechanisms through which sleep architecture affects and is affected by health. Quantitative analysis of the EEG, which shows trait-like characteristics, may hold promise for identifying sleep phenotypes that confer vulnerability to or resilience against disease (e.g., Tucker et al. 2007). This latter point may be especially relevant to behavioral medicine models of disease given that decreased slow-wave sleep and increased EEG spectral power in the fast-frequency beta band have been linked with symptoms of stress and a variety of chronic stressors including job strain, marital dissolution, and bereavement (Cartwright and Wood 1991; Hall et al. 1997; Kecklund and Akerstedt 2004).

Sleep Quality

Sleep quality generally refers to subjective perceptions about one's sleep. The Pittsburgh Sleep Quality Index (PSQI), which is the most widely used self-report sleep instrument and has been translated into over 30 languages, is an example of a "multiple-indicator" measure of sleep quality (Buysse et al. 1989). The PSQI includes 18 retrospective questions about one's sleep over the past month. These questions are used to derive seven subscales (sleep duration, sleep latency, sleep efficiency, sleep disturbance, daytime dysfunction, use of medications for sleep, and overall sleep quality), each of which has a range of 0–3. These subscales may be summed to generate a global measure of subjective sleep quality with a range of 0–21; higher values reflect greater subjective sleep complaints.

In a community-based study of midlife adults without clinical cardiovascular disease, Jennings and colleagues reported that higher PSQI-assessed sleep quality complaints were associated with increased prevalence of the metabolic syndrome (Jennings et al. 2007). Other cross-sectional studies have reported greater subjective sleep quality complaints in patients with hypertension, diabetes, kidney disease, polycystic ovary syndrome, and cancer compared to age- and sex-matched healthy controls (e.g., Liu et al. 2009; Sabbatini et al. 2008; Tasali et al. 2006). Subjective sleep quality complaints may be a consequence of disease. It may also indirectly impact health via health behavior pathways. For instance, subjective perceptions that one's sleep is not sound or restorative may lead to increased daytime caffeine use and increased use of alcohol prior to sleep which, in turn, may negatively impact health and functioning.

Summary

Converging evidence suggests numerous links between specific dimensions of sleep and important indices of health and functioning. The two most prevalent sleep disorders, insomnia and sleep apnea, too have been prospectively linked to adverse health outcomes (see entries for "▶ Obstructive Sleep Apnea"). Yet, little is understood about *how* specific dimensions of sleep or sleep disorders may confer vulnerability or resilience to disease. Identification of the cellular and molecular pathways through which sleep affects and is affected by health is critical to advancing our understanding of the sleep-health relationship in the context of behavioral medicine.

Cross-References

▶ Coffee Drinking, Effects of Caffeine
▶ Sleep Architecture
▶ Sleep Continuity
▶ Sleep Duration
▶ Sleep Quality

References and Further Readings

Akerstedt, T., Knutsson, A., Westerholm, P., Theorell, T., Alfredsson, L., Kecklund, G., et al. (2002). Sleep disturbances, work stress and work hours: A cross-sectional study. *Journal of Psychosomatic Research, 53*, 741–748.

Boivin, D. B. (2000). Influence of sleep-wake and circadian rhythm disturbances in psychiatric disorders. *Journal of Psychiatry & Neuroscience, 25*, 446–458.

Bonnet, M. H., & Arand, D. L. (2003). Clinical effects of sleep fragmentation versus sleep deprivation. *Sleep Medicine Reviews, 7*, 297–310.

Buysse, D. J., Reynolds, C. F., Monk, T. H., Berman, S. R., & Kupfer, D. J. (1989). The Pittsburgh sleep quality index: A new instrument for psychiatric practice and research. *Psychiatry Research, 28*, 193–213.

Cacioppo, J. T., Hawkley, L. C., Berntson, G. G., Ernst, J. M., Gibbs, A. C., Stickgold, R., et al. (2002). Do lonely days invade the nights? Potential social modulation of sleep efficiency. *Psychological Science, 13*, 384–387.

Carrier, J., Land, S., Buysse, D. J., Kupfer, D. J., & Monk, T. H. (2001). The effects of age and gender on sleep EEG power spectral density in the middle years of life (aged 20–60 years old). *Psychophysiology, 38*, 232–242.

Carskadon, M. A., & Dement, W. C. (2005). Normal human sleep: an overview. In M. H. Kryger, T. Roth, & T. Dement (Eds.), *Principles and practice of sleep medicine* (pp. 13–23). Philadelphia: Elsevier/Saunders.

Cartwright, R. D., & Wood, E. (1991). Adjustment disorders of sleep: The sleep effects of a major stressful event and its resolution. *Psychiatry Research, 39*, 199–209.

Dew, M. A., Hoch, C. C., Buysse, D. J., Monk, T. H., Begley, A. E., Houck, P. R., et al. (2003). Healthy older adults' sleep predicts all-cause mortality at 4 to 19 years of follow-up. *Psychosomatic Medicine, 65*, 63–73.

Friedman, E. M., Hayney, M. S., Love, G. D., Urry, H. L., Rosenkranz, M. A., Davidson, R. J., et al. (2005). Social relationships, sleep quality, and interleukin-6 in aging women. *Proceedings of the National Academy of Sciences U S A, 102*, 18757–18762.

Gallicchio, L., & Kalesan, B. (2009). Sleep duration and mortality: A systematic review and meta-analysis. *Journal of Sleep Research, 18*, 148–158.

Hall, M., Buysse, D. J., Dew, M. A., Prigerson, H. G., Kupfer, D. J., & Reynolds, C. F. (1997). Intrusive thoughts and avoidance behaviors are associated with sleep disturbances in bereavement-related depression. *Depression and Anxiety, 6*, 106–112.

Hall, M., Baum, A., Buysse, D. J., Prigerson, H. G., Kupfer, D. J., Reynolds, C. F., et al. (1998). Sleep as a mediator of the stress-immune relationship. *Psychosomatic Medicine, 60*, 48–51.

Hall, M., Vasko, R., Buysse, D. J., Ombao, H., Chen, Q., Cashmere, J. D., et al. (2004). Acute stress affects heart rate variability during sleep. *Psychosomatic Medicine, 66*, 56–62.

Hall, M., Buysse, D. J., Nofzinger, E. A., Reynolds, C. F., & Monk, T. H. (2008). Financial strain is a significant correlate of sleep continuity disturbances in late-life. *Biological Psychology, 77*, 217–222.

Hall, M., Matthews, K. A., Kravitz, H. K., Gold, E. B., Buysse, D. J., Bromberger, J. T., et al. (2009). Race and financial strain are independent correlates of sleep in mid-life women: The SWAN sleep study. *Sleep, 32*, 73–82.

Janackova, S., & Sforza, E. (2008). Neurobiology of sleep fragmentation: Cortical and autonomic markers of sleep disorders. *Current Pharmaceutical Design, 14*, 3474–3480.

Jauch-Chara, K., Schmid, S. M., Hallschmid, M., Born, J., & Schultes, B. (2008). Altered neuroendocrine sleep architecture in patients with type 1 diabetes. *Diabetes Care, 31*, 1183–1188.

Jennings, J. R., Muldoon, M., Hall, M., Buysse, D. J., & Manuck, S. B. (2007). Self-reported sleep quality is associated with the metabolic syndrome. *Sleep, 30*, 219–223.

Jones, B. E. (2005). Basic mechanisms of sleep-wake states. In M. H. Kryger, T. Roth, & W. C. Dement (Eds.), *Principles and practice of sleep medicine* (pp. 136–153). Philadelphia: Elsevier/Saunders.

Kecklund, G., & Akerstedt, T. (2004). Apprehension of the subsequent working day is associated with a low amount of slow wave sleep. *Biological Psychology, 66*, 169–176.

Knutson, K. L., Van Cauter, E., Rathouz, P. J., Yan, L. L., Hulley, S. B., Liu, K., et al. (2009). Association between sleep and blood pressure in midlife: The CARDIA sleep study. *Archives of Internal Medicine, 169*, 1055–1061.

Liu, L., Fiorentino, L., Natarajan, L., Parker, B. A., Mills, P. J., Sadler, G. R., et al. (2009). Pre-treatment symptom cluster in breast cancer patients is associated with worse sleep, fatigue and depression during chemotherapy. *Psycho-Oncology, 18*, 187–194.

Mills, P. J., von Kanel, R., Norman, D., Natarajan, L., Ziegler, M. G., Dimsdale, J. E., et al. (2007). Inflammation and sleep in healthy individuals. *Sleep, 30*, 729–735.

Ohayon, M. M., Carskadon, M. A., Guilleminault, C., & Vitiello, M. V. (2004). Meta-analysis of quantitative sleep parameters from childhood to old age in healthy individuals: Developing normative sleep values across the human lifespan. *Sleep, 27*, 1255–1273.

Opp, M. R. (2006). Sleep and psychoneuroimmunology. *Neurologic Clinics, 24*, 493–506.

Ranjbaran, Z., Keefer, L., Stepanski, E., Farhadi, A., & Keshavarzian, A. (2007). The relevance of sleep abnormalities to chronic inflammatory conditions. *Inflammation Research, 56*, 1–7.

Rasch, B., Dodt, C., Moelle, M., & Born, J. (2007). Sleep-stage-specific regulation of plasma catecholamine concentration. *Psychoneuroendocrinology, 32*, 884–891.

Redwine, L., Dang, J., Hall, M., & Irwin, M. (2003). Disordered sleep, nocturnal cytokines, and immunity in alcoholics. *Psychosomatic Medicine, 65*, 75–85.

Sabbatini, M., Pisani, A., Crispo, A., Nappi, R., Gallo, R., Cianciaruso, B., et al. (2008). Renal transplantation and sleep: A new life is not enough. *Journal of Nephrology, 21*(Suppl 13), S97–S101.

Somers, V. K. (2005). Sleep: A new cardiovascular frontier. *The New England Journal of Medicine, 353*, 2070–2073.

Tartar, J. L., Ward, C. P., Cordeira, J. W., Legare, S. L., Blanchette, A. J., McCarley, R. W., & Strecker, R. E. (2009). Experimental sleep fragmentation and sleep deprivation in rats increases exploration in an open field test of anxiety while increasing plasma corticosterone levels. *Behavioural Brain Research, 197*, 450–453.

Tasali, E., Van Cauter, E., & Ehrmann, D. A. (2006). Relationships between sleep disordered breathing and glucose metabolism in polycystic ovary syndrome. *The Journal of Clinical Endocrinology and Metabolism, 91*, 36–42.

Tucker, A. M., Dinges, D. F., & Van Dongen, H. P. (2007). Trait interindividual differences in the sleep physiology of healthy young adults. *Journal of Sleep Research, 16*, 170–180.

Sleep and Health

Faith S. Luyster
School of Nursing, University of Pittsburgh, Pittsburgh, PA, USA

Synonyms

Sleep deprivation

Definition

Sleep is defined as a reversible state of perceptual disengagement and unresponsiveness to the external environment. Sleep is a complex physiological and behavioral process that is part of every individual's life and a critical determinant of physical and mental health.

Description

It is generally accepted that 7–8 h is the optimal amount of sleep needed per night for adequate daytime functioning and to reduce the risk of developing serious medical conditions. However, many Americans sleep less than 7 h per night and many report sleep difficulties. The percentage of men and women reporting sleeping less than 6 h per night has increased significantly over the last 20 years. Broad societal changes, including longer work hours, shift work, later night life, increased dependence on technology, and a current mindset of "if you snooze, you lose" have contributed to the increases in sleep loss among adults. Sleep loss increases the risk and incidence of diseases that may ultimately result in death. Many of the studies examining sleep duration and adverse health outcomes have found a U-shaped relationship suggesting that too little sleep and too much sleep is detrimental to health. And, between 7 and 8 h of sleep appears to be associated with reduced health risk.

Sleep and Mortality

Growing evidence over the last few decades suggests that progressively shorter (<7 h per night) or longer (>8 h per night) sleep duration is associated with a greater risk of mortality (Cappuccio et al. 2010; Kripke et al. 2002). The mechanisms that underlie these associations are not fully understood. Potential adverse physiologic effects of short sleep duration may contribute to negative health outcomes like cardiovascular disease, diabetes, and obesity, all of which are associated with increased mortality risk. Sleep restriction has been shown to impair glucose tolerance, increase evening cortisol levels, alter sympathetic nervous system activity, reduce leptin levels and increase levels of ghrelin, and increase inflammatory markers. The mechanisms linking long sleep duration with mortality is unknown and may be explained by underlying confounders such as depression, low socioeconomic status, undiagnosed medical disease, poor physical health, and less physical activity.

Sleep and Cardiovascular Disease

Sleeping less than 7 h per night has been found to increase the risk of developing high blood pressure (i.e., hypertension) and elevate blood pressure in those with existing hypertension (Calhoun and Harding 2010). Long sleep duration (≥ 9 h per night) may also increase the risk of hypertension. The effect of insufficient sleep on blood pressure may help to explain the relationship between poor sleep and cardiovascular disease and stroke. Researchers have found both short (<7 h per night) and long (>8 h per night) sleep durations are associated with a greater risk of developing or dying from coronary heart disease and stroke (Cappuccio et al. 2011).

There is also growing evidence of a connection between ▶ "Sleep Apnea" and cardiovascular disease. People with sleep apnea have frequent awakenings at night as a result of repetitive pauses in breathing. This sleep fragmentation and reoccurring drops in oxygen levels in the blood called hypoxemia cause increases in blood pressure during the night that can persist during the daytime and over time can lead to hypertension. People with sleep apnea have an increased risk of developing coronary heart disease, stroke, and heart failure. In a 10-year study, severe sleep apnea was associated with an increased risk of fatal and nonfatal cardiovascular events.

Sleep and Obesity

Numerous studies have reported a link between sleep duration and obesity. For example, researchers have shown that people who sleep less than 6 h per night or more than 8 h per night are more likely to have a higher body mass index and that people who sleep 8 h have the lowest BMI (Cappuccio et al. 2008). Several pathways have been identified that could mediate the relationship between short sleep and increased risk of obesity: alterations in glucose metabolism, appetite control, and energy expenditure. Sleep loss impacts hormones that regulate glucose processing and appetite (Taheri et al. 2004). After sleep loss, the body's tissues are less responsive to insulin (i.e., insulin resistance), a hormone secreted by the pancreas that regulates the level of glucose in the body. As a result, glucose levels in the blood remain high, making it more difficult for the body to use stored fat for energy. Sleep loss also impacts hormones involved in appetite regulation causing people to eat even when they have had an adequate number of calories. Specifically, short sleep lowers levels of leptin, a "full signal" hormone, and increases levels of ghrelin, an appetite stimulant hormone. One night of sleep loss can decrease energy expenditure (i.e., calories burned) during rest.

Sleep and Diabetes

Numerous epidemiological studies have found that short (≤ 6 h per night) and long (≥ 9 h per night) sleep durations are associated with an increased risk of developing type 2 diabetes and impaired glucose tolerance, a precursor to diabetes (Knutson and Van Cauter 2008). Insulin resistance associated with sleep loss can over time compromise the ability of β-cells in the pancreas to release insulin, causing higher than normal levels of glucose in the blood which can lead to type 2 diabetes. In a study of healthy adults, restricting sleep to 4 h per night for six nights led to impaired glucose tolerance.

In addition, sleep apnea is a risk factor for developing type 2 diabetes. Several potential mechanisms explaining how sleep apnea may alter glucose metabolism have been proposed. Sleep fragmentation and hypoxemia associated with sleep apnea can alter autonomic and neuroendocrine function, increase release of inflammatory cytokines, and induce adipokines and thus play a role in altering glucose metabolism.

Sleep and Cancer

Emerging evidence suggests that sleep duration may increase risks of several types of cancer. The first investigation of the association between sleep and breast cancer found women with longer sleep durations (≥9 h per night) had a decreased risk of breast cancer. Subsequent studies have found mixed results with some studies finding an inverse relationship between short sleep duration and risk of breast cancer and one study found no association. Short sleep duration was associated with an increased risk of colorectal cancer in patients undergoing colonoscopy screening and an increased risk of prostate cancer. Epidemiological studies have reported a significantly increased risk of developing a number of malignancies including breast, colon, prostate, and endometrial cancer in night-shift workers. Nocturnal melatonin suppression due to decreased sleep duration or light exposure at night in the case of shift workers may alter the oncostic action of melatonin (Blask 2009).

Sleep and the Immune System

The relationship between sleep and immunity is reciprocal such that infections increase sleep duration and sleep deprivation negatively impacts immune function. Experimental studies have shown that sleep deprivation results in suppression in natural killer cell activity, reductions in interleukin-2 production, increased circulation of pro-inflammatory cytokines such as IL-6, tumor necrosis factor (TNF) α, and reduction of anti-inflammatory cytokines (Bryant et al. 2004). Sleep is needed for optimal resistance to infection. Sleep restriction in healthy adults has been shown to reduce antibody production response to the influenza vaccination. One night of sleep deprivation reduced the formation of specific antibodies to hepatitis A antigens after vaccination. Short sleep duration in the weeks preceding exposure to rhinovirus increased the susceptibility to developing a cold.

Sleep and Neurocognitive Function

It has been established that sleep deprivation impairs cognitive and motor performance (Durmer and Dinges 2005). However, some people are more vulnerable to the effects of sleep loss than others. Sleep deprivation studies have found a wide range of effects on cognitive function including decrements in attention especially vigilance, working and long-term memory, decision making, response inhibition, processing speed, and reasoning (Lim and Dinges 2010). Sleep deprivation results in impairments in psychomotor performance that are comparable to those induced by alcohol consumption at or above the legal limit (Williamson and Feyer 2000). Sleep loss increases the risk of traffic accidents as demonstrated by poor performance on driving simulators after sleep deprivation. In addition to an increased risk for motor vehicle crashes, sleep deprivation and related neurocognitive impairments are associated with work-related injuries and fatal accidents. Sleep apnea is also associated with deficits in cognitive function and accounts for a significant proportion of motor vehicle accidents.

Sleep and Mental Health

Numerous studies have shown a high rate of comorbidity between sleep complaints (e.g., insomnia) and psychiatric disorders, especially mood and anxiety disorders (Staner 2010). This relationship goes beyond mere co-occurrence and is bidirectional since insomnia contributes to the development or exacerbation of depression and anxiety disorders, and affective disorders and their treatments contribute to insomnia (Neckelmann et al. 2007; Sateia 2009). Nondepressed individuals with insomnia have a two times greater risk for developing depression than individuals without sleep difficulties. Sleep problems affect outcomes for patients with depression. Studies report that depressed patients who continue to experience insomnia are at greater risk of relapse and recurrence of depression and risk of suicide.

Conclusions

Sleep loss is a growing public health problem worldwide. The health consequences of a sleepy society are enormous and have a significant economic impact with billions of dollars spent on direct medical costs associated with morbidities and sleep-related injuries and accidents. Sleep deprivation can alter biological processes underlying cardiovascular, metabolic, and immune function. Cumulative long-term effects of sleep loss have been associated with a number of serious health consequences, including cardiovascular disease, obesity, cancer, and type 2 diabetes. Sleep is not a luxury and is as important for health as other health-promoting behaviors like diet and exercise. Public awareness is needed to emphasize and reinforce the essentialness of sleep for health.

Cross-References

▶ Cardiovascular Disease
▶ Glucose: Levels, Control, Intolerance, and Metabolism
▶ Hypertension
▶ Immune Function
▶ Insomnia
▶ Insulin
▶ Sleep
▶ Sleep Apnea
▶ Sleep Duration
▶ Type 2 Diabetes

References and Further Readings

Blask, D. E. (2009). Melatonin, sleep disturbance and cancer risk. *Sleep Medicine Reviews, 13*(4), 257–264.

Bryant, P. A., Trinder, J., & Curtis, N. (2004). Sick and tired: Does sleep have a vital role in the immune system? *Nature Reviews Immunology, 4*, 457–467.

Calhoun, D. A., & Harding, S. M. (2010). Sleep and hypertension. *Chest, 138*(2), 434–443.

Cappuccio, F. P., Taggart, F. M., Kandala, N. B., & Currie, A. (2008). Meta-analysis of short sleep duration and obesity in children and adults. *Sleep, 31*(5), 619–626.

Cappuccio, F. P., D'Elia, L., Strazzullo, P., & Miller, M. A. (2010). Sleep duration and all-cause mortality: A systematic review and meta-analysis of prospective studies. *Sleep, 33*(5), 585–592.

Cappuccio, F. P., Cooper, D., D'Elia, L., Strazzullo, P., & Miller, M. A. (2011). Sleep duration predicts cardiovascular outcomes: A systematic review and meta-analysis of prospective studies. *European Heart Journal, 32*(12), 1484–1492.

Durmer, J. S., & Dinges, D. F. (2005). Neurocognitive consequences of sleep deprivation. *Seminars in Neurology, 25*(2), 117–129.

Knutson, K. L., & Van Cauter, E. (2008). Associations between sleep loss and increased risk of obesity and diabetes. *Annals of the New York Academy of Sciences, 1129*(1), 287–304.

Kripke, D. F., Garfinkel, L., Wingard, D. L., Klauber, M. R., & Marler, M. R. (2002). Mortality associated with sleep duration and insomnia. *Archives of General Psychiatry, 59*(2), 131–136.

Lim, J., & Dinges, D. F. (2010). A meta-analysis of the impact of short-term sleep deprivation on cognitive variables. *Psychological Bulletin, 136*(3), 375–389.

Neckelmann, D., Mykletun, A., & Dahl, A. A. (2007). Chronic insomnia as a risk factor for developing anxiety and depression. *Sleep, 30*(7), 873–880.

Sateia, M. J. (2009). Update on sleep and psychiatric disorders. *Chest, 135*(5), 1370–1379.

Staner, L. (2010). Comorbidity of insomnia and depression. *Sleep Medicine Reviews, 14*(1), 35–46.

Taheri, S., Lin, L., Austin, D., Young, T., & Mignot, E. (2004). Short sleep duration is associated with reduced leptin, elevated ghrelin, and increased body mass index. *PLoS Medicine, 1*(3), e62.

Williamson, A. M., & Feyer, A. M. (2000). Moderate sleep deprivation produces impairments in cognitive and motor performance equivalent to legally prescribed levels of alcohol intoxication. *Occupational and Environmental Medicine, 57*(10), 649–655.

Sleep Apnea

Faith S. Luyster
School of Nursing, University of Pittsburgh, Pittsburgh, PA, USA

Synonyms

Obstructive sleep apnea; Sleep-disordered breathing

Definition

Sleep apnea is a common sleep disorder characterized by repetitive pauses in breathing or very shallow breaths during sleep (Strollo and Rogers 1996; Young et al. 2002). Pauses in breathing, known as apneas, and shallow breathing events, called hypopneas, can last a few seconds to minutes and can occur multiple times during the night. The termination of apneas and hypopneas is associated with a transient arousal from sleep. Sleep disruption due to frequent arousals may lead to excessive daytime sleepiness or fatigue. Loud snoring, witnessed breathing interruptions, and excessive daytime sleepiness are the most common signs of sleep apnea. Obstructive sleep apnea (OSA) occurs when the airway collapses or is blocked during sleep. Central sleep apnea results from temporary loss of ventilatory effort lasting at least 10 seconds and can co-occur with OSA. An evaluation for sleep apnea entails an assessment for signs and symptoms and a detailed craniofacial examination followed by a full night of in-laboratory or portable polysomnography to confirm diagnosis (Epstein et al. 2009). Sleep apnea requires long-term management. Positive airway pressure therapy, oral appliances, and surgery are the most common treatments for sleep apnea, but other behavioral interventions such as weight loss, smoking cessation, body position, and alcohol and sedative cessation, can be useful adjuncts to conventional therapies (Epstein et al. 2009). Untreated sleep apnea can result in a number of negative consequences, including excessive daytime sleepiness and fatigue, psychological symptoms, cognitive and performance impairments, and increased risk for cardiovascular and cerebrovascular disease (Bradley and Floras 2009; Sateia 2003). Decreased vigilance or falling asleep at the wheel increases the risk of motor vehicle crashes in individuals with sleep apnea (Ellen et al. 2006).

Cross-References

▶ Polysomnography
▶ Sleep Fragmentation

References and Further Readings

Bradley, T. D., & Floras, J. S. (2009). Obstructive sleep apnoea and its cardiovascular consequences. *The Lancet, 373*(9657), 82–93.

Ellen, R. L. B., Marshall, S. C., Palayew, M., Molnar, F. J., Wilson, K. G., & Man-Son-Hing, M. (2006). Systematic review of motor vehicle crash risk in persons with sleep apnea. *Journal of Clinical Sleep Medicine, 2*(2), 193–200.

Epstein, L. J., Kristo, D., Strollo, P. J., Friedman, N., Malhotra, A., Patil, S. P., et al. (2009). Clinical guideline for the evaluation, management, and long-term care of obstructive sleep apnea in adults. *Journal of Clinical Sleep Medicine, 5*(3), 263–276.

Sateia, M. J. (2003). Neuropsychological impairment and quality of life in obstructive sleep apnea. *Clinics in Chest Medicine, 24*(4), 249–259.

Strollo, P. J., & Rogers, R. M. (1996). Obstructive sleep apnea. *The New England Journal of Medicine, 334*(2), 99–104.

Young, T., Peppard, P. E., & Gottlieb, D. J. (2002). Epidemiology of obstructive sleep apnea: A population health perspective. *American Journal of Respiratory and Critical Care Medicine, 165*(9), 1217–1239.

Sleep Architecture

Salvatore Insana
Western Psychiatric Institute and Clinic,
Pittsburgh, PA, USA

Definition

Sleep Architecture is the visual representation of the way sleep stages are organized throughout a polysomnographically recorded sleep interval. Sleep Architecture is displayed on a hypnogram plot.

Description

Sleep can be measured with polysomnography (PSG), which consists of multiple measures that include, but are not limited to, electroencephalography (EEG), electrooculography (EOG), and electromyography (EMG) (see for a review Keenan and Hirshkowitz 2011). PSG literally translates to "many" (poly) "sleep" (somno) "writings" (graphy). When sleep is measured with PSG, the measured signals are typically sectioned into 30-s intervals consecutively throughout the entire PSG recording period. These 30-s intervals are termed "epochs." Within each epoch, the PSG-measured signals (from EEG, EOG, and EMG) are cumulatively used to differentiate sleep from wake, and to further classify sleep into different categories that are known as sleep stages.

According to the 2007 American Academy of Sleep Medicine standard practice parameters, sleep can be classified into four stages that include N1, N2, N3, and Rapid Eye Movement (REM) sleep (Iber et al. 2007). The PSG signals are used to identify each individual epoch as a particular sleep stage. The act of using PSG signals to identify each epoch as a particular sleep stage is known as sleep stage scoring. Sleep stage scoring is completed by a trained technician who visually interprets the PSG signals in accordance with standard practice parameters.

Once the entire PSG sleep study is scored, the study is summarized into a clinical report. The clinical report describes the sleep parameters measured (e.g., EEG, EOG, EMG, airflow parameters), sleep scoring data (e.g., lights out clock time, lights on clock time, total sleep time), arousal events (e.g., number of arousals, arousal index), respiratory events (e.g., apnea index, hypopnea index), cardiac events (e.g., average heart rate during sleep), movement events (e.g., number of periodic limb movements during sleep), and summary statements (e.g., findings related to sleep diagnoses, behavioral observations, sleep hypnogram). Of particular relevance to sleep architecture is the sleep hypnogram.

The sleep hypnogram is a summary figure that visually displays the scored wake and sleep stages as they occurred throughout the entire PSG recording period. The sleep hypnogram is formatted with time throughout the entire PSG sleep study as a continuous variable on the X-axis, and the visually scored wake and sleep stages as categorical variables on the Y-axis. The categorical wake and sleep stages are positioned with REM closest to the intersection with the X-axis, followed by N3, N2, N1, and wake in an upward ascending order; however, the order and format of these stages can vary per laboratory (e.g., Fig. 1).

As time progresses throughout the sleep monitoring period, the person being monitored naturally enters and exits the wake and sleep stages that are indicated on the Y-axis. The time spent in a particular stage is represented by a horizontal line adjacent to the respective stage, and the length of that horizontal line reflects the time spent in that particular stage as it corresponds to the "real time" for which the stage occurred – indicated on the X-axis. During a stage transition, the horizontal line turns 90° (right angle) positive or negative to become vertical and adjacent to the newly entered stage – as indicated on the Y-axis; then the line turns 90° (right angle) once again to reach a horizontal position with a length that represents the time spent in that particular stage – indicated on

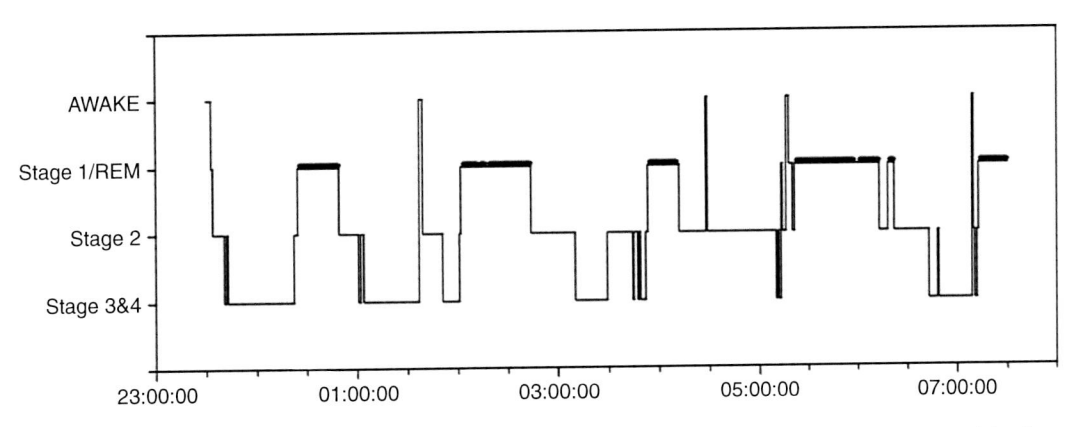

Sleep Architecture, Fig. 1 Sleep hypnogram and sleep architecture during a 20-year-old female's overnight sleep monitoring period

the X-axis. As the different wake and sleep stages fluctuate throughout the night, the hypnogram line appears at different horizontal levels (stage-dependent [Y-axis]), at different lengths on each level (time-dependent [X-axis]); and as the levels shift (stage shift), the horizontal line is connected to the previous and subsequent horizontal level by a vertical line (e.g., elbow connector).

Consequently, the wake and sleep stages represented on a sleep hypnogram resemble the back drop of a city skyline, with continuous geometric cubes and rectangles of different heights and widths that appear to continuously penetrate and retreat from the skyline. The figurative reference to a city skyline has been generally accepted, and has literally generated the term "sleep architecture." Thus, sleep architecture is the visual representation of wake and sleep stages that occurred throughout a polysomnographically recorded sleep interval, and is displayed on a hypnogram plot.

The visual structure of sleep architecture is dependent upon the sleep stage, and the time in the particular sleep stage. Typically, sleep is entered through N1, followed by N2, followed by N3, and then followed by REM – this progressive series is termed a "sleep cycle." The typical sleep cycle occurs throughout sleep at approximately 50-min intervals among infants (Grigg-Damberger et al. 2007) and approximately 90–110-min intervals among adults (Iber et al. 2007). The time spent in the different stages changes throughout the night. The first portion of the night primarily consists of non-REM sleep (i.e., N1, N2, and N3), and the second portion of the night primarily consists of REM sleep.

The sleep architecture displayed on the hypnogram from a normative adult PSG sleep study will display cumulatively longer horizontal lines adjacent to N1, N2, and N3 during the first portion of the night relative to the second portion, and will conversely display cumulatively longer horizontal lines adjacent to REM during the second portion of the night relative to the first portion. A sleep hypnogram will display the sleep stage cyclicity, as well as changes in time spent in particular stages as they occur throughout the recording period – this differs across nights. Since the time spent in different sleep stages generally changes throughout the lifespan (Ohayon et al. 2004), the percentage of time spent in each sleep stage, as reflected in the histogram, can differ by to the age of the person assessed.

Cross-References

▶ Non-REM Sleep
▶ Polysomnography
▶ REM Sleep
▶ Sleep

References and Further Readings

Grigg-Damberger, M., Gozal, D., Marcus, C. L., Quan, S. F., Rosen, C. L., Chervin, R. D., et al. (2007). The visual scoring of sleep and arousals in infants and children. *Journal of Clinical Sleep Medicine, 3*, 201–240.

Iber, C., Ancoli-Israel, S., Chesson, A., Quan, S. F., & American Academy of Sleep Medicine. (2007). *The AASM manual for the scoring of sleep and associated events: Rules, terminology and technical specifications* (1st ed.). Westchester: American Academy of Sleep Medicine.

Keenan, S., & Hirshkowitz, M. (2011). Monitoring and staging human sleep. In M. H. Kryger, T. Roth, & W. C. Dement (Eds.), *Principles and practice of sleep medicine* (5th ed., pp. 1602–1609). St. Louis: Elsevier.

Ohayon, M. M., Carskadon, M. A., Guilleminault, C., & Vitiello, M. V. (2004). Meta-analysis of quantitative sleep parameters from childhood to old age in healthy individuals: Developing normative sleep values across the human lifespan. *Sleep, 27*, 1255–1273.

Sleep Continuity

Elizabeth Mezick
Department of Psychology, University of Pittsburgh, Pittsburgh, PA, USA

Synonyms

Sleep efficiency; Sleep fragmentation; Sleep maintenance

Definition

Sleep continuity refers to the amount and distribution of sleep versus wakefulness in a given sleep period; it includes both sleep initiation and sleep maintenance (Hall et al. in press). Specific indices of sleep continuity may include latency to sleep onset, number of awakenings after sleep onset, total time of wakefulness after sleep onset, and overall sleep efficiency. Sleep continuity is most often assessed using self-report questionnaires (i.e., retrospective reports, morning diaries or logs), wrist actigraphy, or polysomnography.

Sleep continuity declines as part of the normal aging process (Ohayon et al. 2004). Disruptions in sleep continuity are typical among individuals with insomnia and are also commonly reported by or observed in those with mood disorders, anxiety disorders, and substance disorders. Many medical conditions and treatments are also related to disrupted sleep continuity; some of the most common examples include sleep apnea, chronic pain, asthma and respiratory conditions, chronic renal disease, infectious diseases, and cancer. Decreased sleep continuity has been associated with increased inflammatory markers, susceptibility to infection, elevated blood pressure, obesity, presence of metabolic syndrome, diabetes, and cardiovascular disease. Several studies have reported a link between decreased sleep continuity and incident diabetes or incident cardiovascular disease.

Cross-References

▶ Sleep Fragmentation

References and Further Readings

Hall, M., Greeson, J., & Mezick, E. (in press). Sleep as a biobehavioral risk factor for cardiovascular disease. In S. R. Waldstein, W. J. Kop, & L. I. Katzel (Eds.), *Handbook of cardiovascular behavioral medicine*. New York: Springer.

Ohayon, M. M., Carkadon, M. A., Guilleminault, C., & Vitiello, M. V. (2004). Meta-analysis of quantitative sleep parameters from childhood to old age in healthy individuals: Developing normative sleep values across the human lifespan. *Sleep, 27*, 1255–1273.

Sleep Curtailment

▶ Sleep Restriction

Sleep Debt

▶ Sleep Restriction

Sleep Deprivation

Martica H. Hall
Department of Psychiatry, University of Pittsburgh, Pittsburgh, PA, USA

Synonyms

Sleep deprived

Definition

Sleep deprivation generally refers to the total loss of sleep due to experimental manipulations or circumstance.

Description

Sleep deprivation refers to the total loss of sleep. The term is generally used in the context of experimental manipulations which keep individuals (or experimental animals) awake throughout their usual sleep period. Sleep deprivation also occurs in naturalistic conditions such as when a student stays awake all night to study for an exam. Experimental and observational sleep deprivation studies have been used to evaluate the cognitive, behavioral, emotional, and physiological consequences of sleep loss.

Experimental sleep deprivation studies in humans generally deprive participants of 1–3 nights of sleep, resulting in 24–72 h of wakefulness. Experimental animal models can extend sleep deprivation for much longer periods of time (e.g., 2 weeks). In both kinds of studies, electroencephalographic (EEG) monitoring is used to ensure wakefulness, usually through interactions with study staff or procedural manipulations. For example, the classical "disk-over-water" method pioneered by Dr. Allan Rechtschaffen at the University of Chicago involved placing two animals on a rotating disk suspended above water (Rechtschaffen and Bergmann 1995). A barrier divided the disk into half, with the experimental animal on one side of the disk and the yoked animal on the other. When the experimental animal showed EEG signs of sleep, the disk would rotate. If the animal did not wake up, they would fall into the water when they reached the barrier. Through conditioning, the experimental animal would learn to wake up as soon as the disk started to rotate. The yoked animal, on the other hand, would learn to sleep when the disk was *not* rotating. This elegant design allowed experimenters to tease apart the effects of movement and stress associated with older forms of sleep deprivation (e.g., placing the animal on a continuous running wheel with no option for escape) from the effects of sleep deprivation. In human studies, the constant routine protocol, which involves keeping participants in a recumbent position for the duration of the protocol, is used to control for the influence of extraneous factors such as increased movement on study outcomes.

Although individuals may feel that sleep deprivation has no adverse effects on them, experimental evidence suggests that perceptions of resiliency to sleep loss are unfounded. The "disconnect" between subjective perceptions of sleepiness and objective indices of health and functioning in humans has been systematically documented by Dr. David Dinges and his colleagues at the University of California (see Lim and Dinges 2008). More recently, others have demonstrated that one night of total sleep deprivation in healthy young adults is associated with increased blood pressure and amygdala reactivity to negative emotional stimuli (Franzen et al. 2011; Yoo et al. 2007). As a complement to studies in humans, animal models, which allow exquisite control over sleep and wakefulness, have begun to elucidate the influence of sleep deprivation on gene expression, molecular signaling, and synaptic plasticity (e.g., Seugnet et al. 2011; Wang et al. 2010). Taken as a whole, these studies demonstrate that sleep is essential to health and functioning across species.

Cross-References

▶ Gene Expression
▶ Sleep
▶ Sleep and Health

References and Further Readings

Franzen, P. L., Gianaros, P. J., Marsland, A. L., Hall, M., Siegle, G. J., Dahl, R. E., et al. (2011). Cardiovascular reactivity to acute psychological stress following sleep deprivation. *Psychosomatic Medicine, 73*(8), 679–682.

Lim, J., & Dinges, D. F. (2008). Sleep deprivation and vigilant attention. *Annals of the New York Academy of Sciences, 1129*, 305–322.

Rechtschaffen, A., & Bergmann, B. M. (1995). Sleep deprivation in the rat by the disk-over-water method. *Behavioural Brain Research, 69*(1–2), 55–63.

Seugnet, L., Suzuki, Y., Donlea, J. M., Gottschalk, L., & Shaw, P. J. (2011). Sleep deprivation during early-adult development results in long-lasting learning deficits in adult *Drosophila. Sleep, 34*(2), 137–146.

Wang, H., Liu, Y., Briesemann, M., & Yan, J. (2010). Computational analysis of gene regulation in animal sleep deprivation. *Physiological Genomics, 42*(3), 427–436.

Yoo, S. S., Gujar, N., Hu, P., Jolesz, F. A., & Walker, M. P. (2007). The human emotional brain without sleep: A prefrontal amygdala disconnect. *Current Biology, 17*, R877–R878.

Sleep Deprived

▶ Sleep Deprivation

Sleep Duration

Christopher E. Kline
Department of Health and Physical Activity,
University of Pittsburgh, Pittsburgh, PA, USA

Synonyms

Total sleep time

Definition

Sleep duration typically refers to the total amount of sleep obtained, either during the nocturnal sleep episode or across the 24-h period.

Description

Measurement

Sleep duration can be measured via questionnaire, diary, actigraphy, or polysomnography. In population-based epidemiologic studies, single-item self-report measures of sleep duration have often been utilized (e.g., *How many hours of sleep do you obtain on a typical night?*). In clinical and research settings, sleep diaries, actigraphy, and polysomnography provide assessments of sleep duration. Sleep diaries involve the subjective report of sleep duration, typically assessed daily for a minimum of 1 week. Actigraphy provides an objective estimate of sleep/wake status from the detection of bodily movement, whereas polysomnography measures sleep duration through the assessment of multiple physiological signals, including brain, eye, and muscle activity. Although typically correlated, large discrepancies are often noted between subjective and objective measures of sleep duration; in most populations, self-reported sleep duration is overestimated compared to objective measurement (Matthews et al. 2018).

Sleep Duration Across the Lifespan

Sleep is regulated by a complex interaction of homeostatic and circadian factors. The homeostatic process reflects the need for sleep, accumulating during sustained wakefulness and dissipating during sleep. The circadian process, driven by outputs of the circadian pacemaker, promotes wakefulness during the day and evening and promotes sleep during the night, with the peak sleep-promoting signal during the early morning. Thus, circadian signals oppose the rise of homeostatic sleep pressure during the day, allowing for uninterrupted daytime wakefulness. Both circadian and homeostatic processes promote sleep onset, with circadian sleep-promoting signals facilitating continued consolidated sleep despite the gradual dissipation of homeostatic sleep pressure over the course of the night. Aging results in changes in the homeostatic and circadian regulation of sleep, with a phase advance of the circadian wake-promoting signal (i.e., increased signal for wakefulness in the morning but decreased in the evening) and reduced homeostatic drive for sleep (Dijk et al. 1999). As a result, sleep in older adults is commonly phase advanced, of shorter duration, and with greater fragmentation compared to younger adults.

In general, sleep duration decreases from infancy through old age. Sleep duration (per 24 h) averages >13 h during infancy, gradually declining to 8–9 h during late adolescence (Williams et al. 2013). Normative sleep duration then declines throughout adulthood to approximately 6.5 h at 60 years, at which point sleep duration tends to stabilize (Ohayon et al. 2004). However, these average values do not indicate whether sleep need is being met, particularly during development. For instance, although weekday sleep duration decreases throughout childhood and adolescence, weekend sleep duration remains similar from age 5 to 16. This pattern suggests a greater influence of environmental factors (e.g., school schedules) than biological or maturational influences on sleep duration during childhood and adolescence.

Whether sleep duration has changed dramatically over recent decades is controversial. Whereas some studies have documented significant decreases in sleep duration and increased prevalence of short sleep over the past 30–50 years (Ford et al. 2015), others have presented evidence that longitudinal changes in sleep duration have been minimal to nonexistent (Bin et al. 2013; Youngstedt et al. 2016). Moreover, recent work suggests that average adult sleep duration has minimally increased (~1 min/year) over the past 15 years (Basner and Dinges 2018). Other studies estimate that the prevalence of short and long sleep duration (i.e., the extremes of sleep duration that are most strongly associated with health risk) has not appreciably changed over ~30 years (Bonke 2015).

Sleep Duration and Health

Sleep is an essential behavior for memory consolidation, development, and restoration of nervous, immune, skeletal, and muscular systems. Consequently, the amount of sleep obtained has a significant influence on one's health and functioning. Sleep duration is at least partly determined by genetic influences, so interindividual differences in sleep duration are to be expected. Nevertheless, a significant association between sleep duration and health has been consistently documented in epidemiologic research.

The association between sleep duration and health typically has a U-shaped distribution, with the lowest risk associated adverse health outcomes typically observed with a sleep duration of ~7 h for adults (Itani et al. 2017; Jike et al. 2018). Both short and long sleep have been associated with increased risk of mortality and numerous morbidities, including cardiovascular disease (e.g., atherosclerosis), metabolic dysfunction (e.g., type 2 diabetes, obesity), and cognitive impairment. However, the most marked morbidity and mortality risks have been associated with extreme short and long sleep (<5 and >9 h, respectively).

The possible mechanisms by which sleep duration affects health likely differ between short and long sleep duration. Most research has focused on how short sleep may affect health, with blunted hormonal control of appetite, increased inflammatory levels, alterations in hypothalamic-pituitary-adrenal axis and sympathoadrenal activity, and decreased immunity to pathogens observed following short-term experimental sleep restriction (Grandner et al. 2010). Plausible mechanisms linking long sleep duration to excess morbidity and mortality are less clear; however, fatigue, impaired immunity, reduced photoperiod length, and underlying disease have been postulated (Youngstedt and Kripke 2004). However, short and long sleep share some possible mechanisms. Both short and long sleep duration are more common among with those with low socioeconomic status and racial/ethnic minorities. Moreover, sleep complaints and poor health behaviors (e.g., smoking, alcohol, physical inactivity) are more prevalent in short and long sleepers in comparison to those with normal sleep duration.

Sleep Duration Recommendations

In recognition of the growing evidence base on the importance of adequate sleep duration for optimal health, multiple professional organizations have published consensus sleep duration recommendations for children and adults. The American Academy of Sleep Medicine (AASM) recognized that daily sleep need differs across development as they recommended, for example, 12–16 h for infants and 8–10 h for teenagers (Paruthi et al. 2016). For adults, the AASM (along with the Sleep Research Society) recommended sleep duration ≥7 h to promote ideal health (Watson et al. 2015). Recommendations from the American Thoracic Society and National Sleep Foundation were similar to those from the AASM (Mukherjee et al. 2015; Hirshkowitz et al. 2015).

Cross-References

▶ Actigraphy (Wrist, for Measuring Rest/Activity Patterns and Sleep)
▶ Polysomnography
▶ Sleep
▶ Sleep and Health

- Sleep Deprivation
- Sleep Quality
- Sleep Restriction

References and Further Reading

Basner, M., & Dinges, D. F. (2018). Sleep duration in the United States 2003–2016: First signs of success in the fight against sleep deficiency? *Sleep, 41*, zsy012.

Bin, Y. S., Marshall, N. S., & Glozier, N. (2013). Sleeping at the limits: The changing prevalence of short and long sleep durations in 10 countries. *American Journal of Epidemiology, 177*, 826–833.

Bonke, J. (2015). Trends in short and long sleep in Denmark from 1964 to 2009, and the associations with employment, SES (socioeconomic status) and BMI. *Sleep Medicine, 16*, 385–390.

Dijk, D. J., Duffy, J. F., Riel, E., Shanahan, T. L., & Czeisler, C. A. (1999). Ageing and the circadian and homeostatic regulation of human sleep during forced desynchrony of rest, melatonin and temperature rhythms. *Journal of Physiology, 516*, 611–627.

Ford, E. S., Cunningham, T. J., & Croft, J. B. (2015). Trends in self-reported sleep duration among US adults from 1985 to 2012. *Sleep, 38*, 829–832.

Grandner, M. A., Hale, L., Moore, M., & Patel, N. P. (2010). Mortality associated with short sleep duration: The evidence, the possible mechanisms, and the future. *Sleep Medicine Reviews, 14*, 191–203.

Hirshkowitz, M., Whiton, K., Albert, S. M., Alessi, C., Bruni, O., DonCarlos, L., ... Ware, J. C. (2015). National Sleep Foundation's updated sleep duration recommendations: Final report. *Sleep Health, 1*, 233–243.

Itani, O., Jike, M., Watanabe, N., & Kaneita, Y. (2017). Short sleep duration and health outcomes: A systematic review, meta-analysis, and meta-regression. *Sleep Medicine, 32*, 246–256.

Jike, M., Itani, O., Watanabe, N., Buysse, D. J., & Kaneita, Y. (2018). Long sleep duration and health outcomes: A systematic review, meta-analysis and meta-regression. *Sleep Medicine Reviews, 39*, 25–36.

Matthews, K. A., Patel, S. R., Pantesco, E. J., Buysse, D. J., Kamarck, T. W., Lee, L., & Hall, M. H. (2018). Similarities and differences in estimates of sleep duration by polysomnography, actigraphy, diary, and self-reported habitual sleep in a community sample. *Sleep Health, 4*, 96–103.

Mukherjee, S., Patel, S. R., Kales, S. N., Ayas, N. T., Strohl, K. P., Gozal, D., & Malhotra, A. (2015). An official American Thoracic Society statement: The importance of healthy sleep. Recommendations and future priorities. *American Journal of Respiratory and Critical Care Medicine, 191*, 1450–1458.

Ohayon, M. M., Carskadon, M. A., Guilleminault, C., & Vitiello, M. V. (2004). Meta-analysis of quantitative sleep parameters from childhood to old age in healthy individuals: Developing normative sleep values across the human lifespan. *Sleep, 27*, 1255–1273.

Paruthi, S., Brooks, L. J., D'Ambrosio, C., Hall, W. A., Kotagal, S., Lloyd, R. M., ... Wise, M. S. (2016). Recommended amount of sleep for pediatric populations: A consensus statement of the American Academy of sleep medicine. *Journal of Clinical Sleep Medicine, 12*, 785–786.

Watson, N. F., Badr, M. S., Belenky, G., Bliwise, D. L., Buxton, O. M., Buysse, D., ... Tasali, E. (2015). Recommended amount of sleep for a healthy adult: A joint consensus statement of the American Academy of sleep medicine and Sleep Research Society. *Sleep, 38*, 843–844.

Williams, J. A., Zimmerman, F. J., & Bell, J. F. (2013). Norms and trends of sleep time among US children and adolescents. *JAMA Pediatrics, 167*, 55–60.

Youngstedt, S. D., Goff, E. E., Reynolds, A. M., Kripke, D. F., Irwin, M. R., Bootzin, R. R., ... Jean-Louis, G. (2016). Has adult sleep duration declined over the last 50+ years? *Sleep Medicine Reviews, 28*, 69–85.

Youngstedt, S. D., & Kripke, D. F. (2004). Long sleep and mortality: Rationale for sleep restriction. *Sleep Medicine Reviews, 8*, 159–174.

Sleep Efficiency

- Sleep Continuity
- Sleep Fragmentation

Sleep Fragmentation

Elizabeth Mezick
Department of Psychology, University of Pittsburgh, Pittsburgh, PA, USA

Synonyms

Sleep continuity; Sleep efficiency; Sleep maintenance

Definition

Sleep fragmentation typically refers to brief arousals that occur during a sleep period. The American Sleep Disorders Association (1992) defines an arousal as an abrupt shift in electroencephalographic (EEG) frequency (suggestive of an awake state) which is 3 s or greater in duration and which occurs after at least 10 consecutive seconds of sleep. A number of other definitions of arousal have been published or suggested since that time, with some recommending that elements or physiological responses other than EEG frequency be taken into account (e.g., autonomic activation without cortical involvement) (Janackova and Sforza 2008). When assessed with actigraphy, sleep fragmentation may refer to the amount of movement or restlessness in a sleep period. For example, actigraph software programs use algorithms to calculate a sleep fragmentation index, based on the number or proportion of total sleep epochs characterized by movement. When used in a more general sense, sleep fragmentation may also refer to the overall amount and distribution of wakefulness in a sleep period and can be considered the inverse of sleep continuity. For example, some authors have used the term "sleep fragmentation" to describe parameters such as wakefulness after sleep onset and sleep efficiency.

Elevated sleep fragmentation occurs in those with sleep apnea and may correlate with daytime sleepiness. Increased sleep fragmentation as assessed by actigraphy has been associated with a number of physical and psychiatric health outcomes, as well as deficits in neurobehavioral performance. Experimental models of sleep fragmentation, which typically disrupt sleep briefly using auditory, mechanical, or other stimuli, have been used to examine the neurophysiologic, cognitive, and behavioral consequences of fragmented sleep.

Cross-References

► Sleep Apnea
► Sleep Continuity

References and Further Readings

American Sleep Disorders Association Atlas Task Force. (1992). EEG arousals: Scoring rules and examples. *Sleep, 15*, 173–184.

Bonnet, M. H., & Arand, D. L. (2003). Clinical effects of sleep fragmentation versus sleep deprivation. *Sleep Medicine Reviews, 7*, 297–310.

Janackova, S., & Sforza, E. (2008). Neurobiology of sleep fragmentation: Cortical and autonomic markers of sleep disorders. *Current Pharmaceutical Design, 14*, 3474–3480.

Sleep Maintenance

► Sleep Continuity
► Sleep Fragmentation

Sleep Quality

Christopher E. Kline
Department of Health and Physical Activity,
University of Pittsburgh, Pittsburgh, PA, USA

Synonyms

Sleep refreshment; Sleep satisfaction

Definition

Sleep quality is defined as one's satisfaction of the sleep experience, integrating aspects of sleep initiation, sleep maintenance, sleep quantity, and refreshment upon awakening.

Description

Sleep quality is widely recognized as a vital contributor to optimal health and functioning. Yet, despite its common usage, "sleep quality" is a term without a clear definition or operationalization (Ohayon et al. 2017).

Measurement

Measurement of sleep quality is difficult due to its imprecise definition. The construct of sleep quality likely incorporates aspects of sleep quantity, sleep continuity, the feeling of refreshment upon awakening, and daytime sleepiness (Harvey et al. 2008). Many of these aspects cannot be easily measured in an objective fashion. Thus, sleep quality is often assessed with self-reported measures.

Sleep diaries, which track sleep on a daily basis, often assess sleep quality by incorporating a Likert-type rating scale (e.g., 1: *very poor sleep quality*; 5: *very good sleep quality*) or a visual analogue scale (with anchors of *very poor* and *very good* sleep quality) into the diary. Questionnaires, on the other hand, assess sleep quality through the measurement of different domains of the sleep experience. The most widely used questionnaire, the Pittsburgh Sleep Quality Index, is an 18-item instrument with seven components: sleep quality, sleep latency, sleep duration, habitual sleep efficiency, sleep disturbances, sleeping medication use, and daytime dysfunction (Buysse et al. 1989). Another common measure, the Medical Outcomes Study Sleep Scale, assesses six different aspects of sleep: sleep disturbance, sleep adequacy, daytime sleepiness, snoring, awakening with shortness of breath or headache, and sleep quantity (Hays et al. 2005). Scores on both of these measures have been shown to identify individuals who characterize their sleep as being poor in quality.

An alternative approach to measuring sleep quality involves measuring self-reported or objectively recorded sleep parameters related to the magnitude of nocturnal wakefulness, such as sleep onset latency, total wakefulness, sleep efficiency, number of awakenings, or arousals. Moreover, measures of sleep "depth" derived from polysomnography, such as the amount of N1 sleep or N3 sleep (sometimes referred to as "light" and "deep" sleep, respectively), have sometimes been used to characterize sleep quality. However, these parameters often fail to completely capture the essence of sleep quality. In particular, sleep quality should not be considered to be synonymous with the amount of sleep obtained. For example, in comparison to those who report a sleep duration of 7–8 h, poor sleep quality is more prevalent with short and long sleep.

Correlates with Sleep Parameters

Across multiple studies, objective sleep parameters have exhibited only minimal concordance with sleep quality, with sleep efficiency, wakefulness after sleep onset, and total sleep time typically showing the strongest, yet still modest, correlations (Kaplan et al. 2017a, b). While some studies have found that the spectral density of the sleep electroencephalographic (EEG) content correlated with sleep quality (Krystal and Edinger 2008), others have failed to observe a strong link (Gabryelska et al. 2019; Kaplan et al. 2017a). Overall, these findings suggest that sleep quality is a multifaceted construct that cannot be captured by a single surrogate sleep parameter or objective surrogate markers.

Sleep Quality and Health

Poor sleep quality is widespread in modern society. Approximately one-third of adults complain of poor sleep quality, though in most studies, prevalence estimates are based upon insomnia-related symptoms. Poor sleep quality has been associated with increasing age, low socioeconomic status, poor general health, psychological distress, and poor lifestyle behaviors (e.g., high caffeine use, sedentary lifestyle, smoking).

How poor sleep quality may influence future morbidity or mortality risk is less clear. Epidemiologic studies have found that poor sleep quality is predictive of increased risk of metabolic dysfunction and mortality risk (Cappuccio et al. 2010; Kojima et al. 2000). However, most studies have focused on sleep duration rather than sleep quality, perhaps due to the difficulty in concisely defining sleep quality. Interestingly, in studies that have concurrently assessed the health risks of sleep duration and sleep quality, the strongest risk is associated with those reporting poor sleep quality and inadequate sleep duration (Vgontzas et al. 2013), with similar (or greater, in some cases) risk associated with poor sleep quality relative to extreme sleep duration (Bin 2016).

Cross-References

▶ Actigraphy (Wrist, for Measuring Rest/Activity Patterns and Sleep)

- Insomnia
- Polysomnography
- Sleep
- Sleep and Health
- Sleep Architecture

References and Further Reading

Bin, Y. S. (2016). Is sleep quality more important than sleep duration for public health? *Sleep, 39*, 1629–1630.

Buysse, D. J., Reynolds, C. F., III, Monk, T. H., Berman, S. R., & Kupfer, D. J. (1989). The Pittsburgh Sleep Quality Index: A new instrument for psychiatric practice and research. *Psychiatry Research, 28*, 193–213.

Cappuccio, F. P., D'Elia, L., Strazzullo, P., & Miller, M. A. (2010). Quantity and quality of sleep and incidence of type 2 diabetes: A systematic review and meta-analysis. *Diabetes Care, 33*, 414–420.

Gabryelska, A., Feige, B., Riemann, D., Spiegelhalder, K., Johann, A., Białasiewicz, P., & Hertenstein, E. (2019). Can spectral power predict subjective sleep quality in healthy individuals? *Journal of Sleep Research, 28*, e12848.

Harvey, A. G., Stinson, K., Whitaker, K. L., Moskovitz, D., & Virk, H. (2008). The subjective meaning of sleep quality: A comparison of individuals with and without insomnia. *Sleep, 31*, 383–393.

Hays, R. D., Martin, S. A., Sesti, A. M., & Spritzer, K. L. (2005). Psychometric properties of the medical outcomes study sleep measure. *Sleep Medicine, 6*, 41–44.

Kaplan, K. A., Hardas, P. P., Redline, S., & Zeitzer, J. M. (2017a). Correlates of sleep quality in midlife and beyond: A machine learning analysis. *Sleep Medicine, 34*, 162–167.

Kaplan, K. A., Hirshman, J., Hernandez, B., Stefanick, M. L., Hoffman, A. R., Redline, S., ... Zeitzer, J. M. (2017b). When a gold standard isn't so golden: Lack of prediction of subjective sleep quality from sleep polysomnography. *Biological Psychology, 123*, 37–46.

Kojima, M., Wakai, K., Kawamura, T., Tamakoshi, A., Aoki, R., Lin, Y., ... Ohno, Y. (2000). Sleep patterns and total mortality: A 12-year follow-up study in Japan. *Journal of Epidemiology, 10*, 87–93.

Krystal, A. D., & Edinger, J. D. (2008). Measuring sleep quality. *Sleep Medicine, 9*, S10–S17.

Ohayon M., Wickwire E. M., Hirshkowitz M., Albert S. M., Avidan A., Daly F. J., ... Vitiello, M. V. (2017). National Sleep Foundation's sleep quality recommendations: First report. *Sleep Health, 3*, 6–19.

Vgontzas, A. N., Fernandez-Mendoza, J., Liao, D., & Bixler, E. O. (2013). Insomnia with objective short sleep duration: The most biologically severe phenotype of the disorder. *Sleep Medicine Reviews, 17*, 241–254.

Sleep Refreshment

▶ Sleep Quality

Sleep Restriction

Martica H. Hall
Department of Psychiatry, University of Pittsburgh, Pittsburgh, PA, USA

Synonyms

Partial sleep deprivation; Sleep curtailment; Sleep debt

Definition

Sleep restriction generally refers to situational or experimentally induced reductions in overall sleep duration.

Description

Sleep restriction refers to the partial loss of sleep. The term is generally used in the context of experimental manipulations which keep individuals (or experimental animals) awake for some portion of their usual sleep period. Sleep restriction also occurs in naturalistic conditions such as when new parents have to wake repeatedly to care for their newborn child or when an individual purposefully reduces their sleep time in order to meet the competing demands of work, family, or other obligations. Importantly, sleep restriction differs from insomnia in that sleep-restricted individuals do not have an adequate opportunity to sleep whereas individuals with insomnia have sleep difficulties despite adequate opportunity to sleep (see ▶ "Insomnia" entry). Experimental and observational sleep restriction studies have been used to evaluate the cognitive, behavioral, emotional, and physiological consequences of sleep restriction, including the loss of specific components of sleep (e.g., slow-wave sleep).

Dr. Eve Van Cauter and her colleagues at the University of Chicago have been instrumental in highlighting the public health implications of partial sleep restriction, or sleep "curtailment" across the life span (Hanlon and Van Cauter 2011). In a series of carefully controlled studies in healthy young adults, Van Cauter and colleagues demonstrated that sleep restriction is associated with metabolic and endocrine alterations that underlie glucose tolerance, insulin sensitivity, and weight gain. These results are mirrored in epidemiologic studies of obesity and diabetes risk in children and adults (Hanlon and Van Cauter 2011). Other consequences of experimental sleep restriction include decrements in working memory, alterations in inflammatory markers, and decreased testosterone levels in males (Casement et al. 2006; Irwin et al. 2006; Leproult and Van Cauter 2011; Prather et al. 2009). Experimental laboratory studies have also begun to selectively deprive experimental subjects of specific sleep stages to better understand their function. For instance, animal models have been used to identify the neurophysiological mechanisms through which REM sleep regulates learning and memory (Poe et al. 2010). In the only study of its kind conducted to date, Tasali et al. (2008) demonstrated that selective suppression of slow-wave sleep in healthy, lean adults resulted in marked decreases in insulin sensitivity. Importantly, these effects were independent of sleep duration.

Societal trends suggest that large numbers of adults are chronically sleep-restricted. During the work week, they may build up a sleep "debt" and perceive that this debt may be "paid" on non-work nights. Epidemiologic evidence that documents the buildup of sleep debt during the work week and its payment on non-work nights is lacking. Moreover, experimental evidence suggests that multiple, long recovery nights may be necessary to "repay" sleep debt induced by chronic partial sleep restriction (Banks et al. 2010). Although the systematic evaluation of the impact of sleep restriction on indices of health and functioning is in its infancy, the epidemiological and experimental data amassed thus far supports the belief that this is an important public health concern.

References and Further Readings

Banks, S., Van Dongen, H. P., Maislin, G., & Dinges, D. F. (2010). Neurobehavioral dynamics following chronic sleep restriction: dose-response effects of one night for recovery. *Sleep, 33*, 1013–1026.

Casement, M. D., Broussard, J. L., Mullington, J. M., & Press, D. Z. (2006). The contribution of sleep to improvements in working memory scanning speed: A study of prolonged sleep restriction. *Biological Psychology, 72*(2), 208–212.

Hanlon, E. C., & Van Cauter, E. (2011). Quantification of sleep behavior and of its impact on the cross-talk between the brain and peripheral metabolism. *Proceedings of the National Academy of Sciences of the United States of America, 108*(Suppl 3), 15609–15616.

Irwin, M. R., Wang, M., Campomayor, C. O., Collado-Hidalgo, A., & Cole, S. (2006). Sleep deprivation and activation of morning levels of cellular and genomic markers of inflammation. *Archives of Internal Medicine, 166*(16), 1756–1762.

Leproult, R., & Van Cauter, E. (2011). Effect of 1 week of sleep restriction on testosterone levels in young healthy men. *JAMA: The Journal of the American Medical Association, 305*(21), 2173–2174.

Poe, G. R., Walsh, C. M., & Bjorness, T. E. (2010). Cognitive neuroscience of sleep. *Progress in Brain Research, 185*, 1–19.

Prather, A. A., Marsland, A. L., Hall, M., Neumann, S. A., Muldoon, M. F., & Manuck, S. B. (2009). Normative variation in self-reported sleep quality and sleep debt is associated with stimulated pro-inflammatory cytokine production. *Biological Psychology, 82*(1), 12–17.

Spiegel, K., Tasali, E., Penev, P., & Van Cauter, E. (2004). Brief communication: Sleep curtailment in healthy young men is associated with decreased leptin levels, elevated ghrelin levels, and increased hunger and appetite. *Annals of Internal Medicine, 141*(11), 846–850.

Tasali, E., Leproult, R., Ehrmann, D. A., & Van Cauter, E. (2008). Slow-wave sleep and the risk of type 2 diabetes in humans. *Proceedings of the National Academy of Sciences of the United States of America, 105*(3), 1044–1049.

Sleep Satisfaction

▶ Sleep Quality

Sleep Stages 1, 2, 3, and 4

▶ Non-REM Sleep

Sleep Stages 3 and 4

▶ Slow-Wave Sleep

Sleep Study

▶ Polysomnography

Sleep-Disordered Breathing

▶ Sleep Apnea

Slim Disease

▶ Cachexia (Wasting Syndrome)

Slow-Wave Sleep

Salvatore Insana
Western Psychiatric Institute and Clinic,
Pittsburgh, PA, USA

Synonyms

Deep sleep; Delta sleep; N3; Sleep stages 3 and 4

Definition

Sleep can be measured with polysomnography (PSG) (see review, Keenan and Hirshkowitz 2011). Polysomnographically measured sleep behaviors can be classified into distinct categories. Slow-wave sleep (SWS) is a distinct sleep behavior classification. SWS is also known as stage N3 sleep as defined by the 2007 American Academy of Sleep Medicine sleep scoring manual (Iber et al. 2007). SWS is otherwise known as the combination of sleep stages 3 and 4 according to the Rechtschaffen and Kales "classic criteria" (Rechtschaffen and Kales 1968). Other common terms used to describe SWS are "delta sleep" and "deep sleep."

A characteristic component of SWS is the organized pattern of neurological activity that is emitted from the brain as measured by electroencephalography. A component of the organized pattern of neurological activity is the presence of slow waves, otherwise known as delta waves. Slow waves have high amplitude (>75 V) and low frequency (0.5–2 Hz). When slow waves occur during sleep, and present within 20% or more of an epoch, that epoch is classified as SWS, or N3.

Although the true function of sleep and particularly SWS is unknown (e.g., Rector et al. 2009; Siegel 2009), to date the primary explanation is that SWS reflects the homeostatic sleep drive, or one's escalating need for sleep with increasing time awake. This relation is exemplified when One's time spent in SWS increases relative to their time previously spent awake (Bersagliere and Achermann 2010). Thus, SWS is described as the "restorative component" of sleep. Common parasomnias that can occur during SWS are sleep walking and night terrors.

Human Development: Due to developmental changes in infant sleep patterns, typically SWS can be scored by 4–4.5 months post-term (Grigg-Damberger et al. 2007). The percentage of SWS obtained is highest during early-life and decreases from early childhood through old age (Ohayon et al. 2004).

Cross-References

▶ Non-REM Sleep
▶ Polysomnography
▶ REM Sleep

- Sleep
- Sleep Architecture

References and Further Readings

Bersagliere, A., & Achermann, P. (2010). Slow oscillations in human non-rapid eye movement sleep electroencephalogram: Effects of increased sleep pressure. *Journal of Sleep Research, 19*, 228–237.

Grigg-Damberger, M., Gozal, D., Marcus, C. L., Quan, S. F., Rosen, C. L., Chervin, R. D., et al. (2007). The visual scoring of sleep and arousals in infants and children. *Journal of Clinical Sleep Medicine, 3*, 201–240.

Iber, C., Ancoli-Israel, S., Chesson, A., Quan, S. F., & for the American Academy of Sleep Medicine. (2007). *The AASM manual for the scoring of sleep and associated events: Rules, terminology and technical specifications* (1st ed.). Westchester: American Academy of Sleep Medicine.

Keenan, S., & Hirshkowitz, M. (2011). Monitoring and staging human sleep. In M. H. Kryger, T. Roth, & W. C. Dement (Eds.), *Principles and practice of sleep medicine* (5th ed., pp. 1602–1609). St. Louis: Elsevier.

Ohayon, M. M., Carskadon, M. A., Guilleminault, C., & Vitiello, M. V. (2004). Meta-analysis of quantitative sleep parameters from childhood to old age in healthy individuals: Developing normative sleep values across the human lifespan. *Sleep, 27*, 1255–1273.

Rechtschaffen, A., & Kales, A. (1968). *A manual of standardized, techniques and scoring system for sleep stages in human subjects (NIH Publication No. 204)*. Washington DC: US Government Printing Office.

Rector, D. M., Schei, J. L., Van Dongen, H. P., Belenky, G., & Krueger, J. M. (2009). Physiological markers of local sleep. *The European Journal of Neuroscience, 29*, 1771–1778.

Siegel, J. M. (2009). Sleep viewed as a state of adaptive inactivity. *Nature Reviews: Neuroscience, 10*, 747–753.

Small-N

- Outcome for the Single Case: Random Control Index, Single Subject Experimental Design, and Goal Attainment Scale

Smokeless Tobacco

- Tobacco Control

Smoking

- Lifestyle Changes
- Nicotine
- Tobacco Control

Smoking and Health

Elizabeth Baker and Monica Webb Hooper
Department of Psychology, University of Miami, Coral Gables, FL, USA

Synonyms

Cigarette smoking and health; Health consequences of smoking; Smoking and health effects; Tobacco smoking and health

Definition

Health represents a physical, mental, and emotional state of well-being. Health is not simply the absence of disease or sickness but can be defined as a state of optimal wellness.

Cigarette smoking is the act of inhaling smoke from burning tobacco. Cigarette smoking is directly related to a decline in health and various associated health outcomes. There is no safe level of smoking; therefore, for optimal health, tobacco use should be avoided.

Description

The adverse health effects of smoking have been well documented. Each year, smoking causes more deaths than murders, suicides, HIV, drug and alcohol use, and auto accidents combined (Centers for Disease Control and Prevention [CDC] 2009). In the United States, cigarette smoking is responsible for over 443,000 deaths, $96 billion in medical expenditures, and 5.1 million years of potential life lost annually (CDC

2009). In fact, 1 out of 5 Americans will die prematurely from the effects of smoking. Tobacco use is responsible for five to six million deaths per year worldwide (Jha 2009). This makes cigarette smoking the single largest preventable cause of disease and death.

Cigarette smoking causes much of its damage to the body through the inhaled smoke (U.S. Department of Health and Human Services et al. 2010). Cigarettes contain over 7,000 chemical compounds, many of which are toxic and/or carcinogenic. It is the inhalation of these chemicals that leads to increased risks for heart disease, cancer, and stroke (USDHHS 2004). Heart disease is the leading cause of death in the USA and particularly among smokers. Smoking cigarettes causes the heart to work harder by raising heart rate and blood pressure (Erhardt 2009). Additionally, poisonous gases such as carbon monoxide limit the amount of oxygen carried in the blood. This results in a two- to four-fold increased risk of heart attack and stroke (USDHHS 2004). Smoking also causes lung disease such as chronic obstructive pulmonary disease (COPD), which includes emphysema and chronic bronchitis (U.S. Department of Health & Human Services et al. 2010). Indeed, smoking causes about 90% of all deaths from chronic airway obstruction (Forey et al. 2011). There is a well-established link between smoking and multiple cancers including the lung, mouth, throat, stomach, uterus, esophagus, cervix, bladder, and acute myeloid leukemia (USDHHS 2004). Nearly one third of all cancer deaths can be linked directly to cigarette smoking (CDC 2010). People who suffer from chronic diseases such as diabetes and HIV are especially vulnerable to the negative effects of tobacco use. Indeed, smokers with a chronic disease may experience increased complications, longer hospitalizations, interactions with medications, and increased risk of death (CDC 2010).

Smoking also takes a toll on mental health and overall well-being. There is a robust relationship between cigarette smoking and perceived stress (Kassel et al. 2003). Smokers tend to report greater stress levels compared to nonsmokers (Cohen and Williamson 1988). And although smokers believe that cigarette smoking provides stress relief, research suggests that smoking might cause additional stress (Heishman 1999). Smoking is also associated with increased risk of affective disorders, such as anxiety and depression. Smokers with mental health disorders report substantially greater symptom burden and functional disability compared to nonsmokers (Covey 1998; McCloughen 2003; Morissette 2007). Smoking also reduces the effectiveness of a number of medications used to help manage the symptoms of depression and schizophrenia (Goff 1992).

Smoking also affects health in other ways. Compared to nonsmokers, smokers have increased risks of blindness, periodontal disease, deafness, sexual dysfunction, sleeping difficulties, headaches, and premature aging, including wrinkles and damage to the skin (USDHHS 2010). Among men, smoking causes an increased risk of erectile dysfunction (Tengs 2001). Women who smoke have increased risk of hip fractures, infertility, and premature menopause (USDHHS 2001).

Smoking not only affects the health of smokers but also impacts individuals around them (USDHHS 2006). Nonsmokers who are exposed to tobacco smoke inhale many of the same toxins and cancer-causing substances as smokers. Secondhand smoke (or passive smoking) is responsible for numerous health problems among adults, including an increased risk of heart disease and cancer (USDHHS 2006). Women who smoke during pregnancy risk passing on the toxins from cigarettes to their babies. Such exposure leads to increased risk for premature labor, low birth weight, and birth defects (USDHHS 2006). Children and infants also suffer from secondhand smoke exposure including asthma attacks, ear infections, respiratory illness, and sudden infant death syndrome (USDHHS 2006).

There are many immediate and long-term health benefits of smoking cessation (USDHHS 2004). After the last cigarette, a person's heart rate and blood carbon monoxide level drop to normal within hours. Lung function and capacity improves within days. The excess risk of coronary heart disease, cancers of the lung and mouth, and stroke reduce to that of a nonsmoker 1–15 years after quitting smoking (USDHHS 2004). Quitting smoking at any age and despite any existing medical conditions can help improve overall health.

Cross-References

▶ Smoking Cessation

References and Further Readings

Centers for Disease Control and Prevention. (2009). Annual smoking-attributable mortality, years of potential life lost, and productivity losses-United States, 2000–2004. *Morbidity and Mortality Weekly Report, 58*(2), 29–33. Retrieved from http://www.cdc.gov/mmwr/

Centers for Disease Control and Prevention, National Center for Chronic Disease Prevention and Health Promotion. (2010). *Cancer statistics 2010*. Retrieved from http://www.cdc.gov/Features/

Cohen, S., & Williamson, G. (1988). Perceived stress in a probability sample of the United States. In S. Spacapan & S. Oskamp (Eds.), *The social psychology of health: Claremont symposium on applied social psychology* (pp. 31–68). Newbury Park: SAGE.

Covey, L. L. S. C. (1998). Cigarette smoking and major depression. *Journal of Addictive Diseases, 17*(1), 35–46.

Erhardt, L. (2009). Cigarette smoking: An undertreated risk factor for cardiovascular disease. *Atherosclerosis, 205*(1), 23–32. https://doi.org/10.1016/j.atherosclerosis.2009.01.007.

Forey, B., Thornton, A., & Lee, P. (2011). Systematic review with meta-analysis of the epidemiological evidence relating smoking to COPD, chronic bronchitis and emphysema. *BMC Pulmonary Medicine, 11*(1), 36.

Goff, D. C. (1992). Cigarette smoking in schizophrenia: Relationship to psychopathology and medication side effects. *The American Journal of Psychiatry, 149*(9), 1189–1194.

Heishman, S. J. (1999). Behavioral and cognitive effects of smoking: Relationship to nicotine addiction. *Nicotine & Tobacco Research, 1*(2), S143–S147. https://doi.org/10.1080/14622299050011971.

Jha, P. (2009). Avoidable global cancer deaths and total deaths from smoking. *Nature Reviews Cancer, 9*(9), 655–664. https://doi.org/10.1038/nrc2703.

Kassel, J. D., Stroud, L. R., & Paronis, C. A. (2003). Smoking, stress, and negative affect: Correlation, causation, and context across stages of smoking. *Psychological Bulletin, 129*, 270–304. https://doi.org/10.1037/0033-2909.129.2.270.

McCloughen, A. A. (2003). The association between schizophrenia and cigarette smoking: A review of the literature and implications for mental health nursing practice. *International Journal of Mental Health Nursing, 12*(2), 119–129.

Morissette, S. S. B. (2007). Anxiety, anxiety disorders, tobacco use, and nicotine: A critical review of interrelationships. *Psychological Bulletin, 133*(2), 245–272.

Tengs, T. O. (2001). The link between smoking and impotence: Two decades of evidence. *Preventive Medicine, 32*(6), 447.

U.S. Department of Health and Human Services, Centers for Disease Control and Prevention, Coordinating Center for Health Promotion, National Center for Chronic Disease Prevention and Health Promotion, Office on Smoking and Health. (2006). *The health consequences of involuntary exposure to tobacco smoke: A report of the surgeon general*. Atlanta: Author.

U.S. Department of Health and Human Services, Department of Health and Human Services, Centers for Disease Control and Prevention, National Center for Chronic Disease Prevention and Health Promotion, Office on Smoking and Health. (2004). *The health consequences of smoking: A report of the surgeon general*. Atlanta: Author.

U.S. Department of Health and Human Services, Office on Smoking and Health, National Center for Chronic Disease Prevention and Health Promotion. (2010). *How tobacco smoke causes disease: The biology and behavioral basis for smoking-attributable disease: A report of the surgeon general*. Atlanta: Author.

U.S. Department of Health and Human Services, Public Health Service, Office of the Surgeon General. (2001). *Women and smoking: A report of the surgeon general*. Rockville: Author.

Smoking and Health Effects

▶ Smoking and Health

Smoking Behavior

Elizabeth Baker and Monica Webb Hooper
Department of Psychology, University of Miami, Coral Gables, FL, USA

Synonyms

Cigarette smoking; Smoking habits; Smoking topography; Tobacco use

Definition

Smoking behaviors are actions taken by a person that are associated with the burning and inhalation of a substance. Smoking behavior is multifaceted and includes the actual act of smoking, puffing style, depth of inhalation, and rate and frequency of smoking.

Description

The act of smoking consists of several behaviors and is usually applied to tobacco/cigarettes. A smoker is defined as a person who has a lifetime history of smoking 100 cigarettes or more with current smoking on some days or every day. Most people experiment with smoking during adolescence and do not intend to become regular, addicted, or dependent smokers. Environmental or social factors (e.g., peer pressure) often play a role in smoking initiation. Over time, smoking behavior can become a pattern (i.e., habit) and tolerance develops. The next step is the development of dependence, which is indicated by both tolerance and withdrawal symptoms during periods of abstinence from smoking. Finally, people maintain the compulsive (e.g., addictive) behavior largely because of nicotine dependence.

Smoking behavior is based on individual differences. Smoking topography is defined as the unique manner in which an individual smokes a cigarette. In particular, topography includes the quantity of puffs per cigarette, puff volume, velocity, and duration (Scherer 1999). Each of these behaviors is a component of how a cigarette is smoked. On average, smokers ingest less than 1.5 mg of nicotine per cigarette (Jarvis et al. 2001; United States Federal Trade Committee 2000). This amount varies depending on cigarette brand and how an individual smokes a cigarette (Djordjevic 2000). Dependent smokers seek to regulate the amount of nicotine they receive to maintain the desired physical and emotional state and to avoid withdrawal. In general, a smoker takes about 10 puffs per cigarette (Scherer 1999). A smoker can consciously or unconsciously control nicotine intake by the time taken in between puffs (referred to as puff frequency or puff interval). Smokers may also block the ventilation holes in filtered cigarettes to increase nicotine delivery. The depths of inhalation, duration of the puff, and the amount of smoke in a puff (volume) are all characteristics of smoking behavior that impact exposure to the chemicals and toxins in cigarettes and the subsequent damage to the body (Scherer 1999).

The frequency of daily smoking is another aspect of smoking behavior. The Centers for Disease Control [CDC] (2005) reported that 83% of all smokers are daily users. Daily smokers average 20 cigarettes per day (CDC 2005). Intermittent or light smokers do not smoke daily and are thought to be less nicotine dependent. The time to the first cigarette of the day and the frequency of daily smoking are indicators of nicotine dependence. Smoking immediately after waking is one of the best predictors of nicotine dependence. In addition, smoking most of one's cigarettes during the first 2 h of the day is suggestive of dependence (Heatherton 1989). A greater frequency of daily smoking may be related to difficulty quitting smoking.

Smoking behavior is variable and can change depending on the circumstance or day. For instance, puffs per cigarette may decrease while watching television or may increase while listening to another person talking. The number or duration of puffs may also change according to emotional state. Research has found that increased smoking often occurs during times of personal crisis and stressors (Shiffman et al. 1996). Many smokers report increased smoking in social situations such as being in the company of other smokers or while attending parties. Smokers also vary in their handling of cigarettes; some may hold the cigarette in their mouth, while others allow them to burn in ashtrays or between their fingers.

Smoking behavior is complex. Learning models suggest that smoking behavior is maintained by operant conditioning, including positive and negative reinforcement, and classical conditioning, through the repeated pairing of smoking to various physical and emotional states (Wilker 1973). Such learning makes smoking cessation a formidable challenge for most smokers (Patten and Martin 1996).

Cross-References

▶ Behavior Change
▶ Smoking Cessation
▶ Smoking Topography

References and Further Reading

Centers for Disease Control and Prevention. (2005). Cigarette smoking among adults – United States, 2004. *Morbidity and Mortality Weekly Report, 54*(44), 1121–1124. Retrieved 23 November 2011, from http://www.cdc.gov/mmwr/
Djordjevic, M. M. V. (2000). Doses of nicotine and lung carcinogens delivered to cigarette smokers. *Journal of the National Cancer Institute, 92*(2), 106–111.
Heatherton, T. T. F. (1989). Measuring the heaviness of smoking: Using self-reported time to the first cigarette of the day and number of cigarettes smoked per day. *British Journal of Addiction, 84*(7), 791–800.
Jarvis, M. J., Boreham, R., Primatesta, P., Feyerabend, C., & Bryant, A. (2001). Nicotine yield from machine-smoked cigarettes and nicotine intakes in smokers: Evidence from a representative population survey. *Journal of the National Cancer Institute, 93*(2), 134–138. https://doi.org/10.1093/jnci/93.2.134.
Patten, C., & Martin, J. (1996). Does nicotine withdrawal affect smoking cessation? Clinical and theoretical issues. *Annals of Behavioral Medicine, 18*(3), 190–200. https://doi.org/10.1007/BF02883397.
Scherer, G. G. (1999). Smoking behaviour and compensation: A review of the literature. *Psychopharmacology, 145*(1), 1–20.
Shiffman, S., Paty, J., Gnys, M., Kassel, J., & Hickcox, M. (1996). First lapses to smoking: Within-subjects analysis of real-time reports. *Journal of Consulting and Clinical Psychology, 64*(2), 366–379. https://doi.org/10.1037/0022-006X.64.2.366.
United States Federal Trade Committee. (2000). *"Tar," nicotine, and carbon monoxide of the smoke of 1294 varieties of domestic cigarettes for the year 1998.* Retrieved 23 November 2011, from http://www.ftc.gov/reports/tobacco/1998tar%26nicotinereport.pdf
Wilker, A. (1973). Dynamics of drug dependence: Implications of a conditioning theory for research and treatment. *Archives of General Psychiatry, 28*, 611.

Smoking Cessation

Denise de Ybarra Rodríguez and Monica Webb Hooper
Department of Psychology, University of Miami, Coral Gables, FL, USA

Synonyms

Cigarette smoking cessation; Quit smoking; Stop smoking; Tobacco cessation; Tobacco smoking cessation

Definition

Tobacco smoking is defined as the practice of burning and inhaling tobacco. The combustion from the burning allows the nicotine, tar, and other chemicals and toxins to be absorbed through the lungs. Cigarette smoking is the most prevalent form of consuming tobacco. Most national surveys define a current smoker as having smoked at least 100 (5 packs) cigarettes in their lifetime and currently smokes on at least some days.

Cessation refers to a halting or stopping. Smoking cessation refers to the stopping of cigarette use. Smoking cessation may refer to choosing to stop smoking deliberately or become abstinent due to external and/or environmental factors leading to stopping or quitting smoking.

Description

Smoking cessation is the single most important health behavior change a person can make. Since the 1964 Surgeon General's Report concluded that smoking causes cancer, about 50 million people have successfully quit smoking. Approximately 69% of current smokers state that they want to stop, and 52% have made an attempt to quit smoking in the past year (Centers for Disease Control & Prevention [CDC] 2011).

Smoking cessation has major health benefits. The most common causes of death in the United States are cardiovascular disease, cancer, cerebrovascular accidents, and chronic lower respiratory diseases (Kochanek et al. 2011); smoking cessation has been associated with a reduced risk of dying from these diseases (U.S. Department of Health & Human Services [USDHHS] 1990). The benefits of smoking cessation are greater the earlier one quits, though the benefits of quitting can be experienced even after an extended smoking history. For example, after 15 years of smoking cessation, the excess risk of heart disease for a former smoker is equivalent to a never-smoker. With the increasing duration of cessation, the overall rate of cancer mortality approaches that of nonsmokers (USDHHS).

There are several evidence-based smoking cessation methods. Behavioral interventions include brief physician advice to quit, self-help materials, telephone-based interventions, internet-based counseling and support groups, and group and individual counseling (Fiore et al. 2008). Brief physician advice to quit smoking has been demonstrated to increase the likelihood of cessation by 30%. Self-help cessation interventions increase the likelihood of cessation by 20%. Telephone-based interventions increase the likelihood of cessation by 20%, though tobacco quitlines have increased the odds of cessation by up to 60%. Group and individual counseling increase the likelihood of cessation by 30% and 70%, respectively. The U.S. Food and Drug Administration (FDA) has approved seven smoking cessation pharmacotherapies. These include varenicline (marketed as Chantix in the United States and Champix in Canada and Europe), bupropion (marketed as Zyban), transdermal nicotine patches, nicotine gum, nicotine lozenges, nicotine nasal spray, and the nicotine inhaler. Nicotine patches, gum, and lozenges are available in the USA over the counter; varenicline, bupropion, nicotine nasal spray, and the nicotine inhaler require a physician's prescription. Use of nicotine replacement therapies or bupropion doubles the chances of smoking cessation, while recent evidence suggests that varenicline can triple the likelihood of cessation. Using more than one method when trying to quit (e.g., combination of nicotine replacement with counseling or a telephone quitline) further increases the likelihood of cessation, and the likelihood of cessation increases with the number of formats utilized.

There are also smoking cessation methods that are not based on empirical evidence. Indeed, the most common method of attempting to quit is unassisted quitting (going "cold turkey"). However, approximately 90% of unassisted quit attempts fail. Complementary and alternative methods such as acupuncture, acupressure, laser therapy, and hypnotherapy have been evaluated as smoking cessation methods. However, these methods are not more effective than a placebo (Barnes et al. 2010; White et al. 2011).

Public health policy and campaigns have been instrumental in decreasing the prevalence of smoking in the USA. These policies have restricted indoor smoking via clear indoor air acts (e.g., restaurants, airplanes, and workplaces) in most states and have increased taxes on cigarettes. Public health campaigns have utilized mostly media formats to increase knowledge about the dangers of smoking.

Smoking cessation can result in temporary discomfort, known as nicotine withdrawal. When a person quits smoking, they can enter into nicotine withdrawal within 30 min. The peak of withdrawal occurs within 48–72 h for dependent smokers and usually lasts 1–2 weeks if cessation is maintained. Symptoms of nicotine withdrawal include changes in mood (e.g., irritability, anger, depression, sadness, anxiety, and nervousness), desire or craving to smoke, difficulty concentrating, increased appetite, weight gain, insomnia, restlessness, impatience, constipation, dizziness, coughing, and dreaming or nightmares. The use of FDA-approved cessation aids can minimize withdrawal symptoms.

Smoking cessation is greatly encouraged because of the multiple health benefits that follow. Since the dangers of smoking have been identified, the prevalence has declined and leveled off at 20%. Cigarette smoking is the leading cause of preventable death, disease, and disability in the

USA. Multiple methods to achieve smoking cessation exist, though some of these methods have a greater likelihood of success.

Cross-References

- ▶ Cancer and Smoking
- ▶ Lifestyle Changes
- ▶ Smoking and Health
- ▶ Tobacco Control

References and Further Readings

Barnes, J., Dong, C. Y., McRobbie, H., Walker, N., Mehta, M., & Stead, L. F. (2010). Hypnotherapy for smoking cessation. *Cochrane Database of Systematic Reviews*. https://doi.org/10.1002/14651858.CD001008.pub2.

Centers for Disease Control and Prevention. (2011). Quitting smoking among adults-United States, 2001–2010. *Morbidity and Mortality Weekly Report, 60*(44), 1513–1519.

Fiore, M. C., Jaén, C. R., Baker, T. B., Bailey, W. C., Benowitz, N. L., Curry, S. J., et al. (2008). *Clinical practice guideline: Treating tobacco use and dependence*. Rockville: U.S. Department of Health and Human Services. Public Health Service.

Kochanek, K. D., Xu, J., Murphy, S. L., Miniño, A. M., & Kung, H.-C. (2011). Deaths: Preliminary data for 2009. *National Vital Statistics Reports, 59*(4), 1–51.

U.S. Department of Health and Human Services. (1990). *The health benefits of smoking cessation: A report of the surgeon general*. Atlanta: U.S. Department of Health and Human Services, Centers for Disease Control and Prevention, Center for Chronic Disease Prevention and Health Promotion, Office on Smoking and Health.

United States Department of Health and Human Services (USDHHS). (1982). *The health consequences of smoking: Cancer: A report of the surgeon general*. Rockville: USDHHS.

White, A. R., Rampes, H., Liu, J. P., Stead, L. F., & Campbell, J. (2011). Acupuncture and related interventions for smoking cessation. *Cochrane Database of Systematic Reviews, 1*, CD000009. https://doi.org/10.1002/14651858.CD000009.pub3.

Smoking Habits

- ▶ Smoking Behavior

Smoking Prevention

- ▶ Tobacco Control

Smoking Prevention Policies and Programs

Andrea C. Villanti and David B. Abrams
Johns Hopkins Bloomberg School of Public Health, The Schroeder Institute for Tobacco Research and Policy Studies at Legacy, Washington, DC, USA

Synonyms

Tobacco control

Definition

Since up to 80% of smoking initiation has been shown to occur in adolescence, individual and group-level smoking prevention interventions have focused on youth to avert addiction and the long-term health consequences of smoking. A focus of policy efforts for youth prevention has been restricting youth access to tobacco products at the point of purchase. Effective interventions with broader reach to reduce tobacco product initiation among adolescents and adults include policies that increase the unit price of tobacco products and mass media campaigns when combined and coordinated with other interventions.

Description

From 2002 to 2010, the prevalence of past month tobacco use in the United States among those aged 12 and above declined from 30.4% to 27.4%, with stalled reductions in prevalence in the later years. Currently, 23.0% of the population aged 12 or older smokes cigarettes. Patterns in current tobacco and cigarette use and experimentation with smoking cigarettes were similar for middle school and high school students; while overall prevalence has reached a historic low, no overall declines were noted in youth tobacco use for the 2006–2009 period. Among youth, cigarette smoking is more prevalent among whites than blacks and slightly higher among males than females.

Young people are particularly vulnerable to tobacco addiction due to the effect of nicotine on the reward pathways in the developing brain (from in utero to young adulthood). Additionally, some people are at much greater risk of tobacco use due to genetics, poverty, abuse, neglect, trauma, and other comorbid psychological or cognitive factors such as mood disorders, behavioral, conduct, and attention problems. Beyond the individual, there are numerous variables that affect tobacco use, including adult, household and peer behavior, advertising and promotion, availability and price of tobacco products, poverty, unemployment, neighborhood, community, and cultural norms.

Comprehensive national tobacco strategies use a combination of methods to achieve four main goals: (1) to prevent initiation among youth and young adults, (2) to promote quitting among adults and youth, (3) to eliminate exposure to secondhand smoke, and (4) to identify and eliminate tobacco-related disparities among population groups. Since up to 80% of smoking initiation has been shown to occur in adolescence, individual and group-level smoking prevention interventions have focused on youth to avert addiction and the long-term health consequences of smoking. A focus of policy efforts for youth prevention has been restricting youth access to tobacco products at the point of purchase. Recent data indicates increasing initiation in young adults in the USA, possibly due to targeted marketing efforts by the tobacco industry, and signals the need for extended prevention efforts beyond youth. Effective interventions with broader reach to reduce tobacco product initiation among adolescents and adults include policies that increase the unit price of tobacco products and mass media campaigns when combined and coordinated with other interventions.

Individual and School-Based Programs for Youth

For many years, smoking prevention efforts for adolescents were conducted primarily through school-based programs, which have been shown to have positive short-term effects, but little effect on long-term prevention. Early school-based tobacco curricula focused on social influences, training youth to resist social pressures to use tobacco; studies of these interventions have shown that social influences programming alone is not effective in reducing long-term initiation of smoking. More recent school-based programs have achieved greater success by addressing multiple determinants of tobacco use, including communication skills, coping, personal and social competence, and physical consequences of smoking.

Restricting Youth Access to Tobacco Products

Youth access laws prohibit retailers from selling tobacco products to youth under the age of 18. These laws require enforcement to ensure compliance by the many types of retailers selling tobacco products – from street vendors to convenience stores and online distributors. Adolescent access to cigarette vending machines, low enforcement of these laws, and difficulties in confirming age at purchase in online transactions are all barriers to the success of these laws. Studies indicate that youth access laws can slow increases in adolescent smoking and reduce both smoking prevalence and cigarette consumption, but a very high level of retailer compliance is necessary before these changes occur.

Interventions to Increase the Price of Tobacco Products

Tobacco taxation has been hailed as the most effective intervention to reduce demand for and consumption of tobacco products. Increases in tobacco taxes result in increased cigarette prices, and price has been shown to be a key factor in determining both smoking initiation and cigarette consumption among adults and adolescents.

Price elasticity of demand is defined as the percentage change in consumption of a product following a 1% increase in price. Among US adults, estimates of the price elasticity of cigarette demand typically fall between −0.3 and −0.5, relating to a 3% or 5% decrease in consumption, respectively, for a 10% increase in price. Adolescents have been shown to be almost three times more sensitive to cigarette price increases than adults for several reasons, including the following: First, adolescents have been posited to be less addicted to nicotine and more able to reduce or quit smoking following cigarette price increases. Second, adolescents typically have a lower income and spend a larger fraction of their disposable income on cigarettes than adults. Third, adolescents are also likely to be present-oriented and may not be willing to spend the additional money on cigarettes at the expense of other activities. Reductions in adolescent smoking following tobacco tax interventions may also result from fewer smoking peers.

Mass Media Campaigns to Prevent Tobacco Use

Tobacco marketing includes all efforts of the industry to promote tobacco products, and industry marketing has been linked to a variety of smoking behaviors among both adults and youth, notably youth tobacco initiation. Countermarketing is a strategy used by public health agencies to protect individuals who may be susceptible to the influence of tobacco industry marketing – particularly youth – by responding directly to that marketing. Prior to the end of 1999, major statewide comprehensive tobacco control programs in California, Massachusetts, Arizona, Oregon, and Florida included countermarketing media campaigns which were shown to reduce adult and youth smoking; results from evaluations of these interventions indicated that these campaigns had more influence on smoking behavior in younger compared to older adolescents. The 1998 Tobacco Master Settlement Agreement (MSA) in the United States included provisions for reducing youth access to tobacco products and restricted marketing in venues or media attended by youth. Funds were also dedicated from the MSA to create a foundation to develop and deliver national anti-tobacco messages. The truth® campaign, a national tobacco countermarketing effort launched in 2000 by the American Legacy Foundation, has repeatedly been shown to be effective in reducing smoking among adolescents, specifically younger adolescents. Around the same time, tobacco companies developed youth smoking prevention media campaigns which have been shown to be ineffective, and in the case of parent-targeted advertising, to reduce perceptions of smoking-related harm and to increase approval of smoking and intention to smoke among older adolescents.

Future Directions in Smoking Prevention

Passage of the Family Smoking Prevention and Tobacco Control Act in 2009 gave the Food and Drug Administration (FDA) authority to regulate tobacco products and their marketing to protect the public health. One of FDA's first actions was to ban candy flavorings in cigarettes shown to be appealing to youth in order to reduce youth smoking initiation. Other possible regulatory actions aimed at tobacco use prevention include banning menthol in cigarettes, reducing the amount of nicotine in cigarettes to a non-addictive level, and introducing large, graphic warning labels on health effects of tobacco use to cigarette and smokeless tobacco packaging. The national scale of regulatory action through the FDA has the potential to dramatically influence population-level tobacco use and must be complemented by tobacco control efforts at the community, local, and state levels to achieve the maximum impact on prevention.

Summary

Comprehensive tobacco control programs have taken a community-based approach to smoking prevention, using a combination of school-based, policy, educational, and mass media interventions to change the social environment and conditions related to smoking behavior with positive results. Reviews of community-based programs show that coordinated multicomponent interventions reduce smoking among young people more than single strategies alone and that the level of program funding and implementation is critical to the success of these interventions. A population-based health promotion approach that includes media, education, screening, interventions in community settings and policy can provide avenues to address tobacco use more comprehensively. Coordination of policy and program efforts from the local to the national level is needed to enhance the effectiveness of tobacco use prevention interventions.

Cross-References

▶ Smoking and Health
▶ Smoking Behavior
▶ Smoking Cessation
▶ Tobacco Cessation
▶ Tobacco Use

References and Further Readings

American Legacy Foundation. *Youth smoking prevention mass media campaign.* Retrieved from http://www.thetruth.com/

Center for Tobacco Products, Food and Drug Administration. Retrieved from http://www.fda.gov/tobaccoproducts/default.htm

Centers for Disease Control and Prevention. (2007). *Best practices for comprehensive tobacco control programs-2007.* Atlanta: U.S. Department of Health and Human Services, Centers for Disease Control and Prevention, National Center for Chronic Disease Prevention and Health Promotion, Office on Smoking and Health. Retrieved from http://www.cdc.gov/tobacco/stateandcommunity/best_practices/index.htm

Farrelly, M. C., Davis, K. C., Haviland, M. L., Messeri, P., & Healton, C. G. (2005). Evidence of a dose–response relationship between "truth" antismoking ads and youth smoking prevalence. *American Journal of Public Health, 95*(3), 425–431.

Institute of Medicine. (2007). *Ending the tobacco problem: A blueprint for the nation.* Washington, DC: National Academies Press. Retrieved from http://www.iom.edu/Reports/2007/Ending-the-Tobacco-Problem-A-Blueprint-for-the-Nation.aspx

Substance Abuse and Mental Health Services Administration. (2011). *Results from the 2010 National Survey on drug use and health: Summary of national findings.* NSDUH Series H-41, HHS Publication No. (SMA) 11-4658. Rockville: Substance Abuse and Mental Health Services Administration. Retrieved from http://www.samhsa.gov/data/NSDUH/2k10Results/Web/PDFW/2k10Results.pdf

Task Force on Community Preventive Services. (2005). Tobacco. In: S. Zaza, P. A. Briss, & K. W. Harris (Eds.), *The guide to community preventive services: What works to promote health?* (pp. 3–79). Atlanta: Oxford University Press. Retrieved from http://www.thecommunityguide.org/tobacco/index.html

Smoking Profile

▶ Smoking Topography

Smoking Topography

Stefanie De Jesus
Exercise and Health Psychology Laboratory, The University of Western Ontario, London, ON, Canada

Synonyms

Puff topography; Smoking behavior; Smoking profile

Definition

Smoking topography is a representation of the physical characteristics of smoking behavior, such as puff count, puff volume, average flow, puff duration, and interpuff interval.

Description

An individual's interaction with a substance (e.g., tobacco, marijuana) or object (e.g., pipe, e-cigarette) used for smoking is highly complex, multifaceted, and distinct. Smoking topography attributes have been found to be a function of sex, personality, stress level, nicotine yield, cigarette type (i.e., menthol versus non-menthol), ethnicity, and body mass index.

An array of subjective and objective methods exist to measure smoking topography, each differing in accuracy, precision, and feasibility. These include observation, self-report, cigarette weighing, expired carbon monoxide breath levels, and biomarkers (e.g., nicotine, cotinine, or thiocyanate). Specialized instruments (e.g., pressure transducers, flowmeters, and puff analyzers) provide an unrestricted assessment of smoking topography.

Smoking topography has been examined across various disciplines and populations, such as nicotine metabolism, smoking cessation, exercise, adolescents, and individuals with schizophrenia. There is an impetus to further study smoking topography as it is reflective of the rewarding and reinforcing effects of addictive substances, compensation, harm reduction efforts, and exposure to harmful elements and potential carcinogens.

Cross-References

- Cancer and Smoking
- Cessation Intervention (Smoking or Tobacco)
- Nicotine
- Smoking and Health
- Smoking Behavior
- Smoking Cessation

References and Further Readings

Benowitz, N. L. (2001). Compensatory smoking of low-yield cigarettes. In National Cancer Institute (Ed.), *Risks associated with smoking cigarettes with low machine-measured yields of tar and nicotine* (pp. 39–64). Bethesda: US Department of Health and Human Services, National Institutes of Health, National Cancer Institute.

De Jesus, S., Hsin, A., Faulkner, G., & Prapavessis, H. (2015). A systematic review and analysis of data reduction techniques for the CReSS smoking topography device. *Journal of Smoking Cessation, 10*, 12–28. https://doi.org/10.1017/jsc.2013.31.

Shahab, L., West, R., & McNeill, A. (2008). The feasibility of measuring puffing behaviour in roll-your-own cigarette smokers. *Tobacco Control, 17*(Suppl I), i17–i23. https://doi.org/10.1136/tc.2007.021824.

SNP (Pronounced "Snip")

- Single Nucleotide Polymorphism (SNP)

Social Behavior

- Interpersonal Circumplex

Social Capital and Health

Martin Lindström
Department of Clinical Sciences, Malmö, Sweden

Social capital has no direct synonyms. Social cohesion is a broader concept which is *not* directly synonymous with social capital. Social cohesion is a combination of absence of latent social conflict, e.g., in the form of social and economic inequality, ethnic tensions or other forms of polarization, and the presence of strong social bonds measured by levels of trust and reciprocity (i.e., social capital), a strong "civil society" which bridge social divisions, and institutions of conflict management (e.g., a responsive democracy and an independent judiciary) (Kawachi and Berkman 2000).

Definition

The definition of social capital varies by author and academic tradition. Robert Putnam (political science) defines social capital as "features of social organization, such as trust, norms, and networks that can improve the efficiency of society by facilitating coordinated actions" (Putnam 1993). According to James Coleman (sociology), social capital is "...a variety of different entities (that) facilitate certain actions of individuals who are within a structure" (Coleman 1990), while Pierre Bourdieu (sociology) defines it as "...the sum of the resources, actual or virtual, that accrue to an individual or a group by virtue of possessing a durable network" (Bourdieu and Wacquant 1992). The definitions of Putnam, pertaining to the population level of social capital, and Coleman, pertaining to social networks of individuals, have been more commonly used in behavioral medicine and public health than that of Bourdieu, which is closer to the individual level, is less distinct in relation to social support, and also concerns the power structure within social groups and structures. Health as a concept is defined elsewhere.

Description

The social capital concept was first used in 1916 but originates in its modern context in the fields of sociology and political science. Social capital concerns the characteristics of interaction between actors such as individuals, social groups, and organizations rather than the characteristics of actors per se. Social capital includes interpersonal trust, trust in institutions, reciprocity, civic participation, social participation, and social networks which increase cooperation and decrease transaction costs in society.

The first articles concerning social capital and health appeared in international medical and public health journals in the mid-1990s with a fast increase in the number of publications after 1996–1998. From approximately 40 international journal publications in 2001 (Macinko and Starfield 2001), the number of journal publications has increased to 1,179 in 2011 in PubMed only (December 19, 2011). Already in 2001, Macinko and Starfield identified four levels of analysis of social capital and health: the macro (countries, regions), meso (neighborhoods, municipalities), micro (social networks), and psychological (trust) levels (Macinko and Starfield 2001). Putnam's definition of social capital, which includes trust despite Putnam's macro and meso perspectives because the level of trust may be regarded as a trait of populations and countries just as well as a cognitive trait of the individual, has, together with Coleman's definition, had the strongest impact in the behavioral medicine and public health literature, although other authors such as Bourdieu and Portes are also referred to and their definitions also used in empirical studies.

Although Putnam had earlier stated that the area of health and public health was probably a research area not particularly strongly associated with and affected by social capital (Putnam 1993), he 7 years later contended, based on the dramatic increase of results of empirical studies, that health and public health was probably one of the most important areas associated with and affected by social capital (Putnam 2000). Kawachi et al. (1999) suggested four main causal pathways by which social capital may affect health: direct psychological and psychosocial stress pathways, social norms and values which foster health-related behaviors, access to health care and amenities through social networks and contacts, and crime, particularly violent crime (Kawachi et al. 1999).

Kawachi et al. (1997) found in an early ecological study that low levels of social capital were associated with a higher total mortality rate and higher rates of a wide range of major causes of death, including coronary heart disease (CHD), cerebrovascular disease, unintentional injury, and infant mortality (Kawachi et al. 1997). Later epidemiological, ecological, and individual level studies have, just to give some examples, revealed significant associations between low levels of social capital and higher age-adjusted mortality rates, shorter life expectancy, higher mortality and violent crime rates, higher coronary heart disease morbidity and mortality, low birth weight rates, higher incidence rates of a variety of sexually transmitted diseases, low life satisfaction, less happiness, poor self-rated health, poor mental health (measured with the GHQ12 index), poor physical and mental health measured by SF-12, depression, psychiatric morbidity, higher suicide rates, worse chronic conditions, functional limitations (Islam et al. 2006), and health-related behaviors such as lower levels of leisure time physical activity (Lindström et al. 2001). Some studies have investigated associations between vertical social capital, i.e., trust and participation across a well-defined power gradient, and health (Sundquist et al. 2006). Multilevel studies, which mostly include the individual level and one or more contextual levels of analysis, have e.g. shown that low social capital is associated with poor self-rated health and violent crime

(Islam et al. 2006). Multilevel analyses have also demonstrated significant associations between social capital and access to health care (Lindström et al. 2006). Multilevel analyses have increasingly been conducted in order to disentangle the associations between contextual level social capital and individual level health in order to avoid the "ecological fallacy," which denotes the risk of drawing erroneous conclusions concerning individual health from observations of ecological data, and the "individualist fallacy," which denotes the risk of missing associations and effects of neighborhood or other forms of contextual social capital on individual health.

Since social capital is a characteristic of social relations, trust, and cooperation between individuals, groups, and organizations rather than of individuals, one important issue related to social capital and health is to define relevant social contexts for the analysis of the association and impact of contextual social capital on health and health-related phenomena such as health-related behaviors and access to health care and amenities. Most multilevel studies include neighborhoods or other geographic entities as second, third, and so forth levels of analysis. However, one question concerns whether geographic entities are the most relevant social contexts. This discussion is highly relevant because many multilevel studies have shown small or moderate associations between neighborhood and geographic social capital and health of individuals within single countries, while the statistical associations between social capital and health have been stronger and more consistent in individual level studies. Recently, some prospective cohort studies have investigated workplace social capital and found significant effects on, e.g., depression (Kouvanonen et al. 2008). In studies of social capital and school children and adolescents, the family and schools are relevant social contexts in addition to neighborhoods. Putnam suggested already in 2000 that the Internet would become a relevant area for studies of social capital and social networks (Putnam 2000).

Most studies of social capital and health are cross-sectional, i.e., they measure all factors at the same point in time which makes causal inference formally impossible. In many instances, causality may go in both directions. Social capital may, e.g., cause poor mental health, but mental health may also affect social capital in the forms of social participation in social networks, civic participation, and feelings of trust and reciprocity. A few longitudinal studies with panel data including three waves of observations or more have been conducted in recent years (Giordano and Lindström 2011).

Social capital is not always associated with better health. Szreter and Woolcock developed the concepts of bonding, bridging, and linking social capital. Bonding social capital denotes "trusting and cooperative relations between members of a network who see themselves as being similar in terms of their shared social identity," while bridging social capital refers to "relations of respect and mutuality between people who know they are not alike in some sociodemographic (or social identity) sense (differing by age, ethnic group, class, etc.)" (Szreter and Woolcock 2004). While many social networks, associations, and organizations, e.g., youth organizations, sports clubs, and labor unions, manage to combine bonding and bridging social capital, some other, e.g., criminal networks, do not. This phenomenon of exclusion of outsiders and the rest of society is sometimes referred to as "the dark side of social capital," and its effects on health may be detrimental. Linking social capital refers to "norms of respect and networks of trusting relationships between people who are interacting across explicit, formal, or institutionalized power or authority gradients in society" (Szreter and Woolcock 2004).

Critique against the research concerning social capital and health has been expressed by the so-called neo-materialists, who claim that it obscures underlying ideological, political, administrative, and economic determinants of health inequalities and other public health issues. The neo-materialists emphasize the importance of active governments, active welfare politics, and economic preconditions for the realization of public health programs (Navarro 2004).

Cross-References

▶ Cross-Sectional Study
▶ Longitudinal Study
▶ Multilevel Analysis
▶ Social Cohesion
▶ Social Support

References and Further Readings

Bourdieu, P., & Wacquant, L. (1992). *Invitation to reflexive sociology*. Chicago: University of Chicago Press.
Coleman, J. S. (1990). *Foundations of social theory*. Princeton: Harvard University Press.
Giordano, G. N., & Lindström, M. (2011). Social capital and change in psychological health over time. *Social Science and Medicine, 72*, 1219–1227.
Islam, K., Merlo, J., Kawachi, I., Lindström, M., & Gerdtham, U. (2006). Social capital and health: Does egalitarianism matter? A literature review. *International Journal for Equity in Health, 5*, 3.
Kawachi, I., & Berkman, L. (2000). Social cohesion, social capital, and health. In L. Berkman & I. Kawachi (Eds.), *Social epidemiology* (pp. 174–190). Oxford: Oxford University Press.
Kawachi, I., Kennedy, B. P., Lochner, K., & Prothrow-Stith, D. (1997). Social capital, income inequality, and mortality. *American Journal of Public Health, 87*, 1491–1498.
Kawachi, I., Kennedy, B. P., & Wilkinson, R. G. (1999). Social capital and self-rated health: A contextual analysis. *American Journal of Public Health, 89*, 1187–1193.
Kouvanonen, A., Oksanen, T., Vahtera, J., Stafford, M., Wilkinson, R., Schneider, J., et al. (2008). Low workplace social capital as a predictor of depression. The Finnish public sector study. *American Journal of Epidemiology, 167*(10), 1143–1151.
Lindström, M., Hanson, B. S., & Östergren, P. O. (2001). Socioeconomic differences in leisure-time physical activity: The role of social participation and social capital in shaping health related behaviour. *Social Science and Medicine, 52*, 441–451.
Lindström, M., Axén, E., Lindström, C., Beckman, A., Moghaddassi, M., & Merlo, J. (2006). Social capital and access to a regular doctor: A multilevel analysis in southern Sweden. *Health Policy, 79*, 153–164.
Macinko, S., & Starfield, B. (2001). The utility of social capital in research on health determinants. *The Milbank Quarterly, 79*(3), 387–427.
Navarro, V. (2004). Commentary: Is social capital the solution or the problem? *International Journal of Epidemiology, 33*, 672–674.
Putnam, R. D. (1993). *Making democracy work. Civic traditions in modern Italy*. Princeton: Princeton University Press.
Putnam, R. D. (2000). *Bowling alone. The collapse and revival of American community*. New York/London: Simon and Schuster.
Sundquist, J., Johansson, S. E., Yang, M., Sundquist, J., Johansson, S. E., Yang, M., et al. (2006). Low linking social capital as a predictor of coronary heart disease in Sweden: A cohort study of 2.6 million people. *Social Science and Medicine, 62*, 954–963.
Szreter, S., & Woolcock, M. (2004). Health by association? Social capital, social theory, and the political economy of public health. *International Epidemiology, 33*, 650–667.

Social Circumstance

▶ Sociocultural

Social Cohesion

Yori Gidron
SCALab, Lille 3 University and Siric Oncollile, Lille, France

Definition

Social cohesion (SC) refers to the degree to which links between a society's members are strong and the degree to which people in a community share values and goals and are interdependent. Durkehiem conceptualized SC as a major protective variable against adversities including suicide. In his seminal work, Durkheim found that Catholics have lower suicide rates than Protestants, and he attributed this to greater social control and cohesion in the former than among the latter (Pickering and Walford 2000). Kelleher and Daly (1990) found that reduced SC (indexed by reduced marriage rates and increased separations) was among the variables possibly contributing to increased suicide rates in Ireland, between 1970 and 1985. The Dutch sociologist Geert Hofstede conducted the first empirically based quantification of international cultural dimensions in the 1970s in IBM plants around the world. Among his four main cultural dimensions, individualism emerged, which can be seen as the opposite of SC. Individualism from Hofstede's scores does predict on a global level present suicide rates (Gidron and Ferreira 2012). Recent studies have also tested the relationship between SC and various health outcomes, pertinent to behavioral medicine. Chaix et al. (2008) found in Sweden that low SC predicted myocardial infarctions, independent of important demographic variables. More recently, Clark et al. (2011) found that each one point increase in SC predicted a reduction of 53% in deaths attributed to stroke, independent of confounders. SC was assessed individually by six items reflecting social interactions and contacts with neighbors. One mechanism could be that more cohesive societies (such as religious kibbutzim in Israel vs. secular ones) also promote a healthier psychosocial profile – higher sense of coherence and lower hostility levels (Kark et al. 1996). The concept of SC is thus one domain where concepts important in behavioral medicine and sociology may influence health at the more macro level of societies. One type of simple intervention which may increase SC is Walton and Cohen's social belonging method, where people are indirectly shown that others experience similar negative experiences as they do. This was found to raise academic performance in vulnerable or stigmatized people (Walton and Cohen 2007). This could have important implications for preventative medicine and public health. Programs for increasing the sense of belongingness and SC need to be developed and adapted to large-scale social contexts, and their effects on health outcomes can then be empirically examined.

Cross-References

▶ Social Support
▶ Suicide Risk, Suicide Risk Factors

References and Further Readings

Chaix, B., Lindström, M., Rosvall, M., & Merlo, J. (2008). Neighborhood social interactions and risk of acute myocardial infarction. *Journal of Epidemiology and Community Health, 62*, 62–68.

Clark, C. J., Guo, H., Lunos, S., Aggarwal, N. T., Beck, T., Evans, D. A., et al. (2011). Neighborhood cohesion is associated with reduced risk of stroke mortality. *Stroke, 42*, 1212–1217.

Gidron, Y., & Ferreira, O. (2012). *Culture & international suicide rates*. Paper presented at the sixth annual international conference on psychology, May, Athens.

Kark, J. D., Carmel, S., Sinnreich, R., Goldberger, N., & Friedlander, Y. (1996). Psychosocial factors among members of religious and secular kibbutzim. *Israel Journal of Medical Sciences, 32*, 185–194.

Kelleher, M. F., & Daly, M. (1990). Suicide in Cork and Ireland. *British Medical Journal, 157*, 533–538.

Pickering, W. S. F., & Walford, G. (Eds.). (2000). *Durkheim's suicide: A century of research and debate.* London: Psychology Press/Routledge.

Walton, G. M., & Cohen, G. L. (2007). A question of belonging: Race, social fit, and achievement. *Journal of Personality and Social Psychology, 92*, 82–96.

Social Conflict

Orit Birnbaum-Weitzman
Department of Psychology, University of Miami, Miami, FL, USA

Synonyms

Interpersonal conflict; Negative social interaction; Relational distress; Relationship conflict; Social stress

Definition

Social conflict refers to the various types of negative social interactions that may occur within social relationships including, but not limited to, arguments, rejection, criticism, hostility, insensitivity, unwanted demands, and ridicule (Seeman 2001). Social conflict can also escalate to include physical violence. Conflict refers to overt behavior rather than subjective states. It typically results from purposeful interaction among two parties in a competitive setting in which the parties are aware of the incompatibility of positions. Social conflict can extend to different social relationships including those with significant others such as spouses, family members, and friends, as well as less intimate relationships.

Description

Studies on social conflict and interpersonal stress suggest that negative aspects of social interactions including social conflict and social control are inversely related to emotional well-being and health (Miller et al. 2009). There is substantial evidence that interactions marked by acute conflict and negative emotions have direct physiological consequences. Epidemiological studies have linked social isolation, low social support, and high levels of social conflict with morbidity and mortality (Miller et al. 2009). Changes in immune function and elevated inflammation have been suggested as key pathways underlying the association between social conflict and health (Kiecolt-Glaser et al. 2010). Inflammation is a key pathogenic mechanism in many infections and cardiovascular and neoplastic diseases. Recent studies have also linked stressful interpersonal relationships to alterations in gene expression and intracellular signaling mechanisms (Miller et al. 2009).

Consistent evidence also points to the strong relationship between social conflict and psychological distress. Specifically, interpersonal stress and conflict with family and friends has been reliably associated with negative affect, depression, and emotional stress responses (Graham et al. 2007). Depression has been proposed as a particularly important psychological mechanism by which social conflict in close relationships affect immune function (Miller et al. 2009). The literature indicates that social conflict is associated with a range of physiological and psychological mechanisms that are in turn associated with concomitant alterations in the cardiovascular, endocrine, and immune systems. Family conflict and discord and domestic violence have also been linked to suicidal behavior (Van Orden et al. 2010). In drug abusers, interpersonal conflict has been also associated with an increased probability of a history of suicide attempt and ideation (Van Orden et al. 2010).

Social conflict has been assessed using self-report questionnaires about relationship quality and quantity as well as in experimental studies of laboratory-induced marital conflict (Kiecolt-Glaser et al. 2010). To date, there is not one standard measure to assess social conflict. Different types of study designs have been used to assess the impact of social conflict on physical and emotional well-being including correlational studies, experimental studies of couples, and animal studies (see Kiecolt-Glaser et al. 2010). Correlational studies suggest that social isolation, lack of social support, and interpersonal conflict are associated with biological markers of inflammation (i.e., C-reactive protein and interleukin-6). More recent studies have also suggested a plausible link between distressed pair-bond relationships and plasma levels of oxytocin in females and vasopressin in males. However, this research is still preliminary. In other correlation studies, men and women who had recently undergone a marital separation or divorce had poorer immune function than demographically matched married individuals (see Kiecolt-Glaser et al. 2010).

According to Kiecolt-Glaser et al. (1998), being married is not always protective, especially if there is frequent interpersonal conflict in the couple. In experimental studies with married couples, this group of researchers has shown that conflictive social interactions consistently result in heightened blood pressure and heart rate, especially for those with high trait hostility. Conflict discussion tasks are also widely used in marital research by this group and others. Discussion of marital problems has been associated with both immediate and longer term physiological changes related to the degree of negativity or hostility displayed during conflict (see Kiecolt-Glaser et al. 2010). Gender differences have been observed in these studies, with women evidencing greater sensitivity to negative marital interactions than men. Similarly, marital conflict shows a greater impact on health and physiological functioning in older adults compared to young couples. In general, this research suggests that relationships that are stable and long lasting but marked by social conflict have the potential to function as both an acute and chronic stressor that may impact health over an extensive period of time (Kiecolt-Glaser et al. 2010). Relationship conflict and termination can also provoke detrimental health behaviors including disturbed sleep, unhealthy diets, less physical activity, smoking, and greater use of alcohol and other drugs. Thus, relationships characterized by hostility and conflict could have negative health consequences.

The most common social conflict models involving laboratory animals are variations of the resident-intruder model wherein one animal is placed in the home cage of another. Animal studies have shown that social conflict and disruption of social relationships have important immunological and endocrine consequences (Huhman 2006). In rodents, an aggressive social encounter is typically accompanied by elevated levels of stress hormones and changes in cellular and humoral immunity. Exposure to social conflict appears to have long-lasting behavioral and physiological effects not just in defeated/subordinate animals but also in dominant ones that appear to be moderated by developmental level (Huhman 2006). Data from experimental primate models also show that stressful social relationships can exacerbate viral infections by altering gene expression responses to infection. Social conflict models in animals may be useful for studying the physiological concomitants of a number of psychiatric disorders including major depression (see Huhman 2006).

Cross-References

▶ Family Stress
▶ Interpersonal Relationships
▶ Marriage and Health

References and Readings

Graham, J. E., Christian, L. M., & Kiecolt-Glaser, J. K. (2007). Close relationships and immunity. In R. Ader (Ed.), *Psychoneuroimmunology* (pp. 781–798). Burlington, MA: Elsevier Academic Press.

Huhman, K. L. (2006). Social conflict models: Can they inform us about human psychopathology? *Hormones and Behavior, 50*, 640–646.

Kiecolt-Glaser, J. K., Glaser, R., Cacioppo, J. T., & Malarkey, W. B. (1998). Marital stress: Immunologic, neuroendocrine and autonomic correlates. *Annuals of New York Academic Sciences, 840*, 656–663.

Kiecolt-Glaser, J. K., Gouin, J. P., & Hantsoo, L. (2010). Close relationships, inflammation, and health. *Neuroscience and Biobehavioral Reviews, 35*, 33–38.

Miller, G., Chen, E., & Cole, S. W. (2009). Health psychology: Developing biologically plausible models linking the social world and physical health. *Annual Review of Psychology, 60*, 501–524.

Seeman, T. (2001). How do others get under our skin: Social relationships and health. In C. D. Ryff & B. H. Singer (Eds.), *Emotion, social relationships and health* (pp. 189–209). New York: Oxford University Press.

Van Orden, K. A., Witte, T. K., Cukrowicz, K. C., Braithwaite, S. R., Selby, E. A., & Joiner, T. E. (2010). The interpersonal theory of suicide. *Psychological Review, 117*, 575–600.

Social Determinants of Health

▶ Social Factors

Social Ecological Framework

▶ Ecological Models: Application to Physical Activity

Social Ecological Model

▶ Ecological Models: Application to Physical Activity

Social Epidemiology

G. David Batty
Department of Epidemiology and Public Health, University College London, London, UK

Definition

While epidemiology is defined as the study of the distribution and determinants of disease and typically treats social determinants as background to biomedical phenomena, social epidemiology is a sphere of enquiry in its own right. It is distinguished by explicitly investigating social determinants of population distributions of health, disease, and well-being. Social epidemiology was perhaps first coined as a discipline in the 1950s; postgraduate programs in social epidemiology are now offered.

Cross-References

▶ Epidemiology
▶ Socioeconomic Status (SES)

References and Further Reading

Berkman, L., & Kawachi, I. (Eds.). (2000). *Social epidemiology*. New York: Oxford University Press.
Krieger, N. (2001). A glossary for social epidemiology. *Journal of Epidemiology and Community Health, 55*(10), 693–700.

Social Factors

Emily Kothe
School of Psychology, University of Sydney, Sydney, NSW, Australia

Synonyms

Social determinants of health; Socioeconomic status (SES)

Definition

The conditions under which people are born, live, work, and age are collectively known as the social determinants of health. These social factors include both economic and social conditions and are may be responsible for the health inequities both within and between countries.

Description

Research into the social factors underpinning health arose from the dual observations of health disparities both within and between countries. These disparities can be easily (although crudely) demonstrated by way of differences in life expectancy for different groups.

Between-country differences in adult mortality are growing rapidly. Whereas mortality rose in Africa, Central and Eastern Europe between 1970 and 2002, global mortality fell overall during the same period (World Health Organization 2003). These differences in mortality rates are especially stark when comparing life expectancy by country. For example, while the average life expectancy at birth is 89.78 years in Monaco, it is just 29.3 years in Haiti (CIA 2011).

Large differences in morbidity and mortality are also apparent within the same country. For example, in Australia, the life expectancy for Aboriginal and Torres Strait Islanders is approximately 10 years below the national average (Australian Bureau of Statistics 2010).

Study of the social factors that underlie health provides possible mechanisms by which this large health disparity can be understood. The major social factors which influence health include both structural determinants of health, and the conditions of an individual's daily life. Research linking social factors to health outcome has identified a number of key social determinants of health (e.g., Wilkinson and Marmot 2003). These include:

- The social gradient
- Stress
- Early life
- Social exclusion
- Work and unemployment

These factors are thought to influence health both indirectly and directly. In many cases, social factors act in combination to have a cumulative impact on health. For example, while unemployment is known to have a direct influence on health, it is also likely to have an indirect influence on health through its influence on other social factors (e.g., stress).

The Social Gradient

It is widely recognized that poverty is related to high levels of illness and disease. Data consistently shows that the health status of individuals in the poorest countries leads to significantly lower life expectancy and significantly higher risk of disease than that of individuals in richer countries.

The influence of socioeconomic status is also apparent within countries and appears to have an influence on health across the socioeconomic spectrum. This effect, known as the social gradient, shows that even within industrialized countries, both mortality and morbidity are linearly distributed across different levels of socioeconomic advantage and disadvantage. This research suggests that even moderate differences in wealth, and associated social factors, can have an important impact on health status.

For more information, see Social Class.

Early Life

Maternal deprivation and ill-health during pregnancy have both been linked to poor fetal development. Factors such as malnutrition, maternal stress, and inadequate prenatal care all increase the risk of childhood mortality and have profound impacts on health throughout later life.

Research has also linked circumstances during infancy to both physical and mental health in adult life. Social functioning, physical health, and the performance of health-protective behaviors have all been linked to experiences in early life.

For more information, see Maternal Stress; Birth Weight; Child Neglect; Child Development; Stress, Early Life.

Stress

Social and psychological circumstance can have a profound impact on the number of stressors an individual is exposed to and the level of stress that they experience. Increased levels of stress have been linked to increased risk of both morbidity and mortality.

Research suggests that exposure to stressors can have both direct and indirect influences on health. Chronic stress can directly increase risk of disease through its influence on physiological processes such as immune function. However, both acute and chronic stress can also lead to high rates of health-damaging behaviors such as alcohol consumption and smoking.

For more information, see Stress; Stressor.

Social Exclusion

Social exclusion relates to the isolation of certain member within a society and is associated with high rates of disease and mortality. It is most often related to relative poverty, low educational attainment, unemployment, and experiences of stigma and discrimination.

Individuals who experience social exclusion are subject to a pattern of multiple deprivations that prevent them from participating fully in society. This is often characterized by poor access to services, including health care, housing, education, and transport.

For more information, see Social Capital and Health; Stigma.

Work and Unemployment

Research suggests that work and unemployment have separate – but at times overlapping – influences on health.

In general, being unemployed places individuals at increased risk of a number of diseases (e.g., depression and heart disease). The effects of unemployment on health are linked to both material deprivation that may occur due to a lack of income, and to the psychological consequences of being unemployed. The influence of unemployment on health appears to manifest itself even before individuals become unemployed, such that experiencing high levels of job insecurity (in many cases, a precursor of unemployment) can be as harmful to health as being unemployed.

In addition to the role of perceived job security, it appears that there are a range of factors that determine the extent to which employment is health protective. These include:

- Level of job control
- Level of job demand
- Adequacy of rewards for job performance

In particular it appears that professions that are characterized by low control but high demand place workers at increased risk of ill-health. Importantly social support and recognition of job performance, either through higher wages or increased social status, both appear to be health protective.

For more information, see Work-Related Stress.

Social Causation and Social Drift: Explanation of Possible Causal Relationships Between Social Factors and Health

When attempting to understand the influence of social factors on health, it is important to consider the possible causal relationships between these social factors and health. Broadly speaking, there are two possible ways of understanding the causal relationship between these factors. These explanations are described below using the example of the social gradient (Morrison and Bennett 2008).

The first explanation – called social causation – would suggest that low socioeconomic status is causally related to health problems (i.e., that there is something about low socioeconomic status that "causes" ill-health). For example, an individual who experiences being socioeconomically disadvantaged may be exposed to poor living conditions which cause later health problems.

The second explanation – called social drift – would suggest that ill-health is causally related to low socioeconomic status (i.e., that experiencing illness "causes" an individual to lose their socioeconomic position). For example, an individual who has to leave work due to illness may find that without a steady income, they are now socioeconomically disadvantaged.

Longitudinal studies provide evidence for both explanations. For example, studies have consistently shown that low socioeconomic status baseline is a predictor of heart disease at follow-up and that individuals who become unemployed are more likely to suffer from health complaints than individuals who stay employed. On the basis of this evidence, it would appear most likely that social factors and health have a bidirectional relationship (Morrison and Bennett 2008).

Cross-References

- ▶ Birth Weight
- ▶ Child Development
- ▶ Child Neglect
- ▶ Health Care Access
- ▶ Maternal Stress
- ▶ Social Capital and Health
- ▶ Stigma
- ▶ Stress
- ▶ Stress, Early Life
- ▶ Stressor
- ▶ Work-Related Stress

References and Readings

Australian Bureau of Statistics. (2010). *Experimental life tables for Aboriginal and Torres Strait Islander Australians, 2005–2007 (Cat. No. 3302.0.55.003).* Canberra: Author.

CIA. (2011). *The world factbook: Life expectancy at birth.* Retrieved 18 Nov 2010 from https://www.cia.gov/library/publications/the-world-factbook/rankorder/2102rank.html#

Marmot, M. (2005). Social determinants of health inequalities. *The Lancet, 365*(9464), 1099–1104.

Morrison, V., & Bennett, P. (2008). *An introduction to health psychology*. New York: Prentice Hall.

Wilkinson, R. G., & Marmot, M. G. (2003). *Social determinants of health: The solid facts*. Copenhagen: World Health Organization.

World Health Organization. (2003). *World health report 2003: Shaping the future*. Geneva: Author.

Social Health

▶ Racial Inequality in Economic and Social Well-Being

Social Inhibition

Johan Denollet
CoRPS – Center of Research on Psychology in Somatic diseases, Tilburg University, Tilburg, The Netherlands

Synonyms

Behavioral inhibition

Definition

Social inhibition (SI) is a broad personality trait that refers to *the stable tendency to inhibit the expression of emotions and behaviors in social interaction* (Asendorpf 1993). Individuals who are high in SI are more likely to feel inhibited, tense, and insecure when with others. In children, the label *behavioral inhibition* is often used to describe this tendency (Gest 1997).

SI is more closely related to the *interpersonal dimension* of introversion/extraversion than to intrapsychic facets of extraversion such as positive affect or excitement seeking. Infants and children with an inhibited temperament tend to develop into adults who avoid people and situations that are novel or unfamiliar (Schwartz et al. 2003). Hence, individuals who are high in SI try to avoid potential "dangers" involved in social interaction, such as disapproval or criticism by others, through the deliberate inhibition of self-expression (Asendorpf 1993). They tend to experience discomfort in encounters with other people, may keep other people at a distance, and are less likely to actively seek social support.

Interestingly, recent imaging research demonstrates the effect of social inhibition on the *neural coding of threatening signals* in the human brain (Kret et al. 2011). Socially inhibited adults may show greater signal response in the brain to threatening stimuli than adults who are not socially inhibited (Schwartz et al. 2003). Other research also indicates that socially inhibited people tend to overactivate a broad cortical network in the brain when looking at fearful or angry facial and bodily expressions (Kret et al. 2011).

There are several reasons why it is important to account for individual differences in SI in clinical research and practice. First, SI has been related to *difficulties in coping with the challenges of everyday life*. For example, inhibited children may show a delay in establishing a first stable partnership and finding a first full-time job in early adulthood (Asendorpf et al. 2008). Second, socially inhibited individuals may seem quiet on the surface, while they may actually *avoid interpersonal conflict* through excessive control over their emotional and behavioral responses. Third, SI has been associated with an increased long-term *risk of developing internalizing problems* (Asendorpf et al. 2008), including anxiety disorders (Rapee 2002) and other forms of distress (Gest 1997) in adulthood.

SI may also increase the risk of physical health problems. Individuals who are high in SI display physiologic hyperreactivity to stress (Cole et al. 2003), and the active inhibition of emotions induces increased cardiovascular reactivity (Gross and Levenson 1997). In clinical research, SI has been associated with the progression of HIV (Cole et al. 2003) and with an increased risk of adverse cardiac events in patients with heart disease (Denollet et al. 2006).

SI can be reliably *assessed with the 7-item SI measure of the DS14* (Denollet 2005), a scale that was specifically designed to assess this broad and stable tendency to inhibit the expression of emotions and behaviors in social interaction.

Cross-References

▶ Type D Personality

References and Readings

Asendorpf, J. B. (1993). Social inhibition: A general-developmental perspective. In H. C. Traue & J. W. Pennebaker (Eds.), *Emotion, inhibition, and health* (pp. 80–99). Seattle: Hogrefe & Huber.

Asendorpf, J. B., Denissen, J. J., & van Aken, M. A. (2008). Inhibited and aggressive preschool children at 23 years of age: Personality and social transitions into adulthood. *Developmental Psychology, 44*, 997–1011.

Cole, S. W., Kemeny, M. E., Fahey, J. L., Zack, J. A., & Naliboff, B. D. (2003). Psychological risk factors for HIV pathogenesis: Mediation by the autonomic nervous system. *Biological Psychiatry, 54*, 1444–1456.

Denollet, J. (2005). DS14: Standard assessment of negative affectivity, social inhibition, and type D personality. *Psychosomatic Medicine, 67*, 89–97.

Denollet, J., Pedersen, S. S., Ong, A. T., Erdman, R. A., Serruys, P. W., & van Domburg, R. T. (2006). Social inhibition modulates the effect of negative emotions on cardiac prognosis following percutaneous coronary intervention in the drug-eluting stent era. *European Heart Journal, 27*, 171–177.

Gest, S. D. (1997). Behavioral inhibition: Stability and associations with adaptation from childhood to early adulthood. *Journal of Personality and Social Psychology, 72*, 467–475.

Gross, J. J., & Levenson, R. W. (1997). Hiding feelings: The acute effects of inhibiting negative and positive emotion. *Journal of Abnormal Psychology, 106*, 95–103.

Kret, M. E., Denollet, J., Grèzes, J., & de Gelder, B. (2011). The role of negative affectivity and social inhibition in perceiving social threat: An fMRI study. *Neuropsychologia, 49*, 1187–1193.

Rapee, R. M. (2002). The development and modification of temperamental risk for anxiety disorders: Prevention of a lifetime of anxiety? *Biological Psychiatry, 52*, 947–957.

Schwartz, C. E., Wright, C. I., Shin, L. M., Kagan, J., & Rauch, S. L. (2003). Inhibited and uninhibited infants "grown up": Adult amygdalar response to novelty. *Science, 300*, 1952–1953.

Social Integration

▶ Social Support

Social Isolation

▶ Loneliness
▶ Loneliness and Health

Social Marketing

Sara Mijares St. George[1] and Dawn Wilson[2]
[1]Department of Public Health Sciences, University of Miami Miller School of Medicine, Miami, FL, USA
[2]Department of Psychology, University of South Carolina, Columbia, SC, USA

Synonyms

Cause marketing; Noncommercial advertising; Public interest advertising; Public service advertising

Definition

Social marketing is the application of marketing principles to non-tangible "products," including ideas, attitudes, and lifestyle changes. Unlike traditional marketing, the primary goal of social marketing is to improve public health, not to increase the marketer's profitability (Lefebvre and Flora 1988). Specifically, it is a planning and intervention model that targets audiences with marketing technologies to improve health and quality of life (Andreasen 1995). There are five principles addressed in the "marketing mix" of social marketing, known as the "5 Ps:" product, price, place, promotion, and positioning. "Product" is the target behavior (e.g., breastfeeding, healthy eating). "Price" refers to the social, economic, and psychological costs involved in adopting the target behavior. "Place" is the setting, community context, or distribution channels for the product. "Promotion" includes the steps taken to make the audience aware of the ideas, behaviors, and their benefits and may also involve interpersonal communication, media messages, grassroots approaches, special events, and incentives. Lastly, "positioning" describes how the product is framed, namely, to maximize perceived benefits and minimize perceived costs.

Social marketing campaigns using mass media strategies have been effective in promoting positive health behavior outcomes. For example, the Stanford Five-City Project for Heart Disease Prevention, (Farquhar et al. 1985, 1990) which targeted specific audiences, developed a product (i.e., a 6-week quitting contest), and involved local television stations, resulted in a 30% increase in smoking cessation. Similarly, the VERB Campaign (Huhman et al. 2005; Wong et al. 2004) utilized mass media techniques such as advertising on television, on billboards, through a website, and through school- and community-based promotions to increase physical activity in ethnically diverse youth and their parents. While both of the aforementioned social marketing campaigns involved mass media strategies to promote their "products," social marketing campaigns that use interpersonal channels and target the social context may maximize success in promoting health behavior change.

Indeed, effective and sustainable social marketing campaigns are driven largely by social factors (e.g., social norms, social support) and involve the target population in the social marketing processes to increase the integration of the program into established community structures (Bryant et al. 2000). For example, Wilson et al. (2010) used a collaborative community process to develop a social marketing campaign which motivated citizens in a low-income, high-crime community to use a walking path. With the assistance of a communications firm, a community steering committee guided the development of the overall social marketing objectives and approach. One of five key objectives, including increasing perceptions of safety and social connectedness, was targeted each month using corresponding print materials (e.g., a 12-month calendar, matching door hangers). Through grassroots social networking, the program engaged residents to participate in walks with peers, allowing them to feel safe and connected to their neighbors. This study is an example of how involving constituents in the process of social marketing ensures that the approach is tailored and truly fits the needs of the target audience. Furthermore, social marketing campaigns that strategically provide opportunities for interactions between neighbors, friends, and families may influence social norms and support around a particular health behavior and foster a social climate of behavior change.

Cross-References

▶ Health Behaviors
▶ Health Communication
▶ Social Support

References and Readings

Andreasen, A. (1995). *Marketing social change: Changing behavior to promote health, social development, and the environment*. San Francisco: Jossey-Bass.

Bryant, C., Forthofer, M., Landis, D., & McDermott, R. (2000). Community-based prevention marketing: The next steps in disseminating behavior change. *American Journal of Health Behavior, 24*, 61–68.

Farquhar, J., Fortmann, S., MacCoby, N., Haskell, W., Williams, P., Flora, J., et al. (1985). The Stanford five-city project: Design and methods. *American Journal of Epidemiology, 122*(2), 323.

Farquhar, J., Fortmann, S., Flora, J., Taylor, C., Haskell, W., Williams, P., et al. (1990). Effects of communitywide education on cardiovascular disease risk factors: The Stanford five-city project. *Journal of the American Medical Association, 264*(3), 359.

Huhman, M., Potter, L., Wong, F., Banspach, S., Duke, J., & Heitzler, C. (2005). Effects of a mass media campaign to increase physical activity among children: Year-1 results of the VERB campaign. *Pediatrics, 116*(2), e277.

Lefebvre, C., & Flora, J. (1988). Social marketing and public health intervention. *Health Education & Behavior, 15*(3), 299.

Wilson, D. K., Trumpeter, N. N., St. George, S. M., Coulon, S. M., Griffin, S., Van Horn, M. L., et al. (2010). An overview of the "positive action for today's health" (PATH) trial for increasing walking in low income, ethnic minority communities. *Contemporary Clinical Trials, 31*, 624–633.

Wong, F., Huhman, M., Asbury, L., Bretthauer-Mueller, R., McCarthy, S., Londe, P., et al. (2004). VERB™-a social marketing campaign to increase physical activity among youth. *Preventing Chronic Disease, 1*(3), 1–7.

Social Media

▶ Social Networking Sites

Social Network

▶ Family Social Support
▶ Family, Relationships
▶ Social Support

Social Networking Sites

Carly M. Goldstein[1,2] and Anna Luke[3]
[1]The Weight Control and Diabetes Research Center, The Miriam Hospital, Providence, RI, USA
[2]Warren Alpert Medical School, Brown University, Providence, RI, USA
[3]Department of Psychology, Kent State University, Kent, OH, USA

Synonyms

Digital media; Social media; Virtual communities

Definition

Social networking sites, sometimes characterized under the umbrella term social media, are virtual communities or networks that allow individuals, communities, and organizations to create and disseminate user-generated content including but not limited to pictures, videos, text, memes, and profile pages for individuals or groups; social media content has greater virality than other web-based content. By connecting a user's profile (maintained by the social media organization) to other individuals or groups, social networks are formed. Well-known social media sites include Facebook, Myspace, Twitter, Instagram, and Snapchat. When social networking sites were first popularized, the average users were emerging adults, but now users represent a wide range of ages, races, and places of residence.

Description

Social media encompasses all online platforms on which media content is uploaded, and social networking sites are online, dynamic, interaction-based communities where online relationships can be created or maintained. These terms are often used interchangeably and are inherently related.

Social networking sites have undergone rapid and dramatic development since their creation. Emailing, with its ability to connect with others electronically and its inclusion of individualized "profiles" (i.e., email addresses), is considered to be one of the preliminary social network modalities. In the late 1990s, instant communication platforms were developed, such as instant messaging (e.g., AOL Instant Messenger), chat rooms, and online blog communities (e.g., Live Journal). Myspace, LinkedIn, and Facebook, all social networking sites, followed in the early 2000s; they allowed individual users and collective groups to create personalized page profiles from which they could "friend" one another, which adds the other user to the original user's social network. Users could publicly signify their identity and affiliations (e.g., schools, profession) and choose to connect with preexisting acquaintances or reach out to new ones. Although Facebook remains the most popular social networking site to date (Dagan and Beskin 2015), social networking sites that allow users to

Associate Editor responsible for this entry: Dr. Ellen Beckjord comment on shared photographs and videos, such as Instagram and Snapchat, have grown in popularity. Online dating sites are popular, specialized, social networking sites. Most sites allow users to geo-tag posts to indicate their location; content can be aggregated by location.

Social networking sites are used by individuals across the life span, although the most prevalent users are young adults and adolescents (Pagoto et al. 2016), with 92% of teenagers reporting daily Internet access and 71% report using more than one social networking site (Pew Research Center 2015a). Widespread smartphone/tablet ownership has facilitated increased social networking site use from mobile phones: nearly two-thirds of American adults own smartphones, of which approximately 75% reported accessing social networking sites on their phones at least once in the last week (Pew Research Center 2015b).

Although many social networking sites were originally designed to connect with acquaintances, their size, speed, and accessibility have made them increasingly utilized platforms for consumers and corporations to disseminate information, communicate, and coordinate social action (Pagoto et al. 2016). Businesses and researchers have also turned to these sites to advertise products or memberships, collect data on users, and engage with a large sample of diverse consumers and patients. Additionally, Twitter users are more likely to elect sharing their information publicly, making Twitter an innovative and convenient data collection tool (Turner-McGrievy and Beets 2015). Users can also highlight important words or phrases by preceding them with a hashtag (#), a microblogging convention that allows users to see others' messages related to that topic; if many people tweet a common hashtag, such as related to a news sensation or popular artist, the hashtag is prominently featured as "trending" on the site (Gruzd and Haythornthwaite 2013). This potential for virality is a core defining characteristic that differentiates social media content from other Internet content.

Peer-to-peer health care, the use of social networking sites to engage with other patients and health care professionals, is a subtype of electronic health (eHealth) that has become an increasingly popular strategy for individuals to obtain and share information about health conditions and provide social support (Balatsoukas and Kennedy 2015; Pagoto et al. 2016). Beyond benefit to the individual, researchers and community health workers are harnessing the potential power of these sites to deliver prevention messages and intervention to improve health and outcomes through behavior change (Balatsoukas and Kennedy 2015). Social networking-based interventions can reduce barriers of traditional treatment (e.g., scheduling, transportation, social obligations; Pagoto et al. 2016). Messages exchanged between people in a social network may be more influential than messages delivered by an unknown outsider (Maher et al. 2014). These messages may also produce higher patient engagement and retention in interventions (Maher et al. 2014). Social networking sites have been effective in trials targeting smoking, sedentary behavior, weight loss, sedentary behavior, physical activity, and dietary awareness (Cheung et al. 2015; Maher et al. 2014).

Despite numerous advantages, there are many limitations for using social networking sites for research and intervention. While they are capable of quickly spreading useful, correct information, they are equally effective in facilitating the spread of misinformation. This is best illustrated in discussions of childhood vaccinations on social media sites, in which less than 25% of discussants were aware that the majority of evidence supports the safety and efficacy of vaccines (Seymour et al. 2015). Additionally, most health-related studies utilizing social networking sites have not isolated the effects of specific components, and extraneous variables may have influenced the results. Finally, numerous effective in-person interventions are challenging to modify for social networking-based delivery (Pagoto et al. 2016). Modifications may be needed to reach or surpass the success of in-person interventions. Controlled trials with foci on translation of delivery and patient engagement are necessary.

Social networking-based interventions may have massive impacts on health outcomes, but the current evidence is based primarily on qualitative data. Growing evidence with rigorous methodology suggests that virtual communities represent one of the biggest opportunities for research and behavior change of this generation (Eysenbach et al. 2004). Smartphone ownership continues to rise among racial and ethnic minority groups (Pew Research Center 2015c), making social networking-based interventions an exciting opportunity to deliver high-quality behavioral interventions to individuals who are both typically underrepresented in research and often disproportionately affected by chronic health conditions. Research has indicated that the larger a group, the more contagious an idea becomes, highlighting social networking sites as a promising platform to impact healthy behavior changes (Luhmann and Rajaram 2015).

Cross-References

▶ eHealth
▶ Social Marketing

References and Further Readings

Balatsoukas, P., & Kennedy, C. M. (2015). The role of social network technologies in online health promotion: A narrative review of theoretical and empirical factors influencing intervention effectiveness. *Journal of Medical Internet Research, 17*(6), e141. https://doi.org/10.2196/jmir.3662.

Cheung, Y. T. D., Chan, C. H. H., Lai, C. K. J., Chan, W. F. V., Wang, M. P., Li, H. C. W., Chan, S. S. C., & Lam, T. H. (2015). Using whatsapp and facebook online social groups for smoking relapse prevention for recent quitters: A pilot pragmatic cluster randomized controlled trial. *Journal of Medical Internet Research, 17*(10), e238. https://doi.org/10.2196/jmir.4829.

Dagan, N., & Beskin, D. (2015). Effects of social network exposure on nutritional learning: Development of an online educational platform. *JMIR Serious Games, 3*(2), e7. https://doi.org/10.2196/games.4002.

Eysenbach, G., Powell, J., Englesakis, M., Rizo, C., & Stern, A. (2004). Health related virtual communities and electronic support groups: Systematic review of the effects of online peer to peer interactions. *British Medical Journal, 328*(7449), 1–6.

Gruzd, A., & Haythornthwaite, C. (2013). Enabling community through social media. *Journal of Medical Internet Research, 15*(10), e248. https://doi.org/10.2196/jmir.2796.

Luhmann, C. C., & Rajaram, S. (2015). Memory transmission in small groups and large networks: An agent-based model. *Psychological Science, 26*(12), 1909–1917. https://doi.org/10.1177/0956797615605798.

Maher, C. A., Lewis, L. K., Ferrar, K., Marshall, S., De Bourdeaudhuij, I., & Vandelanotte, C. (2014). Are health behavior change interventions that use online social networks effective? A systematic review. *Journal of Medical Internet Research, 16*(2), e40. https://doi.org/10.2196/jmir.2952.

Pagoto, S., Waring, M. E., May, C. N., Ding, E. Y., Kunz, W. H., Hayes, R., & Oleski, J. L. (2016). Adapting behavioral interventions for social media delivery. *Journal of Medical Internet Research, 18*(1), e24. https://doi.org/10.2196/jmir.5086.

Pew Research Center. (2015a). *Teens, social media and technology overview 2015*. Retrieved from http://www.pewinternet.org/2015/04/09/teens-social-media-.technology-2015/

Pew Research Center. (2015b). *The smartphone difference*. Retrieved from http://www.pewinternet.org/2015/04/01/us-smartphone-use-in-2015/

Pew Research Center. (2015c). *Technology device ownership: 2015*. Retrieved from http://www.pewinternet.org/2015/10/29/technology-device-ownership-2015/

Seymour, B., Getman, R., Saraf, A., Zhang, L. H., & Kalenderian, E. (2015). When advocacy obscures accuracy online: Digital pandemics of public health misinformation through an antifluoride case study. *American Journal of Public Health, 105*(3), 517–523. https://doi.org/10.2105/ajph.2014.302437.

Turner-McGrievy, G. M., & Beets, M. W. (2015). Tweet for health: Using an online social network to examine temporal trends in weight loss-related posts. *Translational Behavioral Medicine, 5*(2), 160–166. https://doi.org/10.1007/s13142-015-0308-1.

Social Networks

▶ Social Relationships

Social Norms

▶ Norms

Social Pain

▶ Loneliness

Social Problem-Solving Therapy (SPST)

▶ Problem Solving

Social Processes

▶ Interpersonal Processes

Social Relationships

Kristin J. August[1] and Karen S. Rook[2]
[1]Department of Psychology, Rutgers University, Camden, NJ, USA
[2]Department of Psychology and Social Behavior, University of California Irvine, Irvine, CA, USA

Synonyms

Interpersonal relationships; Social networks; Social ties

Definition

Broadly defined, social relationships refer to the connections that exist between people who have recurring interactions that are perceived by the participants to have personal meaning. This definition includes relationships between family members, friends, neighbors, coworkers, and other associates but excludes social contacts and interactions that are fleeting, incidental, or perceived to have limited significance (e.g., time-limited interactions with service providers or retail employees). Scientists interested in behavioral medicine often emphasize the informal social relationships that are important in a person's life, or the person's social network, rather than formal relationships, such as those with physicians, lawyers, or clergy. Relationship phenomena of interest to scientists encompass both the specific interactions that individuals experience with members of their social networks and the global perceptions of those interactions, which are shaped by past and current interactions with important social network members. The interactions that occur with social network members are often positive, and include the provision of emotional and material support, companionship, and encouragement of health-enhancing behaviors. Interactions with social network members also can be negative, however, and can include insensitive, unresponsive, hurtful, or intrusive actions by others.

Description

A large body of evidence suggests that social relationships are associated with health. Research has linked social relationships to mortality and morbidity (Berkman et al. 2000; Cohen 2004; House et al. 1988a). People with fewer social network ties have been found to have an elevated risk for a number of diseases, including cardiovascular disease and stroke, some forms of cancer, infectious disease, and possibly dementia (Cohen 2004; Uchino 2006). Social relationships also have been linked to the onset and progression of chronic illness, as well as illness adjustment, postsurgical recovery, disability, and survival (e.g., Seeman and Crimmins 2001). Increased confidence in the associations between social relationships and health stems from the fact that the associations emerge not only in large, well-controlled cross-sectional and longitudinal epidemiological studies, but also in experimental studies of humans and animals. Moreover, the strength of these associations is impressive, as evidenced by research suggesting that the effects of social relationships on health are comparable in size to the effects of conventional risk factors, such as smoking (House et al. 1988).

Structural Versus Functional Aspects of Social Relationships

Both structural and functional aspects of social relationships have been distinguished (Berkman et al. 2000). Structural aspects refer to the existence and objective characteristics of social relationships, whereas functional aspects refer to the functions performed by and subjective qualities of social relationships (House et al. 1988b). Structural characteristics of interest to health researchers include the size of a person's social network, the frequency of contact with social network members, and the nature of the role relationships with network members (e.g., family member, friend, coworker). Research has demonstrated that some structural aspects of social relationships, such as social network size and frequency of contact, are related to health. For example, having more social ties and more frequent social interaction has been found to be associated with lower risks for mortality and poor mental and physical health outcomes. Similarly, the marital relationship has been found to be especially consequential for health, relative to other role relationships. Married individuals, compared to unmarried individuals, have a lower prevalence and incidence of both mental and physical health problems and a lower mortality risk (House et al. 1988). Furthermore, research suggests that men may derive more health benefits from marriage than do women. Poor quality marriages, however, and the disruption associated with divorce or widowhood appear to be particularly deleterious to mental and physical health (Burman and Margolin 1992).

Although numerous robust associations between structural aspects of social relationships and health have been documented, functional aspects also need to be examined in order to understand how and why social relationships impact health. The most commonly studied social network function that contributes to health is social support. A great deal of evidence suggests that social support can help to buffer people from the adverse effects of life stress (Cohen 2004; Uchino et al. 1996). Different types of social support have been distinguished (emotional, instrumental, informational), all of which are conceptualized as ways that social network members provide each other with care and aid in times of need. Different types of support are viewed as being important in the context of different stressors, although evidence suggests that emotional support is important across a very broad range of stressors (Cohen and Wills 1985).

Beyond social support, social relationships also serve as sources of companionship, which provides opportunities for enjoyable interaction and camaraderie. The positive affect and relief from stress afforded by companionship, in turn, help to sustain health and well-being (Rook 1987). Social network members also monitor each other's health behavior and intervene to discourage health-compromising behavior, leading researchers to be interested in the health effects of social regulation (or social control; Umberson 1987).

The beneficial functions of social relationships also have been posited to have negative counterparts (Rook 1998). Specifically, social relationships not only can provide support, companionship, and social regulation, but also can fail to provide support or can provide misguided support, can reject or neglect others, and can foster bad, rather than good, health practices. Even though such negative interactions with others are relatively rare, they can take a considerable toll on health and well-being (Rook 1998).

Pathways by Which Social Relationships Influence Health

Understanding the pathways by which social relationships influence health is a key goal for health researchers. Three main pathways have been identified (Berkman et al. 2000; Rook et al. 2010): The first pathway involves psychological processes and conditions associated with social relationships, such as positive and negative emotions, feelings of self-worth and self-efficacy, coping strategies, and depression. The second pathway involves physiological processes, or activation of bodily systems (endocrine, cardiovascular, and immune) in response to various kinds of social interactions. The third pathway involves health behaviors that are fostered by interactions with social network members, including health-enhancing behaviors (e.g., exercise) as well as health-compromising behaviors (e.g., smoking). All three of these pathways have the potential to have independent and joint effects on morbidity and, ultimately, mortality.

Pathways having beneficial health effects. Social support, companionship, and social regulation are believed to affect health through unique mechanisms. Social support is thought to dampen the emotional, physiological (neuroendocrine, cardiovascular, immune), and behavioral effects of stress by improving one's perceived ability to cope with stress (Uchino 2006; Uchino et al. 1996). Companionship, on the other hand, is thought to influence health and well-being by enhancing positive affect and providing a respite from stress (Rook 1987). Positive affect, in turn, has been linked to lower rates of morbidity, fewer symptoms and less pain from health conditions, and greater longevity (Pressman and Cohen 2005). Companionship also may activate physiological processes, such as the release of oxytocin, a neuropeptide that helps to counter harmful stress responses, including release of the stress hormone, cortisol. Social control is believed to affect health through two primary, but opposing, processes (Hughes and Gove 1981). Specifically, social control may discourage health-compromising behaviors and encourage health-enhancing behaviors, thereby contributing to better health and ultimately, a lower risk of mortality. Yet, at the same time, to the extent that social control involves constraints on others' behavior, it may provoke psychological distress, erode feelings of self-efficacy, and kindle relationship tensions. The psychological and relationship costs of social control may thus reduce or cancel the health benefits of social control, although the net effects of social control on health are not yet fully understood (Rook et al. 2010).

Pathways having detrimental health effects. Persistent conflict in social relationships, as well as the absence or loss of social relationships, also impact health through a number of mechanisms. Specifically, recurring strains and conflicts in social relationships lead to repeated activation of physiological systems (e.g., hypothalamic-pituitary-adrenal axis or sympathetic nervous system activity) and impaired immune functioning. These chronically activated and dysregulated physiological systems, in turn, may accelerate disease onset and progression. Additionally, social isolation and loneliness have been linked to negative emotions, chronic stress, cardiovascular activation, low physical activity, and impaired sleep (Cacioppo et al. 2002). Finally, it is important to recognize that social network members sometimes encourage undesirable, rather than desirable, health practices. For example, evidence suggests that adolescents sometimes recruit their peers to use illegal substances or to engage in other risky health behaviors. Thus, conflict and tensions in social relationships, social isolation and loneliness, and undesirable social influence all can increase the risk of disease onset and progression.

Conclusion

It is well established that social relationships are important for health and well-being, and research has identified key aspects of social relationships that warrant consideration in efforts to understand these links with health. The psychological, physiological, and behavioral pathways by which social relationships affect health also are beginning to be understood. As this literature evolves and expands to document patterns that exist across different sociodemographic and lifespan contexts, it may help to inform interventions designed to strengthen social relationships and, in turn, health.

Cross-References

▶ Family and Medical Leave Act
▶ Family Assistance
▶ Family Planning
▶ Family Stress
▶ Family Studies (Genetics)
▶ Family Systems Theory
▶ Family Violence
▶ Family, Caregiver
▶ Family, Income
▶ Family, Relationships
▶ Family, Structure
▶ Loneliness
▶ Psychosocial Characteristics
▶ Psychosocial Factors
▶ Social Capital and Health
▶ Social Cohesion

▶ Social Conflict
▶ Social Factors
▶ Social Stress
▶ Social Support

References and Readings

Berkman, L. F., Glass, T., Brissette, I., & Seeman, T. E. (2000). From social integration to health: Durkheim in the new millennium. *Social Science and Medicine, 51*, 843–857.

Burman, B., & Margolin, G. (1992). Analysis of the association between marital relationships and health problems: An interactional perspective. *Psychological Bulletin, 112*, 39–63.

Cacioppo, J. T., Hawkley, L. C., Crawford, L. E., Ernst, J. M., Burleson, M. H., Kowalewski, R. B., et al. (2002). Loneliness and health: Potential mechanisms. *Psychosomatic Medicine, 64*, 407–417.

Cohen, S. (2004). Social relationships and health. *American Psychologist, 59*, 676–684.

Cohen, S., & Wills, T. A. (1985). Stress, social support, and the buffering hypothesis. *Psychological Bulletin, 98*, 310–357.

House, J. S., Landis, K. R., & Umberson, D. (1988a). Social relationships and health. *Science, 241*, 540–545.

House, J. S., Umberson, D., & Landis, K. R. (1988b). Structures and processes of social support. *Annual Review of Sociology, 14*, 293–318.

Hughes, M., & Gove, W. R. (1981). Living alone, social integration, and mental health. *The American Journal of Sociology, 87*, 48–74.

Pressman, S. D., & Cohen, S. (2005). Does positive affect influence health? *Psychological Bulletin, 131*, 925–971.

Rook, K. S. (1987). Social support versus companionship: Effects on life stress, loneliness, and evaluations by others. *Journal of Personality and Social Psychology, 52*, 1132–1147.

Rook, K. S. (1998). Investigating the positive and negative sides of personal relationships: Through a lens darkly? In B. H. Spitzberg & W. R. Cupach (Eds.), *The dark side of close relationships* (pp. 369–393). Mahwah: Lawrence Erlbaum.

Rook, K. S., August, K. J., & Sorkin, D. H. (2010). Social network functions and health. In R. J. Contrada & A. Baum (Eds.), *The handbook of stress science: Biology, psychology, and health* (pp. 123–136). New York: Springer.

Seeman, T. E., & Crimmins, E. (2001). Social environment effects on health and aging. Integrating epidemiologic and demographic approaches and perspectives. *Annals of the New York Academy of Sciences, 954*, 88–117.

Uchino, B. N. (2006). Social support and health: A review of physiological processes potentially underlying links to disease outcomes. *Journal of Behavioral Medicine, 29*, 377–387.

Uchino, B. N., Cacioppo, J. T., & Kiecolt-Glaser, J. K. (1996). The relationship between social support and physiological processes: A review with emphasis on underlying mechanisms and implications for health. *Psychological Bulletin, 119*, 488–531.

Umberson, D. (1987). Family status and health behaviors: Social control as a dimension of social integration. *Journal of Health and Social Behavior, 28*, 306–319.

Social Resources

▶ Family Social Support
▶ Social Support

Social Stress

Vanessa Juth[1] and Sally Dickerson[2]
[1]Nursing Science, University of California Irvine, Irvine, CA, USA
[2]Pace University, New York, NY, USA

Synonyms

Interpersonal stress or conflict; Societal stress

Definition and Description

Social stress can be broadly defined as a perceived threat that is based on one's relation to or association with another person or group of people. There is great variability in the types of social stress that one may experience. It can arise from interpersonal interactions, such as those with family members, friends, professional colleagues, and strangers; from evaluated performances, including giving a speech in front of an audience; from sharing an experience with someone, such as patients and caregivers dealing with a chronic illness; or from group, community, or societal dynamics, for instance, one's socioeconomic or professional status within a community or society.

Different types of social stress can lead to a range of observable and measurable responses. For instance, socially evaluated performances may lead to negative emotions and self-conscious thoughts. Severe interpersonal social stress, for example, verbal abuse between spouses, may lead to psychological distress (e.g., post-traumatic distress). Workplace social stress can have physiological impacts, including cardiovascular, endocrinological, immunological, and other system responses. Social discrimination, for instance, being treated unfairly or differently due to one's personal characteristics (e.g., gender, race, physical attributes, sexual orientation), can also be linked with negative physiological responses and with risky health behaviors (e.g., substance use, binge eating).

In order to overcome or deal with social stress, people engage in a variety of coping responses. These include active and passive coping strategies in which the individual either engages with or withdraws from the source of the social stress. Active coping strategies include problem-solving strategies (e.g., changing public policy steps to better provide healthcare services for underserved minority groups) and emotion-focused strategies (e.g., verbally communicating one's concerns with a friend about their drug use). Passive coping strategies include avoidant strategies (e.g., ignoring a rude co-worker) and distraction strategies (e.g., taking up exercise to overcome loss of a relationship).

Social stress and its associated responses, as well as the coping strategies used to manage them, can have serious health effects. For instance, acute (e.g., sudden job loss), frequent (e.g., repetitive marital strife), and chronic (e.g., bereavement) social stressors can compromise physiological functioning as well as self-reported physical and mental health conditions. Social stressors can also have long-lasting effects, such that social stress experienced early on in life (e.g., childhood) influences endocrine system responses (e.g., cortisol) to stress in adulthood. Furthermore, social status within a group, community, or society at large (e.g., socioeconomic status) can increase the risk for negative health outcomes and/or behaviors across the lifespan.

Cross-References

▶ Biobehavioral Mechanisms
▶ Psychosocial Factors
▶ Social Conflict
▶ Social Relationships
▶ Social Support
▶ Stress Reactivity

References and Further Reading

Dickerson, S. S., & Kemeny, M. E. (2004). Acute stressors and cortisol responses: A theoretical integration and synthesis of laboratory research. *Psychological Bulletin, 130*, 355–391.

Juth, V., Silver, R. C., & Sender, L. (2015a). The shared experience of adolescent and young adult cancer patients and their caregivers. *Psycho-Oncology, 24*, 1746–1753.

Juth, V., Smyth, J. M., Carey, M., & Lepore, S. (2015b). Social constraints are associated with negative psychological and physical adjustment in bereavement. *Applied Psychology: Health and Well-Being, 7*, 129–148.

Miller, G., Chen, E., & Cole, S. W. (2009). Health psychology: Developing biologically plausible models linking the social world and physical health. *Annual Review of Psychology, 60*, 501–524.

Social Support

John Ruiz[1], Courtney C. Prather[2] and Erin E. Kauffman[2]
[1]Department of Psychology, University of Arizona, Tuscon, AZ, USA
[2]Department of Psychology, University of North Texas, Denton, TX, USA

Synonyms

Moderators/moderating factors; Social integration; Social network; Social resources

Definition

Social support refers to the belief that one is valued, cared for, and loved by others in a social network. Social support can generally be conceptualized as reflecting two broad factors (Cohen and Syme 1985; Cohen and Wills 1985). Structural support reflects properties of the social network and the degree to which a person participates in that network (i.e., social integration). Functional support refers to the ways by which network members aid the individual through tangible assistance or through psychological and emotional buffering. Social support is among the most widely studied and robust psychosocial moderators of health. This entry will expand upon this description, review evidence linking it to health, examine hypothesized mechanisms, and discuss future directions.

Description

Social support is a multicomponent construct reflecting the size, quality, and availability of one's social resources to moderate stress. Social support should be distinguished from conceptually related terms. *Social capital* is a sociological term referring to stock or stored social credit. *Social network* refers to the social collectives or groups to which a person may belong. *Social integration* refers to the degree to which a person is embedded in or a part of a social network. *Relationship* is a descriptor often used to characterize a specific type of social tie.

Social support is generally conceptualized as having structural (i.e., size of the social network, degree of social integration) and functional (i.e., support processes; support received versus support perceived) characteristics. In addition, the quality of support is increasingly recognized as an important moderator of the relationship between support and health. Importantly, relationships are not uniformly positive, with some acting as sources of stress (Uchino 2004).

Measures

Social support is generally measured by self-report. Data sources may include demographic data from hospital, census, or other records; interviews; psychometrically validated instruments; and ad hoc items and measures.

Structural Measures of Support

The simplest of the social integration measures is marital status which is consistently identified as a protective factor in large, prospective studies of mortality. Marital status is a particularly attractive measure as it is a common demographic characteristic and, thus, available for analysis with many kinds of health data. Many researchers are also interested in measuring the size of one's social networks and the degree to which a person is embedded in the networks. One well-validated multicomponent measure of social integration is the Social Network Index (SNI: Berkman and Syme 1979) which provides an aggregate score of social integration by sampling activity in multiple relationships. Lower SNI scores are predictive of a nearly two fold increase in mortality risk. Finally, the literature is replete with numerous ad hoc structural support measures including measures of number of networks, network size, as well as the number of specific kinds of relationships such as friendships, and others.

Functional Measures of Support

Functional measures can be classified into support received and support perceived. Interestingly, measures of received and perceived support tend not to be highly correlated. Measures of received supportive behavior allow assessment of the actual social resources available to an individual. For example, the Inventory of Socially Supportive Behaviors (ISSB: Barrera et al. 1981) is a 40-item structural support measure assessing the frequency with which one receives a variety of supportive actions. Measures of perceived social support assess an individual's beliefs about the social resources available to them. Perceived support measures generally consist of two factors:

beliefs about support available, and satisfaction with level of perceived support. A widely used example of a perceived support measure is Cohen and Wills (1985) Interpersonal Support Evaluation List (ISEL) which assesses perceptions of belonging, tangible support, support appraisals, and confidence in support perceptions.

Quality of Support

Relationship quality has generally been assessed along a single dimension ranging from positive to negative. However, emerging models hypothesize that relationships can have both positive and negative characteristics. The Quality of Relationship Inventory (QRI: Pierce, Baldwin, and Lydon, 1997) is among the most popular multidimensional measures. The 25-item, self-report measure yields discrete support and conflict scales as well as a total quality rating. Several authors have suggested that the relationship quality dimensions of positivity and negativity are orthogonal, yielding four basic relationship types: (1) high positive, low negative (i.e., supportive relationship), (2) low positive, high negative (i.e., conflictual relationship), (3) high positive, high negative (i.e., ambivalent relationship), and (4) low positive, low negative (i.e., benign/irrelevant relationship). The Social Relationships Index (SRI: Uchino 2004) is an example of this multidimensional relationship quality assessment approach. Although health outcome data is limited, this conceptualization appears to be gaining acceptance as a more theoretically sound approach.

Social Support and Health

Social support is among the most robust predictors of disease and all-cause mortality. For example, a recent meta-analysis of 148 studies estimated the effect of social relationships to improve survival rates by 50% (Holt-Lunstad et al. 2010). This effect varied by measurement, with multidimensional measures of social integration associated with more than 90% increase in survival rates. As noted by the authors, the magnitude of the effect of social support on mortality is likely diluted in these studies by unmeasured negative aspects of social relationships (e.g., a conflictual marriage). The results of this meta-analysis extend the work of previous systematic reviews and meta-analyses in identifying that social support is a substantial health and disease moderator with effects equivalent to more traditionally acknowledged risk factors such as cigarette smoking and obesity.

Cardiovascular Disease

The strongest evidence for a protective role of social support on health comes from studies of cardiovascular diseases such as coronary heart disease (CHD) morbidity and mortality (Smith and Ruiz 2002). Multiple prospective studies of initially healthy samples have demonstrated that lower social integration and social support are associated with greater CHD incidence, faster disease progression, risk of myocardial infarction (MI), and greater risk for all-cause mortality. Among persons with diagnosed CHD, lower social support is predictive of significantly greater risk of recurrent MI and death. For example, Welin et al. (2000) found an almost three-fold increased chance of cardiac mortality in post-MI patients with low perceived emotional support at 10-year follow-up. A similar effect size was found by Berkman et al. (1992). Some studies indicate that low social integration is only associated with survival in the most severely isolated of the population. In a review of the literature, Mookadam and Arthur (2004) estimated a two to three times increased risk of 1-year mortality in the socially isolated population, with little health benefits resulting from support systems above this threshold. Moreover, there is some evidence that the beneficial effects of social support on cardiac health are stronger among women and that functional measures of support are more strongly related to cardiac disease compared to structural measures.

Effect sizes for social integration in healthy samples for future development of CHD are comparable to those of more traditional risk factors such as cigarette smoking (Orth-Gomer et al. 1993). Similarly, social integration is as strong a predictor of mortality among clinical populations as traditional risk factors such as cholesterol level, tobacco use, and hypertension in the patient population (Mookadam and Arthur 2004). An important conceptual issue is whether high social support connotes a cardiovascular benefit akin to physical activity or whether it is simply the absence of support that is relevant. In addition, the relative value of structural versus functional support remains an open question. Regardless, the cumulative evidence indicates social support is an important moderator of cardiovascular risk.

Cancer

The relationship between social support and cancer is quite mixed. A recent systematic review of the prospective longitudinal literature concluded that in the context of breast cancer, greater social support was associated with slower disease progression in five of seven well-designed studies. Structural indices were the more commonly used and significant measure of social support in these studies. In contrast, there were no associations between measures of social support and other types of cancer with the paradoxical exception of more social support related to faster cancer progression in a sample of colorectal patients (Villingshoj et al. 2006). A meta-analysis of 87 studies estimated the relative risk of perceived social support and measures of social network size on mortality among cancer patients to be .82 and .80, respectively, suggesting a beneficial effect (Pinquart and Duberstein 2010). Inconsistencies between studies may be partially explained by differences in support types measured and patient needs. The type of support associated with improved prognosis appears to vary by cancer site, with perceived social support representing a stronger predictor for leukemia and lymphoma, whereas breast cancer patients benefit more from have a large number of social ties (Pinquart and Duberstein 2010).

In contrast to the mixed findings regarding physical outcomes, a robust literature supports the beneficial effects of social support on emotional and psychological reactions to cancer and associated treatments. Moreover, cancer is often a shared interpersonal experience – affecting supports as well as patients. A meta-analysis of these *contagion effects* estimated the correlation between patient and caregiver distress is .35 (Hodges et al. 2005). Importantly, partner response to illness affects patient adjustment, particularly in terms of quality of life. The type of coping employed (e.g., positive versus negative), relationship maintenance behaviors, and the amount of communication about the relationship may also be important moderators of couples adjustment.

With respect to interventions, efforts have largely focused on increasing the patient's social network size and opportunity for emotional support. Perhaps the most well known of these interventions was conducted by Spiegel et al. (1989). Women with late-stage metastatic breast cancer were randomized to either supportive group therapy or wait-list control. Findings that women in the treatment condition survived approximately 18 months longer generated interest in the possible healing role of support. Several clinical and prospective trials have failed to replicate these results, fueling doubts about the potential physical benefits of the approach. Regardless, there is substantial effort to translate socially based interventions from bench to bedside where their emotional and quality of life benefits are well recognized.

HIV/AIDS

Conclusions regarding the benefits of social support on physical outcomes in the context of HIV/AIDS are limited by the small number of published studies. A prospective study of HIV-positive men with hemophilia demonstrated that lower levels of perceived support at baseline were predictive of faster decreases in CD4 T-lymphocyte levels, a key marker of AIDS status, over a 4-year follow-up (Theorell et al. 1995). Leserman and colleagues conducted a study of 82 asymptomatic gay men, in which greater satisfaction with social support was associated with slower progression to AIDS, regardless of network size (Leserman et al. 1999). In contrast, other studies have found perceived support to be unrelated to progression to AIDS. More research is needed to adequately evaluate these relationships.

The social environment of the HIV/AIDS population may be uniquely important because of the social stigma associated with the diagnosis (Herek and Glunt 1988). Stigma is associated with both personal distress and hesitancy to self-disclose status to sexual partners, potentiating further transmission of the infection either by the individual or the individual's un-informed sexual partners. A meta-analysis of 21 studies showed that greater perceived social support was associated with increased likelihood of self-disclosing one's HIV-positive status (Smith et al. 2008). Disclosure of HIV status is associated with increased social support within those relationships, indicating that disclosure may be a positive method of eliciting support from others.

Mechanisms

Social support is hypothesized to affect health and well-being through two pathways. The *main effects* hypothesis suggests that having more social resources reduces the chances of exposure to stressful circumstances or the magnitude of threat associated with certain environments. For example, one is likely to be safer walking at night with a large group of friends than when walking alone. Numerous studies have shown that having more social resources (measured as the number of social ties, the degree of social integration, etc.) is predictive of lower disease incidence, better survival following illness, lower all-cause mortality, and greater longevity irrespective of the quality of those relationships. Interestingly, these social resources need not be human to have a beneficial effect. Several studies have demonstrated that having a loving pet is associated with less stress and better survival following disease incidents such as a heart attack.

Social support may also affect health by moderating or reducing the impact of stressful circumstances (i.e., *stress buffering hypothesis*). After a stressful romantic breakup, a friend may comfort you with a hug, by providing you with an opportunity to vent your emotions, or by introducing you to someone new. Substantial laboratory data demonstrates that provision of support reduces self-reported stress and acute physiological responses to lab stressors. For example, individuals who received a note communicating emotional support from a supportive friend experience less blood pressure increase during a subsequent speech task relative to those who receive a note from a less supportive person (Uno et al. 2002). Importantly, the perception of support appears to be more important than the actual provision of support. For example, imagining a supportive tie prior to a stressor results in less cardiovascular reactivity and less self-reported stress (i.e., buffering) compared to imagining an acquaintance (Smith et al. 2004). These findings support the idea that social support, received or perceived, can reduce stressful experiences.

Future Directions

Future research will continue to expand upon conceptual distinctions regarding sources of support and related actions. Longitudinal research is also needed to understand the biobehavioral mechanisms by which social support translates into disease risk. Further, more research is needed to determine whether it is better to have substantial support or simply to not be alone. Finally, emerging social phenomenon such as texting and online social networking through Facebook, Twitter, and other forums presents new challenges for researchers to conceptualize, measure, and gauge as moderators of health.

Cross-References

▶ Psychosocial Factors
▶ Psychosocial Predictors
▶ Psychosocial Variables
▶ Social Capital and Health
▶ Social Cohesion
▶ Social Conflict
▶ Social Factors
▶ Social Relationships

References and Further Readings

Barrera, M., Sandler, I. N., & Ramsay, T. B. (1981). Preliminary development of a scale of social support: Studies on college students. *American Journal of Community Psychology, 9*(4), 435–447.

Berkman, L. F., Leo-Summers, L., & Horwitz, R. I. (1992). Emotional support and survival after myocardial infarction. A prospective, population-based study of the elderly. *Annals of Internal Medicine, 117*(12), 1003–1009.

Berkman, L. F., & Syme, S. L. (1979). Social networks, host resistance, and mortality: A nine-year follow-up study of Alameda County residents. *American Journal of Epidemiology, 109*(2), 186–204.

Cohen, S., & Syme, S. L. (1985). Issues in the study and application of social support. In S. Cohen & S. L. Syme (Eds.), *Social Support and health* (pp. 3–22). San Francisco: Academic Press Inc..

Cohen, S., & Wills, T. A. (1985). Stress, social support, and the buffering hypothesis. *Psychological Bulletin, 98*(2), 310–357.

Herek, G. M., & Glunt, E. K. (1988). An epidemic of stigma: Public reactions to AIDS. *American Psychologist, 43*(11), 886–891.

Hodges, L. J., Humphris, G. M., & Macfarlane, G. (2005). A meta-analytic investigation of the relationship between the psychological distress of cancer patients and their carers. *Social Science & Medicine, 60*(1), 1–12. 1982.

Holt-Lunstad, J., Smith, T. B., & Layton, J. B. (2010). Social relationships and mortality risk: A meta-analytic review. *PLoS Medicine, 7*(7), e1000316–e1000316.

Leserman, J., Jackson, E. D., Petitto, J. M., Golden, R. N., Silva, S. G., Perkins, D. O., et al. (1999). Progression to AIDS: The effects of stress, depressive symptoms, and social support. *Psychosomatic Medicine, 61*(3), 397–406.

Mookadam, F., & Arthur, H. M. (2004). Social support and its relationship to morbidity and mortality after acute myocardial infarction: Systematic overview. *Archives of Internal Medicine, 164*(14), 1514–1518.

Orth-Gomer, K., Rosengren, A., & Wilhelmsen, L. (1993). Lack of social support and incidence of coronary heart disease in middle-aged Swedish men. *Psychosomatic Medicine, 55*, 37–43.

Pierce, T., Baldwin, M. W., & Lydon, J. E. (1997a). A relational schema approach to social support. In G. Pierce, S. Lakey, & B. R. Sarason (Eds.), *Sourcebook of social support and personality* (pp. 19–47). New York: Plenum Press.

Pierce, G. R., Sarason, I. G., Sarason, B. R., & Solky-Butzel, J. A. (1997b). Assessing the quality of personal relationships. *Journal of Social and Personal Relationships, 14*(3), 339–356.

Pinquart, M., & Duberstein, P. R. (2010). Associations of social networks with cancer mortality: A meta-analysis. *Critical Reviews in Oncology/Hematology, 75*(2), 122–137.

Smith, R., Rossetto, K., & Peterson, B. L. (2008). A meta-analysis of disclosure of one's HIV-positive status, stigma and social support. *AIDS Care, 20*(10), 1266–1275.

Smith, T. W., & Ruiz, J. M. (2002). Psychosocial influences on the development and course of coronary heart disease: Current status and implications for research and practice. *Journal of Consulting and Clinical Psychology, 70*(3), 548–568.

Smith, T. W., Ruiz, J. M., & Uchino, B. N. (2004). Mental activation of supportive ties, hostility, and cardiovascular reactivity to laboratory stress in young men and women. *Health Psychology, 23*(5), 476–485.

Spiegel, D., Bloom, J. R., Kraemer, H. C., & Gottheil, E. (1989). Effect of psychosocial treatment on survival of patients with metastatic breast cancer. *Lancet, 2*(8668), 888–891.

Theorell, T., Blomkvist, V., Jonsson, H., Schulman, S., Berntorp, E., & Stigendal, L. (1995). Social support and the development of immune function in human immunodeficiency virus infection. *Psychosomatic Medicine, 57*(1), 32–36.

Uchino, B. N. (2004). *Social support and physical health: Understanding the health consequences of relationships*. New Haven: Yale University Press.

Uno, D., Uchino, B. N., & Smith, T. W. (2002). Relationship quality moderates the effect of social support given by close friends on cardiovascular reactivity in women. *International Journal of Behavioral Medicine, 9*, 243–262.

Villingshoj, M., Ross, L., Thomsen, B. L., & Johansen, C. (2006). Does marital status and altered contact with the social network predict colorectal cancer survival? *European Journal of Cancer (Oxford, England: 1990), 42*(17), 3022–3027.

Welin, C., Lappas, G., & Wilhelmsen, L. (2000). Independent importance of psychosocial factors for prognosis after myocardial infarction. *Journal of Internal Medicine, 247*(6), 629–639.

Social Support at Work

▶ Job Satisfaction/Dissatisfaction

Social Ties

▶ Social Relationships

Societal Stress

▶ Social Stress

Society of Behavioral Medicine

Stephanie Ann Hooker
Department of Psychology, University of Colorado Denver, Denver, CO, USA

Synonyms

SBM

Definition

The Society of Behavioral Medicine (SBM) is a nonprofit organization founded in 1978. The organization strives to be multidisciplinary in nature, creating a dialogue between nursing, public health, psychological, and medical professionals to promote the study of interactions between behavior, biology, and the environment and to apply that knowledge to improve the health and well-being of individuals and communities. This is further illustrated through SBM's vision statement, which is "Better Health Through Behavior Change." In 2011, over 2000 behavioral and biomedical researchers and clinicians were members of SBM.

SBM hosts an annual meeting for its members and other behavioral medicine researchers and clinicians to share recent research findings and clinical strategies. SBM also sponsors two journals, *Annals of Behavioral Medicine* and *Translational Behavioral Medicine: Practice, Policy, and Research*.

References and Readings

Society of Behavioral Medicine. (2011). Society of Behavioral Medicine (SBM). Retrieved July 15, 2011, from http://www.sbm.org.

Sociocultural

Patricia Gonzalez[1] and Orit Birnbaum-Weitzman[2]
[1]Institute for Behavioral and Community Health (IBACH), Graduate School of Public Health, San Diego State University, San Diego, CA, USA
[2]Department of Psychology, University of Miami, Miami, FL, USA

Synonyms

Social circumstance; Sociocultural context; Sociocultural factors; Socioeconomic position; Socioeconomic status (SES)

Definition

"Sociocultural" refers to a wide array of societal and cultural influences that impact thoughts, feelings, behaviors, and ultimately health outcomes. Sociocultural determinants of health and illness encompass socioeconomic status (SES) factors (traditionally assessed by income, education, occupation) and cultural factors. There are several dimensions encompassed by the term, which can include race, ethnicity, ethnic identity, sex, acculturation, language, beliefs and value systems, attitudes, and religion.

Description

Sociocultural factors are salient determinants of health and have been found to be associated with a multitude of health outcomes including health behaviors (e.g., physical activity, diet, health screenings, and health-care utilization) and illness (e.g., cancer, diabetes, cardiovascular disease, and depression). Sociocultural factors are complex and may vary by sex, age, and racial/ethnic groups. In recent years, the term sociocultural has been extensively used in the literature in connection with physical and mental health outcomes.

Social and cultural factors play a central role in preventing illness, maintaining good health, and treating disease. Research has shown that an individual's social environment, family, neighborhood, school, and workplace have a significant impact on health. At the same time, cultural factors influence how physical and mental illness are viewed and diagnosed. A great advance in understanding the determinants of health and disease has been the identification of social and cultural factors influencing them. Social and cultural factors are pertinent not only to understanding individuals' health status but also recognizing the existing health disparities among different populations. In particular, a substantial body of research suggests that social factors stand at the root of health disparities (Marmot 2005).

Some of the most salient sociocultural factors studied in relation to health disparities, including morbidity and mortality, are SES and race/ethnicity. Levels of health within the USA vary dramatically among different social, economic, and racial/ethnic groups. Moreover, considerable research suggests that determinants of health often reflect economic disparities (Braveman et al. 2010). Higher income levels are linked with overall better health, including self-rated health, lower cardiovascular risk factors, and lower mortality (Braveman et al. 2011; Hajat et al. 2011). The incidence and prevalence of many diseases (e.g., cardiovascular disease, arthritis, diabetes, and cervical cancer) increases as SES decreases. In addition, SES differences in mortality have been observed for many causes of death including some cancers, diabetes, and cardiovascular disease. Similarly, individuals with higher SES have greater life expectancy rates than individuals with lower income levels (Braveman et al. 2011). In terms of health status, adults with lower incomes are more likely to report their health status as poor or fair compared with adults with higher incomes (Braveman et al. 2011).

Several explanations have been proposed to account for the association between socioeconomic standing and health. First, economic stability enables individuals to live in safer neighborhoods, access healthier food alternatives, have more leisure time for physical activity, and endure less stress. Second, income impacts access to high-quality health care such that lower SES individuals are less likely to be covered by health insurance and to receive high-quality health care (Braveman et al. 2011). Hence, the uninsured may have less access to preventive services (e.g., health screenings) and early diagnosis. Greater education is also linked with longer life expectancy. Individuals who have completed college have a greater life expectancy (at least 5 years longer) than individuals who have not completed high school (Braveman et al. 2011). Higher education levels are associated with greater knowledge regarding health and feelings of control (Braveman et al. 2011) over different domains of one's life. Therefore, education increases the likelihood that individuals will have the knowledge to prevent illness. As illustrated by these health patterns, SES disparities in health mirror a gradient pattern, with greater social and economic advantage being associated with better health.

Differences in health have also been observed based on race/ethnicity. For example, compared to non-Hispanic Whites, morbidity and mortality rates for cardiovascular disease (CVD) are higher among African-Americans (Payne et al. 2005). Compared to non-Hispanic Whites, African-Americans and Hispanics are more likely to have diabetes (Centers for Disease Control and Prevention 2011). Moreover, ethnic-minority and low-income groups have a disproportionate burden of death and disability as a result of cardiovascular disease. In addition, although significant progress has been made in reducing cancer mortality rates in the USA, decreases in cancer mortality rates in ethnic minorities have been slower compared to non-Hispanic Whites (American Cancer Society 2011).

Culture refers to the shared values, beliefs, and norms held in common by a defined group of people. Within each culture, there is a set of behaviors and values related to health and illness which may vary between different groups, causing differing viewpoints toward illness. Each culture has a set of norms for behavior with related beliefs, knowledge, and customs. Acculturation, a related cultural construct, is often used to explain ethnic disparities in health outcomes. Acculturation as a predictive variable is based on the premise that culturally based knowledge, attitudes, and beliefs influence people to behave in particular ways and to select specific health choices. For limited English proficiency (LEP) individuals, language barriers can contribute to health disparities. For example, LEP individuals may encounter difficulties communicating with medical professionals, understanding printed health information or accessing health-related services due to lack of information about available services (American College of Physicians 2010). Moreover, some individuals may fear jeopardizing their immigration status by using health services. Research also suggests that cultural norms within the USA or Western society contribute to lifestyles and behaviors associated with risk factors for diseases (e.g., cancer, diabetes, cardiovascular disease) (Thomas et al. 2004). Therefore, health behavior interventions must address the target group's belief systems as well as cultural values.

Although the US population is diverse, health policies and interventions are often based on Western cultural assumptions. Often, minimal attention is given to aspects of culture from the perspective of individuals from diverse ethnic or SES membership groups. It is key to acknowledge that social and cultural factors may explain related health behaviors and, in part, elucidate disparities between ethnic/racial and SES groups. More specifically, research findings examined from the perspective of sociocultural differences may provide more meaningful information and help develop innovative intervention strategies for ameliorating some of the disparities in health outcomes and access to health care.

Cross-References

▶ Health Disparities
▶ Socioeconomic Status (SES)

References and Readings

American Cancer Society. (2011). *Cancer facts & figures*. Atlanta: American Cancer Society.
American College of Physicians. (2010). *Racial and ethnic disparities in health care*. Philadelphia: American College of Physicians.
Braveman, P. A., Cubbin, C., Egerter, S., Williams, D. R., & Pamuk, E. (2010). Socioeconomic disparities in the United States: What the patterns tells us. *American Journal of Public Health, 100*, S186–S196.
Braveman, P. A., Egerter, S. A., & Mockenhaupt, R. E. (2011). Broadening the focus: The need to address the social determinants of health. *American Journal of Preventive Medicine, 40*, S4–S18.
Centers for Disease Control and Prevention. (2011). *National diabetes fact sheet: National estimates and general information on diabetes and prediabetes in the United States, 2011*. Atlanta: U.S. Department of Health and Human Services, Centers for Disease Control and Prevention.
Hajat, A., Kaufman, J. S., Rose, K. M., Siddiqi, A., & Thomas, J. C. (2011). Long-term effects of wealth on mortality and self-rated health status. *American Journal of Epidemiology, 173*, 192–200.
Marmot, M. (2005). Social determinants of health inequalities. *The Lancet, 365*, 1099–1104.
Payne, T. J., Wyatt, S. B., Mosley, T. H., Dubbert, P. M., Guiterrez-Mohammed, M. L., Calvin, R. L., et al. (2005). Sociocultural methods in the Jackson Heart Study: Conceptual and descriptive overview. *Ethnicity & Disease, 15*, S6-38–S6-48.
Thomas, S. B., Fine, M. J., & Ibrahim, S. A. (2004). Health disparities: The importance of culture and health communication. *American Journal of Public Health, 94*, 2050.

Sociocultural Context

▶ Sociocultural

Sociocultural Differences

Melissa Walls
Biobehavioral Health and Population Sciences, University of Minnesota Medical School – Duluth, Duluth, MN, USA

Definition

Sociocultural approaches to understanding differences in health call attention to the roles of and potential interdependence between social and cultural factors for health outcomes.

Cultural attitudes, beliefs, values, history, and systems of knowledge are interdependent with the social environment that includes economic status, community and family systems, and interpersonal relationships. Together, sociocultural factors may impact health in numerous ways, such as influencing access/barriers to health care and service utilization preferences/patterns as well as affecting health behaviors such as diet and exercise.

Cross-References

▶ Aerobic Exercise
▶ Sociocultural

Sociocultural Factors

▶ Sociocultural

Socioeconomic Position

▶ Sociocultural
▶ Socio-economic Status

Socio-economic Status

G. David Batty
Department of Epidemiology and Public Health, University College London, London, UK

Synonyms

Socioeconomic position

Definition

Social class is often used by social scientists when the more generic socioeconomic status or socioeconomic position is preferable. Socioeconomic status refers to particular social strata in society and can be measured at a personal or geographical level. For an individual, indicators include occupational social class, occupational prestige, educational attainment, household income, housing tenure, household amenities, and car ownership. For a geographical area, composite measures are often derived from the characteristics of residents in a defined location (Galobardes et al. 2007).

In the context of epidemiology, socioeconomic status has been most commonly related to disease (particularly cardiovascular disease) and disease risk factors (particularly health behaviors such as smoking). Socioeconomic inequalities (variations) in health are essentially universal: with the exception of very few outcomes, poorer health is more common in poorer people. As such, reducing these differentials is a priority for many governments and health agencies.

References and Further Reading

Galobardes, B., Lynch, J., & Davey Smith, G. (2007). Measuring socioeconomic position in health research. *British Medical Bulletin, 81–82*, 21–37.

Socioeconomic Status (SES)

▶ Education, Lack of: As a Risk Factor
▶ Social Factors
▶ Sociocultural

Sodium

▶ Salt, Intake

Sodium Chloride

▶ Salt, Intake

Sodium, Sodium Sensitivity

Jonathan Newman
Columbia University, New York, NY, USA

Definition

Sodium chloride (NaCl), commonly known as salt, is a molecule crucial for fluid balance and free-water homeostasis. However, overconsumption of sodium/salt plays an important role in the development of essential hypertension. Essential hypertension is seen almost exclusively in societies where average daily sodium consumption is greater than 2.3 g. In contrast, hypertension is rare in populations with low-sodium consumption (typically less than 1.2 g/day). These effects of sodium consumption appear independent of other potential causes of essential hypertension, such as obesity.

The blood pressure (BP) responsiveness to variations in sodium intake is known as salt sensitivity.

The change in BP to salt intake varies significantly between individuals and in the same individual at different times.

Salt sensitivity also increases with age and is more prominent in those with diabetes, obesity, and metabolic syndrome.

It may also be more common in African-Americans and other populations, in which excess salt intake may play an important role in the development of hypertension.

There is evidence to suggest that salt-sensitive individuals with normal blood pressure are at a greater risk of developing hypertension and at further risk of hypertension progression and poor blood pressure control. The mechanisms of salt sensitivity are incompletely understood but likely involve a combination of altered salt/water homeostasis, abnormal vascular signaling pathways, and other metabolic abnormalities such as type 2 diabetes and electrolyte abnormalities, such as hypokalemia.

References and Readings

Barba, G., Galletti, F., Cappuccio, F. P., Siani, A., Venezia, A., Versiero, M., Della Valle, E., Sorrentino, P., Tarantino, G., Farinaro, E., & Strazzullo, P. (2007). Incidence of hypertension in individuals with different blood pressure salt-sensitivity: Results of a 15-year follow-up study. *Journal of Hypertension, 25*(7), 1465–1471.

Obarzanek, E., Proschan, M. A., Vollmer, W. M., Moore, T. J., Sacks, F. M., Appel, L. J., Svetkey, L. P., Most-Windhauser, M. M., & Cutler, J. A. (2003). Individual blood pressure responses to changes in salt intake: Results from the DASH-Sodium trial. *Hypertension, 42*(4), 459–467.

Solid Fats

▶ Fat: Saturated, Unsaturated

Somatic Symptom Disorder

▶ Hypochondriasis
▶ Somatization
▶ Somatoform Disorders

Somatic Symptoms

Kurt Kroenke
Department of Medicine, Indiana University, Indianapolis, IN, USA
Regenstrief Institute, Indianapolis, IN, USA
VA HSR&D Center for Implementing Evidence-Based Practice, Indianapolis, IN, USA

Definition

Mental health professionals commonly label bodily symptoms as "somatic" to distinguish them from cognitive, emotional, or other types of non-somatic symptoms (Kroenke 2007a). In contrast, bodily symptoms are more often referred to as "physical" symptoms by those practicing in general medical, surgical and other non-mental health care professions. Somatic symptoms are exceedingly prevalent, accounting for over half of all outpatient encounters. About half of these are pain complaints (e.g., headache, chest pain, abdominal pain, back pain, joint pains), a quarter are upper respiratory (e.g., cough, sore throat, ear or nasal symptoms), and the remainder are non-pain, non-upper-respiratory symptoms (e.g., fatigue, insomnia, dizziness, palpitations).

Description

Epidemiology
About 80% of individuals in the general population experience one or more symptoms each month, of who less than 1 in 4 seek care (Kroenke and Rosmalen 2006). This ubiquitous nature of somatic symptoms mandates that some thresholds be set to distinguish most "persons" who experience common symptoms from the smaller subset of individuals who qualify as "patients." Some thresholds might include severity of the symptom: its duration or persistence; the degree of occupational or social impairment; the level of patient distress, concerns or worries; the decision to seek treatment or use health care; and the direct and indirect financial costs.

An exact medical diagnosis that accounts for the symptom is often not established, with at least one-third of somatic symptoms lacking an adequate physical explanation and referred to by a variety of labels, including functional, idiopathic, atypical, somatoform, or unexplained.

About three-fourths of outpatients presenting with somatic complaints experience improvement within 2 weeks, while 20–25% of symptoms become chronic or recurrent.

Functional Somatic Syndromes
These conditions consist of a cluster of somatic symptoms for which the etiology is poorly understood and include disorders such as irritable bowel syndrome, fibromyalgia, chronic fatigue syndrome, temporomandibular disorder, interstitial cystitis, and others. Experts have questioned whether these are all separate disorders or instead part of a group of poorly explained somatic conditions sharing common features. Supporting the latter, literature syntheses have revealed that these disorders frequently overlap, both at the level of specific syndromes (half to two-thirds of patients with one syndrome also suffer from one or more additional syndromes) as well as in terms of individual symptoms (Kroenke and Rosmalen 2006). Second, they are similar in rates of psychiatric comorbidity, particularly depression and anxiety (Henningsen et al. 2003). Third, functional somatic syndromes respond similarly to certain therapies traditionally considered "psychological" treatments, such as antidepressants and cognitive-behavioral therapy.

Psychological Comorbidity
In patients presenting with poorly explained physical symptoms, a depressive disorder can be diagnosed 50–60% of the time, and an anxiety disorder 40–50% of the time, regardless of the type of symptom. While the specific type of symptom is not particularly important in terms of

predicting depression or anxiety, the number of symptoms is. In two primary care studies involving 1500 patients, those who endorsed 0–1, 2–3, 4–5, 6–8, or ≥ 9 physical symptoms on a 15-symptom scale, the proportion with a depressive or anxiety disorder was 6%, 20%, 33%, 58%, and 80% respectively, suggesting a "dose-response" effect between the number of physical symptoms and the likelihood of psychiatric comorbidity.

Two-thirds of primary care patients with major depression present exclusively with somatic complaints, and half report multiple, unexplained somatic symptoms. Also, depression is present in a quarter to a third of patients referred to medical specialty clinics and, if depressed, referred patients are only about a quarter as likely to have a physical diagnosis established as an explanation for their symptoms triggering the referral. Even disease-specific somatic symptoms (e.g., chest pain in patients with coronary artery disease, dyspnea in patients with pulmonary disease, joint pain in patients with arthritis) are at least as strongly associated with depression and anxiety as they are with objective physiologic measures of the medical disorder (Katon et al. 2007).

Overlap among somatic, anxiety and depressive symptoms (the *SAD triad*) is more common than the "pure" form of any of the three types of symptoms (Löwe et al. 2008). For example, very high levels of depressive, anxiety and somatic symptoms are present in 7%, 8%, and 10% of primary care patients, respectively. However, only 26% of depressed patients have depression alone (i.e., without high levels of anxiety and/or somatic symptoms), 43% of anxious patients have anxiety only, and 46% of patients with high somatic symptom levels have somatization alone. Predictors of psychological comorbidity in patients with somatic symptoms are summarized in Table 1.

Somatoform Disorders

Somatoform disorders currently defined in the American Psychiatric Association's Diagnostic and Statistical Manual, 4th Edition (DSM-IV) include somatization disorder (chronic history of multiple medically unexplained symptoms), conversion disorder (unexplained neurological symptoms), hypochondriasis (preoccupation with having

Somatic Symptoms, Table 1 Predictors of psychological comorbidity in patients with somatic symptoms

Symptom remains medically unexplained after clinical assessment
Multiple symptoms
Three or more unexplained symptoms
Pain symptoms in two or more regions of the body
Multiple functional somatic syndromes
Chronic or recurrent symptom (s)
Excessive health care use
Medication history
Polypharmacy (especially for symptoms)
Poor response of symptoms to multiple medications
Nocebo response (nonspecific adverse effects to multiple medications)
Difficult clinician-patient relationship
Number of S4 predictors[a]
Stress recently
Symptom count is high
Self-rated health is low
Severity of symptom is high

[a]The four S4 predictors are (1) stress in past week (yes/no); (2) Patient reports being "bothered a lot" by five or more symptoms on the PHQ-15 scale of 15 somatic symptoms; (3) self-rated overall health of poor or fair on a 5-point scale (excellent, very good, good, fair, poor); (4) self-rated severity of presenting somatic symptom of ≥ 6 on 0 (none) to 10 (unbearable) scale. The likelihood of a depressive or anxiety disorder with 0, 1, 2, 3, or 4 of these S4 predictors is 8%, 16%, 43%, 69%, and 94%, respectively

a serious medical illness that persists despite medical evaluations and reassurance), body dysmorphic disorder (distorted perceptions of specific bodily features), and chronic pain disorder. However, these are likely to be substantially revised in DSM-V (Kroenke et al. 2007). In particular, criteria for the most common type of somatoform disorder (full and abridged versions of somatization disorder) are likely to rely less on symptom counts or the degree to which symptoms are "medically explained" and more on positive psychological criteria characteristic of somatizing patients (e.g., excessive illness worry and health anxiety, inordinate health care use, catastrophizing).

Measuring Somatic Symptoms

The PHQ-15 is a brief, freely-available scale (www.phqscreeners.com) that measures 15 symptoms that account for more than 90% of non-upper-respiratory symptoms seen in primary care (Kroenke et al. 2010). The PHQ-15 asks patients to rate how much they have been bothered by each symptom during the past month on a 0 ("not at all") to 2 ("bothered a lot") scale. Thus, the total score ranges from 0 to 30, with cutpoints of 5, 10, and 15 representing thresholds for mild, moderate, and severe somatic symptom severity, respectively.

Increasing scores on the PHQ-15 are strongly associated with functional impairment, disability, health care use, and somatoform disorder diagnoses. Also, items on the PHQ-15 overlap better with other validated somatization screeners than any other two screeners do with one another. There is emerging evidence that the PHQ-15 is responsive to treatment.

Treatment

Treatment of somatoform disorders as well as functional somatic syndromes has been recently reviewed (Abbass et al. 2009; Jackson et al. 2006; Kroenke 2007b). In addition to symptom-specific treatments (e.g., analgesics for pain, medications specific to the symptoms for irritable bowel syndrome, medications recently approved for fibromyalgia), the two most evidence-based treatments for both somatoform disorders and functional somatic syndromes are cognitive behavioral therapy and antidepressants, which have a beneficial effect on the somatic symptoms in these conditions independent of their effect on psychological symptoms such as depression and anxiety. Additionally, regular visits with a primary physician, avoidance of excessive testing, and evaluation of new symptoms (but not repeated evaluation of chronic symptoms) is beneficial. A clinical approach to the patient with unexplained somatic symptoms is outlined in Table 2.

Strategies for managing chronic somatization

- Schedule regular, brief appointments that are not related to symptom exacerbations
- Limit extensive diagnostic testing and multiple subspecialty referrals, especially for symptoms previously evaluated
- When new symptoms arise, conduct focused evaluations and testing rather than exhaustive work-ups

Somatic Symptoms, Table 2 Clinical approach to the patient with unexplained somatic symptoms

Initial visit	
Symptom-specific evaluation	Focus the interview and physical examination on the relevant symptom(s) Stratify symptoms into those that are at higher risk of a serious cause (e.g., angina-like chest pain; acute abdominal pain; syncope) and those that are seldom urgent (back pain, fatigue, insomnia). Identify "red flags" of a potentially serious cause (e.g., focal neurologic findings in patient with dizziness or headache; abnormal cardiac exam in patient with syncope)
Probe for symptom-specific concerns and expectations	"Is there anything else you were worried about?" (Serious cause? How long symptom might last?) "Is there anything else you wanted or thought might be helpful?" (Test? subspecialty referral? Specific treatment?)
Consider short-term use of symptom-specific medications (often available over-the-counter)	Simple analgesics for pain Gastrointestinal medications for dyspepsia or constipation Decongestants, antihistamines, cough suppressants for upper respiratory symptoms
Watchful waiting	Have patient follow-up in 2–6 weeks if symptom is not resolved
Follow-up visits	
Psychological screening	Especially for treatable depressive and anxiety disorders (see www.phqscreeners.com) Assess for somatization (PHQ-15 or other scale)
Diagnostic evaluation	Selective testing and/or specialty referral, especially if new unexplained symptom, if findings on interview or examination are worrisome for serious cause, or if patient insists

(continued)

Somatic Symptoms, Table 2 (continued)

Chronic symptom therapies	Pharmacological – analgesics; gastrointestinal medications; antidepressants, other Nonpharmacological – cognitive-behavioral therapy (CBT); other psychological or behavioral therapies; exercise; pain self-management programs; reattribution

- Empathize with the complaint. Do not dispute the reality of the symptom or associated impairment.
- Focus on symptom management/reduction rather than elimination (coping rather than cure).
- Strive for gradual rehabilitation (maximizing function despite the symptom) rather than chronic disability
- Emphasize that referral is for consultation or co-management rather than dismissal (i.e., you are not "dumping" the patient)

Cross-References

▶ Antidepressant Medications
▶ Anxiety Disorder
▶ Chronic Pain
▶ Cognitive Behavioral Therapy (CBT)
▶ Depression: Treatment
▶ Medically Unexplained Symptoms
▶ Pain
▶ Somatization
▶ Somatoform Disorders
▶ Stress
▶ Symptoms

References and Readings

Abbass, A., Kisely, S., & Kroenke, K. (2009). Short-term psychodynamic psychotherapy for somatic disorders: Systematic review and meta-analysis of clinical trials. *Psychotherapy and Psychosomatics, 78*, 265–274.

Dimsdale, J. E., Xin, Y., Kleinman, A., Patel, V., Narrow, W. E., Sirvatka, P. J., & Regier, D. A. (Eds.). (2009). *Somatic presentations of mental disorders: Refining the research agenda for DSM-V*. Arlington: American Psychiatric Association.

Henningsen, P., Zimmermann, T., & Sattel, H. (2003). Medically unexplained physical symptoms, anxiety, and depression: A meta-analytic review. *Psychosomatic Medicine, 65*, 528–533.

Jackson, J. L., O'Malley, P. G., & Kroenke, K. (2006). Antidepressants and cognitive behavioral therapy for symptom syndromes. *CNS Spectrums, 11*, 212–222.

Katon, W., Lin, E., & Kroenke, K. (2007). The association of depression and anxiety with medical symptom burden in patients with chronic medical illness. *General Hospital Psychiatry, 29*, 147–155.

Kroenke, K. (2007a). Somatoform disorders and recent diagnostic controversies. *Psychiatric Clinics of North America, 30*, 593–619.

Kroenke, K. (2007b). Efficacy of treatment for somatoform disorders: A review of randomized clinical trials. *Psychosomatic Medicine, 69*, 881–888.

Kroenke, K., & Rosmalen, J. G. M. (2006). Symptoms, syndromes and the value of psychiatric diagnostics in patients with functional somatic disorders. *Medical Clinics of North America, 90*, 603–626.

Kroenke, K., Sharpe, M., & Sykes, R. (2007). Revising the classification of somatoform disorders: Key questions and preliminary recommendations. *Psychosomatics, 28*, 277–285.

Kroenke, K., Spitzer, R. L., Williams, J. B. W., & Löwe, B. (2010). The patient health questionnaire somatic, anxiety, and depressive symptom scales: A systematic review. *General Hospital Psychiatry, 32*, 345–359.

Löwe, B., Spitzer, R. L., Williams, J. B. W., Mussell, M., Schellberg, D., & Kroenke, K. (2008). Depression, anxiety, and somatization in primary care: Syndrome overlap and functional impairment. *General Hospital Psychiatry, 30*, 191–199.

Somatization

Winfried Rief
Department of Clinical Psychology and Psychotherapy, Philipps University of Marburg, Marburg, Germany

Synonyms

Psychosomatics; Somatic symptom disorder

Definition

Somatization can be defined as "the tendency to experience a variety of somatic symptoms that are usually poorly described by biomedical disease processes"

Description

The term "somatization" goes back to psychodynamic theory and describes the transformation of unconscious conflicts and repressed emotions into somatic symptoms. Later on, Lipowski defined somatization as "a tendency to experience and communicate somatic distress in response to psychosocial stress and to seek medical help for it" (Lipowski 1986). Therefore, this definition postulates that psychosocial stress is the cause for somatization and that seeking medical help is a necessary feature of this syndrome. However, current concepts of somatization use this term more descriptively. According to these modern concepts, somatization could be defined as "the tendency to experience a variety of somatic symptoms that are usually poorly described by biomedical disease processes." In this definition, the presence of multiple somatic complaints is the core feature of somatization.

Somatization itself is not a diagnosis, but is frequently related to the former diagnostic group of "somatoform disorders," which has been reformulated to "Somatic Symptom Disorder" in DSM-5. If multiple somatic symptoms are part of a depressive syndrome or anxiety disorder, the term could be also used. It is not recommended to use the term "somatization" for a postulated association between psychological conflicts and serious medical conditions (e.g., cancer). However, medical conditions like cancer or diabetes can also be associated with multiple medical symptoms that are not explained by the biomedical disease itself. For this subgroup of patients with serious medical conditions, the additional use of the term "somatization" could be appropriate.

Current behavioral-medical concepts prefer the process of "somatosensory amplification" and other perceptual models to describe the development and maintenance of somatization. Somatosensory amplification summarizes the process of focusing attention to bodily perceptions; together with health worries and a catastrophizing style of interpreting bodily perceptions, selective attention leads to an amplified style of perceiving somatic symptoms. If symptoms are chronic, further sensitization processes might be involved. Further details on modern concepts of somatization can be found in Barsky (1992), Henningsen et al. (2018), and Rief and Martin (2014).

Cross-References

▶ Somatoform Disorders

References and Further Readings

Barsky, A. J. (1992). Amplification, somatization, and the somatoform disorders. *Psychosomatics, 33*, 28–34.

Henningsen, P., Gundel, H., Kop, W. J., Lowe, B., Martin, A., Rief, W., Rosmalen, J. G. M., Schroder, A., van der Feltz-Cornelis, C., Van den Bergh, O., & Grp, E.-S. (2018). Persistent physical symptoms as perceptual dysregulation: A Neuropsychobehavioral model and its clinical implications. *Psychosomatic Medicine, 80*(5), 422–431. https://doi.org/10.1097/psy.0000000000000588

Lipowski, Z. J. (1986). Somatization: A borderland between medicine and psychiatry. *Canadian Medical Association Journal, 135*, 609–614.

Rief, W., & Martin, A. (2014). How to use the new DSM-5 diagnosis somatic symptom disorder in research and practice? A critical evaluation and a proposal for modifications. *Annual Review of Clinical Psychology, 10*, 339–367.

Somatoform Disorders

Winfried Rief
Department of Clinical Psychology and Psychotherapy, Philipps University of Marburg, Marburg, Germany

Synonyms

Functional somatic symptoms; Medically unexplained physical symptoms; Somatic symptom disorder

Definition

The common feature of somatoform disorders is the presence of physical symptoms that could indicate a general medical condition, but the physical symptoms are not fully explained by a well-known biomedical disease, by the direct effects of a substance, or by another mental disorder. Somatoform disorders have been replaced by somatic symptom disorders in DSM-5. This group includes somatic symptom disorder, conversion disorder, illness anxiety disorder, and others.

Description

The term "somatoform disorder" has been introduced by DSM-III (*Diagnostic and Statistical Manual of Mental Disorders*, third version) as a category for a group of diagnoses. The common feature of somatoform disorders is the presence of physical symptoms that could indicate a general medical condition, but the physical symptoms are not fully explained by a well-known biomedical disease, by the direct effects of a substance, or by another mental disorder (e.g., panic disorder, depression). Symptoms must cause clinically significant distress or impairment. Somatoform disorders have to be distinguished from factitious disorders and malingering; the physical symptoms in somatoform disorders are not intentional or imagined, but patients perceive these symptoms similar to other physical symptoms caused by medical conditions.

After conceptual critique, the group of somatoform disorders has been replaced by the group of "somatic symptom disorder" (SSD). Again, somatic symptoms are in the core of classifying SSD, but the role of the etiology was discarded, while psychological features such as illness worries, ruminations, and others play a more crucial role. Beyond SSD, illness anxiety disorder, conversion disorder, psychological factors affecting other medical conditions, and factitious disorders are further diagnoses in this category. If pain is the predominant symptom, a diagnoses of somatic symptom disorder with predominant pain can be considered.

While most people suffer from somatic symptoms from time to time, a diagnosis of somatoform disorder or SSD should be only given if the symptoms cause clinically significant distress or impairment. A diagnosis of conversion disorder is justified if people suffer from motor or sensory symptoms or deficits that are not fully accounted by a medical condition. Illness anxiety disorder is considered if illness anxieties (such as in hypochondriasis) are predominant, but somatic symptoms are not significant (such as in SSD). In "Western" cultures, pain symptoms are the most frequent somatic symptoms. If pain duration is longer than 3 months, it should be considered to be chronic. In most cases, chronic pain conditions are not sufficiently understood with pure biomedical approaches, but psychological and social factors have to be also considered.

Somatoform disorders and somatic symptom disorders can develop as a result of the interaction of psychological factors (selective attention to bodily processes, overinterpretation of somatic sensations, illness fears, demoralization) with biomedical factors (e.g., traumatic injuries, car accidents, biological dysregulation of stress and immune responses) and with social factors (c.g., reinforcement of symptom expression by proxies, strong biomedical orientation of health-care systems, fears of doctors to overlook biomedical causes). While somatization typically refers to the experience of multiple medically unexplained symptoms, the concept of somatosensory amplification refers to the self-reinforcing circle of attention to somatic processes, overinterpretation of somatic sensations, intensified physical sensations, and behavioral consequences (Barsky 1992). Modern concepts emphasize perceptual processes (Henningsen et al. 2018). Somatoform disorders and SSD are more prevalent in women than in men. General somatic symptoms can be found in more than 10% of the population (Wittchen and Jacobi 2005).

The classification of "medically explained" versus "medically unexplained" symptoms was found to be unreliable, and medical doctors highly disagree in their ratings about causality of somatic symptoms. Therefore the former concept of somatoform disorders was criticized and accused to further continue a "mind-body separation" instead of favoring a biopsychosocial model. The revision of this category in DSM-5 tries to overcome these shortcomings, but even the new classification bears some problems (Rief and Martin 2014).

To date, no well-founded pharmacological treatment is available for patients with somatoform syndromes. There is some evidence for the use of SSRIs (selective serotonin reuptake inhibitors) in patients with illness anxieties. Psychological interventions (especially behavioral-medical interventions) have been shown to be effective in all groups of somatoform disorders and somatic symptom disorders. However, effect sizes vary substantially, with highest effect sizes for the psychological treatment of illness anxiety, while effect sizes for the treatment of somatization disorder or chronic pain conditions are only in the low to medium range. The rate of overlooked medical conditions that can explain the somatic symptoms does not seem to be increased compared to other mental disorders: long-term studies reveal that less than 10% of patients with somatic symptom disorders must be considered to be misdiagnosed biomedical conditions.

Cross-References

▶ Functional Somatic Syndromes
▶ Somatization
▶ Somatic Symptom Disorder

References and Further Readings

Barsky, A. J. (1992). Amplification, somatization, and the somatoform disorders. *Psychosomatics, 33*, 28–34.
Henningsen, P., Gundel, H., Kop, W. J., Lowe, B., Martin, A., Rief, W., Rosmalen, J. G. M., Schroder, A., van der Feltz-Cornelis, C., Van den Bergh, O., & Grp, Euronet-Soma. (2018). Persistent physical symptoms as perceptual dysregulation: A Neuropsychobehavioral model and its clinical implications. *Psychosomatic Medicine, 80*(5), 422–431. https://doi.org/10.1097/psy.0000000000000588.
Rief, W., & Martin, A. (2014). How to use the new DSM-5 diagnosis somatic symptom disorder in research and practice? A critical evaluation and a proposal for modifications. *Annual Review of Clinical Psychology, 10*, 339–367.
Wittchen, H. U., & Jacobi, F. (2005). Size and burden of mental disorders in Europe – a critical review and appraisal of 27 studies. *European Neuropsychopharmacology, 15*, 357–376.

Spatial Analysis

▶ Geographic Information System (GIS) Technology

Spectral Analysis

▶ Quantitative EEG Including the Five Common Bandwidths (Delta, Theta, Alpha, Sigma, and Beta)

Speech and Language Pathology

▶ Speech and Language Therapy

Speech and Language Therapy

Steven Harulow
Royal College of Speech and Language Therapists, London, UK

Synonyms

Speech and language pathology; Speech therapy; Speech, language, and communication therapy

Definition

Speech and language therapy is an evidence-based discipline that anticipates and responds to the needs of individuals who experience speech, language, communication, or swallowing difficulties. Speech and language therapy works in partnership with individuals and their families and with other professions and agencies to reduce the impact of these often isolating difficulties on well-being and the ability to participate in daily life (Royal College of Speech and Language Therapists 2005).

Speech and language therapists (SLTs) are the lead experts regarding communication and swallowing disorders. This does not mean that others do not work within these areas or that others do not have many skills that may overlap with or complement those of SLTs. Rather, SLTs, through their preregistration education, and later experience, have greater depth and breadth of knowledge and understanding of these clinical areas and associated difficulties. This enables SLTs to lead on the assessment, differential diagnosis, intervention with, and management of individuals with communication and swallowing disorders.

Speech and language therapy assistants and bilingual co-practitioners are integral members of the speech and language therapy team, employed to act in a supporting role under the direction of a professionally qualified SLT.

Description

A wide range of individuals can potentially benefit from speech and language therapy, including:

- Babies with feeding and swallowing difficulties
- Children (from neonates to school age), adolescents, and adults with special needs in communication, communication disability, and/or swallowing disorders associated with diagnosed impairments, genetic and medical conditions, trauma, developmental delays, mental health problems, and learning disability
- Children (from neonates to school age), adolescents, and adults with special needs in the following areas: speech, voice, fluency, language, psychologically based communication disorders, social skills, problem solving, literacy, swallowing functions, and alternative and augmentative communication (AAC)
- Parents and families, caregivers, communication partners, friends, and colleagues of people with communication and swallowing disorders

Speech and language therapists work in and across a variety of settings.

Within education, these settings include:

- Local education authority nurseries and schools (mainstream and special)
- Language and communication units and colleges of further education
- Independent nurseries and schools
- Play groups
- Government-funded initiatives

Within health and social care, settings include:

- Hospitals inpatient and outpatient centers and hospices
- Specialist centers: child development centers, rehabilitation centers, specialist joint consultative clinics
- Primary care: community clinics, community day centers
- Supported living homes
- Mental health services
- Initiatives in areas of social deprivation (such as Sure Start)

Speech and language therapists have an increasing role within the legal system, including within the penal system/prisons, in court tribunals, and as part of adult and child protection services.

They also work in independent practice, as part of social enterprises and for the voluntary/charitable sector.

All speech and language therapy intervention is delivered on the basis of ongoing assessment and review of progress with the individual (and/or carer as appropriate) as measured against targeted outcomes. Various approaches or models of working have been developed to meet the needs of individuals and context.

The following are key principles guiding the provision of services:

- The rights, wishes, and dignities of each individual and their carers are respected at all times.
- Effective intervention is based on a holistic understanding of the individual, including their social, cultural, economic, political, and linguistic context.
- The safety of the individual is paramount.
- Speech and language therapy intervention aims to be efficient and effective, i.e., best results against targeted outcomes within given resources.

Speech and language therapy services may operate at the level of the person (working with individuals); the level of their environment (working with people, processes, or settings); and the level of the wider community (influencing attitude, culture, or practice). The form of intervention will vary according to the changing needs of the individual and contexts.

Benefits

Speech and language therapy can contribute to the following health, educational, and psychosocial benefits:

- Improvement in general health and well-being
- Increased independence
- Improved participation in family, social, occupational, and educational activities
- Improved social and family relationships
- Reduction in the negative effects of communication disability and the harm or distress this may cause to the individual and others
- Reduced risk of surgical intervention and poor nutrition in the case of individuals with swallowing disorders
- Reduced health risks and length of hospital stay through the prevention of respiratory problems associated with swallowing difficulties
- Reduced risk of surgical intervention by maintaining healthy voice mechanisms
- Reduced risk of educational failure
- Reduced risk of social isolation
- Prevention of certain speech, language, and communication disorders

Outcomes

The outcomes of speech and language therapy include:

- Diagnosis of communication and/or swallowing disorders
- Maintenance of optimal communication and/or swallowing abilities
- Improvement in the speech, language, and communication abilities of individuals
- Improved use of existing function
- Reduction of communication anxiety and avoidance
- Provision and use of AAC where oral communication is limited or precluded by a physical condition
- Improvement in interaction and effective social communication
- Increased awareness of others about communication and/or swallowing disorders, intervention, and management
- Improved communication environment
- Greater opportunities for communication
- Improvement in the individual's understanding of the nature and implications of a communication and/or swallowing disorder

In 2010, the Royal College of Speech and Language Therapists (RCSLT) commissioned analysts Matrix Evidence to review the existing evidence and undertake an economic evaluation of the provision of speech and language therapy to four specific client groups. The aim of this was to pinpoint the benefits generated by speech and language therapy in relation to the costs of provision. The result was the UK-wide study "The economic case for speech and language therapy" (Marsh et al. 2010).

The Matrix research aimed to determine the costs and benefits for four common speech and language therapy client groups:

- Adults with dysphagia post stroke
- Adults with aphasia post stroke
- Children with speech and language impairment (SLI)
- Children with autism

Matrix Evidence undertook an evaluation of the costs and benefits of speech and language therapy intervention for each condition and compared either the effects of speech and language therapy with the effects of alternative forms of treatment, or the effects of intensive against less intensive therapy. Specifically, the analysis evaluated:

- Speech and language therapy for stroke survivors with dysphagia compared with "usual" care
- Enhanced NHS speech and language therapy for stroke survivors with aphasia compared with usual NHS therapy
- Enhanced speech and language therapy for children with SLI compared with existing therapy provision
- Enhanced speech and language therapy for children with autism compared with usual SLT treatment

The results of the Matrix report show that speech and language therapy for all four cohorts and conditions represents an efficient use of public resources. The net benefits of the interventions - including health and social care cost savings, quality of life, and productivity gains – are positive and exceed their costs. The report shows the total annual net benefit across aphasia, SLI, and autism is £765 million; it excludes dysphagia from the calculation since the two poststroke conditions are not mutually exclusive.

The RCSLT

Established as the College of Speech Therapists in 1945, the Royal College of Speech and Language Therapists (RCSLT) is the membership organization for UK SLTs, providing and promoting:

- Support and professional leadership for members, including the setting of standards
- Strategic direction for the profession
- Consistent, effective, and accurate professional representation to external bodies and the government
- Heightened public awareness of the medical, social, and emotional effects of communication, eating, drinking, and swallowing difficulties
- Heightened awareness of the contribution of speech and language therapy with the public, government, other professions, and the media

The RCSLT provides leadership so that issues concerning the profession are reflected in public policy and people with communication, eating, drinking, or swallowing difficulties receive optimum care.

Cross-References

▶ Alzheimer's Disease
▶ Brain Injury
▶ Brain Tumor
▶ Chronic Disease Management
▶ Cognitive Impairment
▶ Cost-Effectiveness
▶ Neurological
▶ Neuromuscular Diseases

- Nutrition
- Occupational Therapy
- Rehabilitation
- Stroke Burden

References and Further Reading

For more information, visit the RCSLT website: www.rcslt.org

Marsh, K., Bertranou, E., Suominen, H., Venkatachalam, M. (2010). An economic evaluation of speech and language therapy: Final report. December 2010. *Matrix Evidence*.

Royal College of Speech Therapists Language. (2005). *Communicating quality* (Vol. 3, pp. 2–28). London: RCSLT.

Speech Therapy

- Speech and Language Therapy

Speech, Language, and Communication Therapy

- Speech and Language Therapy

Sperm Donation

- In Vitro Fertilization, Assisted Reproductive Technology
- Surrogacy

Sperm Donor

- In Vitro Fertilization, Assisted Reproductive Technology
- Surrogacy

Spinal Muscular Atrophy

- Neuromuscular Diseases

Spiritual

- Religion/Spirituality

Spiritual Beliefs

Afton N. Kapuscinski
Psychology Department, Syracuse University, Syracuse, NY, USA

Synonyms

Religious beliefs; Spirituality

Definition

The concept of spiritual beliefs is a critical component of the broader terms *spirituality* or *religiousness* and is to some degree inseparable from them. The meanings of these terms, however, remain elusive. In fact, the paramount importance, and difficulty, with defining spiritual concepts has proven a prominent obstacle to establishing a cohesive body of literature. The empirical research is littered with varying, and sometimes incompatible, ways of understanding spiritual constructs (Hill and Pargament 2003; Kapuscinski and Masters 2010). Researchers disagree, for example, regarding the relationship of religiousness and spirituality. This issue takes on special significance when *beliefs* in particular are the subject of consideration because Western notions of religion often differentiate believers from unbelievers based on their convictions (beliefs), rather than behaviors. Historically, spirituality and religiousness were considered to be, if not the same entity, intimately tied to one other. One's personal ideas about and experiences of the sacred were both informed by and occurred in the context of institutional religious beliefs and practices. In recent years, however, a growing minority of Americans have begun to identify themselves as "spiritual but not religious." The distinction often involves the term spiritual being used to signify personal beliefs or experiences of the sacred, apart from traditional religious doctrine and organizations. Interestingly, although most people recognize religion and spirituality as somewhat different concepts, they also see the terms as sharing much in common, including traditional religious concepts of God, Christ, and the church (Zinnbauer et al. 1999).

Some researchers have taken the connotation of spirituality as an individual's internal communion with the transcendent and sharply separated it from the idea of religiousness now defined narrowly as involvement with organized beliefs and practices (Hill and Pargament 2003; Zinnbauer et al. 1999). In some cases, the supernatural or sacred is completely removed from the notion of spirituality or spiritual beliefs, leaving a search for meaning or perspective that is unrelated to the transcendent. Some researchers (Kapuscinski and Masters 2010; Koenig 2010) do not support this separation on several grounds, including that the removal of the sacred creates a somewhat artificial notion of spirituality, devoid of any substance that separates it from mental health variables like optimism and purpose in life. Therefore, the conceptual state of affairs on these topics does not allow spiritual beliefs to be cleanly separated from spirituality or religiousness. All of these concepts overlap significantly.

Nevertheless, despite the overlap, thematic elements in the literature suggest that spiritual beliefs per se may be defined as convictions about self, others, and the world, which emerge from a search for the transcendent or sacred, and include the values regarding lifestyle and moral conduct derived from these convictions. Spiritual beliefs may be roughly synonymous with the notion of spiritual worldview, the basis of which is a belief in the transcendent. Beliefs may or may not include doctrine associated with religious institutions (e.g., that an omnipotent God created the universe, as in the Judeo-Christian tradition).

Description

Most of the questionnaires designed to assess spirituality emphasize beliefs as a critical element of what is measured, and a few, like the Beliefs and Values Scale (King et al., 2006) and the Royal Free Interview for Spiritual and Religious Beliefs (King et al. 2001), focus on beliefs specifically. Thus, consistent with the discussion above, the spiritual beliefs component of religiousness and spirituality (R/S) is strongly embedded in research findings on R/S, even when studies do not claim to focus specifically on beliefs. A wealth of evidence demonstrates that both R/S in general, and sometimes beliefs in particular, influence physical and mental health.

Physical Health

Available research generally indicates a relationship between R/S variables and better physical health and implicates the value of incorporating this aspect of culture into health-promoting interventions. Masters and Hooker (2011) provide an overview of the R/S and health literature. Religious service attendance stands out as a variable that consistently predicts mortality. Frequent attendees are at reduced risk of mortality compared to those who never attended services, even when standard controls are included, and the relationship is especially strong for African Americans. Importantly, this relationship appears to transcend culture, with research demonstrating that R/S serves as a protective factor against mortality in a variety of countries, including non-Western societies such as China and Israel. In this light, it is very important to note that service attendance does not measure spiritual beliefs per se. Nevertheless, the literature also indicates that spiritual beliefs are related to improved outcomes for seriously ill individuals. In cancer patients, for example, spiritual beliefs predict positive psychological adjustment and higher rates of perceived cancer-related growth. Studies also indicate spiritual beliefs and practices may be helpful for cardiac patients, putting them at reduced risk of morbidity, complications, and depression following surgery. However, the relationship between R/S and health is complex, with some studies indicating a detrimental relationship between certain R/S variables and health outcomes. For instance, cardiac patients who viewed God as responsible for their *illnesses* had more difficult recoveries, whereas individuals who attributed their recoveries to God enjoyed better outcomes. Psychologists have theorized several pathways to explain the relationship between R/S and health variables, including the idea that R/S is associated with increased social support, positive coping skills, and the adoption of a healthy lifestyle (e.g., abstinence from smoking and alcohol use, regular exercise, and utilization of preventative health care).

Mental Health

The vast majority of research also indicates a positive association between mental health and spiritual beliefs (Koenig 2010). Individuals scoring higher on measures of spirituality are consistently less likely to have depressive symptoms or disorders, with an effect equivalent in size to that of gender and depression. Similarly, many studies indicate that anxiety is lower for individuals who are more spiritual and that spiritually based interventions result in reduced anxiety. However, the results are mixed – with some research indicating a positive correlation between certain spiritual variables (e.g., spiritual struggle) and anxiety. The relationship between spiritual beliefs and substance use is less ambiguous, with the preponderance of evidence indicating that more spiritual individuals are significantly less likely to engage in substance use, misuse, and abuse.

Despite marked disagreement regarding conceptualization of spiritual constructs, the interaction (whether beneficial or detrimental) of spiritual beliefs with both physical and mental health highlights the significance of recognizing this dimension of human experience in both the science and practice of psychology.

Cross-References

▶ Religion/Spirituality
▶ Spirituality and Health
▶ Spirituality, Measurement of

References and Readings

Hill, P. C., & Pargament, K. I. (2003). Advances in the conceptualization of religiousness and spirituality: Implications for physical and mental health research. *The American Psychologist, 58*, 64–74. https://doi.org/10.1037/0003-066X.58.1.64.

Kapuscinski, A. N., & Masters, K. S. (2010). The current status of measures of spirituality: A critical review of scale development. *Psychology of Religion and Spirituality, 2*, 191–205. https://doi.org/10.1037/a0020498.

King, M., Jones, L., Barnes, K., Low, J., Walker, C., Wilkinson, S., et al. (2006). Measuring spiritual belief: Development and standardization of a beliefs and values scale. *Psychological Medicine, 36*, 417–425. https://doi.org/10.1017/S003329170500629X.

King, M., Speck, P., & Thomas, A. (2001). The royal free interview for spiritual and religious beliefs: Development and validation of a self-report version. *Psychological Medicine, 31*, 1015–1023. https://doi.org/10.1017/S0033291701004160.

Koenig, H. G. (2010). Spirituality and mental health. *International Journal of Applied Psychoanalytic Studies, 7*, 116–122. https://doi.org/10.1002/aps.239.

Koenig, H. G., McCullough, M. E., & Larson, D. B. (Eds.). (2001). *Handbook of religion and health*. New York: Oxford University Press.

Masters, K. S., & Hooker, S. A. (2011). Impact of religion and spirituality on health. In J. Aten, K. O'Grady, & E. Worthington (Eds.), *The psychology of religion and spirituality for clinicians: Using research in your practice* (pp. 357–386). New York: Routledge.

Zinnbauer, B. J., Pargament, K. I., & Scott, A. B. (1999). The emerging meanings of religiousness and spirituality: Problems as prospects. *Journal of Personality, 67*(6), 889–919. https://doi.org/10.1111/1467-6494.00077.

Spiritual Coping

▶ Religious Coping

Spiritual Struggle

▶ Religious Coping

Spirituality

Stephen Gallagher and Warren Tierney
Department of Psychology, Faculty of Education and Health Sciences, University of Limerick, Castletroy, Limerick, Ireland

Synonyms

Religion; Religiosity; Religiousness

Definition

Spirituality is a very unclear concept that has no concrete definition. By its very nature, the concept of spirituality is deeply rooted in religion, yet in contemporary spirituality, there is an incremental divide emerging between religion and spirituality. Therefore, in present-day society, the formation of a dichotomy with spirituality representing the personal, subjective, inner-directed, unsystematic, liberating expression and religion signifying a formal, authoritarian, institutionalized inhibiting expression is being witnessed. Spirituality has also been defined as a subjective and fluid approach to experiences which leads one to search for enlightenment, whereby behaviors are practiced in accordance with these sacred beliefs. Similarly, one can also consider spirituality to be something personal, which is defined by individuals themselves and is mostly likely devoid of the rules and regulations associated with religion.

Description

Pathways Linking Spirituality to Health

Rendering a congruent spiritual outlook on life has been associated with an enhanced quality of life, better mental and physical health, and improved recovery from various illnesses. However, the precise mechanisms behind these relationships remain unclear. This can be partly attributed to several reasons: first, the lack of a clear conceptual definition of what spirituality is; second, researchers using both concepts of religion and spirituality interchangeably; third, measuring both concepts with similar assessments (e.g., denomination and frequency of religious observance) which clearly are not adequate to capture a measure of one's spiritual beliefs; and finally, social acceptance that being spiritual entails performing soothing activities such as meditation, yoga or praying, etc., which may be tied to social interactions. Thus, it is necessary to distinguish social factors involved in these practices from spirituality itself. All of the above make it difficult to draw any firm conclusions; thus, caution must be warranted when interpreting the data from such studies. Nonetheless, a number of pathways linking spirituality and health have been proposed, from direct physiological mechanisms (e.g., immune functioning) to more indirect stress buffering (e.g., coping strategies) and lifestyle choices (e.g., dietary and exercise behaviors coupled to one's spiritual beliefs) (Miller and Thorensen 2003). For example, a positive correlation between spirituality and T-cell percentages in HIV-positive women has been reported, suggestive of a more direct physiological route, while other studies support a more indirect pathway; spiritual beliefs have been found to be linked to lower stress, better nutrition, and more exercise, all of which are associated with positive health indices (Koenig et al. 2001). However, what is more interesting is the strong evidence coming from intervention research; a number of studies have been conducted along this line, but one study found that those taught spiritual meditation had greater decreases in anxiety, negative affect, and frequency of migraine headaches compared to those who practiced internally focused secular meditation, externally focused secular meditation, or muscle relaxation (Wachholtz and Pargament 2009). Taken together, these studies indicate that spirituality influences health and that interventions targeting this concept can bring health benefits.

However, despite these positive benefits, a word of caution is warranted when investigating these relationships as there are also negative health consequences associated with spirituality. For example, a spiritual struggle denotes the anxiety and pressure about spiritual concerns inside oneself, with others, and the godly. Indeed, this spiritual struggle is associated with poor mental and physical health among suffers in some traditional faith practices (Rosmarin et al. 2009); hence, it is sometimes difficult to determine whether spirituality is a resource or a liability and adds to the complexity that already exists in this spirituality-health relationship, which in some instances may not be linear (Gallagher et al. 2015). Further, there have been attempts to adopt the concept of spirituality into an overall definition of health, and some now argue that spiritual health and growth are equally important for quality of life (Sawatzky et al. 2005); thus, spirituality can now be viewed and measured as an endpoint itself.

Measuring Spirituality

Measuring spirituality is a very difficult task due to lack of agreed-upon definition and its close-knit ties with religion. However, there have been some admirable attempts to capture the concept using self-report methods, and some of the measures include the Daily Spiritual Experience Scale (Underwood and Teresi 2002), the Intrinsic Spirituality Scale (Hodge 2003) and the Spiritual Well-Being Scale (Paloutzian and Ellison 1991), and the Theistic Spiritual Outcome Survey (Richards et al. 2005), while the Spiritual Transcendence Scale (Piedmont 1999), the Beliefs and Values Scale (King et al. 2006), and Spiritual Connection Scale (Wheeler and Hyland 2008) offer a conceptualization of spirituality which is nonreligious; these may be useful when one is dealing with individuals who are more inclined to adopt a contemporary view of spirituality.

Cross-References

▶ Religion
▶ Religion/Spirituality
▶ Religiousness/Religiosity
▶ Spiritual Beliefs

References and Further Readings

Gallagher, S., Phillips, A. C., Lee, H. A. N., & Carroll, D. (2015). The association between spirituality and depression in parents caring for children with developmental disabilities: Social support and/or last resort. *Journal of Religion and Health, 54*, 358–370.

Hill, P. C., & Pargament, K. I. (2003). Advances in the conceptualization and measurement of religion and spirituality: Implications for physical and mental health research. *American Psychologist, 58*, 64–74.

Hodge, D. R. (2003). The intrinsic spirituality scale. *Journal of Social Service Research, 30*(1), 41–61.

King, M., Jones, L., Barnes, K., Low, J., Walker, C., Wilkinson, S., et al. (2006). Measuring spiritual belief: Development and standardization of a beliefs and values scale. *Psychological Medicine, 36*(3), 417–425.

Koenig, H. G. (2009). Research on religion, spirituality, and mental health: A review. *Canadian Journal of Psychiatry, 54*, 283–291.

Koenig, H. G., McCullough, M. E., & Larson, D. B. (Eds.). (2001). *Handbook of religion and health*. New York: Oxford University Press.

Miller, W. R., & Thorensen, C. E. (2003). Spirituality, religion, and health: An emerging research field. *American Psychologist, 58*, 24–35.

Paloutzian, R. E., & Ellison, C. W. (1991). *Manual for the spiritual well-being scale*. Nayack: Life Advance.

Peterman, A. H., Fitchett, G., Brady, M. J., Hernandez, L., & Cella, D. (2002). Measuring spiritual well-being in people with cancer: The functional assessment of chronic illness therapy-spiritual well-being scale (FACIT-Sp). *Annals of Behavioral Medicine, 24*, 49–58.

Piedmont, R. L. (1999). Does spirituality represent the sixth factor of personality? Spiritual transcendence and the five-factor model. *Journal of Personality, 67*, 985–1013.

Richards, P. S., Smith, T., Schowalter, M., Richard, M., Berrett, M. E., & Hardman, R. K. (2005). Development and validation of the theistic spiritual outcome survey. *Psychotherapy Research, 15*, 457–469.

Rosmarin, D. H., Pargament, K. I., & Flannelly, K. J. (2009). Do spiritual struggles predict poorer physical/mental health among Jews? *The International Journal for the Psychology of Religion, 19*, 244–258.

Sawatzky, R., Ratner, P. A., & Chiu, L. (2005). A meta-analysis of the relationship between spirituality and quality of life. *Social Indicators Research, 72*, 153–188.

Underwood, L. G., & Teresi, J. A. (2002). The daily spiritual experience scale: Development, theoretical description, reliability, exploratory factor analysis and preliminary construct validity using health-related data. *Annals of Behavioral Medicine, 24*, 22–33.

Wachholtz, M. A. B., & Pargament, K. I. (2009). Migraines and meditation: Does spirituality matter? *Journal of Behavioral Medicine, 3*, 351–366.

Wheeler, P., & Hyland, M. E. (2008). The development of a scale to measure the experience of spiritual connection and the correlation between this experience and values. *Spirituality Health, 9*, 193–217.

Spirituality and Health

Kevin S. Masters
Department of Psychology, University of Colorado Denver, Denver, CO, USA

Synonyms

Faith and health; Religiousness and health

Definition

Spirituality is an elusive term for which definitional consensus has yet to be reached. Many definitions include concepts concerning that which is beyond the material world and may include features of life that are not commonly perceptible by the physical senses. This is sometimes said to include a search for the sacred or belief in the transcendent. Common themes in definitions of spirituality include connectedness or relationship, subjectivity, personal experience, behaviors reflecting sacred or secular beliefs, and belief in something transcendent. This entry regards spirituality as related to health, an area of significantly increased research activity over the last 15–20 years.

Description

Over the last 15–20 years, scholars have become significantly more interested in determining if there is a relationship between spirituality and health, what the strength of this relationship might be, and if the relationship varies depending on the specific dimensions of both spirituality and health under consideration. Clearly both spirituality and health are multidimensional constructs, and thus, any general statement on their relationship will be an oversimplification.

The first major problem that investigators have in this area is, indeed, defining both terms. In this entry, the definitional focus is on spirituality. An important first question pertains to the similarities and differences between religion and spirituality. Most scholars currently agree that they are related, but not synonymous constructs. This understanding diverges from the historic conceptualization that viewed spirituality and religion as indivisible entities but coincides temporally with the increasing secularization of Western culture (Zinnbauer et al. 1999). Compared to spirituality, religion is often viewed as including more organized social or group practices with well-defined rituals, doctrinal creeds, and statements of faith. Spirituality, on the other hand, is thought to be more subjective and personal, lacking in the organizational elements that characterize religion. Shahabi et al. (2002) reported that 10% of individuals in a US national stratified sample classified themselves as spiritual, but not religious. Nevertheless, most highly religious individuals note that their spirituality is pursued within the context of their religion. Further, a common theme for definitions of both religion and spirituality is reference to a higher power, and 70% of spirituality definitions referred to traditional concepts of God, Christ, and the church as constituting what is sacred (Zinnbauer et al. 1997). Based on a review of the nursing literature, Emblen (1992) defined spirituality as "a personal life principle which animates a transcendent quality of relationship with God" (p. 45). More recently, Saucier and Skrzypinska (2006) demonstrated that subjective spirituality and tradition-oriented religiousness are empirically independent and correlate quite distinctly with personality dimensions. It has also been observed that neither spirituality nor religiousness can be simply reduced to a commonly measured personality variable (Piedmont 1999; Saroglou and Muñoz-García 2008; Saucier and Skrzypinska 2006).

Given the definitional problems with spirituality, it is not surprising that there are measurement concerns as well. Recently, Kapuscinski and Masters (2010) reviewed work in this area. They not only observed the lack of definitional consensus and related measurement confusion but also suggested that, given the dearth of lexical studies of spirituality, it is quite likely that the spiritual construct as defined by researchers differs from popular understanding and use of the term.

Clearly, these basic problems limit the extent that strong statements can be made regarding spirituality and health. At this point, most of the research has not focused on spirituality per se, as differentiated from religiousness, but rather has used measures such as religious service attendance as proxies for spirituality or has confounded religion and spirituality often using the R/S naming convention to represent both simultaneously and therefore demonstrate that no attempt at conceptual separation was made. There is significant research suggesting that some practices that are often associated with spirituality or considered behavioral indicators of spirituality can be effective. For example, meditation has a strong history of beneficial findings in the area of stress management and has been an important component in some major lifestyle interventions such as the Ornish Lifestyle Heart Trial (Ornish et al. 1983, 1990). Nevertheless, intervention studies that include a specifically spiritual intervention are almost nonexistent, and observational research, even if longitudinal, is severely limited in considering cause and effect relations. For example, it is clear that people tend to pray more when they are ill (negative relationship with health), but it is quite likely that it is the illness that is "causing" the increase in prayer rather than prayer having a negative impact on health. Investigations on frequency of prayer and health are, at this point, nonconclusive and largely characterized by cross-sectional research designs of self-report data. A few studies have investigated the content of prayer and found that, for example, self-esteem is higher among older adults when they pray, believing that only God knows when and how to best answer prayer (Krause 2004). Krause (2003) also found that prayer for material things did not alleviate the burden of financial strain on physical health. But these are very preliminary findings, and much work in this area remains.

Finally, there are many behavioral and cognitive practices that could be considered either spiritual or not spiritual depending on how they are conceptualized and contextualized. These include concepts such as gratitude, forgiveness, relaxation, compassion, hope, optimism, faith, and connectedness among others. The extent that these may be considered aspects of spirituality depends on many factors notably the extent to which they are conceptualized as aspects of relating to the transcendent or sacred.

Cross-References

▶ Spiritual Beliefs
▶ Spirituality, Measurement of

References and Readings

Emblen, J. D. (1992). Religion and spirituality defined according to current use in nursing literature. *Journal of Professional Nursing, 8,* 41–47. https://doi.org/10.1016/8755-7223(92)90116-G.

Kapuscinski, A. N., & Masters, K. S. (2010). The current status of measures of spirituality: A critical review of scale development. *Psychology of Religion and Spirituality, 2,* 191–205.

Krause, N. (2003). Praying for others, financial strain, and physical health status in late life. *Journal for the Scientific Study of Religion, 42,* 377–391.

Krause, N. (2004). Assessing the relationships among prayer expectancies, race, and self-esteem in late life. *Journal for the Scientific Study of Religion, 42,* 395–408.

Ornish, D., Brown, S. E., Scherwitz, L. W., Billings, J. H., Armstrong, W. T., Ports, T. A., et al. (1990). Can lifestyle changes reverse coronary heart disease? The lifestyle heart trial. *Lancet, 336,* 129–133.

Ornish, D., Scherwitz, L. W., Doody, R. S., Kesten, D., McLanahan, S. M., Brown, S. E., et al. (1983). Effects of stress management training and dietary changes in treating ischemic heart disease. *JAMA, 249,* 54–59.

Piedmont, R. L. (1999). Does spirituality represent the sixth factor of personality? Spiritual transcendence and the five-factor model. *Journal of Personality, 67*, 983–1013. https://doi.org/10.1111/1467-6494.0080.

Saroglou, V., & Muñoz-García, A. (2008). Individual differences in religion and spirituality: An issue of personality traits and/or values. *Journal for the Scientific Study of Religion, 47*, 83–101.

Saucier, G., & Skrzypinska, K. (2006). Spiritual but not religious? Evidence for two independent dispositions. *Journal of Personality, 74*, 1257–1292. https://doi.org/10.1111/j.1467-6494.2006.00409.x.

Shahabi, L., Powell, L. H., Musick, M. A., Pargament, K. I., Thoresen, C. E., Williams, D., et al. (2002). Correlates of self-perception of spirituality in American adults. *Annals of Behavioral Medicine, 24*, 59–68. https://doi.org/10.1207/S15324796ABM2401_07.

Zinnbauer, B. J., Pargament, K. I., Cole, B., Rye, M. S., Butter, E. M., Belavich, T. G., et al. (1997). Religion and spirituality: Unfuzzying the fuzzy. *Journal for the Scientific Study of Religion, 36*, 549–564. https://doi.org/10.2307/1387689.

Zinnbauer, B. J., Pargament, K. I., & Scott, A. B. (1999). The emerging meanings of religiousness and spirituality: Problems as prospects. *Journal of Personality, 67*, 889–919. https://doi.org/10.1111/14676494.

Spirituality, Measurement of

Afton N. Kapuscinski
Psychology Department, Syracuse University, Syracuse, NY, USA

Definition

Quantitative assessment of spirituality, typically in the form of self-report questionnaires.

Description

Measuring spirituality poses a serious challenge to research in the psychology of religion and spirituality. The principal source of difficulty is researchers' inability to reach a consensus on how to define spirituality, especially regarding its relationship to the concept of religiousness (Kapuscinski and Masters 2010). As language in the United States has shifted over the past few decades, such that religion and spirituality are no longer considered to be synonymous, researchers have created instruments intended to measure spirituality as a concept distinct from religiousness. However, the definitions used to generate measures of spirituality are highly diverse, resulting in some instruments that appear to share little overlap in content (Kapuscinski and Masters 2010). For instance, some measures define spirituality using language stemming from traditional religious institutions (e.g., "God"), whereas others include no reference to the transcendent or sacred in their conceptualizations. An additional concern is that some themes in the way researchers tend to understand spirituality stand in contrast to how the term is used in common language by the general public (Hill and Pargament 2003; Zinnbauer et al. 1999). Specifically, researchers tend to sharply divide spirituality from religion, such that religion is considered to be comprised of external behaviors (e.g., religious service attendance) and is associated with formal institutions, whereas spirituality is comprised of personal, inner experience that is separate from organized religion. Further, researchers are inclined to view spirituality as a health-promoting quality associated with positive psychological and societal benefits, and religiousness, in contrast, is perceived to be restrictive and unhealthy. The empirical literature, however, indicates that non-researchers regard the concepts as overlapping considerably and view both religiousness and spirituality as positive qualities. Moreover, researchers' connotations are not consistent with research linking both religion and spirituality to positive mental and physical health outcomes (Masters and Hooker 2011).

Further, theoretical concerns arise regarding the feasibility of quantifying and operationally defining a concept that seems to be, by its nature, highly experiential and personalized. The literature indicates that like researchers, individuals differ in how they understand spirituality (Zinnbauer et al. 1999). Interestingly, the majority of researchers do not consult participants regarding conceptualization of spirituality when developing new measures (Kapuscinski and Masters 2010). Miller and Thoresen (2003) comment that from the believer's perspective, scientists can at best explore mere reflections of spirituality, which approximate but never fully capture its essence.

The disagreement regarding how to conceptualize spirituality is implied by the sheer number of available spirituality instruments. Reviews of measures (Hill and Hood 1999; MacDonald et al. 1995; MacDonald et al. 1999) indicate that over 100 measures exist that are designed to measure a variety of spiritual constructs, including spirituality, intrinsic spirituality, spiritual experiences, spiritual meaning, spiritual development, spiritual transcendence, spiritual transformation, and spiritual well-being. Most measures appear to address interest in or search for the sacred and focus on assessing cognitive (e.g., meaning, beliefs, values) or emotional (e.g., peace, hope, connection) experiences associated with the sacred. Several high-quality measures should be considered as appropriate for use in health psychology research. The FACIT Spiritual Well-Being Scale (Peterman et al. 2002) was designed specifically to assess aspects of spirituality relevant to quality of life for chronically ill individuals. The Daily Spiritual Experiences Scale (Underwood and Teresi 2002) includes language that is relevant to individuals from various faith traditions and has demonstrated a relationship to important health variables such as alcohol consumption and depression. Additionally, the Spiritual Transcendence Scale (Piedmont 1999), which does not include language associated with institutional religion, is noteworthy for its high-quality scale development and validation practices and includes an observer report form. When selecting a measure for use, researchers should carefully consider whether or not the content of scale items is consistent with the conceptualization of spirituality relevant to their study and population of interest.

Cross-References

▶ Spiritual Beliefs
▶ Spirituality
▶ Spirituality and Health

References and Readings

Hill, P. C., & Hood, R. W. (Eds.). (1999). *Measures of religiosity.* Birmingham: Religious Education.

Hill, P. C., & Pargament, K. I. (2003). Advances in the conceptualization of religiousness and spirituality: Implications for physical and mental health research. *American Psychologist, 58,* 64–74. https://doi.org/10.1037/0003-066X.58.1.64.

Kapuscinski, A. N., & Masters, K. S. (2010). The current status of measures of spirituality: A critical review of scale development. *Psychology of Religion and Spirituality, 2,* 191–205. https://doi.org/10.1037/a0020498.

MacDonald, D. A., LeClair, L., Holland, C. J., Alter, A., & Friedman, H. L. (1995). A survey of measures of transpersonal constructs. *Journal of Transpersonal Psychology, 27,* 171–235.

MacDonald, D. A., Friedman, H. L., & Kuentzel, J. G. (1999). A survey of measures of spiritual and transpersonal constructs: Part one – research update. *Journal of Transpersonal Psychology, 31,* 137–154.

Masters, K. S., & Hooker, S. A. (2011). Impact of religion and spirituality on health. In J. Aten, K. O'Grady, & E. Worthington (Eds.), *The psychology of religion and spirituality for clinicians: Using research in your practice* (pp. 357–386). New York: Routledge.

Miller, W. R., & Thoresen, C. E. (2003). Spirituality, religion and health: An emerging research field. *American Psychologist, 58,* 24–35. https://doi.org/10.1037/0003-066X.58.1.24.

Peterman, A. H., Fitchett, G., Brady, M. J., Hernandez, L., & Cella, D. (2002). Measuring spiritual well-being in people with cancer: The functional assessment of chronic illness therapy – spiritual well-being scale (FACIT-Sp). *Annals of Behavioral Medicine, 24,* 49–58. https://doi.org/10.1207/S15324796ABM2401.

Piedmont, R. L. (1999). Does spirituality represent the sixth factor of personality? Spiritual transcendence and the five-factor model. *Journal of Personality, 67,* 986–1013. https://doi.org/10.1111/1467-6494.00080.

Underwood, L. G., & Teresi, J. A. (2002). The daily spiritual experience scale: Development, theoretical description, reliability, exploratory factor analysis and preliminary construct validity using health-related data. *Annals of Behavioral Medicine, 24,* 22–33. https://doi.org/10.1207/S15324796ABM2401_04.

Zinnbauer, B. J., Pargament, K. I., & Scott, A. B. (1999). The emerging meanings of religiousness and spirituality: Problems as prospects. *Journal of Personality, 67*(6), 889–919. https://doi.org/10.1111/1467-6494.00077.

Squamous Cell Carcinoma of the Cervix (SCCC)

▶ Cancer, Cervical

Stages of Change Model

▶ Transtheoretical Model of Behavior Change

Stages-of-Change Model

Jonathan A. Shaffer
Department of Medicine/Division of General Medicine, Columbia University Medical Center, New York, NY, USA

Definition

The Stages-of-Change Model was developed by James Prochaska and Carlo DiClemente as a framework to describe the five phases through which one progresses during health-related behavior change (Prochaska und DiClemente 1983). It is part of their broader Transtheoretical Model, which not only assesses an individual's readiness to act to eliminate a problem behavior but also includes strategies and processes of change to guide the individual through the stages. The Stages-of-Change Model originated in research related to psychotherapy and the cessation of addictive behaviors, such as smoking, alcohol and substance abuse, and issues related to weight management (Buxton et al. 1996). Although Prochaska and DiClemente initially hypothesized that individuals progress linearly through a series of discrete stages of change, researchers now believe that a cyclical or "spiral" pattern more accurately represents how most people change unhealthy behavior over time. Since its development, the Stages-of-Change Model has been related to a variety of problem behaviors, associated with treatment outcomes, and integrated in stage-based interventions. Although most scientists and clinicians agree that the model has heuristic value, it has been criticized by some researchers.

Description

History of the Model

Stage theories have been integral to the field of psychology since its inception and include Freud's and Erikson's psychosexual stages, Kohlberg's stages of moral development, Piaget's stages of cognitive development, and Maslow's hierarchy of needs (Dolan 2005). DiClemente and Prochaska's Stages-of-Change Model uses language similar to Horn. Specifically, Horn hypothesized four stages of change associated with health-related behavior: (1) contemplating change, (2) deciding to change, (3) short-term change, and (4) long-term change (Horn 1976). DiClemente and Prochaska initially identified four stages of changes associated with smoking cessation and maintenance: (1) thinking about change (contemplation), (2) becoming determined to change (decision making), (3) actively modifying behavior and/or environment (action), and (4) maintaining new behaviors (maintenance). Precontemplation was later identified as a separate stage preceding contemplation.

Description of Stages

Precontemplation. The individual in the precontemplation stage has no intention to change his or her behavior in the foreseeable future (Prochaska und Norcross 2001). Although individuals are unaware of their problems, their families, friends, neighbors, and employees are often very aware of these problems. Individuals presenting for treatment in the precontemplation stage generally do so because of pressure from others.

Contemplation. During the contemplation stage, individuals are aware that a problem exists and seriously consider overcoming it. However, they have not yet made a commitment to do so. According to Prochaska and Norcross, individuals often remain stuck in this stage for long periods.

Preparation. The preparation stage combines intention and behavioral criteria. Individuals in the preparation stage intend to enact change in the next month and have unsuccessfully attempted to do so in the past year. These individuals report small behavioral changes, but they have not yet reached a criterion for effective action, such as abstinence from smoking or sufficient weight loss. These individuals do intend to take action in the very near future.

Action. Individuals in the action stage modify their behavior, experiences, and environment in order to overcome their problems. This stage involves the most overt behavioral changes and requires considerable commitment of time and energy. Modifications of the problem behaviors made in this stage are most visible to others and tend to elicit others' recognition. Individuals in this stage must have successfully altered their problem behavior for a period of 1 day to 6 months.

Maintenance. Individuals in the maintenance stage concentrate on preventing relapse and consolidating the gains attended during the previous stage. These individuals must have remained free of their problem behavior and consistently engaged in a new incompatible behavior for more than 6 months.

Termination. Individuals who reach this stage have completed the change process and no longer have to work to prevent relapse. This stage involves total confidence or self-efficacy across all high-risk situations and no temptation to relapse.

Assessing Stages of Change

Multiple ways for measuring stage of change have been proposed and devised, and researchers/clinicians usually assign people to stages on the basis of their responses to questions concerning their prior behavior and current behavioral intentions (Weinstein, Rothman, & Sutton, 1998). A Stages-of-Change Questionnaire has been developed as a brief and reliable instrument for measuring stages of change in psychotherapy and has been adopted to evaluate stages of change for specific problem behaviors (McConnaughy, Prochaska, & Velicer, 1983). This continuous measure includes questions such as "As far as I'm concerned, I don't have problems that need changing" (precontemplation), "I have a problem and I really think I should work on it" (contemplation), "I am working really hard to change" (action), and "I may need a boost right now to help me maintain the changes I've already made" (maintenance). Given that attributes that define the stages of change are mainly internal to the individual (e.g., beliefs, plans, attributions), measurement is often imperfect (Weinstein, Rothman, & Sutton, 1998).

Stages of Change and Specific Health Behaviors

The Stages-of-Change Model has been used to understand a variety of problem behaviors including smoking cessation, cessation of cocaine use, weight control, high-fat food consumption, adolescent delinquent behaviors, risky sexual behaviors, sunscreen use, radon gas exposure, exercise acquisition, mammography screening, and physicians' preventive practices with smokers (Prochaska et al. 1994).

Stage-Based Treatments

The Stages-of-Change Model has been use to aid in treatment planning and to develop stage-based treatments. Prochaska (1991) has argued that a person's stage of change provides proscriptive and prescriptive information about appropriate treatments (Prochaska 1991). For example, those who are in the preparation or action stages presumably benefit from action-oriented therapies, whereas those in the precontemplation or contemplation stages likely may benefit more from insight-oriented, consciousness raising interventions.

Several interventions based on stage-based models of change have been developed to modify risk behaviors. These interventions are tailored to take into account the current stage an individual has reached in the change process in contrast to "one size fits all" interventions. A systematic review of these interventions identified 37 RCTs of such interventions aimed at smoking cessation, promotion of physical activity, dietary change, multiple lifestyle changes, mammography screening, and treatment adherence (Riemsma et al. 2002). The authors of this review concluded that there is little evidence to suggest that stage-based interventions are more effective compared to non-stage-based interventions, no intervention, or usual care. Nonetheless, they recommend additional studies of tailored interventions which involve frequent reassessment of patients' readiness to change. Reviews of stage-based lifestyle interventions in primary care (Van Sluijs, Van Poppel, & Van Mechelen, 2004) and stage-based interventions for smoking cessation (Riemsma et al. 2003) have likewise resulted in limited scientific evidence in support of these interventions.

Revised Stages-of-Change Model

Freeman und Dolan (2001) offered a revised Stages-of-Change Model with five additional changes to more precisely determine a psychotherapy patient's position on the continuum of change (Freeman & Dolan). This revised model has been recommended as a more dynamic and flexible one that provides clinicians with a more experience-centered focus from which to make treatment decisions.

Non-contemplation is the stage during which an individual is not considering or even thinking about changing. These individuals do not actively avoid, resist, or oppose change; they are rather unaware of their need to change or of the effect their behavior has on others. Anti-contemplation involves the process of becoming reactive and violently opposed to the notion of needing change, a response often seen in individuals who are legally mandated to attend treatment or who come to treatment at the urging of their family, friends, or significant others. Freeman and Dolan's precontemplation and contemplation stages are identical to those of Prochaska and DiClemente. Their action planning stage occurs when the clinician and patient have collaboratively developed a treatment focus and treatment plan. Patients in this stage are actively willing to plan change, and next progress to the action stage of Prochaska and DiClemente's model. Prelapse, lapse, and relapse stages may then occur prior to the maintenance stage. During prelapse, an individual experiences overwhelming thoughts, desires, and cravings to engage in the problem behavior. During lapse, the skills needed to maintain the action stage decrease or are ignored. During relapse, the individual returns to the problem behavior. As in Prochaska and DiClemente's model, the maintenance stage occurs when the individual actively works toward maintaining the cessation of the problem behavior.

Evaluation of the Stages-of-Change Model

The Stages-of-Change Model is not without criticism. Those who have criticized the model argue that its inherent concept of discrete stages involves arbitrary distinctions; it falsely assumes that individuals make coherent and stable plans, and it neglects the role of reward, punishment, and associative learning that contribute to the maintenance of problem behaviors (West 2005). Others have found that minimal supportive evidence for the Stages-of-Change Model exists (Whitelaw, Baldwin, Bunton, & Flynn, 2000) and questioned the model's internal validity (Ahijevych und Wewers 1992; Bandura 1997; Farkas et al. 1996), external validity (Clarke und Eves 1997), and ethical difficulties associated with interventions derived from the Stages-of-Change Model (Piper und Brown 1998).

Notwithstanding the criticisms and absence of evidence discussed above, the Stages-of-Change Model provides a pragmatic framework for practitioners and clinical researchers, and it is intuitively appealing to many in the fields of clinical psychology, behavioral medicine, public health, and other fields. Future research promises to offer improved measurement of stages, qualitative case studies of practitioner utilization, and process-based implementation evaluation of the model in various settings (Whitelaw, Baldwin, Bunton, & Flynn, 2000).

Cross-References

▶ Health Beliefs/Health Belief Model
▶ Transtheoretical Model of Behavior Change

References and Readings

Ahijevych, K., & Wewers, M. (1992). Processes of change across five stages of smoking cessation. *Addictive Behaviors, 17*(1), 17–25.

Bandura, A. (1997). Editorial: The anatomy of stages of change. *American Journal of Health Promotion, 12*, 8–10.
Buxton, K., Wyse, J., & Mercer, T. (1996). How applicable is the stages of change model to exercise behaviour? A review. *Health Education Journal, 55*(2), 239–256.
Clarke, P., & Eves, F. (1997). Applying the transtheoretical model to the study of exercise on prescription. *Journal of Health Psychology, 2*(2), 195–207.
Dolan, M. (2005). Stages of change. In A. Freeman et al. (Eds.), *Encyclopedia of cognitive behavior therapy* (pp. 387–390). New York: Springer.
Farkas, A., Pierce, J., Zhu, S., Rosbrook, B., Gilpin, E., Berry, C., et al. (1996). Addiction versus stages of change models in predicting smoking cessation. *Addiction, 91*(9), 1271–1280.
Freeman, A., & Dolan, M. (2001). Revisiting Prochaska and DiClemente's stages of change theory: An expansion and specification to aid in treatment planning and outcome evaluation. *Cognitive and Behavioral Practice, 8*(3), 224–234.
Horn, D. (1976). A model for the study of personal choice health behavior. *International Journal of Health Education, 19*(1), 89–98.
McConnaughy, E., Prochaska, J., & Velicer, W. (1983). Stages of change in psychotherapy: Measurement and sample profiles. *Psychotherapy: Theory, Research & Practice, 20*(3), 368–375.
Piper, S., & Brown, P. (1998). Psychology as a theoretical foundation for health education in nursing: empowerment or social control? *Nurse Education Today, 18*(8), 637–641.
Prochaska, J. (1991). Prescribing to the stage and level of phobic patients. *Psychotherapy: Theory, Research, Practice, Training, 28*(3), 463.
Prochaska, J., & DiClemente, C. (1983). Stages and processes of self-change of smoking: toward an integrative model of change. *Journal of Consulting and Clinical Psychology, 51*(3), 390–395.
Prochaska, J., & Norcross, J. (2001). Stages of change. *Psychotherapy: Theory, Research, Practice, Training, 38*(4), 443.
Prochaska, J., Velicer, W., Rossi, J., Goldstein, M., Marcus, B., Rakowski, W., et al. (1994). Stages of change and decisional balance for 12 problem behaviors. *Health Psychology, 13*, 39–39.
Riemsma, R., Pattenden, J., Bridle, C., Sowden, A., Mather, L., Watt, I., et al. (2002). A systematic review of the effectiveness of interventions based on a stages-of-change approach to promote individual behaviour change. *Health Technology Assessment, 6*(24), 1–231.
Riemsma, R., Pattenden, J., Bridle, C., Sowden, A., Mather, L., Watt, I., et al. (2003). Systematic review of the effectiveness of stage based interventions to promote smoking cessation. *British Medical Journal, 326*(7400), 1175.
Van Sluijs, E., Van Poppel, M., & Van Mechelen, W. (2004). Stage-based lifestyle interventions in primary care: Are they effective? *American Journal of Preventive Medicine, 26*(4), 330–343.
Weinstein, N., Rothman, A., & Sutton, S. (1998). Stage theories of health behavior: Conceptual and methodological issues. *Health Psychology, 17*, 290–299.
West, R. (2005). Time for a change: Putting the transtheoretical (stages of change) model to rest. *Addiction, 100*(8), 1036–1039.
Whitelaw, S., Baldwin, S., Bunton, R., & Flynn, D. (2000). The status of evidence and outcomes in stages of change research. *Health Education Research, 15*(6), 707–718.

Standard Deviation

J. Rick Turner
Campbell University College of Pharmacy and Health Sciences, Buies Creek, NC, USA

Definition

A simple measure of dispersion is the range, the arithmetic difference between the greatest (maximum) and the least (minimum) value in a data set. While this characteristic is easily calculated and useful in initial inspections of data sets, by definition it only uses two of the values in a data set. In a large data set most pieces of numerical information are therefore not used in the calculation of the range, and it is not known whether many data points lie close to the minimum, maximum, or mean, or in any other distribution pattern.

Two more sophisticated measures of dispersion are variance and the standard deviation. These measures are intimately related to each other and take account of all values in a data set. The calculation of variance involves calculating the deviation of each data point from the mean of the data set, squaring these values, and summing them. The process of squaring the deviation is mathematically necessary: If the raw deviations were to be summed they would always sum to zero. However, the squaring process creates the problem that the units of measurement of variance are not the same as the units of measurement of the original data. In the vast majority of cases, the data points in our studies are not simply numbers, but numerical representations of information measured in certain units. For example, a systolic blood pressure measurement of "125" is actually a measurement of 125 millimeters of mercury (mmHg). Since the calculation of variance involves squaring certain values, the variance of a set of blood pressure data points would actually be measured in squared millimeters of mercury, a nonsensical unit.

Fortunately, this problem can be solved by simply calculating the square root of the variance. The resulting value is called the standard deviation (SD), and the unit of measurement of the SD is the same as the unit of measurement of the original data points. The SD is a very commonly presented descriptor in research studies. It is usually presented in conjunction with the mean in the form "mean ± SD."

Cross-References

▶ Variance

Standard Normal (Z) Distribution

J. Rick Turner
Campbell University College of Pharmacy and Health Sciences, Buies Creek, NC, USA

Synonyms

Z distribution

Definition

The Standard Normal distribution, also known as the Z distribution, is one particular form of the Normal distribution in which the mean is zero (i.e., 0) and the variance is unity (i.e., 1). This can be written as ($\mu = 0$, $\sigma = 1$).

Before presenting the Z distribution, it is necessary to discuss the Normal distribution in general. Imagine that the heights of a large number of adult males (or females) are measured and the results plotted as a histogram. Height is plotted in inches on the x-axis and the number of people within each height category is plotted on the y-axis. There would be many more people close to the middle of the histogram than close to either end, since more individuals are close to the mean height, and very few are very tall or very short. Given a large sample and decreasingly thin bars in the histogram (that is, the width of the measurement intervals along the x-axis becomes infinitely small such that the height data become continuous), a curve can be superimposed on this histogram. One particular version of a density curve is called the Normal distribution. This distribution is of considerable interest since height and many physiological variables conform very closely (but not perfectly) to this distribution. Since the word normal is used in everyday language, and since its meaning in Statistics is different and important, the word is written in this entry with an upper case N when it is used in its statistical sense.

The Normal distribution has several notable properties:

- The highest point of the Normal curve occurs for the mean of the population. The properties of the Normal distribution ensure that this point is also the median value and the mode.
- The shape of the Normal curve (relatively narrow or relatively broad) is influenced by the standard deviation (SD) of the data. The sides of the curve descend more gently as the standard deviation increases and more steeply as it decreases.
- At a distance of approximately ±2 SDs from the mean, the slopes of the downward curves change from a relatively smooth downward slope to a curve that extends out to infinity and thus never quite reaches the x-axis. For practical purposes, the curve is often regarded as intercepting the x-axis at a distance of ±3 SDs from the mean, but this is an approximation.

Area Under the Normal Curve

The area under the Normal curve is of considerable interest in the discipline of Statistics. That is, it is of considerable interest to define and quantify the area bounded by the Normal curve at the top and the x-axis at the bottom. This area will be defined as 1.00, or as 100%. Given this interest, the final bullet point in the previous list raised an issue that appears problematic. That is, it appears that, if the two lower slopes of the Normal curve never quite reach the x-axis, the area under the curve is never actually fully defined and can therefore never be calculated precisely. Fortunately, this apparent paradox can be solved mathematically.

The solution is related to the observation that the sum of an infinite series can converge to a finite solution. An example that effectively demonstrates the solution here is the geometric series "1/2 + 1/4 + 1/8 + ... ad infinitum." That is, the series starts with 1/2, and every subsequent term is one half of the previous term. Given this, the terms of the series never vanish to zero. However, the sum of them is precisely 1.00. The proof of this is as follows, where the series is represented as S:

$$S = 1/2 + 1/4 + 1/8 + \ldots ad\, infinitum \quad (1)$$

Both sides of this equation are then multiplied by the same value, namely, 2 (multiplying both sides of an equation by a constant means that the sides are still of equal value):

$$2S = 1 + 1/2 + 1/4 + \ldots ad\, infinitum \quad (2)$$

The value S is then subtracted from both sides (subtracting a constant from both sides of an equation means that the sides are still of equal value). First, consider the left-hand side (LHS) of Eq. 2:

LHS of Eq. 2: $2S - S$, which equals S.

Now consider the right-hand side (RHS) of Eq. 2. Subtracting S from this quantity can be represented as:

RHS of Eq. 2: $(1 + 1/2 + 1/4 + \ldots ad\, infinitum) - S$, which equals what, exactly?

To determine the unknown value we can use Eq. 1, which shows that S is equal to $(1/2 + 1/4 + 1/8 + \ldots ad\, infinitum)$. Therefore, the right-hand side of Eq. 2 can be written as follows:

RHS of Eq. 2: $(1 + S) - S$, which equals 1.

Equation 2 can therefore be rewritten as:

$$S = 1$$

Therefore, despite the initial paradoxical nature of the statement, it can indeed be shown that the sum of an infinite series can converge to a finite solution.

Returning to the topic of immediate interest, i.e., the area under the Normal curve, the statement that the terms of the geometric series never vanish to zero can be reinterpreted in this context as saying that the curves of the Normal curve never intercept the x-axis. Despite this statement, however, an adaptation of the proof just provided shows that the area under the Normal curve is indeed precisely equal to 1.00, or 100%. The visual equivalent of this is that there is indeed a defined area under the Normal curve, bounded by the curve and the x-axis, and the value of this area can be represented as 1.00, or 100%. This can be demonstrated formally using integral calculus. It can also be thought of as analogous to the statement that the probability of all mutually exclusive events must sum to 1.00.

It is of particular interest in Statistics that the means of many large samples taken from a particular population are approximately distributed in this Normal fashion, i.e., they are said to be Normally distributed. This is true even when the population data themselves are not Normally distributed. The mathematical properties of a true Normal distribution allow quantitative statements of the area under the curve between any two points on the x-axis. It was just demonstrated that the total area under the Normal curve is 1, or 100%. It is also of interest to know the proportion of the total area under the curve that lies between two points that are equidistant from the mean. These points are typically represented by multiples of the standard deviation (SD). From the properties of the mathematical equation that governs the shape of the Normal curve, it can be shown that:

- The central 90% of the area under the curve lies between the mean ±1.645 SDs
- The central 95% of the area under the curve lies between the mean ±1.960 SDs
- The central 99% of the area under the curve lies between the mean ±2.576 SDs

The area under the curve is representative of the number of data points falling within that range. That is, the percentage of the area under the curve translates directly into the percentage of data points falling between the two identified points. Of particular relevance for many research studies is that 95% of the area under the curve lies between the mean ±1.960 SDs. The value of 1.960 is often rounded up to 2, leading to the statement in many practical examples in textbooks that 95% of the data points fall within the mean ±2 SDs.

The Z Distribution

The Z distribution is such that the mean and the standard deviation in the immediately preceding statements can be removed, leading to the following statements:

- The central 90% of the area under the curve lies between ±1.645.
- The central 95% of the area under the curve lies between ±1.960.
- The central 99% of the area under the curve lies between ±2.576.

This distribution is used extensively in Statistics, and underpins many more complex statistical procedures (Durham and Turner 2008).

Cross-References

▶ Data
▶ Hypothesis Testing
▶ Median
▶ Mode
▶ Probability
▶ Standard Deviation

References and Further Reading

Durham, T. A., & Turner, J. R. (2008). *Introduction to statistics in pharmaceutical clinical trials*. London: Pharmaceutical Press.

Standardized Tobacco Packaging

▶ Plain Tobacco Packaging

State Anxiety

▶ Anxiety

Static Exercise

▶ Isometric/Isotonic Exercise

Statins

Ken Ohashi
Department of General Internal Medicine, National Cancer Center Hospital, Chuo-ku, Tokyo, Japan

Synonyms

HMG-CoA reductase inhibitors

Definition

Statins, also known as HMG-CoA reductase inhibitors, are a class of cholesterol lowering agents that are prescribed worldwide to hyperlipidemic patients who are at high risk for cardiovascular disease. Statins currently on the market include pravastatin, simvastatin, fluvastatin, atorvastatin, rosuvastatin, and pitavastatin. Statins exert their effect through inhibition of 3-hydroxy-3-methylglutaryl coenzyme A (HMG-CoA) reductase, the rate-limiting enzyme of cholesterol biosynthesis in the liver. In many clinical trials, statins have been beneficial both in the primary and secondary prevention of coronary heart disease. Recent clinical and experimental data suggest that the benefit of statins may extend beyond their lipid lowering effects. Those cholesterol-independent or "pleiotropic" effects of statins involve improving endothelial dysfunction, enhancing the stability of atherosclerotic plaques, decreasing oxidative stress and inflammation, and inhibiting the thrombogenesis.

Cross-References

▶ Hyperlipidemia

---

subjects in a research study to infer the likely responses to the same treatment in the general population of patients who would receive the treatment or intervention if it entered general behavioral medicine practice.

The ultimate purpose of the results from a single behavioral medicine study, such as a randomized clinical trial, is not to tell us precisely what happened in that trial, but to gain insight into likely responses to the behavioral treatment or intervention in patients with the disease or condition of clinical concern who would receive the treatment. Inferential statistics allows us to do this.

The treatment effect calculated from the data in the single study is regarded as the treatment effect point estimate. Confidence intervals are then placed around this point estimate. The range of values between the lower limit and the upper limit of the confidence interval represents a range that covers the true but unknown population treatment effect with a specified degree of confidence.

Cross-References

▶ Hypothesis Testing
▶ Randomized Clinical Trial

Statistical Inference

J. Rick Turner
Campbell University College of Pharmacy and Health Sciences, Buies Creek, NC, USA

Synonyms

Inferential statistics

Definition

Statistical inference is a process of using the precise data and results from a specific group of

---

Statistical Inquiry

▶ Surveys

Statistics

J. Rick Turner
Campbell University College of Pharmacy and Health Sciences, Buies Creek, NC, USA

Definition

For present purposes, the discipline of Statistics (recognized here by the use of an upper case

"S") can be usefully defined as an integrated discipline that is critically and fundamentally important in all of the following activities associated with clinical research in behavioral medicine:

- Identifying a research question that needs to be answered.
- Deciding upon the design of the study, the methodology that will be employed, and the numerical information (data) that will be collected.
- Presenting the design, methodology, and data to be collected in a study protocol. This study protocol specifies the manner of data collection and addresses all methodological considerations necessary to ensure the collection of optimum quality data for subsequent statistical analysis.
- Identifying the statistical techniques that will be used to describe and analyze the data in a section within the protocol or in an associated statistical analysis plan, which should be written in conjunction with the study protocol.
- Describing and analyzing the data. This includes analyzing the variation in the data to see if there is compelling evidence that the treatment is safe and effective. This process includes evaluation of the statistical significance of the results obtained and, very importantly, their clinical significance.
- Presenting the results of a clinical study to the research and clinical communities in conference talks and posters, and in journal publications.

Cross-References

▶ Clinical Decision-Making
▶ Hypothesis Testing
▶ Statistical Inference

Stem Cells

Keiki Kumano
Department of Cell Therapy and Transplantation Medicine, The University of Tokyo, Bunkyo-ku, Tokyo, Japan

Definition

Stem cells are found in all multicellular organisms. They are defined by the ability to renew themselves through mitotic cell division (self-renewal) and to generate all the differentiated cell types of the tissue (multipotency). For this definition, one stem cell divides into one father cell that is identical to the original stem cell and another daughter cell that is differentiated.

The mammalian stem cells are divided into two broad types: embryonic stem cells and adult somatic stem cells. Embryonic stem cells are isolated from the inner cell mass of blastocysts, and adult somatic stem cells that are found in adult tissues. In a developing embryo, stem cells can differentiate into all of the specialized embryonic tissues. The stem cells can become any tissue in the body, excluding a placenta. Only the morula's cells are totipotent, able to become all tissues and a placenta.

In adult organisms, stem cells and progenitor cells act as a repair system for the body, replenishing specialized cells, but also maintain the normal turnover of regenerative organs, such as blood, skin, or intestinal tissues. In addition to the definition described above, adult stem cells are thought to be quiescent within the niche, dividing infrequently to generate one stem cell copy and a rapidly cycling cell (transient amplifying cell). Transient amplifying cells undergo a limited number of cell divisions and differentiate into the functional cells of the tissues.

Recently, the third stem cells, artificially established, induced pluripotent stem cells (iPSCs) are generated. Previously, nuclear transfer of embryo into the adult somatic cells is known to be able to reprogram the somatic cells. These are not adult stem cells but rather reprogrammed cells (e.g., epithelial cells) given pluripotent capabilities. So reprogramming factors are thought to exist in the embryo or embryonic stem cells. Using genetic reprogramming with transcription factors, pluripotent stem cells equivalent to embryonic stem cells have been derived from human adult tissue. Shinya Yamanaka and his colleagues used the transcription factors Oct3/4, Sox2, c-Myc, and Klf4 in their experiments on cells from human faces. Another groups used a different set of factors, Oct4, Sox2, Nanog, and Lin28, and more limited combination of these factors (Oct3/4, Sox2, Klf4 (OSK), OS, only Oct3/4) can reprogram the adult tissue.

Stem cell therapy has the potential to dramatically change the treatment of human disease. A number of adult stem cell therapies already exist, particularly bone marrow transplantation that is used to treat hematological disease (leukemia, lymphoma, etc.). In the future, stem cell therapy will be broadened to treat a wider variety of diseases including cancer, neurological diseases, several inherited diseases, and so on.

Cross-References

▶ Genetics
▶ Hematopoietic Stem Cell Transplantation

Stepped Care Models

Carly M. Goldstein[1,2] and Sarah Jones[3]
[1]The Weight Control and Diabetes Research Center, The Miriam Hospital, Providence, RI, USA
[2]Warren Alpert Medical School, Brown University, Providence, RI, USA
[3]Skidmore College, Saratoga Springs, NY, USA

Synonyms

Adaptive interventions; Minimally intensive interventions

Definition

Stepped care models are minimally intensive care models for treating conditions or changing behaviors. Patients are initially typically provided with an easy-to-disseminate, low-cost, minimally intensive intervention. If this does not produce remission of undesirable symptoms or sufficient behavior change, patients are provided with a slightly more intensive and more costly intervention. This continues until patients receive an intervention that produces the desired outcome. Ideally, each patient receives the least resource-intensive yet most effective treatment they need. Stepped care models require repeated assessments to determine if a treatment is effective (and can be stepped down), too burdensome (and should be stepped down), ineffective (and must be stepped up), when another treatment becomes available and more likely to produce better effects (requiring deimplementation of the current treatment and initiation of the new treatment), or inappropriate/unlikely to produce effects (and must be stepped down or discontinued altogether).

Description

Stepped care models involve the systematic process of care for an individual through stages of treatment meant to address the severity of their condition(s). Stepped care models can take many forms at various steps, such as bibliotherapy, computerized services, medications, and in-person treatment (e.g., cognitive behavioral therapy, a medical procedure).

There is a necessity for resource-efficient psychiatric, behavioral, and medical care. Frequently, individuals encounter insufficiently available care options (Jacobi et al. 2017; Carels et al. 2009). Many individuals do not have the financial means, transportation, or time to get the care they need, they do not have access to high-quality care, or the initial care they receive is insufficient to cause meaningful remission of symptoms; rather than pursue adequate care, they discontinue services or experience crisis requiring higher acuity treatment. Such patterns of care utilization are frequently seen in smoking cessation, psychotherapy for depression or severe mental illness, and weight management.

Stepped care models seek to solve these problems by being a resource-efficient form of care that is accessible, cost-effective, and innovative. Stepped care models have shown clinical and medical benefit for numerous populations and treatment needs. For example, stepped care approaches for weight loss have produced better outcomes or similar weight losses (with lower costs) when compared to standard treatments (Waring et al. 2014). Stepped care approaches have also been found to be effective for the treatment of substance use disorders, including reduced overall drug use (Kidorf et al. 2007).

Stepped care programs may use weekly monitoring and initial assessment data to determine whether a patient needs to step up or down in the stepped care model. Patients may be evaluated for the severity and type of disorder they have, and the patient's preferences are also considered when deciding whether to go into the lowest level of care or higher (Waring et al. 2014; Carels et al. 2009). After treatment initiation, a follow-up assessment of regular symptom monitoring helps the clinician to determine if the original treatment should be transitioned to more intensive treatments, less intensive treatments, or if the treatment should be kept the same, according to how the patient is responding to treatment (Carels et al. 2009).

An example of the stepped model program developed for chronic pain includes pain self-management strategies and cognitive behavioral therapy (CBT). A clinical trial targeted musculoskeletal pain in veterans. In this case, the stepped care model kept participants engaged by including constant contact (biweekly) to check engagement in treatment. Participants were also taught self-management strategies on how to deal with their pain, such as goal setting, positive self-talk, and other relaxation techniques (Bair et al. 2015). Results found that a combination of analgesics, self-management strategies, and CBT effectively reduced the effects of pain on veterans' day-to-day lives (Bair et al. 2015).

The stepped care model has also been effective for weight management. In one program using motivation interviewing (MI), a therapeutic technique used to increase motivation for changes in behavior (Carels et al. 2007), participants met for 45–60 min weekly for MI until they reached their weight loss goal. Participants who were in the stepped care condition lost significantly more weight in comparison to non-stepped care participants. Participants in the stepped care condition also self-reported increased physical activity (Carels et al. 2007). In the context of weight management, the stepped care model may be useful in increasing participation and motivation in weight loss programs.

Stepped care models can be incredibly impactful if adopted. The affordability, accessibility, effectiveness, resource efficiency, and immediacy of care of this model could lead to higher rates of individuals in need receiving treatment without undue stress on the healthcare system.

Cross-References

▶ Agile Science
▶ Health Care System
▶ Multilevel Intervention
▶ Patient-Centered Care

References and Further Readings

Bair, M. J., Ang, D., Wu, J., Outcault, D. S., Sargent, C., Kempf, C., Froman, A., Schmid, A., Damush, T., Yu, Z., Davis, W. L., & Kroenke, K. (2015). Evaluation of stepped care for chronic pain (ESCAPE) in veterans of the Iraq and Afghanistan conflicts: A randomized clinical trial. *JAMA Internal Medicine, 175*(5), 682–689. https://doi.org/10.1001/jamainternmed.2015.97.

Carels, R. A., Darby, L., Cacciapaglia, H. M., Konrad, K., Coit, C., Harper, J., Kaplar, E. M., Young, K., Baylen, A. C., & Versland, A. (2007). Using motivational interviewing as a supplement to obesity treatment: A stepped-care approach. *Health Psychology, 26*(3), 369–374. https://doi.org/10.1037/0278-6133.26.3.369.

Carels, R. A., Wott, C. B., Young, K. M., Gumble, A., Darby, L. A., Oehlhof, M. W., Harper, J., & Koball, A. (2009). Successful weight loss with self-help: A stepped-care approach. *Journal of Behavioral Medicine, 32*(6), 503–509. https://doi.org/10.1007/s10865-009-9221-8.

Jacobi, C., Beintner, I., Fittig, E., Trockel, M., Braks, K., Schade-Brittinger, C., & Dempfle, A. (2017). Web-based aftercare for women with bulimia nervosa following inpatient treatment: Randomized controlled efficacy trial. *Journal of Medical Internet Research, 19*(9). https://doi.org/10.2196/jmir.7668.

Kidorf, M., Neufeld, K., King, V. L., Clark, M., & Brooner, R. K. (2007). A stepped care approach for reducing cannabis use in opioid-dependent outpatients. *Journal of Substance Abuse Treatment, 32*(4), 341–347. https://doi.org/10.1016/j.jsat.2006.09.005.

Waring, M. E., Schneider, K. L., Appelhans, B. M., Busch, A. M., Whited, M. C., Rodrigues, S., Lemon, S. C., & Pagoto, S. L. (2014). Early-treatment weight loss predicts 6-month weight loss in women with obesity and depression: Implications for stepped care. *Journal of Psychosomatic Research, 76*(5), 394–399. https://doi.org/10.1016/j.jpsychores.2014.03.004.

Steptoe, Andrew (1951–)

Mika Kivimaki
Epidemiology and Public Health, University College London, London, UK

Biographical Information

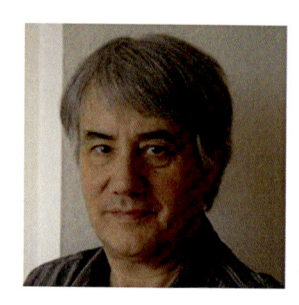

Andrew Steptoe was born in London on April 24, 1951. He is British Heart Foundation Professor of Psychology at University College London, UK, where he is also the Director of the Division of Population Health, a grouping of academic departments including Epidemiology and Public Health, Primary Care and Population Health, Infection and Population Health, and the Medical Research Council Clinical Trials Unit. Steptoe graduated in Natural Sciences from Cambridge in 1972 and completed his Doctorate at Oxford University in 1976. He was appointed lecturer in psychology at St. George's Hospital Medical School in 1977, becoming professor and chair of the Department in 1988. He moved to his present research chair at University College London in 2000, where he is the Director of the Psychobiology Group. Steptoe is also the Director of the English Longitudinal Study of Ageing, a population cohort of older men and women in England.

Major Accomplishments

Steptoe was one of the small group of behavioral medicine specialists, who developed the International Society of Behavioral Medicine (ISBM) in the 1980s. He served as the third President of the ISBM from 1994 to 1996. Additionally, he was the former President of the Society for Psychosomatic Research in the UK. He was the cofounding editor of the *British Journal of Health Psychology* along with Jane Wardle and has served as an associate editor of *Psychophysiology*, the *Annals of Behavioral Medicine*, the *British Journal of Clinical Psychology*, and the *Journal of Psychosomatic Research* and is on the editorial boards of six other journals.

Steptoe is the author of more than 550 journal articles and papers, and author or editor of 17 books, most recently the *Handbook of Behavioral Medicine* (Steptoe 2010) and *Stress and Cardiovascular Disease* (Hjemdahl et al. 2012). His research has addressed many topics in behavioral medicine, including stress and health, socioeconomic status, the determinants of health behavior, health behavior change, cardiovascular disease, respiratory disorders, aging, and positive well-being. His collaborative research with Professor Marmot has focused on understanding the biological processes through which lower socioeconomic status and psychosocial risk factors influence cardiovascular disease risk. This work has involved laboratory studies of the influence of psychosocial factors on cardiovascular, neuroendocrine, and immune function, and naturalistic studies of blood pressure, cortisol, and other biological measures.

Steptoe has advanced our understanding of the psychobiology of health and diseases and the multiple associations between affect and biology in everyday life. He and his team found that people from lower socioeconomic groups tend to suffer the biological effects of stress for longer than more affluent people. This is a potential pathway linking low socioeconomic status with increased risk for coronary heart disease. Further studies by Steptoe's group showed that in some patients, intense episodes of anger and stress occurred in the hours immediately before the onset of chest pain. In experiment settings, episodes of mental stress, similar to those encountered in everyday life, were found to cause transient (up to 4 h) endothelial dysfunction in healthy young individuals. These studies have been important in demonstrating the role of emotional factors in the triggering of coronary ischemia and acute coronary syndromes. Steptoe is also one of the leading scientists on the protective effects of positive affect in physical health.

Steptoe has received many honors for his work. He is a Fellow of the Society of Behavioral Medicine and the Academy of Behavioral Medicine Research in the USA, the Academy of Medical Sciences, the Academy of Learned Societies for the Social Sciences, and the British Psychological Society.

Cross-References

▶ Cardiovascular Disease
▶ Psychological Stress
▶ Socioeconomic Status (SES)
▶ Stress

References and Further Reading

Hjemdahl, P., Rosengren, A., & Steptoe, A. (Eds.). (2012). *Stress and cardiovascular disease*. London: Springer.
Kunz-Ebrecht, S. R., Kirschbaum, C., Marmot, M., & Steptoe, A. (2004). Differences in cortisol awakening response on work days and weekends in women and men from the Whitehall II cohort. *Psychoneuroendocrinology, 29*, 516–528.
Steptoe, A. (Ed.). (2006). *Depression and physical illness*. Cambridge: Cambridge University Press.
Steptoe, A. (Ed.). (2010). *Handbook of behavioral medicine*. New York: Springer.
Steptoe, A., & Appels, A. (Eds.). (1990). *Stress, personal control, and health*. Chichester: Wiley.
Steptoe, A., & Wardle, J. (Eds.). (1994). *Psychosocial processes and health: A reader*. Cambridge: Cambridge University Press.
Steptoe, A., Pollard, T. M., & Wardle, J. (1995). Development of a measure of the motives underlying the selection of food – The food choice questionnaire. *Appetite, 25*, 267–284.
Steptoe, A., Doherty, S., Rink, E., Kerry, S., Kendrick, T., & Hilton, S. (1999). Behavioural counselling in general practice for the promotion of healthy behaviour among adults at increased risk of coronary heart disease: Randomised trial. *BMJ, 319*, 943–947.
Steptoe, A., Cropley, M., Griffith, J., & Kirschbaum, C. (2000). Job strain and anger expression predict early morning elevations in salivary cortisol. *Psychosomatic Medicine, 62*, 286–292.
Steptoe, A., Willemsen, G., Owen, N., Flower, L., & Mohamed-Ali, V. (2001). Acute mental stress elicits delayed increases in circulating inflammatory cytokine levels. *Clinical Science, 101*, 185–192.
Steptoe, A., Wardle, J., & Marmot, M. (2005). Positive affect and health-related neuroendocrine, cardiovascular, and inflammatory processes. *PNAS, 102*, 6508–6512.
Steptoe, A., Hamer, M., & Chida, Y. (2007). The effects of acute psychological stress on circulating inflammatory factors in humans: A review and meta-analysis. *Brain, Behavior, and Immunity, 21*, 901–912.

Stereotypes

▶ Stigma

Steroid Hormones

▶ Estrogen
▶ Steroids

Steroids

Sarah Aldred
School of Sport and Exercise Sciences,
The University of Birmingham, Edgbaston, Birmingham, UK

Synonyms

Steroid hormones

Steroids, Fig. 1 Structure and carbon numbering scheme for cholesterol and other steroids

Definition

A steroid or steroid hormone is a biomolecule derived from cholesterol, with a characteristic structure containing four fused rings (see Fig. 1).

Cholesterol is the precursor for five major classes of steroid hormones: progestagens, glucocorticoids, mineralcorticoids, androgens, and estrogens. These hormones are powerful signaling molecules that are released in order to elicit a specific response.

Androgens, such as testosterone, are responsible for the development of male sex characteristics, whereas estrogens are responsible for the development of female sex characteristics. Dehydroepiandrosterone (DHEA) is the most abundant circulating steroid in humans, and is a precursor for the sex hormones, testerosterone and estradiol. In addition, DHEA is a cortisol antagonist.

Glucocorticoids, such as cortisol, promote the formation of glycogen and inhibit the inflammatory response. They enable humans (and animals) to respond to stress.

Steroids act by interaction with cellular receptors that serve as transcription factors to regulate gene expression. Steroids are incredibly potent and elicit very specific responses due to their interaction with steroid receptors.

Cross-References

▶ Androgen
▶ Cortisol
▶ Estrogen
▶ Inflammation

References and Further Reading

Berg, J. M., Tymoczko, J. L., & Stryer, L. (2002). *Biochemistry* (5th ed.). New York: WH Freeman.
Nussey, S., & Whitehead, S. (2001). *Endocrinology*. Oxford: BIOS Scientific Publishers.

Sterol

▶ Cholesterol

Stigma

Valerie Earnshaw[1] and Stephenie Chaudoir[2]
[1]Department of Public Health, Yale University, New Haven, CT, USA
[2]Department of Psychology, Bradley University, Peoria, IL, USA

Synonyms

Deviance; Discrimination; Prejudice; Stereotypes; Stigmatization

Definition

A stigma is a personal attribute, mark, or characteristic that is socially devalued and discredited (Goffman 1963). A wide variety of attributes are stigmas, including physical illnesses (e.g., HIV/AIDS, tuberculosis, epilepsy), mental illnesses (e.g., schizophrenia, mental disability), social norm violations (e.g., homosexuality, sex work, drug use, obesity), and certain demographic characteristics (e.g., racial/ethnic background, gender, socioeconomic status). People who possess a stigma are perceived and treated negatively by others and ultimately suffer worse physical, psychological, and behavioral outcomes than people who do not possess a stigma.

The following sections describe how certain attributes become socially devalued, how stigma impacts individuals who possess a stigma (i.e., stigmatized people) and who do not possess a stigma (i.e., nonstigmatized people) via a series of stigma mechanisms, and other considerations relevant to stigma. Because HIV/AIDS is one of the strongest stigmas throughout the world and has received a great deal of empirical attention related to stigma (e.g., Aggleton and Parker 2002), it used as the primary example of stigma throughout these sections.

The Social Construction of Stigma

Stigmas are socially constructed (Crocker et al. 1998). In other words, certain attributes become devalued as the result of a social process (Link and Phelan 2001) rather than as the result of innate differences between people who possess the attribute and people who do not possess the attribute. This social process involves stereotyping by associating the attribute with negative characteristics. For example, people living with HIV/AIDS (PLWHA) may be stereotyped to be promiscuous. The social process also involves separating the people who have the attribute into out-group categories. HIV-negative people may view other HIV-negative as part of their social group (i.e., part of "us") but PLWHA as part of a different social group (i.e., part of "them"). Finally, the social process involves experiences of status loss and discrimination by people who have the attribute. PLWHA may not be given medical care because of their HIV-status. Importantly, the social process that results in stigma relies on power. Nonstigmatized people have more power than stigmatized people and use this power to produce and reproduce social inequities and inequalities. This happens in both subtle ways (e.g., stigmatized people being paid systematically less than nonstigmatized people) and blatant ways (e.g., stigmatized people being enslaved by nonstigmatized people).

Because stigma results from a social process, the extent to which an attribute is devalued varies across different social contexts. Social contexts include both individual relationships and cultural contexts. For example, individual people (e.g., friends, family members, employers, and healthcare providers) vary in the degree to which they view HIV/AIDS as a devalued attribute. Similarly, HIV/AIDS may be more devalued in some sociocultural contexts (e.g., Asian cities) than others (e.g., North American cities; Rao et al. 2008). The extent to which an attribute is devalued also varies across time. For example, devaluation associated with HIV/AIDS decreased during the 1990s within the United States (Herek et al. 2002). Taken together, the degree of devaluation associated with a stigma is not universal or fixed; instead, it changes relative to specific social contexts and time periods.

Stigma Mechanisms and Outcomes

Individuals are impacted by stigma via a series of stigma mechanisms. Stigma mechanisms refer to the ways in which people react to either possessing or not possessing a particular stigma (Earnshaw and Chaudoir 2009). Stigma mechanisms, in turn, result in physical, psychological, and behavioral outcomes for both stigmatized and nonstigmatized people. Figure 1 is adapted from the HIV Stigma Framework (Earnshaw and Chaudoir 2009) and shows how stigma leads to stigma mechanisms, which in turn lead to outcomes. Because they represent the link between the social process of stigma and outcomes associated with stigma, stigma mechanisms are often measured by researchers.

Stigma, Fig. 1 Stigma framework

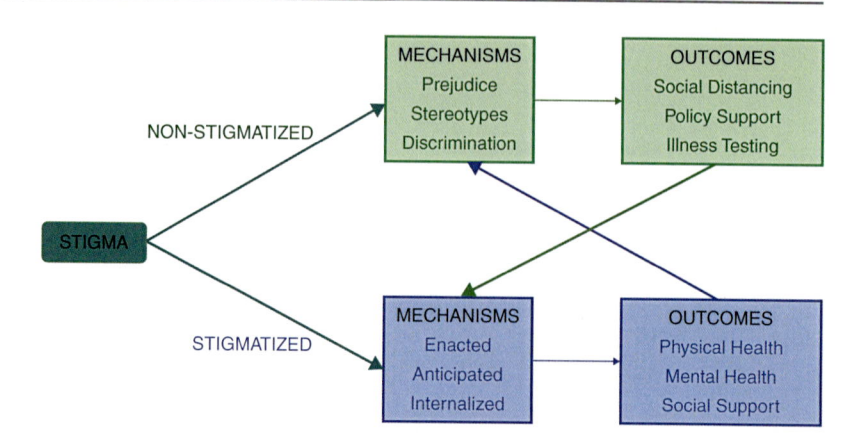

Individuals who do not possess the stigma experience the stigma mechanisms of prejudice, stereotyping, and discrimination. Prejudice refers to negative emotions and feelings toward people who possess the stigma. For example, HIV-negative people may feel disgust toward PLWHA. Stereotypes refer to group-based beliefs about people who possess the stigma. HIV-negative people may believe that PLWHA are mostly gay men. Finally, discrimination refers to behavioral expressions of prejudice directed toward people who possess the stigma. HIV-negative people might refuse to hire, medically treat, or give housing to PLWHA. Although people who do not possess the stigma have more power than people who possess the stigma, people who do not possess the stigma may still suffer negative consequences due to stigma mechanisms. For example, an HIV-negative person who endorses the stereotype that PLWHA are mostly gay men may be less likely to engage in safe sex, be tested for HIV, or seek health care for HIV-related symptoms if they do not identify as a gay man. Consequently, belief in stereotypes can put HIV-negative people at risk for contracting HIV and not receiving treatment.

Individuals who possess the stigma experience the stigma mechanisms of anticipated stigma, enacted stigma, and internalized stigma. Enacted stigma, also called experienced stigma, refers to experiences of prejudice, stereotyping, and/or discrimination. For example, PLWHA may experience social rejection from friends and family members. Anticipated stigma refers to expectations of prejudice, stereotyping, and/or discrimination. PLWHA may expect that they will not be hired by a potential employer. Finally, internalized stigma refers to the endorsement of prejudice and stereotypes associated with one's stigma and applying them to the self. PLWHA may feel that they are dirty due to their HIV status. Further, stigma mechanisms experienced by individuals who do not possess the stigma may impact the outcomes of individuals who do possess the stigma. Discrimination perpetuated by HIV-negative people may be experienced as enacted stigma by PLWHA.

Stigma mechanisms profoundly impact the physical, psychological, and behavioral outcomes of stigmatized individuals. Meta-analytic evidence has shown that stigma mechanisms are associated with decreased physical health (e.g., increased physical illnesses and illness symptoms; Pascoe and Smart Richman 2009) and mental health (e.g., increased depression and decreased self-esteem; Mak et al. 2007). Additionally, stigma mechanisms are associated with maladaptive behaviors which may further undermine the health of stigmatized individuals. For example, stigma mechanisms are related to behaviors such as delayed HIV treatment initiation and non-adherence to medication regimens (Chesney and Smith 1999). Stigma mechanisms are further related to decreased likelihood of disclosure among individuals living with concealable stigmatized identities including HIV/AIDS (Smith et al. 2008).

Other Considerations

Intersectional stigma and layered stigma refer to the possession of multiple stigmas. For example, a gay man living with HIV possesses two stigmas: homosexuality and HIV. Possessing multiple stigmas may exacerbate the impact of stigma on individuals.

Associative stigma, courtesy stigma, and affiliate stigma refer to being connected to someone who possesses a stigma. For example, an HIV-negative man who has a daughter living with HIV/AIDS may experience associative stigma due to his connection to his daughter. People who possess an associative stigma may experience negative outcomes via stigma mechanisms typically reserved for people who possess a stigma.

Concealable stigmas refer to devalued attributes that cannot be seen by others. Examples of concealable stigmas include many physical and mental illnesses and some social norm violations such as homosexuality and drug use. In contrast, visible stigmas refer to devalued attributes that can be seen by others. Examples of visible stigmas include many demographic characteristics such as racial/ethnic background and gender. Whereas people with concealable stigmas can hide their stigma from others in some social interactions, people with visible stigmas cannot.

Cross-References

▶ Discrimination and Health
▶ Health Disparities

References and Readings

Aggleton, P., & Parker, R. (2002). *A conceptual framework and basis for action: HIV/AIDS stigma and discrimination*. Geneva: Joint United Nations Programme on HIV/AIDS.

Allport, G. W. (1954). *The nature of prejudice*. Oxford, UK: Addison-Wesley.

Brewer, M. B., & Brown, R. J. (1998). Intergroup relations. In D. T. Gilbert, S. T. Fiske, & G. Lindzey (Eds.), *The handbook of social psychology* (4th ed., pp. 554–593). Boston: McGraw-Hill.

Chesney, M. A., & Smith, A. W. (1999). Critical delays in HIV testing and care: The potential role of stigma. *The American Behavioral Scientist, 47*, 1162–1174. https://doi.org/10.1177/00027649921954822.

Crocker, J., Major, B., & Steele, C. (1998). Social stigma. In D. T. Gilbert, S. T. Fiske, & G. Lindzey (Eds.), *The handbook of social psychology* (Vol. 2, 4th ed., pp. 504–553). Boston: McGraw-Hill/Distributed exclusively by Oxford University Press.

Earnshaw, V. A., & Chaudoir, S. R. (2009). From conceptualizing to measuring HIV stigma: A review of HIV stigma mechanism measures. *AIDS and Behavior, 13*, 1160–1177. https://doi.org/10.1007/s10461-009-9593-3.

Goffman, E. (1963). *Stigma: Notes on the management of spoiled identity*. New York: Simon & Schuster.

Herek, G. M., Capitanio, J. P., & Widaman, K. F. (2002). HIV-related stigma and knowledge in the United States: Prevalence and trends, 1991–1999. *American Journal of Public Health, 92*, 371–377. https://doi.org/10.2105/ajph.92.3.371.

Jones, E. E., Farina, A., Hastorf, A. H., Markus, H., Miller, D. T., & Scott, R. A. (1984). *Social stigma: The psychology of marked relationships*. New York: W. H. Freeman and Company.

Link, B. G., & Phelan, J. C. (2001). Conceptualizing stigma. *Annual Review of Sociology, 27*, 363–385. https://doi.org/10.1146/annurev.soc.27.1.363.

Major, B., & O'Brien, L. T. (2005). The social psychology of stigma. *Annual Review of Psychology, 56*, 393–421. https://doi.org/10.1146/annurev.psych.56.091103.070137.

Mak, W. W. S., Poon, C. Y. M., Pun, L. Y. K., & Cheung, S. F. (2007). Meta-analysis of stigma and mental health. *Social Science & Medicine, 65*(2), 245–261. https://doi.org/10.1016/j.socscimed.2007.03.015.

Pascoe, E. A., & Smart Richman, L. (2009). Perceived discrimination and health: A meta-analytic review. *Psychological Bulletin, 135*(4), 531–554. https://doi.org/10.1037/a0016059. (Supplemental).

Rao, D., Angell, B., Chow, L., & Corrigan, P. (2008). Stigma in the workplace: Employer attitudes about people with HIV in Beijing, Hong Kong, and Chicago. *Social Science & Medicine, 67*, 1541–1549. https://doi.org/10.1016/j.socscimed.2008.07.024.

Smith, R., Rossetto, K., & Peterson, B. L. (2008). A meta-analysis of disclosure of one's HIV-positive status, stigma and social support. *AIDS Care, 20*(10), 1266–1275. https://doi.org/10.1080/09540120801926977.

Stigmatization

▶ Stigma

Stop Smoking

▶ Smoking Cessation

Strain

▶ Psychological Stress

Stranger Anxiety

▶ Anxiety

Strength Model of Self-Control

▶ Self-Regulatory Capacity

Stress

Kristen Salomon
Department of Psychology, University of South Florida College of Arts and Sciences, Tampa, FL, USA

Synonyms

Anxiety; Distress; Mental stress; Pressure; Psychological stress

Definition

Stress is a transactional process occurring when an event is perceived as relevant to an individual's well-being, has the potential for harm or loss, and requires psychological, physiological, and/or behavioral efforts to manage the event and its outcomes (Lazarus and Folkman 1984). The stimuli or events that cause stress are referred to as stressors (Mason 1975). Stress often results in psychological distress and efforts to cope with the event. Physiological stress responses are often in support of efforts to manage the stressful event and protect the organism from harm (McEwen and Seeman 1999). Stress may not be a uniformly negative experience, as stressful events may also include the potential for benefit and growth (Lazarus & Folkman). Early views of stress focused on physical stress – events that perturb the resting homeostasis of the body, such as changes in temperature or physical injury (McEwen and Seeman 1999). Current views of stress focus heavily on social and psychological sources, with appraisals of the event and the perceived coping resources as key features. Stress may be categorized by its severity, its time course (acute, repeated, or chronic), and degree of control over the stressor. Distinctions also have been made between active coping stressors and passive coping stressors (Obrist 1981). Active coping stressors require overt behavioral action, such as giving a speech or performing a reaction time task, whereas passive coping stressors require that the individual endure without behavioral action, such as watching gruesome photos. Psychological and physiological stress responses have been shown to differ based upon these dimensions (Tomaka et al. 1993).

Cross-References

▶ Coping
▶ Family Stress
▶ Life Events
▶ Perceived Stress
▶ Perceptions of Stress
▶ Physiological Reactivity
▶ Psychological Stress
▶ Stress Responses
▶ Stress, Emotional
▶ Trier Social Stress Test

References and Readings

Cohen, S., Kessler, R. C., & Gordon, L. U. (1995). *Measuring stress: A guide for health and social scientists*. New York: Oxford University Press.

Hobfoll, S. E. (1989). Conservation of resources: A new attempt at conceptualizing stress. *American Psychologist, 44*, 513–524.

Lazarus, R. S., & Folkman, S. (1984). *Stress, appraisal and coping*. New York: Springer.

Mason, J. W. (1975). A historical view of the stress field (Parts I and II). *Journal of Human Stress, 1*, 6–12 & 22–36.

McEwen, B. S., & Seeman, T. (1999). Protective and damaging effects of mediators of stress. Elaborating and testing the concepts of allostasis and allostatic load. *Annals of the NY Academy of Science, 896*, 30–47.

Obrist, P. A. (1981). *Cardiovascular psychophysiology: A perspective*. New York: Plenum Press.

Selye, H. (1956). *The stress of life*. New York: McGraw-Hill.

Tomaka, J., Blascovich, J., Kelsey, R. M., & Leitten, C. L. (1993). Subjective, physiological, and behavioral effects of threat and challenge appraisals. *Journal of Personality and Social Psychology, 65*, 248–260.

Stress and Occupational Health

▶ Psychosocial Work Environment

Stress Appraisals

▶ Perceptions of Stress

Stress Cascade

▶ Neuroendocrine Activation

Stress Diathesis Models

▶ Stress Vulnerability Models

Stress Disorder

▶ Anxiety Disorder

Stress Management

Catherine Benedict
Department of Psychology, University of Miami, Coral Gables, FL, USA

Synonyms

Coping with stress; Relaxation techniques; Stress reduction

Definition

Stress management techniques and interventions can be broadly categorized into skills that are provided via education, relaxation training, psychosocial interventions, and group formats, alone or in combination, that aim to reduce the stress response by targeting coping strategies and relaxation skills.

Description

The deleterious effects of stress on health and well-being are well documented and have led to the incorporation of stress management techniques into many psychosocial treatment protocols, alone or in combination with medical treatments. Chronic stress has been linked to physiologic changes such as neuroendocrine and immune dysregulation, and worsened disease profiles. One of the most prominent associations between stress and poor health has been in the area of cardiovascular risk. For example, evidence suggests that chronic stress is associated with increased sympathetic cardiovascular activity and damage to endothelial functioning, which increases the risk of several cardiovascular conditions, such as arterial hypertension, coronary artery disease, and arrhythmias. Therefore, incorporation of stress management into clinical and research protocols designed to improve health and well-being has become increasingly popular.

The field of stress management is comprised of a variety of methods and techniques. Relaxation skills training methods with the most empirical support include progressive relaxation or progressive muscle relaxation, autogenic training, biofeedback, mental imagery, and other Eastern or Westernized meditation methods. Various cognitive techniques and in some cases, pharmacotherapy, are also part of stress management programs. Other methods that have been incorporated into stress management include listening to relaxing music, massage, aerobic exercise, diaphragmatic breathing, and postural relaxation methods. Some evidence suggests that "active" stress management techniques (e.g., breathing-guided relaxation training) may be more effective in reducing stress symptoms and inducing improved autonomic cardiovascular regulation than "passive" techniques (e.g., massage). Several standardized stress management interventions have been developed and shown to be efficacious in reducing symptoms of stress and improving various indicators of physical and mental health and quality of life. Empirical evidence supports the use of stress management techniques in the treatment of migraines, pain, and other somatic complaints, and have also been used to reduce stress symptoms, improve adjustment, well-being, and quality of life in a range of patient populations, including those diagnosed with type 2 diabetes, coronary heart disease, fibromyalgia, chronic fatigue syndrome (CFS), human immunodeficiency virus (HIV), and cancer.

Stress management intervention strategies range from single session psychosocial treatments to multifaceted treatments involving psychosocial and behavioral modification components. Likewise, intervention aims and target outcomes also range from behavior and lifestyle changes (e.g., diet, exercise, and utilization of stress management techniques) to changes in psychological and physical well-being (e.g., relief of depressive or anxious symptoms, cortisol regulation). It is hypothesized that if one can manage stress effectively, an individual's ability to adopt lifestyle changes that positively impact health outcomes will be maximized. Conversely, chronic stress has been associated with negative lifestyle factors including poor diet, sedentary lifestyle, alcohol and substance use, and poor adherence to medical regimens. Therefore, many stress management programs include medical endpoints such as disease risk factors, disease morbidity, and mortality. For example, stress management interventions in coronary heart disease may include known risk factors as relevant endpoints, such as being overweight or obese, smoking status, blood pressure, cholesterol, lipids, cardiac ischemia (e.g., angina), and number of cardiac events and/or procedures (e.g., myocardial infarction, angioplasty). Endpoints may be measured at proximal, intermediate, or distance time points, depending on the outcome of interest.

Cultural factors have also been shown to be associated with stress and stress management. Although all cultures experience stress and its sequelae, psychosocial sources of stress, the expression of stress symptoms, and the use and acceptability of stress management techniques varies across cultures. For example, evidence suggests that Hispanics are more likely to experience somatic symptoms in response to stress, compared to non-Hispanic Whites. Cultural differences in stress symptoms will likely lead to varying intervention and treatment approaches. Individuals who present with emotional symptoms of stress without a somatic component, for example, receive more treatment in the United States compared to South Korea, a collectivist culture in which individuals are less likely to express signs of emotional distress directly. However, there is no cross-cultural difference between the United States and South Korea in treatment of somatic symptoms of stress, suggesting that treatment methods may be culturally biased.

Stress Management Techniques and Interventions

Many different methods of stress management have been employed with empirical support across a range of populations. Progressive relaxation or progressive muscle relaxation consists of consecutively tensing and relaxing different sets of muscle groups throughout the body, generally starting with the feet and systematically progressing up to the head. Diaphragmatic breathing consists of taking deep breaths in which the diaphragm contracts and the abdomen, rather than the chest, is extended. This type of breathing involves a slow and deep inhalation through the nose, usually to a count of 10, followed by slow and complete exhalation for a similar count; the process is repeated for a preferred number of times to facilitate relaxation. Using mental imagery as a stress management tool involves imagining a scene, place, or event that is considered safe, peaceful, and restful; one that is associated with affective feelings of happiness, job, and contentment. Alternatively, images may involve mental pictures of stress flowing out of the body or being locked away in a padlocked chest. All of the senses are incorporated into the mental imagery exercise and it is encouraged to develop details and complex images that invoke sensual perceptions. The imagined place is used as a retreat from environmental stressors, with the goal of having the body react to imagined scenes of peace and tranquility as if they were real, counteracting the adrenergic effects of stress. These methods have been shown to be beneficial through self-report measures of stress and well-being and physical measures of the body's stress response through biofeedback methods.

Biofeedback is a method that keeps track of the body's physiological responses in real time, generally through machines that measure heart rate, muscle tension, or brain waves. Most often, biofeedback is used as a tool to facilitate control over the stress response sequelae. Individuals are taught to recognize the stress response when it is underway and employ relaxation techniques (e.g., deep breathing, mental imagery, or adaptive cognitive replacement) to calm physiological arousal. Theory and empirical evidence suggest that the real-time feedback of physiological changes in response to stress and the utilization of stress management techniques facilitate learning and adoption of effective relaxation methods into daily life.

Stress Management Programs

Many stress management interventions for clinical populations consist of a combination of methods that frequently incorporate a variety of cognitive and behavioral techniques. For example, cognitive-behavioral stress management (CBSM) interventions have been employed and been shown to have beneficial effects in stressed nonclinical subjects and a range of patient populations. These interventions typically aim to improve adaptive coping and reduce psychological distress through the use of emotion regulation strategies and relaxation training. Didactic training typically addresses stress appraisal and cognitive coping strategies to improve stress management of general- and disease-specific stressors. Often, a psychoeducational component about the nature and consequences of stress and disease processes is also incorporated into intervention protocols. The CBSM protocol consists of a 10-week manualized group intervention in which groups meet for 2 h per week; sessions consist of 90 min of didactic discussion and exercises and 30 min of relaxation training. During the didactic portion of each session, participants are provided information regarding stress awareness, physical responses to stress, and the appraisal process and are taught a variety of cognitive-behavioral techniques designed to manage general- and disease-specific stress. Cognitive techniques include learning to identify cognitive distortions and cognitive restructuring processes (e.g., rational thought replacement), effective coping strategies (e.g., emotional-focused vs. problem-focused coping), and anger management and assertiveness training (e.g., effective communication). Information related to disease physiology, diagnosis, and treatment are also provided and health maintenance strategies are reviewed.

During the relaxation portion, participants are taught a variety of techniques through group relaxation exercises, including progressive muscle relaxation, guided imagery, meditation, and diaphragmatic breathing. Participants are encouraged to practice the techniques at home on a daily basis. The CBSM intervention has been shown to be effective in increasing stress management skills, which has been related to improvements in a number of quality-of-life domains, in HIV, cancer, and CFS populations.

Similarly, some have demonstrated the efficacy of a group-based stress management program that included progressive muscle relaxation training, didactic training in the use of cognitive and behavioral skills to bring awareness to and reduce physiological symptoms of stress (e.g., guided imagery, deep breathing techniques, thought stopping, and recognition of life stressors), and education on the negative effects of stress on health in improving glycemic control in patients with type 2 diabetes. Participants learned stress management techniques in a group-based intervention format and were instructed to practice muscle relaxation at home twice daily with the aid of an audiotape. Specific instructions were given to encourage "mini-practices" (i.e., brief, 30-s versions of a progressive relaxation session) to facilitate the use of stress management and relaxation techniques into daily life. Although similar interventions have been conducted and shown positive effects on blood glucose, findings have been mixed as several others have failed to show a therapeutic effect of stress management on diabetes control.

Mindfulness-based stress reduction (MBSR) is a clinically standardized meditation program, originally developed as a group-based intervention for chronic pain but has since demonstrated efficacy for patients with a range of mental and physical disorders, as well as healthy subjects. The MBSR protocol consists of three different stress management techniques: body scan, which involves focusing on different parts of the body, bringing attention and awareness to sensations and feelings, breath awareness, and relaxation; sitting meditation, which involves focusing on body sensations and breathe, as well as nonjudgmental awareness of the cognitions and the stream of thoughts and distractions that pass through the mind; and Hatha yoga practice, which consists of breathing exercises, stretching, and postural exercises designed to strengthen and relax the musculoskeletal system. The MBSR program is an 8- to 10-week group intervention in which sessions typically last 2.5 h, with an additional single all-day session per course. Homework of at least 45 min a day, 6 days a week, is also encouraged, which may consist of meditation practice, mindful yoga, and/or incorporating mindfulness into daily life. Groups may be either homogenous or heterogeneous with regard to illnesses or presenting problems of participants. Empirical evidence provides consistent and relatively strong effect sizes regarding the efficacy of MBSR on a number of psychological (e.g., depressive and anxiety symptoms, coping style) and physical (e.g., medical symptoms, sensory pain, physical impairment, and functional quality of life) well-being in clinical and nonclinical populations. Clinical populations have included patients diagnosed with anxiety disorders, depression, chronic pain, fibromyalgia, cancer, and stress related to environmental contexts (e.g., medical school, prison life), as well as relatively healthy individuals interested in improving their ability to cope with normal stressors of daily living.

Stress management interventions for healthy and patient populations are promising. However, findings have been mixed and the literature is limited by measurement and research design problems, insufficient information regarding intervention components and protocol fidelity, clinical relevance of statistically significant effects, and feasibility and dissemination concerns regarding the translation of research protocols into clinical practice. Nevertheless, given the detrimental effects of stress on psychological and physical well-being, further research is needed using large-scale, randomized clinical trials, with sound methodological procedures that include objective markers of health and disease status, in addition to self-report measures of psychosocial well-being and functional indicators of distress.

Cross-References

▶ Anger Management

References and Readings

Antoni, M. H., Lechner, S. C., Kazi, A., Wimberly, S. R., Sifre, T., Urcuyo, K. R., Phillips, K., Glück, S., & Carver, C. S. (2006). How stress management improves quality of life after treatment for breast cancer. *Journal of Consulting and Clinical Psychology, 74*(6), 1143–1152.

Blumenthal, J. A., Sherwood, A., Babyak, M. A., Watkins, L. L., Waugh, R., Georgiades, A., Bacon, S. L., Hayano, J., Coleman, R. E., & Hinderliter, A. (2005). Effects of exercise and stress management training on markers of cardiovascular risk in patients with ischemic heart disease. *Journal of the American Medical Association, 293*(13), 1626–1634.

Brown, J. L., & Vanable, P. A. (2008). Cognitive-behavioral stress management interventions for personal living with HIV: A review and critique of the literature. *Annals of Behavioral Medicine, 35*, 26–40.

Chiesa, A., & Serretti, A. (2009). Mindfulness-based stress reduction for stress management in healthy people: A review and meta-analysis. *The Journal of Alternative and Complementary Medicine, 15*(5), 593–600.

Gaab, J., Blattler, N., Menzi, T., Pabst, B., Stoyer, S., & Ehlert, U. (2003). Randomized controlled evaluation of the effects of cognitive-behavioral stress management on cortisol responses to acute stress in healthy subjects. *Psychoneuroendocrinology, 28*, 767–779.

Lehrer, P. M., Carr, R., Sargunaraj, D., & Woolfolk, R. L. (1994). Stress management techniques: Are they all equivalent, or do they have specific effects? *Biofeedback and Self-Regulation, 19*(4), 353–401.

Lehrer, P. M., Woolfolk, R. L., & Sime, W. E. (Eds.). (2007). *Principles and practice of stress management*. New York: Guildford.

Lucini, D., Malacarne, M., Solaro, N., Busin, S., & Pagani, M. (2009). Complementary medicine for the management of chronic stress: Superiority of active versus passive techniques. *Journal of Hypertension, 27*, 2421–2428.

McEwen, B. S. (2007). Physiology and neurobiology of stress and adaptation: Central role of the brain. *Physiological Reviews, 87*, 873–904.

Smith, J. E., Richardson, J., Hoffman, C., & Pilkington, K. (2005). Mindfulness-based stress reduction as supportive therapy in cancer care: Systematic review. *Journal of Advanced Nursing, 52*(3), 315–327.

Surwit, R. S., van Tilburg, M. A., Zucker, N., McCaskill, C. C., Parekh, P., Feinglos, M. N., Edwards, C. L., Williams, P., & Lane, J. D. (2002). Stress management improves long-term glycemic control in type 2 diabetes. *Diabetes Care, 25*(1), 30–34.

Stress Mindset

Jacob J. Keech and Kyra Hamilton
School of Applied Psychology, Menzies Health Institute Queensland, Griffith University, Brisbane, QLD, Australia

Synonyms

Beliefs about stress; Implicit theories; Lay beliefs

Definition

Stress mindset refers to a set of beliefs individuals hold about the consequences of experiencing stress. This includes the belief that stress has enhancing consequences (i.e., a stress-is-enhancing mindset) and the contrasting belief that stress has debilitating consequences (i.e., a stress-is-debilitating mindset) for health and vitality, performance and productivity, and learning and growth (Crum et al. 2013). Stress mindset contrasts with transactional stress appraisal (Lazarus & Folkman 1984); in that the former concerns beliefs about the stress response in general which is theorized to apply across situations, whereas the latter is a single response to a stressor in a particular situation.

Description

Mindsets refer to the beliefs about the malleability of personal qualities that serve as a mental lens or framework through which people make predictions about and judge the meaning of life events (Dweck et al. 1995; Yeager & Dweck 2012). Mindsets are otherwise known as implicit theories in the literature. The term "implicit" is ascribed to these beliefs as they tend not to be explicitly articulated (Dweck et al. 1995; Yeager & Dweck 2012). However, it is not clear whether mindsets are truly implicit and operating outside of conscious awareness, consistent with dual-process theories of cognition and behavior.

Crum et al. (2013) applied the mindset concept to stress research, finding that stress mindset influences a range of stress-related outcomes and is distinct from other important variables in the stress process, such as stressor appraisal and amount of stress. Supporting the notion that stress mindset is a distinct variable in the stress process, Kilby and Sherman (2016) found stress mindset exhibited a moderate correlation with challenge appraisal and no significant correlation with threat appraisal following a mathematics stressor task. They also found no significant difference in stress mindset scores before and after the stressor task, suggesting that stress mindset may not be influenced by stressful events. The potential implicit operation of stress mindset was explored by Keech et al. (2018) using an implicit association test (IAT) based on the single-category procedure (Karpinski & Steinman 2006). Despite the reliability of the test being adequate, the test was not related to any of the outcome variables or the explicit measure of stress mindset. Given this was preliminary research, further studies are needed to understand the processes through which stress mindsets operate.

Mean stress mindset scores across a range of observational studies and experimental studies premanipulation indicate that on average people by default tend to endorse a stress-is-debilitating mindset (Crum et al. 2013, 2017; Keech et al. 2018; Kilby & Sherman 2016; Park et al. 2018). Crum et al. (2013) argue that this is due to public health messages being framed around the requirement of reducing stress to prevent negative consequences. Despite these defaults, several studies have demonstrated that stress mindsets are malleable, with mean mindset scores rising to a level that reflects endorsing a stress-is-enhancing mindset following an experimental manipulation (Crum et al. 2013, 2017).

Measuring Stress Mindset

To date, two self-report measures of stress mindset have been published: the Stress Mindset Measure (SMM; Crum et al. 2013) and the Stress Control Mindset Measure (SCMM; Keech et al. 2018). The SMM is an eight-item scale that examines the extent to which an individual holds a stress-is-enhancing mindset. There is a general and a stressor-specific version. No known studies have been published using the specific version following its initial publication. Crum et al. (2013) describe stress-is-enhancing and stress-is-debilitating mindsets as two ends of a spectrum, and items in the SMM are presented as fixed-enhancing (e.g., "Experiencing stress enhances my performance and productivity") versus fixed-debilitating (e.g., "Experiencing stress debilitates my performance and productivity"). However, many people have non-enhancing experiences of stress, and stress can be both enhancing and debilitating. Preliminary evidence from experimental research also suggests that presenting a balanced view of stress rather than a positive or negative view of stress alone yields lower heart rates and diastolic blood pressure following a laboratory-induced stressor (Liu et al. 2017). Arguing that the polarized approach to measurement of stress mindset diverges from how the construct was conceptualized by Crum et al. (2013) and from mindset theory more broadly (e.g., Dweck et al. 1995; Job et al. 2015), Keech et al. (2018) developed the 15-item SCMM. The SCMM is framed to assess the extent to which an individual holds the mindset that stress "can be" enhancing (e.g., "Stress can be used to enhance your performance and productivity").

Associations Between Stress Mindset and Health-Related Outcomes

Several experimental and correlational studies have observed effects of stress mindset on health and wellbeing, physiological, and affective outcomes in response to laboratory stressor tasks and ecological stress experiences over short periods of time. For example, Crum et al. (2017), in an experimental study examining the influence of stress mindset on a range of outcomes in response to a laboratory stressor, found those who were primed with a stress-is-enhancing mindset exhibited greater positive but not negative affect when anticipating and following the induced stressor. Other studies have examined the association between stress mindset and health and wellbeing outcomes in the context of ecological experiences of stress. Park et al. (2018) found that stress mindset moderated the effect of stressful life events on perceived distress (mediator) and in turn self-control. Keech et al. (2018) found that stress mindset predicted proactive coping behavior under stress, perceived general somatic symptoms, perceived distress, perceived physical health, and, indirectly, psychological wellbeing. Crum et al. (2013) observed a small effect of a stress mindset manipulation on depression and anxiety symptoms from baseline to three days postintervention among company employees.

Two studies have examined the physiological effects of stress mindset when faced with laboratory-induced stressors. Crum et al. (2013) reported that stress mindset moderated the effect of a laboratory-induced stressor on cortisol, yet Crum et al. (2017) found no effect of stress mindset on cortisol in anticipation of, and following, a laboratory-induced stressor. These physiological effects should therefore be interpreted with caution and further research is required to replicate these findings. Crum et al. (2017) also found a quadratic effect of stress mindset on dehydroepiandrosterone sulfate (DHEAS) – a neurosteroid hormone which in reduced levels may increase vulnerability to neurotoxic effects of stress (Maninger et al. 2009) – with those in the enhancing condition experiencing sharper increases and sharper declines in DHEAS prior to and following the laboratory-induced stressor.

Two correlational studies support that stress mindset influences coping responses. Measuring workload anticipation and approach coping daily over five days, Casper et al. (2017) found that employees endorsing a stress-is-enhancing mindset made more approach-coping efforts in anticipation of a high workload. Keech et al. (2018) also found in a cross-sectional study that stress mindset predicted proactive coping behavior under stress.

Providing further evidence to support these notions that beliefs about stress can influence health outcomes, two large national longitudinal studies have found the perception that stress is affecting one's health to be associated with premature death in the United States (Keller et al. 2012) and adverse cardiovascular events in the United Kingdom (Nabi et al. 2013).

How Could Stress Mindset Improve Health?

Keech et al. (2018) proposed a stress beliefs model outlining two mechanisms through which stress mindsets may improve health and wellbeing outcomes. The first of which is that those endorsing more of an enhancing stress mindset would favor more proactive behaviors when coping with stress. The study demonstrated empirically that proactive behavior under stress mediated the influence of stress mindset on psychological wellbeing and perceived stress. Further research is required to evaluate causal links and to examine the role of more emotion-focused coping behaviors under stress in this process.

The second mechanism proposed by Keech et al. (2018) is that those endorsing more of an enhancing stress mindset may interpret the physiological arousal characteristic of the stress response as less adverse than those holding more of a debilitating stress mindset. Keech et al. (2018) provided preliminary empirical support for this process, finding that self-reported perceived general somatic symptoms mediated the effect of stress mindset on psychological wellbeing, perceived stress, and perceived physical health. Further investigation of this process is required. One line of future enquiry is examining whether stress mindsets influence the use of situational cognitive strategies such as arousal reappraisal when under stress (Jamieson et al. 2012).

Conclusion and Future Directions

While preliminary evidence points to positive outcomes being associated with eliciting a stress-is-enhancing mindset prior to the experience of laboratory-induced stressors and ecological stressors over a short period of time, observed effects have been small to medium in magnitude, and it remains unclear whether these mindsets would be activated during the experience of acute and chronic ecological stressors with established links to adverse health outcomes over longer periods of time. Future research should seek to investigate the influence of stress mindset in these contexts to better understand whether these mindsets can be leveraged to meaningfully reduce the impact of stress on health. Further exploration of the mechanisms through which stress mindsets may influence outcomes is also important for maximizing intervention effects and for determining appropriate applications of these interventions.

Cross-References

▶ Lay Beliefs
▶ Perceived Stress
▶ Perceptions of Stress
▶ Stress Management
▶ Stress: Appraisal and Coping

References and Further Reading

Casper, A., Sonnentag, S., & Tremmel, S. (2017). Mindset matters: The role of employees' stress mindset for day-specific reactions to workload anticipation. *European Journal of Work and Organizational Psychology, 26*(6), 798–810. https://doi.org/10.1080/1359432X.2017.1374947.

Crum, A. J., Salovey, P., & Achor, S. (2013). Rethinking stress: The role of mindsets in determining the stress response. *Journal of Personality and Social Psychology, 104*(4), 716–733. https://doi.org/10.1037/a0031201.

Crum, A. J., Akinola, M., Martin, A., & Fath, S. (2017). The role of stress mindset in shaping cognitive, emotional, and physiological responses to challenging and threatening stress. *Anxiety, Stress, and Coping, 30*(4), 379–395. https://doi.org/10.1080/10615806.2016.1275585.

Dweck, C. S., Chiu, C., & Hong, Y. (1995). Implicit theories and their role in judgments and reactions: A word from two perspectives. *Psychological Inquiry, 6*(4), 267–285. https://doi.org/10.1207/s15327965pli0604_1.

Jamieson, J. P., Nock, M. K., & Mendes, W. B. (2012). Mind over matter: Reappraising arousal improves cardiovascular and cognitive responses to stress. *Journal of Experimental Psychology: General, 141*(3), 417–422. https://doi.org/10.1037/a0025719.

Job, V., Walton, G. M., Bernecker, K., & Dweck, C. S. (2015). Implicit theories about willpower predict self-regulation and grades in everyday life. *Journal of Personality and Social Psychology, 108*(4), 637–647. https://doi.org/10.1037/pspp0000014.

Karpinski, A., & Steinman, R. B. (2006). The single category implicit association test as a measure of implicit social cognition. *Journal of Personality and Social Psychology, 91*(1), 16–32. https://doi.org/10.1037/0022-3514.91.1.16.

Keech, J. J., Hagger, M. S., O'Callaghan, F. V., & Hamilton, K. (2018). The influence of university students' stress mindsets on health and performance outcomes. *Annals of Behavioral Medicine, 52*(12), 1046–1059. https://doi.org/10.1093/abm/kay008.

Keller, A., Litzelman, K., Wisk, L. E., Maddox, T., Cheng, E. R., Creswell, P. D., & Witt, W. P. (2012). Does the perception that stress affects health matter? The association with health and mortality. *Health Psychology, 31*(5), 677. https://doi.org/10.1037/a0026743.

Kilby, C. J., & Sherman, K. A. (2016). Delineating the relationship between stress mindset and primary appraisals: Preliminary findings. *SpringerPlus, 5*, 336. https://doi.org/10.1186/s40064-016-1937-7.

Lazarus, R. S., & Folkman, S. (1984). *Stress, appraisal, and coping*. New York: Springer Publishing.

Liu J. J. W., Vickers K., Reed M., Hadad M. (2017). Reconceptualizing stress: Shifting views on the consequences of stress and its effects on stress reactivity. *PLoS ONE, 12*, e0173188

Maninger, N., Wolkowitz, O. M., Reus, V. I., Epel, E. S., & Mellon, S. H. (2009). Neurobiological and neuropsychiatric effects of dehydroepiandrosterone (DHEA) and DHEA sulfate (DHEAS). *Frontiers in Neuroendocrinology, 30*(1), 65–91. https://doi.org/10.1016/j.yfrne.2008.11.002.

Nabi, H., Kivimäki, M., Batty, G. D., Shipley, M. J., Britton, A., Brunner, E. J., . . ., & Singh-Manoux, A. (2013). Increased risk of coronary heart disease among individuals reporting adverse impact of stress on their health: The Whitehall II prospective cohort study. *European Heart Journal, 34*(34), 2697–2705. https://doi.org/10.1093/eurheartj/eht216.

Park, D., Yu, A., Metz, S. E., Tsukayama, E., Crum, A. J., & Duckworth, A. L. (2018). Beliefs about stress attenuate the relation among adverse life events, perceived distress, and self-control. *Child Development, 89*(6), 2059–2069. https://doi.org/10.1111/cdev.12946.

Yeager, D. S., & Dweck, C. S. (2012). Mindsets that promote resilience: When students believe that personal characteristics can be developed. *Educational Psychologist, 47*(4), 302–314. https://doi.org/10.1080/00461520.2012.722805

Stress Reactivity

Wolff Schlotz
Institute of Experimental Psychology, University of Regensburg, Regensburg, Germany

Synonyms

Stress responsivity

Definition

Stress reactivity is the capacity or tendency to respond to a stressor. It is a disposition that underlies individual differences in responses to stressors and is assumed to be a vulnerability factor for the development of diseases.

Description

People respond differently when exposed to the same stressor. Such differences can be observed in all four major stress response domains, namely, physiology, behavior, subjective experience, and cognitive function. Within the physiological domain, two response systems are of particular importance: cardiovascular responses (indicated by blood pressure and heart rate), driven by sympathetic nervous system (SNS) activity, and output of the glucocorticoid hormone cortisol from the adrenal cortex, driven by hypothalamic-pituitary-adrenal (HPA) axis activity. Stress reactivity is assumed to be stable over time, i.e., persons showing high responses at an initial assessment also show high responses when the assessment is repeated at a later time. Stress reactivity can be conceptualized as specific or general. Whereas specific stress reactivity reflects reactivity of a particular response system (e.g., cardiovascular stress reactivity; endocrine stress reactivity; affective stress reactivity), general stress reactivity is indicated by aggregation of responses across domains and/or stressors.

The relevance of stress reactivity for behavioral medicine rests primarily on the assumption that high stress reactivity is assumed to be a vulnerability factor for disease that predicts disease outcome variance independently of well-established risk factors. As early as in the first half of the twentieth century it was proposed that the size of blood pressure responses to placing the hand in cold water (cold pressor test) would indicate the risk of later development of hypertension. More recently, a growing body of evidence from longitudinal studies that used laboratory stress tests support the assumption that cardiovascular stress reactivity is indeed a risk factor for subclinical and clinical cardiovascular disease. This has been shown for both physiological stressors such as the cold pressor test and psychological stressors such as pressure to perform in a social situation (e.g., public speaking). On the basis of this evidence it has been concluded that cardiovascular stress reactivity is a risk factor for cardiovascular disease in addition to the classic risk factors of family history, obesity, smoking, diabetes mellitus, and hypercholesterolemia. As for endocrine stress reactivity, a few longitudinal studies found evidence for associations between endocrine stress reactivity and increased risk for disease. However, this research area is much less developed than that for cardiovascular stress reactivity, and the evidence is less robust. Finally, it has been suggested that endocrine and affective stress reactivity might be a risk factor for the development of mental disorders such as psychosis, depression, and anxiety disorders. Again, research in this area is still relatively scarce and the evidence mostly relies on cross-sectional studies.

In contrast to specific stress reactivity, the concept of general stress reactivity emphasizes generalizability of responses across response systems and stressors. It is based on the notion that stress responses have a common origin in brain areas that mediate activation of the HPA axis and the SNS, as well as behavioral and subjective-emotional responses. In particular, hippocampus, amygdala, and prefrontal cortex are higher central mediators of subjective-emotional responses. These areas are functionally connected to the hypothalamic and brainstem nuclei which are critical in activating the HPA axis and the SNS. If a stressor is processed in higher brain areas, stress responses are expected to show relatively high covariance. This is to be expected for psychological stressors, but less so for physiological stressors. Thus, dissociations between responses systems might reflect individual differences at both levels. In addition, observed physiological stress responses are influenced by peripheral factors such as receptor sensitivity in the periphery or vascular resistance. Although high covariance between response systems would be expected, a number of factors such as different dynamics of the response systems, habituation effects, measurement error, and limited variance due to limited stressor intensity act at attenuating associations between responses.

Complementary to the notion of general stress reactivity, the concepts of individual response specificity (IRS) and stimulus response specificity (SRS) reflect observations of dissociation between response systems or stressors. The concept of IRS describes individual differences in patterns of responses, for example, one person might respond to stressors with a high blood pressure but low cortisol increase, whereas another person might also show a high cortisol increase. SRS describes such response patterns as related to stressors, for example, it has been proposed that the HPA axis in humans is activated by stressors that include social evaluative threat, but not by cognitive effort without that component. In research, it is often difficult to reliably detect general stress reactivity, IRS or SRS response patterns. Although there is now increasing evidence for the concept of general stress reactivity, associations between responses are usually moderate. Therefore, it is important to note that it is not possible to use the stress response in one domain or system as a general indicator of responses in other domains. Although it has been suggested that such dissociations might present useful information about psychobiological responses systems of an individual that could be valuable for behavioral medicine, to date little is known about the stability and implications of response dissociations.

Stress reactivity can be assessed both in the laboratory and in daily life. The major advantage of laboratory stress tests is the high degree of standardization over the conditions implemented. However, stress responses in the laboratory have limited ecological validity, i.e., do not necessarily reflect stress reactivity in daily life. For that reason, ambulatory assessment methods are increasingly used and present the opportunity to assess real-time stress reactivity in daily life for both research and clinical practice. A number of factors influence stress reactivity, with implications for clinical decisions. For example, it is known that stress reactivity is associated with sex, age, ethnicity, personality factors, preexisting disease, and the presence or absence of chronic stress. Due to such moderating factors there is a wide range of associations between stress reactivity and disease outcome. Therefore, the predictive value varies across individuals, making it difficult to use stress reactivity scores in clinical practice. Although the reliability of stress reactivity assessments could be increased by assessing aggregated stress responses in a repeated measure/multiple stressors design, few studies have implemented this design due to the high demands on resources. It would be expected that stronger and more consistent association with disease could be observed with such a design. Finally, an important conclusion from the variety of findings on associations between stress response systems is that, as mentioned above, a single assessment of one response system cannot be used as an indicator for stress responses in other systems. The notion of a consistent "gold-standard" indicator of stress reactivity is not supported by the research literature.

As the assessment of physiological stress responses is relatively expensive and fraught with practical problems, clinicians often rely on retrospective self-reports of individual stress experience to assess stress reactivity. However, such subjective measures of stress experience confound individual stress reactivity with frequency of exposure to daily life stress. Recently, a self-report instrument for the assessment of perceived stress reactivity has been developed and evaluated. Although retrospective self-report methods cannot replace real-time measures, they present an opportunity to assess patients' perceptions of their own stress reactivity in daily life when resources to assess real-time responses are lacking or when such self-observations are of primary interest.

Stress reactivity is assumed to be a consequence of the individual genetic makeup and early environmental factors. Quantitative genetic studies using mainly twin designs have concluded that approximately 50% of the variance in stress responses is due to genetic factors. However, there is some variability of estimates between studies, and the amount of heritability seems to change with repeated exposure to the same stressor. Molecular genetic studies have revealed a number of single gene variants that might influence stress responses in different systems, although many of these effects of candidate genes need replication before valid conclusions can be drawn. In addition to genetic makeup, factors of the environment early in life have been shown to influence stress reactivity. A number of studies suggest that an adverse prenatal environment might exert long-term effects on stress reactivity in the offspring. Similarly, adverse early postnatal environmental factors such as maternal care or abuse have been shown to affect stress reactivity, with consequences for the risk of mental disorder later in life. Animal studies have suggested that such early environmental effects might be mediated by epigenetic changes in specific brain areas.

Despite good evidence for the prediction of cardiovascular disease by cardiovascular stress reactivity, potential pathways and causal chains of effects are unclear. In addition, not all individuals with high cardiovascular stress reactivity later develop cardiovascular disease. This points at another factor implicated in the pathway. It is likely that high stress reactivity leads to disease particularly if a highly stress reactive individual is exposed to chronic stress in daily life (diathesis-stress model). Other areas of discussion are the potential adaptive function of high stress reactivity in an evolutionary context, and the significance of low levels of stress reactivity for the development of diseases and disorders.

Cross-References

▶ General Adaptation Syndrome
▶ Hypothalamic-Pituitary-Adrenal Axis
▶ Individual Differences
▶ Physiological Reactivity
▶ Stress
▶ Stress Responses
▶ Stress Test
▶ Stress Vulnerability Models
▶ Stressor
▶ Sympathetic Nervous System (SNS)

References and Readings

Chida, Y., & Steptoe, A. (2010). Greater cardiovascular responses to laboratory mental stress are associated with poor subsequent cardiovascular risk status: A meta-analysis of prospective evidence. *Hypertension, 55*(4), 1026–1032.

Contrada, R. J., & Baum, A. (Eds.). (2010). *The handbook of stress science: Biology, psychology, and health.* New York: Springer.

Heim, C., & Nemeroff, C. B. (2001). The role of childhood trauma in the neurobiology of mood and anxiety disorders: preclinical and clinical studies. *Biological Psychiatry, 49*(12), 1023–1039.

Kudielka, B. M., Hellhammer, D. H., & Wust, S. (2009). Why do we respond so differently? Reviewing determinants of human salivary cortisol responses to challenge. *Psychoneuroendocrinology, 34*(1), 2–18.

Lovallo, W. R. (2005). *Stress and health: Biological and psychological interactions* (2nd ed.). Thousand Oaks: Sage.

Manuck, S. B., & McCaffery, J. M. (2010). Genetics of stress: Gene-stress correlation and interaction. In A. Steptoe (Ed.), *Handbook of behavioral medicine: Methods and applications* (pp. 455–478). New York: Springer.

Myin-Germeys, I., & van Os, J. (2007). Stress-reactivity in psychosis: Evidence for an affective pathway to psychosis. *Clinical Psychology Review, 27*(4), 409–424.

Phillips, D. I. (2007). Programming of the stress response: A fundamental mechanism underlying the long-term effects of the fetal environment? *Journal of Internal Medicine, 261*(5), 453–460.

Schlotz, W., Yim, I. S., Zoccola, P. M., Jansen, L., & Schulz, P. (2011). The perceived stress reactivity scale: Measurement invariance, stability and validity in three countries. *Psychological Assessment, 23*(1), 80–94.

Treiber, F. A., Kamarck, T., Schneiderman, N., Sheffield, D., Kapuku, G., & Taylor, T. (2003). Cardiovascular reactivity and development of preclinical and clinical disease states. *Psychosomatic Medicine, 65*(1), 46–62.

Ulrich-Lai, Y. M., & Herman, J. P. (2009). Neural regulation of endocrine and autonomic stress responses. *Nature Reviews Neuroscience, 10*(6), 397–409.

Stress Reduction

▶ Stress Management

Stress Response

▶ Immune Responses to Stress
▶ Neuroendocrine Activation
▶ Psychophysiologic Reactivity

Stress Responses

Kristen Salomon
Department of Psychology, University of South Florida College of Arts and Sciences, Tampa, FL, USA

Synonyms

Stress; Stress reactivity

Definition

Stress responses are psychological, physiological, and behavioral responses to an event perceived as relevant to one's well being with some potential for harm or loss and requiring adaptation. Psychological stress responses often include negative emotions, such as anxiety, distress, or anger, although positive emotional states related to feeling challenged and driven may also occur. Cognitive efforts aimed at coping with the stressor, such as planning, distancing, and/or reinterpreting, also occur (Lazarus and Folkman 1984). Physiological stress responses are often those that are in support of coping with or fleeing from the stressor, and protecting the organism from potential harm. These responses include, but are not limited to, changes in heart rate, blood pressure, cortisol, and immune function (Sapolsky 1994). Behavioral stress responses involve actions also aimed at coping with or fleeing from the stressful event, such as actively performing a task or withdrawing effort from a situation perceived as impossible (Lazarus and Folkman 1984).

Cross-References

▶ Coping
▶ Physiological Reactivity

References and Readings

Cacioppo, J. T. (1994). Social neuroscience: Autonomic, neuroendocrine, and immune responses to stress. *Psychophysiology, 31*, 113–128.

Cohen, S., Kessler, R. C., & Gordon, L. U. (1995). *Measuring stress: A guide for health and social scientists.* New York: Oxford University Press.

Lazarus, R. S., & Folkman, S. (1984). *Stress, appraisal and coping.* New York: Springer.

Sapolsky, R. M. (1994). *Why zebras don't get ulcers.* New York: Holt.

Stress Responsivity

▶ Stress Reactivity

Stress Test

Jet J. C. S. Veldhuijzen van Zanten
School of Sport, Exercise and Rehabilitation Sciences, University of Birmingham, Birmingham, UK

Synonyms

Mental stress task; Psychological stress task; Psychological stressor

Definition

Laboratory mental stress tasks are commonly used in behavioral medicine to assess the physiological responses to a standardized stressor in a controlled setting (Turner 1994).

Description

Even though originally it was thought that particularly exaggerated physiological responses to mental stress can be predictive of cardiovascular disease (Obrist 1981), there is now growing evidence that blunted physiological responses can also be associated with poor health (Carroll et al. 2009). Other evidence is available that not the responses to mental stress itself but the physiological recovery upon completion of the stress task can be related with the poor health outcomes (Larsen and Cristenfeld 2011). There is a large body of research that explores the associations between psychological traits (e.g., competitiveness and hostility) and mental disorders (e.g., depression and anxiety) with the individual differences in physiological responses to mental stress (Lovallo 1997). Participants that have been included in these stress studies comprise of young healthy participants, elderly people, and a wide variety of clinical populations. This section will describe the general setup of a laboratory stress task and the most commonly used mental stress tasks in behavioral medicine. Even though the focus will be on mental stress tasks, it is worth noting that physical tests, such as exercise, tilt test, and cold pressor, are also readily used in laboratory settings.

In order to assess the physiological responses to a mental stress task, it is important to assess the resting physiological state of the participant. To quantify the stress response, a reactivity score is calculated, which is the difference between the physiological activity during the stress task and the activity during the rest period (Turner 1994). A typical stress session starts with a resting period of 15–30 min, during which the participant is relaxed. Relaxation can be facilitated by listening to music, reading magazines, or watching a low-stimulating video. This is followed by an explanation of the stress task with, where appropriate, a brief practice session and the actual stress task. Upon completion of the stress task, a recovery period is started, during which the participant is asked again to relax, similar to the baseline rest period. The duration of the recovery period is depending on the variables that are under investigation. Whereas heart rate is known to return to baseline relatively soon after the end of the stress task, changes in other variables, in particular blood-based measures such as cytokines, will not be seen until 30 min or longer (Steptoe et al. 2007). In general, physiological data collection is conducted throughout each of these periods.

When exploring the effects of individual differences in physiological responses to mental stress, it is crucial that the testing procedures are identical between participants (Turner 1994). The conditions in the laboratory, such as temperature and number of experimenters present, but also time of day, should be kept consistent. Care should also be taken to standardize the instructions of the task, which can be done by having the instructions prerecorded. Finally, adherence of the participants to the presession instructions is important. These involve most commonly avoiding strenuous exercise, food, caffeine, and smoking, as well as instructions about the medication which could influence the physiological measurements. The presession instructions are dependent on the physiological measures that are under investigation.

Mental Stress Tasks

Public Speaking – The participant is asked to give a speech in front of an audience and/or a video camera, following a brief preparation period. The topic of speech is psychologically stressful such as "pretend that you are falsely accused of shoplifting and that you have to defend yourself to the shop owner" or "describe your personal strengths and weaknesses" or "describe a recent event that caused anger." The participant will be told that the audience will be critically evaluating the content and delivery of the speech (Van Eck et al. 1996).

Mental Arithmetic – Different varieties are available for mental arithmetic tasks, which include serial subtraction or addition of double-digit numbers or serial addition of single-digit numbers with an element of retention. These tasks, even though not complicated in nature, have been developed to be provocative by adding components of increased time pressure, competition, harassment when a wrong answer is given, and social evaluation (Veldhuijzen van Zanten et al. 2004).

Trier Social Stress Test – This is a combination of mental arithmetic task followed by a public speech, all under conditions of social evaluation.

In addition to the two varieties of mental stress, this task also has a postural component as the speech is conducted while upright (Kirschbaum and Hellhammer 1993).

Computer Games – A variety of computer games have been used to induce stress in participants, which has been mainly conducted in younger participants. These tasks often have a strong component of competition; participants are either directly competing against the experimenter (often in a modified situation to standardize the success rate between participants) or competing against the other participants in the study.

Stroop Color Word Task – The participants are presented with words which describe colors, but the color of the letters is incongruent with the color that the word is written in. For example, the word red is written with yellow ink, and the word yellow is written with red ink. The participant is asked to call out the color of the ink (Stroop 1935).

Mental stress tasks are subject to the effects task novelty and habituation (Turner 1994). For example, even though all of these tasks provoke an increase of heart rate throughout the task, typically, the peak heart rate response is seen at the start of the test. Particularly when a participant is asked to complete the task on different occasions, it is important to maintain the engagement of the participant in each session. It has been shown that the addition of stressful elements such as social evaluation and competition will help to facilitate this. To ensure that the desired levels of stress are obtained, it is common practice to add a measure of self-reported perceptions of the task to each session. These can vary from a simple Likert scale related to perceived stressfulness and difficulty or measures of state stress and anxiety levels both before and after the stress task.

The stress tasks vary in terms of generalizability to real-life settings. Interestingly, an overview of various stress task revealed that public speaking tasks were most consistently effective in inducing myocardial ischemia in patients with coronary heart disease (Strike and Steptoe 2003). It is possible that this is due to the more naturalistic nature of the task than, for example, mental arithmetic or Stroop task. However, care should be taken when interpreting the effectiveness of a certain task to induce physiological changes between studies, as it is hard to compare the stressfulness of tasks between studies. Ambulatory recording techniques are available for the assessment of physiological measurements in real-life setting. Even though these field studies cannot be standardized between participants, it is worth noting that there is evidence that the laboratory cardiovascular responses to mental stress were predictive of ambulatory physiological assessments (Strike and Steptoe 2003).

Cross-References

▶ Cardiovascular Recovery
▶ Immune Responses to Stress
▶ Mental Stress
▶ Psychological Stress
▶ Psychophysiologic Reactivity
▶ Stressor
▶ Trier Social Stress Test

References and Further Reading

Carroll, D., Lovallo, W. R., & Phillips, A. C. (2009). Are large physiological reactions to acute psychological stress always bad for health? *Social and Personality Psychology Compass, 3*, 725–743.

Kirschbaum, C., & Hellhammer, D. H. (1993). The 'Trier Social Stress Test' – A tool for investigating psychobiological stress responses in a laboratory setting. *Neuropsychobiology, 28*, 76–81.

Larsen, B. A., & Cristenfeld, N. J. (2011). Cognitive distancing, cognitive restructuring, and cardiovascular recovery from stress. *Biological Psychology, 86*, 143–148.

Lovallo, W. R. (1997). *Stress & health, biological and psychological interactions*. Thousand Oaks: Sage.

Obrist, P. A. (1981). *Cardiovascular psychophysiology: A perspective*. New York: Plenum Press.

Steptoe, A., Hamer, M., & Chida, Y. (2007). The effects of acute psychological stress on circulating inflammatory factors in humans: A review and meta-analysis. *Brain, Behavior, and Immunity, 21*, 901–912.

Strike, P. C., & Steptoe, A. (2003). Systematic review of mental stress-induced myocardial ischaemia. *European Heart Journal, 24*, 690–703.

Stroop, J. (1935). Studies of interference in serial verbal reactions. *Journal of Experimental Psychology, 18*, 643–662.

Turner, J. R. (1994). *Cardiovascular reactivity and stress.* New York: Plenum Press.

Van Eck, M. M., Nicolson, N. A., Berkhof, H., & Sulon, J. (1996). Individual differences in cortisol responses to a laboratory speech task and their relationship to responses to stressful daily events. *Biological Psychology, 43*, 69–84.

Veldhuijzen van Zanten, J. J. C. S., Ring, C., Burns, V. E., Edwards, K. M., Drayson, M., & Carroll, D. (2004). Mental stress-induced hemoconcentration: Sex differences and mechanisms. *Psychophysiology, 41*, 541–551.

Stress Testing

▶ Exercise Testing

Stress Vulnerability Models

Conny W. E. M. Quaedflieg[1] and Tom Smeets[2]
[1]Faculty of Psychology and Neuroscience, Maastricht University, Maastricht, MD, The Netherlands
[2]Department of Medical and Clinical Psychology, Tilburg School of Social and Behavioral Sciences, Tilburg University, Tilburg, The Netherlands

Synonyms

Stress diathesis models

Definition

Vulnerability models are used to identify factors that are causally related to symptom development. Stress vulnerability models describe the relation between stress and the development of (psycho) pathology. They propose an association between (1) latent endogenous *vulnerability factors* that interact with stress to increase the adverse impact of stressful conditions, (2) *environmental factors* that influence the onset and course of (psycho) pathology, and (3) *protective factors* that buffer against or mitigate the effects of stress on pathological responses.

Description

The prevalence of stress-related mental disorders encompassing mood and anxiety disorders in Europe is above 20%. This morbidity is associated with high health-care costs, disability, and potential mortality. It is widely acknowledged that there are individual differences in how stressful people judge a particular event to be as well as in their ability to cope with adverse stressful life events. While historically stress was said to play an initiating role in the development of pathology, only a minority of people who experience adverse stressful life events go on to develop pathology. To distinguish people who develop pathology from people who do not (i.e., are resilient), vulnerability processes are suggested that predispose individuals to psychopathology when confronted with severe stressors. In the late 1970s, Zubin and Spring were the first to introduce this idea in the field of behavioral medicine by postulating a vulnerability model for schizophrenia. They suggested that humans inherit a predisposition to mental illness but that an interaction between the genetic vulnerability and biological or psychosocial stressors is necessary to develop the disorder. The relationship between predispositional factors (or diathesis) and development of pathology has been described in four basic stress vulnerability models.

Stress Vulnerability Models

The first and most simple stress vulnerability model, the *dichotomous interactive* model, suggests that when predispositional factors are absent, even severe stress will not result in pathology. Instead, it is only when predispositional factors are present that stress may, depending on the severity of the stress, lead to the expression of pathology. Alternatively, the *quasi-continuous* model suggests varying degrees of predisposition with a continuous effect of predispositional factors on pathology once a threshold has been exceeded. The third, more extensive *threshold* model incorporates a specific individual threshold that is determined by the degree of vulnerability and the level of experienced stress. Finally, perhaps the most comprehensive model is the *risk-resilience continuum* model that incorporates different levels of severity of pathology by postulating a continuum that ranges from vulnerability to resilience. This model explicitly emphasizes resiliency characteristics that can make people more resistant to the impact of stress. Note that according to this latter model, even highly resilient individuals might still be at risk for developing pathology when experiencing extreme stress, but their individual threshold will be higher and the symptomatology of post-trauma pathology is likely to be less severe. Collectively, these four models are used to describe the relation between predispositional factors and the development of various pathologies.

Vulnerability Factors

In general, stress vulnerability models postulate that a genetic vulnerability interacts with adverse life events or stressors to produce pathology. This gene-environment interaction with regard to stress and the development of pathology has been most extensively investigated in mood disorders such as depression. Gene-environment interaction studies use monozygotic twin, adoption, and family studies as tools to identify predispositional factors in shared and non-shared environments in order to differentiate genetic from environmental influences. In twin studies, a higher prevalence of pathology in monozygotic twins reared in different environments is used to confirm a genetic predisposition, whereas in adoption studies, the effect of the environment (adoptive parents) can be offset against the effect of genes (biological parents). Using these methods the heritability of major depression, for example, has been estimated at around 40%.

At the neurochemical level, the serotonin (5-HT) system has been implicated in depression. 5-HT regulates among other mood, activity, sleep, and appetite. Accumulating evidence indicates that individuals with a serotonergic vulnerability, manifested in a more sensitive brain serotonergic system, have an increased likelihood of developing mood-related disorders. Specifically, polymorphisms in the 5-HT transporter system (5-HTT) have been associated with stressful life events, a heightened risk for depression, and reactivity to negative emotional stimuli. Individuals carrying two copies of the short variant of the 5-HTT allele (i.e., 5-HTTLPR), a less active gene resulting in fewer 5-HTT transporters, for instance, display an increased sensitivity to the impact of mild stressful life events and an excessive amygdala activity to fearful faces and produce elevated and prolonged levels of cortisol in response to a laboratory stressor compared to individuals with the long variant of the 5-HTT allele. The heritability of the stress hormone response has also been investigated with family studies in relatives of patients with depression using neuroendocrine functioning tests. For example, studies with the dexamethasone suppression test, a drug test used to measure the effectiveness of the negative feedback mechanism of the hypothalamic-pituitary-adrenal (HPA) axis at the level of the pituitary, have found an amplified set point of the HPA axis in relatives of depressed patients compared to healthy controls.

Moreover, 5-HT is also involved in the modulation of the HPA axis and its associated regulatory actions in the secretion of cortisol, the major human glucocorticoid stress hormone. Cortisol binds to two corticosteroid receptors in the brain, namely, the mineralocorticoid receptor (MR) and the glucocorticoid receptor (GR). Two mechanisms of cortisol binding are known. First, cortisol can bind to the hormone response element on DNA to influence gene expression (intracellular MR and GR binding properties). Secondly, cortisol can bind to membrane versions of the corticosteroid receptors to influence glutamate transmission and gene expression in the brain. The MR controls the basal HPA activity through inhibition of the HPA axis, facilitating the selection of adaptive behavioral responses and preventing minor adverse stressful life events to disturb homeostasis. In contrast, the GR promotes recovery after stress as well as the storage of information for future events. The balance between the MR and GR receptors determines the threshold and termination of the HPA axis response to stress. Increased MR expression or functionality has been associated with increased adaptability to cope with stressors. For example, animal studies have demonstrated that increased MR expression contributes to a more adaptive stress response via regulation of the tonic inhibition. Moreover, MRs play a role in memory formation and retrieval during stressful situations, and impaired memory formation alters the appraisal of stressful situations. Likewise, studies have demonstrated that individuals with polymorphisms in the GR gene display higher cortisol responses and inefficient recovery of the HPA axis following standardized laboratory stress tests, thus revealing predisposition factors for stress-related pathology.

Genes can have a direct effect on the development of various brain systems. To illustrate this point, altered gene expression can reduce plasticity in brain circuits regulating mood, anxiety, and aggression, thereby decreasing one's ability to cope with stressful life events. Moreover, genes can bias brain circuits to inefficient information processing which can result in the expression of pathology (e.g., intrusive memories in patients suffering from posttraumatic stress disorder). Genetic polymorphisms are then viewed as vulnerability factors given that they produce an increased sensitivity to the impact of stressful life events. However, it should be kept in mind that replication studies of candidate gene associations in pathology are relatively sparse and that most disorders are polygenetic. Additionally, the net outcome of a stressor is at least in part determined by the individual's personality traits that may be formed by genes, potentially indirectly influencing the selection of environments and thus the risk of exposure to adverse effects.

Lifespan models have examined the relation between early-life stressful events, later stressful life events, and pathology development. Undifferentiated neuronal systems are dependent on early experience during development. It is suggested that early-life stress results in inefficient information processing and sensitization of brain circuits involved in regulating stress reactivity, which may ultimately render people more vulnerable. Different brain structures have specific developmental trajectories resulting in a variety of pathological response after stress across the lifespan. For example, prenatal stress originating from maternal stress or postnatal environmental stress such as the quality of parental care influences the regulation of the HPA axis. Specifically, different early stress experiences result in either a HPA axis hyper- or hypofunction, due to a different regulation of glucocorticoid receptors in the hippocampus. In turn, altered HPA axis activity shapes the activity in prefrontal areas as well as the connectivity between prefrontal areas and the amygdala, which in turn influences the processing of emotions and stress-coping strategies. However, exposure to a manageable stressor during childhood can also desensitize the stress circuits, producing experience-based resilience in which brain systems tend to become less reactive to future stress. Early-life stress can hence be protective in that it can negate or diminish the negative outcomes or alternatively promote adaptive functioning in the context of adverse stressful life events. Additionally, other psychosocial factors during development like social support, parental care, and affective style have been identified as potentially protective factors that can enhance adaptive coping during or after stress. In a similar vein, brain frontal alpha asymmetry has been suggested to bias individuals' affective style and emotion regulation capacities. Specifically, left frontal activation has been linked to approach behavior and suggested to be an indicator of decreased vulnerability to depression, whereas right frontal activation is viewed as a predispositional factor, lowering the threshold for adverse impact of stressful conditions.

In sum, stress vulnerability models underscore that the nature and intensity of the stressor in combination with genetic vulnerability factors, phenotypic vulnerability factors (personality, neuroendocrine reactivity), and both genetic and phenotypic protective (resilience) factors determine the impact and sequela of adverse stressful life events.

Cross-References

- Corticosteroids
- Cortisol
- Family Stress
- Family Studies (Genetics)
- Gene-Environment Interaction
- Glucocorticoids
- Hypothalamic-Pituitary-Adrenal Axis
- Individual Differences
- Quantitative EEG Including the Five Common Bandwidths (Delta, Theta, Alpha, Sigma, and Beta)
- Resilience
- Stress
- Stress Reactivity
- Stress Responses
- Stress Test
- Stress, Caregiver
- Stress, Early Life
- Stress: Appraisal and Coping
- Stressor
- Trier Social Stress Test
- Twin Studies

References and Further Reading

Coan, J. A., & Allen, J. J. B. (2003). The state and trait nature of frontal EEG asymmetry in emotion. In K. Hugdahl & R. J. Davidson (Eds.), *The asymmetrical brain* (pp. 565–616). Cambridge, MA: The MIT Press.

Curtis, W. J., & Cicchetti, D. (2003). Moving research on resilience into the 21st century: Theoretical and methodological considerations in examining the biological contributors to resilience. *Development and Psychopathology, 15*, 773–810.

DeRijk, R. H., & de Kloet, E. R. (2008). Corticosteroid receptor polymorphisms: Determinants of vulnerability and resilience. *European Journal of Pharmacology, 583*, 303–311.

Gotlib, I. H., Joormann, J., Minor, K. L., & Hallmayer, J. (2008). HPA axis reactivity: A mechanism underlying the associations among 5-HTTLPR, stress, and depression. *Biological Psychiatry, 63*, 847–851.

Huizink, A., & De Rooij, S. (2018). Prenatal stress and models explaining risk for psychopathology revisited: Generic vulnerability and divergent pathways. *Development and Psychopathology, 30*(3), 1041–1062. https://doi.org/10.1017/S0954579418000354.

Ingram, R. E., & Luxton, D. D. (2005). Vulnerability-stress models. In B. L. Hankin & J. R. Z. Abela (Eds.), *Development of psychopathology: A vulnerability-stress perspective* (pp. 32–46). Thousand Oaks: Sage.

Lupien, S. J., McEwen, B. S., Gunnar, M. R., & Heim, C. (2009). Effects of stress throughout the lifespan on the brain, behaviour and cognition. *Nature Reviews Neuroscience, 10*, 434–445.

Oitzl, M. S., Champagne, D. L., van der Veen, R., & de Kloet, E. R. (2010). Brain development under stress: Hypotheses of glucocorticoid actions revisited. *Neuroscience and Biobehavioral Reviews, 34*, 853–866.

Stahl, S. M. (2008). *Stahl's essential psychopharmacology: Neuroscientific basis and practical applications* (3rd ed.). New York: Cambridge University Press.

ter Heegde, F., De Rijk, R. H., & Vinkers, C. H. (2015). The brain mineralocorticoid receptor and stress resilience. *Psychoneuroendocrinology, 52*, 92–110.

Van Praag, H. M., de Kloet, E. R., & van Os, J. (2004). *Stress, the brain and depression*. New York: Cambridge University Press.

Zubin, J., & Spring, B. (1977). Vulnerability-a new view of schizophrenia. *Journal of Abnormal Psychology, 86*, 103–126.

Stress, Caregiver

Youngmee Kim[1] and Kelly M. Shaffer[2]
[1]Department of Psychology, University of Miami, Coral Gables, FL, USA
[2]University of Virginia School of Medicine, Charlottesville, VA, USA

Synonyms

Caregiver burden; Caregiver hassle; Caregiver strain

Definition

The stress of caregivers is defined as a feeling experienced when a person thinks that the demands of caregiving exceed the personal and social resources the individual is able to mobilize (Lazarus and Folkman 1984).

Description

An illness affects not only the quality of life of individuals with the disease but also that of their family members and close friends who care for the patients. The stress of caregivers is defined as a feeling experienced when a person thinks that the demands of caregiving exceed the personal and social resources the individual is able to mobilize (Lazarus and Folkman 1984). The caregiver role of family members incorporates diverse aspects involved in dealing with an illness of the relative. This role includes providing the patient with cognitive/informational, emotional, financial/legal, daily activity, medical, and spiritual support, as well as facilitating communication with medical professionals and other family members and assisting in the maintenance of social relationships (Kim and Given 2008). All of these aspects can contribute to caregivers' stress when they perceive it difficult to mobilize their personal and social resources to carry out each of the caregiving-related tasks. Therefore, identifying the gaps between resources available for caregiving and the caregiving demands, unmet needs in caregiving, should be the initial step in the development of programs designed to reduce caregivers' stress and enhance their quality of life.

In addition to assessing the diverse aspects of caregivers' stress and unmet needs, understanding how caregivers' stress varies across the illness trajectory is an important concern (Kim et al. 2010). For example, in the early phase of caregivership, caregivers' stress is often associated with providing informational and medical support to the patients. During the remission phase, dealing with uncertainty about the future, fear that the disease may come back, the financial burden of extended treatment needs of the patients, and changes in social relationships are major sources of caregivers' stress. After the death of the patients, spiritual concerns and psychological and physical recovery efforts from caregiving strain are the challenges caregivers face.

Another important aspect of caregivers' stress is their own unmet needs – things that are not directly related to caring for the patient but represent important personal needs to the caregivers. That is, in addition to caring for the individual with an illness, family caregivers likely have responsibilities for self-care and care for other family members that may have to be set aside or ignored in order to carry out the caregiver role.

This complex construct of caregiver stress has been associated with caregivers' demographic characteristics (Kim et al. 2010; Pinquart and Sörensen 2003, 2005). For example, younger caregivers have reported greater stress in providing psychosocial, medical, financial, and daily activity support during the early phase of the illness trajectory. During the remission years after the illness onset, however, younger caregivers have reported greater stress only in daily activity. Gender has been also an important factor (Kim and Loscalzo 2018). Female caregivers have reported greater stress from dealing with psychosocial concerns of the patients, other family members, and themselves. Ethnic minorities tend to report lower levels of psychological stress but greater levels of physical stress from caregiving. Studies have found mixed associations of caregiver stress to other demographic characteristics, such as education, income, and employment status.

Caregivers' poorer mental health has also been related to higher levels of stress from meeting the medical needs of the patients during the early phase of illness, whereas during remission, poorer mental health has been related to financial stress from caregiving. Furthermore, cancer caregivers' increased risk of poor physical health has recently been recognized by a large epidemiological study using Swedish registries (Ji et al. 2012). This study showed that spouses of persons with cancer, compared with unaffected spouses, were more vulnerable to poor cardiovascular health, including risk of coronary heart disease (13% increase) and stroke (26% increase) up to 20 years after their spouse's cancer diagnosis. Perceived level of stress from providing care has been significantly related to the caregivers' quality of life years later (Kim et al. 2015). Caregivers' depressive symptoms have also shown to be the unique predictor of physical health decline over 6 years (Shaffer et al. 2017). Caregivers who reported higher levels of psychosocial stress from caregiving have shown poorer mental health consistently and strongly across different phases of the illness trajectory.

The physical burden of caregiving, documented in objective measures, has also been considerable. For example, compared with matched non-caregivers, caregivers for a spouse with dementia report more infectious illness episodes, have poorer immune responses to influenza virus and pneumococcal pneumonia vaccines, show slower healing for small standardized wounds, have greater depressive symptoms, and are at greater risk for coronary heart disease (Vitaliano et al. 2003). A recent meta-analysis (2003) concluded that compared with demographically similar non-caregivers, caregivers of dementia patients had a 9% greater risk of health problems, a 23% higher level of stress hormones, and a 15% poorer antibody production. Moreover, caregivers' relative risk for all-cause mortality was 63% higher than non-caregiver controls.

Immune dysregulation has been identified as a key mechanism linking caregiving stress to physical health. Chronically stressed dementia caregivers have numerous immune deficits compared to demographically matched non-caregivers, including lower T-cell proliferation, higher production of immune regulatory cytokines (interleukin-2 [IL-2], C-reactive protein [CRP], tumor necrosis factor-alpha [TNF-α], IL-10, IL-6, D-dimer), decreased antibody and virus-specific T-cell responses to influenza virus vaccination, and a shift from a Th1 to Th2 cytokine response (i.e., an increase in the percentage and total number of IL10+/CD4+ and IL10+/CD8+ cells) (Segerstrom and Miller 2004; Vitaliano et al. 2003). A 6-year longitudinal community study (Kiecolt-Glaser et al. 2003) documented that caregivers' average rate of increase in IL-6 was about four times as large as that of non-caregivers. The mean annual change in IL-6 among former caregivers did not differ from that of current caregivers, even several years after the death of the spouse. There were no systematic group differences in chronic health problems, medications, or health-relevant behaviors that might otherwise account for changes in caregivers' IL-6 levels during the 6 years of the study period (2003).

Another mechanism linking caregiving stress to poor physical health is lifestyle behaviors. Family members with chronic strain from caring for dementia patients increase health-risk behaviors, such as smoking and alcohol consumption (Carter 2002). They also get inadequate rest and inadequate exercise and forget to take prescription drugs to manage their own health conditions, resulting in poorer physical health (Beach et al. 2000; Burton et al. 1997).

In summary, caregiver stress is a multidimensional construct that varies in nature across the illness trajectory. Certain caregivers by their demographic characteristics can be identified as a vulnerable subgroup to greater caregiving stress. Overall, however, caregiving stress takes a considerable toll on the caregivers' mental and physical health. Such effects deserve further systematic study to understand their psychological, biological, and behavioral pathways.

Cross-References

▶ Alzheimer's Disease
▶ Cancer Survivorship
▶ Caregiver/Caregiving and Stress
▶ Daily Stress
▶ Dementia
▶ Family Stress
▶ Family, Caregiver
▶ Family, Relationships
▶ Quality of Life

References and Readings

Beach, S. R., Schulz, R., Yee, J. L., & Jackson, S. (2000). Negative and positive health effects of caring for a disabled spouse: Longitudinal findings from the caregiver health effects study. *Psychology and Aging, 15*(2), 259–271.

Burton, L. C., Newsom, J. T., Schulz, R., Hirsch, C. H., & German, P. S. (1997). Preventive health behaviors among spousal caregivers. *Preventive Medicine, 26*(2), 162–169.

Carter, P. A. (2002). Caregivers' descriptions of sleep changes and depressive symptoms. *Oncology Nursing Forum, 29*(9), 1277–1283.

Ji, J., Zöller, B., Sundquist, K., Sundquist, J. (2012) Increased risks of coronary heart disease and stroke among spousal caregivers of cancer patients. *Circulation, 125*, 1742–1747.

Kiecolt-Glaser, J. K., Preacher, K. J., MacCallum, R. C., Atkinson, C., Malarkey, W. B., & Glaser, R. (2003).

Chronic stress and age-related increases in the proinflammatory cytokine IL-6. *Proceedings of the National Academy of Sciences of the United States of America, 100*, 9090–9095.

Kim, Y., & Given, B. A. (2008). Quality of life of family caregivers of cancer survivors across the trajectory of the illness. *Cancer, 112*(Suppl. 11), 2556–2568.

Kim, Y., & Loscalzo, M. (Eds.). (2018). *Gender in psycho-oncology*. New York, NY: Oxford University Press. ISBN 978-0-19-046225-3.

Kim, Y., Kashy, D. A., Spillers, R. L., & Evans, T. V. (2010). Needs assessment of family caregivers of cancer survivors: Three cohorts comparison. *Psycho-Oncology, 19*, 573–582.

Kim, Y., Carver, C. S., Shaffer, K. M., Gansler, T., & Cannady, R. S. (2015). Cancer caregiving predicts physical impairments: Roles of earlier caregiving stress and being a spousal caregiver. *Cancer, 121*, 302–310.

Lazarus, R. S., & Folkman, S. (1984). *Stress, appraisal and coping*. New York: Springer.

Pinquart, M., & Sörensen, S. (2003). Differences between caregivers and noncaregivers in psychological health and physical health: A meta-analysis. *Psychology and Aging, 18*(2), 250–267.

Pinquart, M., & Sörensen, S. (2005). Ethnic differences in stressors, resources, and psychological outcomes of family caregiving: A meta-analysis. *The Gerontologist, 45*(1), 90–106.

Segerstrom, S. C., & Miller, G. E. (2004). Psychological stress and the human immune system: A meta-analytic study of 30 years of inquiry. *Psychological Bulletin, 130*, 601–630.

Shaffer, K. M., Kim, Y., Carver, C. S., & Cannady, R. S. (2017). Depressive symptoms predict cancer caregivers' physical health decline. *Cancer, 123*, 4277–4285.

Vitaliano, P. P., Zhang, J., & Scanlan, J. M. (2003). Is caregiving hazardous to one's physical health? A meta-analysis. *Psychological Bulletin, 129*, 946–972.

Stress, Early Life

Christine Heim
Institute of Medical Psychology, Charité University Medicine Berlin, Berlin, Germany

Synonyms

Adversity, early life; Trauma, early life

Definition

In order to define early life stress in humans, two main criteria must be considered: (a) the developmental age range that is subsumed under "early life" and (b) the characteristics of the events that would be considered as "stressful" during early life. There is no such generally agreed upon definition (Heim et al. 2003).

Many investigators use an upper age limit to define the early life criterion, usually between 12 and 18 years. An alternative approach is to define the early life period by developmental stage, using, for example, sexual maturation (such as menarche in girls) as a cutoff criterion.

As for the stress criterion, prevailing models suggest that stress is generally experienced when an individual is confronted with a situation, which is appraised as personally threatening and for which adequate coping resources are unavailable. In addition, threats to physiological homeostasis, such as injury or illness, elicit stress responses. Any such situation occurring within the defined developmental period may be classified as early life stress. The most salient forms of early life stress in humans are abuse (sexual, physical, emotional), neglect (emotional, physical), and parental loss (death, separation). Other forms of early life stress include accidents, physical illness, surgeries, natural disasters, and war or terrorism-related events. Less obvious experiences, which pose significant distress on a child, include unstable families, inadequate parental care, dysfunctional relationships between parent and child, and poverty.

Early life stress is often complex, inasmuch as various forms coexist or are associated among each other. While early life stress may be a single event, it more typically occurs as chronic or ongoing adversity in most cases. Taken together, there remains substantial ambiguity in the definition of early life stress in humans (Heim et al. 2003).

Description

It is well established that early life stress, such as childhood abuse, neglect, or loss, dramatically increases the risk for developing a wide range of psychiatric disorders as well as certain medical diseases later in life. Among the major psychiatric disorders, depression and anxiety disorders have been most prominently linked to early life stress. Medical disorders, for which early-life stress induces risk, include ischemic heart disease, lung disease, cancer, gastrointestinal disorders, and chronic fatigue and pain syndromes among others. Early life stress has further been linked to a variety of risk behaviors, including smoking, alcohol, or drug abuse, impulsive behavior, promiscuity, teen pregnancy, and suicide (for further reading, see Anda et al. 2006). Many of the above disorders and risk behaviors are elicited or aggravated by acute stress, and individuals with early life stress experiences have decreased thresholds to exhibit symptoms and risk behaviors even upon mild challenge (Hammen et al. 2000).

The precise mechanisms that mediate the detrimental and persistent impact of early adversity on long-term adaptation and health have been the subject of intense inquiry over decades. Advances from neuroscience research have provided compelling insights into the enormous plasticity of the developing brain as a function of experience. For example, visual sensory input early in life is required for normal development of the visual cortex and perception, and disruptive experiences during such critical periods of plasticity can lead to lifelong and sometimes irreversible damage. The same principle may be applied to stress experiences during critical periods early in life that may permanently impact on the development of brain regions implicated in the regulation of emotion and stress responses (for further reading, see Weiss and Wagner 1998). Enduring effects of early life stress on the brain and its regulatory outflow systems, including the autonomic, endocrine, and immune systems, may then lead to the development of a vulnerable phenotype with increased sensitivity to stress and risk for a range of behavioral and somatic disorders (for further reading, see Heim et al. 2004).

Compelling support for this hypothesis comes from a burgeoning literature of studies in animal models that provide the direct and causal evidence that early adverse experience, such as prolonged maternal separation or naturally occurring low maternal care, leads to structural, functional, and epigenetic changes in a connected network of brain regions that is implicated in neuroendocrine control, autonomic regulation and vigilance, and emotional regulation or fear conditioning. These neural changes converge into lifelong increased physiological and behavioral responses to subsequent stress in animal models (see Heim et al. 2004; Lupien et al. 2009; Meaney 2001). These effects appear to be present across species and in different models of adversity, while the unifying element across studies is timing of the stressor in early life. Particularly intriguing are results from animal studies suggesting that epigenetic changes, stress sensitization, and maternal care behavior are transmitted into the next generation (Francis et al. 1999; Franklin et al. 2010).

Accumulating evidence suggests that these preclinical findings can be translated to humans. For example, adult women with histories of childhood sexual or physical abuse exhibit markedly increased neuroendocrine and autonomic responses to psychosocial laboratory stress, particularly those with depression (Heim et al. 2000). Other alterations in humans with early life stress experiences include glucocorticoid resistance, increased levels of inflammation, increased central corticotropin-releasing hormone activity and decreased activity of the prosocial neuropeptide, oxytocin (Carpenter et al. 2004; Danese et al. 2007; Heim et al. 2008; Heim et al. 2009). A small hippocampus has also been linked to early life stress in humans (Vythilingam et al. 2002). Early adversity has also been found to be associated with epigenetic changes of the glucocorticoid receptor gene in hippocampal tissue obtained by postmortem from suicide victims, leading to reduced glucocorticoid receptor expression and enhanced stress responses (McGowan et al. 2008).

Taken together, these neurobiological and epigenetic changes secondary to early life stress likely reflect risk to develop depression and a host of other disorders in response to additional challenge. In several studies, these changes were not present in depressed persons without early life stress, suggesting the existence of biologically distinguishable subtypes of depression as a function of early life stress (Heim et al. 2004, 2008). These subtypes of depression were also found to be responsive to differential treatments (Nemeroff et al. 2003). Therefore, consideration of early life stress might be critical to guide treatment decisions.

Several genes moderate the link between childhood trauma and adult risk for depression and other disorders, including the serotonin transporter, corticotropin-releasing hormone receptor 1, FK506 binding protein 5, and oxytocin receptor genes. A more recent idea is that such genetic factors might reflect general sensitivity to the environment, inasmuch as persons who are susceptible to the detrimental effects of trauma might also be particularly amenable to the beneficial effects of a positive social environment or early psychological intervention (Binder et al. 2008; Bradley et al. 2008, 2011; for further reading, see Caspi et al. 2010).

References and Readings

Anda, R. F., Felitti, V. J., Bremner, J. D., Walker, J. D., Whitfield, C., Perry, B. D., et al. (2006). The enduring effects of abuse and related adverse experiences in childhood. *European Archives of Psychiatry and Clinical Neuroscience, 256*, 174–186.

Binder, E. B., Bradley, R. G., Liu, W., Epstein, M. P., Deveau, T. C., Mercer, K. B., et al. (2008). Association of FKBP5 polymorphisms and childhood abuse with risk of posttraumatic stress disorder symptoms in adults. *Journal of the American Medical Association, 299*, 1291–1305.

Bradley, R. G., Binder, E. B., Epstein, M. P., Tang, Y., Nair, H. P., Liu, W., et al. (2008). Influence of child abuse on adult depression: Moderation by the corticotropin-releasing hormone receptor gene. *Archives of General Psychiatry, 65*, 190–200.

Bradley, B., Westen, D., Binder, E. B., Jovanovic, T., & Heim, C. (2011). Association between childhood maltreatment and adult emotional dysregulation: Moderation by oxytocin receptor gene. *Development and Psychopathology, 23*(2), 439–452.

Carpenter, L., Tyrka, A., McDougle, C. J., Malison, R. T., Owens, M. J., Nemeroff, C. B., et al. (2004). CSF corticotropin-releasing factor and perceived early-life stress in depressed patients and healthy control subjects. *Neuropsychopharmacology, 29*, 777–784.

Caspi, A., Hariri, A. R., Holmes, A., Uher, R., & Moffitt, T. E. (2010). Genetic sensitivity to the environment: The case of the serotonin transporter gene and its implications for studying complex diseases and traits. *American Journal of Psychiatry, 167*, 509–527.

Danese, A., Pariante, C. M., Caspi, A., Taylor, A., & Poulton, R. (2007). Childhood maltreatment predicts adult inflammation in a life-course study. *Proceedings of the National Academy of Sciences United States of America, 104*, 1319–1324.

Francis, D., Diorio, J., Liu, D., & Meaney, M. J. (1999). Nongenomic transmission across generations of maternal behavior and stress responses in the rat. *Science, 286*, 1155–1158.

Franklin, T. B., Russig, H., Weiss, I. C., Gräff, J., Linder, N., Michalon, A., et al. (2010). Epigenetic transmission of the impact of early stress across generations. *Biological Psychiatry, 68*, 408–415.

Hammen, C., Henry, R., & Daley, S. E. (2000). Depression and sensitization to stressors among young women as a function of childhood adversity. *Journal of Consulting and Clinical Psychology, 68*, 782–787.

Heim, C., Newport, D. J., Heit, S., Graham, Y. P., Wilcox, M., Bonsall, R., et al. (2000). Pituitary-adrenal and autonomic responses to stress in women after sexual and physical abuse in childhood. *Journal of the American Medical Association, 284*, 592–597.

Heim, C., Meinlschmidt, G., & Nemeroff, C. B. (2003). Neurobiology of early-life stress and its relationship to PTSD. *Psychiatric Annals, 33*, 1–10.

Heim, C., Plotsky, P. M., & Nemeroff, C. B. (2004). Importance of studying the contributions of early adverse experience to neurobiological findings in depression. *Neuropsychopharmacology, 29*, 641–648.

Heim, C., Newport, D. J., Mletzko, T., Miller, A. H., & Nemeroff, C. B. (2008). The link between childhood trauma and depression: Insights from HPA axis studies in humans. *Psychoneuroendocrinology, 33*, 693–710.

Heim, C., Young, L. J., Newport, D. J., Mletzko, T., Miller, A. H., & Nemeroff, C. B. (2009). Lower cerebrospinal fluid oxytocin concentrations in women with a history of childhood abuse. *Molecular Psychiatry, 14*, 954–958.

Lupien, S. J., McEwen, B. S., Gunnar, M. R., & Heim, C. (2009). Effects of stress throughout the lifespan on the brain, behaviour and cognition. *Nature Reviews Neuroscience, 10*, 434–445.

McGowan, P. O., Sasaki, A., D'Alessio, A. C., Dymov, S., Labonté, B., Szyf, M., et al. (2008). Epigenetic regulation of the glucocorticoid receptor in human brain associates with childhood abuse. *Nature Neuroscience, 12*, 342–348.

Meaney, M. J. (2001). Maternal care, gene expression, and the transmission of individual differences in stress reactivity across generations. *Annual Reviews in Neuroscience, 24*, 1161–1192.

Nemeroff, C. B., Heim, C., Thase, M. E., Klein, D. N., Rush, A. J., Schatzberg, A. F., et al. (2003). Differential responses to psychotherapy versus pharmacotherapy in patients with chronic forms of major depression and childhood trauma. *Proceedings of the National Academy of Sciences United States of America, 100*, 14293–14396.

Vythilingam, M., Heim, C., Newport, J., Miller, A. H., Anderson, E., Bronen, R., et al. (2002). Childhood trauma associated with smaller hippocampal volume in women with major depression. *American Journal of Psychiatry, 159*, 2072–2080.

Weiss, M. J., & Wagner, S. H. (1998). What explains the negative consequences of adverse childhood experiences on adult health? Insights from cognitive and neuroscience research. *American Journal of Preventive Medicine, 14*, 356–360.

Stress, Emotional

Tamar Mendelson
Mental Health, Johns Hopkins Bloomberg School of Public Health Johns Hopkins University, Baltimore, MD, USA

Synonyms

Emotional distress; Mental stress; Psychological stress; Stress

Definition

Emotional stress involves the experience of negative affect, such as anxiety, in the context of a physiological stress response that includes cardiovascular and hormonal changes. Emotional stress commonly occurs when an individual perceives that he or she does not have adequate personal resources to meet situational demands effectively (Lazarus 1966).

Description

Early conceptions of stress characterized its physical properties, with a focus on the disruption of homeostasis in an organism (Selye 1956). The stress concept subsequently evolved to include a greater emphasis on the influence of psychological factors on the stress process. The term "emotional stress" reflects the fact that the stress process in humans involves a substantial affective component.

Emotional stress includes both negative affect, such as anxiety and distress, as well as a cascade of physiological responses associated with the stress-response system. Physiological responses promote "fight or flight" and include activation of the hypothalamic pituitary adrenal (HPA) axis, which stimulates secretion of cortisol, and activation of the sympathetic nervous system, which increases heart rate (Sapolsky 1994). Behavioral responses may include attempts to flee or avoid the stressor or to actively address it.

Emotional stress can be triggered by various stress exposures, including major life events, chronic stressful situations, and daily hassles. Certain objective features of a stressor influence the likelihood that it will produce emotional stress. For instance, emotional stress is more likely to result from stressors that are not within an individual's control (e.g., a death) and affect central aspects of an individual's life (Dohrenwend 2000).

Individual differences are also critical components in predicting levels of emotional stress, particularly when the stressor is not extremely traumatic. Thus, the same stressor may produce emotional stress in one individual but not in another. Richard Lazarus and Susan Folkman's work has established the importance of appraisal processes in generating or buffering against stress (Lazarus and Folkman 1984). Emotional stress results from an appraisal that the situation is threatening and that efforts to address it effectively are not likely to be successful. In contrast, a sense of positive challenge may arise if the situation is not perceived as overly threatening or if the perceiver feels capable of an effective response. Similarly, a number of other factors can increase risk for, or protect against, emotional stress. These factors include the ability to employ effective coping strategies and the presence of positive social supports (Kessler et al. 1985).

A life course perspective is important for understanding the etiology of vulnerability to emotional stress. Both vulnerability to stress and resilience are likely shaped over the life course by complex interactions of genetic factors, biological mechanisms, and environmental exposures. Emerging research suggests that exposure to stress and adversity during sensitive periods early in the life course (prenatal, early postnatal, childhood) may be especially critical in influencing genetic expression and impacting the developing stress-response system, with long-term effects on vulnerability to emotional stress (Andersen and Teicher 2009; Dudley et al. 2011; Shonkoff et al. 2009).

A key reason for continued interest in the study of emotional stress is its well-documented link with development of both mental and physical disorders. Major depressive disorder and post-traumatic stress disorder are two commonly studied psychiatric sequelae of emotional stress. Emotional stress has also been found to predict cardiovascular disease and other physical health problems (Brotman et al. 2007; Rozanski et al. 1999). Putative mechanisms linking emotional stress with psychiatric and physical disorders include stress-related neurobiological changes (e.g., dysregulation of the HPA axis) and increased cardiovascular reactivity to stress with slow recovery (Chida and Steptoe 2010; Hammen 2005); detailed understanding of these pathways requires more study.

A variety of psychosocial stress management interventions have been developed to reduce emotional stress and prevent its negative effects on health. Such interventions generally aim to enhance positive coping methods, including the use of relaxation techniques, exercise, and cognitive strategies for managing stress. Some stress management interventions have been shown to have positive effects on emotional and physical outcomes (e.g., Blumenthal et al. 2005).

Cross-References

▶ Cardiovascular Disease
▶ Coping
▶ Depression: Symptoms
▶ Relaxation
▶ Stress Reactivity
▶ Stress Responses
▶ Stress Vulnerability Models
▶ Stress, Early Life
▶ Stress: Appraisal and Coping
▶ Stressor
▶ Sympathetic Nervous System (SNS)

References and Readings

Andersen, S. L., & Teicher, M. H. (2009). Desperately driven and no brakes: Developmental stress exposure and subsequent risk for substance use. *Neuroscience and Behavioral Reviews, 33*, 516–524.

Blumenthal, J. A., Sherwood, A., Babyak, M. A., Watkins, L. L., Waugh, R., Georgiades, A., et al. (2005). Effects of exercise and stress management training on markers of cardiovascular risk in patients with ischemic heart disease: A randomized controlled trial. *Journal of the American Medical Association, 293*, 1626–1634.

Brotman, D. J., Golden, S. H., & Wittstein, I. S. (2007). The cardiovascular toll of stress. *Lancet, 370*, 1089–1100.

Chida, Y., & Steptoe, A. (2010). Greater cardiovascular responses to laboratory mental stress are associated with poor subsequent cardiovascular risk status: A meta-analysis of prospective evidence. *Hypertension, 55*, 1026–1032.

Dohrenwend, B. P. (2000). The role of adversity and stress in psychopathology: Some evidence and its implications for theory ad research. *Journal of Health and Social Behavior, 41*, 1–19.

Dudley, K. J., Li, X., Kobor, M. S., Kippin, T. E., & Bredy, T. W. (2011). Epigenetic mechanisms mediating vulnerability and resilience to psychiatric disorders. *Neuroscience and Biobehavioral Reviews, 35*, 1544–1551.

Hammen, C. (2005). Stress and depression. *Annual Review of Clinical Psychology, 1*, 293–319.

Kessler, R. C., Price, R. H., & Wortman, C. B. (1985). Social factors in psychopathology: Stress, coping, and coping processes. *Annual Review of Psychology, 36*, 531–572.

Lazarus, R. S. (1966). *Psychological stress and the coping process*. New York: McGraw Hill.

Lazarus, R. S., & Folkman, S. (1984). *Stress, appraisal, and coping*. New York: Springer.

Rozanski, A., Blumenthal, J. A., & Kaplan, J. (1999). Impact of psychological factors on the pathogenesis of cardiovascular disease and implications for therapy. *Circulation, 99*, 2192–2217.

Sapolsky, R. M. (1994). *Why zebras don't get ulcers.* New York: Holt.

Selye, H. (1956). *The stress of life.* New York: Mc-Graw-Hill.

Shonkoff, J. P., Boyce, W. T., & McEwen, B. S. (2009). Neuroscience, molecular biology, and the childhood roots of health disparities. Building a new framework for health promotion and disease prevention. *Journal of the American Medical Association, 301*, 2252–2259.

Stress, Exercise

Rick LaCaille[1] and Marc Taylor[2]
[1]Psychology Department, University of Minnesota Duluth, Duluth, MN, USA
[2]Behavioral Sciences and Epidemiology, Naval Health Research Center, San Diego, CA, USA

Definition

Exercise is a form of physical activity that involves repeated body movements that are both structured and planned with the intention of maintaining or enhancing one's health or physical fitness. Typically, exercise is characterized as either aerobic or anaerobic with the former emphasizing the use of oxygen for sustained movements such as jogging or swimming, whereas the latter emphasizes the use of muscle glycogen supply and metabolism as sources of energy for higher-intensity activities such as strength and resistance training. Moreover, exercise has been defined in terms of being chronic/regular/habitual or as acute/single bout.

Stress represents a response among biopsychosocial systems in an effort to adapt to a challenge. The nature of the challenge has been delineated along several dimensions, including but not limited to its intensity, duration, frequency, quality, and familiarity. The stress response has been measured in naturally occurring situations as well as in laboratory settings and ranged from self-reported questionnaires to physiological indices of neuroendocrine, heart rate, and blood pressure reactivity.

Description

The health benefits of exercise and physical fitness have been well documented in the literature. In particular, the effects of exercise on reduced morbidity and mortality from cardiovascular disease have received a great deal of attention, in part, due to the association between stress and cardiovascular disease and the potential attenuation of physiological reactivity to stressors. Notably, an acute bout of exercise may also act as a stressor and elicit the same cardiovascular and neuroendocrine responses as psychosocial stressors without the detrimental effects health. As exercise becomes chronic and habitual, the physiological adaptations (e.g., reduced heart rate and blood pressure and increased parasympathetic activity) that occur are thought to yield similar responses and adaptations in the presence of psychosocial stressors. This beneficial adaptation and reduced sensitivity to stress is characterized in the literature as the cross-stressor-adaptation hypothesis. Thus, the effect of exercise on stress response is somewhat paradoxical as it is considered to be both a stressor and a potential modifier of stress. Most investigations of exercise-stress adaptations have relied upon laboratory stressors (e.g., mental arithmetic, public speaking and evaluative scenarios, cold pressor tests, reaction time, Stroop color-word test), cardiorespiratory responses, and cross-sectional designs. Although a number of studies have examined the association between exercise/fitness and psychophysiological stress responses, the findings have been rather mixed even among the reviews and quantitative analyses of the literature.

In an initial meta-analysis of the relationship between aerobic fitness and resistance to stress reactivity by Crews and Landers (1987), the overall effect size across multiple indices was $d = 0.48$ with effects ranging from 0.15 to 0.87. The findings from this review suggested that fitness/exercise training was beneficial in reducing reactivity to stressors with regards to heart rate d = (0.39), diastolic blood pressure d = (0.40), systolic blood pressure d = (0.42), self-reported stress d = (0.57), skin response d = (0.67), and muscle tension d = (0.87). The review has since been criticized for a number of methodological limitations including confounding reactivity with recovery. Later qualitative reviews reported no beneficial effect for fitness on stress reactivity in terms of heart rate, blood pressure, or catecholamine responses, with the effect on stress recovery determined to be inconclusive (Claytor 1991; De Geus and Van Doornen 1993). More recently, Jackson and Dishman (2006) revealed in a meta-analytic review that fitness was associated with a slight increase in stress reactivity to laboratory psychosocial stressors. Notably, a small effect size was present between cardiorespiratory fitness and stress response recovery, indicating that physically fitter individuals appeared to have an enhanced and quicker recovery following their peak stress response. In contrast to these findings, Forcier et al.'s (2006) meta-analytic review examining the effects of aerobic fitness on stress reactivity and recovery revealed that, despite considerable heterogeneity present in the analyses and no significant moderation effects (e.g., gender, stressor intensity), significant effects for exercise/fitness were found for decreased heart rate and systolic blood pressure reactivity. Additionally, a significant effect was found for fitness and heart rate recovery, though no such effect was present for systolic blood pressure. Thus, the findings from this meta-analysis suggest a beneficial attenuated physiological reactivity and improved recovery from psychosocial stressors as a consequence of fitness/chronic exercise. Although the effects between fitness and reactivity/recovery appeared small in magnitude (e.g., 1.8 bpm heart rate reactivity, 3.7 mmHg systolic blood pressure reactivity), the differences are equivalent to 15–25% reductions in reactivity which may still be of clinical importance.

Evidence from a recent meta-analysis (Hamer et al. 2006) examining blood pressure response to a psychosocial stressor suggested that an acute bout of aerobic exercise may result in a significant reduction in reactivity. That is, medium effect sizes revealed that exercise resulted in beneficial attenuated stress reactivity for both diastolic and systolic blood pressure with reductions of a 3.0 mmHg and 3.7 mmHg in diastolic and systolic responses, respectively. The observed effects appeared most robust with psychosocial stressors administered up to 30 min postexercise with moderate to vigorous exercise intensity and durations lasting from 20 min to 2 h. The findings from this review offer the possibility that the effects of acute exercise may account for some of the mixed results from studies examining chronic exercise and blood pressure reactivity because habitually exercising may place an individual in the postexercise "window" more frequently when encountering daily stressors and thereby result in attenuated stress responses.

Although evidence from meta-analytic reviews is lacking, some studies have reported relationships between physical fitness and reduced hypothalamic-pituitary-adrenal (HPA) axis psychosocial stress reactivity, such as cortisol and inflammatory cytokine production. However, the ability to draw solid conclusions in this area is currently limited. With regard to sympathetic-adrenal-medullary responses, the findings appear conflicting as a result of sampling methodology and exercise intensity and durations employed. Some studies have found no effect of fitness on norepinephrine and epinephrine levels, whereas other studies have reported higher norepinephrine levels in the early phases of a stress response or, conversely, an association between lower levels of fitness and an increased norepinephrine response. In animal analogue studies, levels of norepinephrine have been shown to increase in the frontal cortex following an acute bout of exercise, suggesting increased vigilance to threat and reactivity; however, reduced levels have been found in the hypothalamus and hippocampus which suggests diminished stress reactivity.

In summary, although it appears that acute and chronic exercise and fitness may favorably influence an individual's response to psychosocial stress, further research is needed to clarify this relationship. Reviews of the literature suggest that there is a need for greater methodological rigor and reporting as well as examination of potential moderators of exercise-reactivity and exercise-recovery associations.

Cross-References

▶ Benefits of Exercise
▶ Physical Activity and Health
▶ Stress
▶ Stress Reactivity
▶ Stressor

References and Readings

Buckworth, J., & Dishman, R. K. (2002). *Exercise psychology.* Champaign: Human Kinetics.

Claytor, R. P. (1991). Stress reactivity: Hemodynamic adjustments in trained and untrained humans. *Medicine and Science in Sports and Exercise, 23*, 873–881.

Crews, D. J., & Landers, D. M. (1987). A meta-analytic review of aerobic fitness and reactivity to psychosocial stressors. *Medicine and Science in Sports and Exercise, 19*(Suppl), S114–S120.

De Geus, E. J. C., & Van Doornen, L. J. P. (1993). The effects of fitness training on the physiological stress response. *Work and Stress, 7*, 141–159.

Edenfield, T. M., & Blumenthal, J. A. (2011). Exercise and stress reduction. In A. Baum & R. Contrada (Eds.), *The handbook of stress science: Biology, psychology, and health* (pp. 301–319). New York: Springer.

Forcier, K., Stroud, L. R., Papandonatos, G. D., Hitsman, B., Reiches, M., Krishnamoorthy, J., et al. (2006). Links between physical fitness and cardiovascular reactivity and recovery to psychological stressors: A meta-analysis. *Health Psychology, 25*, 723–739.

Hamer, M., Taylor, A., & Steptoe, A. (2006). The effect of acute aerobic exercise on stress related blood pressure responses: A systematic review and meta-analysis. *Biological Psychology, 71*, 183–190.

Hand, G. A., Phillips, K. D., & Wilson, M. A. (2006). Central regulation of stress reactivity and physical activity. In E. Acevado & P. Ekkekakis (Eds.), *Psychobiology of physical activity* (pp. 189–201). Champaign: Human Kinetics.

Jackson, E. M., & Dishman, R. K. (2006). Cardiorespiratory fitness and laboratory stress: A meta-regression analysis. *Psychophysiology, 43*, 57–72.

Sothmann, M. S., Buckworth, J., Claytor, R. P., Cox, R. H., White-Welkley, J. E., & Dishman, R. K. (1996). Exercise training and the cross-stressor adaptation hypothesis. *Exercise and Sport Sciences Reviews, 24*, 267–287.

Stress, Posttraumatic

Viana Turcios-Cotto
Department of Psychology, University of Connecticut, Storrs, CT, USA

Synonyms

PTS

Definition

Posttraumatic stress is a stress reaction characterized by a multitude of symptoms following a traumatic event. Symptoms can be affective, behavioral, cognitive, and/or physiological in nature. These symptoms appear only after exposure to an event that involved a threat to one's physical integrity such as actual or threatened death or serious injury to oneself, witnessing such a threat on another person, or learning of such a threat experienced by a family member or other close person. A traumatic event can come in many forms including but not limited to a natural disaster (e.g., earthquake, tornado), violent personal attack, (e.g., rape, robbery), military combat, terrorist attack, severe automobile accident, or diagnosis of life-threatening illness (American Psychiatric Association [APA] 1994). Although posttraumatic stress is similar to posttraumatic stress disorder (PTSD), a diagnosable psychological condition, it is distinctly different in that the symptoms of posttraumatic stress may not be as severe or as numerous as those of PTSD. Thus, not all of the criteria necessary for diagnosis of PTSD are met, and the symptoms typically do not cause clinically significant distress or impairment in important areas of functioning.

Description

Rates of trauma exposure are unclear, but it is estimated that a majority of people, over 60%, living within the United States have experienced at least one traumatic event (Resick et al. 2008). Some of those affected will develop no signs of distress, whereas some will develop clinically significant, diagnosable signs of distress, and yet others, people experiencing posttraumatic stress, can be categorized as developing subclinical levels of distress. Like many other psychological difficulties, whether or not someone develops significant signs of distress after a traumatic event depends on many variables such as the individual's coping abilities, trauma history, support system, type of traumatic event, intensity of the event, proximity to the event, and so on. Individuals with diminished coping abilities, extensive trauma histories, weak support systems, and who experience more intense and physical traumas closer to their bodies will be at greater risk for suffering from more severe posttraumatic distress (APA 1994; Resick et al. 2008). Since the subclinical population does not warrant a diagnosis and most likely does not seek treatment due to the lack of or low level of impairment, it is difficult to estimate how many are afflicted by posttraumatic stress. However, individuals living with posttraumatic stress experience various difficulties, which can be categorized into groups of affective, behavioral, cognitive, and physiological symptoms.

Affective Symptoms

After a traumatic event, one can feel a variety of stressful emotions as a consequence for days, weeks, or even months after the experience. Intense fear and helplessness are characteristic markers of posttraumatic stress (APA 1994; Beidel and Stipelman 2007; Resick et al. 2008). A person can feel scared that the event might reoccur at any moment and horror that he or she will be unable to stop it from happening again. One might fear for their life and worry that death or severe injury is imminent, creating constant anxiety, and perhaps a sense of a foreshortened future (APA 1994; Beidel and Stipelman, 2007). Some people may react to a traumatic incident with guilt and/or shame, unwilling to talk to others about the incident believing that they are at fault for the event. Sadness and even depression can also arise as a result from experiencing a trauma. This can lead to no longer finding pleasure in activities that the person once enjoyed or in diminished social involvement (Beidel and Stipelman 2007). Lastly, an individual may experience a feeling of anger, manifested through irritability or outbursts (APA 1994). This anger may be focused on the event itself; it may also be geared toward others, perhaps blaming others for the occurrence of the event or fueled by mistrust of others. Overall, the affective symptoms that result from posttraumatic stress are typically negative and can become harmful if they linger for too long.

Behavioral Symptoms

Certain behaviors that were not present before a traumatic event can also surface as a result. Hypervigilance, a constant watchful eye on one's surroundings, is a hallmark behavior used to protect oneself from unexpected threats. This hypervigilance includes heightened sensory sensitivity with an intense, somewhat irrational reaction or an exaggerated startle response (APA 1994; Beidel and Stipelman 2007). For example, an individual who has personally experienced an earthquake may become more aware of slight tremors, flickering lights, rattling windows, or rumbling sounds that others do not notice. These stimuli might arouse fear or anxiety in the individual who might feel as if they are reexperiencing the traumatic event. A person may also purposely work toward not reexperiencing or remembering the event. He or she might avoid certain places, people, smells, sounds, topics of conversation, or anything else that might trigger memories of the incident and may even be unable to recall certain aspects of the event altogether (Beidel and Stipelman 2007; Resick et al. 2008). One might also learn to numb their feelings so that they no longer experience fear, anxiety, or anger as a protective measure from the various affective symptoms that may have developed after the trauma. However, this typically also leads to numbing positive affect such as joy and excitement as well, restricting one's range of affect (APA 1994; Beidel and Stipelman 2007). Avoidance and numbing can further cause a person to become somewhat reclusive and decrease involvement in social situations, resulting in a feeling of detachment or estrangement from friends and family. In general, the behavioral symptoms that appear after a traumatic event are used as coping mechanisms to either protect oneself to keep such an event from reoccurring or to distance oneself from the event that has occurred.

Cognitive Symptoms

There are key cognitions that are representative of those individuals who have experienced a trauma. Most often, there is an overgeneralization of the event and the harm that it caused (Resick et al. 2008). In other words, an individual might believe that harmful or deadly events happen more often and in more places than previously thought. He or she might feel that he or she is always at risk and lacks safety, misappraising minor events or stimuli as much more dangerous than they really are. A victim might lose trust in others and think that others are out to harm him or her, particularly if another human being caused the trauma. Other distorted cognitions about power and control may surface as well (Resick et al.). Such beliefs might be that one has no control or power over events in their daily life, perhaps lowering self-esteem. Another distortion might be self-blame where the victim believes he or she had complete control and power in the situation, bringing the traumatic event upon him or herself. This can result in a feeling of shame or guilt.

Although cognitive symptoms usually only include cognitions or beliefs that a person holds, in the case of posttraumatic stress, they also include ideas, images, and impulses that might materialize in one's mind after a traumatic event. Individuals might have sudden, intrusive memories of images, smells, sounds, etc., of the event flash in his or her mind (APA 1994). The victim might also have distressing dreams about the incident or feel and act as if he or she is reliving the terrible moment (Resick et al. 2008). Due to the many stressors experienced after a traumatic event, concentration may be difficult for individuals with posttraumatic stress.

Physiological Symptoms

Posttraumatic stress causes physiological changes as well. Most notably, there is an increase in heart rate and sweat gland activity. Levels of cortisol may also rise. These symptoms may lead to exhaustion or various serious illnesses such as heart disease (Resick et al. 2008; Sarafino 2008).

Summary

Posttraumatic stress is a psychological stress reaction following a traumatic event. It is characterized by a multitude of affective, behavioral, cognitive, and physiological symptoms that negatively impact an individual. However, the symptoms are not severe enough to cause impairment in social, occupational, or other areas of functioning and therefore do not warrant a diagnosis. Nevertheless, if symptoms become more severe and do not diminish within a month's time, they may be a sign of a diagnosable psychological condition, posttraumatic stress disorder. In such a case, the individual should seek treatment from a professional psychologist or counselor.

Cross-References

▶ Post Traumatic Stress Disorder
▶ Posttraumatic Growth
▶ Stress

References and Readings

American Psychiatric Association. (1994). *Diagnostic and statistical manual of mental disorders* (4th ed.). Washington, DC: Author.

Beidel, D. C., & Stipelman, B. (2007). Anxiety disorders, chapter 11. In M. Hersen, S. M. Turner, & D. C. Beidel (Eds.), *Adult psychopathology and diagnosis* (5th ed., pp. 349–409). Hoboken: Wiley.

Resick, P. A., Monson, C. M., & Rizvi, S. L. (2008). Posttraumatic stress disorder, chapter 2. In D. H. Barlow (Ed.), *Clinical handbook of psychological disorders: A step-by-step treatment manual* (4th ed., pp. 65–122). New York: Guilford Press.

Sarafino, E. P. (2008). Stress – Its meaning, impact, and sources, chapter 3. In E. P. Sarafino (Ed.), *Health psychology: Biopsychosocial interactions* (6th ed., pp. 61–86). Hoboken: Wiley.

Stress: Appraisal and Coping

Susan Folkman
Department of Medicine, School of Medicine,
University of California San Francisco,
San Mateo, CA, USA

Definition

Stress has been defined traditionally either as a *stimulus*, often referred to as a *stressor*, that happens to the person such as a laboratory shock or loss of a job, or as a *response* characterized by physiological arousal and negative affect, especially anxiety. In his 1966 book, *Psychological Stress and the Coping Process* (Lazarus 1966), Richard Lazarus defined stress as a relationship between the person and the environment that is appraised as personally significant and as taxing or exceeding resources for coping. This definition is the foundation of stress and coping theory (Lazarus and Folkman 1984).

Description

Stress and coping theory provides a framework that is useful for formulating and testing hypotheses about the stress process and its relation to physical and mental health. The framework emphasizes the importance of two processes, appraisal and coping, as mediators of the ongoing relationship between the person and the environment. Stress and coping theory is relevant to the stress process as it is experienced in the ordinary events of daily life, major life events, and chronic stressful conditions that stretch out over years.

Appraisal refers to the individual's continuous evaluation of how things are going in relation to his or her personal goals, values, and beliefs. Primary appraisal asks "Am I okay?" Secondary appraisal asks "What can I do?" Situations that signal harm or potential harm that is personally significant and in which there are few options for controlling what happens are appraised as stressful. Stress appraisals include harm or loss, which refer to damage already done; appraisals of threat, which refer to the judgment that something bad might happen; and appraisals of challenge, which refer to something that may happen that offers the opportunity for mastery or gain as well as some risk of an unwelcome outcome. Situations that are appraised as high in personal significance and low in controllability, for example, are usually appraised as threats, and situations that are high in personal significance and high in controllability are more likely to be appraised as challenges.

The concept of appraisal addresses the issue of variability of responses among people experiencing a similar stressor and why a given situation may be more stressful for one person than another. The situation may involve goals, values, or beliefs that are more personally significant for one person than for another, or one person may be better equipped than another to control the situation's outcome. Appraisal-based approaches now dominate the field (Pearlin et al. 1981).

Appraisals generate emotions that vary in quality and intensity according to the person's evaluation of personal significance (primary appraisal) and options for coping (secondary appraisal). Threat appraisals, for example, are often accompanied by fear, anxiety, and worry; harm/loss appraisals are often accompanied by anger, sadness, or guilt; and challenge appraisals are often accompanied by eagerness and excitement as well as a touch of threat.

People experience a complex array of emotions during real-life stressful events, including positive as well as negative emotions (Folkman 1997, 2008). Emotions indicate that something is happening that matters to the individual. Emotions also often signal what the person intends to do. Negative emotions have long been associated with the individual's preparation to approach or avoid, fight or flee (Lazarus 1991). Positive emotions have more recently been examined for their roles in the stress process. Positive emotions, for example, are associated with widened focus of attention, motivating meaning-focused coping, and eliciting social support (Folkman 2008; Fredrickson 1998).

Coping refers to the thoughts and actions people use to manage distress (emotion-focused coping), manage the problem causing the distress (problem-focused coping), and sustain positive well-being (meaning-focused coping). Emotion-focused coping includes strategies such as distancing, humor, and seeking social support that are generally considered adaptive, and strategies such as escape-avoidance, day dreaming, and blaming others that are generally considered maladaptive. Problem-focused coping includes strategies such as information gathering, seeking advice, drawing on previous experience, negotiating, and problem solving. Meaning-focused coping includes strategies such as focusing on deeply held values, beliefs, and goals; reframing or reappraising situations in positive ways; and amplifying positive moments over the course of a day (Folkman and Moskowitz 2000).

Coping is influenced by the person's coping resources including psychological, spiritual, social, environmental, and material resources, and by the nature of the situation, especially whether its outcome is controllable or has to be accepted. Problem-focused coping is used more in situations that are controllable, and emotion-focused coping is used more in situations that have to be accepted. Meaning-focused coping appears to be used more in situations that are chronic and not resolvable, such as in caregiving or serious illness. It is hypothesized that meaning-focused coping becomes more active when initial coping efforts fail to make the situation better (Folkman 2011). Meaning-focused coping sustains other coping efforts and restores coping resources.

People use an array of coping strategies in real-life situations. Most situations involve more than one coping task or goal, each of which requires a coping strategy tailored to that task or goal. And people switch coping strategies when the ones they are using do not have the desired effect. Coping also changes as an encounter unfolds in response to changes in the environment, the situation, or to changes within the person.

Coping effectiveness is determined contextually because effective coping in one situation may be ineffective in another. For instance, distancing may be ineffective when a person should be problem solving or preparing for an upcoming challenge, whereas it may be effective when there is nothing to be done, as when waiting for a test result. Researchers often identify on an a priori basis the outcome that is desired, such as improved mood. In such cases, effective coping is the coping that is associated with the desired outcome.

Another approach to evaluating coping is to examine the goodness of the fit between the appraised options for coping and the choice of coping strategy. Problem-focused coping that is used when the situation is appraised as controllable, for example, would be a good fit, whereas the same form of coping in situation where nothing can be done would be a poor fit. Conversely, distancing that is used when there is nothing that can be done would be a good fit, whereas the same form of coping in a controllable situation that called for attention would be a poor fit.

Like appraisal, coping is key to understanding why the outcomes of given stressful situations can vary from person to person. Two people may cope quite differently with the same stressful situation because of differences in their resources, experiences, motivation, preferences, and skills for coping.

The dynamic quality of the stress process is evident in changes in the appraisal and reappraisal process, the fluidity of emotions, and changes in coping thoughts and actions as an encounter unfolds. The processes are also in reciprocal relationships. An outcome of appraisal and coping at Time 1, such as mood, for example, can become a predictor of appraisal and coping at Time 2.

References and Readings

Folkman, S. (1997). Positive psychological states and coping with severe stress. *Social Science and Medicine, 45*, 1207–1221.

Folkman, S. (2008). The case for positive emotions in the stress process. *Anxiety, Stress, and Coping, 21*, 3–14.

Folkman, S. (Ed.). (2011). *The Oxford handbook of stress, health, and coping*. New York: Oxford University Press.

Folkman, S., & Moskowitz, J. T. (2000). Positive affect and the other side of coping. *American Psychologist, 55*, 647–654.

Fredrickson, B. L. (1998). What good are positive emotions? *Review of General Psychology Special Issue: New Directions in Research on Emotion, 2*, 300–319.

Lazarus, R. S. (1966). *Psychological stress and the coping process*. New York: McGraw Hill.

Lazarus, R. S. (1991). *Emotion and adaptation*. New York: Oxford University Press.

Lazarus, R. S., & Folkman, S. (1984). *Stress, appraisal, and coping*. New York: Springer.

Pearlin, L. I., Lieberman, M. A., Menaghan, E. G., & Mullan, J. T. (1981). The stress process. *Journal of Health and Social Behavior, 22*, 337–356.

Stress-Associated Disorders

▶ Stress-Related Disorders

Stressful Life Event

▶ Psychosocial Factors and Traumatic Events

Stressful Life Events

▶ Life Events

Stress-Induced Asthma

▶ Asthma and Stress

Stress-Induced Disorders

▶ Stress-Related Disorders

Stressor

▶ Psychological Stress

Stress-Related Disorders

Susanne Fischer[1] and Urs M. Nater[2]
[1]Clinical Psychology and Psychotherapy, Institute of Psychology, University of Zurich, Zurich, Switzerland
[2]Department of Psychology, University of Vienna, Vienna, Austria

Synonyms

Stress-associated disorders; Stress-induced disorders

Definition

The term "stress-related disorders" is used in various ways in the scientific literature. A narrow definition includes conditions that are clearly *caused* by stress. Consequentially, merely a handful of (mental) disorders (e.g., posttraumatic stress disorder) are deemed eligible for this label. By contrast, a broad definition includes all illnesses that are somehow adversely *impacted* by stress. This can mean that stress is involved in the predisposition, precipitation, and/or perpetuation of a particular condition. Given that stress exerts negative effects on numerous bodily systems (e.g., the autonomic nervous system, the endocrine system, and the immune system) and on health behaviors (e.g., eating, physical activity, substance use), virtually all mental disorders and a large proportion of somatic diseases can be classified as stress-related disorders according to this definition.

Description

The continuum between conditions in which stress is a causal versus a contributing factor is reflected by the various diagnostic codes for stress-related disorders. In the 11th edition of the International Classification of Diseases (ICD-11; WHO 2018b), stress is most prominently mentioned in "disorders specifically associated with stress" within the mental disorders chapter. This category includes adjustment disorder and posttraumatic stress disorder (PTSD), among other disorders that are triggered by trauma, critical life events, or chronic stress, and is analogous to the category of "trauma- and stressor-related disorders" in the fifth edition of the *Diagnostic and Statistical Manual of Mental Disorders* (DSM-5; APA 2013). In addition, stress is featured as a general "factor influencing health status" at the very end of the ICD-11 and as a "psychological factor affecting disorders or diseases classified elsewhere" within the chapter on mental disorders. These codes are usually used in somatic diseases in which stress is a risk or exacerbating factor (e.g., in cardiovascular or inflammatory diseases).

Stress-related symptoms are highly diverse. When stress is the main factor involved in the development of a particular illness (e.g., in PTSD or adjustment disorder), typical symptoms include depressed mood, anhedonia, problems in concentration, anxiety, irritability, and sleep disturbance. When stress is one among several factors contributing to the development and/or maintenance of a condition (e.g., in somatic symptom disorder or hypertension), any number of these symptoms may be found, in addition to the unique conglomerate of symptoms pertaining to the disease/disorder in question. However, it is often difficult to establish a clear distinction between stress-related symptoms and symptoms of other origins (e.g., a genetic abnormality), especially as stress may exacerbate almost any symptom via its negative effects on stress-responsive bodily systems (e.g., impaired immune functioning) and lifestyle behaviors (e.g., physical inactivity, smoking).

The contribution of stress-related disorders to the global burden of disease is high. Posttraumatic stress disorder alone has a lifetime prevalence of 3.9% (Koenen et al. 2017), and diseases that are adversely affected by stress are among the most debilitating conditions worldwide. According to the WHO (2018a), the top five current causes of disability-adjusted life years (DALYs) and death are ischemic heart disease, stroke, lower respiratory infection, chronic obstructive pulmonary disease (COPD), and road injury. Of these, all three noncommunicable diseases, that is, ischemic heart disease, stroke, and COPD, have direct and indirect links to stress. For instance, a meta-analysis of over 500,000 individuals showed that long working hours (i.e., more than 55 h per week) were directly associated with a significantly increased risk of both ischemic heart disease and stroke (Kivimaki et al., 2015). This can be attributed to physical inactivity and repeated activation of the stress response. Similarly, an extensive meta-analysis confirmed that smoking, which is often used as a means to cope with stress, is a major risk factor for COPD, causing airway obstruction, mucus hypersecretion, and emphysema (Forey et al. 2011).

Depending on the role of stress in the development and/or maintenance of a particular disorder, and depending on the type of stressor involved, different interventions can be applied to alleviate symptom burden. When stress is causal and traumatic (e.g., a rape victim developing PTSD), trauma-focused cognitive behavioral therapy (CBT) should be applied. This treatment comprises prolonged exposure to traumatic cues or memories as well as cognitive restructuring of dysfunctional trauma-related beliefs. In cases where stress is causal, but non-traumatic (e.g., a critical life event or chronic stress triggering an adjustment disorder), the choice of psychological intervention will depend on whether a patient shows symptoms of depression, anxiety, or disturbance of conduct. In the case of depression, behavioral activation or sleep hygiene may prove to be effective, whereas anxiety may best be managed by relaxation exercises or cognitive restructuring, and patients with disturbance of conduct may benefit from social skills training. Finally, when (chronic) stress is a contributing factor, stress management techniques may be a worthy addition to pharmacological or other somatic therapies (e.g., antidepressants for major depressive disorder, surgery after myocardial infarction). Such programs either target the stressor itself (e.g., effort-reward imbalance at work); the individual appraisal of potentially stressful situations, including personality traits that foster stress (e.g., perfectionism); or the immediate consequences of stress (e.g., elevated sympathetic activity, smoking as a coping strategy).

Cross-References

▶ Autonomic Nervous System (ANS)
▶ Cardiovascular Disease
▶ Chronic Obstructive Pulmonary Disease
▶ Cognitive Behavioral Therapy (CBT)
▶ Cognitive Restructuring
▶ Coping
▶ Health Behaviors
▶ Hypertension
▶ Ischemic Heart Disease
▶ Physical Activity
▶ Physical Inactivity
▶ Post Traumatic Stress Disorder
▶ Relaxation Techniques
▶ Smoking
▶ Stress
▶ Stress Disorder
▶ Stress Management
▶ Stress, Posttraumatic
▶ Stress Response

References and Further Readings

APA. (2013). *Diagnostic and statistical manual of mental disorders* (5th ed.). Washington D.C.: APA.

Forey, B. A., Thornton, A. J., & Lee, P. N. (2011). Systematic review with meta-analysis of the epidemiological evidence relating smoking to COPD, chronic bronchitis and emphysema. *BMC Pulmonary Medicine, 11*, 36. https://doi.org/10.1186/1471-2466-11-36.

Kivimaki, M., Jokela, M., Nyberg, S. T., Singh-Manoux, A., Fransson, E. I., Alfredsson, L., et al. (2015). Long working hours and risk of coronary heart disease and stroke: A systematic review and meta-analysis of published and unpublished data for 603,838 individuals. *Lancet, 386*(10005), 1739–1746. https://doi.org/10.1016/S0140-6736(15)60295-1.

Koenen, K. C., Ratanatharathorn, A., Ng, L., McLaughlin, K. A., Bromet, E. J., Stein, D. J., et al. (2017). Posttraumatic stress disorder in the world mental health surveys. *Psychological Medicine, 47*(13), 2260–2274. https://doi.org/10.1017/S0033291717000708.

WHO. (2018a). *Global Health estimates 2016: Deaths by cause, age, sex, by country and by region* (pp. 2000–2016). Geneva: WHO.

WHO. (2018b). International statistical classification of diseases and related health problems (11th revision). Retrieved from https://icd.who.int/browse11/l-m/en.

Stress-Related Growth

▶ Benefit Finding
▶ Perceived Benefits
▶ Posttraumatic Growth

Stroke Burden

Jonathan Newman
Columbia University, New York, NY, USA

Definition

Description

Strokes are one of the leading causes of death and disability: each year, nearly 800,000 Americans experience a new or recurrent stroke. Approximately 600,000 of these are first events and roughly 180,000 are recurrent attacks. In the United States, strokes accounted for 1 out of every 16 deaths in 2004, and more than 50% of the deaths attributable to strokes occurred outside of the hospital. When separated from other cardiovascular diseases, stroke is the third leading cause of death, behind heart disease and cancer. Importantly, strides have been made in reduction of stroke mortality: the stroke death rate has fallen more than 20% from 1994 to 2004. However, important disparities remain. While Hispanic, Latino, American Indian, and Pacific Islander populations have somewhat lower stroke death rates than whites, black men and women continue to have significantly higher stroke death rates than all other populations, and the prevalence of stroke remains higher in minority populations than among whites. Lastly, because women live longer than men, in 2004, women accounted for greater than 60% of stroke deaths in the United States.

In addition to the significant mortality, the morbidity associated with stroke is considerable: more than 25% of stroke survivors older than age 65 are disabled 6 months later. The length of time to recover from a stroke depends on its initial severity. From 50% to 70% of stroke survivors regain functional independence, but 15–30% are permanently disabled, and 20% require institutional care at 3 months after onset. Although 70% of strokes are a first cardiovascular event, 15% of survivors will have a recurrent event within 1 year, and 30% will have a recurrent event within 5 years. The period soon after an acute stroke is associated with the highest rate of stroke recurrence, and the risk of stroke following a transient ischemic attack (TIA) is over 10% for the following 90 days.

The medical costs of stroke are high: the estimated direct and indirect costs of stroke for 2008 are $65.5 billion USD. In comparison, the 2008 costs for coronary heart disease were estimated at $156.4 billion USD, making stroke one of the leading US health-care expenditures. The mean lifetime cost of ischemic stroke is over $140,000 USD, and 70% of the first-year costs following an acute stroke are due to inpatient hospital costs.

Finally, the burden associated with stroke contains an important association with other cardiovascular disease processes and risk. Many risk factors for stroke overlap with those of cardiac and peripheral vascular disease. This overlap has led to the concept of "global risk" for cardiovascular disease in general, of which stroke is one component. High blood pressure is the greatest risk factor for stroke, but factors like smoking, diabetes, and low high-density lipoprotein levels are important risk factors. Depression has been suggested to be an independent risk factor for stroke. The occurrence of a stroke is therefore likely to be the initial manifestation of a global cardiovascular disease process, with high morbidity, mortality, and cost, and risk factors that overlap with traditional cardiovascular risk factor categories.

References and Readings

Asplund, K., Stegmayr, B., & Peltonen, M. (1998). From the twentieth to the twenty-first century: A public health perspective on stroke. In M. D. Ginsberg & J. Bogousslavsky (Eds.), *Cerebrovascular disease pathophysiology, diagnosis, and management* (Vol. 2). Malden: Blackwell. Chap 64.

Rosamond, W. D., Folsom, A. R., Chambless, L. E., Wang, C. H., McGovern, P. G., Howard, G., Copper, L. S., & Shahar, E. (1999). Stroke incidence and survival among middle-aged adults: 9-year follow-up of the Atherosclerotic Risk in Communities (ARIC) cohort. *Stroke, 30*, 736–743.

Rosamond, W., Flegal, K., Furie, K., et al. (2008). Heart disease and stroke statistics-2008 update: A report from the American Heart Association Statistics Committee and Stroke Statistics Subcommittee. *Circulation, 117*, e25–e146.

Stroop Color-Word Test

Mark Hamer
Epidemiology and Public Health, Division of Population Health, University College London, London, UK

Synonyms

Mental stressor; Problem solving

Definition

The Stroop test is commonly used in psychophysiological studies as a problem-solving task to elicit mental stress. The test is an incongruent task that requires participants to identify the name of a color (e.g., "blue," "green," or "red") that is printed in a conflicting color not denoted by the name (e.g., the word "red" printed in blue ink instead of red ink). The task primarily evokes beta-adrenergically driven responses, resulting in increased heart rate and cardiac output. Functional neuroimaging studies of the Stroop effect have consistently revealed activation in the frontal lobe and more specifically in the anterior cingulate cortex and dorsolateral prefrontal cortex, two structures hypothesized to be responsible for conflict monitoring and resolution.

Cross-References

▶ Blood Pressure Reactivity or Responses
▶ Heart Rate

Structural Equation Modeling (SEM)

Maria Magdalena Llabre and William Arguelles
Department of Psychology, University of Miami, Coral Gables, FL, USA

Synonyms

SEM

Definition

Structural equation modeling (SEM) is a multivariate statistical methodology for the estimation of a system of simultaneous linear equations that may include both observed and latent variables. With origins in the path analysis work of the biometrician Sewell Wright and the factor analysis tradition of Charles Spearman, over the past 40 years, SEM has transitioned from a novel methodology for linear models to a mainstream statistical framework for the analysis of latent variable models. SEM-related techniques may be used to examine a wide variety of structures, including causal models, measurement models, growth models, latent classes or mixtures, and combinations of these. The generality and flexibility of SEM, the development of efficient estimation methods, and the availability of computer programs contribute to the utility of this methodology for addressing important research questions in behavioral medicine.

Description

The first step in an SEM analysis is the specification of the model. SEM models are specified via either a system of structural equations or, more commonly, a path diagram. Included in the path diagram are the observed variables to be analyzed, the constructs or latent variables to be inferred, the unobserved but ever-present errors or disturbances, and the ways in which these observed and unobserved variables are related to one another. The path diagram is a valuable tool in itself, helping investigators better understand their research questions and their data. A path diagram forces the investigator to think critically about every variable relevant to the phenomenon under study.

Observed variables (also called indicators) are the variables we measure directly. These could be exogenous (variables whose causes are not included in the model) or endogenous (variables whose causes are posited in the model). *Path analysis* is a special case of SEM in which all variables specified in a model are observed (except for the errors) and assumed to be perfectly reliable. However, when reliability is not perfect and indicators contain measurement error, as is often the case, parameter estimates may be biased. One of the key features of SEM is the possibility of combining multiple observed variables into *latent variables* (the constructs of interest). A latent variable, like a construct, is not observed directly, but is rather inferred from the covariances shared among its corresponding indicators. For example, we could combine multiple measures of depression into a latent variable to improve reliability. Thus, a general SEM model may be viewed as having two components: a structural model (which allows for the specification and testing of relationships among variables) and a measurement model (which offers the advantage of using latent variables to represent constructs of interest, modeling sources of measurement error and bias associated with directly observed variables).

Generally speaking, the purpose of analyzing SEM models is twofold. First, we wish to test whether the specified model fits the data. Second and simultaneously, we want to estimate the parameters of interest and test them for significance. The most common *method of estimation* used by available computer programs is maximum likelihood (ML), performed iteratively to arrive at an admissible solution. ML parameter estimates are unbiased, consistent, efficient, and normally distributed in large samples. Given a particular model specification, this method is used to generate and compare a model-implied variance-covariance matrix to the data-based variance-covariance matrix. ML estimates are those that minimize the discrepancy between those two matrices, and as such, yield parameter values that have the greatest likelihood of having given rise to the sample values obtained, assuming a multivariate normal distribution. The typical output from a computer analysis will have indices of model fit, as well as the parameter estimates, their standard errors, and z-values used to test them for significance.

The primary index used to test model fit is a χ^2 statistic. However, given this statistic's direct dependence on sample size, with large sample sizes, even small differences between the two matrices may yield a significant χ^2 indicative of poor model fit. Several other indices have been developed and proposed as either alternatives or companions to the χ^2 in such cases, including the comparative fit index (CFI), the root mean squared error of approximation (RMSEA), and the standardized root mean residual (SRMR). Beyond overall measures of fit, it is important to make sure that parameter estimates make sense in relation to the problem being investigated.

In terms of the structural aspect of SEM, the *parameters of primary interest* are the path coefficients (or the direct effects among the variables). In SEM, the variances and covariances among the exogenous variables are also estimated, as well as the variances and covariances of the disturbances. In terms of the measurement aspect of SEM, the parameters of primary interest are the factor (or latent variable) loadings, the measurement error variances, and the variances and covariances of the latent variables.

When working within the SEM framework using ML estimation, it is possible to take advantage of its full information capabilities to include all of the available data. Often referred to as full information maximum likelihood (FIML), this approach to *missing data* has been shown to yield unbiased parameter estimates when missingness is related to variables that are accessible for analysis (Little and Rubin 2002; Schafer and Graham 2002). Comparable to multiple imputation, this method is superior to other missing data techniques such as listwise or pairwise deletion, or mean, regression, or hotdeck imputation, particularly when data are not missing completely at random (Enders 2006).

SEM is a large sample methodology and the appropriate sample size must be considered keeping in mind several issues including model complexity, estimation method, and statistical power. With samples less than 100 participants, models must be simple and the variables normally distributed, otherwise problems with model convergence are likely to arise. As a general rule, more complex models or non-normal data will require more participants.

Of note, testing of *alternative models* is necessary to strengthen the causal inferences often associated with SEM. Sometimes researchers improperly assume that models that fit the data represent reality, without recognizing there are always multiple alternative models that fit just as well. Models can be rejected but not proven. It is important to consider design features such as randomization, experimentation, longitudinal designs, instrumental variables, or inclusion of other variables to strengthen model interpretation.

In addition to testing relationships among variables, means and mean structures may be analyzed. For example, multiple groups may be compared with respect to means of latent variables, or mean changes over time may be modeled using *latent growth modeling*. Many other extensions are possible but their description is beyond the scope of this entry. However, this is an active area of research and readers are encouraged to learn more by consulting available textbooks, Web sites, and papers. A very readable conceptual introduction to SEM is provided by Kline (2010). A more detailed presentation of its use in behavioral medicine may be found in Llabre (2010). The Web site for Mplus (Muthen and Muthen 2011) – one of the more popular computer programs – contains a lot of useful information on the basics of SEM, as well as extensions to more complex models.

Cross-References

▶ Hierarchical Linear Modeling (HLM)
▶ Latent Variable
▶ Missing Data
▶ Randomization

References and Readings

Enders, C. K. (2006). Analyzing structural equation models with missing data. In G. R. Hancock & R. O. Mueller (Eds.), *Structural equation modeling: A second course* (pp. 313–344). Greenwich: Information Age Publishing.

Kline, R. (2010). *Principles and practice of structural equation modeling* (2nd ed.). New York: Guilford Press.

Little, R. J., & Rubin, D. B. (2002). *Statistical analysis with missing data* (2nd ed.). Hoboken: Wiley.

Llabre, M. M. (2010). Structural equation modeling in behavioral medicine research. In A. Steptoe (Ed.), *Handbook of behavioral medicine: Methods and applications* (pp. 895–908). New York: Springer.

Muthen, L., & Muthen, B. (1998–2011). *Mplus user's guide*. Los Angeles: Muthen & Muthen.

Schafer, J. L., & Graham, J. W. (2002). Missing data: Our view of the state of art. *Psychological Methods, 7*, 147–177.

Structural Variant

▶ Copy Number Variant (CNV)

Structured Clinical Interview for DSM-IV (SCID)

Ulrike Kübler
Department of Psychology, University of Zurich, Binzmuehlestrasse, Zurich, Switzerland

Definition

The structured clinical interview for DSM-4 (SCID) is a semistructured interview created to make reliable psychiatric diagnoses in adults according to the *Diagnostic and Statistical Manual*, fourth edition (DSM-IV). The SCID has two parts: one for DSM-IV Axis I disorders (SCID-I) and another for DSM-IV Axis II personality disorders (SCID-II).

In order to meet different needs, the SCID-I is available in two versions: the research version (SCID-I-RV; First et al. 2002) and the clinician version (SCID-CV; First et al. 1996). In contrast to the SCID-CV, the SCID-I-RV comprises more disorders, subtypes, severity, and course specifiers and is easier to modify. The SCID-I-RV itself is also available in different versions. The broadest SCID-I-RV version comprises ten self-contained diagnostic modules: mood episodes, psychotic and associated symptoms, psychotic disorders, mood disorders, substance use disorders, anxiety disorders, somatoform disorders, eating disorders, adjustment disorders, and an optional module which allows psychiatric diagnoses that may be of the interviewer's interest, such as the module on acute stress disorder and on minor depressive disorder.

The SCID-I starts with an open-ended overview that includes questions about demographic information, work history, chief complaint, past and present periods of psychopathology, treatment history, and current functioning. This is followed by the diagnostic modules, which are presented in a three-column format: the left-hand column contains the interview questions, the middle column contains the corresponding DSM-IV criteria, and in the right-hand column ratings for the criteria are indicated. Besides rating the presence of the DSM-IV criteria for Axis I disorders, the SCID-I also enables rating of Axis III, IV, and IV of the DSM (see DSM-IV for more details).

The SCID-II (First et al. 1997) is only offered in a single version. It covers the ten standard DSM-IV Axis II personality disorders (avoidant, dependent, obsessive-compulsive, paranoid, schizotypal, schizoid, histrionic, narcissistic, borderline, antisocial personality disorder), as well as personality disorder not otherwise specified, and the appendix categories depressive personality disorder and passive-aggressive personality disorder. The item format and the conventions of the SCID-II are very similar to those of the SCID-I. The SCID-II consists of several questions organized in sections in accordance with the DSM-IV diagnoses for personality disorders. In most cases, the questions correspond accurately with the criteria. To shorten overall administration time, the SCID-II is also provided with a self-report screening questionnaire that is intended to be administered at first. After this questionnaire has been filled out, only those items indicating personality abnormalities need to be inquired in more detail during the interview.

The SCID-II is often used in conjunction with the SCID-I. While administration of SCID-I typically takes between 45 and 90 min, the complete administration time of the SCID-II usually lasts about 1 h. Ideally, the SCID is administered by a trained interviewer familiar with the diagnostic criteria used in the DSM-IV. The SCID can be used in both healthy individuals and psychiatric patients. In individuals with either severe psychotic symptoms or severe cognitive impairments, the administration of the SCID is not recommended.

Overall, the SCID is a widely used assessment tool in both research and clinical settings in many countries. Various versions of the SCID have been translated into multiple languages, including Mandarin, Spanish, French, and German. The psychometric properties of the SCID-I and the SCID-II have been evaluated in several adult populations in numerous investigations, with encouraging results for most Axis I and Axis II disorders (e.g., Lobbestael et al. 2010). Computer-assisted versions of the SCID are also available.

Notably, since October 2015 the Structured Clinical Interview for DSM-5 diagnoses (SCID-5) has been available in English. The SCID-5 can be ordered in two versions: SCID-5-CV (clinician version; comparable with SCID-CV) and SCID-5-PD (personality disorders; comparable with SKID-II). For more information on the SCID-5, the reader is referred to the American Psychiatric Association Publishing website.

References and Further Reading

https://www.appi.org/scid5

American Psychiatric Association. (2000). *Diagnostic and statistical manual of mental disorders* (4th ed.). Washington, DC: Author. Text revision.

First, M. B., Spitzer, R. L., Gibbon, M., & Williams, J. B. W. (1996). *Structured clinical interview for DSM-IV axis I disorders, clinician version (SCID-CV)*. Washington, DC: American Psychiatric Press.

First, M. B., Gibbon, M., Spitzer, R. L., Williams, J. B. W., & Benjamin, L. S. (1997). *Structured clinical interview for DSM-IV axis II personality disorders, (SCID-II)*. Washington, DC: American Psychiatric Press.

First, M. B., Spitzer, R. L., Gibbon, M., & Williams, J. B. W. (2002). *Structured clinical interview for DSM-IV-TR axis I disorders, research version, patient edition. (SCID-I/P)*. New York: Biometrics Research, New York State Psychiatric Institute.

Lobbestael, J., Leurgans, M., & Arntz, A. (2010). Inter-rater reliability of the structured clinical interview for DSM-IV axis I disorders (SCID I) and axis II disorders (SCID II). *Clinical Psychology & Psychotherapy, 18*(1), 75–79. https://doi.org/10.1002/cpp.693.

Study Methodology

▶ Research Methodology

Study Protocol

J. Rick Turner
Campbell University College of Pharmacy and Health Sciences, Buies Creek, NC, USA

Definition

The study protocol is "the most important document in clinical trials, since it ensures the quality and integrity of the clinical investigation in terms of its planning, execution, conduct, and the analysis of the data" (Chow and Chang 2007). The study protocol is a comprehensive plan of action that contains information concerning the goals of the study, details of subject recruitment, details of safety monitoring, and all aspects of design, methodology, and analysis. (In some cases, a Statistical Analysis Plan, associated with and written at the same time as the study protocol, will contain the detailed description of the analyses to be conducted.)

Description

The creation of study protocol requires input from many individuals. Consider a study protocol for a pharmaceutical clinical trial, since this is likely to be more extensive (and complex) than some smaller trials for behavioral medicine interventions and treatments. By considering this more extensive version, one will be able to judge which parts are and are not needed on a case by case basis.

In the case of a pharmaceutical trial, input will be needed from clinical scientists, medical safety officers, study managers, data managers, and statisticians. Consequently, while one clinical scientist or medical writer may take primary responsibility for the protocol's preparation, many members of the study team make important contributions.

The requirements of a study protocol include:

- Objectives (usually primary and secondary objectives). These goals of the study are stated as precisely as possible.
- Measurements related to the drug's safety, and procedures to ensure the safety of all subjects while participating in the trial.
- Inclusion and exclusion criteria. These provide detailed criteria for subject eligibility for participation in the trial.
- Details of the procedures for physical examinations.
- Laboratory procedures. Full details of the nature and timing of all procedures and tests are provided.
- Electrocardiogram (ECG) measurement and any other measurements such as imaging.
- Drug treatment schedule. Route of administration, dosage, and dosing regimen are detailed. This information is also provided for the control treatment.

- In the case of later-phase trials, measurements of efficacy. The criteria to be used to determine efficacy are provided.
- In the case of later-phase trials, details of the method of diagnosis of the disease or condition of clinical concern for which the drug is intended.
- Statistical analysis. The precise analytical strategy needs to be detailed, here and/or in an associated statistical analysis plan.

Inclusion and exclusion criteria are central components of clinical trials. A study's inclusion and exclusion criteria govern which individuals interested in participating in the trial are admitted to the study as subjects. Criteria for inclusion in the study include items such as the following:

- Reliable evidence of a diagnosis of the disease or condition of clinical concern.
- Being within a specified age range.
- Willingness to take measures to prevent pregnancy during the course of treatment. This includes a female in the trial not becoming pregnant (she may be receiving the drug being tested), and a male participating in the trial not causing a female to become pregnant (he may be receiving the drug being tested).

Criteria for exclusion from the study may include:

- Taking certain medications for other medical conditions and which therefore cannot safely be stopped during the trial.
- Participation in another clinical trial within so many months prior to the commencement of this study.
- Liver or kidney disease.

While inclusion and exclusion criteria are typically provided in two separate lists in regulatory documentation, exclusion criteria can be regarded as further refinements of the inclusion criteria. Meeting all the inclusion criteria allows a person to be considered as a study participant, while not meeting any exclusion criteria is also necessary to allow the person to become a participant.

Cross-References

▶ Informed Consent

References and Further Reading

Chow, S.-C., & Chang, M. (2007). *Adaptive design methods in clinical trials: Concepts and methodologies*. Boca Raton: CRC/Taylor Francis.

Study Size

▶ Sample Size Estimation

Subethnic Groups

▶ Ethnicity
▶ Minority Subgroups

Subgroup Heterogeneity

▶ Minority Subgroups

Subject Characteristics

▶ Demographics

Subjective Well-Being

▶ Happiness and Health

Submissiveness

▶ Interpersonal Circumplex

Substance Abuse

▶ Alcohol Abuse and Dependence
▶ Dependence, Drug
▶ Lifestyle Changes

Substance Abuse: Treatment

John Grabowski
Department of Psychiatry, Medical School,
University of Minnesota, Minneapolis, MN, USA

Synonyms

Addiction rehabilitation; Chemical dependency treatment; Drug abuse: treatment; Drug and alcohol treatment; Drug dependence treatment; Drug rehabilitation; Inpatient treatment; Outpatient treatment; Residential treatment

Definition

Treatment refers to a defined, empirically evaluated, data-based intervention intended to manage, remediate, or cure a diagnosed condition, here, impairing or problematic drug use. Historically, there have been two frameworks underpinning substance use treatment, the "disease" and "learning/conditioning" models (Higgins 1997). While some assumptions are divergent and perhaps irreconcilable, a broad integrative view dictates that genetic and other biological factors interact with behavior and environmental factors as composite determinants of substance use disorders. The diagnostic criteria applied to determining need for treatment are found in the International Statistical Classification of Diseases and Related Health Problems (ICD) 10 (*"Mental and behavioral disorders due to psychoactive substance use"–"a wide variety of disorders that differ in severity and clinical form but that are all attributable to the use of one or more psychoactive substances, which may or may not have been medically prescribed"*) and The American Psychiatric Association Diagnostic and Statistical Manual (DSM) IV, (*"Substance Related Disorders"–"The Substance-Related Disorders include disorders related to the taking of a drug of abuse (including alcohol), to the side effects of a medication, and to toxin exposure"*). The intervention may include behavioral, psychological, social, and pharmacological components delivered by skilled practitioners. There is a wide range of self-help and other efforts with little or no documented efficacy that are beyond the purview of this entry as are a number of criminal justice–based interventions.

Description

Underlying Disciplines, Principles, Goals, and Focus

In the public and lay domain, putative treatments for substance use disorders (i.e., "drug abuse" or "addiction") are legend and varied in their underpinnings. However, the core principles for systematic treatment of substance use disorders reside in empirically based interventions of psychology, psychiatry, pharmacology, behavioral science, and neuroscience. Despite diverse theoretical, conceptual, and terminological differences, there are many commonalities in both practice and behaviors and thoughts that are the focus of treatment. Emphasis is typically placed on avoiding drug use–related circumstances (physical or social) and replacing drug-seeking, drug use, and drug-related thoughts with other behaviors (e.g., coping skills, problem-solving skills). The interventions focus on altering biology, behavior, and social interaction through behavioral/psychological and pharmacological techniques. Longer term pharmacotherapy focuses on substituting a therapeutic medication (e.g., methadone) at controlled doses for the drug used (opiate) or a medication blocking (e.g., naltrexone) the effects of the drug used (opiate) with untoward consequences. Each strategy produces blunting or elimination subjective drug effects. Short-term alleviation of withdrawal symptoms or disturbed behavior is achieved with specific symptomatic treatment (e.g., anxiolytics, sedatives, antidepressants, antipsychotics).

Two important considerations in discussion of treatment are the determinants and correlates of the disorders and the not uncommon existence of co-occurring psychiatric/behavioral or medical problems. These may predate or be a consequence of the substance use disorder(s). The most common comorbid condition for treatment is multiple drug use (e.g., cocaine, heroin, alcohol). Next, the psychological/psychiatric diagnoses of problematic drug use or dependence are not uncommon among individuals also diagnosed for schizophrenia, depression, posttraumatic stress disorder, etc. Indeed, observation of common symptoms associated with extreme drug use, for example, disorganization, paranoid ideation, hallucinations, may reveal existence of the other psychiatric condition. Increasing awareness of co-occurrence of other psychiatric conditions with substance use disorders has resulted in extensive research, discussion, and review of conceptualization of treatment. For example, should specialized single interventions be applied to each presenting condition or should integrated treatments be devised? Questions arise as to correlation, association, and causation. Did the substance use cause psychiatric illness or precipitate its onset and reveal its existence or a predisposition? Did the psychiatric illness predispose to drug use, perhaps as a means to self-medicate the underlying condition? Finally, in instances of severe drug use, medical consequences (e.g., respiratory depression, cardiovascular event, accident-induced trauma) rather than psychiatric symptoms may lead to identification of problematic drug use and need for treatment.

Critical in establishing treatment strategies and regimens is understanding that the substance use disorder is the consequence of multiple determinants, some amenable to manipulation or intervention, others not. As with forms of some other common conditions, for example, hypertension, diabetes, obesity, a complex interplay of genetic, biological, behavioral, social, and other environmental factors contributes to the observed disease. However, limits must exist on diagnosis and treatment. Thus, while some patients present with reasonably stable life styles, educational backgrounds, and work histories, others using the same drugs may have limited education and skills. In both cases, systematic focus on diagnosed conditions is essential. However, the myriad collateral circumstances are the purview of other domains (e.g., social service networks, job counselors, educational systems), which can be addressed more effectively, for example, by adept case managers and other experts, rather than health care providers. The two historical models continue to influence the perspective and goals of treatment. Underpinning an integrative behavioral learning perspective is the concept that just as one learns other behaviors (reading, using the internet, sports), one learns to use drugs. The behavior is maintained by biological, behavioral, and social rewards or reinforcers. The treatment strategy is establishment or learning of other behaviors sustained by non-drug reinforcers, while drug seeking and taking are diminished or eliminated. The disease model assumes a "chronic relapsing disease" evidenced when a predisposed individual is exposed to and begins using psychoactive drugs; complete and perpetual abstinence is the goal and relapse is always imminent (Higgins 1997). To the extent that biology underlies behavior, the integrated learning model accounts for genetic and biological differences but focuses on new behaviors and reinforcers rather than the chronicity of disease.

Treatment Settings, Dose, and Costs

Distinct from the intervention is the setting or environment in which treatment is provided. Settings include outpatient (e.g., office, clinics, emergency rooms), inpatient (e.g., hospital facilities), and residential (e.g., community-like living arrangements). The opportunity for access to patients is increased in controlled residential settings and some supplement the professionally driven therapy with a variety of "self-help" activities such as group discussions. Still others may have options for attending work or school. However, many of the same fundamental interventions can be applied in any of these settings. For example, a course of cognitive behavior therapy could be applied weekly in a mental health care practitioner's office, an inpatient facility, a residential care setting, or for that matter a prison. Another dimension of "setting" is whether care is provided to a single patient by a therapist, or with a group of patients, having the therapist interacting with individual members and also facilitating discussion among members. Attempts to match individuals to particular settings for treatment have been flawed and generally ineffective. For example, no data point to advantages of inpatient compared to outpatient care, regardless of severity for treatment of the behavior of substance use itself.

Similarly distinct is the actual amount or "dose" of intervention. Inpatient settings in which the patient resides continuously for days or weeks do not necessarily deliver more, or more efficacious therapeutic care than treatment delivered to a patient residing at home and functioning in her or his natural environment while receiving office-based care a few hours a week. For example, while inpatient or residential care may shield a patient from access to drugs, including alcohol and nicotine, it also prevents them from having exposure to the very environments in which it will be necessary to engage in life without problematic drug use; this exposure is both essential and therapeutic. As an aside, inpatient and residential care are extremely costly strategies that are well beyond the resources of most individuals and, with increasing health cost burdens for society, will be of diminishing importance except in unusual circumstances.

Evaluation and Monitoring

Drug use severity, as determined by substance used, frequency and amount of use, may be critical to determining treatment required. Thorough diagnostics and history determination permit tailoring treatment. An interview method termed Timeline Follow Back (Sobell et al. 1986) permits careful structuring of a history of use. The accepted diagnostic interviews conforming to elements of the DSM or ICD criteria are necessary to determine severity, existence of comorbid conditions, and plausible treatment plans. A collateral finding in many studies of therapeutic interventions for substance use disorders is that individuals presenting with less severe conditions are more successful in treatment. For example, individuals who on entry for evaluation have negative biological screening tests for the drug used (see below) are more likely to continue successfully for a full course of treatment. Comorbid conditions and individual differences in a range of social and environmental circumstances must always be considered.

Both at intake and during treatment, objective measures of determining current use are essential. For alcohol use, this may be a breath test or urine screen. Tobacco smoking can be readily determined using CO monitoring while other tobacco use can be monitored with saliva or urine screens for cotinine, primary metabolite of nicotine. Virtually all other drug use can be monitored with simple and widely available urine screen procedures and this is essential, much as regular blood pressure evaluation is critical in treatment of hypertension or glucose level monitoring is critical to diabetes treatment.

Interventions: Behavioral, Pharmacological, and Combined

Behavioral therapy/psychotherapy and pharmacotherapy are the two broad classes of intervention applied to psychiatric disorders including substance use disorders. Current science points to remarkably effective interventions for specific types of substance use disorders, limited efficacy for some forms of substance use disorders, and for others, little efficacy or even exacerbation of drug use (e.g., olanzapine and cocaine use).

Some therapies are designed primarily to promote understanding of an existing problem or motivate entry into more extended or intensive treatment (e.g., motivational enhancement therapy). Other treatments are intended to provide a systematic course of intervention addressing the gamut of problems linked to substance use disorder and cessation of use (e.g., cognitive behavior therapy, contingency management). Still other interventions are composites with elements incorporated from a number of conceptual and pragmatic frameworks (e.g., community reinforcement approach, matrix model).

There is a clear need to distinguish between treatment of acute drug-related symptoms, notably withdrawal syndromes, and the complex behaviors of drug seeking and drug taking. A patient can achieve a "drug free" state within days by enforced abstinence. Sleep patterns and other biological functions and a variety of disrupted behaviors may stabilize within days or weeks. This normalization does not directly address the problems of drug seeking and drug use; however, for a small minority of individuals, a period of abstinence/cessation, however achieved, may be sufficient. Even this observation may be confounded since these individuals often undergo repeated cessation attempts before achieving behavioral change. For most, some supplemental intervention, ranging from brief, structured therapies to multiple structured sessions, will be required at some point in the drug use career to attain meaningful beneficial outcomes. Indeed, some scientists conceptualize substance use disorders as chronic for many individuals, requiring ongoing treatment and support, similar to obesity (McLellan 2002).

There are several behavioral, or psychotherapy, interventions for which strong supporting data of efficacy exist. One is cognitive behavior therapy; another is contingency management sometimes applied within the broader community-based reinforcement approach; and a third encompassing a range of theoretical frameworks entails variants of "talk therapy." Components or variants exist with labels such as "the matrix model" (Shoptaw et al. 1994), "relapse prevention," and "dialectical behavior therapy." Diverse techniques (e.g., hypnotism, acupuncture) have been incorporated into treatment models with little evidence of added efficacy compared to well-constructed behavioral therapies. All effective non-pharmacological therapies ultimately focus on behavior and thought directed at minimizing or eliminating drug use while increasing the frequency of a range of socially appropriate constructive behaviors. Among adults, these goals are more readily achieved when the individual arrives at therapy with an age and ability appropriate set of social skills, training, job history, and experience. Still, there are times when additional focused therapeutic elements may be included, for example, parenting or marital counseling.

In the realm of pharmacotherapy, opiate replacement therapy (methadone, buprenorphine) provides a clear example of robust and effective treatment applicable to use and dependence ranging from iv heroin use to oral oxycodone use. Some promising data suggest potential efficacy of a similar replacement, or agonist-like strategy for stimulant dependence though there are currently no FDA-approved medications. Possible substitute medications for stimulant dependence include amphetamine analogs. Similarly, while there are currently no approved medications for treatment of marijuana use and dependence, a promising agent that represents substitution or replacement, tetrahydrocannabinol/cannabidiol, is currently being evaluated. A variety of strategies addressing different behaviors and pharmacological mechanisms have been applied to alcohol use (disulfiram, benzodiazepines, naltrexone, acamprosate) with greater or lesser efficacy. Similarly, several medications (nicotine preparations, bupropion, varenicline) have been shown to have varying degrees, but nevertheless modest effectiveness in treatment of tobacco use and nicotine dependence. There are several nicotine preparations (gum or polacrilex, lozenges, nasal spray, patches, inhalers) that alone produce relatively modest rates of cessation across broad populations but have meaningful public health consequences due to the prevalence of tobacco use and the costs of associated diseases. Disulfiram for alcohol dependence has a unique profile: through metabolic interference, it results in high levels of acetaldehyde and induced severe discomfort; integrated into a well-controlled regimen, it can be very effective but is not widely used. Naltrexone and acamprosate appear to have modest effects in reducing alcohol intake or sustaining abstinence. For individuals whose alcohol use is found to be highly correlated with diagnoses of comorbid depression or anxiety, effective treatment may stem from administration of anxiolytics or antidepressants. In some instances, use of two or more medications may be a useful therapeutic approach. A dilemma across most medical and psychiatric is nonadherence or noncompliance with medication regimens. This is particularly true for antagonist medications such as disulfiram and naltrexone.

Ultimately, for many instances of substance use disorders, benefit of joint action of concurrently applied behavioral and pharmacological interventions may be important in all but the least severe cases. This is analogous to treatment of other disorders with clear biological and behavioral determinants. For example, hypertension may be treated with combined behavioral (e.g., exercise, diet) and pharmacological (e.g., ACE inhibitors) interventions. Similarly, depression, while amenable to both behavioral and pharmacological treatments, may be most effectively treated with a combination (e.g., CBT and SSRIs). The need for continuing intervention in treatment of substance use disorders may vary. For example, pharmacotherapy with an effective course of behavior therapy establishing (or reestablishing) alternative behaviors and eliminating drug use may still entail long-term maintenance pharmacotherapy. The latter may be necessitated by biological perturbations that predated or were a consequence of drug use. Here continued medication sustains biological and behavioral stability that would otherwise not be achieved or would only continue with unnecessary behavioral, emotional, or biological burden on the patient. Exemplifying this is treatment of heroin dependence. On completing initial behavioral treatment combined with methadone or buprenorphine maintenance, some patients may successfully undergo gradual reduction in medication dose. In other instances, perhaps more severe and involving many years of heroin use, maintenance pharmacotherapy for years or decades is desirable and warranted. The need for maintenance may reside in engrained perturbations in biology and behavior, resulting from prolonged heroin use. Generally, the costs and inconvenience of maintenance replacement are outweighed by nearly inevitable return to drug dependence and associated dire psychosocial and medical consequences when abstinence without further treatment is undertaken.

Often discussed is the concept of "relapse," "return to drug use," or in some instances, "development of new drug use." Early in treatment (often within days but up to 3–6 months), there may be graded but rapid return to previous baseline levels of use. Some individuals may use a drug a few times, for example, smoke a cigarette, or consume alcohol. They may even engage in periodic use, heavy use, or a binge, but through sustained therapy eventually refrain from further use. The likelihood of return to use greatly decreases after a year. Confounding these general observations are individuals who enter treatment and never use the drug again as well as those who are abstinent for years and then resume use. In some cases, individuals treated for heavy use, for example, heavy alcohol drinking, may resume nominal social use without return to heavy drinking. Here the legal status of a drug is germane. Treatment with a goal of abstinence from cocaine or heroin use has positive implications beyond those related to reducing impairment from drug effects, for example, no risk of incarceration. For those engaged in heavy alcohol use, reduced use may be a realistic, achievable, beneficial goal. However, as with cigarette smoking, the entrenched habitual behavior combined with reinforcing effects of the drug may preclude a goal of moderation. Finally, a small subset of individuals who have well-established behaviors of problematic use may be successfully treated for use of one drug, but at some later date develop similarly problematic use of a different drug. This would reflect reestablishment of drug seeking and taking, but not "relapse" as the word is commonly used. As with any complex disorder with multiple determinants, the core constellation of symptoms, here drug seeking and drug taking, can be addressed directly with supplemental specialty intervention when appropriate.

References and Readings

Higgins, S. T. (1997). Applying learning and conditioning theory to the treatment of alcohol and cocaine abuse. In B. Johnson & J. Roache (Eds.), *Drug addiction and its treatment* (pp. 367–386). Philadelphia: Lippencott-Raven.

McLellan, A. T. (2002). Have we evaluated addiction treatment correctly? Implications from a chronic care perspective. *Addiction, 97*(3), 249–252.

Shoptaw, S., Rawson, R. A., McCann, M. J., & Obert, J. L. (1994). The matrix model of outpatient stimulant abuse treatment: Evidence of efficacy. *Journal of Addictive Diseases, 13*(4), 129–141.

Sobell, M. B., Sobell, L. C., Klajner, F., Pavan, D., & Basian, E. (1986). The reliability of a timeline method for assessing normal drinker college students' recent drinking history: Utility for alcohol research. *Addictive Behaviors, 11*(2), 149–161.

Substance Dependence

▶ Alcohol Abuse and Dependence

Substance H

▶ Histamine

Substance Use Disorders

▶ Dependence, Drug

Success

▶ Attribution Theory

Successful Aging

Barbara Resnick
School of Nursing, University of Maryland, Baltimore, MD, USA

Synonyms

Optimal aging

Definition

Successful aging has been addressed and discussed repeatedly with at least 29 different definitions articulated from both cross-sectional and longitudinal research studies. Common themes across all of this work describe successful aging as the absence of physical and mental disability. Generally, successful aging is noted to occur when the individual has perceived "good health."

Description

Successful Aging

The concept of successful aging emerged in the late 1980s and early 1990s as a departure from the loss-focused geriatric and gerontological research that preceded the concept. In their groundbreaking 1987 article, Human Aging: Usual and Successful, Rowe and Kahn argued that the cognitive and physiological losses documented in the literature as age-related changes were mischaracterizations of the natural aging process. "We believe that the role of aging per se in these losses has often been overstated and that a major component of many age-associated declines can be explained in terms of lifestyle, habits, diet, and an array of psychosocial factors extrinsic to the aging process."

Definition

Successful aging has been addressed and there are at least 29 different definitions articulated from both cross-sectional and longitudinal research studies. Common themes across all of this work consider successful aging as the absence of physical and mental disability and perceived "good health." In addition, successful aging has increasingly been associated with resilience and maintenance of an active lifestyle and having good supportive relationships. Everyone has the opportunity to age successfully. From the outside, objectively, this may look very different across people. For some, aging successfully is still working at age 98. For others, it is sitting quietly in a room in assisted living and reliving past memories reviewing very rich, fulfilling lives.

More important than the absolute state of health of the individual is the notion of one's conceptualization and acceptance of his or her health status. Acceptance of changes and optimization of physical and mental health are the most critical aspects of aging successfully. Changes that occur as part of normal aging must be accepted, addressed, and adjusted to. Vision changes that occur starting around age 40 provide the first experience adults have to cope with and age successfully. Successful adaptation includes buying reading glasses over the counter as needed or getting eye examinations and vision testing done and getting new glasses! Increasingly baby boomers carry small lights with magnification to read restaurant menus, telephone books, and other pertinent information. Other changes, such as painful degenerative joint disease, are not so easily or commonly recognized, accepted, and adjusted to. It is being able to accept and adjust to changes that are at the core of successful aging.

As noted, resilience is central to successful aging. The word "resilience" comes from the Latin world "salire," which means to spring up and the word "resilire" means to spring back. Resilience, therefore, refers to the capacity to spring back from a physical, emotional, financial, or social challenge. Being resilient indicates that the individual has the human ability to adapt in the face of tragedy, trauma, adversity, hardship, and ongoing significant life stressors. Resilient individuals are able to adapt to all types of situations, especially with regard to social functioning, morale, and somatic health, and are less likely to succumb to illness. That is, a resilient individual may still get ill but will respond in a way in which he or she optimizes recovery, maintenance, or even death in a way that defines resilience. Resilience, as a component of the individual's personality, develops and changes over time through ongoing experiences with the physical and social environment. Resilience can, therefore, be perceived as a dynamic process that is influenced by life events and challenges. Increasingly, there is evidence that resilience is related to motivation, specifically the motivation to age successfully and to recover from physical or psychological traumatic events.

Resilience research has helped to uncover the many factors or qualities within individuals that are associated with resilience. These include such things as positive interpersonal relationships, incorporating social connectedness with a willingness to extend oneself to others, strong internal resources, having an optimistic or positive affect, keeping things in perspective, setting goals and taking steps to achieve those goals, high self-esteem, high self-efficacy, determination, and spirituality which includes purpose of life, religiousness or a belief in a higher power, creativity, humor, and a sense of curiosity. Strengthening any of these factors will help individuals to become more resilient when faced with a challenge.

Older women who have successfully recovered from orthopedic or other stressful events describe themselves as resilient and determined and tend to have better function, mood, and quality of life than those who are less resilient. These are the women who at 97 engage in rehabilitation services post–hip fracture to their fullest ability and then following discharge home are insistent on getting back on their exercise equipment at the gym. Resilience has also been associated with adjustments following the diagnosis of dementia, widowhood, management of chronic pain, and overall adjustment to the stressors associated with aging. Thus, it is through resilience he or she adjusts, adapts, and addresses the physical, emotional, and mental challenges that are to be anticipated as one ages.

Older adults accrue a lifetime of experiences through which resilience develops. Resilient individuals generally age successfully. A resilient older adult is exemplified by such things as accepting the loss of a spouse; symptoms associated with an acute medical event; or a fracture and responding with determination to recover and grow through the experience. He or she does not waste energy on complaining about what has happened but rather on pooling the resources needed to overcome the challenging event.

Resilience alone is not sufficient to assure successful aging. It is believed that all individuals have the innate ability to be resilient and return to homeostasis successfully and to transform, change, and grow, regardless of age. He or she must, however, summon motivation in the face of adversity to be resilient. Thus, motivation may be present independent of resilience, but resilience depends on being motivated to successfully reintegrate. Resilient reintegration requires increased energy, or motivation, for resilience to successfully occur.

Motivation comes from within and is based on an inner urge that moves or prompts a person to action. This is in contrast to resilience which is stimulated in response to adversity or challenge. Motivation refers to the need, drive, or desire to act in a certain way to achieve a certain end. We do not need to be challenged to be motivated. We do have to be motivated to respond, with resilience, to a challenging event. There are some factors that are associated with both resilience and motivation such as determination, self-efficacy, being open and willing to experience new things, and social supports. The capacity to be resilient and/or motivated is present in everyone and choices are made in the face of routine and challenging situations to be motivated and/or resilient. Motivation related to engaging in physical activities may be high for some individuals while others are motivated to sit in a chair or lie in a bed. Conversely, some older adults are motivated to take classes in a senior center while others refuse to even consider this and are motivated to sit daily and watch television alone. Some individuals are resilient with regard to physical challenges but cannot cope with challenges associated with finances or cognitive changes. Thus, there are traits and characteristics of individuals associated with resilience and motivation as well as external factors that can impact resilience and motivation as individuals respond to challenges or activities within their lives.

Resilience, unlike motivation, relies on the individual experiencing a life challenge or some type of adversity. These challenges may be developmental challenges such as those associated with normal aging (e.g., vision changes), or they maybe social and/or economic challenges such as those experienced by the loss of employment, the loss of a spouse, or a move into an assisted living facility. Conversely, motivation is not dependent on an adverse event or challenge; rather motivation is a necessary component for all activity. Routine personal care activities such as bathing and dressing require motivation, as do making plans to have dinner with a friend or play cards. Resilience would be required, however, when he or she is faced with bathing and dressing challenges following a wrist fracture.

Keys to Aging Well

An individual has the ability to be resilient as long as he or she is motivated to do so. The first step in the process is to engage in appropriate health promotion activities, particularly exercise. Due to the changes that can occur with aging, underlying physical capability will vary among older individuals. For some individuals, maintaining a regular exercise program will involve running for 40 min on the treadmill. For others, it may be walking within their apartment building or long-term care facility, doing a sitting exercise program, or swimming or walking in the water. There is, however, an exercise program that matches each individual's needs. This is critically important to appreciate and recognize. The benefit of physical activity for older adults should not focus on preventing cardiovascular disease and managing blood pressure to prevent a stroke. Rather, it should be geared toward the mental health benefits associated with physical activity as well as the sense of achievement and physical benefit of maintaining function and improving balance and strength.

Successful Aging Guidelines

Meta-analytic reviews provide strong evidence to support the many benefits of exercise including decreased risk of coronary heart disease and stroke; decreased progression of degenerative joint disease; prevention of osteoporosis of the lumbar spine; decreased incidences of falls; increased gait speed if the activity is of sufficient intensity and dosage; improved cognitive function in sedentary older adults and in those with dementia; a modest benefit in quality of life for frail older adults; and a positive association with successful aging. Current guidelines from the American College of Sports Medicine and the American Heart Association recommend that all older adults engage in moderately intense aerobic exercise for 30 min daily at least 5 days a week or vigorous exercise 20 min a day, 3 days a week. In addition, each should do eight to ten strength training exercises, 10–15 repetitions of each exercise two to three times per week. These exercises are well described in a book published by the National Institute of Aging, *Exercise: A Guide from the National Institute of Aging*. For older adults at risk for falling, balance exercise is also recommended. It is not known, however, what dose of exercise is needed for each individual to age successfully. For some, a walk to get the mail is sufficient psychologically to constitute an exercise program. For others, one activity a day (e.g., playing bridge, going to dinner) makes them feel successful and engaged. The focus should be on helping the individual understand what successful aging means to them and helping them develop a plan to achieve that.

Unfortunately, all too many older adults assume that they cannot exercise or engage actively in routine life activities and social activities because of underlying disease, pain, shortness of breath, or other limiting symptoms. Health outcomes can be achieved at even relatively low levels of exercise intensity, particularly for those who have previously been sedentary. Thus, initiation of physical activity even at 1-min intervals is an important step to successful aging. Adjustments can be made to engage them in social activities via chair positioning that will help them maintain independence in public or remain comfortable to sit for a game of bridge or an evening eating with friends. Solving these challenges is part of the necessary resilience needed to age successfully. Health-care providers can serve as sources to help with overcoming such challenges and barriers.

In addition to physical activity, mental stimulation may also be important for successful aging. In a recent meta-analysis, there was not statistical support to indicate that cognitive stimulation through structured programs prevents or slows the progression of Alzheimer's disease. The current research, however, is limited by a lack of consensus on what constitutes the most effective type of cognitive training, insufficient follow-up times, a lack of matched active controls, and few outcome measures showing changes in daily functioning, global cognitive skills, or a decrease in disease progression. Keeping actively engaged mentally through volunteer work or activities within one's own living space certainly will build resilience and likewise assure successful aging. Opportunities abound for such activities, however, as with physical activity the older individual must be motivated to initiate and engage in these activities.

Older adults should be encouraged to move beyond their level of comfort and engage in new and different activities to stimulate their minds and their bodies. If playing bridge or doing a crossword puzzle is lifelong acquired skill, newer activities such as learning a new language or playing an instrument will provide important mind stimulation and encourage plasticity and growth.

The Health-Care Provider's Role in Successful Aging

Informing young and older adults about the ways in which to age successfully is the first step toward facilitating successful aging for any individual. There are ways in which to measure resilience and motivation, although at a clinical level they will not necessarily direct interventions. Thus, the best approach is to motivate individuals toward resilient behaviors.

Cross-References

▶ Aging
▶ Elderly
▶ Exercise
▶ Geriatric Medicine
▶ Gerontology
▶ Physical Activity

References and Readings

Boardman, J., Blalock, C., & Button, T. (2008). Sex differences in the heritability of resilience. *Twin Research and Human Genetics, 11*(1), 12–27.

Bonanno, G., Galea, S., Bucciarelli, A., & Vlahov, D. (2007). What predicts psychological resilience after disaster? The role of demographics, resources, and life stress. *Death Studies, 31*(10), 863–883.

Chow, S., Hamagani, F., & Nesselroade, J. (2007). Age differences in dynamical emotion-cognition linkages. *Psychology and Aging, 22*(4), 765–780.

Hardy, S., Concato, J., & Gill, T. (2002). Stressful life events among community-living older persons. *The Journal of General Internal Medicine, 17*(11), 832–838.

Hardy, S., Concato, J., & Gill, T. (2004). Resilience of community-dwelling older persons. *Journal of the American Geriatrics Society, 52*(2), 257–262.

Harris, P. (2008). Another wrinkle in the debate about successful aging: The undervalued concept of resilience and the lived experience of dementia. *International Journal of Aging and Human Development, 67*(1), 43–61.

Hegney, D., Buikstra, E., Baker, P., Rogers-Clark, C., Pearce, S., Ross, H., et al. (2007). Individual resilience in rural people: A Queensland study, Australia. *Rural and Remote Health, 7*(4), 620–625.

Hicks, G., Simonsick, E. M., Harris, T. B., Newman, A. B., Weiner, D. K., Nevitt, M. A., & Tylavsky, F. A. (2005). Trunk muscle composition as a predictor of reduced functional capacity in the health, aging and body composition study: The moderating role of back pain. *The Journal of Gerontology Series A, Biological Sciences and Medical Sciences, 60*(11), 1420–1424.

Karoly, P., & Ruehlman, L. (2006). Psychological "resilience" and its correlates in chronic pain: Findings from a national community sample. *Pain, 123*(1–2), 90–97.

Lee, H., Brown, S., Mitchell, M., & Schiraldi, G. (2008). Correlates of resilience in the face of adversity for Korean women immigrating to the US. *Journal of Immigrant and Minority Health, 10*(5), 415–422.

O'Connell, R., & Mayo, J. (1998). The role of social factors in affective disorders: A review. *Hospital & Community Psychiatry, 39*, 842–851.

Ong, A., Bergeman, C., Bisconti, T., & Wallace, K. (2006). Psychological resilience, positive emotions, and successful adaptation to stress in later life. *Journal of Personality and Social Psychology, 91*(4), 730–749.

Resnick, B., Orwig, D., Zimmerman, S., Simpson, M., & Magaziner, J. (2005). The exercise plus program for older women post hip fracture: Participant perspectives. *The Gerontologist, 45*(4), 539–544.

Rossi, N., Bisconti, T., & Bergeman, C. (2007). The role of dispositional resilience in regaining life satisfaction after the loss of a spouse. *Death Studies, 31*(10), 863–883.

Sanders, A., Lim, S., & Sohn, W. (2008). Resilience to urban poverty: Theoretical and empirical considerations for population health. *American Journal of Public Health, 98*(6), 1101–1106.

Wagnild, G., & Young, H. (1993). Development and psychometric evaluation of the resilience scale. *Journal of Nursing Measurement, 1*(2), 165–177.

Werner, E., & Smith, R. (1992). *Overcoming the odds: High risk children from birth to adulthood*. Ithaca: Cornell University Press.

Sudden Cardiac Death

▶ Cardiac Death
▶ Death, Sudden

Suicidal Ideation, Thoughts

Orit Birnbaum-Weitzman[1] and Mariam Dum[2]
[1]Department of Psychology, University of Miami, Miami, FL, USA
[2]Jackson Memorial Hospital, Miami, FL, USA

Synonyms

Suicidal impulses; Suicidal thoughts

Definition

Suicidal ideation refers to thoughts or impulses of engaging in behavior intended to end one's life (Nock et al. 2008). Suicidal ideation should be distinguished from suicidal plan, which refers to the formulation of a specific method through which one intends to die, and from suicide attempt, which refers to an actual engagement in potentially self-injurious behavior in which there is at least some intent to die (Nock et al. 2008).

Description

Ongoing suicidal ideation is a chronic risk factor and has been considered predictive of suicidal behavior especially if accompanied with severe hopelessness, prior suicide attempts, not having a child under 18 years old living at home, and a history of alcohol and drug abuse (Tishler and Reiss 2009). Suicidal ideation represents an important phase in the suicidal process and often precedes suicide attempts or completed suicide. However, not all patients experiencing suicidal ideation attempt suicide (Weissman et al. 1999). While approximately 10–20% of the population across diverse countries report suicidal ideation and 3–5% have made a suicide attempt at some time in their life, only 0.01% will complete suicide (Kessler et al. 2005). Acute risk factors including severe anxiety, agitation, and severe anhedonia are most predictive of whether someone will commit suicide in inpatients (Tishler and Reiss 2009; Bostwick and Rackley 2007).

Physical as well as mental health problems have been associated with suicidal ideation. Patients with chronic medical illnesses, such as HIV and cancer, and especially those experiencing physical pain are more likely to report suicidal thoughts (Tang and Crane 2006). Certain medical illnesses, such as neurological disorders and some cancers, appear to have higher rates of suicidal ideation and suicide compared to other medical disorders (Hugues and Kleespies 2001). A higher prevalence of suicidal ideation has been observed in patients experiencing pain associated with a variety of medical conditions including migraines, musculoskeletal pain, fibromyalgia, and arthritis (Tang and Crane 2006). Research suggests that the location and type of pain as well as the intensity and duration of the pain may have implications for the risk of suicidal ideation (Tang and Crane 2006). In addition, sleep-onset insomnia associated with pain is also a significant discriminator of the presence or absence of suicidal ideation (Tang and Crane 2006).

Research in the elderly suggests that physical illness plays an important role in suicidal ideation and behavior (Szanto et al. 2002). In the elderly with physical illness, untreated or undertreated physical pain, anticipatory anxiety regarding the progression of the physical illness, fear of dependence, and fear of burdening the family have been reported as the major contributing factors for suicidal ideation (Szanto et al. 2002). For all age groups, social isolation is considered another important risk factor that has been shown to be associated with suicidal ideation.

Sociodemographic factors including age and income level have also been associated with suicidal ideation (Kessler et al. 2005). In general, younger age, lack of education, and unemployment have been associated with higher rates of suicidal ideation and may represent an increased risk associated with social disadvantage (Nock et al. 2008). For all age groups, social isolation is considered another important risk factor that has been shown to be associated with suicidal ideation (Van Orden et al. 2010).

Prior suicide attempts and the presence of a psychiatric disorder are the most consistently reported risk factors associated with suicidal ideation and behavior (Nock et al. 2008). Mood disorders such as anxiety and particularly depression significantly increase the risk of suicidal ideation in the general population and in medical patients in particular. Suicidal ideation has also been associated with other mental illnesses including severe anxiety, psychotic and personality disorders, and alcohol and substance abuse (Van Orden et al. 2010). A number of psychological processes have been found to exacerbate suicidal ideation. Specifically, findings from cross-sectional as well as longitudinal studies have attested to the role of hopelessness and helplessness, feelings of defeat and entrapment, deficits in problem solving abilities, and avoidant coping in the development of suicidal ideation (Van Orden et al. 2010; Nock et al. 2008; Szanto et al. 2002).

The presence of suicidal ideation in a clinical or medical setting typically requires a thorough risk assessment including chronic and acute risk factors as well as the frequency, intensity, and duration of suicidal thoughts (see Tishler and Reiss 2009 for prevention in medical settings).

References and Readings

Kessler, R. C., Berglund, P., Borges, G., Nocke, M., & Wang, P. S. (2005). Trends in suicide ideation, plans, gestures, and attempts in the United States, 1990–1992 to 2001–2003. *JAMA: The Journal of the American Medical Association, 293*, 2487–2495.

Nock, M. K., Borges, G., Bromet, E. J., Cha, C. B., Kessler, R. C., & Lee, S. (2008). Suicide and suicidal behavior. *Epidemiologic Reviews, 30*, 133–154.

Szanto, K., Gildengers, A., Mulsant, B. H., Brown, G., Alexopoulus, G. S., & Reynoldsm, C. F. (2002). Identification of suicidal ideation and prevention of suicidal behavior in the elderly. *Drugs & Aging, 19*, 11–24.

Tang, N. K., & Crane, C. (2006). Suicidality in chronic pain: A review of the prevalence, risk factors, and psychological links. *Psychological Medicine, 36*, 575–586.

Tishler, C. L., & Reiss, N. S. (2009). Inpatient suicide: Preventing a common sentinel event. *General Hospital Psychiatry, 31*, 103–109.

Van Orden, K. A., Witte, T. K., Cukrowicz, K. C., Braithwaite, S. R., Selby, E. A., & Joiner, T. E. (2010). The interpersonal theory of suicide. *Psychological Review, 117*, 575–600.

Weissman, M. M., Bland, R. C., Canino, G. J., Greenwald, S., Hwu, H. G., Joyce, P. R., et al. (1999). Prevalence of suicide ideation and suicide attempts in nine countries. *Psychological Medicine, 29*, 9–17.

Suicidal Impulses

▶ Suicidal Ideation, Thoughts

Suicidal Thoughts

▶ Suicidal Ideation, Thoughts

Suicide

Mariam Dum[1] and Orit Birnbaum-Weitzman[2]
[1]Jackson Memorial Hospital, Miami, FL, USA
[2]Department of Psychology, University of Miami, Miami, FL, USA

Synonyms

Deliberate self-harm; Self-directed violence; Self-Inflicted injurious behavior; Self-murder

Definition

Suicide is the act of intentionally ending one's own life. The definition of suicide reflects three important components (Rudd et al. 2001): (a) that the person died, (b) that the person's behavior caused death, and (c) that the person intended to cause his or her own death. While intentionality is the most precise characteristic that distinguishes those who have died by suicide and those who had died by other causes, its assessment remains controversial.

Description

Suicide is a major public health problem, and reports from the World Health Organization (WHO) indicate that suicide is projected to become an increasingly important contributor to the global burden of disease over the coming decades. Suicide is the 11th leading cause of death among all ages in the United States and the 13th leading cause of death worldwide. Suicide rates vary significantly cross-nationally (Center for Disease Control and Prevention 2007). In general, rates are highest in Eastern Europe and lowest in Central and South America, with the United States, Western Europe, and Asia falling in the middle. Epidemiological surveys showed that 2.7% of the US population has made a suicide attempt (Nock et al. 2008). Most individuals that attempt suicide die during their first suicide attempt (Nock et al. 2008). Within medical settings, according to Joint Commission on Accreditation of Healthcare Organizations (JCAHO 2010), suicide ranks among the five top most frequent sentinel events in hospitals. Seeking help from mental health professionals can assist in the reduction of distressing psychological symptoms. However, according to a recent review, while 45% of people who successfully committed suicide contacted a primary care provider within 1 month of their death, only 20% contacted mental health services within the same time period (Lauma et al. 2002).

Rudd et al. (2001) provide in their book a good description on a number of psychiatric, psychological, demographic, and biological variables have been recognized as suicide risk factors. The presence of one or more psychiatric problem is a central variable explaining suicide acts. At least 90% of individuals who have died from suicide have had at least one psychiatric disturbance. In addition, past suicide attempts, history of childhood abuse, and family history of suicide are associated with increased risk of suicide. Other variables that contribute to suicide risk are psychological variables, such as hopelessness, impulsivity, problem-solving deficits, and perfectionism. In terms of demographic variables, men are more likely to die by suicide than are women. Death by suicide is more common in older, lower socioeconomic status, and veterans. Similarly, non-Hispanic White individuals have a higher rate of suicide than individuals from other ethnical background. In addition, individuals who are unemployed, single, divorced, or widowed are also at a higher risk. Biological variables have also been found to be associated with suicide behaviors. Family, twin, and adoption studies have found evidence for heritable risk of suicidality. Biological factors related to lower levels of serotonin metabolites in the cerebrospinal fluid, higher serotonin receptor binding in platelets, and fewer presynaptic serotonin transporter sites were found in individuals who died by suicide. In addition, biological factors that inhibit impulsive behaviors, such as greater postsynaptic serotonin receptors in specific brain areas, such as the prefrontal cortex, have been associated with suicide behaviors.

The high rate of medical illness among individuals who committed suicide shows that both mental disorders and physical illness are important risk factors. Research shows variability in the risk of suicide according to the type of medical diagnosis. According to Hughes and Kleespies (2001), medical illnesses such as AIDS, cancer, chronic pain, end-stage renal diseases, severe neurological disorders, and chronic obstructive pulmonary disease have been correlated with increased risk of suicide. In contrast, they reported that other medical conditions including sclerosis, heart transplant, hypertension, rheumatoid arthritis, neoplasms, and cervix and prostate cancer have not been associated with increased risk. Studies have shown that at least one quarter of inpatients that have committed suicide in medical/surgical units did not report any previous psychiatric history (JCAHO 2010). Furthermore, suicide among these patients tends to happen within the first 2 weeks of their initial diagnosis (JCAHO 2010). This highlights the need of assessing suicidality in individuals who have chronic medical problems or who have been recently diagnosed with a life-threatening illness. Additionally, significant differences have been found between individuals who have completed suicide in inpatient psychiatric facilities and inpatient medical units. According to these studies, individuals who committed suicide in medical units tend to be older, their death did not include careful planning, and their means of committing suicide were significantly more violent (Nock et al. 2008).

In contrast to the vast literature on variables associated with suicide, there are some studies that have identified protective factors. Protective factors are those that decrease the probability of suicide in the presence of elevated risk. Rudd et al. (2001) summarized some of the most consistent findings in the literature are supportive social network or family, reasons for living, and religious beliefs. Being pregnant and having young children in the home are also protective against suicide.

Clinical providers face the difficulty of recognizing individuals at risk of committing suicide as no single factor is sufficient to trigger or protect an individual from a suicidal act. Suicide warning signs are the earliest detectable signs or symptoms that indicate high risk for suicide in the near term (i.e., within minutes, hours, or days before the suicidal act; Rudd et al. 2001). They provide immediate cues to loved ones or clinical providers of the imminent risk of attempting to end one's life. Some suicide warning signs include hopelessness, anger, dramatic changes in mood, acting recklessly or engaging in risky activities, reports of feeling trapped, increased alcohol or drug use, withdrawal from loved ones, agitation or anxiety, and drastic sleep changes (Rudd et al. 2001).

Due to the difficulty of preventing and recognizing suicide, the assessment of suicide risk should be completed in a standardized and systematic way. In addition to assessing risk and protective factors, as well as warning signs to understand the risk level of an individual, suicide ideation, suicide plan, intent to act, previous suicide attempts, and the medical lethality of means need to be considered. When assessing suicide risk, it is important to differentiate between chronic risk and acute risk (Rudd et al. 2001). Chronic risk involves the presence of risk factors. Acute risk is determined by suicide ideation, intention, and a suicide plan in combination with warning signs. Acute risk can be further classified into low, moderate, and high. Low acute risk involves the presence of suicide thoughts with no specific plan, intent, or behavior. Moderate acute risk involves the presence of suicide ideation and a plan without intent or behavior. High acute risk refers to the presence of persistent suicide ideation and a specific plan with the intent to die.

References and Readings

Centers for Disease Control and Prevention. (2007). Web-based injury statistics query and reporting system (WISQARS). Retrieved June 20, 2011, from Centers for Disease Control and Prevention, National Center for Injury and Prevention Control Website: http://www.cdc.gov/ncipc/WISQARS

Hughes, D., & Kleespies, P. (2001). Suicide in the medically ill. *Suicide and Life Threatening Behaviors, 31*, 48–59.

Joint Commission on Accreditation of Healthcare Organizations. (2010). *Sentinel event statistics data*. Retrieved June 20, 2011, from the Joint Commission Website: http://www.jointcommission.org/sentinel_event_statistics_quarterly/

Lauma, J. B., Martin, C. E., & Pearson, J. L. (2002). Contact with mental health and primary care providers before suicide: A review of the evidence. *The American Journal of Psychiatry, 159*(6), 909–916.

Nock, M. K., Borges, G., Bromet, E. J., Cha, C. B., Kessler, R. C., & Lee, S. (2008). Suicide and Suicidal Behavior. *Epidemiologic Reviews, 30*, 133–154.

Rudd, M. D., Joiner, T., & Rajab, M. H. (2001). *Treating suicide behavior: An affective, time-limited approach*. New York: Guilford Press.

Wenzel, A., Brown, G. K., & Beck, A. T. (2009). *Cognitive therapy for suicide patients: Scientific and clinical applications*. Washington, DC: American Psychological Association.

Suicide Risk, Suicide Risk Factors

Yori Gidron
SCALab, Lille 3 University and Siric Oncollile, Lille, France

Definition

Death from suicide in 1998 was ranked by the World Health Organization (WHO) as the 12th leading cause of mortality worldwide. Suicide is the cause of death of one million people a year worldwide (Lineberry 2009). Suicide has been committed via several methods, which vary across geographic regions (Ajdacic-Gross et al. 2008). It is a main cause of death in later adolescence (ages 15–24 years; Shields et al. 2006).

The main difficulty in suicide prevention is its prediction because it constitutes a rare event and because of the multiple risk factors of suicide. These include situational factors such as social stressors and life events (e.g., unemployment, poverty), psychological factors such as hopelessness and hostility, biological factors (e.g., reduced brain-derived neurotrophic factor, protein kinase A; Dwivedi and Pandey 2011), and mere access to means of suicide (e.g., arms). One main difficulty in predicting suicidal behavior is the reliance on self-reported instruments, where people either conceal their real replies or are unaware of them. Furthermore, most studies in this domain have been retrospective and thus carry multiple sources of bias including survivors' and family members' attempt to find an explanation rather than the real cause.

Conversely, some recent studies have shown that assessing implicit associations between the "self" and "life" versus "death," with the Implicit Association Test, predicted suicidal behavior beyond what was detected by traditional risk factors (e.g., depression, past attempts, clinicians' ratings; Nock et al. 2010). Similarly, attention biases to suicide-related words relative to neutral words, using the "emotional Stroop," predicted suicidal behavior better than traditional risk factors (Cha et al. 2010). More research needs to utilize such instruments to identify additional suicide risk factors assessed in such indirect manners. Often, an accumulation of risk factors occurs, culminating in the tragic event. To conclude, explicit and implicit psychosocial factors and biological and situational factors serve as risk factors for suicide and need to be considered in the important attempt to prevent this severe health outcome. Given that recent studies mentioned here found that attention bias to suicide-related concepts predicted risk of suicide, future studies may also wish to test whether targeting such biases via attention-modification training, which was found to reduce mental problems (e.g., Heeren et al. 2015), may also prevent suicide in people with known suicide risk factors.

Cross-References

▶ Hopelessness
▶ Suicide

References and Further Readings

Ajdacic-Gross, V., Weiss, M. G., Ring, M., Hepp, U., Bopp, M., Gutzwiller, F., et al. (2008). Methods of suicide: International suicide patterns derived from the WHO mortality database. *Bulletin of the World Health Organization, 86*, 726–732.

Cha, C. B., Najmi, S., Park, J. M., Finn, C. T., & Nock, M. K. (2010). Attentional bias toward suicide-related stimuli predicts suicidal behavior. *Journal of Abnormal Psychology, 119*, 616–622.

Dwivedi, Y., & Pandey, G. N. (2011). Elucidating biological risk factors in suicide: Role of protein kinase A. *Progress in Neuropsychopharmacology and Biological Psychiatry, 35*, 831–841.

Heeren, A., Mogoaşe, C., Philippot, P., & McNally, R. J. (2015). Attention bias modification for social anxiety: A systematic review and meta-analysis. *Clinical Psychology Review, 40*, 76–90.

Lineberry, T. (2009). Suicide rates in 2009. Do the economy and wars have an effect? *Minnesota Medicine, 92*, 49–52.

Nock, M. K., Park, J. M., Finn, C. T., Deliberto, T. L., Dour, H. J., & Banaji, M. R. (2010). Measuring the suicidal mind: Implicit cognition predicts suicidal behavior. *Psychological Science, 21*, 511–517.

Shields, L. B., Hunsaker, D. M., & Hunsaker, J. C., 3rd. (2006). Adolescent and young adult suicide: A 10-year retrospective review of Kentucky medical examiner cases. *Journal of Forensic Sciences, 51*, 874–879.

Sulcus

▶ Brain, Cortex

Summary Data

▶ Aggregate Data

Sun Exposure

Yori Gidron
SCALab, Lille 3 University and Siric Oncollile, Lille, France

Definition

Sun exposure refers to the amount and manner in which people expose themselves to sunlight. This is a highly complex parameter for quantification, as it relies on self-report and its effects depend on multiple environmental and personal factors, as well as on frequency and location of exposure on the body. Most skin cancers are related to sun exposure, and a great majority of exposure to sun takes place before adulthood, making children and adolescents central target groups for assessment and prevention of sun exposure and skin cancers. Multiple studies have linked sun exposure to various cancers, particularly to skin cancer. In a review of 57 studies, intermittent sun exposure and history of burns were related to risk of melanoma. In contrast, high occupational sun exposure was inversely related to melanoma. Furthermore, factors such as country of study seem to moderate effects of sun exposure on melanoma, suggesting that effects of sun exposure depend on geographical factors as well. Indeed, geographic latitude synergistically interacts with history of sunburn in relation to occurrence of melanoma (Gandini et al. 2005). A major cause of melanoma due to sun exposure is ultraviolet light (Armstrong and Kricker 1993). Various questionnaires exist for assessing sun exposure, which consider the manner and duration of sun exposure, context (working vs. nonworking days), and cumulating measures in relation to various time frames (years or one's life time; Kricker et al. 2005). Importantly, to achieve greater test-retest reliability, it may be beneficial to assess sun exposure in relation to activities (e.g., with family, at work) rather than in relation to specific time periods (Yu et al. 2009). In children, important social factors related to usage of sun protective agents include parental reminders (Donavan and Singh 1999). Furthermore, in children, sun protective behavior decreases with age though sun exposure increases with age, possibly reflecting greater peer pressure and reduced parental control in older children (Pichora and Marrett 2010). Thus, sun exposure reflects a major and complex cause of various skin cancers and must be properly assessed and better controlled in attempt to prevent skin cancers. Future studies may wish to identify the social pressures people face concerning sun exposure and the cognitive barriers people have about protection from sun exposure, which could be then targeted by "psychological inoculation," an evidence-based cognitive method with far stronger effects than health education only (Duryea et al. 1990).

Cross-References

▶ Cancer Screening/Detection/Surveillance

References and Further Readings

Armstrong, B. K., & Kricker, A. (1993). How much melanoma is caused by sun exposure? *Melanoma Research, 3*, 395–401.

Donavan, D. T., & Singh, S. N. (1999). Sun-safety behavior among elementary school children: The role of knowledge, social norms, and parental involvement. *Psychological Reports, 84*, 831–836.

Duryea, E. J., Ransom, M. V., & English, G. (1990). Psychological immunization: Theory, research, and current health behavior applications. *Health Education & Behavior, 17*(2), 169–178.

Gandini, S., Sera, F., Cattaruzza, M. S., Pasquini, P., Picconi, O., Boyle, P., et al. (2005). Meta-analysis of risk factors for cutaneous melanoma: II. Sun exposure. *European Journal of Cancer, 41*, 45–60.

Kricker, A., Vajdic, C. M., & Armstrong, B. K. (2005). Reliability and validity of a telephone questionnaire for estimating lifetime personal sun exposure in epidemiologic studies. *Cancer Epidemiology, Biomarkers & Prevention, 14*, 2427–2432.

Pichora, E. C., & Marrett, L. D. (2010). Sun behaviour in Canadian children: Results of the 2006 national sun survey. *Canadian Journal of Public Health, 101*, 14–18.

Yu, C. L., Li, Y., Freedman, D. M., Fears, T. R., Kwok, R., Chodick, G., et al. (2009). Assessment of lifetime cumulative sun exposure using a self-administered questionnaire: Reliability of two approaches. *Cancer Epidemiology, Biomarkers & Prevention, 18*, 464–471.

Supervisory Attentional System

▶ Executive Function

Supplication

▶ Prayer

Supportive Care

▶ Palliative Care

Suprachiasmatic Nucleus

▶ Hypothalamus

Supraoptic Nucleus

▶ Hypothalamus

Surgery

▶ Cancer Treatment and Management

Surgical Resection

▶ Cancer Treatment and Management

Surrogacy

Miranda Montrone[1] and Kerry Sherman[2]
[1]Counselling Place, Glebe, Sydney, NSW, Australia
[2]Department of Psychology, Centre for Emotional Health, Macquarie University, Sydney, NSW, Australia

Synonyms

ART, Assisted reproductive technology; Commissioning parent; Cross-border reproductive care; Egg donation; Egg donor; Embryo donation; Gestational carrier; ICSI; Infertility; Intended parent; IVF; Sperm donation; Sperm donor; Surrogate mother

Definition

A surrogacy arrangement is one in which, before the child is conceived, the commissioning parent/s (also known as intended parent/s) and the surrogate mother (also known as gestational carrier, or birth mother) and her partner (if she has one) agree that the surrogate will become pregnant with the intention that the child will, at birth, be given into the care of the commissioning parent/s to raise as their own.

Description

Common reasons for surrogacy include absence of the uterus (such as hysterectomy for women or men without a female partner), congenital malformation of the uterus, or a medical condition that compromises pregnancy making it unsafe for the commissioning woman (intended mother) or her prospective baby. Surrogate conception may occur in a number of ways including where the genetic material is provided by both commissioning parents or by one only of them, by both the surrogate mother and her partner or by one only of them, or by third-party donors (egg, sperm, or embryo) who are not involved in the actual surrogacy arrangement. A surrogacy arrangement can take the form of a natural process, through the surrogate's self-insemination, or occur at an in vitro fertilization (IVF) clinic through assisted reproductive technology. Surrogacy, as practiced worldwide, is primarily IVF or gestational surrogacy that does not involve any genetic material of the surrogate or her partner but may involve third-party donor gametes. Insemination surrogacy (also known as genetic, traditional, or partial surrogacy) is less common.

The availability and conditions of surrogacy arrangements vary according to the jurisdiction in which the arrangement takes place (Jadva 2016). For example, in the USA, gestational surrogacy is primarily undertaken through IVF clinics with the gestational carrier being financially compensated for her contractual participation in the surrogacy arrangement. In comparison, in countries such as Australia and New Zealand, only altruistic surrogacy is legally permitted, with mostly gestational surrogacy (Hammarberg et al. 2011). In the UK surrogacy is altruistic, with both gestational and genetic insemination surrogacy (Van den Akker 2007). Commercial surrogacy has also been available in a number of developing countries including India (Lamba et al. 2018), Thailand, Mexico, Cambodia, and more recently, Greece and Ukraine. In many of these countries, the commissioning parents mostly originate from the developed world, with the surrogates having significantly less agency over decisions in the surrogacy arrangement, with subsequent legal and ethical implications. One of the greatest challenges arises from this type of cross-border surrogacy where there is uncertainty regarding the status of the parent and the child, particularly when considering the legal aspects of citizenship (Crockin 2013).

Despite the conception process being relatively straightforward medically, the psychological and social implications of surrogacy are complex. Social relationships between the surrogate and commissioning parents vary from close family or friends, to those where there is no prior or anticipated subsequent relationship between the surrogate and the child born of the surrogacy arrangement. For many intended parents, the point of surrogacy may reflect years of physical, emotional, and financial stressors in the unsuccessful quest to conceive through IVF-type techniques. This, is turn, may lead the intended parents to be over vigilant and anxious about the surrogate's well-being throughout the pregnancy (Greenfeld 2014). It is critical that the capacity of the commissioning woman to manage the emotional challenges is considered prior to engaging in the surrogacy arrangement, including the challenges of having another woman carrying her baby. Potential conflicts may also arise between the intended parents and the surrogate from differences in values and preferences regarding diet, medications, delivery options, and even termination options, if required. Variations in the amount of contact that intended parents expect to have with the surrogate during the pregnancy and whether or not the surrogate will maintain contact antenatally can be sources of conflict, particularly as the expectations of all involved parties may fluctuate with changing circumstances surrounding the surrogacy. Trust is clearly a key factor underlying successful surrogacy arrangements, pointing to the need for adequate pre-surrogacy counselling and education for all involved parties (Fuchs and Berenson 2016). In best medical and psychological practice, counselling should address four key principles relating to the best interests of the child born of the surrogacy arrangement; the surrogate's ability to make free and informed decisions; the requirement that the surrogate be free of exploitation; and a requirement for legal clarity about the resulting parent-child relationship, including documented information of genetic and birth history (Hammarberg et al. 2011).

There is no universally agreed standard for implications counselling in surrogacy. Professional psychological counselling may be provided through a treating IVF clinic, or it may be provided by a mental health professional independent of the treating clinic. There may be a requirement for in-depth psychological assessment and screening such as is required in the USA for gestational carriers and egg (oocyte) donors (Fuchs and Berenson 2016). In some countries, such as Australia, there may be pre-surrogacy psychosocial assessment of all parties to the surrogacy arrangement including the intended parents. In the UK pre-surrogacy counselling of all parties is recommended, but not mandated (Norton et al. 2015). Overall, there is more intensive and comprehensive attention to the psychosocial issues in countries such as the USA, UK, Australia, Canada, and New Zealand, with less being provided in countries such as Ukraine, Greece, Mexico, India, Thailand, and Cambodia.

With increasing uptake of surrogacy arrangements worldwide, there is a need to consider the short- and long-term outcomes for all parties concerned. In general, surrogates appear to score within the normal range on personality tests and to have medically and psychologically healthy pregnancies (Klock and Covington 2015). The greatest psychological challenge for surrogates appears to be at the time for the surrogate to hand over the child following the birth (Jadva 2016). Regarding the adjustment of children born of surrogates, one systematic review of 55 studies reported that by 10 years of age, these children had similar levels of psychological functioning as children naturally conceived and those conceived through assisted reproductive technology (ART) (Söderström-Anttila et al. 2016). The findings from one study of gay men parenting a child conceived through surrogacy further support the view that this practice has no adverse effects on child health outcomes (Carone et al. 2018). Moreover, it appears that disclosure to the child about the surrogacy arrangement is common in such families, reflecting a greater level of openness within the family than has been found in children conceived from other assisted third-party reproduction (Ilioiv et al. 2017). Despite a growing literature in this area, unfortunately there is limited high-quality research, with few studies providing adequate control groups and sample sizes and most studies having low-response rates questioning the generalizability of these findings (Söderström-Anttila et al. 2016). Clearly, there is an urgent need for more methodologically rigorous investigations regarding the psychosocial correlates and consequences of individuals involved in surrogacy arrangements.

Cross-References

▶ Assisted Reproductive Technology
▶ Infertility
▶ Infertility and Assisted Reproduction: Psychosocial Aspects
▶ Infertility-Related Stress
▶ In Vitro Fertilization
▶ In Vitro Fertilization, Assisted Reproductive Technology

References and Further Reading

Carone, N., Lingiardi, V., Chirumbolo, A., & Baiocco, R. (2018). Italian gay father families formed by surrogacy: Parenting, stigmatization, and children's psychological adjustment. *Developmental Psychology, 54*(10), 1904–1916.

Crockin, S. L. (2013). Growing families in a shrinking world: Legal and ethical challenges in cross-border surrogacy. *Reproductive Biomedicine Online, 27*(6), 733–741.

Fuchs, E. L., & Berenson, A. B. (2016). Screening of gestational carriers in the United States. *Fertility and Sterility, 106*(6), 1496–1502.

Greenfeld, D. A. (2014). Use of gestational carriers: Psychological aspects. In J. M. Goldfarb (Ed.), *Third party reproduction: A comprehensive guide* (pp. 79–83). New York: Springer.

Hammarberg, K., Johnson, L., & Petrillo, T. (2011). Gamete and embryo donation and surrogacy in Australia: The social context and regulatory framework. *International Journal of Fertility and Sterility, 4*(4), 176–183.

Ilioiv, E., Blake, L., Jadva, V., Roman, G., & Golombok, S. (2017). The role of age of disclosure of biological origins in the psychological wellbeing of adolescents conceived by reproductive donation: A longitudinal study from age 1 to age 14. *Journal of Child Psychology and Psychiatry, 58*(3), 315–324.

Jadva, V. (2016). Surrogacy: Issues, concerns and complexities. In S. Golombok, R. Scott, J. B. Appleby, M. Richards, & S. Wilkinson (Eds.), *Regulating reproductive donation* (pp. 126–139). Cambridge: Cambridge University Press.

Klock, S. C., & Covington, S. N. (2015). Results of the Minnesota multiphasic personality inventory-2 among gestational surrogacy candidates. *International Journal of Gynecology & Obstetrics, 130*, 257–260.

Lamba, N., Jadva, V., Kadam, K., & Golombok, S. (2018). The psychological well-being and prenatal bonding of gestational surrogates. *Human Reproduction, 33*(4), 646–653.

Norton, W., Crawshaw, M., Hudson, N., Culley, L., & Law, C. (2015). A survey of UK fertility clinics' approach to surrogacy arrangements. *Reproductive Biomedicine Online, 31*, 327–338.

Söderström-Anttila, V., Wennerholm, U.-B., Loft, A., Pinborg, A., Aittomäki, K., Bente Romundstad, L., & Bergh, C. (2016). Surrogacy: Outcomes for surrogate mothers, children and the resulting families – A systematic review. *Human Reproduction Update, 22*(2), 260–276.

Van den Akker, O. B. (2007). Psychosocial aspects of surrogate motherhood. *Human Reproduction Update, 13*(1), 53–62.

Surrogate

▶ In Vitro Fertilization, Assisted Reproductive Technology

Surrogate Decision Making

Howard Sollins
Attorneys at Law, Shareholder at Baker Donelson in the BakerOber Health Law Group, Baltimore, MD, USA

Synonyms

Proxy

Definition

Surrogate Decision Making

If an individual is unable to make decisions about personal health care, some other individual can be authorized to provide direction. Such a person is called the surrogate decision maker, a proxy, or some other term specific to the type of authorization. For example, under an advance directive, the decision maker is typically an "agent"; under a durable power of attorney for health care, the decision maker is the "attorney in fact" (although in slang, some health-care providers refers to such persons as "the POA"); an individual may be judicially appointed as a "guardian," or state law may identify certain next of kin or other close persons as eligible to serve as a surrogate. State law will determine the role of domestic partners in the absence of an advance directive appointing someone as an agent.

Each type of surrogate or proxy has a scope of authority to make health-care decisions for an individual depending on the source of the surrogate or proxy's authority and state law. For example, the surrogate may have broad authority to consent to health care and to refuse or direct the withdrawal of health care but with limitations if the care is life-sustaining. An agent under an advance directive from an individual may have immediate, broader authority to direct the withholding or withdrawal of life-sustaining treatment than a surrogate acting only under state law. Guardians may nor may not need court approval for certain actions involving life-sustaining treatment.

Surrogates or proxies appointed by the individual patient have decision making priority. Where there is no such person, state law determines the process for consulting with next of kin or others, which can include close friends, potentially in an order of hierarchy as to who priority, and how to resolve disagreements among those with the same level of relationship. Where there are no such persons or there is an irreconcilable disagreement, a judicial guardianship may be needed. Ethics committees or Patient Care Advisory Committees are examples of bodies within a health-care facility that can be very helpful in gathering an evaluating information about an individual's clinical condition, treatment options and prognosis, previously expressed wishes, interpretations of available documents, varying points of view, and related considerations.

In a recent study, it was noted that surrogate decision making is often required for older Americans at the end of life. Among a sample of 4246 deaths of respondents in the Health and Retirement Study, proxies reported that 42.5% of these individuals needed decision making about medical treatment before death; 70.3% of subjects lacked the capacity to make those decisions themselves and, overall, 29.8% required decision making at the end of life but lacked decision-making capacity. These findings suggest that more than a quarter of elderly adults may need surrogate decision making before death.

Cross-References

▶ End-of-Life Care

References and Readings

Silveira, M. J., Kim, S. Y. H., & Langa, K. M. (2010). Advance directives and outcomes of surrogate decision making before death. *The New England Journal of Medicine, 362*, 1211–1218.

Surrogate Mother

▶ Surrogacy

Surveys

Seppo Laaksonen
University of Helsinki, Helsinki, Finland

Synonyms

Micro data collection and analysis system; Opinion poll; Statistical inquiry

Definition

Survey is a methodology and a practical tool used to collect, handle, and analyze in a systematic way information from individuals. These individuals or micro units can be of various types, such as people, households, hospitals, schools, businesses, or other corporations. The units can be simultaneously available from two or more levels such from households and their members. Information in surveys may be concerned various topics such as people's personal characteristics, their behavior, health, salary, attitudes and opinions, incomes, poverty and housing environments, or characteristics and performance of businesses. Survey research is unavoidably interdisciplinary, although the role of statistics is most influential since the data for surveys is constructed in a quantitative form. Correspondingly, many survey methods are special statistical applications. However, surveys exploit substantially many other sciences such as informatics, mathematics, cognitive psychology, and theory of submatter sciences of each survey topic.

Basic Survey Concepts

A key concept in surveys is *target population* the universe of which should be exactly determined and realistic. It is possible that there are more than one target population (e.g., hospitals of certain types and their clients during a specific period). Before determining a strict target population, a researcher can have in mind *population of interest*, but this is often too difficult to reach, and hence, a realistic population is chosen. For example, more or less heavy alcohol drinkers may be interest for a researcher, but such people cannot be found from any data source. Respectively, such a target population is not realistic, but fortunately, one can try with a larger target population where there are also nondrinkers or light drinkers. The study itself can, among others, concentrate on those heavy drinkers, and results are correct if there are in data enough such people in order to get appropriate results. This requires also that we have a good frame and *frame population* from which reasonable data are downloaded. A drawback is that although the frame seems to be ideal, it includes such people who do not belong to our realistic target population, nevertheless, and secondly, we cannot get responses from all selected people due to *nonresponse*. Thus, when designing data collection, it is necessary to predict nonresponse and other gaps as well as possible in order to get enough respondents for the study.

Sampling

Survey data can cover the whole target population, but if it is large, it is rational to use sampling. This leads to plan an optimal sampling design. The design may be more or less complex. The simplest one is to use completely random selection in which case every frame unit has an equal *inclusion probability* to be selected in the sample. Such a design is rarely rational since the data collection may be too expensive or such a frame is not available. For these reasons, the most common strategy in people surveys is in the first stage, to select so-called *clusters* (small areas, service houses, households), and in the second stage, the desired sample units (target people, clients, household members) are to be interviewed and studied. This strategy is called *two-stage sampling*, but *three-stage sampling* is also applied. These both strategies lead to *probability sampling* that is definitely a valid method. Naturally, next steps must have been done successfully too.

Two- and three-stage samplings are generally called multistage sampling, but if the study units are selected directly from the frame, it is one-stage sampling, but this term is not much used. In contrast, the term *element sampling* is common. Multistage sampling is *hierarchical* in its nature, that is, we approach to study units by stage by stage. This strategy is different from *multiphase sampling* in which case after one sample selection, a new sample from the first sample has been selected. This is much used in *panels* in which case the second or the consecutive samples have been selected even with 100% from those who have responded in the first phase. This panel approach gives opportunity to follow respondents over time. It is common in health, poverty, and living condition research, for instance. Panel designs can be very complex too. *Rotating design* is much used when needed to analyze data both *cross-sectionally* (for a specific time point or time period) and *longitudinally* (for following individuals over time). Long panels might be hard to do well, and there can be met too much nonresponse that leads a worsening data quality.

Two-phase sampling is also useful when analyzing how respondents differ from nonrespondents. This information is necessary for survey quality documentation, but it can be used also for improving the quality. The second phase could in this case lead to draw a subsample of the nonrespondents, and then attempts to get some information from them. Naturally, this is not easy since they are reluctant, but most nonrespondents still are willing to answer to some simple but key questions of the survey.

Moreover, it is often advantageous to exploit *stratification* in surveys. This leads to create a number of strata that are like subpopulations. Sampling designs for each stratum may be similar or different. The main varying point is maybe that the sample size has been allocated for each stratum so that the research targets are satisfied ideally. Typically, the relative sample size is larger for a smaller stratum population and smaller for a larger population, respectively. This is due to an ordinary target to get about as accurate estimates (results) for each stratum.

Data Collection Tools and Methods

Data collection is not ready after selection a sample (or the full data). Three other major tasks are needed: (1) design the questionnaire, (2) decide the data collection mode (mail or phone or face-to-face interviewing or web or mixed mode such as web plus phone), (3) collect supported data (auxiliary) both for sampling and further data handling. Such data are required both from respondents and nonrespondents. *Auxiliary data* are very advantageous for adjusting *sampling weights* from the initial ones. Consequently, the bias in estimates will be reduced.

Data Cleaning and Analysis

Survey data should be cleaned before starting the analysis. In addition to computing the sampling weights, the following tasks are needed: data editing, imputation of missing data, data documentation (called metadata), data collection process documentation (called paradata), and selection of a good IT format (e.g., SPSS or SAS). The sampling design strategy is necessary to correctly take into account in the analysis.

Cross-References

▶ Clusters
▶ Cohort Study
▶ Data
▶ Internet-Based Studies
▶ Interview
▶ Multivariate Analysis
▶ Odds Ratio
▶ Participation Bias
▶ Population Stratification
▶ Probability
▶ Randomization
▶ Regression Analysis
▶ Retrospective Study

- ▶ Sample Size Estimation
- ▶ Selection Bias
- ▶ Standard Deviation
- ▶ Statistics
- ▶ Study Methodology

References and Readings

Bethlehem, J. G. (2009). *Applied survey methods: a statistical perspective* (375 pp). Hoboken: Wiley.

de Leeuw, E. D., Hox, J. J., & Dillman, D. A. (Eds.). (2009). *International handbook of survey methodology*. New York\London: Lawrence Erlbaum Associates \Taylor and Francis Group. 549 pp.

Surwit, Richard S.

James A. Blumenthal
Department of Psychiatry and Behavioral Sciences, Duke University Medical Center, Durham, NC, USA

Biographical Information

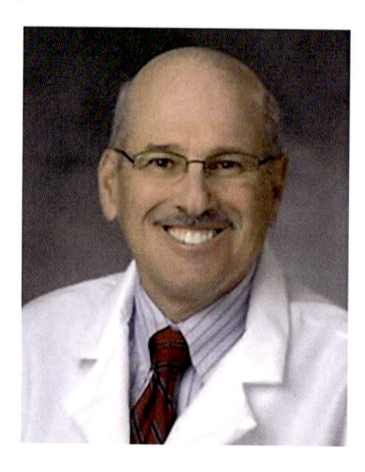

Richard S. Surwit received his B.A. from Earlham College and Ph.D. in clinical psychology from McGill University. He completed a postdoctoral fellowship in psychophysiology at Harvard University and joined the Duke faculty in 1977. He is currently professor of medical psychology and vice chair for research in the Department of Psychiatry and Behavioral Science at Duke University Medical Center, Durham, NC.

Major Accomplishments

Surwit's early work focused on the utility of biofeedback in the treatment of medical disorders, including Raynaud's disease and hypertension, and he was instrumental in establishing one of the first clinical biofeedback facilities in the country. Over the course of a long and productive career, his scientific contributions range from basic research on the use of mouse models to examine genetic and behavioral interactions in the development of obesity to clinical investigations of the effects of stress and hostility on glucose metabolism and diabetes. He also pioneered the use of computers in the medical management of such chronic diseases as diabetes and congestive heart failure. He has received multiple grants from the National Institutes of Health, private foundations, and industry to support his research program. He has played a key administrative role in the Department of Psychiatry and Behavioral Sciences at Duke University as vice chair for research and is a former president of the Society of Behavioral Medicine. He also has served on the editorial boards of such journals as *Health Psychology*, the *Journal of Consulting and Clinical Psychology*, *Obesity*, and *Metabolism*. He is the recipient of numerous awards and honors including the Research Career Award in Health Psychology from the American Psychological Association.

Cross-References

▶ Diabetes

Sustainability

▶ Ecosystems, Stable and Sustainable

Dr. Surwit recently received the Distinguished Scientist Award from the Society of Behavioral Medicine.

Sympathetic

▶ Autonomic Balance
▶ Heart Rate Variability

Sympathetic Nervous System (SNS)

Michael Richter[1] and Rex A. Wright[2]
[1]Department of Psychology, University of Geneva, Geneva, Switzerland
[2]Department of Psychology, College of Arts and Sciences, University of North Texas, Denton, TX, USA

Definition

The sympathetic nervous system (SNS) is one of two main branches or subsystems of the autonomic nervous system (ANS). It originates in the thoracic and upper lumbar segments of the spinal cord and commonly – but not always – yields peripheral adjustments that are complementary to those produced by its counterpart, the parasympathetic nervous system (PNS).

Description

The sympathetic nervous system is one of two main branches or subsystems of the autonomic nervous system, the physical system responsible for unconsciously maintaining bodily homeostasis and coordinating bodily responses. Working with the second main branch, the parasympathetic nervous system, the sympathetic nervous system regulates a wide range of functions such as blood circulation, body temperature, respiration, and digestion. Sympathetic activation commonly leads to adjustments on organs and glands that are complementary to those produced by parasympathetic activation and suitable for high activity ("fight and flight" as opposed to "rest and digest"). Examples of high-activity adjustments are constriction of blood vessels in the skin, dilation of blood vessels in the skeletal muscles and lungs, and increased heart rate and contraction force. Although sympathetic adjustments tend to complement parasympathetic adjustments, they do not always. For example, both sympathetic nervous system arousal and parasympathetic nervous system arousal increase salivary flow, although to different degrees and yielding different compositions of saliva.

Basic functional units of the sympathetic nervous system are preganglionic and postganglionic neurons. Preganglionic neurons have cell bodies in the thoracic and upper lumbar segments of the spinal cord and axons that extend to cell bodies of postganglionic neurons. Postganglionic neurons have cell bodies that are clustered in the so-called ganglia and relatively long axons that innervate target organs and glands. The major neurotransmitters of the sympathetic nervous system are acetylcholine and norepinephrine. Acetylcholine is the neurotransmitter of all preganglionic neurons. Stimulation of cholinergic receptors of the nicotinergic subtype located on the cell bodies of the postganglionic neurons by acetylcholine leads to an opening of nonspecific ion channels. This opening permits transfer of potassium and sodium ions, which depolarizes the postganglionic cell and initiates an action potential. Norepinephrine is the neurotransmitter of most sympathetic postganglionic neurons and stimulates adrenergic receptors lying on targeted visceral structures. All adrenergic receptors are coupled with G-proteins, but transmission pathways depend on the receptor subtype. Activation of alpha-1 receptors changes the calcium concentration in the cell, which in turn triggers the specific effect on the targeted visceral structure. Alpha-2 and beta receptors trigger visceral responses by affecting cAMP production in the cell. Specific effects depend on the receptor subtype and on the innervated visceral structure. For instance, stimulation of alpha-1 receptors on blood vessels of skeletal muscles leads to vasoconstriction and reduced blood flow, whereas stimulation of alpha-1 receptors on the radial pupil muscle leads to muscle contraction and increased pupil size. Stimulation of beta-2 receptors on the heart leads to increased heart rate and contraction force, whereas stimulation of beta-2 receptors on skeletal muscle blood vessels leads to vasodilation and increased blood flow.

In working jointly with the parasympathetic nervous system, the sympathetic nervous system does not function in an all-or-none fashion, but rather activates to different degrees. Depending on the affected visceral structure and situation, it may be more or less active than the parasympathetic nervous system. Shifts in the magnitude of sympathetic and parasympathetic influence can occur locally within a single visceral structure (e.g., the eye) or across visceral structures, with local shifts occurring to meet highly specialized demands (e.g., a change in ambient light) and global shifts adapting the body to large-scale environmental changes (e.g., the appearance of a substantial physical threat). Autonomic control is maintained by structures in the central nervous system that receives visceral information from an afferent (incoming) nervous system. A key central nervous system structure is the hypothalamus, which integrates autonomic, somatic, and endocrine responses that accompany different organism states.

Cross-References

▶ Acetylcholine
▶ Autonomic Activation
▶ Autonomic Balance
▶ Autonomic Nervous System (ANS)
▶ Epinephrine
▶ Parasympathetic Nervous System (PNS)

References and Further Readings

Berne, R. M., Levy, M. N., Koeppen, B. M., & Stanton, B. A. (2004). *Physiology* (5th ed.). St. Louis: Mosby.
Cacioppo, J. T., & Tassinary, L. G. (1990). *Principles of psychophysiology: Physical, social, and inferential elements*. New York: Cambridge University Press.
Cacioppo, J. T., Tassinary, L. G., & Berntson, G. G. (2000). *Handbook of psychophysiology* (2nd ed.). New York: Cambridge University Press.
Ganong, W. F. (2005). *Review of medical physiology* (22nd ed.). New York: McGraw-Hill.
Levick, J. R. (2009). *An introduction to cardiovascular physiology* (5th ed.). London: Hodder.

Sympathetic Nervous System (SNS) Activation

▶ Sympatho-adrenergic Stimulation

Sympatho-adrenergic Stimulation

Sabrina Segal
Department of Neurobiology and Behavior, University of California, Irvine, CA, USA

Synonyms

Adrenergic activation; Sympathetic nervous system (SNS) activation

Definition

Activation of one of the three branches (the sympathetic nervous system) of the autonomic nervous system via disruption of physiological homeostasis which results in the release of epinephrine/adrenaline and norepinephrine/noradrenaline from the adrenal medulla.

Description

The sympatho-adrenomedullary (SAM) system is one of two major components of the stress system. Stress activates the sympathetic nervous system and the goal of this response is to return the individual to physiological homeostasis. Epinephrine release from the adrenal medulla causes physiological alterations in cardiovascular tone, respiration rate, and blood flow to the muscles. Epinephrine does not cross the blood–brain barrier, but acts indirectly on the brain via the vagus nerve, which projects to the nucleus of the solitary tract (NTS), resulting in noradrenergic projections to the amygdala, as well as other brain regions. The release of epinephrine and norepinephrine from the adrenal medulla increases blood glucose levels and enhances alertness, learning, and memory.

Cross-References

▶ Norepinephrine/Noradrenaline

References and Readings

Cannon, W. B. (1914). The interrelations of emotions as suggested by recent physiological research. *The American Journal of Psychology, 25*(2), 256–282.

Chrousos, G. P., & Gold, P. W. (1992). The concepts of stress and stress system disorders. Overview of physical and behavioral homeostasis. *Journal of the American Medical Association, 267*(9), 1244–1252.

Hollenstein, T., McNeely, A., Eastabrook, J., Mackey, A., & Flynn, J. (2011). Sympathetic and parasympathetic responses to social stress across adolescence. *Developmental Psychobiology.* https://doi.org/10.1002/dev.20582.

Sherwood, L. (2008). *Human physiology: From cells to systems* (7th ed., p. 240). Stamford: Cengage Learning.

Tilders, F. J. H., & Berkenbosch, F. (1986). CRF and catecholamines; their place in the central and peripheral regulation of the stress response. *Acta Endocrinology, 113*, S63–S75.

Symptom Magnification Syndrome

Karen Jacobs
Occupational Therapy, College of Health and Rehabilitation Science, Sargent College, Boston University, Boston, MA, USA

Synonyms

Learned symptom behavior; Maladaptation of symptom behaviors to chronic illness; Malingering; Martyr behavior; Secondary gain

Definition

Symptom magnification is a self-destructive, socially reinforced behavioral response pattern consisting of reports or displays of symptoms which function to control the life of circumstances of the sufferer.

Description

Symptom magnification syndrome (SMS) may be described as a conscious or unconscious self-destructive learned pattern of behavior which is maintained through social reinforcement and typically controls the individual's life activities. SMS may be labeled "malingering" or exaggerated psychological complaints which can be associated with individuals who are seeking financial compensation or a secondary gain, e.g., increased attention from a family member, from symptom reporting. The validity scales of the Minnesota Multiphasic Personality Inventory-2 (MMPI-2) are widely used for the detection of exaggerated psychological complaints.

Cross-References

▶ Psychosocial Adjustment
▶ Psychosocial Predictors
▶ Psychosocial Variables
▶ Psychosocial Work Environment
▶ Psychosomatic
▶ Psychosomatic Disorder
▶ Somatic Symptoms
▶ Somatization
▶ Somatoform Disorders

References and Readings

Kopel, S., Walders-Abramson, N., MsQuaid, E., Seifer, R., Koinis-Mitchell, D., Klein, R., et al. (2010). Asthma symptom perception and obesity in children. *Biological Psychology, 84*, 135–141.

Matheson, L. N. (1986). *Work capacity evaluation: Systematic approach to industrial rehabilitation.* Anaheim: Employment and Rehabilitation Institute of California.

Matheson, L. N. (1987). *Symptom magnification casebook.* Matheson: Employment and Rehabilitation Institute of California.

Theodore, B., Kishino, N., & Gatchel, R. (2008). Biopsychosocial factors that perpetuate chronic pain, impairment, and disability. *Psychological Injury and Law, 1*, 182–190.

Tsushima, W., & Tsushima, V. (2009). Comparison of MMPI-2 validity scales among compensation-seekin Caucasian and Asian American medical patients. *Assessment, 16*, 159–164.

Symptom Scale

Yori Gidron
SCALab, Lille 3 University and Siric Oncollile, Lille, France

Synonyms

Symptoms Inventory

Definition

Symptom scales are psychometric instruments aimed at assessing the frequency or severity of any type of symptom associated with a mental or physical health condition. Development of symptom scales requires the same type of rigor as any other self-report instrument requires, including tests of internal reliability and test-retest reliability and face, concurrent, construct, and predictive validity. Questions on such scales can be asked in relation to a specific time frame (e.g., the present moment, the past week) and in relation to certain severity levels. For example, in the assessment of pain symptoms, patients may be asked to rate their level of average and worse pain in a given time frame. Finally, some scales also ask the extent to which certain symptoms interfere with one's daily functioning, as is often done in the domain of quality of life or pain. Another issue is whether the scale includes items concerning general symptoms or disease-specific symptoms. One of the earliest developed psychological symptom scales is the Symptom Checklist 90 (SCL-90) which was designed to assess psychological symptoms for evaluating the outcomes of mental health interventions and for research purposes. The symptoms are assessed in relation to the past 7 days and are categorized into nine dimensions (e.g., psychoticism, depression). Its internal reliability is adequate (e.g., Cronbach's alpha of 0.77–0.90 on its dimensions). Its concurrent, construct, and predictive validities have been shown as well. A physical symptom scale is the Patient Health Questionnaire 15 (PHQ-15; Kroenke et al. 2002). This scale assesses 15 common physical symptoms including stomach, back, head, and chest pains, dizziness, shortness of breath, etc. Scores on the PHQ-15 correlate with functional status and with health-care utilization. Numerous other instruments exist for assessment of various psychiatric symptoms including depression, anxiety, and post-traumatic stress disorder and for disease-specific symptoms. The latter include symptom scales of upper respiratory infections (Orts et al. 1995), the Rose chest pain questionnaire (Rose et al. 1977), and many others. More recently, Baxter et al. (2011) developed a brief pictorial scale for assessing nausea in children which can be used for pediatric oncological treatments. Symptom scales are a basic element in diagnosis and monitoring of treatment effects and in research in many health disciplines including medicine and behavior medicine. However, it is noteworthy to consider the limitations of symptom scales, as in most self-report scales. These include reporting biases, memory, and lack of self-awareness. One important factor known to underlie reporting biases is neuroticism or negative affectivity, which, when elevated, often leads to inflated symptom reporting and needs to be considered when patients complete symptom scales (Watson and Pennebaker 1989).

Cross-References

▶ Somatic Symptoms

References and Further Readings

Baxter, A. L., Watcha, M. F., Baxter, W. V., Leong, T., & Wyatt, M. M. (2011). Development and validation of a pictorial nausea rating scale for children. *Pediatrics, 127*, e1542–e1549.

Kroenke, K., Spitzer, R. L., & Williams, J. B. (2002). The PHQ-15: Validity of a new measure for evaluating the severity of somatic symptoms. *Psychosomatic Medicine, 64*, 258–266.

Orts, K., Sheridan, J. F., Robinson-Whelen, S., Glaser, R., Malarkey, W. B., & Kiecolt-Glaser, J. K. (1995). The reliability and validity of a structured interview for the assessment of infectious illness symptoms. *Journal of Behavioral Medicine, 18*, 517–529.

Rose, G., McCartney, P., & Reid, D. D. (1977). Self-administration of a questionnaire on chest pain and intermittent claudication. *British Journal of Preventive & Social Medicine, 31*, 42–48.

Watson, D., & Pennebaker, J. W. (1989). Health complaints, stress, and distress: Exploring the central role of negative affectivity. *Psychological Review, 96*, 234–254.

Symptom-Limited Exercise Test

▶ Maximal Exercise Stress Test

Symptoms

Tana M. Luger
Department of Psychology, University of Iowa, Iowa City, IA, USA

Synonyms

Indicators

Definition

Symptoms are physical sensations or changes in internal state that a person recognizes, interprets, and reports (Pennebaker 1982). Although symptoms are a key indicator of disease, it has been shown that perceived symptoms do not always correspond with objective, physiological pathology. Thus, researchers have sought to examine the various factors that can influence the perceptual processing and attributing of physical symptoms.

Because perception involves attention to certain cues while ignoring others, a person is more likely to recognize symptoms if their external world is not supplying them with information or distractions (Pennebaker 1982). For example, a person with a boring job is more likely to report symptoms than one with a fast-paced job. The assumption is that the person with the boring job can focus more attention on his internal, physical state rather than managing the external.

There is much evidence that people selectively search for information when interpreting their symptoms. People tend to focus on information which either confirms their expectations or shows the potential symptoms to be benign (Leventhal et al. 1998; Pennebaker 1982). Situational cues may also influence a person's search for information. For example, a recent outbreak of influenza in one's town may make a person more sensitive to his physiological changes and more likely to interpret his symptoms as signs of the flu. Previous experience with similar symptoms may also prime a person to attribute symptoms as being indicators of a particular disease (Jemmott III et al. 1988).

Finally, researchers have found that individual differences like gender, age, and personality can affect the amount that people report symptoms (Pennebaker 1982). For example, women tend to report more physical symptoms than men, older adults report more than young adults, and those high in the personality trait of negative affectivity report more than those high in positive affectivity. One reason suggested for these differences are differing tendencies to focus on one's internal state, resulting in more attention and recognition of symptoms.

Cross-References

▶ Cognitive Appraisal
▶ Common-Sense Model of Self-regulation
▶ Illness Cognitions and Perceptions

References and Readings

Jemmott, J. B., III, Croyle, R. T., & Ditto, P. H. (1988). Commonsense epidemiology: Self-based judgments from laypersons and physicians. *Health Psychology, 7*, 55–73.

Leventhal, H., Leventhal, E. A., & Contrada, R. J. (1998). Self-regulation, health, and behavior:

A perceptual-cognitive approach. *Psychology & Health, 13*, 717–733.

Pennebaker, J. W. (1982). *The psychology of physical symptoms*. New York: Springer.

Symptoms Inventory

▶ Symptom Scale

Syndrome X

▶ Metabolic Syndrome

Syntocinon (Synthetic Forms)

▶ Oxytocin
▶ Oxytocin, Social Effects in Humans

Syringe Exchange Programs

▶ Needle Exchange Programs

Systematic Bias

▶ Bias

Systematic Desensitization

Alan Kessedjian[1] and Faisal Mir[2]
[1]Clinical Psychologist, Birmingham, UK
[2]School of Sport and Exercise Sciences, University of Birmingham, Edgbaston, Birmingham, UK

Synonyms

Graded exposure counterconditioning

Definition

Systematic desensitization or graded exposure is a behavioral intervention commonly used in the treatment of phobias and other anxiety-related disorders. Individuals with phobias tend to possess irrational fears of stimuli such as heights, close spaces, dogs, and snakes. In order to cope, the individual avoids such stimuli. Since escaping from the phobic object reduces anxiety temporarily, the individual's behavior to reduce the perceived fear is negatively reinforced. The aim of systematic desensitization is to overcome this avoidance by gradually exposing individuals to the phobic stimulus until their anxiety to the fear is extinguished (Sturmey 2008).

Description

Joseph Wolpe (1915–1997)

Joseph Wolpe was a South African-born American doctor. During his work as a medical officer, Wolpe's task was to treat soldiers who were diagnosed with "war neurosis" which is now referred to as post-traumatic stress disorder. It was argued at the time that by talking about their war experiences would lead to a resolution of their symptoms. However, this was not found to be the case, and Wolpe became increasingly disillusioned by Freud's psychoanalytic therapy. It was this which served as a catalyst for Wolpe to discover other more effective treatment strategies (Wolpe 1973).

Wolpe began to investigate behavioral strategies through laboratory experiments. One of his concepts was reciprocal inhibition by which anxiety is inhibited by a feeling which is incompatible such as relaxation (Wolpe 1961). He pioneered the intervention assertiveness training and deciphered that this approach was useful for people who were anxious about social situations. As they learned assertiveness skills, this assisted to minimize the anxiety associated with such situations and in turn relaxed. As this proved to be highly fruitful, it further led to the development of systematic desensitization (Wolpe 1973).

Systematic Desensitization

It was discovered that fears could be learned through the behavioral model of classical conditioning (see ▶ "Classical Conditioning"). Therefore, Wolpe (1973) sought to eliminate the fear response generated by the stimulus and replace it with a competing response of relaxation. The notion of systematic desensitization was based upon two principles of conditioning. The first was that an individual could not produce two different responses to stimuli such as fear and relaxation. Secondly, classical conditioning often involves stimulus generalization which refers to stimuli which are similar and lead to the learned response of fear (Sturmey 2008).

During the process of systematic desensitization, the therapist works in conjunction with the person who has a phobia to ascertain the exact stimulus which triggers the phobia. Next, the individual is taught relaxation-inducing techniques often related to a cue for relaxing. After this stage, the therapist and individual develop a list of fear-evoking stimuli, ranging from very mild to very intense anxiety. This list is referred to as a hierarchy of fears as the stimulus items are listed in order of the intensity of fear they evoke. Then, working gradually the therapist attempts to recondition the person so that the stimuli in the hierarchy become associated with a relaxed response rather than fear. Once the individual can eventually confront the stimulus which originally evoked the greatest anxiety and remains relaxed, then the phobia has been effectively extinguished (Sturmey 2008).

Systematic desensitization has been found to be highly effective in the treatment of phobias (Clark 1963), sexual disorders (Obler 1973), and traumatic nightmares (Schindler 1980).

Cross-References

▶ Anxiety Disorder
▶ Behavior Change
▶ Behavior Modification
▶ Behavioral Intervention
▶ Behavioral Therapy
▶ Classical Conditioning
▶ Cognitive Behavioral Therapy (CBT)

References and Further Reading

Clark, D. F. (1963). The treatment of monosymptomatic phobia by systematic desensitization. *Behaviour Research and Therapy, 1*(1), 63–68.

Obler, M. (1973). Systematic desensitization in sexual disorders. *Journal of Behavior Therapy and Experimental Psychiatry, 4*(2), 93–101.

Schindler, F. E. (1980). Treatment by systematic desensitization of a recurring nightmare of a real life trauma. *Journal of Behavior Therapy and Experimental Psychiatry, 11*(1), 53–54.

Sturmey, P. (2008). *Behavioral case formulation and intervention: A functional analytic approach*. Chichester: Wiley.

Wolpe, J. (1961). The systematic desensitization treatment of neuroses. *The Journal of Nervous and Mental Disease, 132*(3), 189–203.

Wolpe, J. (1973). *The practice of behavior therapy* (2nd ed.). New York: Pergamon Press.

Systematic Review

J. Rick Turner
Campbell University College of Pharmacy and Health Sciences, Buies Creek, NC, USA

Definition

Systematic reviews present a descriptive assessment of a collection of original research articles related to a specific research question. These reviews "collate, compare, discuss, and summarize the current results in that field" (Matthews 2006). Campbell et al. (2007) noted that "It has now been recognised that to obtain the best current evidence with respect to a particular therapy all pertinent clinical trial information needs to be obtained." This "overview process" (Campbell et al. 2007) has led to many changes in the way clinical trial programs are developed. They have become an integral part of evidence-based medicine, impacting decisions that affect patient care.

A considerable problem in writing such reviews is the retrieval of all relevant publications in the behavioral medicine literature, although the advent of computerized searchable databases has made this task much less arduous.

While such a narrative review can be very useful in its own right, it can also be the first step in a two-step process that also includes conducting a meta-analysis. This provides a statistical (quantitative) answer, whereas the authors' conclusions in a systematic review will largely be qualitative.

Cross-References

▶ Meta-analysis

References and Further Reading

Campbell, M. J., Machin, D., & Walters, S. J. (2007). *Medical statistics: A textbook for the health sciences* (4th ed.). Chichester: Wiley.

Matthews, J. N. S. (2006). *Introduction to randomized controlled clinical trials* (2nd ed.). Boca Raton: Chapman & Hall/CRC Press.

Systems Theory

Afton N. Kapuscinski
Psychology Department, Syracuse University, Syracuse, NY, USA

Definition

An approach to science that emphasizes unity and wholeness (von Bertalanffy 1968) and views factors that influence phenomena as mutually affecting each other at various levels of complexity.

Description

Systems theory, which became popular in the mid-twentieth century, developed in opposition to some of the philosophical assumptions that permeated the sciences across a variety of disciplines (von Bertalanffy 1968). Specifically, systems theory opposed the idea that knowledge about the universe is best obtained through a perspective rooted in notions of reductionism, mechanism, and objectivism (Midgley 2000). Mechanism assumes that the universe and all phenomena contained within it can be likened to machines, composed of parts that operate in predictable, logical ways. Therefore, traditional scientific theory and methodology seeks to reduce complex phenomena to the functions of the smallest possible parts (reductionism), assuming that such analysis will yield complete understanding and ultimately control, in the area under study (Midgley 2000). For example, a reductionistic approach to psychology may pose that all behavior can ultimately be traced to genetic endowment or chemical reactions occurring at the level of individual brain cells.

Systems theorists, however, argue that the search for simple, linear, cause and effect relationships between variables may lead to the neglect of developing more holistic, comprehensive conceptual models (Midgley 2000), leaving the field of psychology impoverished in a couple of ways. First, mechanistic and reductionist approaches may struggle to explain emergent properties of systems, that is, those qualities of a system that cannot be explained merely as the sum of its individual parts (Bertalanffy 1968), such as the human capacity for agency, creativity, or love. Even the concept of life itself cannot be explained by the activity of individual cells (Bertalanffy), but emerges from a complex system of interacting cells. Second, reductionistic scientific disciplines tend to exist in relative isolation from each other, without attempts at integration that may benefit the individual field, as well as facilitate broader societal improvement. Since system thinking views the boundaries between disciplines as somewhat unnecessary and artificial, a behavioral medicine investigator working from a systems perspective may draw from many sciences to obtain a more holistic understanding of a given topic. Therefore, in contrast to the "zooming in" approach of reductionism, systems thinking values panning outward to examine different levels of contextual factors that may be influencing and be influenced by a particular aspect of a system – including concepts across disciplines.

Ecological models of health behavior (see Sallis et al. 2008) are a good example of research grounded in systems thinking. These models assume multiple influences on health behaviors at various levels, with influences interacting across the levels (Sallis et al. 2008). For example, consider the problem of cardiovascular disease.

A systemic approach to reducing the incidence of cardiovascular disease would aim to target a variety of factors that are interacting to determine one's degree of risk for developing the condition, including biological (e.g., hypertension, high cholesterol), psychological (e.g., hostility), social (interpersonal relationships and support), and behavioral (e.g., diet, exercise, medication compliance) contributors. Such conceptualization in behavioral medicine is often referred to as taking a biopsychosocial approach, a form of systems thinking. A systemic model would also examine contextual factors that affect the individual, such as health care utilization or level of education, which may influence the individual's exposure to preventative medicine and information about healthy eating habits. Further, the approach would likely be mindful of broader social and economic concerns (e.g., unemployment rate, racial inequality) that may, in turn, influence one's access to these resources and thus would also be considered relevant to intervention efforts. These types of ecological models have been developed to further understanding of various health behaviors such as physical activity, tobacco control, and diabetes management (Sallis et al. 2008).

Just as systems theory questions the validity of boundaries between disciplines, it also disputes the boundary between scientists and their objects of study (Midgley 2000). Systems theorists reject the position that one can passively observe reality, standing separate from the object of study, but holds that scientists interact with these objects to actively create reality and interpret observations based on the lens through which they view them (von Bertalanffy 1968). If objectivism is not possible and scientists can never capture "reality," then theories and methodologies become "ways of seeing" that are full of value (Midgley 2000). A critical implication of this shift in thinking is the possibility for theoretical pluralism, wherein investigators value contributions from various perspectives and types of research.

Influence on Psychotherapy

The principles inherent in the systems approach have influenced important shifts in the way psychotherapists understand the process of facilitating client change. First, there has been a shift away from the traditional psychoanalytic approach, which viewed the therapist as a relatively objective figure who could successfully remove his or her self from the process, providing the patient with a "blank screen" on which to project unconscious material for interpretation by the therapist. Modern psychoanalytic approaches, such as the object relations or two-person paradigms, assert that the therapist cannot avoid revealing the self and influencing the therapeutic encounter so as to create it along with the patient (Levenson 1995). When viewing the therapeutic relationship as a system, the interaction between the therapist and patient, including the therapists' behaviors and feelings, becomes critically important and should be considered to aid case formulation and planning interventions. Since a change in any part of a system affects the whole of the system (von Bertalanffy 1968), the therapist's attempts to foster a healthy relationship can encourage improved interpersonal functioning in the patient (Levenson 1995). Second, systems theory gave rise to another popular paradigm for understanding individual and family dysfunction, known as family systems theory. Family systems theory holds that an individual's or family's distress cannot be understood fully by looking at any one person in isolation, but must be viewed as the symptom of problematic patterns of interactions within the larger family structure (Smith-Acuña 2010). Systems therapists therefore seek to improve the functioning of the family as a unit.

Cross-References

▶ Ecological Models: Application to Physical Activity
▶ Family Systems Theory

References and Readings

Breunlin, D. C., Schwartz, R. C., & Mac Kune-Karrer, B. (2001). *Metaframeworks: Transcending the models of family therapy*. San Francisco: Wiley.
Levenson, H. (1995). *Time-limited dynamic psychotherapy: A guide to clinical practice*. New York: Basic Books.

Midgley, G. (2000). *Systemic intervention: Philosophy, methodology and practice.* New York: Plenum.
Sallis, J. F., Owen, N., & Fisher, E. B. (2008). Ecological models of health behavior. In K. Glanz, B. K. Rimer, & K. Viswanath (Eds.), *Health behavior and health education: Theory, research and practice* (pp. 465–485). San Francisco: Wiley.
Smith-Acuña, S. (2010). *Systems theory in action: Applications to individual, couple, and family therapy.* Hoboken, NJ: Wiley.
von Bertalanffy, L. (1968). *General systems theory.* London: Penguin.

Systolic Blood Pressure (SBP)

Annie T. Ginty
School of Sport and Exercise Sciences,
The University of Birmingham, Edgbaston,
Birmingham, UK

Synonyms

Blood pressure

Definition

Systolic blood pressure is the force exerted by blood on arterial walls during ventricular contraction measured in millimeters of mercury (see Tortora and Grabowski 1996). It is the highest pressure measured; normal range for systolic blood pressure is <120 mmHg.

Cross-References

▶ Blood Pressure
▶ Blood Pressure Classification
▶ Blood Pressure, Measurement of
▶ Diastolic Blood Pressure (DBP)

References and Further Reading

Tortora, G. J., & Grabowski, S. R. (1996). *Principles of anatomy and physiology* (8th ed.). New York: Harper Collins College.

Tachycardia

Lois Jane Heller
Department of Biomedical Sciences, University of Minnesota Medical School – Duluth, Duluth, MN, USA

Definition

The word "tachycardia" means rapid heart rate. This condition is more precisely defined as a heart rate that is above the age-adjusted range of normal heart rates (see Table 1). Children normally have higher heart rates than adults and can tolerate rapid heart rates more easily.

Description

Normal Determinants of Heart Rate

Heart rate is normally established by the rate of spontaneous generation of an electrical signal (action potential) by "pacemaker" cells located in the sinoatrial (SA) node of the heart (in the wall of the right atrium near the entry of the superior vena cava) (Mohrman and Heller 2011). These electrical signals are normally generated at a rate of 60–100 beats per min in a human adult. They are propagated from the SA node through the atrial and ventricular muscle cells in a set pathway that stimulates contraction in a pattern that optimizes pumping of blood from the heart. Most other cardiac muscle cells have the potential to act as pacemakers, but the SA nodal cells drive the heart at a slightly faster rate than any of these other "latent" pacemakers.

The normal fluctuations in heart rate that occur in response to normal changes in the body's metabolic demands are accomplished by altering autonomic neural influences on the SA nodal pacemaker cells from the parasympathetic and sympathetic nervous system. Increased sympathetic activity causes an increase in heart rate whereas increase in parasympathetic activity causes a decrease in heart rate.

Symptoms of Tachycardia

A person with significant tachycardia may or may not be aware that their heart rate is fast without actually measuring their pulse rate (Valentin et al. 2008). However, tachycardia often results in a feeling of light-headedness, dizziness, tunnel vision, or fainting. Other symptoms may include muscle weakness, nervousness, sweating, pallor, or a feeling of fullness in the chest. The cause of many of these symptoms is often related to a decrease in arterial blood pressure and therefore blood flow to the brain and other tissues.

Physiological Cause of the Symptoms

The amount of blood that the heart pumps in a minute is called the cardiac output (Mohrman and Heller 2011). This is determined by the volume of blood ejected in each beat *(stroke volume)* and the number of beats per minute *(heart rate)*:

© Springer Nature Switzerland AG 2020
M. D. Gellman (ed.), *Encyclopedia of Behavioral Medicine*,
https://doi.org/10.1007/978-3-030-39903-0

Tachycardia, Table 1 Age-associated upper limit to normal human heart rates. (Adapted from Greene 1991)

Less than 1 year	~170 bpm
1–2 years	~150 bpm
3–5 years	~135 bpm
6–12 years	~130 bpm
12–15 years	~120 bpm
15 years through adulthood	~100 bpm

Cardiac output = stroke volume × heart rate

One might predict from this equation that the cardiac output would increase whenever heart rate increased. This is true over the normal range of heart rates. However, when the heart rate exceeds this normal range, the cardiac output may actually fall. There are three primary reasons for this: (1) There is insufficient time between beats to allow the heart to fill adequately. (2) The coronary circulation to the cardiac muscle may be compromised by the compressive forces in the ventricular wall associated with each individual beat. (3) The energy requirements for the heart increase enormously and may not be met by the compromised coronary blood flow.

Physiological Causes of Tachycardia

1. *Atrial Tachycardia or Supraventricular Tachycardia* (i.e., associated with a narrow QRS complex on an ECG) (Valentin et al. 2008). This condition is more common than ventricular tachycardia (see below) and can often be successfully treated. It is often uncomfortable and alarming to the individual, but does not usually portend immediate, possibly fatal consequences.
   (a) *Sinus Tachycardia* – Elevated sympathetic neural activity or an increase in circulating catecholamines stimulates the normal pacemaker cells in the SA node to fire at a very rapid rate and this electrical signal is then carried via normal pathways through the entire heart.
   (b) *Ectopic Atrial Pacemakers* – Atrial cells that are not part of the SA node can sometimes become irritable and generate electrical signals that spread throughout the cardiac tissue.
   (c) *AV Nodal Reentrant Tachycardia* – This is a conduction defect rather than a pacemaker defect. In this case, a rapid heart rate may result from an abnormal portion of conduction pathway usually found in the AV node in which the electrical signal circles back on itself to rapidly re-excite the downstream tissue.
   (d) *Atrial Flutter* – An ectopic pacemaker or reentrant pathway in the atria evokes in a very rapid atrial rate such that AV node fails to conduct every signal. The atria may beat three or more times for each ventricular beat. The ventricular rate may be faster than normal or within the normal range but the atrial rate is faster.
   (e) *Atrial Fibrillation* – The atrial conduction pathways become disorganized and the normal synchronized excitation of the atrial tissue is disrupted. Electrical signals are initiated and conducted in bizarre patterns, resulting in unpredictable intermittent conduction through the AV node. This results in an irregular ventricular rhythm that may, on the average, be faster than normal (tachycardia), normal, or slower than normal (bradycardia).
2. *Ventricular Tachycardias* (i.e., associated with wide QRS complex on an ECG). This is a more serious condition than atrial tachycardia and needs immediate attention. The heart is still operating as a pump but the possibility of a sudden deterioration to ventricular fibrillation is high.
   (a) *Ectopic Ventricular Pacemakers* – Ventricular cells can sometimes become irritable and generate electrical signals that spread throughout the cardiac tissue. This may occur if blood flow to a portion of the ventricular wall is inadequate and the tissue becomes ischemic.
   (b) Ventricular Reentrant Pathways – In this case, a rapid heart rate may result from abnormal conduction of the electrical signal through a small portion of ventricular

muscle such that the electrical signal circles back on itself to rapidly re-excite the cardiac tissue. Because all cardiac muscle cells are electrically connected, this rapidly firing small group of cells can drive the ventricles at a fast rate.

Cross-References

▶ Arrhythmia
▶ Maximal Exercise Heart Rate

References and Readings

Greene, M. G. (Ed.). (1991). *The Harriet Lane handbook* (12th ed.). St Louis: Mosby Yearbook.

Mohrman, D. E., & Heller, L. J. (2011). *Cardiovascular physiology* (Lange series 7th ed.). New York: McGraw-Hill.

Valentin, F., O'Rourke, R. A., Walsh, R. A., & Poole-Wilson, P. (2008). *Hurst's the heart* (12th ed.). New York: McGraw-Hill.

Tailored Communications

Celette Sugg Skinner
Clinical Sciences, The University of Texas Southwestern Medical Center at Dallas
Harold C. Simmons Cancer Center, Dallas, TX, USA

Synonyms

Tailored health behavior change interventions

Definition

> "Tailored communications are any combination of information intended to reach one specific person, based on characteristics unique to that person, related to the outcome of interests, and derived from an individual assessment" (Kreuter and Farrell 2000).

Description

Background

The field of behavioral medicine studies how behaviors affect health and medical conditions, as well as how behaviors can be changed. Good behavior-change interventions are, of course, guided by strong health behavior theories that elucidate factors (variables) affecting individuals' behaviors. One of most basic of these, the Health Belief Model (HBM), was developed in the 1950s when the US public health service consulted with psychologists to understand why people were not availing themselves of free tuberculosis screenings. This simple model delineates three major factors (or theoretical constructs) affecting whether people take a health action. They must feel susceptible to a health threat serious enough to warrant attempts to reduce the risk, believe that changing their behavior would reduce their risk, and overcome perceived barriers to behavior change (Champion and Skinner 2008). Individuals can vary widely on these beliefs. One's threat perception may be low whereas another may perceive the threat but not believe the behavior change would have benefit for lowering it. Among those who perceive barriers to behavior change, specific types of barriers may vary widely. For example, not having a ride to a screening site is very different from not being able to afford screening or of being afraid the screen would find a problem.

Message Customization

Face-to-face communications are usually customized for different people. For example, nurses seeking to facilitate medication adherence communicate with different patients differently, depending on factors influencing *that persons'* behavior. The message differs when talking with someone who cannot remember to take the pills versus someone avoiding the medication due to side effects. But only recently did this kind of message customization become possible in mass-produced media such as print and video. From the 1950s through the 1980s, mass-media communications such as brochures and videos were developed to address an array of variables, with the hope that at least some of the message components would be relevant to most audience members.

Mass-Produced Tailored Communications

In the 1980s, the rise of micro-computing capabilities opened possibilities for mass-producing communications that retained advantages of customized face-to-face interactions. These "tailored communications" are reminiscent of tailor-made clothing that is based on numerous measurements taken by the tailor before beginning his work. Tailored communications begin with measures of people's behavior-influencing factors such as the HBM variables of perceived risks and beliefs about the behavior's benefits and barriers. The "fabric" of tailored communications is distinct text, audio, or graphic components that are "sewn" together to fit the measurements of a particular message recipient.

In their 2000 book, *Tailored Health Messages; Customizing Communication with Computer Technology* Kreuter, Farrell et al. provide this elegant definition of tailored communications: "any combination of information intended to reach one specific person, based on characteristics unique to that person, related to the outcome of interests, and derived from an individual assessment." Continuing the clothing analogy, this definition distinguishes between tailored and targeted communications, as follows. *Tailored communications* – and tailored clothing – are intended to fit one individual. *Targeted communications* – and off-the-rack clothing – are intended to fit any one of a group sharing some common characteristics (e.g., men who wear a size 40 long, like pinstripes, and shop in a certain price range). Targeted messages are usually directed to a particular demographic group (i.e., African American church members) and address factors known to be important for *many* members of that group. In contrast, tailored communications are based on individual-level assessment of theory-based behavior-influencing variables, with a unique combination of messages assembled for each individual within the group (Kreuter and Skinner 2000).

The original rational for tailoring was that tailored communications would be more noticeable and compelling and less burdensome because they are streamlined to only include content relevant to the recipient. According to Petty and Cacioppo (Petty et al. 1981), the more personal involvement with the message, the more careful consideration (i.e., "central processing") and elaboration on the message which, in turn, increases likelihood of attitude and behavior change.

Early Trials of Tailored Print Communications

Several initial randomized trials compared printed communications that were v. were not tailored on theory-derived behavior-influencing variables (Skinner et al. 1999). Three of these, targeting mammography screening (Skinner et al. 1994), smoking cessation (Strecher et al. 1994), and dietary change (Campbell et al. 1994), were conducted among primary-care patients who completed telephone surveys and were randomly assigned to receive tailored or non-tailored printed newsletters. In addition to age, race, and risk factors, messages in the tailored letters directly addressed variables such as the recipients' perceived risk, benefits and barriers, their stage of behavior adoption, characteristics such as age, race, and risk factors and, for smokers, causal attributions for past failed quite attempts. In each of these three studies, the non-tailored letter version addressed a number of factors that had been shown to influence people's behaviors, in general. For example, the non-tailored mammography letter was adapted from a letter from US Surgeon General's office mailed to women who requested information about breast cancer screening. Because these three trials were designed to compare tailored versus non-tailored *content*, the tailored letters did not include statements such as "the information was prepared especially for you," as have later studies. Tailored and non-tailored letters looked very much alike. They were printed in black and white on two-column 8½ × 11 paper and included a head-and-shoulders line drawing. Therefore, it is remarkable that recipients of the tailored letters were more likely to report remembering and reading their letters. Receipt of a tailored letter was also associated with behavior change (Campbell et al. 1994), at least among important subgroups (Skinner et al. 1994; Strecher et al. 1994). Indeed, of the seven initial comparisons of tailored versus. non-tailored print communications, six (Skinner et al. 1999) found more behavior change among tailored recipients.

Movement Toward Different Comparisons

Given these impressive results from studies comparing tailored versus similar non-tailored print, and with tailoring technology expanding rapidly, tailoring researchers moved on to different comparisons. Studies tested tailored communications as an adjunct to other intervention components such as self-help smoking manuals, and compared tailored messages delivered through different media, such as tailored print versus tailored telephone counseling (Champion et al. 2007; Rimer et al. 2002), tailored on different types of variables (Kreuter et al. 2005), and with and without booster doses (Skinner 2006). Even within the tailored print medium, researchers moved beyond the newsletter format to tailored booklets and magazines with tailored features such as cartoons and advice columns (Rimer et al. 2002; Kreuter et al. 2005). Because there were so many kinds of comparisons of different tailoring approaches and for different target behaviors, data do not exist from head-to-head comparisons of every feature (e.g., more vs. less content, fewer vs. more graphics). As reported in a 1998 review of the "first generation" of tailored communications, these various comparisons showed mixed results, and "when (tailored print communications) are only one component of a complex intervention strategy without a factorial design, it is more difficult to isolate their relative contribution to the overall intervention effect" (Skinner et al. 1999, p 296). Nonetheless, this initial review and several others published subsequently (Kreuter and Farrell 2000; Kroeze et al. 2006; Revere and Dunbar 2001; Rimer and Glassman 1999) reported that tailoring seems to "work" both for attracting and retaining attention and for facilitating behavior change. Further, delivering tailored messages via print plus another medium such as telephone generally is more effective than tailored print alone.

Interactive "Real-Time" Tailoring

Original print-tailored interventions collected questionnaire data and then used that entire "batch" of data to put together specific messages that, depending on algorithms, were selected from a library of potential messages. More recently, CD-ROMs, DVDs, and the internet have allowed for interactive tailoring based on data collected during program use rather than in questionnaire form before the intervention is delivered. For example, a DVD or CD-ROM can ask a question about barriers to behavior change, then immediately show videos, selected from a tailored video library, that address the specific barriers named by the user (Skinner et al. 2011). Some web-based programs provide tailored content based on pre-determined algorithms, others allow users to "self-tailor" by selecting any content of interest to them. As described in Lustria et al. 2009 review of computer-tailored health interventions delivered over the web, these interventions "have involved a great diversity of features and formats," and "further outcome research is needed to enhance our understanding of how and under what conditions computer-tailoring leads to positive health outcomes in online behavioral interventions" (Lustria et al. 2009, p. 156). Therefore, as with the print-tailored communications, it is difficult to draw conclusions across studies.

Conclusions and Challenges

One problem in understanding findings and implications of tailored communication intervention studies is that journals often severely limit the amount of space for intervention descriptions. As a result, we have many statistics associated with the intervention outcomes, but we know little about the interventions themselves. In other words, we may learn that "it worked" without knowing exactly what "it" was or with what "it" was compared. Tailoring researchers have, therefore, recently called for new reporting standards through which intervention studies will report similar descriptions and metrics, which should help in evaluation and dissemination of best practices in tailored interventions (Harrington and Noar 2011).

In summary, communication interventions that are tailored to include theory-based messages relevant to individual recipients, based on data collected from them, are generally better than non-tailored communications in drawing the attention of message recipients and facilitating their health behavior change. However, questions still remain about optimal amounts and types of tailoring for different behavioral targets and through different media.

Cross-References

▶ Health Behavior Change
▶ Health Behaviors
▶ Health Beliefs/Health Belief Model
▶ Health Communication
▶ Health Risk (Behavior)
▶ Stages-of-Change Model

References and Readings

Campbell, M. K., DeVellis, B. M., Strecher, V. J., Ammerman, A. S., DeVellis, R. F., & Sandler, R. S. (1994). Improving dietary behavior: The effectiveness of tailored messages in primary care settings. *American Journal of Public Health, 84*, 783–787.

Champion, V. L., & Skinner, C. S. (2008). The health belief model. In K. Glanz, B. K. Rimer, & K. Viswanath (Eds.), *Health behavior and health education: Theory, research and practice* (4th ed., pp. 45–65). San Francisco: Jossey-Bass.

Champion, V., Skinner, C. S., Hui, S., Monahan, P., Juliar, B., Daggy, J., et al. (2007). The effect of telephone versus print tailoring for mammography adherence. *Patient Education and Counseling, 65*, 416–423.

Harrington, N. G., & Noar, S. M. (2011). Reporting standards for studies of tailored interventions. *Health Education Research, 27*(2), 331–342.

Kreuter, M. W., & Farrell, D. (2000). *Tailoring health messages: Customizing communication with computer technology*. Mahwah: Lawrence Erlbaum.

Kreuter, M. W., & Skinner, C. S. (2000). Tailoring: What's in a name? *Health Education Research, 15*, 1–4.

Kreuter, M. W., Skinner, C. S., Holt, C. L., Clark, E. M., Haire-Joshu, D., Fu, Q., et al. (2005). Cultural tailoring for mammography and fruit and vegetable intake among low-income African-American women in urban public health centers. *Preventive Medicine, 41*, 53–62.

Kroeze, W., Werkman, A., & Brug, J. (2006). A systematic review of randomized trials on the effectiveness of computer-tailored education on physical activity and dietary behaviors. *Annals of Behavioral Medicine, 31*, 205–223.

Lustria, M. L., Cortese, J., Noar, S. M., & Glueckauf, R. L. (2009). Computer-tailored health interventions delivered over the Web: Review and analysis of key components. *Patient Education and Counseling, 74*, 156–173.

Petty, R. E., Cacioppo, J. R., & Goldman, R. (1981). Personal involvement as a determinant of argument-based persuasion. *Journal of Personality and Social Psychology, 41*, 847–855.

Revere, D., & Dunbar, P. J. (2001). Review of computer-generated outpatient health behavior interventions: Clinical encounters "in absentia". *Journal of the American Medical Informatics Association, 8*, 62–79.

Rimer, B. K., & Glassman, B. (1999). Is there a use for tailored print communications in cancer risk communication? *Journal of the National Cancer Institute Monographs, 25*, 140–148.

Rimer, B. K., Halabi, S., Skinner, C. S., Lipkus, I. M., Strigo, T. S., Kaplan, E. B., et al. (2002). Effects of a mammography decision-making intervention at 12 and 24 months. *American Journal of Preventive Medicine, 22*, 247–257.

Skinner, C. S. (2006). Tailored interventions for screening mammography: When is a booster dose important? *Patient Education and Counseling, 65*, 87–94.

Skinner, C. S., Strecher, V. J., & Hospers, H. (1994). Physicians' recommendations for mammography: Do tailored messages make a difference? *American Journal of Public Health, 84*, 43–49.

Skinner, C. S., Campbell, M. K., Rimer, B. K., Curry, S., & Prochaska, J. O. (1999). How effective is tailored print communication? *Annals of Behavioral Medicine, 21*, 290–298.

Skinner, C. S., Buchanan, A., Champion, V., Monahan, P., Rawl, S., Springston, J., et al. (2011). Process outcomes from a randomized controlled trial comparing tailored mammography interventions delivered via telephone vs. DVD. *Patient Education & Counseling, 85*, 308–312.

Strecher, V. J., Kreuter, M., Den Boer, D. J., Kobrin, S., Hospers, H. J., & Skinner, C. S. (1994). The effects of computer-tailored smoking cessation messages in family practice settings. *Journal of Family Practice, 39*, 262–270.

Tailored Health Behavior Change Interventions

▶ Tailored Communications

Teens

▶ Williams LifeSkills Program

Telehealth

▶ eHealth and Behavioral Intervention Technologies

Telehealth Cost-Effectiveness

▶ eHealth Cost-Effectiveness

Telencephalon

▶ Brain, Cortex

Telephone Coaching

▶ Williams LifeSkills Program

Telepsychology

▶ Online Therapy and E-Counselling

Telomere and Telomerase

A. Janet Tomiyama[1] and Elissa S. Epel[2]
[1]Rutgers University, New Brunswick, NJ, USA
[2]Department of Psychiatry, Weill Institute for Neurosciences, University of California, San Francisco, CA, USA

Definition

Telomeres are noncoding repeat DNA sequences (consisting of TTAGGG) that cap the ends of eukaryotic chromosomes. Telomerase is an enzyme that adds basepairs to telomeres.

Description

Like the plastic tips that protect shoelaces from unravelling, telomeres protect DNA material. When cells divide, the enzymes that replicate the chromosomes are unable to do so fully. The main purpose of telomeres is to form a buffer so that genetic material is not lost in this process. With each cell division, telomeres can shorten, and when telomeres become critically short, a cell undergoes senescence (cell arrest). Telomeres also function to protect chromosomes from genomic instability, end-to-end chromosome fusion, less efficient cell division, loss of ability for cell replenishment, and apoptosis or cell death (Blackburn 2000).

Because of these important functions, telomeres are related to a number of health outcomes and disease states. Shorter telomere length is associated with chronic diseases of aging such as cardiovascular disease, cancer development, and Alzheimer's disease, and is related to earlier mortality. Telomere length is also thought to be an indicator of biological, rather than chronological, age (Epel 2009).

Telomere length is associated with a number of psychosocial factors. For example, depression, higher perceived stress, longer stress duration, caregiving, lower socioeconomic status, pessimism, childhood adversity, and lower subjective well-being are correlated with shorter telomere length. Health behaviors such as smoking, lack of physical activity, and repeated dieting as well as altered metabolic states such as obesity and insulin resistance are also linked with shorter telomere length (Lin et al. 2009).

Telomerase is the enzyme that adds base pairs back onto telomeres. This serves to protect telomeres from shortening. Recent work suggests telomerase may have future applications for antiaging therapies as evidenced by telomerase knockout mice displaying reversed aging with telomerase treatment (Jaskelioff et al. 2010).

Telomerase, like telomeres, appears to be responsive to psychological states, and may serve to protect cells under stress. Exposure to acute stress (Epel et al. 2010) as well as states of chronic psychosocial adversity are associated with high telomerase. Because telomerase levels change more dynamically than telomere length, psychosocial interventions such as meditation (Jacobs et al. 2010) and comprehensive lifestyle changes (Ornish et al. 2008) have been tested in preliminary studies as a potential treatment to increase telomerase, with promising results.

Cross-References

▶ Aging
▶ Alzheimer's Disease
▶ Cardiovascular Disease
▶ Chromosomes
▶ Depression
▶ Insulin Resistance
▶ Lifestyle Changes
▶ Meditation
▶ Obesity
▶ Pessimism
▶ Physical Activity
▶ Smoking and Health
▶ Socioeconomic Status (SES)
▶ Subjective Well-Being

References and Readings

Blackburn, E. H. (2000). Telomere states and cell fates. *Nature, 408*, 53–56.
Epel, E. (2009). Telomeres in a life-span perspective: A new "psychobiomarker?". *Current Directions in Psychological Science, 18*, 6–10.
Epel, E. S., Lin, J., Dhabhar, F. S., Wolkowitz, O. M., Puterman, E., Karan, L., et al. (2010). Dynamics of telomerase activity in response to acute psychological stress. *Brain, Behavior, and Immunity, 24*, 531–539.
Jacobs, T. L., Epel, E. S., Lin, J., Blackburn, E. H., Wolkowitz, O. M., Bridwell, D. A., et al. (2010). Intensive meditation training, immune cell telomerase activity, and psychological mediators. *Psychoneuroendocrinology, 36*(5), 664–681.
Jaskelioff, M., Muller, F. L., Paik, J., Thomas, E., Jian, S., Adams, A. C., et al. (2010). Telomerase reactivation reverses tissue degeneration in aged telomerase-deficient mice. *Nature, 469*, 102–106.
Lin, J., Epel, E., & Blackburn, E. (2009). Telomeres, telomerase, stress, and aging. In G. G. Benton & J. T. Cacioppo (Eds.), *Handbook of neuroscience for the behavioural sciences*. New York: Wiley.

Ornish, D., Lin, J., Daubenmier, J., Weidner, G., Epel, E., Kemp, C., et al. (2008). Increased telomerase activity and comprehensive lifestyle changes: A pilot study. *The Lancet Oncology, 9*, 1048–1057.

Temporal

▶ Brain, Cortex

Temporal Self-Regulation Theory

Peter A. Hall
Faculty of Applied Health Sciences, University of Waterloo, Waterloo, ON, Canada

Synonyms

Dual process models of health behavior; Dual systems models

Definition

Temporal self-regulation theory (TST; Hall and Fong 2007; Hall and Marteau 2014) is a theoretical framework for explaining individual health behavior. TST posits that health behavior is proximally determined by three factors: *intention strength*, *behavioral prepotency*, and *executive function*. The latter two constructs are theorized to have direct influences on behavior and also to moderate the intention-behavior link. Specifically, intentions are proposed to have a stronger influence on behavioral performance in the presence of stronger executive function and/or when the behavioral prepotency is weak. Also included in the model is consideration of ecological context in the form of contingencies supplied to the behavior by the social and physical environment (i.e., *ambient temporal contingencies*). In the TST model, *intention strength* is a function of anticipated connections between one's behavior and salient outcomes (i.e., *connectedness beliefs*); the valence of the latter can range from negative (i.e., costs) to positive (i.e., benefits). These beliefs are weighted hyperbolically by temporal proximity (i.e., *temporal valuations*), as assumed by intertemporal choice theory. For example, the perceived self-relevant contingencies for making a healthy dietary choice might include eventual benefits (e.g., improved appearance, better health status), but more temporally proximal – therefore more heavily influential-immediate costs (e.g., inconvenience, monetary costs, time costs). The sum of the perceived contingencies weighted by their respective temporal proximities should determine intention strength to make a healthy dietary choice, according to the TST model.

Description

The aim of the TST is to explain variability in health behavior in a manner that is sensitive to biological capacities for self-control (i.e., executive function), motivation level, and the ecological context in which the behavior takes place. Given the complexities of the model and the fact that it crosses many levels of analysis (from biological to social to ecological), it is expected that the model is not typically testable in its entirety. Rather, individual components of the model may be tested individually or in relation to each other (e.g., hypothesized moderating effects), ideally using experimental paradigms.

The TST model was initially offered as an improvement over traditional models of individual health behavior which posited that behavior was most proximally determined by social cognitive variables, without direct or indirect links to neurobiological resources. While TST preserves the central role of intention strength, it adds two important moderating and direct effects on health behavior performance: (1) *executive function (EF)* and (2) *behavioral prepotency* (BPP).

EFs are commonly ascribed to operation of the prefrontal cortex and associated neural systems implicated in the neurobiology of self-control (Miller and Cohen 2001). BPP is the psychological inertia of a given behavior, by virtue of frequent past performance in similar contexts or via the presence of strong cues (which may be social or visceral in nature) to perform the behavior at a given time. The combination of EF and BPP determines the likelihood that intentions will be translated into behavior, and each also has direct influences on behavior itself regardless of intention.

Additional components of TST that differentiate it from its predecessors are (1) an explicit focus on temporal proximity of behavioral contingencies as determinants of their relative potency and (2) a consideration of ecological factors as causal agents in health behavior performance. These two components are conceptually linked, as ecological contexts often determine what kinds of consequences (positive, neutral, or negative) are experienced following performance of a behavior, as well as the relative proximity of those consequences (immediate vs. long term).

The primary contribution of the TST model has been to provide some basis for understanding the possibility of brain-behavior relationships as being partial determinants of health behavior trajectories and to provide an interface for individual models of health behavior with ecological and social-level determinants of behavior. Given that intention strength (Armitage and Connor 2001) and behavioral prepotency (Wood and Neal 2007) are among the most well-established determinants of behavior in the extant research literature, the construct within TST that has required the most empirical justification is the inclusion of biologically based EF. The importance of EF as a causal determinant of health-related behaviors has been underscored in recent years with the advent of epidemiological, observational, and experimental findings from diverse fields of research (see Hall and Marteau 2014 for a review).

Cross-References

▶ Executive Function
▶ Self-Regulatory Capacity
▶ Theory

References and Further Readings

Armitage, C. J., & Connor, M. (2001). Efficacy of the theory of planned behaviour: a meta-analytic review. *British Journal of Social Psychology, 40*, 471–499.

Hall, P. A., & Fong, G. T. (2007). Temporal self-regulation theory: A model for individual health behavior. *Health Psychology Review, 1*, 6–52.

Hall, P. A., & Marteau, T. M. (2014). Executive function in the context of chronic disease prevention: Theory, research and practise. *Preventive Medicine, 68*, 44–50.

Miller, E. K., & Cohen, J. D. (2001). An integrative theory of prefrontal cortex function. *Annual Review of Neuroscience, 24*, 167–202.

Wood, W., & Neal, D. T. (2007). A new look at habits and the interface between habits and goals. *Psychological Review, 114*, 843–863.

Tension

▶ Affect Arousal

Terminal Care

▶ End-of-Life Care
▶ Palliative Care

Tertiary Care

▶ Clinical Settings

Testicular Neoplasms

▶ Cancer, Testicular

Testoid

▶ Androgen

Thanatophobia

▶ Death Anxiety

Thanksgiving

▶ Prayer

The KIHD Study, in Finnish also: SVVT (Sepelvaltimotaudin vaaratekijätutkimus)

▶ Kuopio Ischemic Heart Disease Risk Factor Study

Theories of Behavior Change

▶ Intervention Theories

Theory

Julia Allan
School of Medicine and Dentistry, University of Aberdeen, Aberdeen, Scotland, UK

Synonyms

Conjecture; Model

Definition

A theory is a coherent set of statements or ideas used to organize, generalize, explain, and predict phenomena. Theories are based on observations, experimentation, and abstract reasoning, and play a fundamental role in scientific research.

Theories must (a) successfully describe and explain existing observations, (b) make predictions about future observations, and (c) be falsifiable, that is, they must be refutable by some conceivable event or observation.

While not directly verifiable, theories gain support as empirical evidence accumulates in their favor, particularly if such evidence results from "risky" predictions where the outcome could conceivably have been different (Popper 1963/2004). An accumulation of contradictory empirical evidence results in the theory being abandoned, modified, or superseded by a new theory. This dynamic process of testing, evaluation, and change allows research to move forwards toward the "truth." Theories provide a shared language for researchers to use, enabling the development of a cumulative science. The most useful theories are those that make specific and relevant predictions that can be tested in a straightforward manner.

Prominent theories in behavioral medicine cover a range of domains and include the Transactional Theory of Stress and Coping (Lazarus und Folkman 1984), Type D Personality (Denollet et al. 1996), the Theory of Planned Behavior (Ajzen 1991), and the Common Sense Model of Self-Regulation of Health and Illness (Leventhal et al. 1992).

Cross-References

▶ Causal Diagrams
▶ Hypothesis Testing

References and Readings

Ajzen, I. (1991). The theory of planned behaviour. *Organizational Behavior and Human Decision Processes, 50*, 179–211.
Denollet, J., Sys, S. U., Stroobant, N., Rombouts, H., Gillebert, T. C., & Brutsaert, D. L. (1996). Personality as independent predictor of long term mortality in patients with coronary heart disease. *Lancet, 347*, 417–421.
Lazarus, R. S., & Folkman, S. (1984). *Stress, appraisal and coping*. New York: Springer.
Leventhal, H., Diefenbach, M., & Leventhal, E. A. (1992). Illness cognition: Using common sense to understand treatment adherence and affect cognition interactions. *Cognitive Therapy and Research, 16*, 143–163.
Popper, K. R. (1963/2004). *Conjectures and refutations: The growth of scientific knowledge*. London: Routledge.

Theory of Reasoned Action

Lara LaCaille
Department of Psychology, University of Minnesota Duluth, Duluth, MN, USA

Definition

The Theory of Reasoned Action (TRA; Ajzen und Fishbein 1980; Fishbein und Ajzen 1975) and its extension, the Theory of Planned Behavior (TPB; Ajzen 1985, 1991), are cognitive theories that offer a conceptual framework for understanding human behavior in specific contexts. In particular, the theory of planned behavior has been widely used to assist in the prediction and explanation of several health behaviors.

Description

According to the initial Theory of Reasoned Action, an intention to engage in a certain behavior is considered the best predictor of whether or not a person actually engages in that behavior. Intentions, in turn, are predicted by attitudes and subjective norms. That is, the more positively a person regards a certain behavior or action and the more they perceive the behavior as being important to their friends, family, or society, the more likely they are to form intentions to engage in the behavior. Azjen, however, noted the importance of a behavior being under volitional control in both forming intentions and engaging in the actual behavior. Therefore, he added perceived behavioral control to the model, which is now known as the Theory of Planned Behavior. See Fig. 1.

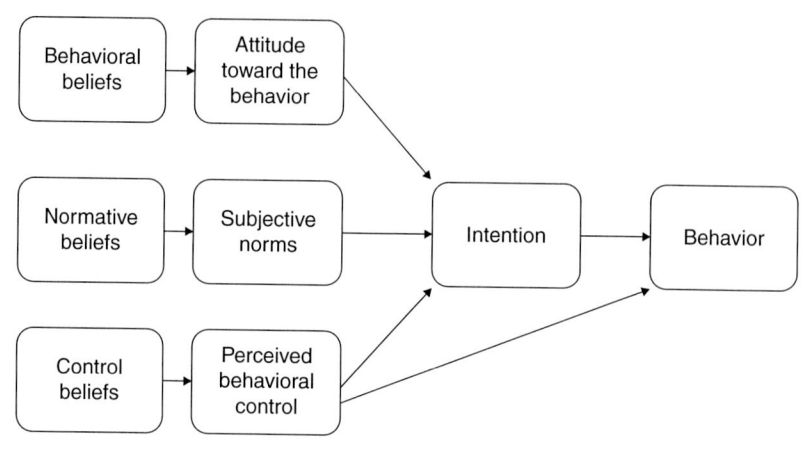

Theory of Reasoned Action, Fig. 1 Theory of planned behavior

Description of the Theoretical Factors

Behavioral beliefs and attitudes: A person first forms beliefs about the outcomes of a given behavior (e.g., "If I exercise, I will improve my health, lose weight, and be more attractive"). These beliefs contribute to his or her attitude or evaluation of the outcome of the behavior (e.g., "Being healthy and attractive is good/valuable"). The more favorable the attitude, the stronger the intention.

Normative beliefs and subjective norms: Normative beliefs refer to a person's perception about the expectations of important others (e.g., "My friends think I should exercise"). These beliefs contribute to the perception of social pressure and contribute to motivation to comply (e.g., "I feel pressured to exercise and I want to fit in with my friends"). The more powerful the perceived norm/pressure, the stronger the intention.

Control beliefs and perceived behavioral control: A person forms beliefs about the factors that may facilitate or be barriers to engaging in the specific behavior (e.g., "I have time before work, I have access to a gym, and I am physically able to exercise"). These beliefs lead to a perception of behavioral control or sense of ease/difficulty in engaging in the behavior (e.g., "I will be able to exercise"). Although many researchers have used the terms self-efficacy and perceived behavioral control interchangeably, including Ajzen (1991), these concepts are not quite synonymous. Whereas self-efficacy reflects individuals' beliefs about their competence or internal control, perceived behavioral control also incorporates other external/environmental factors (e.g., time, resources, social support). The greater the perceived behavioral control, the stronger the intention and the greater the likelihood of engaging in the behavior.

Intention: Intentions refer to peoples' plan of action and represent their expressed motivation to perform the behavior.

Evaluation of the Model

Meta-analytic reviews have supported the predictive efficacy of the TPB model for both behavioral intentions and behaviors (Armitage und Conner 2001; Godin und Kok 1996; Sheeran 2002). The theory typically accounts for about 40–50% of the variance in intentions and 20–40% of the variance in behavior. The relative importance of each of the three factors (attitudes, norms, perceived behavioral control) varies across behaviors and situations. Subjective norms are usually the weakest predictor, though this may reflect measurement issues or people's denial of the effects of social pressures. With regard to health behaviors, the model is better at predicting some behaviors (exercise, condom use, drug use, and cigarette smoking) than others (weight loss and dietary behavior, clinical and screening behavior, oral hygiene; see Godin & Kok). Intentions are usually more potent than perceived behavioral control in predicting health behaviors, suggesting that such behaviors are largely driven by personal motivation.

Although TPB is widely used and offers one of the most robust set of predicators of human behavior, it has been criticized for failing to include emotional variables, such as perceptions of threat, mood, and affect, which may limit is predictive power, particularly with certain health behaviors. It has been argued that many behaviors are not rational and that one's affect may be counter to one's cognitions about engaging in a particular behavior. Thus, attitude may be shaped by affect in addition to beliefs. Another criticism of the TRA/TPB model is that the majority of research testing the theory has been correlational (cross-sectional or longitudinal, typically with brief follow-up periods). The experimental studies testing the theory have provided less support for the model (Webb und Sheeran 2006).

Measurement of the Theory of Planned Behavior Constructs

It is common practice to assess each of the constructs with only one or two items, though multi-item measures are often recommended. Differences in the way the constructs are assessed have led to confusion and may account for some of the variation between studies (see Armitage und Conner (2001) for a meta-analytic review of such differences).

Attitude: Attitude is typically assessed via the use of semantic differential scales that tap into both affective and cognitive attitude. Pairs of adjectives (reflecting a positive and negative component of an attitude) that have relevance to the health behavior being studied are provided as anchors. For example, "To me, engaging in regular exercise is..." [*unpleasant-pleasant; unsatisfying-satisfying*(affective); *harmful-beneficial; useless-useful* (cognitive)].

Subjective norms: When assessing subjective norms, it is recommended to measure both injunctive norms (what others think) and descriptive norms (what others actually do). Social groups are often identified as peers, family, friends, or important people. Examples of items include the following: "People who are important to me think I should exercise regularly" (injunctive); "My friends exercise regularly" (descriptive). Items are usually measured using a 7-point Likert scale.

Perceived behavior control: Perceived behavioral control is often measured with Likert-scale items assessing both internal control (i.e., self-efficacy), such as "I am confident that I can exercise regularly," a perception of ease/difficulty of engaging in the behavior, such as "It is easy for me to exercise," and perception of control, such as "How much personal control do you feel you have over engaging in regular exercise?" In general, measures of self-efficacy account for the most added variance to intentions.

Intentions: Many researchers assess intentions with one Likert-scale item, such as "I intend to engage in regular exercise for the next 3 months." Although intentions tend to be highly reliable, additional items may strengthen the measurement of this construct. Items are sometimes phrased as, "I will try to...," "I plan to...," and "I will make an effort to...." This construct has also been assessed with questions related to self-prediction (e.g., "It is likely that I will engage in regular exercise over the next 3 months"), though such a conceptualization probably incorporates perceived behavioral control.

Behavior: Behavior is often assessed via self-report, but observed behavior is clearly preferred. The TPB model typically predicts more of the variance in self-reported behavior than observed behavior.

Specific recommendations and guidelines for developing questionnaires for use in a particular study are offered by Ajzen (see http://people.umass.edu/aizen/tpb.html), Fishbein und Ajzen (2010), Godin und Kok (1996), and the National Cancer Institute (see http://cancercontrol.cancer.gov/brp/constructs/index.html).

Cross-References

▶ Attitudes
▶ Self-efficacy

References and Readings

Ajzen, I. (1985). From intentions to action: A theory of planned behavior. In J. Kuhl & J. Beckman (Eds.), *Action control: From cognitions to behaviors* (pp. 11–39). New York: Springer.

Ajzen, I. (1991). The theory of planned behavior. *Organizational Behavior and Human Decision Processes, 50*, 179–211.

Ajzen, I. (n.d.) *Theory of planned behavior*. Retrieved 6 July, 2011 from http://people.umass.edu/aizen/tpb.html

Ajzen, I., & Fishbein, M. (1980). *Understanding attitudes and predicting social behavior*. Englewood Cliffs: Prentice-Hall.

Armitage, C. J., & Conner, M. (2001). Efficacy of the theory of planned behavior: A meta-analytic review. *British Journal of Social Psychology, 40*, 471–499.

Fishbein, M., & Ajzen, I. (1975). *Belief, attitude, intention and behavior: An introduction to theory and research*. Reading: Addison-Wesley.

Fishbein, M., & Ajzen, I. (2010). *Predicting and changing behavior: The reasoned action approach*. New York: Psychology Press.

Godin, G., & Kok, G. (1996). The theory of planned behavior: A review of its applications to health-related behaviors. *American Journal of Health Promotion, 11*(2), 87–98.

National Cancer Institute, US National Institutes of Health. (n.d.) *Health behavior constructs: Theory, measurement, and research*. Retrieved 6 July, 2011 from http://cancercontrol.cancer.gov/brp/constructs/index.html

Sheeran, P. (2002). Intention-behaviour relations: A conceptual and empirical review. In W. Stroebe & M. Hewstone (Eds.), *European review of social psychology* (Vol. 12, pp. 1–36). London: Wiley.

Webb, T. L., & Sheeran, P. (2006). Does changing behavioral intentions engender behavior change? A meta-analysis of the experimental evidence. *Psychological Bulletin, 132*, 249–268.

Therapy, Family and Marital

Ashley K. Randall[1] and Guy Bodenmann[2]
[1]College of Integrative Sciences and Arts, Arizona State University, Tempe, AZ, USA
[2]Department of Psychology, University of Zurich, Zurich, Switzerland

Synonyms

Couple therapy; Family therapy; Interventions therapy

Definition

Both family and marital therapy are branches of psychotherapy that aim to facilitate positive change, by addressing the dyad and family as a whole. Broadly, these branches of psychotherapy help teaching communication and problem-solving techniques in an effort to ameliorate distress.

Description

There are a wide range of therapeutic interventions that work with families and couples during times of distress. The goal of each therapeutic approach is to alleviate the distress, to strengthen dyadic and family resources, and to improve well-being of the couple or family members. Although family and couple therapies can be applied with various techniques or theoretical approaches, there are common approaches that have been shown effective in alleviating family distress, such as behavioral family and couple therapy.

Family Therapy Techniques

Therapeutic techniques for families are grounded in family systems theory, which states that each member of the family is interconnected and one cannot just treat one family member independently (Segrin and Flora 2005). The most common family therapy techniques address adolescent concerns in respect to the family dynamic.

Below, we review some of the commonly used therapies.

Bowen's family approach. Bowen's family systems theory views behavior within the family as an emotional unit. This theory operates under the balance of two forces: togetherness and individuality, whereby too much of any one force can create an imbalance in the system. Bowen's approach also uses eight concepts that aim to explain family development and functioning: (1) differentiation of self, (2) triangles, (3) nuclear emotional process, (4) family projection process, (5) multigenerational transmission process,

(6) sibling position, (7) emotional cutoff, and (8) societal emotion process. Some of the main goals of therapy include reframing the family problem as a multigenerational problem that is caused by factors outside the individual and to lower the family "emotional turmoil" (Bowen 2004; Bowen Center for the Study of the Family 2011).

Structural family therapy (*SFT*). SFT is a way to address problems within the family by looking at the invisible rules or boundaries which help its functioning (family rules). The role of the therapist is to manipulate the therapy session in a way to accelerate change in the family, for example, by changing the seating of each family member. This helps the family members see the unbalance of the family system and the dysfunctional patterns that have developed (Minuchin 1974).

Brief strategic family therapy (*BSFT*). BSFT aims to improve and change the family interaction patterns that have led to the disruptive behaviors in adolescents. Specifically, BSFT targets children between the ages of 6 and 17 that display or are at risk for developing behavior, conduct, and substance abuse problems. Specifically, BSFT focuses on inappropriate family alliances, poor boundaries (open vs. closed), and allows the parents to recognize the adolescent is not necessarily the cause for familial problems but the expression of dysfunctional family patterns (Szapocznik and Williams 2000).

Functional family therapy (*FFT*). FFT is an intervention program that focuses on adolescents with disruptive behavior problems (conduct, alcohol, and/or substance abuse). The goal is to reduce the problem behavior while using an individualized nonjudgmental attitude, focusing on strengths and protective factors specific to each client. This intervention can be implemented in a variety of settings such as schools, probation and aftercare systems, and well as in mental health facilities (Alexander and Parsons 1982).

Multisystemic therapy (*MST*). MST is an intensive family- and community-based treatment program that focuses on the entire "world" of chronic and violent juvenile offenders – their homes and families, schools and teachers, neighborhoods and friends (Heneggler et al. 1998).

Other techniques, such as contextual therapy, focal family therapy, systemic therapy, and symbolic-experimental family therapy have also been used in family therapy (see Gurman and Kniskern 1991, for an overview).

Marital Therapy

Traditional behavioral couple therapy (*TBCT*). TBCT attempts to increase the level of reinforcing exchange between the two partners. This approach classically aims at teaching more effective communication and problem-solving skills that will enhance the ability of the couple to effectively communicate as well as minimize punishment and maximize reward (Jacobson and Christensen 1994; Jacobson and Margolin 1979).

Cognitive behavioral couple therapy (*CBCT*). CBCT takes the basic principles of TCBT and incorporates partner's relationship assumptions, standards, expectancies, and attributions that contribute to the relationship distress (Baucom et al. 1998; Epstein and Baucom 2002).

Integrated behavioral couple therapy (*IBCT*). ICBT also takes the basic principles of CBCT and expands them to emphasize interventions aimed at increasing acceptance. The three components, empathetic joining, tolerance building, and detachment from the problem, are focused at enhancing the couple's ability to appreciate the differences in their marriage (Christensen et al. 1995; Jacobson and Christensen 1998).

Emotion-focused couple therapy (*EFCT*). EFCT focuses on inner emotional experiences in combination with self-reinforcing interactions, based on adult attachments and attachment bonds. Therapists in this approach try to (1) access and reprocess the emotional experience of the partners' and (2) restructure the partner's interaction patterns. Partners are thought to learn new aspects about themselves and develop a more functional pattern of interaction with their partner that is cohesive with their specific attachment needs (Greenberg and Johnson 1988; Johnson and Greenberg 1985).

Integrated systematic couple therapy (ISCT). The specific goal of ISCT is not to resolve all of the issues causing distress but rather instigated a reversal of the negative interaction. ISCT is based on procedures from family and marital systems therapy and primarily targets the problem at the interaction level. Specifically, ISCT tries to initiate a reversal in the "fight cycle" by changing the meaning attributed to the situation. Empirical evidence exists for the efficacy of ISCT showing greater maintenance of marital satisfaction and goal attainment after the intervention (Greenberg and Goldman 1985).

Insight-oriented therapy (IOMT). IOMT focuses on the interpretation of underlying intrapersonal and interpersonal dynamics between the couple partners contributing to the marital distress. IOMT also examines developmental issues, interactions, expectations, and maladaptive relationship patterns that may exist in the relationship. The role of the therapist is to guide the couple to gain a better understanding and clarification of each partner's unconscious feelings and beliefs that may be affecting the relationship (Snyder and Wills 1989; Wills 1982).

Coping-oriented couple therapy (COCT). COCT is based on stress and coping research in couples and cognitive behavioral couple therapy. It aims to enhance communication, problem-solving, and dyadic coping in both partners (Bodenmann 2007, 2010). A main focus lies on dyadic coping and building mutual intimacy and understanding. A key element of this approach is the three-phase method. By means of this method the therapist aims to enhance mutual understanding for each partner's personal functioning (that becomes most evident in stressful situations) and its impact on the close relationship as well as the enhancement of mutual support that matches personal needs of the partner. Overall, this approach fosters (a) understanding for each partner's personality, (b) mutual dyadic coping, and (c) mutual intimacy, trust in the partner, cohesion, and emotional security (Table 1).

Prevention Programs

Several evidence-based programs aim to prevent marital distress (e.g., Couples Communication Program (CCP); Miller et al. 1983; Premarital-Relationship Enhancement Program (PREP): Markman et al. 1994, Couples Coping Enhancement Training (CCET); Bodenmann and Shantinath 2004).

Efficacy of Marital and Family Therapy

The efficacy of family and couple therapies are well documented (Dunn and Schwebel 1995; Shadish and Baldwin 2005) including substantial mean effect sizes which demonstrate the effectiveness in relieving distress ($d = .74-.95$; Shadish et al. 1993; $d = .50-1.30$; Shadish and Baldwin 2003). Prior research has shown that approximately 70% of couples seeking evidence-based couple therapy report an improvement after therapy (Baucom et al. 1998; Christensen and Heavey 1999), and more recent numbers suggest 46–56% of couples show significant clinical improvement (Christensen et al. 2010).

Application to Behavioral Medicine

Family and marital therapy techniques have been used to alleviate distress within the family, stemming from things such as communication issues or family dynamics. Nevertheless, some of these therapeutic approaches have been used for a range of behavioral and physical health problems (see Snyder et al. 2006 for a review). Additionally, CanCOPE is an education program developed for people facing cancer (personally or within the family). The focus of this program is to strengthen the resources within the family so that they can more effectively deal with the realities of cancer management (Scott et al. 2004). Family-based obesity treatment programs have also been developed, and show that child–parent interactions can influence the outcome of obesity treatment (Temple et al. 2006). Osterman, Sher, Hales, Canar, Singla and Tilton (2003) encourage health psychologists to incorporate more of a couple's perspective into illness, so that the partner can facilitate health-promoting attitudes and behaviors.

Therapy, Family and Marital, Table 1 Marital and family therapies

Marital and family therapies	Goal	Content
Family therapies		
Bowenian Family Therapy	Individuals are encouraged to look at the view they play in the family system, patterns of emotional reactivity, and interlocking triangles. In addition, the goal is to decrease anxiety	Examines how the family may operate as an "emotional system" using key concepts such as: triangles, differentiation of the self, emotional cutoff, and sibling position
Structural Family Therapy (SFT)	Address the problem in functioning within a family, in an attempt to restructure the family system's rules to become more flexible (Minuchin 1974)	Therapist helps to show family how their family system may be unbalanced and to help the family see the dysfunctional patterns they have created. SFT also helps families move toward an understanding of how the behavior has developed into a positive feedback loop
Brief Strategic Family Therapy (BSFT)	Aims to improve family interaction and change family interaction patterns that have led to disruptive behaviors in adolescents (e.g., conduct problems, delinquency, and drug abuse) (Szapocznik and Williams 2000)	BSFT operates on five basic concepts: (1) *context* – the behavior cannot be understood outside the context to which it occurs; (2) *systems* – the family is an interconnected entity that cannot be understood by just examining one member; (3) *structure* – provides the habitual and repetitive patterns of family interaction; (4) *strategy* – interventions tend to be practical, problem-focused, and planned; and (5) *content versus process* – the therapist's focus is on **how** the family members' interaction, not **what** the family members discuss, is the problem
Functional Family Therapy (FFT)	Family intervention program for adolescents with disrupting behavior problems (conduct, alcohol, and/or substance abuse). The goal is to reduce the problem behavior while using an individualized nonjudgmental attitude, focusing on strength/protective factors that are linked to each client (Alexander and Parsons 1982; Alexander et al. 2000)	FFT operates on five major components: (1) *engagement phase* – the goal of this phase is to demonstrate a desire to listen and help. The therapist focuses on immediate responsiveness and maintains a strength-based focus; (2) *motivational phase* – the goals of this phase include creating a positive motivational context that will facilitate change, minimizing hopelessness, and changing the meaning of the family context to promote change; (3) *relational assessment* – the focus of this phase is on intra- and extra-familial context (e.g., values, interaction patterns, and sources of resistance, resources, and limitation); (4) *behavior change phase* – this phase helps build coping patterns, such as teaching communication as well as training conflict resolution; and (5) *generalization phase* – this phase focuses on extending positive family functions and helps the family plan for relapse prevention (e.g., using other family and community members for support)
Multisystemic Therapy (MST)	Intensive family and community-based treatment program that focuses on violent and criminal youth behavior (Heneggler et al. 1998)	MST views the child/adolescent embedded within interconnected systems: family, peers, school, neighborhood, and community/culture. Focus is on increasing parenting skills: spending time with children, teaching communication techniques and how to develop boundaries/discipline, and teaching skills on how to deal with conflict. Help adolescents participate in positive activities (sports or extracurricular clubs) and create a supportive social network among family, peers, and community to maintain change

(continued)

Therapy, Family and Marital, Table 1 (continued)

Marital and family therapies	Goal	Content
Couple therapies		
Traditional Behavioral Couple Therapy	Attempts to increase the level of reinforcing exchange between partners. Minimize punishment and maximize reinforcement (Jacobson and Margolin 1979; Jacobson and Christensen 1994)	Help couples identify positive behaviors that they can do for one another (e.g., show more affection). Help guide couples to engage in these behaviors and acknowledge when they occur (e.g., to give praise)
Cognitive Behavioral Couple Therapy (CBCT)	Examined the evidence about their thoughts about their partner	Use of cognitive restructuring strategies to modify different types of dysfunctional cognitions. Examine the interplay between thoughts, emotions, and behavior
	Alter assumptions and standards, couple evaluates consequences of living according to their standards and assumptions about their partner (Baucom et al. 1998; Epstein and Baucom 2002)	
Integrated Behavioral Couple Therapy (IBCT)	To help the couple think about the problem and identify feelings associated with that issue before one can accept them (Christensen et al. 1995; Jacobson and Christensen 1998)	Educate couples that partners need to learn a way to alter negative emotional responses that make them and their partners unhappy. Teaches couple new ways to resolve problems and emotions through three steps: (1) Empathetic joining, (2) tolerance building, and (3) detachment from the problem
Emotion-Focused Couple Therapy (EFCT)	Conceptualizes distress in adult romantic relationships in terms of attachment theory. Focus on re-establishing attachment bonds (Johnson and Greenberg 1985; Greenberg and Johnson 1988)	(1) Identify the negative interaction cycle of the conflict, (2) access unacknowledged feelings, (3) reframe the problem(s) in terms of underlying feelings, (4) promote identification with disowned needs and aspects of self, (5) promote acceptance by each partner; (6) facilitate the expression of needs and wants to restructure the interaction based on the new understandings, (7) establish the emergence of new solutions (cycles), and (8) consolidate new positions
Integrated Systematic Couple Therapy (ISCT)	Try to change meaning attributed to situation that caused distress. Aims to initiate a reversal in the "fight cycle" (self-perpetuating negative cycles that lead to changes in behavior) (Greenberg and Goldman 1985)	(1) Define the issue presented, (2) identify the negative interactional cycle, (3) attempt restructuring, (4) reframe the problem using positive connotation followed by prescribing the symptom, (5) restrain using "go slow" and dangers of improvement, (6) consolidate the frame, and (7) prescribe a relapse
Insight-Oriented Marital Therapy (IOMT)	Emphasis is on the interpretation of underlying intra- and interpersonal dynamics that influence relationship distress (Wills 1982; Snyder and Wills 1989)	Focus on expectations, interactions, and maladaptive relationship rules using clarification and interpretation, to highlight unconscious feelings, beliefs, or thoughts causing the marital discord
Copying-Oriented Couple Techniques (COCT)	Teach couples the notion the better the partners *together* can cope with stress, the higher their chance for optimal marital satisfaction and stability (Bodenmann et al. 2008)	Focus on educating the couple about the effects stress has on the relationship. Couples become aware of the influence of environmental factors on their close relationship. Focus on teaching dyadic copying that goes beyond the traditional models of interpersonal communication and social support in close relationships

Cross-References

▶ Family Stress

References and Readings

Alexander, J. F., & Parsons, B. V. (1982). *Functional family therapy.* Monterey: Brooks/Cole.

Alexander, J. F., Pugh, C., Parsons, B. V., & Sexton, T. L. (2000). *Functional family therapy* (2nd ed.). Boulder: Center for the Study and Prevention of Violence, University of Colorado.

Baucom, D. H., Shoham, V., Mueser, K. T., Daiuto, A. D., & Stickle, T. R. (1998). Empirically supported couple and family interventions for marital distress and adult mental health problems. *Journal of Consulting and Clinical Psychology, 66,* 53–88.

Bodenmann, G. (2007). Dyadic coping and the 3-phase-method in working with couples. In L. VandeCreek (Ed.), *Innovations in clinical practice: Focus on group and family therapy* (pp. 235–252). Sarasota: Professional Resources Press.

Bodenmann, G. (2010). New themes in couple therapy: The role of stress, coping and social support. In K. Hahlweg, M. Grawe, & D. H. Baucom (Eds.), *Enhancing couples. The shape of couple therapy to come* (pp. 142–156). Cambridge, MA: Hogrefe Publishing.

Bodenmann, G., & Shantinath, S. D. (2004). The Couples Coping Enhancement Training (CCET): A new approach to prevention of marital distress based upon stress and coping. *Family Relations, 53*(5), 477–484.

Bodenmann, G., Plancherel, B., Beach, S. R. H., Widmer, K., Gabriel, B., & Meuwly, N. (2008). Effects of coping-oriented couples therapy on depression. A randomized clinical trial. *Journal of Consulting and Clinical Psychology, 76,* 944–954.

Bowen, M. (2004). Family psychotherapy in office practice. *Family Systems, 7*(1), 29–44.

Bowen Center for the Study of the Family. (2011). Bowen family therapy. Retrieved October 2011 from: www.thebowencenter.org

Christensen, A., & Heavey, C. L. (1999). Interventions for couples. *Annual Review Psychology, 50,* 165–190.

Christensen, A., Jacobson, N. S., & Babcock, J. C. (1995). Integrative behavioral couple therapy. In N. S. Jacobson & A. S. Gurman (Eds.), *Clinical handbook of marital therapy* (2nd ed., pp. 31–64). New York: Guilford Press.

Christensen, A., Atkins, D. C., Baucom, B., & Yi, J. (2010). Marital status and satisfaction five years following a randomized clinical trial comparing traditional versus integrative behavioral couple therapy. *Journal of Consulting and Clinical Psychology, 78,* 225–235.

Dunn, R. L., & Schwebel, A. I. (1995). Meta-analytic review of marital therapy outcome research. *Journal of Family Psychology, 9,* 58–68.

Epstein, N. B., & Baucom, D. H. (2002). *Enhanced cognitive-behavioral therapy for couples: A contextual approach.* Washington, DC: American Psychological Association.

Greenberg, L. S., & Goldman, A. (1985). *Integrated systemic couples' therapy: A treatment manual.* Unpublished manuscript, University of British Columbia, Vancouver, Canada.

Greenberg, L. S., & Johnson, S. M. (1988). *Emotionally focused therapy for couples.* New York: Guilford Press.

Gurman, A. S., & Kniskern, D. P. (1991). *Handbook of family therapy* (Vol. I and II). New York: Brunner & Mazel.

Henegler, S. W., Schoenwald, S. K., Borduin, C. M., Rowland, M. D., & Cunningham, P. B. (1998). *Multisystemic treatment of antisocial behavior in children and adolescents.* New York: Guilford Press.

Jacobson, N. S., & Christensen, A. (1994). *Traditional behavioral couple therapy manual.* Unpublished manuscript, University of Washington.

Jacobson, N. S., & Christensen, A. (1998). *Acceptance and change in couple therapy: A therapist's guide to transforming relationships.* New York: Norton.

Jacobson, N. S., & Margolin, G. (1979). *Marital therapy: Strategies based on social learning and behavior exchange principles.* New York: Brunner/Mazel.

Johnson, S. M., & Greenberg, L. S. (1985). Emotionally focused couples therapy: An outcome study. *Journal of Marital and Family Therapy, 11,* 313–317.

Markman, H. J., Stanley, S., & Blumberg, S. L. (1994). *Fighting for your marriage: Positive steps for preventing divorce and preserving a lasting love.* San Francisco: Jossey Bass.

Miller, S., Wackman, D. B., & Nunnally, E. W. (1983). Couple communication: Equipping couples to be their own best problem solvers. *The Counseling Psychologist, 11,* 73–77.

Minuchin, S. (1974). *Families and family therapy.* Cambridge, MA: Harvard University Press.

Osterman, G. P., Sher, T. G., Hales, G., Canar, W. J., Singla, R., & Tilton, T. (2003). *Physical illness.* New York: Guilford Press.

Scott, J. L., Halford, W. K., & Ward, B. (2004). United we stand? The effects of a couple-coping intervention on adjustment to breast or gynecological cancer. *Journal of Consulting and Clinical Psychology, 76,* 1122–1135.

Segrin, C., & Flora, J. (2005). Theoretical perspectives on family communication: Family systems theory. In *Family communication* (pp. 28–33). Mahwah: Erlbaum.

Shadish, W. R., & Baldwin, S. A. (2003). Meta-analysis of MFT interventions. *Journal of Marital and Family Therapy, 29,* 547–570.

Shadish, W. R., & Baldwin, S. A. (2005). Effects of behavioral marital therapy: A meta-analysis of randomized controlled trials. *Journal of Consulting and Clinical Psychology, 73*, 6–14.

Shadish, W. R., Montgomery, L. M., Wilson, P., Wilson, M. R., Bright, I., & Okwumabua, T. (1993). Effects of family and marital psychotherapies: A meta-analysis. *Journal of Consulting and Clinical Psychology, 61*, 992–1002.

Snyder, D. K., & Wills, R. M. (1989). Behavioral vs. insight oriented marital therapy: A controlled comparative outcome study. *Journal of Consulting and Clinical Psychology, 57*, 39–46.

Snyder, D. K., Castellani, A. M., & Whisman, M. A. (2006). Current status and future directions in couple therapy. *Annual Review of Psychology, 57*, 317–344.

Szapocznik, J., & Williams, R. A. (2000). Brief strategic family therapy: Twenty-five years of interplay among theory, research and practice in adolescent behavior problems and drug abuse. *Clinical Child and Family Psychology Review, 3*(2), 117–134.

Temple, J. L., Wrotniak, B. H., Paluch, R. A., Roemmich, J. N., & Epstein, L. H. (2006). Relationship between sex of parent and child on weight loss and maintenance in a family-based obesity treatment program. *International Journal of Obesity, 30*, 1260–1264.

Wills, R. M. (1982). *Insight oriented marital therapy* [Treatment manual]. Unpublished manuscript, Wayne State University, Detroit.

Therapy, Occupational

Jennifer Creek[1], Kit Sinclair[2] and Cecilia W. P. Li-Tsang[3]
[1]Occupational Therapist, Guisborough, North Yorkshire, UK
[2]School of Medical and Health Sciences, Tung Wah College, Kowloon, Hong Kong, China
[3]Department of Rehabilitation Sciences, The Hong Kong Polytechnic University, Kowloon, Hong Kong, China

Synonyms

Ergotherapy; Occupational therapist

Definition

Occupational therapy is a profession that works with people of all ages and abilities, helping them to perform those tasks and roles essential to productive living. The primary goal is to assist people to participate satisfactorily in the things they want and need to do, such as: taking care of themselves and others; working; volunteering, and participating in hobbies, interests, and social events. Occupational therapists are concerned with all the activities that make up the pattern of people's lives, and with people's capacity to carry out those activities in ways that support their health and well-being.

Description

For occupational therapists, the concept of *occupation* goes beyond paid work to encompass everything that people do in their daily lives, including self-care, domestic activities, interactions with others, work, and leisure activities. Occupational therapists understand that occupation is fundamental to survival, to development and learning across the lifespan, to social relations, to individual health and well-being, and to the well-being of communities. Occupation enables the development and integration of bodily systems, promotes socialization, and verifies the individual's identity as a contributing member of society.

Occupational therapy intervention is a complex, dynamic process that comprises multiple practices and is undertaken within particular contexts. Intervention does not follow a standard process but is specific to particular clients, contexts, and environments. The approach taken, the goals of intervention and the techniques employed by the occupational therapist are strongly influenced by the social context in which the therapist is working, the work setting, government policies and standards, local norms and procedures, and the available research evidence.

Through the therapeutic use of everyday activities, occupational therapists work to mitigate the effects of disease or injury and prevent secondary disability. They also help people to manage and live with long-term health conditions, such as arthritis, diabetes, and cancer. The focus of intervention is not on the person's diagnosis, impairment, or functional limitations but on the impact that illness, disability, or environmental factors can have on someone's ability to carry out expected daily activities. Activity and occupation are both the goal of occupational therapy and the main therapeutic tool. Three of the ways that occupational therapists help people to participate in the occupations they need and want to do are by enhancing people's own knowledge and life skills, adapting environments to better support occupation, and finding new ways of doing activities.

The occupational therapist works not only with a person's functional problems but also with the *meaning* of restricted activity to his or her life. This has been called a two-body practice because occupational therapy is concerned both with the physical body and with the whole person, including social, cultural, and psychological aspects.

The knowledge base that supports a two-body practice is necessarily broad and varied. Occupational therapists have a deep understanding of the importance of activity and occupation in people's lives and additionally draw on relevant knowledge from the biological, medical, psychological, social, and technological sciences. Areas of knowledge include theory, research, policy, and legislation. In most countries, occupational therapy entry-level education is a Bachelors, Masters, or Doctoral degree.

Occupational therapy is practiced in a wide range of public, private, and voluntary sector settings, although most occupational therapists work in the fields of health and social care. They work with people of all ages, who have functional problems arising from physical, psychological, social, educational, economic, or other difficulties. Examples of occupational therapy practices include: helping children to achieve their developmental milestones, working with communities to develop disaster preparedness and response strategies, and assisting older people to reduce the risk of falls.

Occupational therapy clients may be individuals, groups of people, communities, health and social care agencies, or other organizations. Individual clients may be hospital or community patients, schoolchildren, workers, compensation claimants, caregivers, homeless people, or anyone who is experiencing occupational dysfunction. Group clients can be families, co-workers, paid carers, or groups of patients. Some occupational therapists work in the areas of public health, primary care, occupational health, or health promotion. They may work in the field of law as expert witnesses or consultants, for example, carrying out assessments to ascertain the level of disability sustained following an accident.

Occupational therapists work in a wide range of settings. Their major role is in habilitation and rehabilitation; helping people to gain or regain the ability to perform their occupations and preventing secondary disability. However, they also contribute to the treatment of, and early recovery from, injury and disease. They are engaged in health promotion and disease prevention with populations at risk. They work with those who have long-term or deteriorating health conditions, assisting them to remain active for as long as possible and slowing down the decline of functional ability. Increasingly, occupational therapists are working with older people to promote their health and well-being through activity. Those occupational therapists who work with marginalized and displaced persons, such as refugees and homeless people, employ a human rights perspective.

Occupational therapists are experts in assessing function in the activities of daily life, including personal care, mobility, domestic activities, social interactions, education, leisure, and work. When a person is unable to perform the activities of daily life to an acceptable standard, the occupational therapist can assist him or her to relearn the necessary skills, develop new skills, or adapt activities so that they are within the individual's capabilities. The occupational therapist can also recommend augmentative and assistive technology, communication aids and equipment, and environmental modifications to support function or compensate for loss of function.

An expert occupational therapist is able to engage with people within their own environments, to identify the activities that have meaning and relevance for them, and to work in partnership to devise individually tailored interventions. The occupational therapist works in collaboration with individuals, families, care givers, employers, teachers, co-workers, colleagues, and others to develop and deliver relevant and effective interventions. As far as possible, people are engaged as active partners in the process and interventions are carried out within people's own living and working environments.

Occupational therapy has relevance for everyone who is experiencing occupational dysfunction, and it is practiced in many countries throughout the world. Services are contextualized to local culture, resources, occupations, and needs. In most countries, it is regulated as a health profession. The worldwide professional body for occupational therapy is the World Federation of Occupational Therapists (WFOT): member countries all have a national professional body and full member countries also have at least one occupational therapy education program approved by the WFOT.

References and Further Reading

American Association of Occupational Therapists. www.aota.org/About-Occupational-Therapy.aspx. Accessed 29 Aug 2018.

Australian Occupational Therapy Association. http://aboutoccupationaltherapy.com.au. Accessed 29 Aug 2018.

Mattingly, C. (1994). Occupational therapy as a two-body practice: the body as machine. In C. Mattingly & M. H. Fleming (Eds.), *Clinical reasoning: forms of inquiry in a therapeutic practice*. Philadelphia: FA Davis.

Nhunzvi, C., & Galvaan, R. (2017). Defining occupational therapy. In S. A. Dsouza, R. Galvaan, & E. L. Ramugondo (Eds.), *Concepts in occupational therapy: understanding Southern Perspectives* (pp. 103–109). Manipal: Manipal University Press.

Pentland, D., Kantartzis, S., Clausen, M. G., & Witemyre, K. (2018). *Occupational therapy and complexity: defining and describing practice*. London: Royal College of Occupational Therapists.

Therapy, Physical

▶ Physical Therapy

Thoughts

▶ Cognitions

Thriving

▶ Perceived Benefits

Thrombosis

▶ Coagulation of Blood

Tinnitus

Linda C. Baumann[1] and Alyssa Ylinen[2]
[1]School of Nursing, University of Wisconsin-Madison, Madison, WI, USA
[2]Allina Health System, St. Paul, MN, USA

Synonyms

Ringing in the ears

Definition

Tinnitus is a condition characterized by the perception of sound in the ears or head without the presence of an external source. Tinnitus itself is not a disease, but a symptom that can result from a number of different causes. Sounds heard can manifest in many different ways such as low to high pitched, heard in one or both ears, heard as a single noise or competing noises, or be heard intermittently or continuously. Sounds have been described as ringing, buzzing, blowing, humming, hissing, whooshing, hissing, and whistling among many others. Mild forms of tinnitus are very common and experienced by most people at some point in their lives. More severe forms, however, are less common and can lead to chronic sleep disturbance, anxiety, and depression.

Description

Tinnitus is generally categorized into two types: subjective tinnitus and objective tinnitus. Objective tinnitus is the less common of the two types, and sound is not only heard by the patient but also audible to other people, most often a clinician listening with a stethoscope or an ear tube. Pulsatile tinnitus is a common example of objective tinnitus. It is caused by muscle contractions or audible blood flow in arteries or veins (e.g., bruits) close to the inner ear that resonate as rhythmic pulsing in the ear. Subjective tinnitus is the most common form and is heard exclusively by the patient. This type of tinnitus has many causes and pathologies.

Although tinnitus is most often associated with abnormalities of the auditory or central nervous systems, it can also be caused by nonauditory etiologies. These include hypertension and cardiovascular disease, hypo- and hyperthyroidism, stress and fatigue, temporomandibular joint (TMJ) disorder, poor diet and physical inactivity, and wax buildup in the outer ear putting pressure on the tympanic membrane. Exposure to excessive noise is also a common cause of tinnitus, which can precede hearing loss and should therefore be an indicator of the need for protection from excessive noise exposure. Tinnitus associated with abnormalities of the auditory or central nervous systems including middle ear infections; damage to the inner ear; disorders that affect the central nervous system such as meningitis, encephalitis, and stroke; head and neck trauma; surgical injury; tumors affecting the acoustic nerve (cranial nerve VIII); Meniere's disease (an inner ear disorder characterized by hearing loss vertigo and tinnitus); and vestibular schwannoma (e.g., acoustic neuroma). Over 200 ototoxic medications are associated with inducing tinnitus. These medications include aspirin, some antibiotics, diuretics, cancer chemotherapy drugs, and quinine.

With many causes of tinnitus, treatment of the underlying disease often alleviates symptoms. Drug therapies include benzodiazepines, anticonvulsants, antidepressants, vasodilators, tranquilizers, and antihistamines. Acamprosate, a drug used to treat alcohol dependence, has shown to have potential as a treatment, as well as zinc and gabapentin. Antiarrhythmic agents such as lidocaine have also shown to have tinnitus-suppressing qualities.

Hearing aides are another modality shown to benefit patients. Loss of hearing often increases awareness of tinnitus, and a hearing aid, which amplifies external sound, often helps mask the perception of tinnitus. Wearable sound generators or tinnitus maskers are also used. These devices fit into the ear much like a hearing aid and deliver low-level sound directly into the ear.

Cochlear implant is a treatment used in patients whose tinnitus is accompanied by severe hearing loss. Electrical and magnetic stimulation treatments include transcranial magnetic stimulation and trans-electrical nerve stimulation. Cognitive behavioral therapy treatments include tinnitus retraining therapy (TRT), tinnitus activities treatment, sound therapies, auditory discrimination therapy, and neurofeedback. Alternative therapies for tinnitus have included acupuncture, hypnosis, craniosacral therapy, antioxidants, vitamin, and herbal remedies.

References and Further Readings

Langguth, B., Hajak, G., Kleinjung, T., Cacace, A., & Moller, A. R. (Eds.). (2007). *Tinnitus: Pathophysiology and treatment*. Amsterdam: Elsevier.

Tinnitus. (2010a). *American academy of otolaryngology-head and neck surgery*. Retrieved 18 Feb 2011, from http://www.entnet.org/HealthInformation/tinnitus.cfm

Tinnitus. (2010b). *Medline plus medical encyclopedia*. Retrieved 18 Feb 2011, from http://www.nlm.nih.gov/medlineplus/ency/article/003043.htm

Tinnitus. (2010c). *National Institutes of Health: NIDCD*. Retrieved 18 Feb 2011, from http://www.nidcd.nih.gov/health/hearing/tinnitus

Tinnitus and Cognitive Behavior Therapy

Gerhard Andersson
Department of Behavioural Science and Learning,
Linköping University, Linköping, Sweden

Synonyms

Hearing disturbances; Perception of internal noise (false)

Definition

Tinnitus is an auditory perceptual phenomenon that is defined as the conscious perception of internal noises without any outer auditory stimulation. The sounds may be very loud and bizarre, and the most common ones are heard like a high-pitched musical tone or a rushing sound like escaping steam or air. Other descriptions can be more complicated such as metallic sounds, multiple tones of varying frequencies, and mixtures between buzzing and ringing.

Tinnitus is in most cases a temporary sensation, which many people have experienced at least sometime in their life. However, it may develop into a chronic condition, and prevalence figures show that at least 10–15% of the general population have tinnitus. Fortunately, most persons do not have severe tinnitus. Only about 1–3% of the adult population has severe tinnitus, in the sense that it causes marked disruption of everyday activities, mood changes, reduced quality of life, and disrupted sleep patterns. Tinnitus has been reported in children, but in its severe form, it is more common in adults and in particular in the elderly.

Tinnitus is known to occur in association with almost all the dysfunctions that involve the human auditory system. This includes damage to the middle ear, the cochlea, the audiovestibular cranial nerve, and pathways in the brain from cochlear nucleus to primary auditory cortex. A common distinction is often made between so-called objective (somatosounds, which can actually be heard from the outside) and subjective tinnitus (that are heard only by the afflicted person). Objective tinnitus represents a minority of cases. Subjective tinnitus has been linked to sensorineural hearing loss, caused by various deficits such as age-related hearing loss and noise exposure. Links to other conditions such as temporomandibular joint dysfunction have also been found. Tinnitus has been explained as the result of increased neural activity in the form of increased burst firing or as a result from pathological synchronization of neural activity. Other suggested mechanisms are hypersensitivity and cortical reorganization. With the advent of modern imaging techniques, it has been observed that tinnitus involves certain areas of the brain, particularly those that are related to hearing and processing of sounds. Some involvement of the brain's attentional and emotional systems has also been seen (Cacace 2003).

Description

Distress and Tinnitus

What distinguishes mild from severe tinnitus is not easily established, apart from variations in subjective ratings of intrusiveness and loudness. In particular, in attempts to determine the handicap caused by tinnitus, it has not been possible to make the determination using the characteristics of the tinnitus itself (e.g., loudness, pitch, etc.). However, psychological factors are of major importance in determining the severity of tinnitus, and this has been observed in both clinical and epidemiological studies.

The problems experienced by tinnitus patients can be divided into four categories: hearing difficulties including noise sensitivity, emotional consequences, concentration problems, and insomnia. In addition, there might be interpersonal consequences and occupational difficulties (e.g., for a musician, admitting tinnitus can be regarded as a sign of weakness).

Hearing loss is the most common symptom that goes together with tinnitus and that can in itself be a great problem. Another common problem is noise sensitivity, which in its severe form can develop into hyperacusis, which is sensitivity to everyday sounds not regarded as loud by most people.

In its severe form, tinnitus is strongly associated with lowered mood and depression. Suicide caused by tinnitus is however rare. Most cases reported have had comorbid psychiatric disturbances. Anxiety, and in particular anxious preoccupation with somatic sensations, is an aggravating factor, and stress is often mentioned as a negative factor for tinnitus and in particular in association with major adverse life events, but the evidence for this notion is weak. Personality factors have been investigated, and associations have been reported between degree of optimism and tinnitus distress (Andersson 1996) and between perfectionism and tinnitus distress (Andersson et al. 2005a).

Tinnitus patients often report difficulties with concentration, for example, with reading. Often this is perceived as auditory intrusions while trying to hold concentration on a task. Until recently, there have been few attempts to measure tinnitus patients' performance on tests of cognitive functioning, but recent research implies a role of the working memory system (Hallam et al. 2004). Another line of research has focused on the role of selective information processing. Finally, sleep problems represent a significant element in tinnitus patients' complaints and are often a driving reason for seeking help.

Theories

Among the most influential psychological theories on why tinnitus becomes annoying is Hallam et al.'s (1984) habituation model of tinnitus, which presents the notion that tinnitus annoyance is caused by lack of habituation, and the neurophysiological model by Jastreboff and coworkers (Jastreboff 1990), which is a classical conditioning model where the tinnitus signal is conditioned to aversive reactions such as anxiety and fear. The latter model puts less emphasis on conscious mechanisms involved in tinnitus perception. Other researchers have endorsed a cognitive-behavioral conceptualization of tinnitus, suggesting a major role for thoughts and beliefs regarding tinnitus (Andersson 2002).

In clinical settings, management of tinnitus involves taking history of its characteristics such as onset, loudness, character, fluctuations, and severity. Audiological and neuro-otological measurements such as pure-tone audiometry, otoscopy, and brain stem audiometry are also included in routine assessment to exclude treatable conditions (Andersson et al. 2005b).

Treatments

There is a long history of attempts to cure tinnitus, but surgical and pharmacological interventions have been largely without any success. When the aim is to reduce the suffering, treatment outcome is more promising, and psychologically informed treatments have been found to be helpful in randomized trials (Andersson and Lyttkens 1999).

Among the psychosocial treatments, cognitive-behavioral therapy (CBT) is the most researched alternative. As for other medical conditions such as chronic pain, CBT for tinnitus distress is directed at identifying and modifying maladaptive behaviors and cognitions by means of behavior change and cognitive restructuring. The focus is on applying techniques such as applied relaxation in real-life settings. An overview of the techniques used in CBT for tinnitus is presented in the Table. There is now evidence from randomized trials that CBT can be effective for alleviating the distress caused by tinnitus in adults (e.g., Hesser et al. 2011), including a trial on the use of CBT with older adults, and also that it works in a self-help format presented via the Internet (Kaldo et al. 2008). However, while the effects are promising, there is room for more improvement, and tinnitus is a typical example of an area where multidisciplinary input is necessary. Most recent development in CBT for tinnitus is to incorporate treatment procedures from acceptance and commitment therapy (ACT; Hayes et al. 1999).

Conclusion

Tinnitus is a poorly understood phenomenon, and while the role of psychological factors is widely acknowledged, there is yet little research on basic mechanisms such as information processing bias, the role of psychopathology, and the influence of the tinnitus sound on working memory capacity. While there are few cases of tinnitus for which surgical and medical interventions might help, in most cases, there is no cure in the sense that the tinnitus sound will not disappear. However, longitudinal fluctuations of both loudness and severity of tinnitus have been observed, and health psychologists could benefit in the pursuit of an explanation why it is that tinnitus becomes bothersome only for a proportion of individuals. When it comes to methods to lessen the distress and to cope with the adverse consequences, such as lowered mood and sleep difficulties, CBT is a promising approach. However, the dissemination of CBT into audiological hospital settings has been slow, and there are very few clinical psychologists working with tinnitus. Self-help methods are promising and could at least partly solve that problem, and there is also much to be done regarding preventive work as noise-induced hearing loss is the cause of tinnitus in one third of cases with recent onset of tinnitus (Table 1).

Tinnitus and Cognitive Behavior Therapy, Table 1 Overview of cognitive-behavioral treatment for tinnitus

Case formulation
Structured clinical interview following audiological screening
Questionnaire assessment
Treatment rationale and information
Treatment presented in 6–10 sessions
Applied relaxation (1. progressive relaxation, 2. short progressive relaxation, 3. cue-controlled relaxation, and 4. rapid relaxation)
Positive imagery
Sound enrichment by means of external sounds
Hearing tactics and advice regarding noise sensitivity
Modification of negative thoughts and beliefs
Behavioral sleep management
Advice regarding concentration difficulties, exercises of concentration (mindfulness)
Exposure to tinnitus
Advice regarding physical activity
Relapse prevention
Follow-up
Interview and questionnaires

Cross-References

▶ Cognitive Behavioral Therapy (CBT)

References and Readings

Andersson, G. (1996). The role of optimism in patients with tinnitus and in patients with hearing impairment. *Psychology and Health, 11*, 697–707.

Andersson, G. (2002). Psychological aspects of tinnitus and the application of cognitive-behavioral therapy. *Clinical Psychology Review, 22*, 977–990.

Andersson, G., Airikka, M.-L., Buhrman, M., & Kaldo, V. (2005a). Dimensions of perfectionism and tinnitus distress. *Psychology, Health & Medicine, 10*, 78–87.

Andersson, G., Baguley, D. M., McKenna, L., & McFerran, D. J. (2005b). *Tinnitus: A multidisciplinary approach*. London: Whurr.

Andersson, G., & Lyttkens, L. (1999). A meta-analytic review of psychological treatments for tinnitus. *British Journal of Audiology, 33*, 201–210.

Cacace, A. T. (2003). Expanding the biological basis of tinnitus: Cross-modal origins and the role of neuroplasticity. *Hearing Research, 175*, 112–132.

Hallam, R. S., McKenna, L., & Shurlock, L. (2004). Tinnitus impairs cognitive efficiency. *International Journal of Audiology, 43*, 218–226.

Hallam, R. S., Rachman, S., & Hinchcliffe, R. (1984). Psychological aspects of tinnitus. In S. Rachman (Ed.), *Contributions to medical psychology* (Vol. 3, pp. 31–53). Oxford: Pergamon Press.

Hayes, S. C., Strosahl, K. D., & Wilson, K. G. (1999). *Acceptance and commitment therapy*. New York: Guilford Press.

Hesser, H., Weise, C., Zetterqvist Westin, V., & Andersson, G. (2011). A systematic review and meta-analysis of randomized controlled trials of cognitive-behavioral therapy for tinnitus distress. *Clinical Psychology Review, 31*(4), 545–553.

Jastreboff, P. J. (1990). Phantom auditory perception (tinnitus): Mechanisms of generation and perception. *Neuroscience Research, 8*, 221–254.

Kaldo, V., Levin, S., Widarsson, J., Buhrman, M., Larsen, H. C., & Andersson, G. (2008). Internet versus group cognitive-behavioral treatment of distress associated with tinnitus. A randomised controlled trial. *Behavior Therapy, 39*, 348–359.

Tiredness

▶ Fatigue

Tissue Repair

▶ Wound Healing

Tobacco

▶ Nicotine

Tobacco Advertising

Reiner Hanewinkel and Matthis Morgenstern
Institute for Therapy and Health Research, Kiel, Germany

Synonyms

Tobacco marketing; Tobacco promotion

Definition

Tobacco advertising is a form of communication by the tobacco industry with the aim of promoting tobacco products (typically cigarettes) and use. Different forms of advertising can be classified into "above the line" (ATL) and "below the line" (BTL) advertising. ATL advertising is traditional mass media advertising in print, television, radio, in cinemas, and on billboards. BTL advertising focuses more on specific target groups and uses less traditional advertising methods, such as sponsoring, promotion, event marketing, point-of-sale displays, product placements, direct marketing, ambient marketing, viral marketing, or brand stretching. Most research on the effects of tobacco advertising focuses on ATL advertising. However, the importance of BTL tobacco advertising is growing in the light of bans or partial bans of traditional tobacco advertising in most countries.

Description

A fundamental premise for the tobacco industry to spend money into tobacco advertising is the assumption that it is effective. The term "effective" can refer to different levels or "outcomes." It can either mean that tobacco advertising increases the market share of a specific brand, given a fixed market size for tobacco products. It can also mean that tobacco advertising increases or stabilizes the market size, by recruiting new smokers and by stimulating current smokers not to quit or ex-smokers to relapse. Empirical research conducted by non-industry-funded researchers has mainly focused on the latter interpretation of effectiveness, which is the one with high impact from a public health perspective.

One type of study in this field has analyzed changes in the global or country-specific tobacco market size dependent on advertising spending or dependent on changes in tobacco policy (e.g. implementation of advertising bans). These studies are usually time series or interrupted time-series designs and use highly aggregated data. While many of the early econometric studies found no association between aggregate cigarette advertising spending and total market sales, there are also studies that found positive relations, especially if the aggregation of the data was reduced (Saffer and Chaloupka 2000). Studies that compare countries with and without advertising bans or that conduct comparisons within a country before and after an advertising ban often find that bans reduce overall consumption of tobacco (Quentin et al. 2007). The effect is stronger in countries with comprehensive bans compared to partial bans.

A second type of studies uses individual-level data, looking at the effects of tobacco advertising on smoking behavior, mostly of young people. These studies are either experimental and quasi-experimental studies or cross-sectional and longitudinal observational studies. The effect of tobacco advertising is usually studied in terms of individual exposure to tobacco advertising. This is some form of induced exposure in the experimental studies or a measure of self-reported advertising exposure in the observational studies.

Measures of exposure can be direct (e.g., advertising recall, brand recall, notice of advertising, liking of advertising, ownership of promotional items) or indirect (e.g., television screen times, reception and liking of specific television programs, movies, sports, or magazines). A 2006 systematic review of the empirical evidence based on individual-level studies found 29 studies from 5 continents with more than 300,000 participants (DiFranza et al. 2006). The authors concluded that there is strong evidence for a link between exposure to tobacco promotion and tobacco use of children and adolescents. Applying Hill's criteria for judging the likelihood of a causal relationship between exposure and behavior, the authors found that many of Hill's criteria of causation were fulfilled (Hill 1965). They found that (1) children are exposed to tobacco promotion before the initiation of tobacco use (criterion temporality), (2) exposure increases the risk for initiation (criterion strength), (3) greater exposure results in higher risk (criterion dose–response), (4) the increased risk is robust (criterion consistency), (5) the risk is scientifically plausible (criterion plausibility), and (6) no other explanation can account for the evidence (criterion analogy). A recent study additionally confirmed the Hill criterion "specificity" (Hanewinkel et al. 2011).

It is less explicitly studied *how* this effect is mediated, i.e., how tobacco advertising leads to an increase in market size. However, tobacco advertising is not systematically different from other forms of advertising and can, therefore, be conceptualized within broader psychological and marketing theories. Most psychological theories of advertising can be classified as "hierarchy of effects" models (Vakratsas and Ambler 1999). These models suggest that advertising is not directly influencing behavioral responses, but that the effects are always mediated by a mental process. In the broadest sense, this mental process is a change in object valence, the object being the brand, the product, the product group, or the advertising itself. The most common models used to explain the effects of advertising are based on the information processing approach (McGuire 1976). They assume that people are persuaded by the contents of the advertising and consciously follow a cognitive path which is mediated by preferences, attitudes, norms, and beliefs about the advertised object. Newer variants of these models are the so-called dual-process models which conceptualize two routes of information processing, a central route and a peripheral route (Eagly and Chaiken 1993; Petty and Cacioppo 1986). The central route is activated if advertising contents are thoughtfully elaborated and recipients have high involvement and attention. On the peripheral route, information is less thoughtfully processed (low involvement) which happens if advertisings are consumed rather casually. Recipients with low involvement are more influenced by peripheral or emotional characteristics of the advertising (e.g., attractiveness of the source, colors, music). Most recent psychological theories even go a step further and assume that conscious mental processes are not a necessary precondition for behavioral influences (Bargh 2002; Harris et al. 2009). From this perspective, advertising is a form of behavioral priming that automatically affects the perceiver. The term "automatic" implies that the consumer does not have to be aware of having seen the advertising and also does not have to be aware that she/he responded to it. Such conceptions of advertising effects have, of course, strong implications for prevention strategies as it may be very difficult to counteract unconscious advertising effects.

Cross-References

▶ Tobacco Control
▶ Tobacco Use

References and Readings

Bargh, J. A. (2002). Losing consciousness: Automatic influences on consumer judgment, behavior and motivation. *Journal of Consumer Research, 29*(2), 280–286.

DiFranza, J. R., Wellman, R. J., Sargent, J. D., Weitzman, M., Hipple, B. J., & Winickoff, J. P. (2006). Tobacco promotion and the initiation of tobacco use: Assessing the evidence for causality. *Pediatrics, 117*(6), e1237–e1248.

Eagly, A. H., & Chaiken, S. (1993). Process theories of attitude formation and change: The elaboration likelihood model and heuristic systematic models. In A. H. Eagly & S. Chaiken (Eds.), *The psychology of attitudes* (pp. 305–325). Fort Worth: Harcourt Brace Jovanovich.

Hanewinkel, R., Isensee, B., Sargent, J. D., & Morgenstern, M. (2011). Cigarette advertising and teen smoking initiation. *Pediatrics, 127*(2), e271–e278.

Harris, J. L., Bargh, J. A., & Brownell, K. D. (2009). Priming effects of television food advertising on eating behavior. *Health Psychology, 28*(4), 404–413.

Hill, A. B. (1965). The environment and disease: Association or causation? *Proceedings of the Royal Society of Medicine, 58*, 295–300.

McGuire, W. J. (1976). Some internal psychological factors influencing consumer choice. *Journal of Consumer Research, 2*(4), 302–319.

Petty, R. E., & Cacioppo, J. T. (1986). *Communication and persuasion: Central and peripheral routes to attitude change*. New York: Springer.

Quentin, W., Neubauer, S., Leidl, R., & Konig, H. H. (2007). Advertising bans as a means of tobacco control policy: A systematic literature review of time-series analyses. *International Journal of Public Health, 52*(5), 295–307.

Saffer, H., & Chaloupka, F. (2000). The effect of tobacco advertising bans on tobacco consumption. *Journal of Health Economics, 19*(6), 1117–1137.

Vakratsas, D., & Ambler, T. (1999). How advertising works: What do we really know? *Journal of Marketing, 63*(1), 26–43.

Tobacco Cessation

▶ Smoking Cessation

Tobacco Control

Pekka Puska
National Institute for Health and Welfare (THL), Helsinki, Finland

Synonyms

Secondhand smoke; Smokeless tobacco; Smoking; Smoking cessation; Smoking prevention; Tobacco policy

Definition

Tobacco control includes all measures aiming at the reduction of tobacco use and of its harmful consequences in the population.

Thus tobacco control includes measures aiming at both prevention and cessation of the use of all tobacco products – both smoking and the use of smokeless tobacco.

Description

Introduction

The great health risks from smoking have been convincingly shown since the 1950s. It is now known that all forms of tobacco use, both smoking and the use of smokeless tobacco, i.e., are both addictive and potentially lethal. Scientific evidence confirms that smokers have significantly elevated risks of death from many cancers, cardiovascular and respiratory diseases, and many other fatal conditions US Department of Health and Education and Welfare 1972). The harmful effects of secondhand smoke have also long been convincingly established (Öberg et al. 2011).

Tobacco is a highly addictive substance that directly kills half of its users, as well as non-smokers exposed to secondhand smoke. There is no safe form of tobacco use or no safe level of exposure to secondhand smoke.

It is estimated that currently about one billion of men (nearly 50% of adult men) and about 250 million women (over 10% of women) in the world smoke. Smoking rates among men seem to have peaked but among women still increasing on global scale.

Tobacco kills currently annually some six million people (about 10% of world deaths) and with current trends some eight million people annually by 2030. Of the tobacco deaths, some three-fourths occur in low- and middle-income countries and generally proportionally more among lower socioeconomic segments of the population. The economic costs of tobacco-related harms are enormous: both the direct costs to health services and the indirect societal costs (Eriksen et al. 2014).

Health professionals started to warn about the harmful consequences of tobacco use already in the 1950s. Because of the disinformation and lobbying of the big tobacco industry, policy actions to reduce tobacco use started much later, generally only in the 1980s and the 1990s. A milestone was the adoption of the WHO Framework Convention on Tobacco Use, FCTC, in 2003 WHO 2003). Currently some 180 countries have ratified the convention that is a pioneering example of the use of international law in the field of public health. FCTC covers all the main elements of tobacco control.

Elements of Tobacco Control

Reduction of Demand for Tobacco
Education and communication: This includes comprehensive educational and public awareness programs on the health risks and on the addictive nature of tobacco products and exposure to tobacco smoke. This includes also effective training programs on tobacco control to health workers, to other professional and community groups dealing potentially with tobacco control, as well as to decision-makers.

Tobacco cessation: Stopping tobacco use is often very difficult because of strong physical addiction to nicotine and to the social dependence to the habit. During the last few decades, pharmacological and nonpharmacological (psychological, educational) methods have been developed to effectively help smokers and other tobacco users to quit the habit. Tobacco control policies include measures to provide tobacco users access to cessation services.

Elimination of tobacco advertising and promotion: An important background for the global tobacco epidemic is the powerful push from the multinational tobacco industry in the form of effective advertising, promotion, sponsorship, and lobbying of decision-makers. Thus an important component of tobacco control is a comprehensive ban on advertising, promotion, and sponsorship. Here an international agreement is especially important because of the cross border spreading of advertising. It is also important to eliminate false or misleading messages about the tobacco products.

Price and tax measures: Price is an important aspect of the use of any product. Accordingly price and tax measures are effective and important means of reducing tobacco consumption, in particular among young persons.

Regulation on the contents of tobacco products: Although there is no safe tobacco products, authorities can introduce regulations on testing, measuring, and levels of the contents and emissions of tobacco products. This can also include introduction of self-extinguishing cigarettes to reduce fires. National legislation can also regulate tobacco product disclosures.

Smoke-free environments: Exposure to tobacco smoke, especially indoors, is a health risk to everybody and especially to vulnerable population groups like children. At the same time, smoke-free environments discourage initiation and continuation of smoking. Thus important elements of any tobacco control policies include the prohibition of smoking in indoor workplaces, public transport, indoor public places, and also in other public places (e.g., stadia).

Packaging and labeling of tobacco products: Tobacco product packages and labels should not promote the product by any false, misleading, or deceptive messages. Such messages may include terms like "low tar," "light," "ultralight," or "mild." Tobacco products should carry large and clear health warnings in text or in form of pictures. Recently also generic tobacco packages have been proposed.

Reduction of the Supply of Tobacco
Sale to minors: An important part of tobacco-related health work is the prevention of tobacco use among children and youth and moving the possible initiation to as late as possible. Thus sale of tobacco to minors should be prohibited, and this legislation is well enforced, e.g., by requiring the purchaser to provide appropriate evidence of age. Vending machines should be placed so that minors cannot buy from them. Regulations should also prohibit sale of tobacco products by minors, as well as sale of individual or small cigarette packets.

Illicit trade: Surprisingly the big part of tobacco used in the world is smuggled, manufactured illicitly, or counterfeited. Thus elimination of illicit trade of tobacco products is important, and an issue in which international collaboration by authorities is especially needed.

Economic alternatives to tobacco business: The reduction of tobacco use calls also for the reduction of tobacco growing. Thus alternatives for tobacco growing should be encouraged, as well as also other viable alternatives for tobacco-related work.

Other Aspects of Tobacco Control

Research, monitoring, and surveillance: Although the scientific base of tobacco control is very strong, further research is needed in several areas. It is also important that every country has also its own research on aspects of its special features. Monitoring of tobacco use trends in the population and its subgroups is crucial. It is also important to monitor many aspects of determinants and process of tobacco use as well as activities related to tobacco control.

Exchange of information: For the international collaboration and the reporting of the FCTC, the implementation exchange of tobacco control-related information is needed. This includes, e.g., information on legislative, administrative, and other tobacco control measures, as well as information on tobacco use trends.

International collaboration in scientific, technical, and legal fields of tobacco control: Because of the global nature of the tobacco epidemic, the tobacco control calls for strong international collaboration, much assisted by the international FCTC-related work.

Implementation of International Tobacco Control

The FCTC Convention Secretariat published in 2014 a summary report on the global progress in implementation of the FCTC (2014). The report concluded that the implementation of the Convention has progressed steadily since the entry in force in 2005, but the implementation levels vary substantially between different policy measures. Overall, countries report high implementation rates for measures on packaging and labeling, sales to minors, and education, training, and public awareness. Rates remain low in areas like disclosure of marketing expenditures or programs for tobacco use cessation.

The implementation of tobacco control measures varies across different regions of the world. Also comparability of reports from different countries varies both concerning implementation measures and tobacco use data.

Overall there seems to be notable progress in introduction and implementation of various tobacco control measures in most parts of the world. After 10 years of existence of the Convention, the Secretariat has commissioned an assessment of the global impact of FCTC by a group of independent experts.

Cross-References

▶ Health Promotion and Disease Prevention
▶ Public Health
▶ Risk Factors and Their Management
▶ Smoking Prevention Policies and Programs

References and Further Readings

Eriksen, M., McKay, J., Schluger, N., Gomeshtapeh, F. I., & Drope, J. (2014). *The tobacco Atlas*. Atlanta: American Cancer Society.
FCTC. (2014). *Global progress report 20124 on report on implementation of the WHO Framework Convention on Tobacco Control*. Geneva: The Convention Secretariat.
Öberg, M., Jaakkola, M., Woodward, A., Peruga, A., & Pruss-Ustun, A. (2011). Worldwide burden of disease from exposure to second-hand smoke: A retrospective analysis of data from 192 countries. *The Lancet, 377*, 139–146.
US Department of Health, Education and Welfare. (1972). The health consequences of smoking. A report of the surgeon general: 1972. DHEW Publication No. (HSM) 72–7516. Washington, DC.
WHO. (2003). *WHO framework convention on tobacco control*. Geneva: World Health Organization.

Tobacco Marketing

▶ Tobacco Advertising

Tobacco Policy

▶ Tobacco Control

Tobacco Promotion

▶ Tobacco Advertising

Tobacco Smoking and Health

▶ Smoking and Health

Tobacco Smoking Cessation

▶ Smoking Cessation

Tobacco Use

▶ Smoking Behavior

Tonic REM

▶ REM Sleep

Total Cholesterol

▶ Lipid

Total Cholesterol in the Blood

▶ Lipid, Plasma

Total Sleep Time

▶ Sleep Duration

Touch

▶ Massage Therapy

Traditional Chinese Medicine

▶ Acupuncture

Trail-Making Test

Romola S. Bucks
School of Psychological Science, The University of Western Australia (M304), Perth, WA, Australia

Synonyms

Trails

Definition

This term refers to a widely used test assessing organized visual search, planning, attention, set shifting, cognitive flexibility, and divided attention (Rabin et al. 2005): all capacities thought to be executive in nature. Originally developed by Partington in 1938 (Partington and Leiter 1949), it was first published as part of the *Army Individual Test Battery* (1984). The test is currently available in public domain (see Lezak et al. 2004; Strauss et al. 2006) and revised versions (e.g., Reynolds 2002; Salthouse et al. 2000) and as part of a number of assessment batteries (e.g., Delis et al. 2001).

The standard trail-making test (TMT) contains two parts: Trails A and Trails B, which usually take no more than 5–10 min to complete. In Trails A, the participant draws lines to connect consecutively numbered circles, drawn on a single A4 sheet (1-2-3...). In Trails B, the participant connects consecutively numbered and lettered circles, alternating between them (e.g., 1-A-2-B-3...) on a second sheet. The participant is asked to connect the numbers, or numbers and letters, as fast as possible without lifting the pencil from the sheet. Revised versions (e.g., Delis et al. 2001; Reynolds 2002; Salthouse et al. 2000) usually contain an equivalent to Trails B, plus up to four other subtests designed to help the assessor distinguish the cause(s) of difficulties in the switching task, such as number or letter sequencing, visual scanning, or motor deficits.

The main performance measure is time taken to complete the sequence, but errors are commonly recorded as they can also be clinically useful (Lezak et al. 2004) and some variants score the number of items completed in a fixed period of time (Salthouse et al. 2000). Because of the significant motor requirements of the task, normative data are often age stratified (e.g., Mitrushina et al. 1999; Tombaugh 2004; see e.g., Hester et al. 2005, for difference and ratio norms). Education-based norms are also recommended (Tombaugh 2004).

Trails A is thought to rely most markedly on processing speed and tracking skills, whereas Trails B is thought to require more executive skills because it requires shifting between sequences (Kortte et al. 2002), inhibition, and visual working memory (Fellows et al. 2017). Indeed, fMRI evidence supports this view: Zakzanis et al. (2005) found greater left frontal activation in the dorsolateral prefrontal cortex during Trails B than Trails A.

Three methods of comparing Trails A and B are commonly employed: total time to complete Trails A subtracted from total time to complete Trails B (B–A); the ratio of Trails B to Trails A (B/A); or a residual representing the difference between Trails B performance predicted using Trials A (B.A; Fellows and Schmitter-Edgecombe 2015; Salthouse 2011). Evidence suggests that the ratio or the residual may be clearer indices of executive function by controlling for baseline motor, speed, visual tracking, age, and sequencing differences (Arbuthnott and Frank 2000; Salthouse 2011).

Both parts of the TMT are highly sensitive to dementia and brain injury, including Parkinson's (Goldman et al. 1998) and Alzheimer's disease (Chen et al. 2000). Importantly, deficits in TMT performance predict everyday activities of daily living difficulties (Bell-McGinty et al. 2002), including medication management (Fellows et al. 2017) and mortality (Vazzana et al. 2010) and may indicate preclinical Alzheimer's dementia (Chen et al. 2000).

Cross-References

▶ Executive Function
▶ Neuropsychology

References and Further Reading

Arbuthnott, K., & Frank, J. (2000). Trail making test, part B as a measure of executive control: Validation using a set-switching paradigm. *Journal of Clinical and Experimental Neuropsychology, 22*, 518–528.

Bell-McGinty, S., Podell, K., Franzen, M., Baird, A. D., & Williams, M. J. (2002). Standard measures of executive function in predicting instrumental activities of daily living in older adults. *International Journal of Geriatric Psychiatry, 17*, 828–834.

Chen, P., Ratcliff, G., Belle, S. H., Cauley, J. A., DeKosky, S. T., & Ganguli, M. (2000). Cognitive tests that best discriminate between presymptomatic AD and those who remain nondemented. *Neurology, 55*, 1847–1853.

Delis, D., Kaplan, E., & Kramer, J. (2001). *Delis–Kaplan executive function scale*. San Antonio: The Psychological Corporation.

Fellows, R. P., & Schmitter-Edgecombe, M. (2015). Between-domain cognitive dispersion and functional abilities in older adults. *Journal of Clinical and Experimental Neuropsychology, 37*, 1013–1023.

Fellows, R. P., Dahmen, J., Cook, D., & Schmitter-Edgecombe, M. (2017). Multicomponent analysis of a digital trail making test. *Clinical Neuropsychologist, 31*, 154–167.

Goldman, W. P., Baty, J. D., Buckles, V. D., Sahrmann, S., & Morris, J. C. (1998). Cognitive and motor functioning in Parkinson disease: Subjects with and without questionable dementia. *Archives of Neurology, 55,* 674–680.

Hester, R. L., Kinsella, G. J., Ong, B., & McGregor, J. (2005). Demographic influences on baseline and derived scores from the trail making test in healthy older Australian adults. *Clinical Neuropsychologist, 19,* 45–54.

Kortte, K. B., Horner, M. D., & Windham, W. K. (2002). The trail making test, part B: Cognitive flexibility or ability to maintain set? *Applied Neuropsychology, 9,* 106–109.

Lezak, M. D., Howieson, D. B., Loring, D. W., Hannay, H. J., & Fischer, J. S. (2004). *Neuropsychological assessment* (4th ed.). New York: Oxford University Press.

Mitrushina, M. N., Boone, K. L., & D'Elia, L. (1999). *Handbook of normative data for neuropsychological assessment.* New York: Oxford University Press.

Partington, J. E., & Leiter, R. G. (1949). Partington's pathway test. *Psychological Service Center Bulletin, 1,* 9–20.

Rabin, L. A., Barr, W. B., & Butler, L. A. (2005). Assessment practices of clinical neuropsychologists in the United States and Canada: A survey of INS, NAN, APA division 40 members. *Archives of Clinical Neuropsychology, 20,* 33–65.

Reynolds, C. R. (2002). *Comprehensive trail-making test.* Austin: PRO-ED.

Salthouse, T. A. (2011). What cognitive abilities are involved in trail-making performance? *Intelligence, 39,* 222–232.

Salthouse, T. A., Toth, J., Daniels, K., Parks, C., Pak, R., Wolbrette, M., & Hocking, K. (2000). Effects of aging on the efficiency of task switching in a variant of the trail making test. *Neuropsychology, 14,* 102–111.

Strauss, E., Sherman, E. M. S., & Spreen, O. (2006). *A compendium of neuropsychological tests: Administration, norms, and commentary.* New York: Oxford University Press.

Tombaugh, T. N. (2004). Trail making test A and B: Normative data stratified by age and education. *Archives of Clinical Neuropsychology, 19,* 203–214.

Vazzana, R., Bandinelli, S., Lauretani, F., Volpato, S., Lauretani, F., Di Iorio, A., et al. (2010). Trail making test predicts physical impairment and mortality in older persons. *Journal of American Geriatrics Society, 58,* 719–723.

Zakzanis, K. K., Mraz, R., & Graham, S. J. (2005). An fMRI study of the trail making test. *Neuropsychologia, 43,* 1878–1886.

Trails

▶ Trail-Making Test

Trait Anger

Judith Carroll
Cousins Center for Psychoneuroimmunology,
University of California, Los Angeles, CA, USA

Synonyms

Hostile affect; Hostility

Definition

Trait anger is described as a dispositional characteristic where one experiences frequent anger, with varying intensity (e.g., mild irritability, intense rage), and is often accompanied by related negative emotions such as envy, resentment, hate, and disgust (Buss 1961; Siegman and Smith 1994). There is considerable construct overlap between hostile dispositions and trait anger, making it difficult to disentangle. Martinn et al. (2000) have proposed a three-factor model of trait anger, which includes the anger-related affect, behavior (i.e., aggression), and cognitions (i.e., cynicism), similar to several of the subscales of the Cook-Medley Hostility Scale (Barefoot et al. 1989). A frequently used measure of trait anger is the Spielberger State-Trait Anger Expression Inventory (STAXI), which measures trait anger as having a proneness to experiencing anger either as a general tendency (*Anger temperament*), or with provocation (*Anger Reactions*) (Spielberger 1988; Spielberger and Sydeman 1994). Furthermore, Speilberger describes three different styles of anger expression: (1) showing anger emotions (*Anger-Out*), (2) preventing anger from being expressed but still experiencing it internally (*Anger-In*), or (3) having the initial affective response but then regulating it well (*Anger-Control*) (Spielberger 1988).

Behavioral medicine research has documented associations of trait anger, and the related constructs of hostility, with greater cardiovascular disease incidence and progression (al'Absi and Bongard 2006; Chida and Steptoe 2009; Miller et al. 1996; Siegman and Smith 1994; Smith et al. 2004). Although poor health behaviors are thought to partially explain these associations (Everson et al. 1997; Siegman and Smith 1994), it is also likely that this trait disposition contributes to worse health through the repeated emotionally driven activation of the neuroendocrine stress response and its associated downstream biological effects, including increases in blood pressure, inflammation, and oxidative stress (Carroll et al. 2010, 2011; Greeson et al. 2009; Smith and Gallo 1999; Suarez et al. 1998). Further work is needed to better define the mechanisms of this association.

Cross-References

▶ Anger, Measurement
▶ Hostility, Cynical
▶ Hostility, Measurement of

References and Further Readings

al'Absi, M., & Bongard, S. (2006). Neuroendocrine and behavioral mechanisms mediating the relationship between anger expression and cardiovascular risk: Assessment consideration and improvements. *Journal of Behavioral Medicine, 29*, 573–591.

Barefoot, J. C., Dodge, K. A., Peterson, B. L., Dahlstrom, G., & Williams, R. B. (1989). The cook-medley hostility scale: Item content and ability to predict survival. *Psychosomatic Medicine, 51*, 46–57.

Buss, A. H. (1961). *The psychology of aggression.* New York: Wiley.

Carroll, J. E., Marsland, A. L., Jenkins, F., Baum, A., Muldoon, M. F., & Manuck, S. B. (2010). A urinary marker of oxidative stress covaries positively with hostility among midlife community volunteers. *Psychosomatic Medicine, 72*(3), 273–280.

Carroll, J. E., Low, C. A., Prather, A. A., Cohen, S., Fury, J. M., Ross, D. C., et al. (2011). Negative affective responses to a speech task predict changes in interleukin (IL)-6. *Brain, Behavior, and Immunity, 25*, 232–238.

Chida, Y., & Steptoe, A. (2009). The association of anger and hostility with future coronary heart disease: A meta-analytic review of prospective evidence. *Journal of the American College of Cardiology, 53*(11), 936–946.

Everson, S. A., Kauhanen, J., Kaplan, G. A., Goldberg, D. E., Julkunen, J., Tuomilehto, J., et al. (1997). Hostility and increased risk of mortality and acute myocardial infarction: The mediating role of behavioral risk factors. *American Journal of Epidemiology, 146*(2), 142–152.

Greeson, J. M., Lewis, J. G., Achanzar, K., Zimmerman, E., Young, K. H., & Suarez, E. C. (2009). Stress-induced changes in the expression of monocytic beta2-integrins: The impact of arousal of negative affect and adrenergic responses to the anger recall interview. *Brain, Behavior, and Immunity, 23*(2), 251–256.

Martinn, R., Watson, D., & Wan, C. K. (2000). A three-factor model of trait anger: dimensions of affect, behavior, and cognition. *Journal of Personality, 68*, 869–897.

Miller, T. Q., Smith, T. W., Turner, C. W., Guijarro, M. L., & Hallet, A. J. (1996). A meta-analytic review of research on hostility and physical health. *Psychological Bulletin, 119*, 322–348.

Siegman, A. W., & Smith, T. W. (Eds.). (1994). *Anger, hostility, and the heart.* Hillsdale: Erlbaum.

Smith, T. W. (1992). Hostility and health: Current status of a psychosomatic hypothesis. *Health Psychology, 11*(3), 139–150.

Smith, T. W., & Gallo, L. C. (1999). Hostility and cardiovascular reactivity during marital interaction. *Psychosomatic Medicine, 61*(4), 436–445.

Smith, T. W., Glazer, K., Ruiz, J. M., & Gallo, L. C. (2004). Hostility, anger, aggressiveness, and coronary heart disease: An interpersonal perspective on personality, emotion, and health. *Journal of Personality, 72*(6), 1217–1270.

Spielberger, C. D. (1988). *Manual for the state-trait anger expression inventory (STAXI).* Odessa: Psychological Assessment Resources.

Spielberger, C., & Sydeman, S. J. (1994). State-trait anxiety inventory and state-trait anger expression inventory. In M. E. Maruish (Ed.), *The use of psychological testing for treatment planning and outcome assessment* (pp. 292–321). Hillsdale: Erlbaum.

Suarez, E. C., Kuhn, C. M., Schanberg, S. M., Williams, R. B., Jr., & Zimmermann, E. A. (1998). Neuroendocrine, cardiovascular, and emotional responses of hostile men: The role of interpersonal challenge. *Psychosomatic Medicine, 60*(1), 78–88.

Trait Anxiety

Yori Gidron
SCALab, Lille 3 University and Siric Oncollile, Lille, France

Synonyms

Neuroticism

Definition

Trait anxiety refers to the stable tendency to attend to, experience, and report negative emotions such as fears, worries, and anxiety across many situations. This is part of the personality dimension of neuroticism versus emotional stability. Trait anxiety also manifests by repeated concerns about and reporting of body symptoms. Trait anxiety is characterized by a stable perception of environmental stimuli (events, others' statements) as threatening. Trait-anxious people often experience and express also state anxiety, in situations in which most people do not experience such responses. This bias is thought to reflect a cognitive-perceptual bias. At the perceptual level, there is an over-attentional bias to threatening stimuli. At the cognitive level, there is a distorted negative interpretation of information congruent with and fostering anxious responses. Finally, at the level of memory, there is over-recall of threatening information. These three biases are common in people with a trait-anxious personality type and have important etiological roles in various types of affective disorders (Mathews and Macleod 2005). Trait anxiety is commonly assessed with the State-Trait Anxiety Inventory – trait version (Spielberger et al. 1970) – though other instruments exist as well. An indirect measure of anxiety was developed using the implicit association test – IAT. Indeed, the Anxiety-IAT correlated with self-reported anxiety but outperformed the latter in predicting various criteria (Egloff and Schmukle 2002). Trait anxiety is an important predictor and moderator in behavior medicine. For example, trait anxiety predicts functional recovery following spine surgery, risk of posttraumatic stress disorder, as well as adaptation to and risk of death following myocardial infarction (e.g., Szekely et al. 2007). These relationships could occur since trait anxiety is related to various coping strategies and to various neurophysiological responses. For example, high trait-anxious people demonstrate greater activity in the amygdala and reduced activity in the inhibitory dorsal anterior cingulate cortex, during extinction of fear responses (Sehlmeyer et al. 2011). This brain pattern can explain their increased vulnerability for psychological disorders and adaptation problems. As such, this psychological trait deserves attention in research and clinical applications of behavior medicine. The underlying causes, mechanisms for contributing to poor health outcomes, and ways for reducing the consequences of trait anxiety are important avenues of research for the benefit of clinical practice.

Cross-References

▶ Anxiety and Heart Disease
▶ Anxiety and Its Measurement
▶ Anxiety Disorder

References and Further Readings

Egloff, B., & Shmukle, S. C. (2002). Predictive validity of an implicit association test for assessing anxiety. *Journal of Personality and Social Psycholology, 83*, 1441–1455.

Mathews, A., & MacLeod, C. (2005). Cognitive vulnerability to emotional disorders. *Annual Review of Clinical Psychology, 1*, 167–195.

Sehlmeyer, C., Dannlowski, U., Schöning, S., Kugel, H., Pyka, M., Pfleiderer, B., et al. (2011). Neural correlates of trait anxiety in fear extinction. *Psychological Medicine, 41*, 789–798.

Spielberger, C. D., Gorsuch, R. L., & Lushene, R. E. (1970). *Manual for the state-trait anxiety inventory.* Palo Alto: Consulting Psychologists Press.

Székely, A., Balog, P., Benkö, E., Breuer, T., Székely, J., Kertai, M. D., et al. (2007). Anxiety predicts mortality and morbidity after coronary artery and valve surgery- a 4-year follow-up study. *Psychosomatic Medicine, 69*, 625–631.

Traits

▶ Personality

Trans Fats

▶ Fat, Dietary Intake
▶ Trans Fatty Acids

Trans Fatty Acids

Leah Rosenberg
Department of Medicine, School of Medicine,
Duke University, Durham, NC, USA

Synonyms

Trans fats

Definition

Trans fatty acids are unsaturated fatty acids with one double bond in the *trans* structural configuration as opposed to the *cis* conformation. These differences in conformation likely have consequences in the development of atherosclerosis secondary to diets rich in trans fatty acids. Dyslipidemia and adverse health outcomes have been linked to frequent consumption of *trans* fatty acids. While *trans* fatty acids do appear in nature, the vast majority in industrialized-world diets are manufactured to promote shelf life stability and enhance flavor in prepared foods. Preventative approaches to cardiovascular disease prevention and management include elimination of *trans* fatty acid consumption (Curhan and Mitch 2007). Certain municipalities, such as New York City, have recently enacted prohibitions against the use of *trans* fatty acids in restaurant food.

References and Readings

Curhan, G. C., & Mitch, W. E. (2007). Chapter 53-Diet and kidney disease. In *Section IX – Conservative and pharmacologic management of kidney disease* (Brenner and Rector's the kidney) (8th ed.). Philadelphia: Saunders.

Transactional Model

▶ Cognitive Appraisal

Transcendental Meditation

Alan M. Delamater
Department of Pediatrics, University of Miami Miller School of Medicine, Miami, FL, USA

Synonyms

Attention training; Concentration; Contemplation; Meditation; Mental training

Definition

Transcendental meditation (TM) is a meditation technique that has its origins in the ancient Vedic tradition of India. In the 1960s, Maharishi Mahesh Yogi introduced this meditative technique to the western world in a simple, nonreligious fashion, and since then TM has been practiced by millions of people worldwide. A considerable amount of research has been conducted on the effects of TM on physiological and psychological outcomes. Overall, the results of this research indicate that the practice of TM has beneficial effects in individuals with chronic health conditions as well as healthy people.

TM is classified as a concentrative meditation technique. The method consists of twice-daily 20 min practice in which the individual focuses on their mantra which is individually prescribed by a certified instructor. The individual is instructed to sit in a relaxed posture in a quiet environment and focus on the silent repetition of their mantra in their mind to the exclusion of other thoughts or feelings.

As concentration deepens, feelings of calm or tranquility are experienced. Research has shown that when individuals practice this type of meditation, they experience a restful hypometabolic state in which their respiration, heart-rate, blood pressure, muscle tension, and other indicators of sympathetic nervous system activation all decrease. This state of hypometabolic, restful alertness has been termed "the relaxation response." The relaxation response can be reliably elicited by the repetition of a mental stimulus (e.g., a mantra) while the individual adopts a relaxed mental attitude in a quiet environment.

Cross-References

▶ Meditation
▶ Mindfulness
▶ Relaxation

References and Readings

Anderson, J. W., et al. (2008). Blood pressure response to transcendental meditation: A meta-analysis. *American Journal of Hypertension, 21*(3), 310–316.
Benson, H. (1975). *The relaxation response*. New York: Morrow.
Chandler, H. M., et al. (2005). Transcendental meditation and postconventional self-development: A 10-year longitudinal study. *Journal of Social Behavior and Personality, 17*(1), 93–121.
Dillbeck, M. C., & Orme-Johnson, D. W. (1987). Physiological differences between transcendental meditation and rest. *American Psychologist, 42*, 879–881.
Goleman, D. (1988). *The varieties of the meditative experience*. New York: Tarcher.
Mahesh Yogi, M. (1963). *Transcendental meditation*. New York: New American Library.
Paul-Labrador, M., et al. (2006). Effects of randomized controlled trial of transcendental meditation on components of the metabolic syndrome in subjects with coronary heart disease. *Archives of Internal Medicine, 166*, 1218–1224.
So, K. T., & Orme-Johnson, D. W. (2001). Three randomized experiments on the holistic longitudinal effects of the transcendental meditation technique on cognition. *Intelligence, 29*(5), 419–440.
Walton, K. G., et al. (2004). Review of controlled clinical research on the transcendental meditation program and cardiovascular disease: Risk factors, morbidity, and mortality. *Cardiology in Review, 12*(5), 262–266.

Transducer

Yori Gidron
SCALab, Lille 3 University and Siric Oncollile, Lille, France

Synonyms

Biophysical converter

Definition

In physics, a transducer is a device or system which converts one type of energy to another type. In biology, this term can refer to cells or intracellular elements which transform one form of input or signal to another. Both are applicable for behavior medicine. Looking at devices, transducers are found in any machine which measures bodily parameters and depicts them electronically. A device measuring heart rate or pulse can detect changes in light passing through blood vessels, which reflect amount of blood as a function of one's heart rate. These changes in light are sensed, for example, by photoresistors, which are then translated to changes in electrical energy (current), which is then translated to digital numbers reflecting the rate of change in heart rate. The photoresistor constitutes the transducer in this case. Such devices are pivotal in medical diagnosis and in psychophysiological research. Another example of a device would be a galvanic skin conductance measure, which detects changes in electrical conductance of the skin, which reflects sympathetic activity and input into the skin. The conductance is translated into a digital representation, to reflect sympathetic activity. This too is used in psychophysiological research on stress responses.

Biologically, numerous transducers exist in the pathways of the sensory system and in cells. In the eyes, for example, the retina contains numerous photoreceptor cells that contain molecules called opsins. These photoreceptor cells synapse onto neuronal pathways and, via signal transducers, convert light energy detected by the opsins to neuronal energy, for visual processing in the brain. In the auditory system, sound reaches the middle ear after being channeled by the ear's shape. The eardrum and bones carry vibrations to the inner ear, where physical movements are transformed to fluid movement in the cochlea. This fluid movement excites hair cells in the basilar membrane that generates, via transduction, neuronal signals to the auditory cortex for higher auditory processing. Another example is the neuroendocrine transducer, where a neuron, for example, in the pituitary gland, translates electrical stimulation in its input to secretion of hormones at its output. In recent years, the vagus nerve has been found to be a pivotal neuroimmune transducer since its paraganglia express receptors for interleukin-1, an inflammatory signal (Ek et al. 1998). Upon signaling by that cytokine, neuronal information is carried to the brain via acetylcholine, the major vagal neurotransmitter, thus translating immune to nerve information, which then triggers several negative feedback anti-inflammatory loops (Tracey 2009). Transducers also play major roles in diseases. In cancer, for example, among multiple intracellular signaling pathways, the signal transducer and activator of transcription 3 (STAT3) is a transcription factor which is active upon extracellular activation by many signals including cytokines and growth factors. STAT3 plays a role in cell apoptosis and growth. In some cancers, constant activity of STAT3 is related to procarcinogenic activity and to poor prognosis (e.g., Alvarez et al. 2006). Thus, transducers are omnipresent in the body (or in devices) and are crucial for communication between the body and the external world as well as between different types of signals inside the body, in relation to health and disease.

Cross-References

▶ Psychophysiological

References and Further Readings

Alvarez, J. V., Greulich, H., Sellers, W. R., Meyerson, M., & Frank, D. A. (2006). Signal transducer and activator of transcription 3 is required for the oncogenic effects of non-small-cell lung cancer-associated mutations of the epidermal growth factor receptor. *Cancer Research, 66*, 3162–3168.

Ek, M., Kurosawa, M., Lundeberg, T., & Ericsson, A. (1998). Activation of vagal afferents after intravenous injection of interleukin-1beta: Role of endogenous prostaglandins. *Journal of Neuroscience, 18*, 9471–9479.

Tracey, K. J. (2009). Reflex control of immunity. *Nature Reviews Immunology, 9*, 418–428.

Trans-fatty Acids

▶ Fat: Saturated, Unsaturated

Transfer RNA

▶ RNA

Transformational Coping

▶ Posttraumatic Growth

Translational Behavioral Medicine

Bonnie Spring[1], Angela Fidler Pfammatter[2], Sara A. Hoffman[3] and Jennifer L. Warnick[4]
[1]Department of Preventive Medicine, Feinberg School of Medicine, Northwestern University, Chicago, IL, USA
[2]Feinberg School of Medicine, Northwestern University, Chicago, IL, USA
[3]Feinberg School of Medicine, Northwestern University, Evanston, IL, USA
[4]University of Florida, Gainesville, FL, USA

Synonyms

Implementation; Integrated behavioral medicine research, practice, policy; Research to practice translation

Definition

"Translation" is the process of adapting theoretical principles and empirical findings from research so that these can be applied in the real-world contexts of clinical and public health practice (Sung et al. 2003; Westfall et al. 2007; Woolf 2008). In translational behavioral medicine (TBM), knowledge from the basic psychosocial, behavioral, and biomedical sciences is applied to develop behavioral interventions to improve health, evaluate the effectiveness of those interventions, and study how to improve their implementation in practice and policy. The overarching objective of TBM is to advance, integrate, and actualize knowledge from the research, practice, and policy arenas to improve the health of individuals and communities. To advance progress in translating behavioral science knowledge to improved health, a new scholarly professional journal, *Translational Behavioral Medicine: Practice, Policy, Research*, was established in 2011 by the Society of Behavioral Medicine, with founding editor, Dr. Bonnie Spring.

Description

In 2001, the Institute of Medicine (IOM) published a report on the quality of health care in the United States. The IOM noted the chasm between the health care Americans receive and the kind they should receive. They attributed this gap largely to inadequate translation of scientific discoveries into actual practices. An oft-cited statistic is that it takes 15–20 years for a scientific discovery to influence clinical practice (Balas and Boren 2000). Moreover, even when a research-supported treatment does become recognized as a best practice, adherence across practitioners is highly variable.

The translation process proceeds through a series of phases, as illustrated in the conceptual model by Westfall et al. (2007), shown in Fig. 1. The first translational phase (T1) utilizes knowledge obtained from the study of basic biological, psychosocial, and behavioral processes to inform the development and refinement of promising health interventions. T1 research, sometimes called "bench to bedside," provides the first link from basic science to human clinical application. The second translational phase (T2), sometimes called "bench to trench," is concerned with evaluating the efficacy and effectiveness of interventions under conditions that become progressively less controlled and more representative of the general population and usual practice settings. The third translational phase (T3) is sometimes called dissemination and implementation (D & I). T3 research examines how to facilitate the uptake of evidence-based (research-supported) interventions into routine, day-to-day provision of clinical care and public health services. In contrast to T1, which concerns developing interventions, and T2, which concerns determining whether interventions work, T3 research examines how to get effective interventions widely implemented in real-world settings.

T1 Translation

The earliest work of T1 translation is focused on developing the intervention; later work is focused on optimizing or refining it. The ideas that

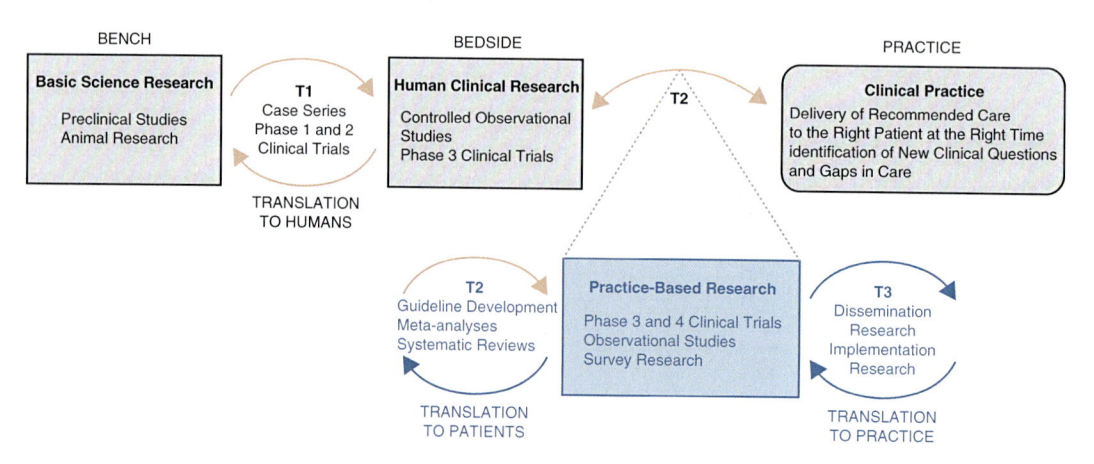

Translational Behavioral Medicine, Fig. 1 Translational research phases from the NIH roadmap (Reprinted with permission from Westfall et al. (2007))

underlie behavioral medicine interventions tend to originate from one of two fields: epidemiology and basic biopsychosocial sciences. The field of origin then influences the research designs initially implemented to develop a candidate intervention. Whereas epidemiologists commonly apply observational approaches, basic behavioral and psychosocial scientists are more likely to implement experimental methods.

Intervention Development

A simple form of naturalistic observational research design is a *case series* (or clinical series). In a case series to develop a new treatment, a single individual or small group of individuals is observed (either prospectively or retrospectively using recorded information). The aim is to detect whether an association exists between exposure to putative therapeutic elements and a clinical event (e.g., symptom improvement or remission). Usually applied in the earliest phases of treatment development, a series of cases may be gathered to establish "proof of concept" that a new treatment holds sufficient promise to warrant further study. An advantage of case series studies is that they capture clinical events in a naturalistic context. Disadvantages are that case studies examine small, highly selected samples of people who may be atypical. Also, case series can demonstrate only correlation, not causation.

In contrast to a naturalistic observational approach, when using *experimental methods*, the researcher manipulates one or more independent variables to determine the effects on a dependent variable. These methods lend themselves well to the needs of basic scientists who study fundamental questions about mechanisms that underlie human functioning. Basic behavioral scientists usually approach intervention development by hypothesizing that probing a particular psychosocial or biobehavioral mechanism will have a beneficial effect on the health outcome of interest. Because experimental methods are ideally suited to carry out such work, they have become a cornerstone of research on the science of behavior change. Such work endeavors to build interventions from the ground up based on an understanding of how and why humans function as they do. Once an early prototype intervention has been assembled, a type of experiment called a phase I clinical trial can be conducted to pilot test the safety, feasibility, acceptability, and optimal dosing of a potential intervention. Typically, phase I trials are conducted with small samples of participants, who are relatively free of complex medical histories.

Intervention Optimization

Behavioral medicine interventions usually combine multiple treatment components that are brought together as a package haphazardly, rather than systematically. For example, an intervention to promote physical activity might aggregate individual coaching delivered by an exercise physiologist together with provision of a free gym membership, a wrist worn accelerometer that detects and wirelessly transmits physical activity data to the participant's smartphone, and incentives for wearing the accelerometer and meeting activity goals. The developer's reason for bundling intervention components into a single treatment package is usually to produce the strongest possible treatment effect and the largest benefit on the targeted health outcome when the developed intervention is formally evaluated in a randomized controlled trial. However, choosing to test a treatment package before evaluating its individual components can prove disadvantageous for long-term treatment implementation. The available toolbox of behavioral interventions is filled with compound, multi-session treatments that received limited uptake because the multi-component intervention proved too complex and expensive for the health-care system to implement and too burdensome for patients to fully engage. Because only the complete treatment package has been evaluated, it remains unclear which treatment components produced the positive effect, whether some treatment elements are inert and could be eliminated (potentially reducing costs), and whether the dose and timing of the delivery of other components is optimal. Subsequent "dismantling" studies are needed to address those questions and evaluate more efficient versions of treatment delivery, but those are rarely undertaken.

In contrast, *multiphase optimization strategy* (*MOST*), adapted from engineering science, is a methodology designed to build new interventions from the ground up by first optimizing and evaluating the contribution of individual intervention components (Collins et al. 2007). Questions about the intensity, timing, or duration of treatment components are examined in experiments that vary them systematically. MOST follows a sequential, stepped approach to intervention development. The first step (screening) is to establish a conceptual, theoretical model of how the eventual intervention should produce benefit and to apply the model to derive the potential intervention components. The second step (refining) involves experimenting to examine the impact of individual intervention components. That stage may be followed by further experimentation to refine and optimize the components (e.g., by modifying their dose, timing, or delivery channel). Once the individual treatment components are optimized, the third step is to assemble the treatment package (the beta intervention) and confirm its efficacy via a randomized controlled trial (RCT). If the trial proves successful, the fourth step is releasing the new intervention and further testing its effectiveness in real-world settings. Note that the MOST approach delays the RCT of a treatment package until after the intervention has been systematically optimized. A key feature of the MOST strategy is that each subsequent version of the intervention will have been engineered and empirically validated to be superior to the previous one on whatever optimization parameter the interventionist desires.

A first phase of optimizing an intervention in MOST is usually to select intervention components that target the key mechanisms specified by the conceptual model. Next, a *factorial experiment* may be conducted to estimate the effect size associated with each component. The choice of which components to include in the treatment package can then be optimized. If, for example, cost-effectiveness is the optimization goal, then each included component can be chosen based on what has been learned about its effect size and its cost. The aim is to compile the treatment package that produces the maximum change attainable for a given level of financial resources. The treatment package could also be optimized for temporal efficiency, such that the components produce the maximal cardiovascular health benefit that a primary care nurse can accomplish in her five available minutes of clinic time per patient. Alternatively, the intervention can be optimized for reach, e.g., to maximize the number of low-income adults that can be exposed to an intervention with available resources. By optimizing for a specific context, MOST emphasizes the careful, efficient management of resources to increase the implementation of scientifically grounded practices.

The rationale for conducting a factorial experiment in the MOST framework is in some sense to optimize the best "one-size-fits-all" treatment that can be made available for the average patient given particular contextual constraints. This strategy accords with contemporary evidence-based practice process policy by initially offering patients the treatment or intervention that has the strongest overall empirical support for efficacy and effectiveness, regardless of cost considerations (Spring and Neville 2010). However, since health-care resources are never unlimited, and since both individual and contextual variability are evident in how individuals respond to an intervention, a different research design in the MOST framework also can be applied.

The *sequential multiple assignment randomized trial* (*SMART*) is a research design that allows the researcher to learn how to adapt interventions by identifying what intervention works for whom and at what time (Almirall et al. 2014). SMART trials are well suited to establish evidence-based practice policy to manage the health of a population. The aim of a SMART trial is to derive decision rules for how to modify intervention over time in order to respond to variability in the treatment response. The SMART trial examines tailoring variables that have the potential to be useful for determining when or to whom an intervention should be optimally delivered. As the tailoring variable changes, the SMART design implements multiple random assignments over the course of the trial. Hence, the yield from a SMART trial is a set of decision rules that specify how best to make changes in the intervention to adapt optimally to variation in the outcome. The stepped series of decision rules that will comprise the intervention to emerge from a SMART can be triggered by time, by a change in a variable of interest, or by attaining a criterion on a variable. For example, the first randomization in a SMART design could be conducted in order to learn whether low-intensity or moderate-intensity activity is the optimal starting goal to assign a physical activity intervention to treat frailty. The second randomization might test whether it is more effective to maintain or to step up treatment intensity if the patient fails to improve within a predetermined period.

In contrast to a tailoring variable like changes in frailty or weight loss that unfold gradually over time, some important health outcomes change more rapidly. Examples include mood, stress, concentration, or willingness to exercise, which can fluctuate many times per day. In such cases, decision rules are needed to determine when, how, and what to deliver to people so that the intervention will arrive at a time and in a format when they need it and will use it. Microrandomized trials can be implemented to formulate decision rules needed to craft such *just-in-time adaptive interventions* (*JITAI*) (Nahum-Shani et al. 2014; Klasnja et al. 2015). The JITAI's decision rules operate on real-time information to select and trigger an appropriate intervention to the individual at the right time. For example, a microrandomized trial might deliver an exercise prompt or no exercise prompt in the morning and in the evening while tracking whether the person exercised in the hour immediately following the microrandomization. If the exercise prompt triggers increased physical activity, compared to no prompt, in the morning but not the evening, the researcher would conclude that time of day is a useful tailoring variable and would implement a decision rule that only delivers exercise prompts in the morning. If the exercise prompt triggers greater activity than no prompt at both times of day, then time of day would prove not to be a useful tailoring variable, and the decision rule would specify that exercise can be prompted at either time of day.

Ideally, both initial intervention development and intervention optimization should occur during T1 translation before the developed intervention is subjected to evaluation in a clinical trial. Doing so allows intervention's mechanisms of action, its selection of treatment components, and its decision rules regarding which components to administer, when, and to whom to be systematically developed before the trial.

T2 Translation

The T2, "bench to trench," translational phase is concerned with evaluating the efficacy and effectiveness of interventions under conditions that become progressively less controlled and more representative of the general population and usual practice settings. T2 research introduces phase II and III clinical trials to test the efficacy and effectiveness of developed and optimized interventions. Phase II clinical trials evaluate the efficacy of an intervention for the treatment of a specific, circumscribed problem. Efficacy testing is performed under optimal conditions; for example, in an academic medical setting, employing highly trained research staff as interventionists, and involving patients without co-occurring health conditions. Phase III trials move past the highly controlled conditions and are often called studies of effectiveness (in contrast to efficacy) because they involve more "real-world," less highly selected settings, interventionists, and patients. For example, local staff in a community setting may deliver an intervention as part of their regular job duties to most of their patients with the target health problem. Such trials impose few exclusion criteria and enroll patients even if they have comorbidities.

Randomized controlled trials (*RCTs*) are the gold standard method of testing whether a treatment works. After screening for inclusion and exclusion criteria, patients are randomly assigned to one of two or more treatments, such that neither they nor the interventionist knows the treatment prior to randomization. In a two-group design, participants in one group receive the active intervention (e.g., smoking cessation treatment), and participants in the other group receive a control intervention (e.g., general health education) that is comparable in some elements (e.g., credibility, contact time) but inert in the active elements (e.g., specific skills training) thought responsible for the treatment's effect. The primary outcome might change from baseline in the number of study participants who smoke. Because the group allocation is concealed until randomization has occurred, neither investigator nor patient can influence the treatment assignment, so that participants have an equal chance of being assigned to either the intervention or the control group. This enables researchers to eliminate any bias that might otherwise occur in the group assignment.

Two different randomization procedures are employed in RCTs. They are (1) fixed allocation randomization (which includes simple, blocked, or stratified randomization) and (2) adaptive randomization (which includes baseline adaptive or response-adaptive randomization). Simple randomization is analogous to repeated fair coin tossing. However, this procedure is prone to creating imbalanced group sizes. Blocked randomization (also referred to as permuted block randomization) instead ensures that at no time during the randomization will the difference between group sizes be large, and at some points, groups will be equal. Stratified randomization helps to ensure the even distribution of certain factors (e.g., gender) between the groups and conditions. In adaptive randomization, the probability of being randomized to different groups changes as the study progresses. Altering the randomization procedure can help to overcome imbalances based on differences in participants' baseline characteristics (i.e., baseline adaptive randomization) or based on their responses at a later point in the study (i.e., response-adaptive randomization).

In RCTs testing drug treatments, the use of identical appearing pills to contain active and inactive agents makes it possible to keep both participants and study personnel naïve to group assignment, a state of affairs referred to as double blind. When only participants are naive, the trial is described as being single blind. Blinding participants and personnel to study conditions helps to ensure that treatment effects are due to the intervention, rather than person-level factors (e.g., knowledge or expectancies about the treatment or outcome). However, double blinding is rarely feasible in trials of behavioral interventions: Both patients and interventionists usually know which treatment is being given. One important form of blinding that does remain feasible is blinding of outcome assessors. When blinded, the assessors who evaluate study outcomes are unaware of whether patients belong to the treatment or the control group.

RCTs are the gold standard for evaluating treatments because this design surpasses others in its internal validity. This means that outcome differences between the study groups can be attributed to the treatment because the researchers held constant other extraneous variation between groups. The presence of the control group enables the researcher to account for shared influences, such as being repeatedly assessed or receiving attention from professionals. Equally important is the need to establish treatment fidelity, i.e., that the intended intervention was delivered as planned. Fidelity is induced by training and supervising therapists to follow a treatment protocol (i.e., a treatment manual or algorithm) and is monitored to ensure that critical intervention elements are delivered. The RCT's internal validity permits researchers to make causal inferences, that is, to attribute between group differences in patient outcomes to variation in the treatment. Its drawbacks are that RCTs are expensive and time-consuming to implement and that random assignment of study participants to conditions is not always feasible. Just as an RCT's validity is compromised by low-quality design or execution, its utility is undermined by incomplete reporting. To facilitate comprehensive, uniform reporting of RCTs, most scholarly journals in health have adopted the international CONSORT guidelines, which guide the information to be reported when publishing a RCT (Moher et al. 2010).

In some cases, randomization of participants to intervention conditions is infeasible (or impossible), and *quasi-experimental designs* need to be used. These designs gained popularity with the development of advanced statistical procedures to control for the effect of extraneous variables associated with group membership. In essence, these procedures help researchers to overcome some of the limitations of non-randomization. Suppose, for example, a researcher wished to study the effect of cigarette taxation policy on the prevalence of smoking. Ideally, one would randomize state legislatures to tax on cigarettes at different rates. However, that would not be feasible. Therefore, instead of being randomized, states will be grouped into those that tax cigarettes at more versus less than $1.00 per pack. Quasi-experimental designs are more susceptible than RCTs to confounding variables that may affect the outcomes of interest. In this case, we will find that the prevalence of smoking is lower in states that impose higher cigarette taxes. However, there are other demographic, geographic, and sociocultural differences besides cigarette taxation between states that have the highest and lowest prevalence of cigarette smoking. For instance, Minnesota, Massachusetts, and Rhode Island, three states that have among the lowest smoking rates, tax cigarette taxes at least $3.00 per pack. In contrast, Kentucky, Missouri, and Tennessee, several states with the highest smoking rates levy a cigarette tax per pack between $0.17 and $0.62. In addition to their lower tax rates, Kentucky and Missouri are states where tobacco is grown and manufactured. Hence, it will not be possible to determine whether it is the imposition of differing cigarette taxes or other extraneous differences that account for the observed variation in smoking prevalence.

The advantage of quasi-experimental designs is that they are broadly applicable and easy to implement. For policy interventions or other contexts that preclude randomization, quasi-experimental designs may be the only option available. Their disadvantage is that non-randomization prevents researchers from being able to make causal inferences about what generated the outcomes, particularly because confounding variables (both measured and unmeasured) offer alternative explanations.

T3 Translation

The T3, or dissemination and implementation (D & I) phase of translation, incorporates both primary and secondary research, such as the creation of systematic evidence reviews and practice guidelines. Unlike primary research, which involves the collection of new data, systematic evidence reviews are secondary research that cull and combine information from prior reports. The science of systematic reviewing is in itself a sophisticated and evolving field with many nuances that surround the unbiased acquisition of publications, extraction and analysis of data, and interpretation of results. Systematic reviews offer a means to evaluate whether the evidence about a treatment's effectiveness is strong and consistent enough to warrant widespread application in practice. If the data are plentiful and the studies sufficiently similar, a systematic review can provide evidence about whether a treatment's effects are broadly generalizable. In other words, the review can indicate whether there are boundary conditions or types of people for whom the treatment is less helpful or even contraindicated. The comprehensive, unbiased evidence base analyzed for a systematic review affords an excellent grounding from which experts can formulate practice guidelines. The dissemination of evidence-based guidelines conveys best research-tested practices to clinicians and policy makers.

D & I studies also include primary research evaluating how to facilitate the uptake of evidence-based (research-supported) interventions into routine, day-to-day provision of clinical care and public health services. In contrast to T1 and T2, which concern determining whether interventions work (and for whom), T3 research examines how to get effective interventions widely implemented in real-world settings. The aim of primary D & I research is to identify and learn how to overcome barriers at the practitioner, institutional, and system levels that keep effective interventions from being used. Barriers may include limitations in clinician training or skills, lack of available resources for training, competing institutional priorities, or policy barriers (e.g., lack of insurance reimbursement).

Cross-References

▶ Evidence-Based Behavioral Medicine (EBBM)
▶ Research to Practice Translation

References and Further Reading

Abernethy, A. P., & Wheeler, J. L. (2011). True translational research: Bridging the three phases of translation through data and behavior. *Translational Behavioral Medicine, 1*(1), 26–30. https://doi.org/10.1007/s13142-010-0013-z.

Almirall, D., Nahum-Shani, I., Sherwood, N. E., & Murphy, S. A. (2014). Introduction to SMART designs for the development of adaptive interventions: With application to weight loss research. *Translational Behavioral Medicine, 4*(3), 260–274.

Balas, E. A., & Boren, S. A. (2000). Managing clinical knowledge for health care improvement. In J. Bemmel & A. T. McCray (Eds.), *Yearbook of medical informatics 2000: Patient-centered systems* (pp. 65–70). Stuttgart: Schattauer Verlagsgesellschaft mbH.

Collins, L. M., Murphy, S. A., & Strecher, V. (2007). The multiphase optimization strategy (MOST) and the sequential multiple assignment randomized trial (SMART): New methods for more potent eHealth interventions. *American Journal of Preventive Medicine, 32*(5), S112–S118. https://doi.org/10.1016/j.amepre.2007.01.022.

Dougherty, D., & Conway, P. H. (2008). The "3T's" road map to transform US health care: The "how" of high-quality care. *JAMA: The Journal of the American Medical Association, 299*, 2319–2321.

Hopewell, S., Dutton, S., Yu, L., Chan, A., & Altman, D. (2010). The quality of reports of randomized trials in 2000 and 2006: Comparative study of articles indexed in PubMed. *BMJ, 340*, c1432.

Klasnja, P., Hekler, E. B., Shiffman, S., Boruvka, A., Almirall, D., Tewari, A., & Murphy, S. A. (2015). Microrandomized trials: An experimental design for developing just-in-time adaptive interventions. *Health Psychology, 34*(S), 1220.

Moher, D., Hopewell, S., Schulz, K., Montori, V., & Gotzsche, P. (2010). Consort 2010 explanation and elaboration: Updated guidelines for reporting parallel group randomized trials. *BMJ, 340*, c869.

Nahum-Shani, I., Spring, B., Smith, S. N., Collins, L. M., Witkiewitz, K., Tewari, A., & Murphy, S. A. (2014). Just–in-time adaptive interventions (JITAIs): Key components and design principles for ongoing health behavior support. *Annals of Behavioral Medicine*, 1–17.

Spring, B. (2011). Translational behavioral medicine: A pathway to better health. *Translational Behavioral Medicine, 1*(1), 1–3.

Spring, B., & Neville, K. (2010). Evidence-based practice in clinical psychology. In D. Barlow (Ed.), *Oxford handbook of clinical psychology* (pp. 128–149). New York: Oxford University Press.

Sung, N. S., Crowley, W. F., Jr., Genel, M., Salber, P., Sandy, L., Sherwood, L. M., Johnson, S. B., Catanese, V., Tilson, H., Getz, K., Larson, E. L., Scheinberg, D., Reece, E. A., Slavkin, H., Dobs, A., Grebb, J., Martinez, R. A., Korn, A., & Rimoin, D. (2003). Central challenges facing the national clinical research enterprise. *JAMA: The Journal of the American Medical Association, 289*(10), 1278–1287.

Westfall, J. M., Mold, J., & Fagnan, L. (2007). Practice-based research-"Blue Highways" on the NIH roadmap. *JAMA: The Journal of the American Medical Association, 297*(4), 403–406.

Woolf, S. H. (2008). The meaning of translational research and why it matters. *JAMA: The Journal of the American Medical Association, 299*(2), 211–213.

Translational Research

▶ RE-AIM Guidelines
▶ Research to Practice Translation

Transmethylation

▶ Methylation

Transtheoretical Model of Behavior Change

James O. Prochaska
Clinical and Health Psychology, University of Rhode Island, Kingston, RI, USA

Synonyms

Stages of change model

Definition

The Transtheoretical Model (TTM) construes behavior change as an intentional process that unfolds over time and involves progress through a series of six stages of change (Prochaska et al. 1992). TTM integrates principles and processes of change from across leading theories, hence the name Transtheoretical.

Description

Precontemplation (not ready) is the initial stage in which individuals are not intending to take action in the foreseeable future, usually assessed as the next 6 months.

People can be in this stage due to a lack of awareness of the health consequences of a behavior.

Or, they can be demoralized about their abilities to change, like millions of people who have tried to lose weight multiple times in multiple ways. This stage is often misunderstood to mean that these people do not want to change.

The history of demoralized individuals indicates that they want to change, but they have given up on their abilities to change.

Contemplation (getting ready) is the stage in which individuals are intending to change in the next 6 months, but not immediately in the next month. These individuals are more aware of the benefits or pros of changing but can also be acutely aware of the cons, such as having to give up some of their favorite foods or having to risk failure. Decisional conflict between the pros and cons can lead to profound ambivalence reflected in the motto: "When in doubt, don't act." With smokers intending to quit for good in the next 6 months, without help, less than 50% will quit for 24 h in the next 12 months.

In the Preparation (ready) stage, individuals are intending to take action in the next month. Their number one concern is, "If I act, will I fail?" The emphasis here is helping them to be well-prepared, because people know in growing up, the better prepared they are in academics or athletics, the more likely they are to reach their goal.

In the Action stage, change is typically overt and observable, with individuals having quit smoking, started exercising, or practicing stress management. This is the busiest stage, where people have to work the hardest to keep from regressing or returning to an earlier stage. Many people believe the worst risks for relapse will be over in a few days or few weeks. We find that people who progress through Action work the hardest for about 6 months, which happens to represent the steepest part of relapse curves across addictions (Prochaska and DiClemente 1983). So, Action is defined as 6 months being risk-free and we encourage individuals to think of this time as the behavior medicine equivalent of life-saving surgery. Following such surgery, would they give themselves 6 months to recover? Will they let others know they will not be at their best and will need more support? This is the type of priority needed to progress through this tough time.

Maintenance is the stage in which people are free from their problem for 6 months to 5 years. People are considered cured from cancer after 5 years without symptom remission. For many people, it may take 5 years to get free from behavioral causes of cancer. During this stage, individuals do not have to work as hard, but they do have to be prepared to cope with the most common causes of relapse. These causes are times of distress, when people are anxious, depressed, lonely, bored, or stressed. Average Americans cope with such distress by increasing unhealthy habits. We try to prepare people to cope with such temptations through healthy alternatives, like talking with a supportive person, walking, or relaxing.

Termination is the stage in which people are totally confident that they are never going back to their high-risk behavior and have no temptation to return. We have found that of alcoholics and smokers in their first 5 years of abstinence, about 20% have reached this criterion (Snow et al. 1992). These people can put all of their change efforts into enhancing other aspects of their lives. But, for many it may mean a lifetime of maintenance. The ideal goal is to have a new healthy behavior be automatic and under stimulus control, like taking an aspirin every day at the same time and place.

Applying TTM usually begins by assessing which stage the patient is in and then helping them set a realistic goal for now, like progressing to the next stage. Research shows that if we try to pressure patients to progress quickly from Precontemplation to Action, there can be unforeseen consequences of dropping out of treatment, stopping until treatment is over and then quickly relapsing, or simply lying.

What are the principles for helping patients progress from Precontemplation to Contemplation? A meta-analysis of the pros and cons of changing for 48 health behaviors revealed some remarkable results from 120 datasets from studies from 10 countries in 9 languages (Hall and Rossi 2008). The cons are clearly greater than the pros in Precontemplation (PC) and the pros are clearly higher in Contemplation (C). So, the first principle of progress is to raise the pros. With sedentary individuals, we might ask them if they like bargains and tell them that if so, physical activity (PA) is the bargain basement of behaviors. There is no other behavior from which they can get as many benefits as PA. We would ask them to list all the benefits that they believe they could get from regular PA, chart their list, and then challenge them to try to double the list. Most have five or six and we tell them there are over 70 scientific benefits and we only want them to find five more (Prochaska and Prochaska 2016). If we see the list going up, it is like seeing cholesterol or blood pressure coming down. We know our behavior medicine is working.

In Contemplation (C), the pros and cons are exactly tied, reflecting their profound ambivalence. From C to Preparation (PR), the cons come down, so the second principle is to help lower the cons. The number one con for PA is time, so some individuals lower this con by riding a lifecycle where they can multitask and read or review an article for work, read a book for pleasure, or catch up on the news. Others may volunteer to help coach their kid's soccer team and at the same time, get some PA, be with their child, do community service, meet more parents, and have fun. Fortunately, the cons have to decrease only half as much as the pros increase, so we put twice as much emphasis on raising the pros.

In the Preparation stage, the pros clearly outweigh the cons, so individuals are not encouraged to take action until they have a favorable profile. Once in the Action stage, they can use their growing list of pros to put other principles and processes of change into operation. When they write down on their "To-Do" list, "walking for my heart" they are making a daily commitment based on the process of self-liberation from Existential Therapy. When they look at the list they are cued to action based on stimulus control from Behavior Therapy. When they scratch off their list, they are reinforcing themselves based on Skinnerian Theory. As they move from one pro to the next each week, like walking for my weight, my sleep, my self-esteem, my immune system, and my sex life, after a while they may be running. Over time, they are using PA to affirm so much of their body, selves, and others based on self-reevaluation from Cognitive Behavior Theory and Self-Psychology.

This description illustrates how different principles and processes are applied to produce progress at different stages of change. This integrative approach led to the development of computer-tailored interventions (CTIs) by which individuals are assessed on TTM variables related to their current stage. Their assessment is compared to a normative database, and they can be given feedback on how they are applying principles and processes of change compared to peers who make the most progress. Over time, they can be given feedback compared to themselves, such as "Congratulations, you have progressed two stages, which means you have about tripled the chances you will be taking effective action in the next few months."

Such CTIs have been found in randomized population trials to be effective with a growing range of problems, including smoking, exercise, diet, stress, depression, bullying, partner violence, and medication adherence. The percentage of those in the Action or Maintenance stage at long-term follow-up ranges from about 25% for smoking (Prochaska et al. 2001) to about 45% for exercise and diet (Prochaska et al. 2008), to over 65% for stress (Evers et al. 2006) and medication adherence (Johnson et al. 2006). These results are with populations in which typically the majority, like 80%, would be labeled as unmotivated or not ready to change when we proactively reached out to them at home, school, work, or in clinics to offer them help matched to their personal needs. The results can be remarkably robust with very comparable outcomes with smoking, for example, with adolescents and older smokers, Hispanic and African-American smokers, and smokers with mental illness (Velicer et al. 2007).

Similar interventions have been found to be just as effective when we treat populations for three or four behaviors at the same time (Prochaska et al. 2006). Individuals working on one behavior are just as effective as those working on two who are just as effective as those working on three. But, very few people are taking action on more than one behavior at a time because they are not ready. So, they can be progressing through early stages on two behaviors, for example, while they are working to maintain action on another single behavior.

One exciting development in simultaneously changing multiple behaviors is the phenomenon of coaction. Coaction is the increased probability that individuals who take action on one behavior (like exercise) are likely to take action on a second behavior (like diet). We have found that significant coaction typically occurs only in our TTM treatment groups (e.g., Paiva et al. 2012; Johnson et al. 2014; Mauriello et al. 2010) and not in control groups, suggesting it is likely to be treatment induced.

With a population of 1400 employees in a major medical setting, the study of Prochaska et al. (2008) made available online modular TTM computerized-tailored interventions or three motivational interviewing (a psychotherapeutic approach designed to enhance motivation for positive change) telephonic or in-person sessions for each of four behaviors (smoking, inactivity, BMI >25, and stress). Patients chose which behaviors to target and how much time and effort to spend on any behavior. At 6 months, both treatments outperformed the Health Risk Intervention (HRI), which included feedback on the person's stage for each risk and guidance on how they could progress to the next stage.

With a population of 1800 students recruited from eight high schools in four states, Mauriello et al. (2010) applied a second-generation strategy with exercise as the primary behavior. Students received three online sessions of fully tailored CTIs. The secondary behaviors of fruit and vegetable intake and limited television watching alternated between moderate and minimal (stage-only) tailoring. Over the course of the 6-month treatment, there were significant treatment effects in each of the three behaviors, but only changes in fruit and vegetable intake were sustained at 12 months. Significant coaction was found for each pair of behaviors in the treatment group but none in the control group. The amount of coaction decreased after treatment, suggesting that longer treatment may be needed for this age population where health risk behaviors tend to increase.

Mauriello et al. (2016) also successfully tested the concept of healthy pregnancy with women on Medicaid at Community health Clinics as they worked on multiple behaviors of stress management, smoking cessation, and healthy eating. As with any theory, effective applications may be limited more by our creativity than by the ability of the theory to drive significant research and effective interventions.

Prochaska et al. (2012) recruited 3391 adults from 39 states who were at risk for lack of exercise and ineffective stress management. This study involved a strategy for multiple tailored behavior change. One treatment group received a fully tailored TTM online for the primary behavior of stress management and minimal tailoring for exercise. A second group received three sessions of optimally tailored telephonic coaching for exercise and minimal tailoring for stress. In this study, the TTM exercise coaching outperformed the TTM online stress management, which outperformed the controls. Also, the exercise coaching produced significant effects on healthy eating and depression management, which were not treated. Finally, the same order of effective treatment was found for enhancing five domains of well-being: emotional health, physical health, life evaluation, thriving, and overall well-being. This study represents the greatest impact to date on decreasing health risk behaviors and increasing health and well-being; over time the outcomes will have much greater impact on populations with multiple risk behaviors who have the highest risk for mortality, disabilities, lost productivity, and increased health care costs (Prochaska 2008).

References and Further Reading

Evers, K. E., Prochaska, J. O., Johnson, J. L., Mauriello, L. M., Padula, J. A., & Prochaska, J. M. (2006). A randomized clinical trial of a population and transtheoretical model-based stress-management intervention. *Health Psychology, 25*, 521–529.

Hall, K. L., & Rossi, J. S. (2008). Meta-analytic examination of the strong and weak principles across 48 health behaviors. *Preventive Medicine, 46*, 266–274.

Johnson, S. S., Driskell, M. M., Johnson, J. L., Dyment, S. J., Prochaska, J. O., Prochaska, J. M., et al. (2006). Transtheoretical model intervention for adherence to lipid-lowering drugs. *Disease Management, 9*, 102–114.

Johnson, S. S., Paiva, A., Mauriello, L., Prochaska, J. O., Redding, C. A., & Velier, W. F. (2014). Coaction in multiple behavior change interventions: Consistency across multiple studies on weight management & obesity prevention. *Health Psychology, 33*(5), 475–480.

Mauriello, L. M., Ciavatta, M. M. H., Paiva, A. L., Sherman, K. J., Castle, P. H., Johnson, J. L., & Prochaska, J. M. (2010). Results of a multi-media multiple behavior obesity prevention program for adolescents. *Preventive Medicine, 51*, 451–456.

Mauriello, L. M., Van Marter, D. F., Umanzor, C. D., Castle, P. H., & de Aguiar, E. L. (2016). Using mhealth to deliver behavior change interventions within prenatal care at community health centers. *American Journal of Health Promotion, 30*(7), 554–562.

Paiva, A. L., Prochaska, J. O., Hui-Qing Yin, H., Redding, C. R., Rossi, J. S., Blissmer, B., Robbins, M. L., Velicer, W. F., Lipschitz, J., Amoyal, N. R., Babbin, S. F., Creeden, C. L., Sillice, M. A., Fernandez, A., McGee, H., & Horiuchi, S. (2012). Treated individuals who progress to action or maintenance for one behavior are more likely to make similar progress on another behavior: Coaction results of a pooled data analysis of three trials. *Preventive Medicine, 54*, 331–334.

Prochaska, J. O. (2008). Multiple health behavior research represents the future of preventive medicine. *Preventive Medicine, 46*, 281–285.

Prochaska, J. O., & DiClemente, C. C. (1983). Stages and processes of self-change of smoking: Toward an integrative model of change. *Journal of Consulting and Clinical Psychology, 51*, 390–395.

Prochaska, J. O., & Prochaska, J. M. (2016). *Changing to thrive: Using the stages of change to overcome the top threats to your health and happiness*. Center City: Hazelden Publishing.

Prochaska, J. O., DiClemente, C. C., & Norcross, J. C. (1992). In search of how people change: Applications to the addictive behaviors. *American Psychologist, 47*, 1102–1114.

Prochaska, J. O., Norcross, J. C., & DiClemente, C. C. (1994). *Changing for good*. New York: Morrow. Released in paperback by Avon, 1995.

Prochaska, J. O., Velicer, W. F., Fava, J. L., Rossi, J. S., & Tsoh, J. Y. (2001). Evaluating a population-based recruitment approach and a stage-based expert system intervention for smoking cessation. *Addictive Behaviors, 26*, 583–602.

Prochaska, J. J., Velicer, W. F., Prochaska, J. O., Deluschi, K. I., & Hall, S. M. (2006). Comparing intervention outcomes in smokers with single versus multiple behavior risks. *Health Psychology, 25*, 380–388.

Prochaska, J. O., Butterworth, S., Redding, C. A., Burden, V., Perrin, N., Leo, M., . . ., Prochaska, J. M. (2008). Initial efficacy of MI, TTM tailoring and HRI's with multiple behaviors for employee health promotion. *Preventive Medicine, 45*, 226–231.

Prochaska, J. O., Ever, K. E., Castle, P. H., Johnson, J. L., Prochaska, J. M., Rula, E. Y., . . ., Pope, J. E. (2012). Enhancing multiple domains of well-being by decreasing multiple health risk behaviors: A randomized clinical trial. *Population Health Management, 15*, 276–286.

Snow, M. G., Prochaska, J. O., & Rossi, J. S. (1992). Stages of change for smoking cessation among former problem drinkers: A cross-sectional analysis. *Journal of Substance Abuse, 4*, 107–116.

Velicer, W. F., Redding, C. A., Sun, X., & Prochaska, J. O. (2007). Demographic variables, smoking variables, and outcome across five studies. *Health Psychology, 26*(3), 278–287.

Trauma, Early Life

▶ Stress, Early Life

Traumatic Brain Injury

Mary Spiers and Emily W. Reid
Department of Psychology, Drexel University, Philadelphia, PA, USA

Synonyms

Brain damage; Brain injury; Brain trauma; Concussion; Head injury.

E. W. Reid: deceased.

Definition

Traumatic brain injury (TBI) is an acquired brain injury resulting in diffuse brain damage. Injury is caused by the direct impact of an external force or whiplash, which results in a rapid acceleration or deceleration of the brain against the skull. The rapid movement causes neurons to shear and tear, and the impact of the brain against the skull can result in bruising and bleeding. The trauma can cause secondary complications such as ischemia, increased blood pressure, or ruptured blood vessels. The impairments caused by TBI depend on its severity. Due to the diffuse nature of the injury, a variety of cognitive, emotional, and behavioral changes are often seen.

Description

Epidemiology of Traumatic Brain Injury

The CDC estimates that 1.5–2 million people suffer a traumatic brain injury (TBI) every year in the United States (Faul et al. 2010). Of those, an estimated 80% are mild in severity, 10% are moderate, and the remaining 10% have severe injuries (Kraus et al. 1996). A small proportion (estimated 275,000) are hospitalized, whereas 1.4 million are treated and released (Faul et al. 2010). This is likely to be an underestimate of incidence as many do not go to the emergency room, and it is estimated that 1.6–3.8 million sports-related TBIs occur each year, of which many are treated on the field and do not seek emergency room assistance (Brain Trauma Foundation 2011). Approximately 2% of the US population currently live with disabilities from TBI and represent a significant public health challenge (Brain Trauma Foundation 2011).

The majority of TBIs are caused by falls (35.2%), motor vehicle accidents (17.3%), striking or being struck by or against an object (16.5%), and assaults (10%) (Faul et al. 2010). Another common cause for military personnel is blast-related injury. Approximately 52,000 deaths each year are due to traumatic brain injury with motor vehicle accidents resulting in the largest number of fatalities (31.8%) (Faul et al. 2010).

TBI is the leading cause of death and disability for children and adults under the age of 44 (Brain Trauma Foundation 2011). Those most vulnerable to TBI are children, ages 0–4; older adolescents, ages 15–19; and adults over 65 years old. However, the number of emergency room visits for ages 0–14 is twice as many as those for adults over 65 years of age (Faul et al. 2010). Across all age groups, men sustain at least twice as many head injuries as women (Faul et al. 2010), and males, ages 0–4, have the highest rates of TBI-related emergency visits, hospitalizations, and deaths.

TBI also has a strong economic impact. In a 1998 consensus report from NIH, an estimated $9–10 billion were spent on new TBI cases each year ("Consensus Conference," 1999). Financially, the lifelong care for a person with a TBI is estimated to be between $600,000 and $1.9 million (Elias and Saucier 2006). The NIH acknowledges that these are likely underestimates of the actual cost, as these numbers do not reflect the lost earnings, costs to social services systems, and the value of time and forgone earnings of family members who care for persons with TBI (Elias and Saucier 2006). Further complications to care include insurance coverage, access to care, ability to navigate the health system, and available family and community support ("Consensus Conference," 1999).

Mechanism of Injury

Traumatic brain injury results either from object penetration or from rapid acceleration or deceleration of the brain resulting in the classifications of open head and closed head injuries.

Open or Penetrating Head Injury

In an open or penetrating head injury, the skull and the covering of the brain, or meninges, are ruptured. These injuries occur when an object (e.g., bullet, knife, bone fragment) lodges or passes through the brain. Because the brain is exposed, infection is a concern. Also, because penetrating head injuries may create more focal damage than in a closed head injury, the pattern of behavioral deficits is dependent on location of injury. After-effects of the initial injury, including swelling and bleeding, may cause more global, though usually time-limited, effects due to intracranial pressure or inflammatory response.

Closed Head Injury

The majority of head injuries are closed head injuries. These injuries occur by either direct impact or whiplash and may be caused by, for example, motor vehicle accidents, sports-related concussions, falls, and war-related blast injuries. The brain undergoes a rapid acceleration or deceleration or both but without skull penetration.

Contusions and/or hematomas may be seen at the location of impact (i.e., coup) and the opposite side of the brain (i.e., contre-coup) owing to the acceleration and deceleration of the brain against the skull. Despite the location of impact, a pattern of diffuse injury is likely to occur, impacting the frontal lobes and temporal poles because of the jagged surface of the tentorial plates that hold those brain structures in place. The physical forces may shear, tear, and rupture neurons, blood vessels, and the meninges, or covering, of the brain.

Diffuse axonal injury (DAI) may occur with shearing or tearing of neurons, often as a result of head rotation or rapid deceleration. Consequently, the axon damage can result in fewer axonal connections and/or less efficient transmission from one axon to another (Lux 2007). The neurons most vulnerable to this type of strain are those with long axons, usually white-matter tracts that connect distant brain regions. DAI produces two types of cell death, necrosis and apoptosis, which are the leading contributors to brain damage in closed head injuries. Both impede axonal transport, induce atypical metabolic changes, and cause the axon to swell. In DAI, the damage is widespread, regional, multifocal, and at times global, and the course of damage may change over time. The swelling leads to detachment downstream from other neurons. This pattern of deafferentation is considered to affect more neurons than those identified as originally damaged. Although the brain's plasticity does allow for new axonal growth in living neurons, spurious growth can cause additional complications by forming undesirable connections leading to behavioral disturbances.

Consequences of Traumatic Brain Injury

The neuropsychological and behavioral consequences of TBI are related to injury characteristics and severity. The injury characteristics of importance in the acute phase are length of loss of consciousness (LOC) and length of emergence into consciousness with accompanying degree of posttraumatic amnesia (PTA), characterized by confusion and disorientation. For example, LOC ranges from none to brief LOC in concussion and mild traumatic brain injury (MTBI) to weeks in severe head injury. Emergence into consciousness ranges from minutes to hours in MTBI to weeks to days in severe head injury. Corresponding recovery of neuropsychological functioning can range from days to years.

LOC and coma are directly associated with an injury to those areas of the brain, typically the lower brain stem and reticular activating system (RAS), that are involved in maintaining consciousness and arousal. Coma falls along a continuum related to depth of responsiveness and is typically assessed at regular intervals after an injury via the Glasgow Coma Scale (GCS) (Teasdale and Jennett 1974). The GCS assesses best motor, verbal, and eye opening response at one point in time. Scores range from 15 (can obey motor commands, is oriented, and eyes are open) to 3 (flaccid motor response, no verbal response, and no eye opening). Medically, coma is defined as a score of 3–8, which typically corresponds to a severe brain injury. Greater mortality is typically associated with scores below 7. Although initial severity of GCS is an important prognostic indicator for survival, other indicators, such as number of days to reach a GCS of 15, and length of PTA are added predictors for long-term neuropsychological outcome. Duration of PTA and education appear to be two of the best predictors of long-term functional outcome. On measures of global functioning and disability, those who had less education preinjury or a longer period of PTA had poorer outcomes 10 years after the injury (Ponsford et al. 2008).

The recovery from coma is a process of "emergence" in which greater awareness of environmental stimuli occurs. Characteristic of traumatic brain injury is a loss of recall for the actual impact event. Since the injured person does not recall the event, he or she cannot usually give a reliable account of the length of LOC. This period of PTA is characterized by confusion and disorientation and typically includes both retrograde and anterograde amnesia. Retrograde amnesia is the impairment in the retrieval of information for events preceding the injury. Conversely, anterograde amnesia is impairment in encoding new memories after the injury.

The difference in diagnosis between mild, moderate and severe head injuries relates both to immediate injury severity as rated by the GCS and time related to resolution of symptoms. For example, MTBI is characterized by a GCS score of 13–15 and a fairly rapid resolution of LOC (less than 30 min) and PTA (less than 24 h). Moderate-level brain injuries are characterized by a GCS of 9–12, LOC between 30 min and 24 h, and PTA between 1 and 7 days. Severe head injuries are those with a GCS of 3–8, LOC longer than a day, and PTA longer than 7 days.

Neuropsychological Consequences of TBI
The neuropsychological consequences of TBI may include a number of deficits. However, those deficits that correspond to frontal and temporal injuries, as well as diffuse axonal injuries are most common. Specifically, these include difficulties in attention, memory, and language functions, executive dysfunction, and emotionality.

Regardless of injury severity, attentional deficits are common after TBI. Reports include a feeling of mental slowness, difficulty following conversations, losing a train of thought, and trouble with multitasking (Gronwall 1987; Van Zomeren and Brouwer 1994). The most universal consequence is a reduced ability to process information (McCullagh and Feinstein 2005). Therefore, when tasks become more complex, reaction time becomes slower. As a result, a TBI sufferer may not appear cognitively impaired in simpler routine assessments, but the deficits may become more evident in the multicomponent tasks of daily life (Granacher 2008; Lux 2007). Deficits are seen across all types of attention processing, including selective, sustained, and divided attention with particular problems on tasks that require controlled rather than automatic processing (Park et al. 1999).

In addition to attention and working memory difficulties, a deficit in episodic memory is a hallmark feature of TBI (Richardson 2000). Memory impairment is one of the most frequent (Arcia and Gualtieri 1993; King et al. 1995) and long-lasting complaints with significant deficits found in many people 10 years postinjury (Zec et al. 2001) and poor employment prognosis 7 years postinjury (Brooks et al. 1987). Furthermore, TBI patients tend to have impairments in prospective memory, or remembering to perform an intended action, which may lead to forgetting appointments, payment of bills, and medication taking (Kinsella et al. 1996). Adding further difficulty, patients tend to be less aware of their memory difficulties than those around them (McCullagh and Feinstein 2005).

Those with TBI may also experience language and communication difficulties. Speech tends to be less productive and efficient, with less content in longer discourse, and with greater fragmentation (Hartley and Jensen 1991). Additionally, language difficulties may include trouble naming objects and, to a lesser extent, comprehension of complex commands (Levin et al. 1976; Sarno et al. 1986).

Deficits in executive functioning influence functional, emotional, and social outcomes after TBI. The term "executive functioning" refers to higher-order capabilities that include goal setting, planning, initiating, sequencing, reasoning abilities, decision making, inhibiting responses, self-monitoring, and self-regulation (Stuss and Levine 2002). Since these processes underlie many daily and social skills, such as impulse control, judgment, creativity, emotional regulation, and moral judgment, routine testing might not detect the degree of impairment evident in these areas (Zillmer et al. 2008). Verbal fluency tests, as a measure of executive dysfunction, however, consistently show impairment for TBI patients because they require organization of verbal retrieval and recall, self-monitoring aspects of cognition, and effortful self-initiation and inhibition of responses. (Henry and Crawford 2004)

Emotional and behavioral complications are common after TBI and often lead to depressed and anxious mood, impulsivity, agitation, and amotivation (Vaishnavi et al. 2009). Mood disturbances are considered the most common psychiatric complication of TBI and are often the most difficult adjustment for those who care for the TBI patient (Rosenthal et al. 1998). Approximately 10–60% of patients are depressed, reporting feelings of hopelessness, worthlessness, and anhedonia (Hurley and Taber 2002). Also, they display somatic symptoms, such as sleep disturbances, reduced initiation, fatigue, and changes in appetite. TBI patients have reduced participation in leisure activities and have difficulty engaging in new hobbies (Rosenthal et al. 1998). Mood disturbances can cause significant emotional distress in patients with TBI, contributing to the disruption of social relationships.

In sum, while a pattern of neuropsychological deficits in TBI may show common features, the evaluation of any particular individual should include a consideration of the unique injury location and severity features in a context of previous levels of education, work, and social history.

Cross-References

▶ Brain Damage
▶ Brain, Injury
▶ Neuropsychology

References and Readings

Arcia, E., & Gualtieri, C. T. (1993). Association between patient report of symptoms after mild head injury and neurobehavioural performance. *Brain Injury, 7,* 481–489.

Brain Trauma Foundation. (2011). Facts about TBI in the USA. Retrieved March 3, 2011, from https://www.braintrauma.org/tbi-faqs/tbi-statistics/

Brooks, N., McKinlay, W., Symington, C., Beattie, A., & Campsie, L. (1987). Return to work within the first seven years of severe head injury. *Brain Injury, 1,* 5–19.

Consensus Conference Writing Group. (1999). Consensus conference. Rehabilitation of persons with traumatic brain injury. NIH consensus development panel on rehabilitation of persons with traumatic brain injury. *Journal of the American Medical Association, 282*(10), 974–983. jcf90001(pii).

Elias, L. J., & Saucier, D. M. (2006). *Neuropsychology: Clinical and experimental foundations.* Boston: Pearson/Allyn & Bacon.

Faul, M., Xu, L., Wald, M. M., & Coronado, V. G. (2010). Traumatic brain injury in the United States: Emergency department visits, hospitalizations and deaths 2002–2006. Retrieved March 3, 2011, from www.cdc.gov/TraumaticBrainInjury

Granacher, R. P. (2008). *Traumatic brain injury: Methods for clinical and forensic neuropsychiatric assessment* (2nd ed.). Boca Raton: CRC Press/Taylor & Francis Group.

Gronwall, D. (1987). *Advances in the assessment of attention and information processing after head injury in neurobehavioral recovery from head injury.* New York: Oxford University Press.

Hartley, L. L., & Jensen, P. J. (1991). Narrative and procedural discourse after closed head injury. *Brain Injury, 5*(3), 267–285.

Henry, J. D., & Crawford, J. R. (2004). A meta-analytic review of verbal fluency performance in patients with traumatic brain injury. *Neuropsychology, 18*(4), 621–628. https://doi.org/10.1037/0894-4105.18.4.621.

Hurley, R. A., & Taber, K. H. (2002). Emotional disturbances following traumatic brain injury. *Current Treatment Options in Neurology, 4*(1), 59–75.

King, N. S., Crawford, S., Wenden, F. J., Moss, N. E., & Wade, D. T. (1995). The rivermead post concussion symptoms questionnaire: A measure of symptoms commonly experienced after head injury and its reliability. *Journal of Neurology, 242*(9), 587–592.

Kinsella, G., Murtagh, D., Landry, A., Homfray, K., Hammond, M., & O'Beirne, L. (1996). Everyday memory following traumatic brain injury. *Brain Injury, 10*(7), 499–507.

Kraus, J. F., McArthur, D. L., Silverman, T. A., & Jayaraman, M. (1996). Epidemiology of brain injury. In R. K. Naravan, J. E. Wilberger, & J. T. Povlishock (Eds.), *Neurotrauma.* New York: McGraw-Hill.

Levin, H. S., Grossman, R. G., & Kelly, P. J. (1976). Aphasic disorder in patients with closed head injury. *Journal of Neurology, Neurosurgery & Psychiatry, 39*(11), 1062–1070.

Lux, W. E. (2007). A neuropsychiatric perspective on traumatic brain injury. *Journal of Rehabilitation Research and Development, 44*(7), 951–962.

McCullagh, S., & Feinstein, A. (2005). Cognitive changes. In J. M. Silver, T. W. McAllister, & S. C. Yudofsky (Eds.), Textbook of traumatic brain injury (1stst ed., p. 321). Washington, DC: American Psychiatric.

Park, N. W., Moscovitch, M., & Robertson, I. H. (1999). Divided attention impairments after traumatic brain injury. *Neuropsychologia, 37*(10), 1119–1133. S0028393299000342[pii].

Ponsford, J., Draper, K., & Schonberger, M. (2008). Functional outcome 10 years after traumatic brain injury: Its relationship with demographic, injury severity, and cognitive and emotional status. *Journal of International Neuropsychological Society, 14*(2), 233–242. https://doi.org/10.1017/S1355617708080272.

Richardson, J. (2000). *Clinical and neuropsychological aspects of closed head injury.* East Sussex: Psychology Press.

Rosenthal, M., Christensen, B. K., & Ross, T. P. (1998). Depression following traumatic brain injury. *Archives*

- *of Physical Medicine and Rehabilitation, 79*(1), 90–103.
- Sarno, M. T., Buonaguro, A., & Levita, E. (1986). Characteristics of verbal impairment in closed head injured patients. *Archives of Physical Medicine and Rehabilitation, 67*(6), 400–405.
- Stuss, D. T., & Levine, B. (2002). Adult clinical neuropsychology: Lessons from studies of the frontal lobes. *Annual Review of Psychology, 53*, 401–433. https://doi.org/10.1146/annurev.psych.53.100901.13522053/1/401[pii].
- Teasdale, G., & Jennett, B. (1974). Assessment of coma and impaired consciousness. A practical scale. *Lancet, 2*, 81–84.
- Vaishnavi, S., Rao, V., & Fann, J. R. (2009). Neuropsychiatric problems after traumatic brain injury: Unraveling the silent epidemic. *Psychosomatics, 50*(3), 198–205. https://doi.org/10.1176/appi.psy.50.3.198.
- Van Zomeren, A., & Brouwer, W. (1994). *Clinical neuropsychology of attention*. New York: Oxford University Press.
- Zec, R. F., Zellers, D., Belman, J., Miller, J., Matthews, J., & Femeau-Belman, D. (2001). Long-term consequences of severe closed head injury on episodic memory. *Journal of Clinical and Experimental Neuropsychology, 23*(5), 671–691.
- Zillmer, E. A., Spiers, M. V., & Culbertson, W. C. (2008). *Principles of neuropsychology* (2nd ed.). Belmont: Thomson/Wadsworth.

Treatment of Fatigue

▶ Fatigue

Trier Social Stress Test

Lisa Juliane Weckesser[1], Robert Miller[1] and Clemens Kirschbaum[2]
[1]Faculty of Psychology, Technische Universität Dresden, Dresden, Germany
[2]Department of Psychology, Faculty of Psychology, Technische Universität Dresden, Dresden, Germany

Synonyms

Laboratory stress protocol; Psychosocial stress; Stress

Definition

The Trier Social Stress Test is a standardized protocol for the reliable induction of acute psychosocial stress responses under laboratory conditions.

Description

Stress is a critical determinant of mental health (Van Hedger et al. 2017). Since impairments in mental health often manifest or aggravate in response to acute stress, investigating acute stress responses might reveal mechanisms that promote the transition from health to stress-related health impairments (Zänkert et al. 2019). To do this under standardized laboratory conditions, the Trier Social Stress Test (TSST) has been developed (Kirschbaum et al. 1993).

The TSST protocol consists of four components of 5 min each, i.e., instruction, preparation, free speech (covered as job interview), and mental arithmetic (totaling 20 min; Kirschbaum et al. 1993). In its most recent version, it requires three employees, one of whom functions as experimenter and two as mixed-gender jurors trained to withhold any positive or negative feedback during the whole procedure (i.e., stay neutral). A separate room equipped with two desks (one for the jurors, one for the participant), a watch with seconds hand, a video camera, and a microphone placed approx. 1 m in front of the jurors' table is additionally required. Before entering the TSST room, the experimenter asks the participant for which position he/she would hypothetically apply for (without providing any further information about the TSST). In front of the microphone, he/she informs the participant about the upcoming tasks (preparation, speech and mental arithmetic). Regarding the preparation, the participant is told that he/she may take notes about his/her speech but may not use them while giving the speech. Concerning the free speech, the participant is instructed to present only personality traits which qualify him/her for the position in question (but not any information usually provided in a curriculum vitae). After giving this instruction, the experimenter leaves the room, and the participant takes a seat at the second table to prepare his/her speech. Henceforth, only the opposite-sex juror speaks to the participant, with the same-sex juror being responsible for camera operation. After exactly 5 minutes, one juror starts the camera, the other asks the participant to step in front of the microphone and give the free speech. Most participants have little more to say after approx. 2 minutes. Only after 20 s of silence, the juror asks the participant to continue with the speech as there is still time available. After making this request repeatedly without producing any speech response, the participant is asked a standardized question (e.g., about strengths and weaknesses). After 5 min of speaking, the participant is instructed to stop and continue with the mental arithmetic task comprising of a continuous serial subtraction of 17 from 2043 and to start anew from the initial number with every error he/she is made aware of. After 5 min of mental arithmetic, the participant is asked to stop and leave the room, in front of which he/she is awaited by the experimenter (for further assessments).

If the TSST protocol is implemented as described, it induces psychosocial stress responses in more than 70% of participants (Miller et al. 2013; Zänkert et al. 2019). These responses are characterized by the perception of threat to one's own social esteem or status, uncontrollability, and unpredictability (more detailed information is provided below), as well as by the activation of the sympathetic-adrenal-medullary (SAM) system and the hypothalamic-pituitary-adrenal (HPA) axis (i.e., two key stress response systems; Dickerson and Kemeny 2004; Koolhaas et al. 2011). Social-evaluative threat, unpredictability, and uncontrollability are monitored by self-report measures (peaking in anticipation of or during the TSST exposure; Campbell and Ehlert 2012; Hellhammer and Schubert 2012). Usually, SAM system activity is characterized by plasma (nor) epinephrine or salivary amylase concentrations as well as heart rate (variability), blood pressure, and electrodermal activity (peaking during TSST exposure and returning to resting values within the first 10 min after TSST cessation; Kirschbaum et al. 1993; Schommer et al. 2003; Ulrich-Lai and Herman 2009). HPA axis activity is mostly characterized by plasma or salivary cortisol (peaking 10 to 25 min after TSST cessation and returning to resting values within 90 min after TSST cessation) or less frequently by plasma adrenocorticotropic hormone or corticotropin-releasing hormone concentrations (wherein the latter two hormones finally lead to cortisol secretion; Kirschbaum et al. 1993; Schommer et al. 2003). Although the TSST induces alterations in many other systems as well, such as the low-grade inflammation in the innate immune system (Rohleder 2019), most of the TSST literature so far has focussed on acute HPA axis activity as indicated by cortisol concentrations in healthy as well as participant samples (Goodman et al. 2017; Miller and Kirschbaum 2019; Van Hedger et al. 2017; Zänkert et al. 2019).

This focus on HPA axis activity was largely based on findings showing that the HPA axis, unlike the SAM system, is only reliably activated in response to anticipated or perceived uncontrollability, unpredictability, or social-evaluative threat, but not in response to any physical or appetitive stimulation (de Souza Vale et al. 2010; Dickerson and Kemeny 2004; Hackney 2006; Hamilton et al. 2009; Krueger et al. 1998; Lovallo et al. 1990). This makes the HPA axis one if not the most specific stress response system to date and qualifies its humoral end product cortisol as an ideal analyte to quantify acute stress responses (Koolhaas et al. 2011). Importantly, the TSST affects all three components required for HPA axis activation: unpredictability (esp. of the tasks and their duration), uncontrollability (esp. of the juries' response and thus the outcome of the fictitious job interview), and social-evaluative threat (esp. through the presence of the jury and camera, as well as the risk of negative judgment and subsequent loss of social esteem or status; Dickerson and Kemeny 2004; Kirschbaum et al. 1993; Zänkert et al. 2019). These properties make the TSST superior to alternative stress-induction protocols, which is reflected in higher peak cortisol concentrations and longer recovery periods (that enable the reliable assessment of outcome variables) or the existence of first evidence confirming its external validity (Dickerson and Kemeny 2004; Henze et al. 2017; Zänkert et al. 2019).

The frequent and successful employment of the TSST in young adult populations has stimulated its adaptation for specific participant samples (e.g., children, retirees, psychiatric patients, and groups; Brenner et al. 2009; Buske-Kirschbaum et al. 1997; Kudielka et al. 1998; von Dawans et al. 2011) as well as the development of standardized control protocols (that do not reliably affect any of the aforementioned indicators of acute stress responses; Het et al. 2009; Wiemers et al. 2013). The TSST is therefore one of the most powerful tools to induce acute stress responses (with HPA axis activity) in the laboratory and thus well-suited to investigate stress-related alterations in health behavior or outcome measures (that comprises HPA axis activity itself; Kudielka et al. 2009; Zänkert et al. 2019).

The frequent use of the TSST has also enabled the identification of moderators of HPA axis activation or peak cortisol concentrations using meta-analytical methods (Dickerson and Kemeny 2004; Goodman et al. 2017; Miller and Kirschbaum 2019). Among these, gender, age (Miller and Kirschbaum 2019), oral contraceptive intake (Liu et al. 2017), glucose status (Gonzalez-Bono et al. 2002), and previous experience with the TSST (Kudielka et al. 2006; Petrowski et al. 2012; Schommer et al. 2003; Wüst et al. 2005) seem to be among the strongest moderators of TSST-induced HPA axis activity or peak cortisol concentrations (whereby high age, male sex, no oral contraceptive intake, high glucose availability, and no previous experience with the TSST are associated with higher peak cortisol concentrations than the respective control condition). Gender of the jurors, pre-TSST acclimation time, and the valence of the jurors' feedback appear to be the strongest methodological moderators of HPA axis activity or peak cortisol concentrations (with mixed-gender juries, acclimation times between 15 and 30 min, and neutral feedback inducing higher peak cortisol concentrations than the respective control condition; Goodman et al. 2017). Less important for HPA axis activity or peak cortisol concentrations – but of utmost importance to increase the comparability across different studies and laboratories using the TSST – seem to be time of the day, the number of jurors, and venepuncture prior to TSST exposure (Goodman et al. 2017). Taken together, the completion of TSST studies in the afternoon with two mixed-gender jurors, no venepuncture, and the administration of a glucose-containing beverage (e.g., 200 ml grape juice) directly before TSST exposure is recommended along with the highest possible adherence to the above described TSST procedure and documentation of any protocol deviation (further recommendations are given in Gonzalez-Bono et al. 2002; Zänkert et al. 2019).

Despite its advantages and the high amount of accumulated knowledge about the TSST, further research is needed especially with respect to its transfer to scanning or virtual reality environment (with the existing adaptations still inducing comparably low and/or less reliable HPA axis activation or cortisol peak concentrations; Jönsson et al. 2010; Pruessner et al. 2008; Smeets et al. 2012) and the still lacking explanation of systematic differences in the TSST-induced peak cortisol concentrations between different study populations (that is not attributable to the abovementioned participant-related or methodological moderators; Miller and Kirschbaum 2019).

Cross-References

- Biomarkers
- Cortisol
- Stress
- Stress Response

References and Further Readings

Brenner, K., Liu, A., Laplante, D. P., Lupien, S., Pruessner, J. C., Ciampi, A., Joober, R., & King, S. (2009). Cortisol response to a psychosocial stressor in schizophrenia: Blunted, delayed, or normal? *Psychoneuroendocrinology, 34*(6), 859–868.

Buske-Kirschbaum, A., Jobst, S., Wustmans, A., Kirschbaum, C., Rauh, W., & Hellhammer, D. (1997). Attenuated free cortisol response to psychosocial stress in children with atopic dermatitis. *Psychosomatic Medicine, 59*(4), 419–426.

Campbell, J., & Ehlert, U. (2012). Acute psychosocial stress: Does the emotional stress response correspond with physiological responses? *Psychoneuroendocrinology, 37*(8), 1111–1134.

de Souza Vale, R. G., Rosa, G., Júnior, R. J. N., & Dantas, E. H. M. (2010). Cortisol and physical exercise. In A. Esposito & B. Vito (Eds.), *Cortisol: Physiology, regulation and health implications* (pp. 129–138). New York: Nova Science Publisher.

Dickerson, S. S., & Kemeny, M. E. (2004). Acute stressors and cortisol responses: A theoretical integration and synthesis of laboratory research. *Psychological Bulletin, 130*(3), 355–391.

Gonzalez-Bono, E., Rohleder, N., Hellhammer, D. H., Salvador, A., & Kirschbaum, C. (2002). Glucose but not protein or fat load amplifies the cortisol response to psychosocial stress. *Hormones and Behavior, 41*(3), 328–333.

Goodman, W. K., Janson, J., & Wolf, J. M. (2017). Meta-analytical assessment of the effects of protocol variations on cortisol responses to the Trier social stress test. *Psychoneuroendocrinology, 80*, 26–35.

Hackney, A. C. (2006). Stress and the neuroendocrine system: The role of exercise as a stressor and modifier of stress. *Expert Reviews in Endocrinology and Metabolism, 1*(6), 783–792.

Hamilton, L. D., Rellini, A. H., & Meston, C. M. (2009). Cortisol, sexual arousal, and affect in response to sexual stimuli. *The Journal of Sexual Medicine, 5*(9), 2111–2118.

Hellhammer, J., & Schubert, M. (2012). The physiological response to Trier social stress test relates to subjective measures of stress during but not before or after the test. *Psychoneuroendocrinology, 37*(1), 119–124.

Henze, G. I., Zänkert, S., Urschler, D. F., Hiltl, T. J., Kudielka, B. M., Pruessner, J. C., & Wüst, S. (2017). Testing the ecological validity of the Trier social stress test: Association with real-life exam stress. *Psychoneuroendocrinology, 75*, 52–55.

Het, S., Rohleder, N., Schoofs, D., Kirschbaum, C., & Wolf, O. T. (2009). Neuroendocrine and psychometric evaluation of a placebo version of the "Trier Social Stress Test". *Psychoneuroendocrinology, 34*(7), 1075–1086.

Jönsson, P., Wallergård, M., Österberg, K., Hansen, Å. M., Johansson, G., & Karlson, B. (2010). Cardiovascular and cortisol reactivity and habituation to a virtual reality version of the Trier social stress test: A pilot study. *Psychoneuroendocrinology, 35*(9), 1397–1403.

Kirschbaum, C., Pirke, K. M., & Hellhammer, D. H. (1993). The "Trier Social Stress Test" – A tool for investigating psychobiological stress responses in a laboratory setting. *Neuropsychobiology, 28*, 76–81.

Koolhaas, J. M., Bartolomucci, A., Buwalda, B., de Boer, S. F., Fluegge, G., Korte, S. M., Meerlo, P., Murison, R., Olivier, B., Palanza, P., Richter-Levin, G., Sgoifo, A., Steimer, T., Stiedl, O., van Dijk, G., Wöhr, M., & Fuchs, E. (2011). Stress revisited: A critical evaluation of the stress concept. *Neuroscience and Biobehavioral Reviews, 35*(5), 1291–1301.

Krueger, T., Exton, M. S., Pawlak, C., von zur Muehlen, A., Hartmann, U., & Schedlowski, M. (1998). Neuroendocrine and cardiovascular response to sexual arousal and orgasm in men. *Psychoneuroendocrinology, 23*(4), 401–411.

Kudielka, B. M., Hellhammer, J., Hellhammer, D. H., Wolf, O. T., Pirke, K. M., Varadi, E., Pilz, J., & Kirschbaum, C. (1998). Sex differences in endocrine and psychological responses to psychosocial stress in healthy elderly subjects and the impact of a 2-week dehydroepiandrosterone treatment. *The Journal of Clinical Endocrinology & Metabolism, 83*(5), 1756–1761.

Kudielka, B. M., Von Känel, R., Preckel, D., Zgraggen, L., Mischler, K., & Fischer, J. E. (2006). Exhaustion is associated with reduced habituation of free cortisol responses to repeated acute psychosocial stress. *Biological Psychology, 72*(2), 147–153.

Kudielka, B. M., Hellhammer, D. H., & Wüst, S. (2009). Why do we respond so differently? Reviewing determinants of human salivary cortisol responses to challenge. *Psychoneuroendocrinology, 34*(1), 2–18.

Liu, J. J. W., Ein, N., Peck, K., Huang, V., Pruessner, J. C., & Vickers, K. (2017). Sex differences in salivary cortisol reactivity to the Trier social stress test (TSST): A meta-analysis. *Psychoneuroendocrinology, 82*, 26–37.

Lovallo, W. R., Pincomb, G. A., Brackett, D. J., & Wislon, M. F. (1990). Heart rate reactivity as a predictor of neuroendocrine responses to aversive and appetitive challenges. *Psychosomatic Medicine, 52*, 17–26.

Miller, R., & Kirschbaum, C. (2019). Cultures under stress: A cross-national meta-analysis of cortisol responses to the Trier social stress test and their association with anxiety-related value orientations and internalizing mental disorders. *Psychoneuroendocrinology, 105*, 147–154.

Miller, R., Plessow, F., Kirschbaum, C., & Stalder, T. (2013). Classification criteria for distinguishing cortisol responders from nonresponders to psychosocial stress: Evaluation of salivary cortisol pulse detection in panel designs. *Psychosomatic Medicine, 75*(9), 832–840.

Petrowski, K., Wintermann, G. B., & Siepmann, M. (2012). Cortisol response to repeated psychosocial stress. *Applied Psychophysiology Biofeedback, 37*(2), 103–107.

Pruessner, J. C., Dedovic, K., Khalili-Mahani, N., Engert, V., Pruessner, M., Buss, C., Renwick, R., Dagher, A., Meaney, M. J., & Lupien, S. J. (2008). Deactivation of the limbic system during acute psychosocial stress: Evidence from positron emission tomography and functional magnetic resonance imaging studies. *Biological Psychiatry, 63*(2), 234–240.

Rohleder, N. (2019). Stress and inflammation – The need to address the gap in the transition between acute and chronic stress effects. *Psychoneuroendocrinology, 105*, 164–171.

Schommer, N. C., Hellhammer, D. H., & Kirschbaum, C. (2003). Dissociation between reactivity of the hypothalamus-pituitary-adrenal axis and the sympathetic-adrenal-medullary system to repeated psychosocial stress. *Psychosomatic Medicine, 65*(3), 450–460.

Smeets, T., Cornelisse, S., Quaedflieg, C. W. E. M., Meyer, T., Jelicic, M., & Merckelbach, H. (2012). Introducing the Maastricht acute stress test (MAST): A quick and non-invasive approach to elicit robust autonomic and glucocorticoid stress responses. *Psychoneuroendocrinology, 37*(12), 1998–2008.

Ulrich-Lai, Y. M., & Herman, J. P. (2009). Neural regulation of endocrine and autonomic stress responses. *Nature Reviews Neuroscience, 10*(6), 397–409.

Van Hedger, K., Bershad, A. K., & de Wit, H. (2017). Pharmacological challenge studies with acute psychosocial stress. *Psychoneuroendocrinology, 85*, 123–133.

von Dawans, B., Kirschbaum, C., & Heinrichs, M. (2011). The Trier social stress test for groups (TSST-G): A new research tool for controlled simultaneous social stress exposure in a group format. *Psychoneuroendocrinology, 36*(4), 514–522.

Wiemers, U. S., Schoofs, D., & Wolf, O. T. (2013). A friendly version of the Trier social stress test does not activate the HPA axis in healthy men and women. *Stress, 16*(2), 254–260.

Wüst, S., Federenko, I. S., Van Rossum, E. F. C., Koper, J. W., & Hellhammer, D. H. (2005). Habituation of cortisol responses to repeated psychosocial stress – further characterization and impact of genetic factors. *Psychoneuroendocrinology, 30*(2), 199–211.

Zänkert, S., Bellingrath, S., Wüst, S., & Kudielka, B. M. (2019). HPA axis responses to psychological challenge linking stress and disease: What do we know on sources of intra- and interindividual variability? *Psychoneuroendocrinology, 105*, 86 97.

Triglyceride

Chad Barrett
Department of Psychology, University of Colorado, Denver, CO, USA

Synonyms

Lipid

Definition

Triglycerides are a type of lipid (fat) which consist of glycerol and three molecules of fatty acid and are found in blood plasma and fat tissue. They are derived from fats and carbohydrates that are consumed. When calories are consumed, the body converts any calories not immediately used by tissues into triglycerides and transports them into fat cells for storage. Hormones regulate the release of triglycerides from fat tissues in order to provide energy for the body between meals. If the body uses fewer calories than are consumed in a day, then the surplus of calories can cause elevated levels of triglycerides (Welson 2006).

According to the American Heart Association, the normal level of triglycerides is less than 150 mg/dL and the optimal level of triglycerides is 100 mg/dL or lower. Borderline high levels range from 150 to 199 mg/dL; high levels range from 200 to 499 mg/dL; very high levels range from 500 mg/dL and above. Elevated levels of triglycerides are often the result of being overweight, physically inactive, smoking, excessive consumption of alcohol, and diets high in fat and carbohydrates. High levels of triglycerides have been linked to atherosclerosis (hardening of the arteries) and increased risk of heart disease, stroke, metabolic syndrome (Triglycerides 2010; What Your Cholesterol Levels Mean 2011), and Alzheimer's disease (Altman and Rutledge 2010). Interventions to lower triglycerides typically involve changes in lifestyle such as losing weight, adopting a more heart-healthy diet consisting of less fats and foods with added sugars, engaging in regular exercise, quitting smoking, and reducing alcohol consumption (Haffner et al. 2005; Graves and Miller 2003; Triglycerides 2010). Omega-3 fatty acids can also help reduce triglyceride levels and reduce the risk of cardiovascular diseases and possibly even strokes (Kris-Etherton et al. 2002).

Cross-References

▶ Cardiovascular Disease
▶ Cardiovascular Disease Prevention
▶ Cholesterol

References and Readings

Altman, R., & Rutledge, J. C. (2010). The vascular contribution to Alzheimer's disease. *Clinical Science, 119*, 07–421. Retrieved from http://www.ncbi.nlm.nih.gov/pubmed/20684749.

Graves, K. D., & Miller, P. M. (2003). Behavioral medicine in the prevention and treatment of cardiovascular disease. *Behavior Modification, 27*, 3–25.

Haffner, S., Temprosa, M., Crandall, J., Fowler, S., Goldberg, R., Horton, E., et al. (2005). Intensive lifestyle. Intervention or metformin on inflammation and coagulation in participants with impaired glucose tolerance. *Diabetes, 54*, 1566–1572.

Kris-Etherton, P. M., Harris, W. S., & Appel, L. J. (2002). Fish consumption, fish oil, omega-3 fatty acids and cardiovascular disease. *Circulation, 106*, 2747–2757. Retrieved from http://circ.ahajournals.org/content/106/21/2747.full.

Triglycerides. (2010). Retrieved October 10, 2011, from http://www.heart.org/HEARTORG/GettingHealthy/NutritionCenter/Triglycerides_UCM_306029_Article.jsp

Welson, L. T. (2006). *Triglycerides and cholesterol research*. New York: Nova.

What your cholesterol levels mean. (2011). Retrieved October 10, 2011, from http://www.heart.org/HEARTORG/Conditions/Cholesterol/AboutCholesterol/What-Your-Cholesterol-Levels-Mean_UCM_305562_Article.jsp

tRNA

▶ RNA

Tumor Necrosis Factor-Alpha (TNF-Alpha)

Nicolas Rohleder
Department of Psychology, Brandeis University, Waltham, MA, USA

Synonyms

Cachectin

Definition

Tumor necrosis factor-alpha (TNF-alpha) belongs to the group of pro-inflammatory cytokines. Cytokines are chemical messenger molecules of the immune system, and the group of pro-inflammatory cytokines characterizes molecules that are secreted in response to inflammatory stimuli, and further promote inflammatory responses in target cells. The cytokine now known as tumor necrosis factor-alpha was first discovered as a molecule that appeared to be essential in the wasting syndrome associated with bacterial infection, and therefore initially referred to as cachectin. At the same time, another molecule was discovered that induced pronounced necrosis of certain tumors in organisms infected by gram-negative bacteria. This molecule turned out to be identical to cachectin, and both were then called tumor necrosis factor-alpha (Beutler and Cerami 1989; Pennica et al. 1984).

TNF-alpha is one of the major products secreted by macrophages that are activated by inflammatory stimuli, and it acts through a family of different receptors that have some structural similarities and are present as transmembrane proteins on a variety of target cells. There are two different categories of receptors, based on their effect on the target cell. The first category is characterized by intracellular signals preceding programmed cell death; these are most likely the receptors that mediate the tumor necrotic effects of TNF. The second category induces pro-inflammatory effects, for example, by stimulation of proliferation or transcription of further inflammatory mediators. On a systemic level, TNF-alpha plays a notable role in sepsis and in the induction of septic shock. Similar to the interleukins (IL)-6 and −18, TNF-alpha does also act on nonimmune tissues such as endothelial cells, adipocytes, muscle cells, the liver, and the gastrointestinal tract (Beutler and Bazzoni 1998; Hehlgans and Pfeffer 2005).

Of note, along with IL-1, TNF-alpha is an important mediator of CNS effects of peripheral inflammation. TNF-signaling into the CNS has been shown to activate the hypothalamus-pituitary-adrenal axis, to induce hyperalgesia, to reduce food intake, and to contribute to the well-described sickness behavior response (e.g., Besedovsky et al. 1991; Watkins et al. 1995). This immune-to-CNS signaling function of TNF-alpha and other inflammatory cytokines plays an essential role in the control of peripheral inflammation during infectious and inflammatory diseases, and disruption of this loop leads to death in animal models of inflammatory diseases (Sternberg 2006).

TNF-alpha and other inflammatory cytokines are further important as targets of CNS-to-immune signaling, and serve as a link between CNS states with disease-relevant pathophysiological factors. Inflammatory cytokine production is modulated by the sympathetic nervous system and the hypothalamus-pituitary-adrenal axis, and pro-inflammatory cytokines in blood are sensitive to acute and chronic stress, and found increased in depression and posttraumatic stress disorder (e.g., Rohleder et al. 2009, 2010; Steptoe et al. 2007). Inflammatory cytokines also increase with age and have been found to predict later life morbidity and mortality (e.g., Bruunsgaard et al. 2003).

Cross-References

▶ Depression
▶ Inflammation
▶ Post Traumatic Stress Disorder
▶ Psychoneuroimmunology
▶ Stress

References and Readings

Besedovsky, H. O., del Rey, A., Klusman, I., Furukawa, H., Monge Arditi, G., & Kabiersch, A. (1991). Cytokines as modulators of the hypothalamus-pituitary-adrenal axis. *The Journal of Steroid Biochemistry and Molecular Biology, 40*(4–6), 613–618.

Beutler, B., & Bazzoni, F. (1998). TNF, apoptosis and autoimmunity: A common thread? *Blood Cells, Molecules & Diseases, 24*(2), 216–230.

Beutler, B., & Cerami, A. (1989). The biology of cachectin/TNF – a primary mediator of the host response. *Annual Review of Immunology, 7*, 625–655.

Bruunsgaard, H., Ladelund, S., Pedersen, A. N., Schroll, M., Jorgensen, T., & Pedersen, B. K. (2003). Predicting death from tumour necrosis factor-alpha and interleukin-6 in 80-year-old people. *Clinical and Experimental Immunology, 132*(1), 24–31.

Hehlgans, T., & Pfeffer, K. (2005). The intriguing biology of the tumour necrosis factor/tumour necrosis factor receptor superfamily: Players, rules and the games. *Immunology, 115*(1), 1–20.

Pennica, D., Nedwin, G. E., Hayflick, J. S., Seeburg, P. H., Derynck, R., Palladino, M. A., et al. (1984). Human tumour necrosis factor: Precursor structure, expression and homology to lymphotoxin. *Nature, 312*(5996), 724–729.

Rohleder, N., Marin, T. J., Ma, R., & Miller, G. E. (2009). Biologic cost of caring for a cancer patient: Dysregulation of pro- and anti-inflammatory signaling pathways. *Journal of Clinical Oncology, 27*(18), 2909–2915.

Rohleder, N., Wolf, J. M., & Wolf, O. T. (2010). Glucocorticoid sensitivity of cognitive and inflammatory processes in depression and posttraumatic stress disorder. *Neuroscience and Biobehavioral Reviews, 35*(1), 104–114.

Steptoe, A., Hamer, M., & Chida, Y. (2007). The effects of acute psychological stress on circulating inflammatory factors in humans: A review and meta-analysis. *Brain, Behavior, and Immunity, 21*(7), 901–912.

Sternberg, E. M. (2006). Neural regulation of innate immunity: A coordinated nonspecific host response to pathogens. *Nature Reviews: Immunology, 6*(4), 318–328.

Watkins, L. R., Goehler, L. E., Relton, J., Brewer, M. T., & Maier, S. F. (1995). Mechanisms of tumor necrosis factor-alpha (TNF-alpha) hyperalgesia. *Brain Research, 692*(1–2), 244–250.

TV Viewing

▶ Screen Time

Twin Studies

Jennifer Wessel
Public Health, School of Medicine, Indiana University, Indianapolis, IN, USA

Definition

The classic twin study builds on the fact that there are two kinds of twins that provide contrasting degrees of genetic relationship in siblings of the same age and family circumstances. Monozygotic (MZ) twins, or identical twins, have identical copies of all their genes. In contrast, dizygotic (DZ) twins, or fraternal twins, share, on average, only half of their genes by descent, as do ordinary siblings.

If there are genetic influences on the phenotype of interest, the MZ correlation will exceed that for the DZ twins. The greater the influence of the genes in determining individual differences in the phenotype, i.e., the greater the proportion of phenotypic variance attributable to genetic differences, the greater the difference between the MZ and DZ correlations will be. With some simplification of assumptions, twice the difference between the MZ and DZ correlations can be taken as an estimate of the heritability of the trait.

If genetic influences are the only cause of familial aggregation, if there is no nonadditive genetic variation, and if mating is random with respect to the characteristic under study, the correlation for DZ twins would be expected to be half that for MZ twins. However, if there are significant nonadditive genetic influences or there is significant competition between the twins or other contrast effects that accentuate the genetic differences of siblings, the DZ correlation may be less than half the MZ correlation. Conversely, assortative mating (like marrying like) or imitative or cooperative effects within the sibship, e.g., cooperative involvement in smoking or drinking behavior, may cause the DZ correlation to exceed half the MZ correlation.

Environmental influences on the phenotype of interest have two distinct characteristic consequences. First, if there are environmental influences that are shared by siblings growing up in the same home, e.g., socioeconomic status or parenting style, the MZ and DZ correlations will reflect this source of familial aggregation to the same extent. In the absence of genetic influences, these shared environmental influences would lead to equal MZ and DZ correlations. If there are genetic influences present, the shared environment will raise the DZ correlation relative to the MZ correlation. Another point to consider is individual environmental influences. If there are significant environmental influences that are unique to individuals, e.g., significant personal life events, familial aggregation will be attenuated and the MZ and DZ correlations will be reduced, although their relative magnitudes will continue to reflect the importance of genetic versus shared environmental causes of familial aggregation.

Historically, the twin study design has been a key tool for understanding behavioral genetics, but the use of twins has expanded to facilitate our understanding of the genetic contribution to a number of complex traits and diseases.

Cross-References

▶ Dizygotic Twins
▶ Monozygotic Twins

References and Further Reading

Nussbaum, R. L., Mc Innes, R. R., & Willard, H. F. (2001). *Genetics in medicine* (6th ed.). Philadelphia: W.B. Saunders Company.

Spector, T. D., Snieder, H., & MacGregor, A. J. (2000). *Advances in twin and sib-pair analysis* (1st ed.). London: Greenwich Medical Media.

Type 1 Diabetes

▶ Insulin-Dependent Diabetes Mellitus (IDDM)

Type 1 Diabetes Mellitus

Luigi Meneghini
Diabetes Research Institute, University of Miami, Miami, FL, USA

Synonyms

Autoimmune diabetes mellitus; Insulin-dependent diabetes mellitus (IDDM); Juvenile diabetes

Definition

Type 1 diabetes (T1DM) is an elevation in blood glucose due to insufficient production of insulin thought to result from cell-mediated autoimmune destruction of insulin-producing pancreatic beta cells. Autoimmunity is manifested by mononuclear cell invasion of islets (insulitis) and the production of islet-specific antibodies, such as GAD (Glutamic Acid Decarboxylase), IA-2 autoantibodies and ICA (Islet Cell Antibodies), detectable in ~85% of newly diagnosed patients. Genetic, environmental, and possibly other unknown factors contribute to disease susceptibility, which is most commonly manifested in the teenage years (hence the former designation of juvenile diabetes).

If not replaced, absolute insulin deficiency in T1DM results in severe hyperglycemia and diabetic ketoacidosis (DKA), which if left untreated can prove fatal (hence the designation insulin-dependent diabetes mellitus). Insulin replacement ideally takes the form of basal/bolus insulin therapy, delivered either via multiple daily insulin injections or an insulin pump infusion. Poorly controlled type 1 diabetes can lead to, among other complications, nephropathy (kidney damage manifested by excess protein in the urine) and end-stage kidney failure, retinopathy potentially leading to decreased visual acuity, and neuropathy and the risk of diabetic foot infections or ulcerations. Long-standing diabetes is also associated with increased risk for heart disease, stroke, and peripheral vascular disease. Maintaining good glycemic control, as reflected by an HbA1c of less than 7%, will prevent many of the chronic complications of the disease.

Cross-References

▶ Diabetes

References and Readings

Joslin, E. P., & Kahn, C. R. (2005). *Joslin's diabetes mellitus* (14th ed.). Philadelphia: Lippincott Williams & Willkins.

Type 2 Diabetes

▶ Type 2 Diabetes Mellitus

Type 2 Diabetes Mellitus

Elizabeth R. Pulgaron[1] and Alan M. Delamater[2]
[1]Department of Pediatrics, University of Miami, Miami, FL, USA
[2]Department of Pediatrics, University of Miami Miller School of Medicine, Miami, FL, USA

Synonyms

Non-insulin-dependent diabetes mellitus; Type 2 diabetes

Definition

In type 2 diabetes mellitus (T2D), high blood glucose (or hyperglycemia) is the result of the pancreas producing insufficient quantities of insulin due to beta-cell dysfunction, as well as insulin resistance. Peripheral insulin resistance, in which cells resist the action of insulin at the receptor level, occurs early in the disease course. Initially this is compensated for by increased production of insulin, or hyperinsulinemia. Over time, however, insulin secretion declines, and hyperglycemia results. There is no single cause of T2D, although it is generally accepted to be the result of genetic, physiologic, and lifestyle factors, including obesity and physical inactivity.

Most cases of diabetes worldwide are due to T2D. Obesity and family history are well-known correlates of T2D, with over 85% of individuals being either overweight or obese at diagnosis, and most having a positive family history of T2D. The incidence of T2D is increasing dramatically, particularly among children and youth, most likely attributable to the increase in obesity among youth. This increasing incidence is expected to continue in the future unless significant prevention efforts are successfully implemented at the population level.

T2D is generally managed by prescription of oral medications such as Metformin to help reduce blood glucose, but insulin is also used in the treatment of T2D. Because of the association of obesity with insulin resistance, weight loss is another important goal of treatment, achieved through lifestyle modification of dietary habits and physical activity. The health complications associated with poorly controlled diabetes, whether from type 1 or T2D, include cardiovascular disease, renal disease, blindness, and limb amputations. Thus, management of T2D constitutes an important public health issue. In the past, T2D was referred to as non-insulin-dependent diabetes or adult onset diabetes. However, now that T2D is diagnosed at earlier ages in the life course and treatment often does utilize insulin, T2D is the accepted term.

Cross-References

▶ Insulin Resistance
▶ Type 1 Diabetes

References and Readings

Joslin, E. P., & Kahn, C. R. (2005). *Joslin's diabetes mellitus* (14th ed.). Philadelphia: Lippincott Williams & Willkins.
Kaufman, F. R. (2002). Type 2 diabetes mellitus in children and youth: A new epidemic. *Journal of Pediatric Endocrinology and Metabolism, 15*, 737–744.

Type 2 Diabetes Prevention

▶ Diabetes Prevention Program

Type A Behavior

Shin-ichi Suzuki[1] and Yoshihiko Kunisato[2]
[1]Faculty of Human Sciences, Graduate School of Human Sciences, Waseda University, Tokorozawa-shi, Saitama, Japan
[2]School of Human Sciences, Senshu University, Kawasaki, Kanagawa, Japan

Definition

The type A behavior pattern is a personality type that is considered a risk factor for coronary artery disease. It was described by Friedman and Rosenman in 1959. The type A behavior pattern is a complex set of actions and emotions and is characterized by floating hostility, a sense of time urgency, impatience, intense achievement drive, and a desire for recognition and advancement (Friedman 1996). A behavior pattern is associated with inadequacy and low self-esteem (Friedman 1996).

The association between type A behavior pattern and coronary artery disease has been examined for many decades; strong epidemiological evidence for this association exists. However, successive studies have failed to find an association between type A behavior pattern and coronary artery disease. From these findings, hostility was hypothesized to be the main psychosocial predictor of coronary artery disease instead of the global type A behavior pattern (Razzini et al. 2008; Trigo et al. 2005).

The type A behavior pattern was originally assessed by structured interview. The interviewer must have training to ask the questions in an interview format before administering them. In addition, self-report questionnaires have been developed. For example, the Bortner Rating Scale and Framingham Type A Scale assess the type A behavior pattern. Although self-report questionnaires have been used widely, Friedman (1996) noted that inconsistencies in the association between type A behavior pattern and coronary artery disease were caused by assessment methods including self-report questionnaires and structured interview. Friedman proposed the type A videotaped clinical examination (VCE) to detect physical signs of type A behavior patterns; it was valid for diagnosis of type A behavior patterns. The VCE method has predictive validity for myocardial infarctions.

Modifications of the type A behavior pattern were proposed and summarized by Friedman (1996). The modifications of the type A behavior pattern consisted of components including self-esteem enhancement and modifications of floating hostility and sense of time urgency. Friedman et al. (1986) conducted a large randomized clinical trial to examine the effects of type A modification group therapy for myocardial infarction male patients. Their results showed that the recurrence rate of coronary artery disease in a treatment group was lower than that of a control group.

Cross-References

- ▶ Behavioral Medicine
- ▶ Coronary Artery Disease
- ▶ Coronary Heart Disease
- ▶ Health Psychology
- ▶ Hostility, Cynical
- ▶ Personality
- ▶ Trait Anger

References and Further Reading

Friedman, M. (1996). *Type a behavior: Its diagnosis and treatment*. New York: Plenum Press.

Friedman, M., & Rosenman, R. H. (1959). Association of specific overt behavior pattern with blood and cardiovascular findings; blood cholesterol level, blood clotting time, incidence of arcus senilis, and clinical coronary artery disease. *Journal of the American Medical Association, 169*, 1286–1296.

Friedman, M., Thoresen, C. E., Gill, J. J., Ulmer, D., Powell, L. H., Price, V. A., et al. (1986). Alteration of type A behavior and its effect on cardiac recurrences in post myocardial infarction patients: Summary results of the recurrent coronary prevention project. *American Heart Journal, 112*, 653–665.

Razzini, C., Bianchi, F., Leo, R., Fortuna, E., Siracusano, A., & Romeo, F. (2008). Correlations between personality factors and coronary artery disease: From type A behaviour pattern to type D personality. *Journal of Cardiovascular Medicine (Hagerstown, Md.), 9*, 761–768.

Trigo, M., Silva, D., & Rocha, E. (2005). Psychosocial risk factors in coronary heart disease: Beyond type A behavior. *Revista Portuguesa de Cardiologia, 24*, 261–281.

Type D Personality

Johan Denollet
CoRPS – Center of Research on Psychology in Somatic diseases, Tilburg University, Tilburg, The Netherlands

Synonyms

Distressed personality type

Definition

The Type D (distressed) personality refers to *a general propensity to psychological distress* (Denollet et al. 2010) *that is defined by elevated scores on two broad personality traits*, negative affectivity (NA), and *social inhibition* (SI). NA refers to the tendency to experience negative emotions across time and situations, and SI to the tendency to inhibit the expression of emotions and behaviors in social interaction (Denollet 2005).

Description

Individuals with a Type D personality are more likely to report *feelings of dysphoria, tension, and worry* (Denollet 2005). On an interpersonal level, Type D individuals tend to feel *insecure and inhibited* in the company of others, fearing rejection and disapproval (Denollet). Although these individuals may experience emotional difficulties, this may not be acknowledged by others given their inhibited behavior. Type D individuals are less likely to express their true thoughts and feelings and may keep other people at a distance.

A number of studies have reported that Type D was associated with an increased risk of *mortality and other adverse events in cardiac patients*, even after statistical adjustment for measures of depression or anxiety. In 1996, a paper published in the Lancet was one of the first reports on Type D personality as an independent predictor of mortality in patients with heart disease (Denollet et al. 1996). A meta-analytic review that summarized the findings from Type D studies that were published over a 15-year period (1995–2009) concluded that this personality profile may be related to adverse health outcomes in patients with a cardiovascular condition (Denollet et al. 2010). Another independent meta-analytic review confirmed that Type D was associated with adverse health outcomes among patients with cardiovascular disorder (O'Dell et al. 2011). There are also null studies that found no effect of Type D personality on mortality in patients with heart failure (Coyne et al. 2011; Pelle et al. 2010) or other cardiac conditions (Grande et al. 2011). However, depression or anxiety also failed to predict prognosis in these null studies.

The *prevalence* of Type D among patients with cardiovascular disease largely ranges between 25% and 35%. Type D personality and its two components, NA and SI, can be reliably assessed with the *DS14 self-report scale* (Denollet 2005). The 14 items of the DS14 are rated on a five-point Likert scale, ranging from 0 (false) to 4 (true) and are divided into NA and SI subscales. The seven NA items cover the tendency to experience feelings of dysphoria, anxiety, and irritability. The seven SI items cover social discomfort, reticence, and lack of social poise. These personality measures have good internal consistency and are stable over time. Due to its brevity and the simplicity of the items, completing the DS14 takes only a few minutes and comprises little burden to patients. The DS14 has been validated in multiple languages, making it widely applicable. In the International HeartQoL study of 6,222 patients with ischemic heart disease, cross-cultural measurement equivalence was demonstrated for the Type D scale in 21 countries (Kupper et al. 2012).

Type D research is based on the notion that (a) research should examine *the way traits combine* in the determination of disease, and that (b) the *delineation of subtypes* may help to identify groups of patients who share a set of relevant characteristics in terms of clinical course. Only those individuals scoring positive on both NA and SI are classified as "Type D." Type D caseness is determined by a cutoff score ≥ 10 on both the NA and SI subscales. Some have argued that Type D personality is more accurately represented as a *dimensional* rather than as a *categorical* construct (Ferguson et al. 2009). The Type D construct does not infer a true taxon that is defined by discontinuity between groups on an underlying dimension; rather, individuals belong only probabilistically to Type D and non-Type D subgroups (Denollet et al. 2010). Therefore, dimensional and categorical approaches to Type D personality do not need to be mutually exclusive, but rather represent two different ways of capturing psychological tendencies of individuals (Chapman et al. 2007).

General distress, shared across anger, depression, and anxiety, partly accounts for the link between mind and heart (Denollet and Pedersen 2009). The Type D personality profile identifies *individuals who are particularly vulnerable to this adverse effect of general distress*. Hence, Type D personality is not a concurrent of standard psychological risk factors such depression, anxiety, or stress, but rather aims at the early identification of individuals who are inclined to experience these manifestations of distress over a longer period of time. At first glance, depression and Type D personality may appear quite similar, but there are some clear differences. While depression reflects psychopathology, Type D represents a normal personality construct. Accordingly, a narrative review of 29 studies showed that Type D personality and depression are distinct manifestations of psychological distress, with different and independent cardiovascular effects (Denollet et al. 2010). It is not surprising that there is some overlap between Type D and the neuroticism and extraversion traits of the Five Factor Model of personality. However, Type D still predicts health outcomes after controlling for these traits (Denollet et al.), and both the Five Factor and Type D models are related to health outcomes in primary care patients (Chapman et al. 2007).

Several biological and behavioral pathways may *explain the link* between Type D and health outcomes. Potential *biological pathways* associated with Type D personality include elevated levels of the stress hormone cortisol (Molloy et al. 2008), elevated biomarkers of inflammation (Conraads et al. 2006; Einvik et al. 2011), decreased capacity to repair vascular damage (Van Craenenbroeck et al. 2009), and reduced heart rate recovery after exercise (von Känel et al. 2009). Type D has also been related to cardiovascular effects during experimental stress, including higher cardiac output (Williams et al. 2009) and blood pressure (Habra et al. 2003), and lower heart rate variability (Martin et al. 2010).

Behavioral pathways may also mediate the relationship between Type D personality and adverse health outcomes (Williams et al. 2008). In the International HeartQoL study of cardiac patients from 21 different countries, Type D was associated with a higher prevalence of hypertension, smoking, and a sedentary lifestyle (Kupper et al. 2012). In the general population, Type D has also been linked to unhealthy behaviors such as smoking and physical inactivity (Einvik et al. 2011; Hausteiner et al. 2010). Type D individuals may show reluctance to consult clinical staff for cardiovascular symptoms (Schiffer et al. 2007), and are not likely to seek care for their mental problems (Williams et al. 2008). In the medical care for patients with chronic condition, *adherence to treatment* may be of particular importance. Type D has been associated with poor adherence to treatment in patients with cardiac (Williams et al. 2011) and sleep (Broström et al. 2007) disorders.

Type D personality has been mainly studied in cardiovascular patients, but there is evidence to suggest that Type D personality can also provide relevant information in *other populations* as well. Type D has been related to poor patient-reported health outcomes in patients with *other conditions*. In cancer survivors, for example, Type D personality has been associated with impaired quality of life and poor mental health (Mols et al. 2012). In the *general population*, Type D individuals have been shown to have an increased risk for clinically significant depression, panic disorder, and alcohol abuse (Michal et al. 2011). In this study, Type D was also robustly associated with major stressors such as traumatic events and social isolation. These authors concluded that Type D as a frequent disposition is of high relevance for health care (Michal et al. 2011). In other studies of individuals without cardiovascular disease, Type D personality was related to unhealthy behaviors such as smoking and low physical activity (Einvik et al. 2011; Hausteiner et al. 2010).

The evidence so far seems to indicate that patients with a Type D personality profile are at increased risk of for a multitude of adverse health outcomes, particularly in the context of cardiac disease. However, there still are a number of unresolved issues. Evidence suggests that social inhibition modulates the adverse effect of negative emotions on cardiac prognosis (Denollet et al. 2006) but more research is needed to test this model. Although to date the optimal treatment and the applicability of counseling options for Type D individuals are still unknown, screening may identify these high-risk patients. Overall, the findings of Type D research support the simultaneous use of specific and general measures of distress in cardiovascular research and practice. In this context, *screening for Type D personality with the DS14* (Denollet 2005) may be useful to improve clinical research and practice in the context of cardiovascular disease and other chronic conditions.

Cross-References

▶ Negative Affectivity
▶ Social Inhibition

References and Readings

Broström, A., Strömberg, A., Mårtensson, J., Ulander, M., Harder, L., & Svanborg, E. (2007). Association of type D personality to perceived side effects and adherence in CPAP-treated patients with OSAS. *Journal of Sleep Research, 16*, 439–447.

Chapman, B. P., Duberstein, P. R., & Lyness, J. M. (2007). The distressed personality type: Replicability and general health associations. *European Journal of Personality, 21*, 911–929.

Conraads, V. M., Denollet, J., De Clerck, L. S., Stevens, W. J., Bridts, C., & Vrints, C. J. (2006). Type D personality is associated with increased levels of tumor necrosis factor (TNF)-alpha and TNF-alpha receptors in chronic heart failure. *International Journal of Cardiology, 113*, 34–38.

Coyne, J. C., Jaarsma, T., Luttik, M. L., van Sonderen, E., van Veldhuisen, D. J., & Sanderman, R. (2011). Lack of prognostic value of type D personality for mortality in a large sample of heart failure patients. *Psychosomatic Medicine, 73*, 557–562.

Denollet, J. (2005). DS14: Standard assessment of negative affectivity, social inhibition, and type D personality. *Psychosomatic Medicine, 67*, 89–97.

Denollet, J., & Pedersen, S. S. (2009). Anger, depression and anxiety in cardiac patients: The complexity of individual differences in psychological risk. *Journal of the American College of Cardiology, 53*, 947–949.

Denollet, J., Sys, S. U., Stroobant, N., Rombouts, H., Gillebert, T. C., & Brutsaert, D. L. (1996). Personality as independent predictor of long-term mortality in patients with coronary heart disease. *The Lancet, 347*, 417–421.

Denollet, J., Pedersen, S. S., Ong, A. T., Erdman, R. A., Serruys, P. W., & van Domburg, R. T. (2006). Social inhibition modulates the effect of negative emotions on cardiac prognosis following percutaneous coronary intervention in the drug-eluting stent era. *European Heart Journal, 27*, 171–177.

Denollet, J., Schiffer, A. A., & Spek, V. (2010). A general propensity to psychological distress affects cardiovascular outcomes: Evidence from research on the type D (distressed) personality profile. *Circulation: Cardiovascular Quality and Outcomes, 3*, 546–557.

Einvik, G., Dammen, T., Hrubos-Strøm, H., Namtvedt, S. K., Randby, A., Kristiansen, H. A., et al. (2011). Prevalence of cardiovascular risk factors and concentration of C-reactive protein in type D personality persons without cardiovascular disease. *European Journal of Cardiovascular Prevention and Rehabilitation, 18*, 504–509.

Ferguson, E., Williams, L., O'Conner, C., Howard, S., Hughes, B. M., Johnston, D. W., et al. (2009). A taxometric analysis of Type D personality. *Psychosomatic Medicine, 71*, 981–986.

Grande, G., Romppel, M., Vesper, J. M., Schubmann, R., Glaesmer, H., & Herrmann-Lingen, C. (2011). Type D personality and all-cause mortality in cardiac patients – Data from a German cohort study. *Psychosomatic Medicine, 73*, 548–556.

Habra, M. E., Linden, W., Anderson, J. C., & Weinberg, J. (2003). Type D personality is related to cardiovascular and neuroendocrine reactivity to acute stress. *Journal of Psychosomatic Research, 55*, 235–245.

Hausteiner, C., Klupsch, D., Emeny, R., Baumert, J., Ladwig, K. H., & the KORA Investigators. (2010). Clustering of negative affectivity and social inhibition in the community: Prevalence of Type D personality as a cardiovascular risk marker. *Psychosomatic Medicine, 72*, 163–171.

Kupper, N., Pedersen, S. S., Höfer, S., Saner, H., Oldridge, N., & Denollet, J. (2012). Cross-cultural analysis of type D (distressed) personality in 6222 patients with ischemic heart disease: A study from the International HeartQoL Project. *International Journal of Cardiology*. in press.

Martin, L. A., Doster, J. A., Critelli, J. W., Lambert, P. L., Purdum, M., Powers, C., et al. (2010). Ethnicity and type D personality as predictors of heart rate variability. *International Journal of Psychophysiology, 76*, 118–121.

Michal, M., Wiltink, J., Grande, G., Beutel, M. E., & Brähler, E. (2011). Type D personality is independently associated with major psychosocial stressors and increased health care utilization in the general population. *Journal of Affective Disorders, 134*, 396–403.

Molloy, G. J., Perkins-Porras, L., Strike, P. C., & Steptoe, A. (2008). Type D personality and cortisol in survivors of acute coronary syndrome. *Psychosomatic Medicine, 70*, 863–868.

Mols, F., Thong, M. S., de Poll-Franse, L. V., Roukema, J. A., & Denollet, J. (2012). Type D (distressed) personality is associated with poor quality of life and mental health among 3080 cancer survivors. *Journal of Affective Disorders, 136*, 26–34.

O'Dell, K. R., Masters, K. S., Spielmans, G. I., & Maisto, S. A. (2011). Does type D personality predict outcomes among patients with cardiovascular disease? A meta-analytic review. *Journal of Psychosomatic Research, 71*, 199–206.

Pelle, A. J., Pedersen, S. S., Schiffer, A. A., Szabó, B. M., Widdershoven, J. W., & Denollet, J. (2010). Psychological distress and mortality in systolic heart failure. *Circulation: Heart Failure, 3*, 261–267.

Schiffer, A. A., Denollet, J., Widdershoven, J. W., Hendriks, E. H., & Smith, O. R. (2007). Failure to consult for symptoms of heart failure in patients with a type D personality. *Heart, 93*, 814–818.

Van Craenenbroeck, E. M., Denollet, J., Paelinck, B. P., Beckers, P., Possemiers, N., Hoymans, V. Y., et al. (2009). Circulating CD34 + KDR + endothelial progenitor cells are reduced in chronic heart failure patients as a function of Type D personality. *Clinical Science, 117*, 165–172.

von Känel, R., Barth, J., Kohls, S., Saner, S., Znoj, H., Saner, G., et al. (2009). Heart rate recovery after exercise in chronic heart failure: Role of vital exhaustion and type D personality. *Journal of Cardiology, 53*, 248–256.

Williams, L., O'Connor, R. C., Howard, S., Hughes, B. M., Johnston, D. W., Hay, J. L., et al. (2008). Type D personality mechanisms of effect: The role of health-related behavior and social support. *Journal of Psychosomatic Research, 64*, 63–69.

Williams, L., O'Carroll, R. E., & O'Connor, R. C. (2009). Type D personality and cardiac output in response to stress. *Psychology and Health, 24*, 489–500.

Williams, L., O'Connor, R. C., Grubb, N., & O'Carroll, R. (2011). Type D personality predicts poor medication adherence in myocardial infarction patients. *Psychology and Health, 26*, 703–712.

U

Understanding

▶ Empathy

Unexplained Patient Complaints

▶ Medically Unexplained Symptoms

Unexplained Symptoms

▶ Medically Unexplained Symptoms

Unintentional Nonadherence

Tavis S. Campbell, Jillian A. Johnson and Kristin A. Zernicke
Department of Psychology, University of Calgary, Calgary, AB, Canada

Synonyms

Noncompliance

Definition

Unintentional nonadherence refers to a non-deliberate alteration in treatment (e.g., medications, exercise, diet). Unintentional nonadherence includes forgetting, poor manual dexterity, lack of understanding of requirements, losing medications, or not being able to afford treatment (DiMatteo, 2004). Unlike intentional nonadherence that is more strongly related to individuals' beliefs, unintentional nonadherence is more strongly related to demographics and clinical variables, such as age, socioeconomic factors, and stage of illness (DiMatteo, 2004).

Cross-References

▶ Noncompliance

References and Readings

DiMatteo, R. M. (2004). Variations in patients' adherence to medical recommendations: A quantitative review of 50 years of research. *Medical Care, 42*(3), 200–209.

Horne, R. (2007). Adherence to treatment. In S. Ayers, A. Baum, & C. McManus (Eds.), *Cambridge handbook of psychology, health and medicine* (pp. 417–423). Cambridge, MA: Cambridge University Press.

Wroe, A. I. (2002). Intentional and unintentional nonadherence: A study of decision making. *Journal of Behavioural Medicine, 25*(4), 355–372.

© Springer Nature Switzerland AG 2020
M. D. Gellman (ed.), *Encyclopedia of Behavioral Medicine*,
https://doi.org/10.1007/978-3-030-39903-0

Unipolar Depression

Amy Wachholtz[1] and Elizabeth Gleyzer[2]
[1]Department of Psychology, University of Colorado Denver, Denver, CO, USA
[2]Department of Psychology, William James College, Newton, MA, USA

Synonyms

Depressive episode; Dysthymia; Major depressive disorder; Persistent depressive disorder

Definition and Description

Unipolar depression is a mood disorder characterized by either persistent feelings of sadness or emptiness or by diminished interest or pleasure in activities (anhedonia). These symptoms are often accompanied by a combination of emotional/cognitive and vegetative symptoms. Emotional/cognitive symptoms involve those that are related to how a person processes information, e.g., depressed mood, feeling worthless or excessively guilty, feeling helpless, hopelessness, irritability, anhedonia, difficulty thinking or decreased concentration, or suicidal ideation. Vegetative symptoms are those symptoms that are directly related to the body, e.g., insomnia/hypersomnia, dysregulated eating, fatigue, or decreased energy. Functional impairment caused by depression can range from mild to moderate to severe (American Psychiatric Association [APA] 2013).

Etiology

Physiology, psychology and personality, genetics and family history, social environment, and life circumstances all play a role in a person's vulnerability to depression. It is unknown exactly how depression develops and the etiology is usually multifactorial and varies for every patient. Depression is a disorder that involves brain structures, neurotransmitters, and cognitive and emotional processes.

Diagnosis

A physician, psychiatrist, psychologist, or other mental health professional can diagnose a patient with depression. In order to be diagnosed as depression, symptoms must be unremitting for more than 2 weeks and must include either depressed mood or anhedonia (APA 2013). Five additional emotional and vegetative criterion symptoms must be present. When diagnosing, clinicians consider duration of symptoms, symptom history, degree of functional impairment, and treatment history. While all people occasionally experience sadness, feeling "blue," or mood swings, it is important to note that depression affects important areas of a patient's life, such as social or occupational functioning, and is of greater severity than normative emotional responses. Individuals with depression may each present somewhat differently. Some patients may report irritability, tearfulness, somatic complaints, psychomotor agitation or slowing, social withdrawal, anger, or a combination of such symptoms.

The course of depression is often episodic, with symptoms remitting for a time and then returning (National Institute for Health and Care Excellence [NICE] 2009). When depressive symptoms are present and unremitting for more than 2 years and do not meet full criteria for depression, it is called persistent depressive disorder, or dysthymia (APA 2013).

The term unipolar depression is used to differentiate between this disorder and *bipolar depression* which involves periods of mania in addition to depression. The term depression is also differentiated from an *adjustment disorder* (see ▶ "Adjustment Disorders in Health"), which may include feeling depressive symptoms due to a specific life change (e.g., job loss, divorce, recent cancer diagnosis) or *bereavement* due to the loss of a loved one. However, both adjustment disorder and bereavement may progress to unipolar depression if symptoms are present for a prolonged period of time.

Comorbidity with Medical Disorders

Unipolar depression is associated with increased medical morbidity (Carney et al. 1995) and may be seen in conjunction with a number of physical health issues (see ▶ "Comorbidity") including chronic pain, cancer, physical trauma, cardiac issues (heart attack), inflammatory bowel disease, diabetes, HIV/AIDS, chronic health concerns (see ▶ "Maladaptation of Symptom Behaviors to Chronic Illness"), and terminal stage illnesses. Patients with both depression and medical illness may have more severe symptoms of both (National Institute of Mental Health [NIMH] 2015). Chronic medical conditions and comorbid depression are associated with increased symptom reporting, amplification of severity of symptoms, and increased medical care costs (Katon and Ciechanowski 2002). And patients with chronic illnesses are at a higher risk for depression than the general population (Cassano and Fava 2002).

Depression and the chronic stress that often accompanies affective disorders have a negative effect on immune function through overproduction of proinflammatory cytokines (Kiecolt-Glaser and Glaser 2002). In immunocompromised patients, depression may contribute to prolonged or repeated infection and delayed healing due to inhibited immune responses (Kiecolt-Glaser and Glaser 2002).

Conversely, the presence of medical issues may also increase the risk of developing depression (Krishnan et al. 2002). Disruption of physiological systems such as endocrine, cardiovascular, or immune systems in medically ill patients can contribute to the development or recurrence of depression (Glannon 2002). For example, vitamin B12 deficiency can result in depressive symptoms (Tiemeier et al. 2002). Patients with an underactive thyroid, a condition called hypothyroidism, are susceptible to symptoms of depression (Kirkegaard and Faber 1998). Even those with subclinical hypothyroidism are at an increased risk of developing depression (Haggerty et al. 1993). Some patients with depression may show thyroid dysfunction such as lower levels of thyroid-stimulating hormone (TSH) and another thyroid hormone, T_3 (Stipčević et al. 2008). Because of thyroid hormones' role in mood and cognition (Bauer et al. 2008), symptoms of hypothyroidism manifest in some patients as fatigue, depressed mood, appetite changes, fluctuations in weight, or memory difficulties (Hueston 2001) and may overlap with symptoms of depression. Depression can have an impact on cognition, especially in older adults. Depression can also mimic symptoms of dementia in older individuals. Depression may also be a precursor to dementia. In patients with mild cognitive impairment (MCI), depression is a risk factor for development of dementia (Modrego and Ferrández 2004). Overlapping symptoms of depression and dementia or MCI, such as cognitive slowing, lack of interest, loss of energy, and difficulty concentrating, may lead to misdiagnosis if not fully assessed.

When patients present in a medical setting, diagnosis of depression must take into account potential overlapping somatic symptoms such as fatigue, change in appetite, cognitive deficits, decreased concentration, and sleep difficulties. Additionally, some medications used to treat medical disorders can mimic or trigger depressive symptoms such as beta blockers and interferon treatments.

Treatment

The goal of all treatments for depression is to alleviate depressive symptoms and to help patients return to a normal level of functioning. Patients with depression may respond to some treatments and not others. Therefore, many clinicians are trained to offer a variety of treatment options that cater to the patient's presentation and symptom history. Common treatments for depression include cognitive-behavioral psychotherapy, interpersonal therapy, behavioral activation, antidepressant medications, or a combination of these treatments. Of the nonpharmacological options, cognitive-behavioral therapy (CBT) is most frequently recommended as an evidence-based approach to treatment. CBT is a model of therapy in which the patient and clinician work collaboratively to identify negative thoughts, beliefs, behaviors, and interpretations that contribute to depressed mood. The clinician helps the patient develop skills to counteract problematic cognitive processes and behaviors and replace them with a repertoire of coping strategies (National Collaborating Centre for Mental Health [NCCMH] 2010). CBT treatment has been found to create similar neural activity changes in the brain as antidepressants using fMRI assessments, but CBT treatment effects continue after the cessation of treatment. In contrast, fMRI studies show that those treated with medication alone tend to return to baseline activity levels soon after treatment ends (DeRubeis et al. 2008).

Current commonly used classes of antidepressant medications include selective serotonin reuptake inhibitors (SSRIs), tricyclic antidepressants (TCAs), monoamine oxidase inhibitors (MAOIs), serotonin and norepinephrine reuptake inhibitors (SNRIs), norepinephrine and dopamine reuptake inhibitors (NDRIs), and tetracyclic antidepressants. There are also a number of complementary treatments that are gaining empirical research support for use in combination with traditional approaches to enhance treatment outcomes. These include treatments such as exercise therapy, light therapy, vitamin B and D supplements, acupuncture, and hypnosis.

Adherence

A common symptom of depression is lack of motivation and energy which can often interfere with a patient's ability to adhere to his or her medical regimen (see ▶ "Disease Management"). Medically ill patients with comorbid depression may have difficulty taking their prescribed medication on time, keeping medical appointments, carrying out activities of daily living and maintaining general self-care. Patients with depression are three times more likely to struggle with treatment adherence than non-depressed patients (DiMatteo et al. 2000). Depression can also complicate the course of treatment for many medical conditions. Patients may be slower to return to work, report higher levels of stress, and struggle to adhere to doctor recommendations such as diet and exercise (DiMatteo et al. 2000).

Conclusion

Unipolar depression is a mood disorder that is characterized by low mood, loss of interest or pleasure in previously enjoyable activities, and other emotional, cognitive, physical, and behavioral symptoms. The diagnosis of depression depends on the severity of symptoms, duration, and degree of functional impairment. Other mental health disorders such as bipolar disorder and adjustment disorder may present with depressive symptoms but are diagnostically differentiated by additional symptom criteria. Depression frequently co-occurs with medical illness. Depression effects endocrine, gastrointestinal, and immune system functioning and can complicate wound healing and medical treatment. Depression is also associated with poorer medical outcomes in patients such as those with cardiovascular issues. Some illnesses, such as hypothyroidism, can present with depressive symptoms and clinicians should take care making a diagnosis when assessing for overlapping symptoms. Medically ill patients with comorbid depression may struggle with adherence to treatment recommendations due to the nature of depressive symptoms such as amotivation, lack of energy, hopelessness, and poor self-efficacy. Available treatments for unipolar depression include antidepressant medications, psychotherapies such as cognitive-behavioral therapy, and other complimentary treatments that are gaining empirical support. While many treatments are effective in helping patients regain normal functioning and remission of symptoms, not all patients respond equally to treatment. Therefore, catering treatment to a patient's unique symptom presentation, considering comorbidities and symptom and treatment history, and accounting for the patient's medical status will help improve patient outcomes.

Cross-References

▶ Adjustment Disorders in Health
▶ Comorbidity
▶ Dementia
▶ Disease Management
▶ Maladaptation of Symptom Behaviors to Chronic Illness

References and Further Reading

American Psychiatric Association. (2013). *Diagnostic and statistical manual of mental disorders* (5th ed.). Washington, DC: Author.

Bauer, M., Goetz, T., Glenn, T., & Whybrow, P. C. (2008). The thyroid-brain interaction in thyroid disorders and mood disorders. *Journal of Neuroendocrinology, 20*(10), 1101–1114.

Carney, R. M., Freedland, K. E., Eisen, S. A., Rich, M. W., & Jaffe, A. S. (1995). Major depression and medication adherence in elderly patients with coronary artery disease. *Health Psychology, 14*(1), 88.

Cassano, P., & Fava, M. (2002). Depression and public health: An overview. *Journal of Psychosomatic Research, 53*(4), 849–857.

Dayan, C. M., & Panicker, V. (2013). Hypothyroidism and depression. *European Thyroid Journal, 2*(3), 168–179.

DeRubeis, R. J., Siegle, G. J., & Hollon, S. D. (2008). Cognitive therapy vs. medications for depression: Treatment outcomes and neural mechanisms. *Nature Reviews: Neuroscience, 9*, 788–796.

DiMatteo, M. R., Lepper, H. S., & Croghan, T. W. (2000). Depression is a risk factor for noncompliance with medical treatment: Meta-analysis of the effects of anxiety and depression on patient adherence. *Archives of Internal Medicine, 160*(14), 2101–2107.

Dwight, M. M., Kowdley, K. V., Russo, J. E., Ciechanowski, P. S., Larson, A. M., & Katon, W. J. (2000). Depression, fatigue, and functional disability in patients with chronic hepatitis C. *Journal of Psychosomatic Research, 49*(5), 311–317.

Glannon, W. (2002). The psychology and physiology of depression. *Philosophy, Psychiatry, & Psychology, 9*(3), 265–269.

Haggerty, J. J., Jr., Stern, R. A., Mason, G. A., Beckwith, J., Morey, C. E., & Prange, A. J., Jr. (1993). Subclinical hypothyroidism: A modifiable risk factor for depression? *The American Journal of Psychiatry, 150*(3), 508.

Hueston, W. J. (2001). Treatment of hypothyroidism. *American Family Physician, 64*(10), 1717–1724.

Irwin, M., Patterson, T., Smith, T. L., Caldwell, C., Brown, S. A., Gillin, J. C., & Grant, I. (1990). Reduction of immune function in life stress and depression. *Biological Psychiatry, 27*(1), 22–30.

Katon, W., & Ciechanowski, P. (2002). Impact of major depression on chronic medical illness. *Journal of Psychosomatic Research, 53*(4), 859–863.

Kiecolt-Glaser, J. K., & Glaser, R. (2002). Depression and immune function: Central pathways to morbidity and mortality. *Journal of Psychosomatic Research, 53*(4), 873–876.

Kirkegaard, C., & Faber, J. (1998). The role of thyroid hormones in depression. *European Journal of Endocrinology, 138*(1), 1–9.

Krishnan, K. R. R., Delong, M., Kraemer, H., Carney, R., Spiegel, D., Gordon, C., et al. (2002). Comorbidity of depression with other medical diseases in the elderly. *Biological Psychiatry, 52*(6), 559–588.

Lustman, P. J., Clouse, R. E., & Carney, R. M. (1989). Depression and the reporting of diabetes symptoms. *The International Journal of Psychiatry in Medicine, 18*(4), 295–303.

Modrego, P. J., & Ferrández, J. (2004). Depression in patients with mild cognitive impairment increases the risk of developing dementia of Alzheimer type: A prospective cohort study. *Archives of Neurology, 61*(8), 1290–1293.

National Collaborating Centre for Mental Health (UK). (2010). Depression: The treatment and management of depression in adults (updated edition). British Psychological Society. Retrieved from http://www.ncbi.nlm.nih.gov/pubmed/22132433

National Institute for Health and Care Excellence (UK). (2009). Depression in adults: Recognition and management (NICE guidelines CG90). Retrieved from http://www.nice.org.uk/guidance/CG90

Stipčević, T., Pivac, N., Kozarić-Kovačić, D., & Mück-Šeler, D. (2008). Thyroid activity in patients with major depression. *Collegium Antropologicum, 32*(3), 973–976.

Sullivan, M., LaCroix, A., Spertus, J., & Hecht, J. (2000). Effects of anxiety and depression on function and symptoms in patients with coronary heart disease: A 5-year prospective study. *The American Journal of Cardiology, 86*, 1135–1140.

Tiemeier, H., Van Tuijl, H. R., Hofman, A., Meijer, J., Kiliaan, A. J., Breteler, M. M. (2002). Vitamin B12, folate, and homocysteine in depression: The Rotterdam Study. *American Journal of Psychiatry, 159*(12), 2099–2101.

U. S. Department of Health and Human Services, National Institutes of Health, National Institute of Mental Health. (2015). *Depression* (NIH Publication No. 34625). Retrieved from https://www.nimh.nih.gov/health/publications/depression/depression-booklet_34625.pdf

Uomoto, J. M., & Esselman, P. C. (1995). Psychiatric disorders and functional disability in outpatients with traumatic brain injuries. *The American Journal of Psychiatry, 152*(10), 1493–1499.

Walker, E. A., Gelfand, M. D., Gelfand, A. N., Creed, F., & Katon, W. J. (1996). The relationship of current psychiatric disorder to functional disability and distress in patients with inflammatory bowel disease. *General Hospital Psychiatry, 18*(4), 220–229.

Waraich, P., Goldner, E. M., Somers, J. M., & Hsu, L. (2004). Prevalence and incidence studies of mood disorders: A systematic review of the literature. *Canadian Journal of Psychiatry, 49*, 124–138.

United States Department of Labor

▶ Job Classification

Units of Nature

▶ Ecosystems, Stable and Sustainable

Univariate Analysis

J. Rick Turner
Campbell University College of Pharmacy and Health Sciences, Buies Creek, NC, USA

Definition

Univariate analyses analyze one outcome variable at a time.

Cross-References

▶ Multivariate Analysis

References and Further Reading

Campbell, M. J., Machin, D., & Walters, S. J. (2007). *Medical statistics: A textbook for the health sciences* (4th ed.). Chichester: Wiley.

Unprotected Sex

▶ Sexual Risk Behavior

Upper Respiratory Infection (Mild)

▶ Common Cold

Upper Respiratory Infection (Mild): Cause

▶ Common Cold: Cause

Upper Respiratory Infection (Mild): The Stress Factor

▶ Common Cold: The Stress Factor

Urothelial Carcinoma of the Bladder

▶ Cancer, Bladder

Usability Evaluation

▶ Usability Testing

Usability Testing

Colleen Stiles-Shields[1,2] and Enid Montague[3]
[1]Loyola University, Chicago, IL, USA
[2]Northwestern University, The University of Chicago, Chicago, IL, USA
[3]DePaul University, Northwestern University, Chicago, IL, USA

Synonyms

Usability Evaluation

Definition

Usability testing is a systematic evaluation of a product with the ultimate goal of improving the product's design.

Description

Usability evaluation can be conducted by experts, without or with potential end users; this entry focuses on the latter. Through systematic observation of a planned task or scenario carried out by an actual or potential user, usability testing is a method of evaluation that involves testing users' interactions with a product and system to improve design (Usability.gov). This process is intended to ensure that a technology is intuitive and easy to use, with the importance ranging from lifesaving (e.g., in use of hospital equipment) to convenience (e.g., saving time on a task; (Tullis and Albert 2008). This process also provides actionable answers to questions that are critical for organizations, researchers, clinicians, etc., which are developing or using products. Usability standards have been developed and validated by the International Standards Organization (ISO), specifying the necessary information to take into account when evaluating the usability of an evaluated product (Tullis and Albert 2008).

In an effort to increase the visibility of software usability, the US National Institute of Standards and Technology (NIST) developed and validated a Common Industry Format (CIF) for reporting methodologies and results of usability testing (Stanton 2015). The CIF defines a consistent method of carrying out usability tests and makes a distinction between "formative" and "summative" usability tests. Formative tests are typically carried out during the development of a product with the test administrator and participant present, to shape or improve the product. The outputs from a formative test typically include a list of usability problems and recommendations for redesign. In contrast, summative tests are usually carried out at the end of a development stage, with the possible goals of (1) measuring/validating the usability of a product; (2) answering the question: "How usable is this product"; (3) comparing against competitor products or usability metrics; or (4) generating data to support marketing claims about usability. These tests are typically conducted in a usability lab with the participant working alone to minimize confounding variables. The outputs from a summative test typically include empirical, statistical measures of usability such as success rates, average time to complete a task, and number of errors.

Usability testing is often iterative, applying a "test, fix, test" paradigm to the development of a product. For formative and qualitative evaluation, testing is often completed with a sample of about five users evaluating each new iteration (Lewis 1994; Nielsen and Landauer 1993; Tullis and Albert 2008). For summative and quantitative evaluation, more participants are usually needed to achieve statistical significance. With relatively small sample sizes for each iteration, usability testing provides a systematic evaluation of research questions that require the measurement of human behavior in an interaction with a technology or product (Tullis and Albert 2008).

Data Usability is not measured directly, but metrics of usability are collected. Usability metrics include the time needed to complete a task, level of satisfaction, number of errors, etc. All usability metrics must be: (1) indirectly or directly measurable, and (2) quantifiable (Tullis and Albert 2008). Usability metrics differ from other metrics because usability metrics reveal information about an interaction between a user and a technology. How this interaction is defined is typically measured via five primary attributes of usability: (1) learnability, the ease with which a user can accomplish tasks upon initial encounter; (2) efficiency, how accurately and completely a user can complete tasks in a given time; (3) memorability, how easily and proficiently a user can complete tasks after a delay in use; (4) errors, how frequently a user makes and how easily a user can recover; and (5) satisfaction, how pleasant a user finds a product (Nielsen 1993).

Surveys and Questionnaires When possible, validated surveys should be included during usability tests. A variety of validated surveys exist to measure different measures related to usability, such as ease of use, satisfaction, and usefulness (Davis 1989; Lin et al. 1997; Lund 2001). Surveys can be used after usability tasks, or at the conclusion of the entire test (when appropriate). Not all usability surveys are appropriate for every test objective, so care should be taken to choose the correct measures. Simply disseminating a survey to a user is not considered usability testing. Rather, testing with users involves developing research questions, tasks, collecting usability measures, observing behavior, and identifying usability problems. Surveys can assist with the process of identifying usability problems, but measures on surveys alone will not direct the researcher to the usability problems.

Limitations Results from usability testing are not meant to be generalizable to other products, users, or contextual situations. The potential for bias in usability testing is a limitation in usability testing, but only when tests are not well designed; most biases are reduced with selecting the appropriate test for the product, sound sampling, and test design. Snyder (2006) argued that biases in usability testing can be minimized, but not eliminated. Therefore, possible biases must be considered in findings (Snyder 2006). Tullis and Albert (2008) generalize usability testing biases into six categories: (1) participants; (2) the types of tasks selected for evaluation; (3) the method of evaluation; (4) the artifact used for testing; (5) the physical environment; and (6) the moderator(s) (Tullis and Albert 2008). These general categories must be considered when interpreting the findings of usability testing and researchers should attempt to address these biases in the design of usability testing studies.

Strengths Metrics resulting from usability testing provide many benefits to the development and understanding of products. First, usability testing adds structure to the design process, highlighting overall issues that could lead to costly repairs (Bevan 2009). Indeed, it removes the need to make design decisions from an uninformed or "gut-feeling" perspective. Further, the metrics demonstrate if improvement is actually made as a result of design changes from one iteration to the next. Second, these data can often be collected quickly, without the need to test a product for several weeks or months (Tullis and Albert 2008). Third, usability testing research questions specify what needs to be learned about the user experience. This specificity can lead to explicit data to address questions of usability. Finally, evaluating the usability of a product to address any notable issues increases the likelihood the product will be used (Tullis and Albert 2008). Indeed, users are less likely to engage with a product that is difficult or perceived as a mismatch with user needs (Chiu and Eysenbach 2010; Price et al. 2014). Usability testing provides multiple strengths to the design and use of a product.

Cross-References

▶ Scenario-Based Design

References and Further Reading

Bevan, N. (2009) *"Usability." Encyclopedia of database systems* (pp. 3247–3251). New York: Springer.

Chiu, T. M., & Eysenbach, G. (2010). Stages of use: Consideration, initiation, utilization, and outcomes of an internet-mediated intervention. *BMC Medical Informatics and Decision Making, 10*(73). https://doi.org/10.1186/1472-6947-10-73.

Davis, F. D. (1989). Perceived usefulness, perceived ease of use, and user acceptance of information technology. *MIS Quarterly, 13*(3), 319–340.

Lewis, J. R. (1994). Sample sizes for usability studies: Additional considerations. *Human Factors, 36*(2), 368–378.

Lin, H. X., Choong, Y. Y., & Salvendy, G. (1997). A proposed index of usability: A method for comparing the relative usability of different software systems. *Behaviour and Information Technology, 16*(4/5), 267–278.

Lund, A. M. (2001). Measuring usability with the USE questionnaire. *STC Usability SIG Newsletter, 8*(2), 3–6.

Nielsen, J. (1993). *Usability engineering*. New York: Academic.

Nielsen, J., & Landauer, T. K. (1993). A mathematical-model of the finding of usability problems. *Human Factors in Computing Systems*, 206–213.

Price, M., Yuen, E. K., Goetter, E. M., Herbert, J. D., Forman, E. M., Acierno, R., & Ruggiero, K. J. (2014). mHealth: A mechanism to deliver more accessible, more effective mental health care. *Clinical Psychology & Psychotherapy, 21*(5), 427–436. https://doi.org/10.1002/cpp.1855.

Snyder, C. (2006). *Bias in usability testing*. Paper presented at the Boston Mini-UPA Conference, Natick, MA.

Stanton, B. (2015). *Industry usability reporting*. Retrieved from https://www.nist.gov/itl/iad/industry-usability-reporting.

Tullis, T., & Albert, B. (2008). *Measuring the user experience: Collecting, analyzing, and presenting usability metrics*. Burlington: Morgan Kaufmann Publishers.

Usability.gov. Usability testing. *Methods*.

User-Centered Design Approaches

▶ Scenario-Based Design

Usual Care

Manjunath Harlapur[1] and Daichi Shimbo[2]
[1]Center of Behavioral Cardiovascular Health, Division of General Medicine, Columbia University, New York, NY, USA
[2]Center for Behavioral Cardiovascular Health, Columbia University, New York, NY, USA

Synonyms

Control group of a randomized trial; Usual care arm

Definition

Although the definition of usual care has not been standardized, it can include the routine care received by patients for prevention or treatment of diseases.

Description

In cardiology, the type of routine care can vary by disease type and severity, the practice in which the patient is seen, health care system, and individual physician. Major task forces such from the American College of Cardiology and American Heart Association have published guidelines on the diagnosis, prevention, and treatment of several cardiovascular diseases. These guidelines are based on expert opinion as well as on the strength of the evidence. The purpose of these guidelines is to ensure that these recommendations are disseminated to the practicing cardiology community, as the type and quality of diagnostic, preventive, and treatment strategies widely varies.

In randomized trials, there has been some debate about the advantages and disadvantages of including a usual care arm as a control group. The Declaration of Helsinki states that the "benefits, risks, burdens, and effectiveness of a new method should be tested against those of the best current prophylactic, diagnostic, and therapeutic methods." In theory, it makes sense that in a randomized controlled trial, the usual care arm should be defined by the "best current" method available. The main advantage, of course, is to test the intervention against what is currently available in evidence-based clinical practice. However, there has been disagreement on what should constitute "usual" care in a randomized controlled trial. First, in the community, usual care can sometimes include suboptimal or older practices. Thus, whether "usual care" should really be changed to "optimal care" or "evidence-based care" remains unclear. Second, the outcome in the usual care arm may be affected by the Hawthorne effect. It is difficult to blind the physicians and the patients to being in the usual care arm. The physicians or the patients may improve or modify their behavior after finding out that they are not in the active intervention arm. Third, because physician treatment patterns vary, the components of the usual care arm and their effects on the outcome are difficult to quantify. Some investigators have advocated for proposing a standardized treatment plan for patients randomized to the usual care arm. Further, differences between the active intervention arm and the usual care arm could be minimized if the usual care arm contains the proposed intervention. Finally, the types and nature of treatment typically given by physicians in the usual care arm could change during the study period.

For example, in the Antihypertensive and Lipid-Lowering Treatment to Prevent Heart Attack Trial (ALLHAT-LLT), 10,355 persons, aged 55 years or older with hypertension and moderately elevated low-density lipoprotein cholesterol levels, were randomized in an unblinded fashion to pravastatin (a statin) or to usual care. During a mean follow-up of 5 years, there was no significant difference in all-cause mortality or coronary heart disease events. ALLHAT-LLT was unique as it was one of the few trials that did not show the beneficial effects of statin therapy on cardiovascular events in patients who were at risk for future events. The reasons for the lack of difference in outcomes between the two arms are unknown, but the inclusion of a usual care arm as a control group may have played a role. For example, ALLHAT-LLT was conducted during a period that several other randomized trials of statin therapy were published. Thus, over time, physicians could have treated patients in the control arm with statin therapy. In fact, there was a steady increase in the use of statins in the usual care arm: 8.2% at year 2, 17.1% at year 4, and 26.1% at year 6. In addition to statins, other treatments in the usual care arm could have played a role. For example, physicians could have disproportionately recommended non-pharmacologic strategies (i.e., exercise, diet, and weight reduction) to their patients in the usual care arm as well. Given that the types of and intensity of the treatments in the usual care arm were likely variable, ultimately, these reasons remain speculative. Overall, ALLHAT-LLT is one example of the potential limitations, described above that may be associated with a usual care arm.

Cross-References

▶ Randomized Clinical Trial
▶ Randomized Controlled Trial

References and Further Reading

ALLHAT Officers and Coordinators for the ALLHAT Collaborative Research Group. (2002). Major outcomes in moderately hypercholesterolemic, hypertensive patients randomized to pravastatin vs usual care: The antihypertensive and lipid-lowering treatment to prevent heart attack trial (ALLHAT-LLT). *Journal of the American Medical Association, 288,* 2998–3007.

Smelt, A. F., et al. (2010). How usual is usual care in pragmatic intervention studies in primary care? An overview of recent trials. *British Journal of General Practice, 60*(576), e305–e318.

Usual Care Arm

▶ Usual Care

Uutela, Antti

Born: *March 27, 1946*

Antti Uutela
Department for Lifestyle and Health, National Institute for Health and Welfare, Helsinki, Province of Uusimaa, Finland

Biographical Information

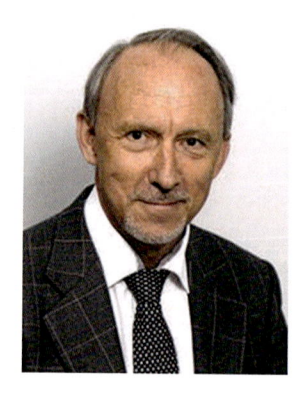

Antti Uutela was born in Tammela, Finland, on March 27, 1946. He is Doctor of Social Sciences (social psychology) from the University of Helsinki. Retired from the position of research professor and department director at the National Public Health Institute (THL) Department of Lifestyle and Participation in 2014, he works currently as course teacher at the Universities of Helsinki and Tampere and as visiting scientist to the National Institute for Health and Welfare. He was professor of public health at the University of Tampere, Finland, 2009–2013. Earlier in his career, he worked as researcher at the Academy of Finland, as lecturer and assistant professor at University of Helsinki, and chief of laboratory at the National Public Health Institute (KTL), respectively.

Uutela was educated as a cognitive social psychologist with a special interest in the link of attitudes and behavior. The latter and interest in practical applications of social psychology led him to start working with health-related applications in 1975, first at the Department of Social Psychology, and from 1980 at the Department of Public Health of the Helsinki University. In 1986, Uutela established a connection to the National Public Health Institute (KTL) and to the Finrisk Study. This contact was to become a signpost for his later professional career, which also included project membership in the Health 2000 Study.

When accepting the position of chief of the new Health Behavior Research Unit at National Public Health Institute (KTL) in 1994, Uutela started to look for possibilities of establishing a national member society associated with the International Society of Behavioral Medicine. This emerged rapidly, and he became the founding president of the Finnish Section of Behavioral Medicine, a section of Finnish Society of Social Medicine in 1994, the year when the section was also accepted as a full member of ISBM. Uutela has been a member of the Board of the Finnish Section till 2008.

Currently Uutela is member of the Swedish Society of Behavioral Medicine and the Society of Behavioral Medicine. He has been active in the International Society of Behavioral Medicine in several officer positions and organization of international meetings since 1996. He was the president of ISBM from 2004 to 2006, president-elect from 2002 to 2004, immediate past president and chair of the Awards Committee from 2006 to 2008, and chair of the Finance Committee of ISBM (2008–2012). He started his officer career in ISBM by becoming the treasurer of society for the period 1996–2002. On several occasions, he has represented the Finnish Section in the Governing Council. Dr. Uutela has belonged to the Editorial Board of IJBM from 1996 onward and been a program committee member for ISBM international congresses in 1996–2006, chair of the local organizing committee (ICBM, Helsinki 2002), and program track chair (1996–2000). He was the poster session chair for the 2008 and 2010 international meetings.

In addition to his work in behavioral medicine, Uutela has been involved in academic research and education, in several national and international committees and expert duties in health promotion, including program chair of the Nordic Public Health Conference in 2011. He was the president of the Finnish Society of Sport Sciences LTS and a board member of the Foundation for Sport and Health Sciences (LIKES) in 1999–2011.

Major Accomplishments

Upon becoming the unit chief at KTL, Uutela assumed leadership of the working age and senior citizens' lifestyle monitoring research, which produced information for public health planning and evaluation in the general population, its subgroups and regionally. This monitoring system is one of the oldest in the world, an excellent basis for evaluation and planning of national health policy and national and international lifestyle statistics. The system has given rise to similar systems, e.g., in the Baltic countries of Europe. Uutela led the study of several projects funded by the Academy of Finland related to socioeconomic health inequalities and health promotion. From 2001 to 2014, he has participated and led intervention studies in the Good Old Age in Lahti region (GOAL) community intervention framework aimed at improving functional capacity of the aging population and preventing type 2 diabetes. He was in charge of the nutrition intervention study focusing on Finnish male conscripts (2005–2015) and also contributed to the upper primary school nutrition intervention at the National Public Health Institute. Dr. Uutela has more than 350 publications.

During his ISBM presidency, Uutela worked actively to broaden the global basis of the society: Asia, Central and Eastern Europe, and Middle and Southern America were especially targeted. In June 2005, the Governing Council of ISBM gathered in Mexico City in association with the Latin-American Regional Meeting in Behavioral Medicine. The Central European Society of Behavioral Medicine held a network meeting in Targu Mures, Romania, in November 2005. Contacts between ISBM and South America were strengthened during the president's visit to Caracas, Venezuela, in association with the Third Venezuelan Congress of Behavioral Medicine in October 2005. A Thai

Forum of Behavioral Medicine was held in Bangkok in December 2005 as a gateway to the 2006 ICBM there. Uutela with his fellow executives worked toward improvement of the administration and budgeting of ISBM. As an important item, in 2006, special funds in ISBM budgeting were devoted to developmental funds of ISBM to increase chances for global development and participation of behavioral medicine. The highly successful Bangkok ICBM, with Brian Oldenburg and Marc Gellman as program chairs and Naiphinich Kotchabhakdi as chair of local organization, led to acceptance of the Central-Eastern Society of Behavioral Medicine as an ISBM member and to a change of by-laws regarding individual membership.

Dr. Uutela is a Knight, First Class, of the Order of the Lion of Finland from 2012, and he has been granted with the Golden Cross of Sports and Sports Culture of Finland in 2013.

V

Validity

J. Rick Turner
Campbell University College of Pharmacy and Health Sciences, Buies Creek, NC, USA

Definition

The primary objective of an experimental or nonexperimental research study is to obtain a valid estimate of the treatment effect of interest. Validity can be divided into considerations of internal validity and external validity (Rothman et al. 2008).

Both experimental and nonexperimental studies require consideration to be paid to study design, data acquisition, data management, and analysis. If all of these are of optimum quality and there are no imperfections in the study, the study is deemed valid and the correct result is provided. Any imperfections lead to bias of various types.

Internal validity addresses the validity of inferences concerning the source population, and external validity addresses the validity of inferences to the general population, an issue also known as generalizability.

Cross-References

▶ Bias
▶ Confounding Influence
▶ Experimental Designs
▶ Generalizability
▶ Nonexperimental Designs
▶ Statistical Inference

References and Further Reading

Kleinbaum, D. G., Sullivan, K. M., & Barker, N. D. (2007). *A pocket guide to epidemiology*. New York: Springer.

Rothman, K. J., Greenland, S., & Lash, T. L. (2008). Validity in epidemiologic studies. In K. J. Rothman, S. Greenland, & T. L. Lash (Eds.), *Modern epidemiology* (3rd ed., pp. 128–147). Philadelphia: Lippincott Williams & Wilkins.

Variability

▶ Dispersion
▶ Variance

Variance

J. Rick Turner
Campbell University College of Pharmacy and Health Sciences, Buies Creek, NC, USA

Synonyms

Variability

Definition

Variance is a sophisticated measure of dispersion that takes into account the position of every data point about a central value, typically the mean. It is therefore a measure of the variability within a data set.

Imagine the following data set: 6, 8, 10, 12, and 14. The mean is the sum of all the values divided by the total number of values, i.e., 50/5 = 10. How can we find a measure that will capture the totality of the dispersion of the numbers around the mean? An initial thought is to calculate the arithmetic distance each number, or score, lies from the mean, and sum these values. This leads to the following: −4, −2, 0, 2, and 4, the sum of which is 0. That is, the total deviation of the scores from the mean is 0.

This is actually true for any such calculation for any data set. The mathematics of calculating the mean ensures that the sum of the deviations of any set of scores from its mean is always zero. So, this strategy does not help convey the degree of dispersion around a central value.

However, one extra step takes us to a useful strategy: This involves squaring all of the deviations. Given that a negative number multiplied by another negative number produces a positive value, we now get the following for our original data set: 16, 4, 0, 4, and 16, which sum to 40. This value is known as the sum of squares. If most of the scores in a data set tend to be close to the mean, the sum of squares (the variance) will be relatively low. The converse is true when most of the scores tend to be relatively further away from the mean. It is therefore possible to have two data sets with identical means and yet very different sums of squares.

One further step is required to calculate the variance: The sum of squares is divided by the value that is one less than the number of scores in the data set. This value is called the degrees of freedom, and is discussed in the entry titled ▶ "Degrees of Freedom." In this case, the sum of squares, 40, is divided by (5−1), i.e., 4. The variance is therefore 10, which is coincidentally the same as the mean in this case.

In most cases, one further step will be taken: the standard deviation will be calculated as the square root of the variance, as discussed in the entry titled ▶ "Standard Deviation."

Cross-References

▶ Degrees of Freedom
▶ Standard Deviation

Vascular Abnormalities, Function

Jonathan Newman
Columbia University, New York, NY, USA

Description

Vascular function can be described as the function of the vascular endothelium, the monolayer of cells lining the intimal surface of the entire circulatory system. The surface of the vascular endothelium in one individual is enormous and has been estimated to contain roughly 3×10^{13} cells, covering the surface of more than six tennis courts. This section will review the cardinal domains of vascular function in cardiovascular disease; will describe putative pathogenic abnormalities in vascular function, and will briefly review measures to assess vascular function.

The regulation of vascular tone and hemostasis/coagulation are two primary domains of vascular function important in the pathogenesis of cardiovascular disease (CVD). There are other physiologically important vascular functions, including complex metabolic properties and the regulation of vascular permeability, but these domains are outside of this review. The regulation of vascular tone is a delicate balance of opposing vasoconstrictive and vasodilatory functions. The endothelial cells lining the vasculature have vasodilatory and vasoconstrictive properties and synthesize some local active molecules that have both local and systemic effects on vascular tone. The vasoconstrictive and vasodilatory properties of the endothelium that help maintain normal hemodynamics are a crucial portion of the response to local (vascular trauma, compromise) or systemic (congestive heart failure, hypertension) abnormalities. Vasodilation and vasodilatory function is reviewed elsewhere (see ▶ "Vasodilation, Vasodilatory Functions"). Vasoconstriction is mediated in part by the endothelium-derived molecules endothelin-1, thromboxane-A_2, and platelet activating factor. Importantly, the vasodilatory and vasoconstrictive properties of the endothelium also have anti- and prothrombotic activities, respectively. This leads to delicate balance of vascular function in which the vasodilatory properties also promote blood fluidity through the inhibition of coagulation, whereas the vasoconstrictive properties of the endothelium promote platelet activation and hemostasis. Thus, the regulation of vascular tone interacts crucially with the other primary domain of vascular function, coagulation, and hemostasis, and in most normal circumstances, the endothelium constitutively expresses an antithrombotic surface to the blood that inhibits platelet aggregation and clot formation. When the endothelium is activated or compromised, however, it is capable of quickly becoming prothrombotic, activating platelets and promoting coagulation.

Given its importance, a number of different modalities have been developed and investigated to assess vascular function.

There are, however, two main categories of assessment.

The first and "gold standard" methodology is coronary angiography (catheterization) to measure coronary circulation with infusion of vasoactive medications, such as adenosine, to measure coronary blood flow and resistance.

However, this technique is invasive, expensive, and not without risk.

Therefore, relying on the principle that endothelial dysfunction is a systemic disorder, vascular function can be measured in other arterial beds in a less invasive manner.

The most widely studied method is flow-mediated dilation (FMD) of the brachial artery using high-resolution ultrasound.

During the measurement of FMD, brachial artery diameter is measured before and after an increase in wall stress induced by reactive hyperemia (increased blood flow) seen following inflation of a sphygmomanometer cuff proximal to the brachial artery for 5 min at high pressures, up to 200 mmHg.

The amount of dilation seen largely reflects endothelial function and the availability of important vasodilatory molecules, such as nitric oxide (NO).

FMD is predictive of the extent and severity of coronary atherosclerosis and is an independent predictor of prognosis.

Brachial artery FMD is also moderately correlated with coronary artery FMD.

However, FMD is operator dependent and requires significant training.

It is also influenced by catecholamines, levels of hormones such as estrogen and progesterone, stress level, and sleep deprivation.

Further, it remains unclear whether the assessment of FMD provides information that is additional to traditional risk factors.

A recent technology that utilizes similar methods of assessing changes following reactive hyperemia is finger-pulse plethysmography.

This technology relies on changes in pulse wave amplitude following reactive hyperemia in the finger.

These changes in amplitude are filtered, amplified, displayed, and stored, and a threshold has been identified that may have utility in identifying endothelial dysfunction within the coronary circulation.

Measurement of both brachial FMD and finger-pulse plethysmography has largely been restricted to research use, but investigation into the potential clinical applications of these modalities is ongoing.

References and Readings

Gori, T., Parker, J. D., & Manzel, T. (2010). Flow-mediated constriction: Further insight into a new measure of vascular function. *European Heart Journal, 32*, 784–787.

Lerman, A., & Zeiher, A. M. (2005). Endothelial function: Cardiac events. *Circulation, 111*, 363–368.

Moncada, S., & Higgs, E. A. (Eds.). (2006). *The vascular endothelium*. New York: Springer.

Munzel, T., Sinning, C., Post, F., Warnholtz, A., & Schulz, E. (2008). Pathophysiology, diagnosis and prognostic implications of endothelial dysfunction. *Annals of Medicine, 40*, 180–196.

Vascular Endothelial Growth Factor (VEGF)

Alexandra Erdmann and Erin S. Costanzo
Department of Psychiatry, Carbone Cancer Center, University of Wisconsin-Madison, Madison, WI, USA

Definition

Vascular endothelial growth factor (VEGF) is a key regulatory molecule that promotes growth of new blood vessels. VEGF plays an important role in normal physiological processes that require increased vascularization to bring oxygen and nutrients to tissues, including embryonic and postnatal development and wound healing (Ferrara et al. 2003). VEGF can also contribute to disease processes. For example, upregulation of VEGF has been linked to development of intraocular neovascular syndromes, inflammatory disorders, and brain edema, among others (Ferrara et al. 2003). VEGF also plays a critical role in tumor growth and development. Specifically, VEGF recruits endothelial cells to the tumor site, allowing for growth of capillary networks that enable tumor development by increasing the supply of oxygen and nutrients essential for cell division and growth (Antoni et al. 2006; Ferrara et al. 2003). The vascularization of a tumor in its early stages allows the mass to grow beyond a critical point and to eventually metastasize, or spread through the circulatory system to other tissues and organs (Kerbel 2000). Consequently, anti-VEGF agents have been developed for cancer treatment, with promising results from recent clinical trials (e.g., Escudier et al. 2007).

Of relevance to behavioral medicine, there is evidence that stress can affect VEGF production. Specifically, stimulation of in vitro ovarian, melanoma, and nasopharyngeal tumor cell lines with stress hormones such as norepinephrine, epinephrine, and cortisol leads to increased production of VEGF. Effects appear to occur via β-adrenergic signaling pathways and can be moderated by β-blockers, such as propranolol (Lutgendorf et al. 2003; Yang et al. 2006, 2009). These results suggest a potential pathway by which stress-related psychosocial factors may affect tumor development and progression. New investigations are determining the extent to which β-blockers may be promising therapeutic options (Costanzo et al. 2011). These studies pinpoint a physiological pathway by which behavioral interventions targeting stress may have the potential to improve cancer outcomes.

Cross-References

▶ Cancer, types of
▶ Cortisol

- Cytokines
- Epinephrine
- Ovarian Cancer
- Stress

References and Readings

Antoni, M. H., Lutgendorf, S. K., Cole, S. W., Dhabhar, F. S., Sephton, S. E., McDonald, P. G., et al. (2006). The influence of bio-behavioural factors on tumour biology: Pathways and mechanisms. *Nature Reviews Cancer, 6*, 240–248.

Costanzo, E. S., Sood, A. K., & Lutgendorf, S. K. (2011). Biobehavioral influences on cancer progression. *Immunology and Allergy Clinics of North America, 31*, 109–132.

Escudier, B., Pluzanska, A., Koralewski, P., Ravaud, A., Bracarda, S., Szczylik, C., et al. (2007). Bevacizumab plus interferon alfa-2a for treatment of metastatic renal cell carcinoma: A randomized, doubleblind phase III trial. *Lancet, 370*, 2103–2111.

Ferrara, N., Gerber, H., & LeCouter, J. (2003). The biology of VEGF and its receptors. *Nature Medicine, 9*, 669–676.

Kerbel, R. (2000). Tumor angiogenesis: Past, present, and the near future. *Carcinogenesis (London), 21*, 505–515.

Lutgendorf, S. K., Cole, S., Costanzo, E., Bradley, S., Coffin, J., Jabbari, S., et al. (2003). Stress-related mediators stimulate vascular endothelial growth factor secretion by two ovarian cancer cell lines. *Clinical Cancer Research, 9*, 4514–4521.

Yang, E. V., Kim, S. J., Donovan, E. L., Chen, M., Gross, A. C., Webster Marketon, J. I., et al. (2009). Norepinephrine upregulates VEGF, IL-8, and IL-6 expression in human melanoma tumor cell lines: Implications for stress-related enhancement of tumor progression. *Brain, Behavior, and Immunity, 23*, 267–275.

Yang, E. V., Sood, A. K., Chen, M., Li, Y., Eubank, T. D., Marsh, C. B., et al. (2006). Norepinephrine up-regulates the expression of vascular endothelial growth factor, matrix metalloproteinase (MMP)-2, and MMP-9 in nasopharyngeal carcinoma tumor cells. *Cancer Research, 66*, 10357–10364.

Vascular Headache

- Migraine Headache

Vasoconstriction

Leah Rosenberg
Department of Medicine, School of Medicine, Duke University, Durham, NC, USA

Definition

Vasoconstriction is the process by which smooth muscle causes contraction and narrowing along the vessel length. The mechanism of vasoconstriction is mediated by intracellular calcium levels and a variety of calcium-binding proteins, particularly calmodulin (Barrett et al. 2010).

Vasoconstriction is a physiologic cardiovascular regulatory mechanism that has essential functions throughout the body. Vasoconstriction may be triggered locally in the vasculature or from afar by upstream mediators in response to a variety of physical and emotional stimuli. It is also an example of autoregulation, when organism homeostasis is maintained through balance of vasoconstriction and vasodilatory mechanisms. While most changes are in response to blood flow of the vascular bed or an intrinsic reaction to stretch, there are many other stimuli that induce acute and chronic changes. In the event of vascular injury or compression, there is local response thought to be mediated by serotonin released by platelets that have accumulated proximate to the injured tissue. In addition to serotonin, there are a variety of other vasoconstrictor proteins that have systemic effects.

Several mechanisms have been developed to measure vasoconstriction in the central as well as peripheral vasculature. These are mostly utilized in research settings and have been put into mainstream clinical practice. However, the noninvasive measurement of vascular tone may soon prove to have indications for identifying patients at increased risk for complications like heart attack and stroke.

Cross-References

▶ Coronary Vasoconstriction

References and Readings

Barrett, K. E., Barman, S. M., Boitano, S., & Brooks, H. (2010). Chapter 33. Cardiovascular regulatory mechanisms. In K. E. Barrett, S. M. Barman, S. Boitano, & H. Brooks (Eds.), *Ganong's review of medical physiology* (23rd ed.). New York: McGraw-Hill.

Vasodilation, Vasodilatory Functions

Jonathan Newman
Columbia University, New York, NY, USA

Definition

Vasodilation refers to the opening or enlargement of blood vessels as a result of relaxation in the smooth muscle cells lining the arteries and to a lesser extent, the veins of the human body. Vasodilation is largely the reverse of the vasoconstriction, which refers to the narrowing of the same blood vessels throughout the human body.

Description

In general, vasodilation leads to a decrease in resistance in that vascular structure and a subsequent increase in blood flow. This relationship can be illustrated by examining the hemodynamic relationships of total peripheral resistance (TPR). Total peripheral resistance is equal to the difference between mean arterial pressure (MAP) and mean venous pressure (MVP), divided by the cardiac output (CO), represented by the equation: TPR = (MAP − MVP)/CO. In general, resistance in tubular structures, like blood vessels, is inversely proportional to the radius of that tube (blood vessel) raised to the 4th power (Resistance = $1/radius^4$). Therefore, any increase in the radius of a blood vessel produces a significant decrease in the resistance of the vessel in question. In general, vasodilation works to decrease TPR through the actions of local and systemic factors that relax the smooth muscle cells in and around arteries and arterioles, increasing the size of blood vessels through a change in their radius.

Vasodilation plays an important role in the maintenance of body temperature through the vasodilation of superficial blood vessels and the release of heat into the cooler air surface surrounding the human body. Vasodilation is mediated by local or paracrine factors secreted by the endothelial cells themselves such as nitric oxide, bradykinin, potassium, and adenosine diphosphate (a breakdown product of working muscles). Vasodilatory function has an important role in the pathophysiology and treatment of cardiovascular disease and impaired vasodilation, and vasodilatory function has been demonstrated to be an important component of atherosclerotic coronary artery disease (see ▶ "Vascular Abnormalities, Function"). Impaired vasodilation is thought to reflect reduced nitric oxide bioavailability. Further, the promotion or stimulation of vasodilation with different cardioactive medications has proven therapeutic benefit in conditions such as mitral regurgitation, aortic regurgitation, hypertension, coronary artery disease, and congestive heart failure.

In general, the stimulation of vasodilation may help to reduce the amount of regurgitant blood flow seen in aortic and mitral regurgitation. Acutely, intravenous vasodilation in these conditions may reduce ventricular pressures and increase forward flow, potentially improving ventricular function. It is not clear if the hemodynamic improvement seen with vasodilator use in regurgitant valvular lesions is due to the reductions in blood pressure alone or through a combination of factors. In heart failure, the use of vasodilators encompasses both arterial and venous vasodilation, typically with agents such as hydralazine (arteriolar dilation) and nitrates (venodilation). The next effect of the use of these two vasodilators is to reduce the amount of a forward (preload) and "backward" (afterload) pressure on the heart, thereby reducing myocardial work and improving function. The antihypertensive effect of vasodilators is due mostly to the reduction arterial tone and therefore blood pressure. In coronary disease, nitrates can have profound anti-ischemic effects through their actions as both arterio- and venodilators, though the main effects of vasodilation in patients with coronary disease may be through decreasing ventricular filling (preload) which decreases wall tension, cardiac work, and hence myocardial oxygen demand, and may in turn lessen anginal symptoms.

In conclusion, vasodilation and vasodilatory function is an important component in both normal cardiovascular function and in the pathogenesis of disease. As described, the promotion of vasodilation is a useful therapeutic target for the treatment of a wide range of cardiovascular diseases.

Vasopressin

George J. Trachte
Academic Health Center, School of Medicine-Duluth Campus, University of Minnesota, Duluth, MN, USA

Background

Vasopressin has numerous behavioral influences such as reinforcing bonding between mating pairs, enhancing memory, and promoting aggressive behavior. It also regulates the osmolarity of blood and influences blood pressure.

Physiological Relevance

Vasopressin is essential for bond formation in a number of species. Mating bonds occurring in normally monogamous rodents are ablated by blockade of brain vasopressin V_{1a} receptors. Vasopressin is suspected to have a similar role in humans. Memory also is enhanced by vasopressin in a number of species but the physiological relevance to memory remains to be determined in humans. Finally, vasopressin constricts blood vessels to elevate blood pressure and this action is important in hypovolemic states.

Vasopressin is present in all terrestrial animals, presumably to concentrate urine to retain water. Vasopressin absence results in a condition called diabetes insipidus, characterized by excretion of large volumes of dilute urine and the need to consume large quantities of water to survive.

Vasopressin actions are mediated by at least three separate receptors termed V_{1a}, V_{1b}, and V_2. The V_{1a} receptor mediates vasoconstrictor effects of vasopressin whereas V_2 receptors mediate the renal effects to concentrate urine. Both V_{1a} and V_{1b} receptors are present in the brain and account for behavioral effects of vasopressin. Receptor mutations in both mice and humans have greatly assisted in defining the roles of the receptor subtypes in various vasopressin actions.

Control of Release/Secretion

Vasopressin is synthesized in the supraoptic and paraventricular nuclei of the hypothalamus and is transported to the posterior pituitary gland within magnocellular neurons. It is synthesized as a 168 amino acid preprohormone that is converted to a 145 amino acid prohormone with the 9 amino acids of the amino terminal representing the final vasopressin molecule. Vasopressin is stored in the posterior pituitary and released in response to plasma hyperosmolarity, sexual activity, or hypotension.

Localization/Molecular Biology

The preprovasopressin gene is located on chromosome 20 in humans and expressed in hypothalamic nuclei. Vasopressin receptors are expressed in high levels in brain regions associated with emotional regulation or sensory integration, such as the amygdala and thalamus.

Behavioral Actions

Vasopressin has at least three prominent behavioral actions, including promotion of pair bonding, improvement of memory, and increased aggression toward sexual rivals. The pair bonding data are derived primarily from monogamous rodents who fail to develop pair bonds when vasopressin V_{1a} receptors are blocked. Similar actions are suspected in humans and vasopressin is referred to as a "bonding" hormone. Memory also is improved in humans and other species by vasopressin infusions, whereas, V_{1a} receptor antagonists impair memory. Finally, vasopressin increases aggression in males toward other males with this behavior attributable to the V_{1b} receptor in rodents.

Alterations in V_{1a} receptor levels have been associated with autism and schizophrenia whereas V_{1b} receptor mutations have been associated with excessive aggression in humans. Excessive aggression also correlates with high cerebrospinal vasopressin concentrations.

Ultimately, vasopressin is viewed as a monogamy hormone, enhancing bonding with a mate and children while reinforcing protective or aggressive behaviors.

Vegetative Nervous System

▶ Autonomic Nervous System (ANS)

Venereal Diseases

▶ Sexually Transmitted Diseases (STDs)

Ventromedial Nucleus

▶ Hypothalamus

Video Applications

▶ Williams LifeSkills Program

Videogames

▶ Health Gaming

Vigilance

▶ Coffee Drinking, Effects of Caffeine

Viral Hepatitis

▶ Hepatitis C and Cognitive Functioning

Virtual Communities

▶ Social Networking Sites

Virtual Humans

▶ Digital Relational Agents

Virtual Reality

Carly M. Goldstein[1,2] and Stephanie P. Goldstein[2]
[1]The Weight Control and Diabetes Research Center, The Miriam Hospital, Providence, RI, USA
[2]Warren Alpert Medical School, Brown University, Providence, RI, USA

Synonyms

Artificial environment; Artificial intelligence; Computerized simulation; VR

Definition

Virtual reality is computer technology that approximates virtual worlds, allowing the user to explore and interact in a reality or a sci-fi environment. It may include augmentative devices like headsets or handsets, but some virtual reality is available solely on a desktop or laptop computer (e.g., Second Life). Well-known virtual reality programs include Sega VR, Google Street View, and Oculus Rift. For the purposes of behavioral medicine, virtual reality can be used to foster self-management, provide psychoeducation or exposure exercises, and practice behavioral skills.

Description

Virtual reality can include haptic systems, which send vibrations into the hands or body to create the illusion of grabbing, touching, or movement. The tactile information is frequently called force feedback. Some systems include multi-room displays, allowing the user to walk through space to explore and interact. Hardware that composes the system typically includes gyroscopes, small and large screens, motion sensors, headphones, and processors. Augmented reality, a related term, blends what the user sees in real life with the virtual experience. Social media platforms (e.g., Instagram, Snapchat, Facebook) use augmented reality to create special effects when the user takes a picture or video; these are frequently referred to as filters or face lenses. Virtual worlds consist of a platform that allows individuals to create virtual representations of themselves (i.e., avatars) that are capable of interaction and exploration.

One of the earliest virtual reality systems was the View-Master; paper and film cartridges were inserted into a set of viewing goggles. Users could see a still scene mapped on top of their visible world. Another early technology was the Aspen Movie Map created at Massachusetts Institute of Technology in 1978; it allowed users to walk through Aspen, Colorado, in different seasons. In 1992, Louis Rosenberg created Virtual Fixtures, which was a body-like system that enabled sight, sound, and touch for the US Air Force. These early developments informed the virtual realities available today.

There are several modern-day VR platforms such as PlayStation VR, HTC VR, and Oculus Rift. Oculus Rift has received attention for its quality and value (as it was purchased for $2 billion by Facebook to support its development). Oculus Rift was released on March 28, 2016, and consists of a headset display with position tracking system and 3D audio capability with headphones. It is primarily used for gaming and entertainment and has had no formal use in the healthcare industry yet.

Virtual reality is used in medical training, armed forces training, marketing, fine arts, video games, and entertainment. Surgeons have used virtual reality to practice risky operations and to model intricate vascular structures. It is also used in occupational health to safely test hazardous processes, like disease containment.

In a patient population, virtual reality has been most widely used to facilitate exposure in treatments of anxiety (Powers and Emmelkamp 2008). Virtual reality has also been used, although less extensively, in medical settings to assist patients in coping with medical procedures and operations (Robertson et al. 2017). In the developing field of neurorehabilitation, it has been evaluated as a modality for enhancing cognitive and motor performance in patients with cerebral palsy, stroke, and traumatic brain injury using force feedback and practicing a variety of activities in low-risk, naturalistic environments (Dascal et al. 2017). This is an especially valuable application as the world's population continues to age and be affected by cognitive impairment, which can limit independence and quality of life.

Virtual reality has been implemented in hospital settings to facilitate distraction among patients with acute and chronic pain (Garcia-Palacios et al. 2015; Murray et al. 2009; van Twillert et al. 2007). Hopefully, similar interventions can be translated to aid healthcare providers in treating opioid abuse and dependence in other patients with chronic pain (Wiederhold et al. 2014). Virtual reality has also been used with cancer patients to reduce cancer-related psychological symptoms during chemotherapy and other painful procedures with children and adults (Chirico et al. 2016). Research has evaluated several uses of virtual reality to address obesity and disordered eating through simulations that target body image, exposure to cues that trigger binge eating, and practice making healthy eating decisions (Marco et al. 2013; Riva et al. 2000; Thomas et al. 2015). There have also been preliminary investigations on the use of virtual reality to facilitate cue exposure in conjunction with cognitive behavioral treatment for tobacco (Culbertson et al. 2012) and alcohol use disorders (Lee et al. 2009).

As evidenced by a growing body of literature in this area, there are several advantages to using virtual reality in behavioral medicine that include the power to control stimulus presentation and response measurement, safe assessment of hazardous situations, generalization of learning, standardization of protocol, and increased user participation (Schultheis and Rizzo 2001). There are also presently numerous limitations to using virtual reality in behavioral medicine. First, virtual reality systems are very costly to make, and the necessary costs typically far exceed funds provided by many departments or grant mechanisms. Additionally, behavioral medicine professionals are rarely trained in how to communicate with developers, who are usually completely naïve to behavioral medicine concepts. It may also be difficult to disseminate a large volume of hardware for an adequately powered research trial and many research trials can suffer from methodological flaws (McCann et al. 2014). Conversely, virtual reality that solely uses desktop computers may underwhelm patients with more impressive expectations if their expectations are not managed at the start of use. Finally, patients may have limited exposure to using the necessary technology if specialized hardware is a part of the system. Future virtual reality interventions for behavioral medicine topic areas should be feasible, cost-efficient, and innovative. These interventions should build on the literature of successful applications in anxiety disorders and medical training.

Virtual reality is poised to have a significant impact on the field of behavioral medicine and patient care, but current progress has been thwarted by costs and a lack of history of developers and behavioral medicine specialists' collaboration. Forays into behavioral medicine thus far have been fruitful, and future advances should model the successes seen in virtual reality to other applications like surgery, gaming, and occupational health. Given the recent commercial availability of Oculus Rift, Facebook's acquisition of the company for a large sum, and the virtual/augmented reality being built into to commonplace technologies (e.g., smartphone) and marketing campaigns, the role of virtual reality is expanding not only in everyday life but also in chronic disease management and patient care. Virtual reality is becoming a part of common popular culture, and this technology acceptance can be applied to helping communities become healthier and thrive.

Cross-References

▶ Behavior Therapy
▶ Digital Health Coaching
▶ Digital Relational Agents
▶ Online Therapy and E-Counselling
▶ Self-Management
▶ Telehealth

References and Further Reading

Burdea Grigore, C., & Coiffet, P. (1994). *Virtual reality technology*. London: Wiley-Interscience.
Chirico, A., Lucidi, F., De Laurentiis, M., Milanese, C., Napoli, A., & Giordano, A. (2016). Virtual reality in health system: Beyond entertainment. A mini-review on the efficacy of VR during cancer treatment. *Journal of Cellular Physiology, 231*(2), 275–287.
Culbertson, C. S., Shulenberger, S., De La Garza, R., Newton, T. F., & Brody, A. L. (2012). Virtual reality cue exposure therapy for the treatment of tobacco dependence. *Journal of Cyber Therapy and Rehabilitation, 5*(1), 57–64.
Dascal, J., Reid, M., IsHak, W. W., Spiegel, B., Recacho, J., Rosen, B., & Danovitch, I. (2017). Virtual reality and medical inpatients: A systematic review of randomized, controlled trials. *Innovations in Clinical Neuroscience, 14*(1–2), 14–21.
Garcia-Palacios, A., Herrero, R., Vizcaíno, Y., Belmonte, M. A., Castilla, D., Molinari, G., ..., & Botella, C. (2015). Integrating virtual reality with activity

management for the treatment of fibromyalgia: Acceptability and preliminary efficacy. *Clinical Journal of Pain, 31*(6), 564–572.

Gigante, M. A. (1993). Virtual reality: Definitions, history and applications. In R. A. Earnshaw, M. A. Gigante, & H. Jones (Eds.), *Virtual reality systems* (pp. 3–14). London: Academic.

Lee, S. H., Han, D. H., Oh, S., Lyoo, I. K., Lee, Y. S., Renshaw, P. F., & Lukas, S. E. (2009). Quantitative electroencephalographic (qEEG) correlates of craving during virtual reality therapy in alcohol-dependent patients. *Pharmacology, Biochemistry, and Behavior, 91*(3), 393–397.

Marco, J. H., Perpina, C., & Botella, C. (2013). Effectiveness of cognitive behavioral therapy supported by virtual reality in the treatment of body image in eating disorders: One year follow-up. *Psychiatry Research, 209*(3), 619–625.

Mazuryk, T., & Gervautz, M. (1996). *Virtual reality, history, applications, technology and future* (pp. 1–72). Vienna: Institute of Computer Graphics, Vienna University of Technology.

McCann, R. A., Armstrong, C. M., Skopp, N. A., Edwards-Stewart, A., Smolenski, D. J., June, J. D., ..., & Reger, G. M. (2014). Virtual reality exposure therapy for the treatment of anxiety disorders: An evaluation of research quality. *Journal of Anxiety Disorders, 28*(6), 625–631.

Murray, C. D., Pettifer, S., Howard, T., Patchick, E., Caillette, F., & Murray, J. (2009). Virtual solutions to phantom problems: Using immersive virtual reality to treat phantom limb pain. In C. D. Murray (Ed.), *Amputation, prosthesis use, and phantom limb pain* (pp. 175–196). New York: Springer.

Parsons, T. D., & Rizzo, A. A. (2008). Affective outcomes of virtual reality exposure therapy for anxiety and specific phobias: A meta-analysis. *Journal of Behavior Therapy and Experimental Psychiatry, 39*(3), 250–261.

Powers, M. B., & Emmelkamp, P. M. (2008). Virtual reality exposure therapy for anxiety disorders: A meta-analysis. *Journal of Anxiety Disorders, 22*(3), 561–569.

Riva, G., Bacchetta, M., Baruffi, M., Rinaldi, S., Vincelli, F., & Molinari, E. (2000). Virtual reality-based experiential cognitive treatment of obesity and binge-eating disorders. *Clinical Psychology & Psychotherapy, 7*(3), 209–219.

Robertson, A., Khan, R., Fick, D., Robertson, W. B., Gunaratne, D. R., Yapa, S., ..., & Rajan, R. (2017). The effect of virtual reality in reducing preoperative anxiety in patients prior to arthroscopic knee surgery: A randomised controlled trial. In: 2017 I.E. 5th international conference on serious games and applications for health (SeGAH), IEEE, Perth, pp. 1–7.

Schultheis, M. T., & Rizzo, A. A. (2001). The application of virtual reality technology in rehabilitation. *Rehabilitation Psychology, 46*(3), 296–311.

Stone, R. (2001). Haptic feedback: A brief history from telepresence to virtual reality. In R. Murray-Smith (Ed.), *Haptic human–computer interaction* (Vol. 2058, pp. 1–16). Heidelberg: Springer.

Thomas, J. G., Spitalnick, J. S., Hadley, W., Bond, D. S., & Wing, R. R. (2015). Development of and feedback on a fully automated virtual reality system for online training in weight management skills. *Journal of Diabetes Science and Technology, 9*(1), 145–148. https://doi.org/10.1177/1932296814557326.

van Twillert, B., Bremer, M., & Faber, A. W. (2007). Computer-generated virtual reality to control pain and anxiety in pediatric and adult burn patients during wound dressing changes. *Journal of Burn Care & Research, 28*(5), 694–702.

Wiederhold, B. K., & Wiederhold, M. D. (2005). *Virtual reality therapy for anxiety disorders: Advances in evaluation and treatment*. Washington, DC: American Psychological Association.

Wiederhold, B. K., Riva, G., & Wiederhold, M. D. (2014). How can virtual reality interventions help reduce prescription opioid drug misuse? *Cyberpsychology, Behavior and Social Networking, 17*(6), 331–332.

Visceral Adiposity

▶ Central Adiposity

Visceral Nervous System

▶ Autonomic Nervous System (ANS)

Visible Difference

▶ Body Image and Appearance-Altering Conditions

Visualization

▶ Guided Imagery

Vital Exhaustion

Douglas Carroll
School of Sport and Exercise Sciences,
The University of Birmingham, Edgbaston,
Birmingham, UK

Definition

Vital exhaustion is a prodromal constellation of symptoms including physical exhaustion and feelings of hopelessness preceding major coronary heart disease events such as myocardial infarction.

Description

Vital exhaustion was a concept first proposed by Appels some 25 years ago. Appels argued that exhaustion was not simply premonitory to cardiac events, reflecting established pathology and representing early warnings, the historic clinical view. Rather, he contended that the syndrome of vital exhaustion was casually related to subsequent events. The causal pathway was hypothesized to be the neuroendocrine mechanisms typically invoked as the link between psychosocial exposures and heart disease. Support for a causal role for vital exhaustion was gleaned from a number of subsequent observational epidemiological studies demonstrating an association between measure of exhaustion and subsequent all-cause mortality and cardiac disease mortality and morbidity. Unfortunately, such evidence is necessarily only indicative and provides insufficient surety of the direction of causation. Reverse causation, where heart disease that has not yet been formally diagnosed leads to symptoms of exhaustion, must remain a possibility. A growing literature illustrates how the inflammatory processes implicated in atherosclerosis may contribute to feeling of fatigue and depression. In addition, confounding by some unmeasured or poorly measured variable in these observational studies cannot be wholly dismissed.

The proper test of causation is intervention: a randomized control trial, whether patients are randomly allocated to a exhaustion treatment invention or to a condition in which no such treatment is available. Some 5 years ago, Appels and his colleagues reported the outcome of such an intervention. Participants were over 700 cardiac disease patients who had undergone successful angioplasty, a procedure for the surgical repair of block coronary arteries. Patients were randomized to a 6-month exhaustion intervention comprising among other things relaxation training and stress management, or to usual care. At the 18-month, but not the 6-month, follow-up, fewer intervention than usual care patients reported feeling exhausted and fewer were depressed. However, the intervention did not reduce the likelihood of patients having a recurrent cardiac disease event.

Cross-References

▶ Depression
▶ Heart Disease

References and Further Reading

Appels, A., & Mulder, P. (1989). Fatigue and heart disease. The association between "vital exhaustion" and past, present, and future heart disease. *Journal of Psychosomatic Research, 33*, 727–738.

Appels, A., Bar, F., van der Pol, G., Erdman, R., Assman, M., Trijsburg, W., et al. (2005). Effects of treating exhaustion in angioplasty patients on new coronary events. Results of the randomised Exhaustion Intervention Trial (EXIT). *Psychosomatic Medicine, 67*, 217–223.

Carroll, D., Phillips, A. C., & Macleod, J. (2006). Intervening for exhaustion. *Journal of Psychosomatic Research, 61*, 9–10.

Vital Status

▶ Mortality

Vitality

Christiane A. Hoppmann[1] and Denis Gerstorf[2]
[1]Department of Psychology, University of British Columbia, Vancouver, BC, Canada
[2]Institute of Psychology, Humboldt University, Berlin, Germany

Definition

The concept of active life expectancy revolves around the fundamental question of how many of the years added to life through advances in average life expectancy are spent in reasonably good health. A comprehensive and multifaceted view of health considers a variety of different physical, mental, and psychological health aspects.

Description

Overview

Human life expectancies have almost doubled over the last century. As a result, an unprecedented number of individuals can expect to reach old age. This historically new situation challenges us to better understand the factors that may contribute to vitality in old age. This entry aims to shed light on two important questions: First, it introduces the concept of active life expectancy to address the fundamental question of how many of those years added to life are spent in reasonably good health. Second, it argues for a comprehensive multifaceted view on vitality in old age that takes into account important psychological variables, including well-being, social engagement, and cognitive functioning. It concludes by alluding to key challenges that this line of work has to confront in the future.

Active Life Expectancy

Recent increases in human life expectancies and longevity are a great achievement, due to many different factors including improved public health and medical advances in Western countries (▶ Longevity). Those demographic trends also pose important societal challenges such as the question whether the gains in quantity of life are accompanied by gains in (or at least maintenance of) quality of life. A central construct in this regard is active (or healthy) life expectancy, which is frequently defined as the number of years individuals can expect to live without chronic disability (Crimmins et al. 1996). Research using this concept has advanced our knowledge regarding segments of the population who benefit or who are excluded from such trends. This line of inquiry has also helped put some of the earlier enthusiasm about increasing longevity into perspective. For example, although women can typically expect to live longer than men, they often spend a greater portion of their lives in disabling conditions. Likewise, individuals with higher socioeconomic status do not only live longer, but they also enjoy old age in better health than individuals with lower socioeconomic status. Moreover, there are notable racial differences in active life expectancies with African Americans typically spending more years with disabilities than non-Blacks in the United States (Crimmins et al. 1996). More generally, research on active life expectancy has revealed important insights into which demographic strata can be expected to spend the years added to life in reasonably good health and which strata do not.

Apart from identifying key population-level predictors of vitality, this line of research has also fueled important discussions about big-picture trends. Different propositions have been put forward regarding future changes in morbidity-mortality dynamics. The probably most prominent example is the compression of morbidity hypothesis (Fries 1980), according to which increases in active life expectancy occur at a faster rate than increases in life expectancy. As a consequence, the years people spend in ill health are compressed into an increasingly shorter period at the very end of life. Conversely, other scholars have proposed that further increases in longevity would result in increased disease prevalence, ultimately leading to an expansion of morbidity (Gruenberg 1977). Thirty years later, the verdict is still out. It appears as if individual perceptions of the years spent in good health are indeed increasing at the population level. In contrast, trends for the years spent in disability differ by severity. Years spent with severe disabilities are declining, whereas years spent with less severe forms are on the rise (Christensen et al. 2009). More generally, some researchers are skeptical about the possibility to successfully compress morbidity (e.g., Crimmins et al. 1996) whereas others report promising findings regarding delayed disabilities among more recently born cohorts of older adults (e.g., Manton et al. 2008). Taken together, the epidemiological literature has posed big-picture questions regarding how increasing longevity impacts disease prevalence and has raised awareness to tremendous heterogeneity in how well older adults from different backgrounds can expect to live their last years of life.

Psychological Indicators of Vitality

A comprehensive understanding of vitality in old age fundamentally depends on how health is defined. Specifically, it has been proposed that the time is due to move away from disease-centered definitions of health (Ryff and Singer 2000). For example, the WHO defines health as "a state of complete physical, mental and social well-being" (Official Records of the World Health Organization 1948). This definition dovetails with notions of successful aging that emphasize the importance of older adults maintaining their cognitive and physical functioning as well as actively engaging with life (Rowe and Kahn 1997). To provide a more holistic account of health with aging, social scientists have thus embarked on a search for psychological factors that contribute to a more comprehensive understanding of vitality in old age that goes beyond the mere absence of disease. For example, it has been shown that emotional well-being is closely linked with physical health (Pressman and Cohen 2005). In a similar vein, social relationships seem to be associated with older adults' physical and mental health (Hoppmann and Gerstorf 2009), and associations between cognitive functioning and physical health in old age are a well-established research finding (Schaie 2005). Hence, psychological research promises to broaden the scope of what constitutes vitality in old age by pointing to the important role of such diverse factors as emotional well-being, motivational processes, and cognition.

In addition to such normative accounts of vitality, there is also a rich literature on interindividual differences in self-regulatory processes. Importantly, this line of research takes into account that older adults may be able to maintain their well-being when confronted with losses in functional health. For example, it has been shown that strategies of selective optimization with compensation, self-efficacy, and control processes are positively associated with health in old age (e.g., Baltes and Smith 2004; Seeman et al. 1999; Wrosch et al. 2004).

Identifying key psychological factors that distinguish older adults who spend their final years in reasonably good health from those who suffer from disease is important because it allows us to move beyond a recognition of well-established risk factors of late-life disability (e.g., being male, low socioeconomic status, member of a minority) that are in fact unalterable. Hence, recognizing that psychological constructs are key ingredients of or central contributors to vitality in old age may offer important insight into factors that may be amenable to intervention and where growth might be possible until old age (Ryff and Singer 2000).

Future Directions

In a final step, we would like to highlight two key societal challenges that are intrinsically linked with the concept of vitality. First, it is going to become increasingly important to recognize the practical implications of (changes in) vitality. For example, many developed countries currently face a heated debate about whether or not to increase mandatory retirement age. Importantly, it seems as if more flexible and individualized retirement decisions are necessary so as to accommodate the specific needs of the aging population. Some older adults may simply not be well enough to continue working beyond age 65, whereas other

65+ year olds may benefit from staying in the work force for longer and would profit from work-related cognitive stimulation and social participation (Pinquart and Schindler 2007).

Second, it is well possible that positive secular trends that have repeatedly been reported for earlier points in life such as retirement age may be offset or even reversed in more advanced ages or at the end of life. In fact, there is empirical evidence that later-born cohorts may experience steeper end-of-life declines in cognitive abilities than earlier-born cohorts (Gerstorf et al. 2011). One way to interpret such results is that members of later-born cohorts may have survived diseases that would have resulted in death among members of earlier-born cohorts. However, the previously higher levels of (cognitive) functioning were not maintained for this manufactured survival time (Olshansky et al. 2002). More generally, it remains unclear if it will ultimately be possible to successfully compress morbidity into increasingly shorter time periods at the end of life. We have to keep in mind that humans were not designed to enjoy such long post-reproductive lives as it is often the case today and that chance plays a much greater role in determining health during the post-reproductive as compared to the reproductive years of life (Finch and Kirkwood 2000).

Cross-References

▶ Longevity

References and Readings

Baltes, P. B., & Smith, J. (2004). Lifespan psychology: From developmental contextualism to developmental biocultural co-constructivism. *Research in Human Development, 1*, 123–144.
Christensen, K., Doblhammer, G., Rau, R., & Vaupel, J. W. (2009). Ageing populations: The challenges ahead. *Lancet, 374*, 1196–1208.
Crimmins, E. M., Hayward, M. D., & Saito, Y. (1996). Differentials in active life expectancy in the older population of the United States. *Journals of Gerontology: Series B, Psychological Sciences and Social Sciences, 51*, 111–120.
Finch, C. E., & Kirkwood, T. B. L. (2000). *Chance, development, and aging*. New York: Oxford University Press.
Fries, J. F. (1980). Aging, natural death, and the compression of morbidity. *New England Journal of Medicine, 303*, 1369–1370.
Gerstorf, D., Ram, N., Hoppmann, C. A., Willis, S. L., & Schaie, K. W. (2011). Cohort differences in cognitive aging and terminal decline in the Seattle Longitudinal Study. *Developmental Psychology, 47*(4), 1026–1041.
Gruenberg, E. F. (1977). The failures of success. *Milbank Memorial Fund Quarterly/Health and Society, 55*, 3–24.
Hoppmann, C., & Gerstorf, D. (2009). Spousal interrelations in old age – A mini review. *Gerontology, 55*(449), 459.
Manton, K. G., Gu, X., & Lowrimore, G. R. (2008). Cohort changes in active life expectancy in the U.S. elderly population: Experience from the 1982–2004 national long-term care study. *Journals of Gerontology: Series B, Psychological Sciences and Social Sciences, 63*, 269–281.
Olshansky, S. J., Hayflick, L., & Carnes, B. A. (2002). Position statement on human aging. *Journals of Gerontology Series A: Medical and Biological Sciences, 57A*, B292–B297.
Pinquart, M., & Schindler, I. (2007). Changes of life satisfaction in the transition to retirement: A latent-class approach. *Psychology and Aging, 22*, 442–455.
Pressman, S. D., & Cohen, S. (2005). Does positive affect influence health? *Psychological Bulletin, 131*, 925–971.
Rowe, J. W., & Kahn, R. L. (1997). Successful aging. *The Gerontologist, 37*, 433–440.
Ryff, C. D., & Singer, B. (2000). Interpersonal flourishing: A positive health agenda for the new millennium. *Personality and Social Psychology Review, 4*, 30–44.
Schaie, K. W. (2005). *Developmental influences on intelligence: The Seattle longitudinal study*. New York: Oxford University Press.
Seeman, T. E., Unger, J. B., McAvay, G., & Mendes de Leon, C. F. (1999). Self-efficacy beliefs and perceived declines in functional ability: MacArthur Studies of Successful Aging. *Journals of Gerontology: Series B, Psychological Sciences and Social Sciences, 54B*, P214–P222.
World Health Organization. (1948). *Official records*, No. 2. New York.
Wrosch, C., Schulz, R., & Heckhausen, J. (2004). Health stresses and depressive symptomatology in the elderly: A control-process approach. *Current Directions in Psychological Science, 13*, 17–20. American Psychological Society.

VO$_2$max Test

▶ Maximal Exercise Stress Test

Vocal Group

▶ Singing and Health

Vocational Assessment

Jeong Han Kim
Department of Clinical Counseling and Mental Health, Texas Tech University Health Science Center, Lubbock, TX, USA

Synonyms

Career assessment; Career evaluation; Vocational evaluation

Definition and Description

Vocational assessment is a continuing process for systematically gathering and synthesizing valid information of the individuals' needs that is relevant to the career goal. Although incidental and casual sources of data have influence, it is a proactive and intentional activity. To provide a brief but sufficient introduction to vocational assessment, this chapter addresses (1) unique characteristics of vocational assessment, (2) assessment types, (3) labor market analysis, (4) assessor's role and function, (5) disability accommodation, and (6) multicultural concerns.

Characteristics of Vocational Assessment

The unique characteristic of vocational assessment is that the constructs relevant to vocational assessments are multidimensional and include both innate (e.g., personality, intelligence) and learned dispositions (e.g., value, interest, character, transferable skills). When the assessment is used to determine service eligibility or the qualification for a job, the nature of vocational assessment is diagnostic. On the other hand, when it used for general career guidance and planning, the nature of assessment is more evaluative. Evaluation and assessment often used interchangeably; however, in specific, two terms are not identical. The term evaluation has a broader meaning with the emphasis on the collaborative relationship, while assessment is often used for the purpose of diagnosis.

Types of Vocational Assessment

Vocational assessment can be classified broadly into the following type: (1) achievement and intelligence, (2) aptitude test, (3) personality, (4) career interest, (5) work values, and (6) transferable skills.

First, in achievement and intelligence, norm-referenced standardized tests are often used as it provides an individual's achievement/intelligence in comparison to the norm population. Assessment in this area includes the Wide Range Achievement Test, Wechsler Adult Intelligence Scale, Woodcock-Johnson Intelligence Test, and so on.

Second, aptitude tests measure one's capability to perform a certain task without pre-owned knowledge and often include General Aptitude Test Battery (GATB), the Minnesota Clerical Test, and Career Ability Placement Survey.

Third, personality assessment provide information regarding a pattern of an individual behavior in a certain situation. For example, it provides supplemental information (e.g., social/peer relationship, problem solving style), but the need must be carefully determined depending on the client's situation.

Fourth, career interest test is often built based on career theory such as Holland's Hexagon (Holland 1997) that include Realistic (do-ers), Investigative (thinker), Artistic (creator), Social (helper), Enterprising (persuader), and Conventional (organizer). Results from career interest test are often associated with the six occupational areas in terms of designing career plan and intervention. Commonly used career interest inventories are Career Assessment Inventory, Career Occupational Preference System Inventory, the Strong-Campbell Interest Inventory, and the Minnesota Vocational Interest Inventory.

Fifth, work values are traits and qualities that an individual search in the career (Zunker 2016) and reflects individual's attitude, beliefs, and feelings in regard to specific occupation (Ros et al. 1999).

Sixth, transferrable skills are developed through various life experiences such as previous career, education, and social interaction and often include skills in communication, time management, dependability, problem-solving, and conflict resolution. Transferrable skills are important in that those skills can be used in various job setting (Bolton and Parker 2001).

In addition, work sample and situational assessment are often administered for an individual with disabilities. Work samples are designed to provide a reference point to objectively evaluate individual's capability to perform a certain job task. Examples include, but not limited to, assessment of client performance level in dexterity, spatial perception, mechanical assembly skills, physical and mobility training, and eye-hand-foot coordination. Situational assessment is given in a real employment setting, allowing an evaluator can gather on-the-job related data. Work samples and situation assessment are relatively more often used with persons with disabilities (Szymanski and Parker 2010).

Labor Market Information

Results from the vocational assessment often related to the labor market information. Three most common labor market databases are Occupational Information Network (O'NET), *Dictionary of Occupational Titles* (DOT), and *Occupational Handbook* (OOT). These database offer information, but not limited to, on the job task/description, technology skills, knowledge, work activities, work context, qualification, wage, projected growth, and job opening.

Role and Function

Various roles and functions are required. First of all, a test administer should be aware of issues relevant to test anxiety. Being professionally considerate so that a client can freely show their assets, strengths, and weakness at their best is important. Such competency is particularly important in semi- or unstructured assessment as in some cases an individual is not able to make a sound judgment on their capacity and interest. In regard to that, basic counseling skills such as probing, listening, and attending skills are always important. In a situation when families or others are involved in vocational assessment, facilitating communication is a function expected to test administered. Although assessment is often used for the purpose of diagnosis and evaluation of certain disposition, assessment itself also has therapeutic function. It is because assessment increases self-awareness, important in career development. Besides these skills, abilities to become accurate, constructive, objective, comprehensive, and considerate are important qualities recommended for career assessment.

Disability Accommodation

Equity is important in the assessment and requires that appropriate assessment be available to all individuals with disability in accessible manner. It further indicates the importance of focusing on ability, not the disability, of an individual. Disability accommodation is important in ensuring equity and often includes extended time, alternative format (reading instruction instead of written instruction), letting an individual answer verbally depending on their disability types, and modifications of standardized test. As equitable does not mean ideal, it is important to individualize test accommodation. To do so, vocational assessor and evaluator need to understand the physical and functional aspects of disability in relation to assessment. The use of accommodation also needs to be taken into consideration for proper interpretation (Ekstrom and Smith 2002).

Multicultural Concerns

Cultural competency is important in that a construct tested in the assessment may have different meaning across cultures. Although the use of instrument with construct equivalence and cross-cultural validity is important, in reality, it is not always easy to prepare such an instrument. At minimum to be culturally responsive, test administers are recommended to improve professional competencies in their cultural knowledge, self-awareness on their own bias and prejudice (Sue and Sue 2013), and culturally relevant skills. As culture is not a fixed-term and changes over time, there is no endpoint in the development of cultural competency. It is ideal for test administer to see cultural competence from a virtue perspective and to deliver their best effort in a consistent manner.

Cross-References

▶ Readiness for Return-to-Work (RRTW)

References and Further Readings

Bolton, B. F., & Parker, R. M. (2001). *Handbook of measurement and evaluation in rehabilitation*. Austin: PRO-ED, Inc..

Ekstrom, R. B., & Smith, D. K. (2002). *Assessing individuals with disabilities in educational, employment, and counseling settings*. Washington: American Psychological Association.

Holland, J. L. (1997). *Making vocational choices: A theory of vocational personalities and work environments* (3rd ed.). Odessa: Psychological Assessment Resources.

Ros, M., Schwartz, S. H., & Surkiss, S. (1999). Basic individual values, and the meaning of work. Applied Psychology-An International Review, 48, 49–71.

Sue, W. D., & Sue, D. (2013). *Counseling the culturally diverse: Theory and practice*. New Jersey: Wiley.

Szymanski, E. M., & Parker, R. M. (2010). *Work and disability*. Austin: PRO-ED, Inc..

Zunker, V. G. (2016). *Career counseling: A holistic approach*. Belmont: Brooks/Cole.

Vocational Evaluation

▶ Vocational Assessment

Vocational Rehabilitation

Michiel F. Reneman[1] and Douglas P. Gross[2]
[1]Department of Rehabilitation Medicine, University of Groningen, University Medical Center Groningen, Groningen, The Netherlands
[2]Department of Physical Therapy, University of Alberta, Edmonton, AB, Canada

Definition

Vocational rehabilitation (VR) is defined as a multiprofessional evidence-based approach to optimize work participation that includes various services and activities provided in different settings to working age individuals with health-related impairments, limitations, or restrictions in work functioning (Escorpizo et al. 2011). While this definition is comprehensive, it is also quite complex. In simple language, VR can also be defined as "anything that helps someone with a health problem to stay at, return to, and remain in work" (Waddell et al. 2008b).

Description

A comprehensive review of VR for workers with common health problems highlighted that VR for workers with chronic musculoskeletal pain conditions (CMPC) can be effective for promoting work outcomes (Waddell et al. 2008b). Work outcomes may be very diverse and includes staying at work, modified work, temporarily or permanently working, returning to work (RTW) or a combination of these. For years the strongest evidence was on low back pain, but recent evidence shows that the same principles apply to most common CMPC such as neck, shoulder, or arm pain/complaints. It was also demonstrated that from a societal perspective, VR in patients with CMSC has a good business case, indicating that society as a whole may benefit from investment in VR. Although estimates vary, a ratio of 1:5 was mentioned: for every currency unit invested in VR, the societal return will be fivefold (Waddell et al. 2008b). An overview of evidence of effectiveness for VR for other health conditions is outside the scope of this entry. Effective principles, as described below, however, may also apply to VR in other health conditions.

VR principles and interventions are fundamentally the same for work related and other comparable (nonwork related) health conditions, irrespective of whether they are classified as injury, condition, or disease. Healthcare has a key role, but VR is not a matter of healthcare alone. Employers also have a key role – there is strong evidence that proactive company approaches to sickness, including temporary provision of modified work and accommodations, are effective and cost-effective (Franche et al. 2005), although there is less evidence on VR in small and medium enterprises. Overall, the evidence shows that effective VR depends on work- and worker-focused healthcare and accommodating workplaces; both are necessary as they are interdependent and must be coordinated simultaneously (Waddell et al. 2008b).

Stepped-Care Approach and Differential Care

The concept of early intervention is central to vocational rehabilitation, because the longer a worker is off work, the greater the obstacle to return to work and the more challenging vocational rehabilitation becomes. It is simpler, more effective, and cost-effective to prevent people with a health condition from developing long-term sickness absence. A "stepped-care approach" starts with monodisciplinary, low-intensity, low-cost interventions which will be adequate for most sick or injured workers (e.g., physical therapy, education, RTW coaching), and provides progressively more intensive and structured interventions for those who need additional help to return to work, such as multidisciplinary VR. This approach allocates resources most appropriately and efficiently to meet individual and payers' needs. Effective VR depends on communication and coordination between the key players – particularly the individual, healthcare, and the workplace.

Given that VR is about helping people with health problems stay at, return to, and/or remain in work, the question is how to make sure that everyone of working age receives the help they require. This should start from the needs of people with health problems at various stages; build on the evidence about effective interventions; and consider potential resources and the practicalities of how these interventions might be delivered. From this perspective, there are three broad types of workers, who are differentiated mainly by duration out of work, and who have correspondingly different needs: workers who are absent short term (less than 6 weeks), intermediate (between 6 weeks and 12 months), and long term (more than 3 months) (Franche et al. 2005). There is also a fourth type of worker that has recently started to gain attention: those workers who manage to stay at work despite a health condition (de Vries et al. 2012).

For workers with subacute disorders and sick leave for more than 4–8 weeks, multidisciplinary VR programs in occupational settings may be an option to offer to workers who need additional help to return to work. However, within the stepped care approach, diagnostic triaging is needed to screen those who can benefit and to screen out those who will not benefit, for example whose course of recovery may still be considered favorable without health care interventions. At this stage, the advice for VR will be a trade-off between prognosis, costs, and benefits. Those with a prognosis that is unfavorable based on bio-, psycho-, or social factors may, even though the time off work may be limited, may still be advised to follow vocational rehabilitation. The "risk" that the individual worker will regain normal work without help care interventions, because of the favorable prognosis based purely on limited time off work, should be weighed against the risk of not regaining work because of unfavorable other prognostic factors ("too much, too soon, too costly" vs. "too late"). At this point in time, however, validated instruments to assist with these decisions are unavailable.

Multidisciplinary Vocational Rehabilitation

For workers who are out of work more than about 6 months, multidisciplinary VR is recommended (Waddell et al. 2008b; Airaksinen et al. 2006). There is strong evidence that multidisciplinary VR is effective to facilitate work outcomes (Waddell et al. 2008b; Airaksinen et al. 2006). However, there are also major challenges that accompany VR. Even though its effectiveness has been established, the effect sizes are rather modest (Waddell et al. 2008b; Airaksinen et al. 2006). This means that the average worker will benefit somewhat from VR, but there is a large variety of results: from no benefit at all, to complete recovery of work outcomes. Theoretically, average effect sizes should increase when workers who will not benefit from these programs will not be offered such a program, or should be offered a different program that will provide better results. This requires reliable and valid screening tools that would be able to differentiate, but these tools are presently in development stages.

Multidisciplinary VR is delivered in many different shapes and forms. Literature describes a huge variety of content, disciplines, and dosage, and the optimum components for each individual worker is currently unknown. It is currently regarded as one of the main challenges in this field. It requires a set of diagnostic instruments that can validly distinguish subgroups of workers in need of specific content ("what works for whom"). Perhaps because of the absence of these instruments, many VR programs contain a more or less standard mix of content (mostly consisting of physical exercises, cognitive behavioral therapy or principles, education, graded activities) delivered by more or less standard disciplines (physical therapy, occupational therapy, psychology), with durations varying from a few hours/weeks to 100 h or more delivered over several months (Waterschoot et al. 2014). Theoretically, content, disciplines, and dosage that add nothing to the results can be removed from these programs, leading to similar effectiveness and improved cost-effectiveness. However, at this point, strong evidence-based recommendations for specific content (van Tulder et al. 2006) or dosage (Waterschoot et al. 2014) cannot be given.

Effective Principles

Even though detailed recommendations about effective components of VR cannot be given, effective principles can be derived from the literature. Realizing that differences exist between jurisdictions with all its different barriers and facilitators, these principles can be used to tailor VR to the needs of the individual worker and within the context of work. An overarching principle is that it depends on work-focused healthcare and accommodating workplaces. To make a real and lasting difference, both need to be addressed and coordinated. The main principles are (Main et al. 2008): the presence of a return to work (RTW) coordinator, the principle of graded activity and graded exposure to work, including modified work, and a biopsychosocial orientation of the VR team.

Most VR programs benefit from RTW coordinator or case manager, who serves as liaison between the worker, the work, health care, benefits office, and other stakeholders. The effectiveness of communication between health care and the workplace has been established (Franche et al. 2005). The role of RTW coordinator as key to the program's success, and the competencies of the RTW coordinator may be more important than professional background (Gardner et al. 2010).

The second principle for VR is that of graded activity and graded exposure to work, including modified work. During VR, the worker should increase activities according to schedule that the worker and the VR team codevelop. This plan involves a gradual progressing of activities, regardless of daily fluctuations in pain intensity. "Activities" may involve exercise, physical activities, and sports activities, but also work related activities. Preferably, if jurisdictions allow for this, this should involve modified work (Franche et al. 2005). Modifications can be duties, tasks, hours, days, etc., based on shared decision by the worker and supervisor, often guided by the RTW coordinator (Lambeek et al. 2010). If modified work is not an option, VR programs may involve simulated work activities performed at the rehabilitation clinic. These simulated work activities should follow the same principles of codevelopment and gradual increase of workload towards a predefined endpoint.

As a general principle, the VR team and its members typically embrace the biopsychosocial model to guide their functional diagnostic and treatment approach (Waddell et al. 2008b). One of the key principles of VR is to address dysfunctional beliefs and behavior. There is extensive clinical evidence that symptoms may originate from a health condition, but the development of chronic symptoms and disability also depends on psychosocial factors. There is now broad agreement that understanding and management of human illness and disability must take account of biological, psychological, *and* social dimensions – a biopsychosocial model. It is an individual-centered model that considers the person, their health problem, *and* their social context: biological refers to the physical or mental health condition; psychological recognizes that personal/psychological factors also influence functioning; social recognizes the importance of the social context, pressures, and constraints on illness behavior and functioning. These elements are often described and dealt with separately. In reality, functioning depends on complex interactions between the individual, the health condition, and the environment in a dynamic social process over time (Waddell et al. 2008a; Bartys et al. 2017).

Cross-References

▶ Occupational Rehabilitation
▶ Return to Work

References and Further Reading

Airaksinen, O., Brox, J. I., Cedraschi, C., Hildebrandt, J., Klaber-Moffett, J., Kovacs, F., et al. (2006). Chapter 4. European guidelines for the management of chronic nonspecific low back pain. *European Spine Journal, 15*(Suppl 2), S192–S300.

Bartys, S., Frederiksen, P., & Bendix, T., Burton, K. (2017). System influences on work disability due to low back pain: An international evidence synthesis. *Health Policy, 121*(8), 903–912. https://doi.org/10.1016/j.healthpol.2017.05.011

Escorpizo, R., Reneman, M. F., Ekholm, J., Fritz, J., Krupa, T., Marnetoft, S. U., et al. (2011). A conceptual definition of vocational rehabilitation based on the ICF: Building a shared global model. *Journal of Occupational Rehabilitation, 21*(2), 126–133.

Franche, R. L., Cullen, K., Clarke, J., Irvin, E., Sinclair, S., Frank, J., et al. (2005). Workplace-based return-to-work interventions: A systematic review of the quantitative literature. *Journal of Occupational Rehabilitation, 15*(4), 607–631.

Gardner, B. T., Pransky, G., Shaw, W. S., Nha Hong, Q., & Loisel, P. (2010). Researcher perspectives on competencies of return-to-work coordinators. *Disability and Rehabilitation, 32*(1), 72–78.

Lambeek, L. C., Bosmans, J. E., Van Royen, B. J., Van Tulder, M. W., Van Mechelen, W., & Anema, J. R. (2010). Effect of integrated care for sick listed patients with chronic low back pain: Economic evaluation alongside a randomised controlled trial. *British Medical Journal, 341*, c6414.

Main, C., Sullivan, M. J. L., & Watson, P. J. (Eds.). (2008). *Pain management; practical applications of the biopsychosocial perspective in clinical and occupational settings* (2nd ed.). London: Elsevier Limited.

van Tulder, M., Becker, A., Bekkering, T., Breen, A., del Real, M. T., Hutchinson, A., et al. (2006). Chapter 3. European guidelines for the management of acute nonspecific low back pain in primary care. *European Spine Journal, 15*(Suppl 2), S169–S191.

de Vries, H. J., Reneman, M. F., Groothoff, J. W., Geertzen, J. H., & Brouwer, S. (2012). Factors promoting staying at work in people with chronic nonspecific musculoskeletal pain: A systematic review. *Disability and Rehabilitation, 34*(6), 443–458.

Waddell, G., Burton, K., & Aylward, M. (2008a). A biopsychosocial model of sickness and disability. *The Guides Newsletter*, Chicago: American Medical Association, 1–13.

Waddell, G., Burton, A. K., & Kendall, N. A. S. (Eds.). (2008b). *Vocational rehabilitation – What works, for whom, and when? Report for the Vocational rehabilitation Task Group.* London: TSO.

Waterschoot, F. P., Dijkstra, P. U., Hollak, N., de Vries, H. J., Geertzen, J. H., & Reneman, M. F. (2014). Dose or content? Effectiveness of pain rehabilitation programs for patients with chronic low back pain: A systematic review. *Pain, 155*(1), 179–189.

VR

▶ Virtual Reality

Vulnerabilities

▶ Cardiovascular Risk Factors

W

Waist Circumference

▶ Waist Girth
▶ Waist Size

Waist Circumference (WC)

Tavis S. Campbell, Jillian A. Johnson and Kristin A. Zernicke
Department of Psychology, University of Calgary, Calgary, AB, Canada

Synonyms

Girth

Definition

Waist circumference (WC) is considered a measure of the relative health risk associated with excess abdominal fat. Abdominal fat contains higher amounts of visceral fat, a fat that is produced by the liver, turned into cholesterol, and released into the bloodstream where it can form plaque on artery walls. Excess abdominal fat is associated with high cholesterol, high blood pressure, and cardiovascular disease.

Waist circumference may be a better indicator of obesity-related diseases than body mass index (BMI) (Cawley 2006), especially among certain populations (e.g., elderly persons). Certain ethnic groups are genetically predisposed to store more fat in the abdomen, even at healthy weights (e.g., non-Hispanic blacks, people of Asian descent).

It is measured by first locating the upper hipbone and lowest rib, followed by placing the end of a measuring tape between these two points and wrapping horizontally around the abdomen.

Men with a waist circumference greater than 102 cm (40 in.) and women with a waist circumference exceeding 88 cm (35 in.) are considered to be at increased risk for developing obesity-related health problems, including type II diabetes, hypertension, and cardiovascular disease.

Cross-References

▶ Body Mass Index

References and Readings

Cawley, J. H. (2006). *Beyond BMI: The value of more accurate measures of fatness and obesity in social science research*. Cambridge, MA: National Bureau of Economic Research.

Heart and Stroke Foundation (2010, January). *Healthy waists*. Retrieved April 8, 2011 from http://www.heartandstroke.com/site/c.ikIQLcMWJtE/b.3876195/

National Heart Lung and Blood Institute (2011, April). *Assessing your weight and health risk*. Retrieved April 8, 2011 from http://www.nhlbi.nih.gov/health/public/heart/obesity/lose_wt/risk.htm

© Springer Nature Switzerland AG 2020
M. D. Gellman (ed.), *Encyclopedia of Behavioral Medicine*,
https://doi.org/10.1007/978-3-030-39903-0

Waist Girth

Christopher Shaw
Deakin University, Melbourne, VIC, Australia

Synonyms

Waist circumference

Definition

Waist girth is related to abdominal visceral fat and predicts a number of disease risk factors associated with obesity.

Description

Obesity which is explained by an increase in body fat is associated with a clustering of risk factors known as the metabolic syndrome and originates from an imbalance between energy intake and energy expenditure. However, there is substantial evidence that body fat distribution rather than total fat mass per se plays a more important role in the development of such risk factors. Gynoid obesity (commonly referred to as "pear shaped") reflects adipose tissue accumulation around the hips and buttocks, whereas android obesity (more commonly referred to as "apple shaped") reflects increased abdominal fat deposition. Android obesity increases with age, is more prominent in males, and poses a significantly greater risk for the development of hypertension, dyslipidemia, insulin resistance, atherosclerosis, type 2 diabetes, coronary artery disease, and certain types of cancer and higher rates of mortality than gynoid obesity. Girth measurements can be used to assess such differences in body fat distribution, and measurement of waist girth specifically represents abdominal obesity. Therefore, it may be a more relevant measure for anyone looking to use simple anthropometric measurements to predict the risk of obesity-related diseases across populations or in response to interventions over time. A variety of gender and age-specific equations are also available to predict body fat percentage from waist girth measurements.

The measurement of waist girth can be used in conjunction with hip circumference to measure waist-hip ratio which is a common method used to predict many health hazards associated with obesity. However, waist girth is more predictive of obesity-related risk factors than waist-to-hip ratio as it is a more accurate reflection of deep visceral adipose tissue (Roche et al. 1996). Furthermore, waist girth measurements also correlate well with the gold standard CT or MRI techniques for the measurement of visceral abdominal fat. The reason that this adipose tissue site is such a risk factor is complex but is likely related to it being more active to lipolytic stimuli such as catecholamines, expression of adrenoreceptors and receptors for insulin, glucocorticoids, and testosterone. Abdominal fat also expresses and releases a multitude of peptides and inflammatory cytokines which are also likely to be involved.

The standardized measurement of waist girth is described by the American College of Sports Medicine (*ACSM's Guidelines for Exercise Testing and Prescription*, 2006). Measurements should be made with a flexible, inelastic tape without compression of the subcutaneous adipose tissue. Measurements should be performed with the participant standing with their feet together and arms by their side. A horizontal measure is then taken at the narrowest part of the torso, typically between the bottom of the ribs and the iliac crest. Duplicate measures should be taken and repeated if the variation exceeds 5 mm.

Waist girth alone, or in combination with other anthropometric measures, has been used to classify and evaluate disease risk. However, different cut off points have been suggested depending on the specific population studied. For example, a waist circumference over 99 cm for males and over 89 cm for females is associated with a high risk for the development of obesity-related disease

(American College of Sports Medicine 2006). Further, a disease risk classification is also available taking into account both BMI and waist circumference (see McArdle et al. 2001). This describes a higher risk of disease when a BMI over 25 kg/m^2 is combined with a waist circumference greater than 102 or 88 cm for males and females, respectively.

Cross-References

▶ Waist Circumference
▶ Waist Size

References and Further Reading

American College of Sports Medicine. (2006). *ACSM's guidelines for exercise testing and prescription* (7th ed.). Philadelphia: Lippincott Williams & Wilkins.

McArdle, W. D., Katch, F. I., & Katch, V. L. (2001). *Exercise physiology: Energy, nutrition and human performance* (5th ed.). Philadelphia: Lippincott Williams & Wilkins.

Roche, A. F., Heymsfield, S. B., & Lohman, T. G. (1996). *Human body composition*. Champaign: Human Kinetics.

Waist Size

Kazuo Hara
Department of Metabolic Diseases, Graduate School of Medicine, The University of Tokyo, Bunkyo-ku, Tokyo, Japan

Synonyms

Waist circumference

Definition

There are several lines of evidence that suggest subjects with a large waist size are at increased risk of developing type 2 diabetes and cardiovascular diseases, even after adjustment for body mass index (BMI), an indicator of total adiposity (Hu et al. 2007; Winter et al. 2008; Yusuf et al. 2005). The large waist size reflects accumulation of excess abdominal fat, also known as central obesity, and is reported to be a primary risk factor for glucose intolerance, dyslipidemia, and high blood pressure, which together is now defined as metabolic syndrome (Kadowaki et al. 2006). Therefore, the measurement of waist size is essential for the screening of metabolic syndrome. Two international definitions for metabolic syndrome are currently used in daily practice, one provided by the International Diabetes Federation (IDF) (IDF Worldwide Definition of the Metabolic Syndrome) and the other by the National Cholesterol Education Program (NCEP) (Expert Panel on Detection, Evaluation, and Treatment of High Blood Cholesterol in Adults 2001). The former criterion requires waist size above a certain cut point for a diagnosis of metabolic syndrome, whereas the latter one does not require a large waist size if the subject has three or more of the following: raised fasting plasma glucose concentrations, elevated blood pressure, elevated levels of triglycerides, and/or reduced levels of high-density lipoproteins.

The IDF recommends that the cut point for waist size used to define central obesity should vary according to ethnic group, and they proposed the following European-specific cut points for waist size: 94 and 80 cm for men and women, respectively (Alberti et al. 2005). Nonetheless, further extensive investigations must be performed before more suitable cut points can be established for use in clinical practice to accurately predict cardiovascular diseases.

The method of measurement must also be standardized. Waist size is usually measured at a level midway between the lowest rib and the iliac crest (Han et al. 1995). However, the waist size is measured at the umbilical level in some countries, such as Japan, for screening metabolic syndrome (Matsuzawa 2005). It is essential that the subjects being measured are not holding their breath and that the tape measure is not at an angle around their waist.

Cross-References

▶ Obesity
▶ Waist to Hip Ratio

References and Further Reading

Alberti, K. G., Zimmet, P., Shaw, J., & IDF Epidemiology Task Force Consensus Group. (2005). The metabolic syndrome – A new worldwide definition. *Lancet, 366*(9491), 1059–1062.

Expert Panel on Detection, Evaluation, and Treatment of High Blood Cholesterol in Adults. (2001). Executive summary of the third report of the national cholesterol education program (NCEP) expert panel on detection, evaluation, and treatment of high blood cholesterol in adults (adult treatment panel III). *Journal of American Medical Association, 285*(19), 2486–2497.

Han, T. S., van Leer, E. M., Seidell, J. C., & Lean, M. E. (1995). Waist circumference action levels in the identification of cardiovascular risk factors: Prevalence study in a random sample. *British Medical Journal, 311*(7017), 1401–1405.

Hu, G., Tuomilehto, J., Silventoinen, K., Sarti, C., Männistö, S., & Jousilahti, P. (2007). Body mass index, waist circumference, and waist-hip ratio on the risk of total and type-specific stroke. *Archives of Internal Medicine, 167*(13), 1420–1427.

IDF Worldwide Definition of the Metabolic Syndrome. Retrieved form http://www.idf.org/idf-worldwide-definition-metabolic-syndrome

Kadowaki, T., Yamauchi, T., Kubota, N., Hara, K., Ueki, K., & Tobe, K. (2006). Adiponectin and adiponectin receptors in insulin resistance, diabetes, and the metabolic syndrome. *Journal of Clinical Investigation, 116*(7), 1784–1792.

Matsuzawa, Y. (2005). Metabolic syndrome – Definition and diagnostic criteria in Japan. *Journal of Atherosclerosis and Thrombosis, 12*(6), 301.

Winter, Y., Rohrmann, S., Linseisen, J., Lanczik, O., Ringleb, P. A., Hebebrand, J., et al. (2008). Contribution of obesity and abdominal fat mass to risk of stroke and transient ischemic attacks. *Stroke, 39*(12), 3145–3151.

Yusuf, S., Hawken, S., Ounpuu, S., Bautista, L., Franzosi, M. G., Commerford, P., et al. (2005). Obesity and the risk of myocardial infarction in 27,000 participants from 52 countries: A case-control study. *Lancet, 366*(9497), 1640–1649.

Waist to Hip Ratio

Kazuo Hara
Department of Metabolic Diseases, Graduate School of Medicine, The University of Tokyo, Bunkyo-ku, Tokyo, Japan

Synonyms

WHR

Definition

The waist hip ratio (WHR) is the ratio of waist circumference to hip circumference. It was reported that the mortality and the risk of coronary artery disease are positively correlated with WHR both in men and women (Lapidus et al. 1984; Larsson et al. 1984). It is well documented that subjects with high WHR and upper body obesity present insulin resistance (Peiris et al. 1986). According to the standard defined by World Health Organization (WHO) in 1999 about metabolic syndrome, in which type 2 diabetes mellitus, glucose tolerance, and insulin resistance are required items, obesity is defined as WHR >0.9 in men and WHR >0.85 in women (World Health Organization 1999).

Cross-References

▶ Obesity
▶ Waist Size

References and Further Reading

Lapidus, L., Bengtsson, C., Larsson, B., Pennert, K., Rybo, E., & Sjöström, L. (1984). Distribution of adipose tissue and risk of cardiovascular disease and death: A 12 year follow up of participants in the population study of women in Gothenburg, Sweden. *British Medical Journal, 289*, 1257–1261.

Larsson, B., Svardsudd, K., Welin, L., Wilhelmsen, L., Björntorp, P., & Tibblin, G. (1984). Abdominal adipose tissue distribution, obesity, and risk of cardiovascular disease and death: 13 year follow up of participants in the study of men born in 1913. *British Medical Journal, 288*, 1401–1404.

Peiris, A. N., Mueller, R. A., Smith, G. A., Struve, M. F., & Kissebah, A. H. (1986). Splanchnic insulin metabolism in obesity. Influence of body fat distribution. *Journal of Clinical Investigation, 78*(6), 1648–1657.

World Health Organization. (1999). *Definition, diagnosis and classification of diabetes mellitus and its complication. Part 1: Diagnosis and classification of diabetes mellitus*. Geneva: Department of Non-communicable Disease Surveillance.

Warmth

▶ Interpersonal Circumplex

Water Pill

▶ Diuretic

Ways of Coping Checklist (WCCL)

Susan Folkman
Department of Medicine, School of Medicine, University of California San Francisco, San Mateo, CA, USA

Definition

The Ways of Coping Checklist (WCCL) is a measure of coping based on Lazarus and Folkman's (1984) stress and coping theory. The WCCL contains 66 items that describe thoughts and acts that people use to deal with the internal and/or external demands of specific stressful encounters. Usually the encounter is described by the subject in an interview or in a brief written description saying who was involved, where it took place, and what happened. Sometimes a particular encounter, such as a medical treatment or an academic examination, is selected by the investigator as the focus of the questionnaire. Subjects respond on a 4-point Likert scale (0 = does not apply and/or not used; 3 = used a great deal), the extent to which the item was used in the specific stressful encounter.

Subscales

Factor analysis of data from a study of stressful encounters reported by a community sample of middle-aged married couples indicated eight scales: planful problem-solving, positive reappraisal, seeking social support, distancing, self-controlling, escape-avoidance, accepting responsibility, and confrontive coping (Folkman et al. 1986). The eight scales use 50 of the 66 items. The additional items are retained on the WCCL because some investigators find them useful. Subsequent factor analyses indicated variability in factor structure. Some factors such as planful problem-solving, positive reappraisal, escape-avoidance, and distancing are relatively stable. Other factors such as self-controlling, accepting responsibility, seeking social support, and confrontive coping are less stable. For a critical review of the WCCL, see Schwarzer and Schwarzer (1996).

Scoring

There are two systems for scoring the WCCL. The "Raw Score" method is to sum the ratings for each scale. This method provides a score for amount of each type of coping used in the specified event.

The "Relative Score" method, introduced by Vitaliano et al. (1987), controls for the variability in scale length. Relative scores are computed by first obtaining the mean item score for each scale. Once the mean effort (ME) is obtained for each scale, the relative effort is calculated by dividing the ME for the particular scale by the sum of the MEs for each of the scales.

Interpretation

The WCCL is descriptive, not diagnostic. Typically, scores are correlated with outcomes of interest, such as depressive symptoms, distress, positive mood, or a relevant behavior.

Investigators ask if there are population norms for comparison purposes. Stress and coping theory (Lazarus and Folkman 1984) views coping as contextual, which means that there is no "standard" amount of coping that can be used as a norm. For example, certain types of coping (e.g., planful problem-solving) are used more in situations that are controllable while other types (e.g., distancing) are used more in situations that have to be accepted.

The Ways of Coping Checklist can be obtained through Mind Garden Publishers (www.mindgarden.com).

References and Readings

Folkman, S., Lazarus, R. S., Gruen, R. J., & DeLongis, A. (1986). Appraisal, coping, health status, and psychological symptoms. *Journal of Personality and Social Psychology, 50*, 571–579.

Lazarus, R. S., & Folkman, S. (1984). *Stress, appraisal, and coping*. New York: Springer.

Schwarzer, R., & Schwarzer, C. (1996). A critical survey of coping instruments. In M. Zeidner & N. S. Endler (Eds.), *Handbook of coping: Theory, research, applications* (pp. 107–132). Oxford, UK: Wiley.

Vitaliano, P. P., Maiuro, R. D., Russo, J., & Becker, J. (1987). Raw versus relative scores in the assessment of coping strategies. *Journal of Behavioral Medicine, 10*, 1–18.

Wearable Fitness Trackers

▶ Physical Activity Monitors

Web-Based Studies

▶ Internet-Based Studies

Weight

▶ Body Mass Index
▶ Lifestyle Changes

Weight Loss

▶ Lifestyle Changes

Weight Loss Surgery

▶ Bariatric Surgery

Weight: Control, Gain/Loss/Reduction, Maintenance, Monitoring

Shuji Inada
Department of Stress Science and Psychosomatic Medicine, Graduate School of Medicine, The University of Tokyo, Tokyo, Japan

Definition

Weight is the mass of one's body. Weight is usually measured by a scale in kilograms, which are base units of mass in the international systems of unit. Weight is used as barometer of adiposity or condition of nutrition or index of growth in children. Weight is useful for intrapersonal comparisons, while body mass index (in adults) or Rohrer's index (in children), which is adjusted for body height, is used for interpersonal comparisons. Weight is also applied for index of water balance in patients who have water imbalance such as congestive heart failure or renal failure.

Since weight measured by a scale is affected by meal, urine, and stool, it is better to measure on the same time after bladder emptying and defecation.

Description

Weight Control

Weight control is to keep, increase, or decrease one's weight within a certain range. Weight category is classified with body mass index as follows (also see ▶ "Body Mass Index") (Table 1).

Since overweight and obese population is increasing, "weight control" often means "weight loss." Weight control is essential to prevention and treatment of many diseases, especially of metabolic disease (Must et al. 1999; Strazzullo et al. 2010).

Weight Gain/Loss/Reduction/Maintenance

Weight gain/loss depends on an energy balance under a normal water balance. Energy intake is usually derived from food intake. Energy consumption includes basal metabolism, consumption for physical activity, and consumption for thermogenesis. Energy intake exceeding energy consumption results weight gain, and energy consumption exceeding energy intake results weight loss.

Diet is the most important for weight reduction, and exercise is often combined with diet. Exercise alone has minimal effect for body weight (Franz et al. 2007). Sibtramine and Orlistat are approved by FDA for use in obesity patients (see ▶ "Obesity: Prevention and Treatment"). Bariatric surgery is performed to severe obese patients (see ▶ "Bariatric Surgery").

Behavioral therapy is applied to weight management and achieves preferable short-term outcome. Behavioral management of obesity includes self-monitoring of diet, physical activity, and/or body weight; stimulus control; cognitive restructuring; goal setting; and problem solving (Johnston et al. 2007).

Maintenance of reduced weight is more difficult than weight reduction. Some regain of weight is inevitable for nonsurgical weight-loss therapy (Franz et al. 2007).

Monitoring

Self-monitoring is an important element of behavioral weight-loss program. Self-monitoring of dietary intake, physical activity, and/or body weight achieves self-evaluation of the weight-loss behavior, one's awareness of weight and behavior, and self-reinforcement of preferable behavior (Burke et al. 2011). While paper-pencil diaries are conventionally used for self-monitoring, internet-based diaries or PDA-based diaries are recently developed for easier recording and less-biased data recording (Burke et al. 2011; Fukuo et al. 2009).

Weight: Control, Gain/Loss/Reduction, Maintenance, Monitoring, Table 1 The international classification of adult underweight, overweight, and obesity according to BMI (WHO 2006)

Classification	Principal cutoff point
Underweight	<18.5
Normal	18.5–24.99
Overweight	25–29.99
Obese class I	30–34.99
Obese class II	35–39.99
Obese class III	>40

Cross-References

▶ Bariatric Surgery
▶ Basal Metabolic Rate
▶ Body Mass Index
▶ Obesity: Prevention and Treatment
▶ Self-monitoring

References and Readings

Burke, L. E., Wang, J., & Sevick, M. A. (2011). Self-monitoring in weight loss: A systemic review of the literature. *Journal of American Dietetic Association, 111*, 92–102.

Franz, M. J., vanWormer, J. J., Crain, A. L., Boucher, J. L., Histon, T., Caplan, W., et al. (2007). Weight-loss outcomes: A systematic review and meta-analysis of weight-loss clinical trials with a minimum 1-year follow-up. *Journal of American Dietetic Association, 107*, 1755–1767.

Fukuo, W., Yoshiuchi, K., Ohashi, K., Togashi, H., Sekine, R., Kikuchi, H., et al. (2009). Development of a hand-held personal digital assistant-based food diary with food photographs for Japanese subjects. *Journal of American Dietetic Association, 109*, 1232–1236.

Johnston, C. A., Tyler, C., & Foreyt, J. P. (2007). Behavioral management of obesity. *Current Atherosclerosis Reports, 9*, 448–453.

Must, A., Spadano, J., Coakley, E. H., Field, A. E., Colditz, G., & Dietz, W. H. (1999). The disease burden associated with overweight and obesity. *Journal of American Medical Association, 282*, 1523–1529.

Strazzullo, P., D'Elia, L., Cairella, G., Garbagnati, F., Cappuccio, F. P., & Scalfi, L. (2010). Excess body weight and incidence of stroke meta-analysis of prospective studies with 2 million participants. *Stroke, 41*, e418–e426.

WHO. (2006). *Global database on body mass index*. Retrieved January 31, 2011, from http://apps.who.int/bmi/index.jsp

Weighted Sample

Jane Monaco
Department of Biostatistics, The University of North Carolina at Chapel Hill, Chapel Hill, NC, USA

Definition

In a weighted sample, not all sample observations contribute equally to the estimate of a population parameter.

Investigators are often interested in estimating quantities (such as means, counts, or proportions) in a population by using a representative sample selected from that population. Probability samples, defined as samples in which each sampling unit has a known, nonzero probability of selection based on the sampling design, allow investigators to compute estimates of population parameters. The most straightforward type of probability sampling design, a simple random sample (SRS), is a selection method in which each sample has the same probability of being selected. In an SRS, the probability of selection of each member in the population is the same.

The estimation of the population mean is straightforward for the SRS design. Let n = sample size, N = population size. Also, let $\{Y_1, \ldots, Y_N\}$ be the population values and $\{y_1, \ldots, y_n\}$ be the sample values. We define the overall sampling fraction as $f = \frac{n}{N}$. Then $\bar{Y} = \frac{1}{N}\sum_{i=1}^{N} Y_i$ the population mean, can be estimated by the statistic,

$$\bar{y} = \frac{1}{n}\sum_{i=1}^{n} y_i$$

Under this SRS design, each sample observation, y_i, contributes equally to the estimate, $\bar{y}$, of the population mean.

More complicated sampling designs, such as stratified sampling, may be chosen by investigators for various reasons including potential efficiency and the ability to use different sampling methods for different strata. In stratified sampling, the population is grouped by some characteristic (such as gender, geographic location, or age category), and a sample is selected within each subgroup separately. In this stratified design, the probability of selecting an individual is likely not the same for all individuals, but rather depends on the individual's subgroup (stratum). For example, in a study of illicit drug use among adolescents in a particular city, the population could be stratified into two age groups, middle school and high school. The probability of selection of a particular student will depend on the sample size and population size within that student's age group. Therefore, the sample statistics using a stratified design must be weighted to account for the unequal selection probability of observations.

To compute a weighted sample mean for a stratified sample, first consider the partition of the population into H mutually exclusive strata. Let N_h = the population size in the hth stratum, n_h = the sample size in the hth stratum so that $N = \sum_{h=1}^{H} N_h$ and $n = \sum_{h=1}^{H} n_h$. The stratum specific sampling fraction is $f_h = \frac{n_h}{N_h}$. We can compute each stratum-specific mean, $\bar{y}_h$, as the average of the n_h units in the hth stratum. The weighted sample mean is computed as weighted sum of the stratum specific means: $\bar{y}_w = \frac{1}{N} \sum_{h=1}^{H} N_h \bar{y}_h$. This weighted sample mean can be shown to provide an unbiased estimate of the population mean, $\bar{Y}$.

Cross-References

▶ Probability

References and Further Reading

Foreman, E. K. (1991). *Survey sampling principles.* New York: M. Dekker.
Kish, L. (1965). *Survey sampling.* New York: Wiley.
Korn, E. L., & Graubard, B. I. (1995). Examples of differing weighted and unweighted estimates from a sample survey. *The American Statistician, 49*(3), 291–295.

Weiss, Stephen M.

Stephen M. Weiss
Department of Psychiatry and Behavioral Sciences, Miller School of Medicine, University of Miami, Miami, FL, USA

Biographical Information

Stephen Weiss was born in northern New Jersey on June 17, 1937. He received his B.A. in Psychology from the University of Maryland (1959) and his Master's (AM) in Psychology from Temple University (1961). He completed his clinical psychology internship and residency in the Department of Medical Psychology at the University of Oregon Medical School (1962–1963) and received his PhD in Psychology (doctoral minor: Cultural Anthropology) from the University of Arizona (1965). Returning to school after nearly 30 years, he completed his MPH in International Health at Johns Hopkins University School of Hygiene and Public Health in 1993.

Weiss has had several "careers" over the past 45+ years. He began his academic career with appointments including the following: assistant professor, University of Arizona (1964–1967); assistant professor, Johns Hopkins University School of Medicine (1967–1970); associate professor and professor (adjunct), Uniformed Services University of the Health Sciences (1978–1993); and adjunct appointments at the Johns Hopkins University School of Hygiene and Public Health (1976–1998) and the NIH Graduate School (Foundation for Advanced Education in the Sciences) (1979–1994). During "intermissions" in his academic career, Weiss spent 5 years (1969–1974) with the US peace corps (including 2 years in the Ivory Coast in West Africa as director of Training for Africa) as deputy director to the Family Health International AIDS Control and Prevention Project (1991–1993) and nearly 20 years at NIH, directing the behavioral medicine program at the National Heart, Lung and Blood Institute (NHLBI: 1974–1991) and as senior advisor at the National Institute of Mental Health (1993). He joined the faculty of the University of Miami School of Medicine in late 1993 as professor in the Department of Psychiatry and Behavioral Sciences, serving as vice chair for research from 2002 to 2009.

Major Accomplishments

Throughout his career(s), Weiss has focused his professional and scientific energies on one principal issue: to better understand how biological, behavioral, and psychosocial factors *interact* in the etiology, treatment, and prevention of chronic illness.

The first 30 years were focused on cardiovascular health and disease. Beginning with his doctoral dissertation, "Psychological Adjustment Following Open Heart Surgery," he continued this work at Johns Hopkins University School of Medicine and subsequently at NHLBI. His program development mandate at NIH enabled him to advance the "biobehavioral" perspective in behavioral and biomedical science venues. For example, when he arrived at NIH (1974), there was *very* little biobehavioral research related to the prevention and control of chronic disease. Upon becoming acquainted with the NIH system of "peer review," it became obvious that one of the principal reasons for this concerned the *lack* of "peer review" for grant applications attempting to combine biological and behavioral perspectives. He demonstrated the need for a "Behavioral Medicine" study section to the senior officials responsible for grant review by screening over 7,000 grant applications from a single review cycle and identifying over 50 applications requiring both behavioral and biomedical review expertise. Established the following year (Joseph Matarazzo was the first Chair), the Behavioral Medicine study section soon proved its relevance to the NIH mission and was permanently chartered after a 3-year trial period.

During this same period, Weiss, with the active participation of a small group of similarly inclined "biobehaviorists" (e.g., Neal Miller, Joseph Matarazzo, Redford Williams, Neil Schneiderman, Gary Schwartz, Herbert Benson, Margaret Chesney, Thomas Coates, and Judith Rodin to name but a few), convened several conferences and workshops which stimulated the establishment of the fields of behavioral medicine (e.g., the Yale Conference on Behavioral Medicine; the Institute of Medicine/National Academy of Sciences Working Group on Behavioral Medicine) and health psychology (e.g., the Arden House Conference on Education and Training in Health Psychology).

These activities led to the formation and growth of several professional organizations (including the Society of Behavioral Medicine; the Academy of Behavioral Medicine Research; the Division of Health Psychology of the American Psychological Association; the International Society of Behavioral Medicine). He served as President of each of these organizations and was instrumental in establishing new scientific journals representing these areas during his stewardship of these organizations (e.g., *Journal of Behavioral Medicine; Annals of Behavioral Medicine; Health Psychology; International Journal of Behavioral Medicine*).

Discussions between Weiss and David Hamburg, president of the Institute of Medicine of the National Academy of Sciences, in the late 1970s concerning the importance of the biobehavioral perspective in understanding the multifaceted, multilayered nature of chronic illness stimulated two major "health and behavior" efforts by the Institute of Medicine (IOM) to highlight the need for expanding NIH research efforts in this area. Two seminal volumes were published by the IOM Committee on Health and Behavior over a 20-year period synthesizing important scientific findings and providing direction for future research. Weiss served as consultant to this Committee, as well as being invited to provide testimony to several related IOM committees in the ensuing years.

During the 1980s, Weiss became active in international health scientific exchanges, participating as scientific liaison to the US-USSR Scientific Exchange in Cardiovascular Behavioral Medicine for over 10 years, and in a similar capacity with the US-Israel Scientific Exchanges on Hypertension and Coronary Heart Disease. He returned to the Johns Hopkins University School of Hygiene and Public Health to complete the MPH in International Health, a course of study that had important implications for his professional career direction. During this program, he became acutely aware of the growing catastrophe of the HIV/AIDS pandemic, particularly in the developing world. Based on this experience (and his newly minted MPH degree), he set out to explore what role he might play in challenging this public health disaster in Africa, where he had spent 2 years in the early 1970s working with the US peace corps.

Retiring from the NIH in 1991, Dr. Weiss began to search for a meaningful professional direction in HIV/AIDS. He spent 2 years with Family Health International and NIMH in HIV/AIDS administrative and program advisory capacities. Recognizing the major differences in the epidemics in the developed vs. developing worlds, he realized that new and unique approaches would be required to establish effective prevention strategies for HIV transmission. It took several years, however, before sufficient momentum was achieved in scientific circles to stimulate the NIH to establish an aggressive extramural research program in the search for new barriers to sexual transmission of the virus.

The advent of the female condom and growing interest in chemical barriers (microbicides) stimulated the need for a "critical mass" of research to answer important questions of safety, efficacy, acceptability, and effectiveness of these new sexual barrier products. Designation of HIV/AIDS as a "threat to our national security" by former President Clinton produced a "sea change" in the federal government's willingness to invest in international studies and demonstration projects to contain the epidemic in the developing world.

The critical need to develop *acceptable* barrier products for the varied populations at high risk of HIV infection suggested that biological efficacy must be coupled with product acceptability studies to ultimately demonstrate the effectiveness and impact of such strategies in containing the epidemic. He received NIH funding to address many of these issues in the USA, Africa, and India. In addition to being P.I. on two large-scale US trials of behavioral interventions with HIV+ women, over the last 16 years, he also has been funded to conduct several studies in Zambia with HIV+ and HIV− men, women, and couples and also to serve as PI, Co-PI, Protocol Co-Chair, and site investigator for an additional five studies on sexual risk reduction and medication adherence in Zambia, South Africa, and India.

Since settling in Miami nearly 20 years ago, Weiss has continued to lead an active professional life. Nonetheless, he still has made time for his passion for flying (commercial license, instrument, multiengine, with over 5,600 flight hours), as well as the occasional fishing trip on his small boat. He has four grown children and nine growing grandchildren, whom he and his wife, Deborah, visit regularly, thanks to his aging, but trusty, Beech Bonanza. He has served as mentor to many junior faculty, residents, and fellows within the medical school through his "Grantsmanship 101" seminar and open invitations to join his research program. He has authored/coauthored over 120 papers, monographs, and scientific reviews, in addition to 10 edited volumes on health and behavior. He currently serves on the editorial boards of several scientific journals and health publications and regularly participates as a reviewer on NIH study sections.

When asked what the single most influential factor in his professional preparation was, Weiss answered with one word: *mentorship*. He attributes the guidance he received from strong mentors like Joe Matarazzo and Neal Miller, his psychologist role models during graduate training, as instrumental in preparing him for the many challenges he has faced in his varied, multifaceted professional journey.

Cross-References

▶ Behavioral Medicine
▶ HIV Infection

References and Readings

Jones, D. L., Weiss, S. M., Chitalu, N., et al. (2008). Acceptability and use of sexual barrier products and lubricants among HIV-seropositive Zambian men. *AIDS Patient Care and STDs, 22*, 1015–1020.

Kapiga, S., Kelly, C., Weiss, S., Daley, T., Peterson, L., Leburg, C., et al. (2009). Risk factors for incidence of sexually transmitted infections among women in South Africa, Tanzania and Zambia: Results from HPTN 055 study. *Sexually Transmitted Diseases, 36*(4), 199–206.

Lopez, E. J., Jones, D. L., Villar-Loubet, O. M., Arheart, K. L., & Weiss, S. M. (2010). Violence, coping, and consistent medication adherence in HIV-positive couples. *AIDS Education and Prevention, 22*, 61–68.

Schneiderman, N., Weiss, S. M., & Kaufmann, P. G. (Eds.). (1989). *Handbook of research methods in cardiovascular behavioral medicine*. New York: Springer.

Schwartz, G., & Weiss, S. (1977). What is behavioral medicine. *Psychosomatic Medicine, 39*(6), 377–381.

Weiss, S. M. (1966). Psychological adjustment following open heart surgery. *The Journal of Nervous and Mental Disease, 143*(4), 363–368.

Weiss, S. M., Fielding, J., & Baum, A. (Eds.). (1991). *Perspectives in behavioral medicine: Health at work* (p. 219). Hillsdale: Erlbaum.

Weiss, S. M., Jones, D. L., Lopez, M., Villar-Loubet, O., & Chitalu, N. (2011a). The many faces of translational research: A tale of two studies. *Translational Behavioral Medicine, 1*, 327–330.

Weiss, S. M., Tobin, J. N., Antoni, M., Ironson, G., Ishii, M., Vaughn, A., et al. (2011b). Enhancing the health of women living with HIV: The SMART/EST women's project. *International Journal of Women's Health, 3*, 63–77.

Welfare

▶ Well-Being: Physical, Psychological, and Social

Well-Being

▶ Williams LifeSkills Program

Well-Being Technologies

▶ Quality of Life Technologies

Well-Being: Physical, Psychological, and Social

Sarah D. Pressman[1], Tara Kraft[2] and Stephanie Bowlin[2]
[1]Psychology and Social Behaviour, University of California, Irvine, CA, USA
[2]Department of Psychology, University of Kansas, Lawrence, KS, USA

Synonyms

Happiness; Health; Positive emotions; Welfare; Wellness

Definition

Well-being is a multifaceted construct best described as a state of physical, psychological, and social health.

Description

Well-being is a broad term that encompasses what it means to be functioning as a healthy person across multiple domains. Although words like "well-being (WB)," "health," and "happiness" permeate scientific literature, they are frequently variably defined from one study to the next, with many researchers relying on a single construct, such as "happiness" or "high quality of life" to provide an adequate definition. Rather than constricting WB to one equivocal definition, a review of the literature suggests that it is most comprehensively defined and productively discussed as a combination of the following three components: psychological well-being (PsWB), social well-being (SWB), and physical well-being (PWB).

Psychological Well-Being (PsWB)

Psychological well-being (PsWB) and "happiness" have historically been synonymous and equally indefinite in literature across academic disciplines. Contemporary scientific definitions of PsWB, however, encompass three substantial, coherent domains: emotional experience, cognitive evaluation of life satisfaction, and human flourishing (e.g., Diener et al. 2002; Keyes et al. 2002). Although PsWB is frequently referred to as synonymous with subjective WB (a cognitive evaluation of satisfaction with life), some models of PsWB consider cognitive evaluation a related yet distinct subcomponent of a larger construct of PsWB. Both models will be further discussed below.

Early in the study of emotion, Bradburn (1969) clarified that the absence of negative emotion does not indicate the presence of positive emotion;

thus, experiencing both frequent positive emotion and infrequent negative emotion is essential to *feeling* "happy." Instruments to measure positive and negative emotion at both the short-term "state" and long-term "trait" level ask individuals to rate the degree to which they experience a range of emotions, varying in valence (e.g., happy vs. sad) and arousal (e.g., excitement vs. calm) and have led to valuable research on emotion. For example, Fredrickson's (2001) notable "broaden and build" theory states that positive emotions increase WB by broadening our cognitive range and building lasting resources that can be utilized in times of need. For example, when experiencing positive emotion, individuals are able to identify a wider range of activities they would like to engage in and are more likely to set and reach goals. Furthermore, the manipulation and natural expression of positive emotion in experimental settings has been shown to improve post-stress cardiovascular recovery, possibly resulting in protective effects against the negative physiological consequences of stress.

As outlined above, PsWB frequently involves and is debatably defined as a cognitive evaluation of satisfaction with life (for a review, see Diener et al. 1999) partnered with positive and negative emotion ratings. This model of PsWB is based on ratings of WB from the respondent's own perspective. For example, although an outside person may judge circumstances to be unfortunate, if a respondent reports high life satisfaction, he or she has high subjective WB. Furthermore, this model assumes that this report has some amount of stability over time; however, reports can vary with momentary experience and events. Measures connecting these two evaluative components are associated with many positive outcomes, such as hope, optimism, and greater income. Interestingly, twin studies have revealed correlations between genes and PsWB, indicating a possible genetic influence on the "set point" for happiness. Since a variety of factors (e.g., genetics, culture, age, gender, emotional experience) can influence life satisfaction ratings, Diener and colleagues have suggested that "happiness" is best understood through a discussion of the factors that influence subjective WB.

Ryff (1989) has differentially argued that PsWB includes happiness ("hedonic" WB or the experience of pleasure) and "eudaimonic" WB. Eudaimonic WB is concerned with human flourishing and encompasses constructs related to engagement with and evaluation of challenging life events, including self-acceptance, purpose and meaning in life, sense of mastery over one's environment, positive interpersonal relationships, personal growth, and autonomy. Proponents of this approach argue that this combination of factors provides a more complete picture of happiness or "optimal" WB than emotional or cognitive/evaluative WB components alone and have found this optimal balance to increase with age, education, and the presence of certain personality characteristics (i.e., high extraversion and conscientiousness). While Ryff's work suggests that a comprehensive discussion of PsWB must consider the combination of factors that influence both subjective WB and human flourishing more broadly, it is somewhat problematic when contemplating research questions attempting to determine the critical components of WB. For example, interpersonal relationships (a component of eudaimonic WB) may have independent pathways (e.g., neuroanatomy, hormonal) to PWB as compared to more emotional constructs within eudaimonia (e.g., autonomy, acceptance) whose paths may have more in common with hedonic measures. It seems important then to consider these subcomponents and their differential mechanisms separately in order to understand how PsWB "gets under the skin" to alter physical health.

Social Well-Being (SWB)

Humans are inherently social creatures who evolved in groups that helped ensure the survival of the species. As a result, there is a deeply engrained need to belong and feel supported. When these social needs are met, individuals experience SWB. There is no firmly agreed upon definition of SWB, but generally it can be considered to be a *multifactorial* construct that includes different components of the social environment that when evaluated together result in an overall positive assessment of one's social life. No single measure completely captures SWB, and as a result, many different types of social characteristics must be considered.

The most basic measures of the social environment are collected via integration measures that assess the extent to which people feel like they belong to their communities. This is typically measured by measures that enumerate important social roles (e.g., spouse, close friend). This work has a rich history dating back to the industrial revolution when Durkheim noted that individuals were more likely to commit suicide upon leaving their families for industrial positions in other cities. Since then, the finding that isolated individuals are at risk for detrimental health outcomes is one of the most pervasive and robust in health psychology. For example, an early study from Alameda County, CA (Berkman and Syme 1979), revealed that those who lacked ties to others were up to three times more likely to die over a 9-year follow-up. Broader social networks (e.g., online networks of friends) are generally less strongly tied to WB since the presence of distant social contacts has less of an immediate and regular impact on one's life. What seems to be critical is the support and resources that your network provides. Related then is the concept of social support or the perception that emotional and objective resources (e.g., information, tangible aid) are available if and when negative events occur. Research has indicated that those who report having support in times of need have lower physiological stress responses, better immune function, and overall better health and resilience to health problems, resulting in broad WB benefits.

Other work focuses more closely on the perception and quality of social ties. For example, loneliness is an indicator of low SWB but can be relatively independent from objective network size. The hallmark of loneliness is not being alone but the accompanying distress related to the *perception* of isolation. The relationships approach would state that SWB is present when an individual can have satisfactory close relationships and also shows evidence of secure attachment (i.e., a strong emotional bond between two people). If a romantic partner is missing or an individual is insecurely attached, then high SWB would not be expected. There are a number of other related constructs, such as feelings of love and intimacy, social acceptance, and measures of social conflict and hostility, that are also tied to positive and negative appraisals of WB. When considering these feelings and perceptions or relationships, it is critical to also consider differences in social needs. For example, individuals high in extraversion will have greater needs for regular social contact than someone low on this personality trait. By definition, extraverts feel "better" when in the presence of social others and may therefore require greater interaction to achieve SWB as compared to their more introverted counterparts.

Finally, the social milieu contributes to SWB. Groups (e.g., clubs, volunteer groups, religious organizations) provide important feelings of belongingness, support, and contribution, which promote SWB. Those individuals who endorse group membership roles as well as those who report engaging in various social activities generally have higher WB. Beyond close groups, the broader environment also impacts SWB. Social capital describes the resources available to individuals through their membership in their community (e.g., civic associations, civic engagement, perceptions of trust, and sharing in the community). Higher social capital leads to belonging and increased social participation and has been tied to crime prevention and better societal health. This type of social engagement is critical for SWB as it likely has a trickle-down effect onto many of the previously discussed measures.

From the above examples, it is clear that SWB arises from a number of places. It is unlikely that any one characteristic uniquely predicts SWB. It is also important to consider the interaction between internal factors (e.g., attachment style, personality) and external characteristics of the social environment. Two individuals may live in the same social environment yet experience their social world in different manners, illustrating the importance of individual perception. Future research should consider which components are most critical to SWB and study more closely the interactions between different measurement types in terms of how they predict WB outcomes.

Physical Well-Being

Physical health researchers generally adhere to a medical model that conceptualizes health as the absence of disease, despite the definition in 1948 by the World Health Organization for health as "a state of complete physical, mental and social WB and *not* merely the absence of disease or infirmity." Physical well-being (PWB) then, is something more than "not sick" and may even reflect individuals realizing their fullest wellness potential, as echoed by the model of positive health by Seligman (2008). Compatible with the PWB model, the wellness continuum model (Sheridan and Radmacher 1992) anchors one end of their model by disease, disability, and death and the other end by optimal human functioning where a person is maximally healthy, has resources for resisting disease, and is capable of experiencing joy (Sheridan and Radmacher 2003). If the medical model idea of health were captured in the continuum model, it would end at the neutral/zero point with no room or definition of WB beyond "disease absent." Despite multiple models suggesting that there is something beyond the absence of illness, health is still primarily measured by the presence or absence of symptoms, illness and disease, physiological markers, and reports of physical health typically topping off at "I feel very healthy." Reports of positive physical functioning beyond this "zero" mark are not typically gathered by health practitioners or researchers.

To determine *objective* wellness, researchers and practitioners frequently rely on assessments of biomarkers to determine disease status and risk. These might include factors like immune function, endocrine hormones, or cardiovascular function, which are important indicators of disease status. While there are general guidelines about what levels indicate "healthy" functioning, these are not frequently tied to current WB. For example, someone may be hypertensive as assessed by blood pressure readings, be a genetic carrier of a serious disease, or even have a blocked artery, but still report feeling healthy and asymptomatic. Furthermore, while biological markers are *possible* correlates of physical health, conclusive statements often cannot be drawn based on physiological measures alone (e.g., lowered immune cell counts). This raises the importance of *subjective* assessments of health when considering PWB.

Self-rated health (SRH), a formalized measure of subjective health, has been used in research studies and suggests that individuals have insight into their health beyond the capabilities of biological measurement tools. Specifically, the commonly used Short-Form Health Survey (SF-36; Ware and Sherbourne 1992) asks questions such as, "In general, would you say your health is excellent, very good, fair, or poor?" Several of these questions take into account individual perspectives concerning what "health" means to the individual and even ask for reports comparative to the past. Additionally, questions such as "Have you felt calm/peaceful/full of pep/happy?" are tapping physical health via constructs that influence reports of PWB but are not direct physical measures. Interestingly, poor SRH is independently associated with increased mortality in diverse socioeconomic groups, age groups, in men and women, over time, even after accounting for objective health status at baseline (e.g., Lekander et al. 2004). Researchers are now investigating whether these nonspecific "sickness" symptoms (weakness, listlessness, decreased motivation) are mediated by stress-induced dysfunctional immune patterns (e.g., high inflammation). Given that positive traits and events are tied to healthy immune function (for further reading, see Pressman and Cohen 2005), it is plausible that positive reports of SRH are occurring via generalized positive feelings that alter the perception of the body and that these positive feelings are representative of an objectively healthy physiology.

At this point, the full mapping of these connections with SRH, biomarkers, emotion, and objective longitudinal health outcomes has not been done.

Problematic in definitions based on biomarkers and disease indicators is determining whether individuals suffering from chronic illness can have high PWB. Based on biological assessment, if an individual is diagnosed with cancer, they have low PWB. However, cancer patients frequently survive their cancer, find benefit in the experience of their illness, build relationships with others, and become optimistic about their future. During treatment, they will clearly experience poor PWB (e.g., side effects of radiation or chemotherapy); however, at some point, they will begin to recover. Self-report measures of PWB may be able to track this based on changes in perceptions of symptoms and health; however, biological measures may be more deficient at determining at what point the person's PWB is on the positive end of the spectrum (i.e., it is unlikely that PWB can be measured by a simple assessment of circulating cancer cells). To truly understand WB in this population and many others, it is clear that there is a need for PWB tools that assess both "harder" biological outcomes partnered with "softer" self-report measures.

Conclusions and Future Directions

Although themes of happiness, physical health, and social involvement have long been studied in philosophy, social psychology theory, and cultural analysis, it has only been in the last 10 years that WB has seen an upswing in interdisciplinary scientific study. Because of this, the scientific community is still working on definitions and operationalizations of critical constructs in the field. Currently, significant overlap exists between WB measures making it difficult to separate and understand these constructs. For example, individuals with serious illness by definition have poor PWB, but it is also likely that PsWB and SWB additionally suffer since illness will block engagement in activities that promote these WB types. Similarly, current measures of depression and loneliness frequently include questions tapping *both* PsWB and SWB revealing the extent to which these constructs overlap. Measures need to be improved to reflect the specific underlying components of WB in order to better understand the unique ways that these different WBs impact one another as well as outside outcomes. Finally, it is also critical to consider that in many cases, there is benefit to the overlap of these constructs. When considering interventions to improve PWB, it is frequently via SWB (e.g., support) and PsWB (e.g., relaxation) that impressive improvements are seen, ranging from physiological alterations to increased life span. There is clearly therapeutic value to considering ALL types of WB and the interrelations that they have with one another. A thorough understanding of the underlying constructs of WB will enable scientists, health professionals, and individuals of all walks of life to better promote and increase WB at multiple levels, with implications for both personal health and public policy decisions.

Cross-References

▶ Emotions: Positive and Negative
▶ Happiness and Health
▶ SF-36

References and Further Reading

Berkman, L. F., & Syme, L. (1979). Social networks, host resistance, and mortality: A nine-year follow-up study of Alameda County residents. *American Journal of Epidemiology, 109*, 186–204.

Bradburn, N. M. (1969). *The structure of psychological well-being*. Chicago: Aldine.

Cacioppo, J. T., & Patrick, B. (2008). *Loneliness: Human nature and the need for social connection*. New York: W.W. Norton.

Cohen, S., Underwood, L. G., & Gottlieb, B. H. (2000). *Social support measurement and intervention: A guide for health and social scientists*. New York: Oxford University Press.

Diener, E., Suh, E. M., Lucas, R. E., & Smith, H. L. (1999). Subjective well-being: Three decades of progress. *Psychological Bulletin, 125*, 276–302.

Diener, E., Lucas, R. E., & Oishi, S. (2002). Subjective well-being: The science of happiness and life satisfaction. In C. R. Snyder & S. J. Lopez (Eds.), *Handbook of positive psychology* (pp. 63–73). New York: Oxford University Press.

Fredrickson, B. L. (2001). The role of positive emotions in positive psychology: The broaden-and-build theory of positive emotions. *American Psychologist, 56*, 218–226.

Fredrickson, B. (2002). Positive emotions. In C. R. Snyder & S. J. Lopez (Eds.), *Handbook of positive psychology* (pp. 120–134). New York: Oxford University Press.

Keyes, C. L. M., Shmotkin, D., & Ryff, C. D. (2002). Optimizing well-being: The empirical encounter of two traditions. *Journal of Personality and Social Psychology, 82*, 1007–1022.

Lekander, M., Elofsson, S., Neve, I. M., Hansson, L. O., & Unden, A. L. (2004). Self-rated health is related to levels of circulating cytokines. *Psychosomatic Medicine, 66*, 559–563.

Lyubomirsky, S., King, L., & Diener, E. (2005). The benefits of frequent positive affect: Does happiness lead to success? *Psychological Bulletin, 131*, 803–855.

Pressman, S. D., & Cohen, S. (2005). Does positive affect influence health? *Psychological Bulletin, 131*, 925–971.

Putnam, R. D. (1985). *Bowling alone: The collapse and revival of American community*. New York: Simon & Schuster.

Ryff, C. (1989). Happiness is everything, or is it? Explorations on the meaning of psychological well-being. *Journal of Personality and Social Psychology, 57*, 1069–1081.

Seligman, M. E. P. (2008). Positive health. *Applied Psychology, 57*, 3–18.

Sheridan, C. L., & Radmacher, S. A. (1992). *Health psychology: Challenging the biomedical model*. New York: Wiley.

Sheridan, C. L., & Radmacher, S. A. (2003). Significance of psychosocial factors to health and disease. In L. A. Schein, H. S. Bernard, H. I. Spitz, & P. R. Muskin (Eds.), *Psychosocial treatment for medical conditions: Principles and techniques*. New York: Brunner-Routledge.

Ware, J. E., & Sherbourne, C. D. (1992). The MOS 36-item short-form health survey (SF-36): I. Conceptual framework and item selection. *Medical Care, 30*, 473–483.

Wellbutrin®

▶ Bupropion (Wellbutrin, Zyban)

Wellness

▶ Well-Being: Physical, Psychological, and Social

Wellness Coaching

▶ Digital Health Coaching

Whitehall Study

Mark Hamer
Epidemiology and Public Health, Division of Population Health, University College London, London, UK

Definition

The original Whitchall study of British civil servants began in 1967 and showed a steep inverse association between social class, as assessed by grade of employment, and mortality from a wide range of diseases. The Whitehall II study was later established in 1985 to identify causal pathways linking socioeconomic position to pathophysiological changes and clinical disease. The Whitehall II is an ongoing prospective cohort study of 10,308 British white-collar workers employed in the civil service (Marmot et al. 1991). The study is primarily interested in the pathways explaining social inequalities via characteristics of the work environment, such as job strain, and health-related behaviors including physical activity, smoking, and diet. Data are collected at regular intervals through a combination of self-administered questionnaires and clinical examination. In the 20 years separating the two studies, there has been no diminution in social class difference in morbidity: there remains an inverse association between employment grade and prevalence of common diseases such as heart disease, cancer, and respiratory diseases. Self-perceived health status and symptoms are worse in participants from lower-status jobs. There are also clear employment-grade differences in health-risk behaviors including smoking, diet, and exercise, in economic circumstances, in possible effects of early-life environment as reflected by height, in social circumstances at work (e.g., monotonous work characterized by low control and low satisfaction), and in social supports. These key findings appear to partly explain the social disparities in health (Stringhini et al. 2010). The Whitehall II study currently has available data for nearly 30 years of follow-up, and many of the participants are now in their seventh and eighth decades of life. Thus, the focus of the study is gradually shifting toward aging since many of the participants are now retired from full-time employment.

Social position can be viewed as an indicator of chronic lifetime stress exposure since people of lower social status tend to experience adverse psychosocial factors including greater financial strain, lower control at work, chronic neighborhood and domestic stresses, and more limited social networks. The Whitehall psychobiology studies have been conducted in healthy subsamples ($N = 250-500$) of the main study cohort, in 2001 and 2006, and were specifically undertaken to examine the biological processes that might explain the association between psychosocial stress and coronary heart disease (Hamer et al. 2010; Steptoe et al. 2002). In these studies, healthy men and women from the Whitehall II cohort (stratified by grade of employment as a marker of social status) underwent psychophysiological stress testing involving measurement of cardiovascular and biological responses to laboratory-induced mental stressors. Results suggested that lower social status individuals were characterized not so much by heightened cardiovascular responsiveness, but by impaired poststress recovery, or sustained activation after termination of stressors. Results from the most recent study have suggested that stress responsivity is also associated with subclinical coronary atherosclerosis. Population-based psychophysiological studies with detailed biological measures have contributed to a better understanding about stress and disease pathways.

Cross-References

▶ Heart Disease and Cardiovascular Reactivity
▶ Psychophysiologic Reactivity
▶ Psychophysiologic Recovery

References and Further Reading

Hamer, M., O'Donnell, K., Lahiri, A., & Steptoe, A. (2010). Salivary cortisol responses to mental stress are associated with coronary artery calcification in healthy men and women. *European Heart Journal, 31*, 424–429.

Marmot, M. G., Davey Smith, G., Stansfeld, S., Patel, C., North, F., Head, J., et al. (1991). Health inequalities among British civil servants: The Whitehall II study. *Lancet, 337*, 1387–1393.

Steptoe, A., Feldman, P. J., Kunz, S., Owen, N., Willemsen, G., & Marmot, M. (2002). Stress responsivity and socioeconomic status: A mechanism for increased cardiovascular disease risk? *European Heart Journal, 23*, 1757–1763.

Stringhini, S., Sabia, S., Shipley, M., Brunner, E., Nabi, H., Kivimaki, M., et al. (2010). Association of socioeconomic position with health behaviors and mortality. *Journal of the American Medical Association, 303*, 1159–1166.

Whole Health

▶ Integrative Medicine

Whole-Genome Association Study (WGAS)

▶ Genome-Wide Association Study (GWAS)

WHR

▶ Waist to Hip Ratio

Williams LifeSkills Program

Virginia P. Williams[1] and Redford B. Williams[2]
[1]Williams LifeSkills, Inc., Durham, NC, USA
[2]Department of Psychiatry and Behavioral Sciences, Division of Behavioral Medicine, Duke University, Durham, NC, USA

Synonyms

Cognitive-behavioral stress management training; Coping skills training; Hardiness; Heart patients; Incarcerated youths; Online training; Pastors; Resilience; Resilience training; Teens; Telephone coaching; Video applications; Well-being

Definition

Williams LifeSkills is a protocol-driven manualized training program that aims to improve stress coping and interpersonal relationship skills. It focuses on acquiring ten skills in two categories: (1) six skills for handling problematic situations (logkeeping, think before you act to decide between action and deflection, deflection, problem-solving, assertion, and saying no) and (2) four skills for improving relationships with others and oneself (speaking, listening, empathy, and increasing positives over negatives). The program has been evaluated in several clinical trials, with resulting evidence of its efficacy on psychosocial and biological markers. There are several delivery options. The initial standard was face-to-face workshops of 5–12 participants, with a trained facilitator. The video version consists of a 70-min video covering the ten skills, with an accompanying workbook; this video/workshop can be incorporated into a workshop or used as a stand-alone intervention, with or without telephone coaching by a trained facilitator. There is also an online version, either freestanding or with submission of exercises. One-on-one coaching is another option. The initial program has been expanded to include a number of specialized versions that maintain focus on the ten skills: for caregivers with a relative with Alzheimer's, teens delivered by high school teachers, a specialized teen version for incarcerated youths, pastors who otherwise are usually supporting others, and heart patients.

Description

The Williams LifeSkills copyrighted program evolved over the last two decades as a means of translating research by Redford Williams and others (Williams 2008) that has documented the health-damaging effects of psychosocial factors like hostility/anger, depression, social isolation, job stress, and stressful life situations into a behavioral intervention that can reduce levels, and hopefully the health-damaging effects, of these psychosocial risk factors. Williams LifeSkills, Inc., was founded as a commercial entity in 1996 by Redford and Virginia Williams with the goals of developing and refining this behavioral intervention, doing research to test its efficacy and effectiveness in both controlled and observational clinical trials, and marketing behavioral intervention products shown to work in this research. The founders of Williams LifeSkills have written three books for a lay audience that also serve to describe the program as it evolved (Williams and William 1993, 1997, 2006). While the programs are presented as wellness training for increasing participants' effectiveness in the increasingly stress-filled modern world, they also provide a first-level intervention for individuals with mild to moderate anxiety, depression, and hostility. The intervention has also been used with outpatients with a wide variety of diagnoses, both to help them cope with their illness and to reduce distress over other issues in their lives.

The face-to-face workshop has been used extensively in the United States, Brazil, Singapore, Hungary, and China. Intervention groups are quite varied in these varied settings: some examples are medical students, college students, heart patients, corporate employees, pastors, and health professionals. High school and middle school students, as well as young violent offenders, also have been incorporated into a general intervention for heart patients in Germany. Facilitators are initially trained for at least 5 days, spending the first 2 days as participants and the last 3 days focusing on practicing supervision of the interactive sections of the program. There is an accompanying participant text (about 40 pages long) and a workbook (about 15 pages long), so the text can either be given to a participant or used again. Participants begin by learning to write up log entries, emphasizing the objective facts, their thoughts and feelings, behaviors, and consequences. They then apply their own examples to practice the other skills. The program thus involves iteration without repetition, since new layers of training are being added. Facilitators are trained to encourage participation, within a set of ground rules, and to emphasize improvement through practice, rather than aiming for perfection. The entire program is designed to fit together, with algorithms to address which skills to apply. As a result, the program can be used in almost any situation a participant might face.

The generic LifeSkills program has also been adapted for specific groups. The LifeSkills course for caregivers focuses on a special video created to address problems particular to caring for someone with a disabling memory disorder. A 121-page workbook accompanies the video. Also part of the program is a manual for five sessions of telephone coaching by a LifeSkills facilitator. All of the materials are oriented to the ten LifeSkills. There is an adaptation for teens in which the emphasis is on issues faced by teens. There is an extensive Facilitator's Manual for high school teachers, which is incorporated into the week-long training that prepares them to deliver the training to students in the high school setting. Teens can either report a personal log entry or draw a role-playing card. Separate packets of cards accompany each skill. Teens have a special text and workbook. The teen program has been modified for incarcerated teens. The same general format is used as in the school program, but the role-playing cards are different. Some of the illustrations and workbook examples also are modified. In the United States, prison educators are trained to be the facilitators. In China, the program is being tested, using psychiatrists and psychologists as facilitators. The program for medical personnel has assumed different forms in the United States, Hungary, and China. The program for heart patients also has assumed different forms in the United States and Singapore (also adapted a number of clinical trials that have documented the efficacy of the LifeSkills program in its various forms in the United States and Canada). The first study to document benefits of an early version – based on *Anger Kills* (Williams and William 1993) – of the LifeSkills workshop was a small randomized controlled trial (RCT) in males following a heart attack. Results showed that hostility after the end of training as assessed by both structured interview and questionnaire and resting diastolic blood pressure were reduced significantly more in patients in the active arm than those randomized to usual care (Gidron et al. 1999). Both these improvements were maintained or enhanced at follow-up 2 months later. Because this study was conducted in Canada, it was possible to do a follow-up assessment of the clinical course over the 6 months post-training. Compared to usual care, men in the active arm showed significant reductions in both hospital stay and medical care costs over the 6 months follow-up (Davidson et al. 2007). Another RCT evaluating benefits of the LifeSkills video found significantly larger reductions in both trait anxiety and perceived stress among the active arm participants compared to those randomized to wait list control, both 2 weeks after the end of training and after 6 months follow-up (Kirby et al. 2006). In an RCT evaluating the LifeSkills workshop augmented by the LifeSkills video, hypertensive employees of a large urban medical center who were randomized to LifeSkills training showed significantly larger, clinically significant decreases in systolic blood pressure compared to those receiving usual care according to JNC-7 guidelines (Clemow et al. 2018). A controlled (alternating assignment to active vs. wait list arms), clinical trial of the LifeSkills video adapted for use by caregivers of a relative with Alzheimer's disease showed that those in the LifeSkills for Caregivers video arm, who also received weekly telephone coaching calls, showed significantly larger decreases in depressive symptoms, trait anxiety, perceived stress, and systolic and diastolic blood pressure that were maintained or enhanced at 6 months follow-up (Williams et al. 2010). In addition to replicating findings of psychosocial improvement following LifeSkills training, this study extends the demonstration of benefits to include a potential biological mechanism whereby stress damages health – higher blood pressure.

The LifeSkills program has also been adapted for use in Singapore, China, and Hungary. In Singapore, Bishop et al. (2005) conducted a RCT of the LifeSkills workshop in a sample of 59 male Singaporean (60% Chinese) patients following coronary bypass surgery. In addition to robust improvements with regard to both negative and positive psychosocial risk factors, blood pressure and heart rate at both rest and in response to anger recall were significantly decreased in men randomized to LifeSkills workshop training, with all improvements maintained or enhanced at 3 months follow-up. Effect sizes for these psychosocial and cardiovascular improvements in the LifeSkills workshop arm were moderate to large. In China the focus to date has been on students (Li et al. 2012; Chen et al. 2013; Zhang et al. 2015). In Hungary, an observational trial of the LifeSkills workshop by Stauder et al. (2010) found that distressed persons in the Budapest metro area who participated in the workshop showed a pattern of psychosocial improvements that is remarkably similar to those observed by Bishop et al. (2005) on the other side of the world. Effect sizes in Hungary were similarly moderate to large. Dr. Stauder and colleagues at Semmelweis University in Budapest are now conducting RCTs of the LifeSkills workshop in workplace settings in Hungary. A large-scale study in the northwest section of Hungary is now underway to train 6000 teachers in 300 schools in LifeSkills, with additional modules on conflict training, aggression management and prevention, bullying management and prevention, motivation increase, and burnout prevention in the school setting.

Evidence for the effectiveness of Williams LifeSkills products in real-world settings comes from two observational trials. In one, conducted by Campo et al. (2008), second-year medical students who participated in the WLSR workshop over a 2-day period showed significant reductions in hostility and in the use of placating and avoidant responses in difficult patient scenarios following the training. In contrast, a comparison group of second-year students the following year who did not receive WLSR training showed slight increases in both hostility and placating and avoidant responses. In an observational trial of the LifeSkills workshop among employees of one of our corporate clients, at the end of training, there were significant decreases in depressive symptoms and state and trait anxiety and increased social support; except for social support, all these improvements were maintained or enhanced at follow-up 6 months later (Williams et al. 2009).

The LifeSkills reach continues to expand, since the skills acquired contribute to resiliency and hence can be applied across a broad range of situations where potential high stress needs to be inoculated against.

Cross-References

▶ Alzheimer's Disease
▶ Cognitive Behavioral Therapy (CBT)
▶ Coping
▶ Hardiness and Health
▶ Internet-Based Interventions
▶ Resilience

References and Further Reading

Bishop, G. D., Kaur, D., & Tan, V. L. M. (2005). Effects of a psychosocial skills training workshop on psychophysiological and psychosocial risk in patients undergoing coronary artery bypass grafting. *American Heart Journal, 150*, 602–609.

Campo, A. E., Williams, V., Williams, R. B., Segundo, M. A., Lydston, D., & Weiss, S. M. (2008). Effects of LifeSkills training on medical students' performance in dealing with complex clinical cases. *Academic Psychiatry, 32*(3), 188–193.

Chen, C., Li, C., Wang, H., Joun, J., Zhou, J.-S., & Want, X.-P. (2013). Cognitive behavioral therapy to reduce overt aggression behavior in Chinese young male violent offenders. *Aggressive Behavior, 40*(4), 329–336.

Clemow, L. P., Pickering, T. G., Davidson, K. W., & Liriano, C. (2009). Multi-component stress management for hypertensives: For whom does it work best? *Psychosomatic Medicine, 71*, A-127.

Clemow, L. P., Pickering, T. G., Schwartz, J., Williams, V. P., Shaffer, J. A., Williams, R. B., & Gerin, W. (2018). Stress management in the workplace for employees with hypertension: A randomized controlled trial. *Translational Behavioral Medicine, 8*(5), 761–770.

Davidson, K. W., Gidron, Y., Mostofsky, E., & Trudeau, K. J. (2007). Hospitalization cost offset of a hostility intervention for coronary heart disease patients. *Journal of Consulting and Clinical Psychology, 75*, 657–662.

Gidron, Y., Davidson, K. W., & Bata, I. (1999). The short-term effects of a hostility-reduction intervention on male coronary heart disease patients. *Health Psychology, 18*, 416–420.

Kirby, E. D., Williams, V. P., Hocking, M. C., Lane, J. D., & Williams, R. B. (2006). Psychosocial benefits of three formats of a standardized behavioral stress management program. *Psychosomatic Medicine, 68*, 816–823.

Li, C., Chu, F., Wang, H., & Wang, X.-p. (2012). Efficacy of Williams LifeSkills training for improving psychological health: A pilot comparison study of Chinese medical students. *Asia-Pacific Psychiatry, 6*(2), 161–169.

Stauder, A., Konkolÿ Thege, B., Kovács, M. E., Balog, P., Williams, V. P., & Williams, R. B. (2010). Worldwide stress: Different problems, similar solutions? Cultural adaptation and evaluation of a standardized stress management program in Hungary. *International Journal of Behavioral Medicine, 17*, 25–32.

Williams, R. B. (2008). Psychosocial and biobehavioral factors and their interplay in coronary heart disease. *Annual Review of Clinical Psychology, 4*, 349–365.

Williams, R. B., & William, V. P. (1993). *Anger kills: Seventeen strategies for controlling the hostility that can harm your health*. New York: Times Books. Trade paperback edition published by Harper-Collins, Spring, 1994.

Williams, V. P., & Williams, R. B. (1997). *LifeSkills: 8 Simple ways to build stronger relationships, communicate more clearly, improve your health, and even the health of those around you*. New York: Times Books/Random House. Paperback, Apr 1999.

Williams, R. B., & Williams, V. P. (2006). *In control*. New York: Rodale Books.

Williams, V. P., Brenner, S. L., Helms, M. J., & Williams, R. B. (2009). Coping skills training to reduce psychosocial risk factors for medical disorders: A field trial evaluating effectiveness in multiple worksites. *Journal of Occupational Health, 51*, 437–442.

Williams, V. P., Bishop-Fitzpatrick, L., Lane, J. D., Gwyther, L. P., Ballard, E. L., Vendittelli, A. P., et al. (2010). Video-based coping skills to reduce health risk and improve psychological and physical well-being in Alzheimer's disease family caregivers. *Psychosomatic Medicine, 72*(9), 897–904.

Zhang, S., Wang, H., Chen, C., Zhou, J. G., & Wang, X.-P. (2015). Efficacy of Williams LifeSkills training in improving psychological health of Chinese male juvenile violent offenders. *Neuroscience Bulletin, 31*(1), 53–60.

Williams Redford B. Jr.

Redford B. Williams
Department of Psychiatry and Behavioral Sciences, Division of Behavioral Medicine, Duke University, Durham, NC, USA

Biographical Information

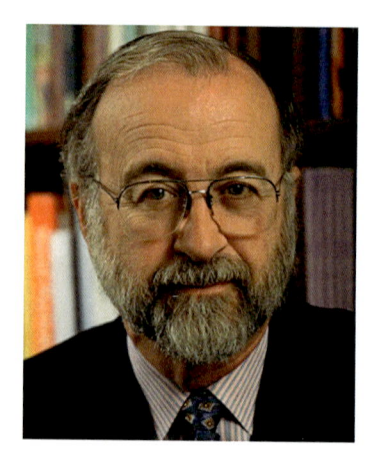

Redford B. Williams, Jr., was born in Raleigh, NC, on December 14, 1940. Following graduation from Northampton High School in Eastville, Virginia, in June 1959, he entered Harvard College, receiving his A.B.. degree in 1963. He married Virginia Carter Parrott in 1963, and they have two children and three grandchildren. Williams received his M.D. degree from Yale in 1967, where he completed his internship and residency in internal medicine in 1970. Following 2 years as a clinical associate at NIMH in Bethesda, MD, he was appointed assistant professor in the Departments of Psychiatry and Medicine at Duke University Medical Center, Durham, NC, in 1972, advancing to the rank of professor in 1978. Since 1985, he has been director of the Behavioral Medicine Research Center at Duke. He was named Head, Division of Behavioral Medicine in the Department of Psychiatry and Behavioral Sciences at Duke in 1990. In 1991, he was appointed professor of Psychology at Duke and adjunct professor of Epidemiology in the School of Public Health at the University of North Carolina, Chapel Hill. He has served on several Medical Center committees over the years, including the Awards Committee (Chair), the Conflict of Interest Committee, and the Department of Psychiatry and Behavioral Sciences Appointments, Promotion, and Tenure Committee. Williams has been continuously funded by the NIH since receiving a Research Scientist Development Award from NIMH in 1974; he has been principal investigator on a program project grant from the NHLBI that began in 1986, continuing till April, 2015. In 1996, he collaborated with Virginia Parrott Williams to found Williams LifeSkills, Inc., a company with the mission of developing, testing, and marketing behavioral intervention products aimed at reducing the health-damaging effects of psychosocial risk factors such as hostility, depression, and social isolation. Williams has served as the president of the leading scientific societies in the field of psychosomatic/behavioral medicine, including the Society of Behavioral Medicine (1983–1984), the American Psychosomatic Society (1992–1993), the Academy of Behavioral Medicine Research (1995–1996), and the International Society of Behavioral Medicine (2006–2008). He was the inaugural recipient of the Society of Behavioral Medicine's Distinguished Scientist Award (1992). Williams is grateful for the mentorship he has received from George Goethals, Stan King, and John Spiegel at Harvard; Pat McKegney and Mickey Willard at Yale; Irv Kopin and Lyman Wynne at NIMH; Bud Busse and Saul Schanberg at Duke; and numerous colleagues and students at each step along the way over the years.

Major Accomplishments

Beginning with publication of two papers in 1965–1967 reporting effects of interview variables on blood pressure reactivity that were found in his research as a medical student at Yale, Williams has been continuously engaged in research aimed at identifying psychosocial factors that increase risk of cardiovascular disease and the biobehavioral mechanisms that mediate that risk. In the mid-1970s, following training in the assessment of type A behavior by Ray Rosenman and Meyer Friedman, Williams began a still ongoing project that initially pinpointed hostility as the toxic core of the type A behavior pattern. Working over the ensuing years with his Duke psychiatry and cardiology colleagues, Williams has made important contributions to our understanding of the role played by psychosocial factors such as hostility, depression, social isolation, and low socioeconomic status in the pathogenesis and course of cardiovascular disease, as well as the role of mediators such as increased sympathetic and HPA axis function, decreased parasympathetic function, and unhealthy lifestyle behaviors.

In the mid-1980s, Williams began the process of translating research findings on the health-damaging effects of psychosocial risk factors into behavioral interventions to prevent and/or ameliorate those effects. He has collaborated with his spouse of 48 years, Virginia Parrott Williams, to develop the Williams LifeSkills coping skills training program and evaluate its effects on psychosocial risk factors and biobehavioral mechanisms. Published clinical trials have documented a broad range of benefits of this program: decreased levels of hostility, anger, depression, anxiety, and perceived stress; decreased levels of blood pressure and heart rate at rest and during lab challenge; and increased levels of satisfaction with social support and satisfaction with life. These benefits persist over 6 months after the end of training and have been observed in distressed groups like patients following coronary artery bypass surgery and caregivers of a relative with Alzheimer's disease and in diverse cultural settings ranging from the USA to Singapore, to China, and to Hungary.

Beginning in the late 1990s, Williams has extended the focus of his research to include a search for genetic variants that increase one's vulnerability to the effects of environmental stressors on psychosocial risk factors and biobehavioral mechanisms. Based on his hypothesis that dysregulated central nervous system, serotonin plays an important role in the clustering of psychosocial and biobehavioral risk factors in certain individuals; this work focused initially on genes that regulate serotonin functions. A typical finding emerging in this ongoing work is an association between the more functional long allele of the serotonin promoter 5HTTLPR polymorphism and increased cardiovascular reactivity to acute mental stress, suggesting that the long allele will be associated with increased risk of coronary heart disease – a prediction that has been confirmed in three independent case-control studies in Asia and Europe. Williams and his colleagues at Duke and elsewhere are currently working to test the hypothesis that genetic variants found associated – whether directly or via gene x environment interactions – with predisease endophenotypes such as increased neuroendocrine, sympathetic nervous system, and cardiovascular reactivity to stress, and increased expression of the metabolic syndrome are also associated with incidence of cardiovascular disease and/or type 2 diabetes in large cohorts of both healthy persons and persons with coronary heart disease.

Another important contribution over the years has been Williams' mentoring of students and postdoctoral fellows who have gone on to make their own important contributions to the field of behavioral medicine: Norman Anderson, Gary Bennett, James Blumenthal, Beverly Brummett, Shin Fukudo, Jim Lane, Linda Luecken, Marcellus Merritt, Len Poon, and Ed Suarez.

Cross-References

▶ Williams LifeSkills Program

References and Readings

Anderson, N. B., Muranaka, M., Williams, R. B., Lane, J. D., & Houseworth, S. J. (1988). Racial differences in blood pressure and forearm vascular responses to the cold face stimulus. *Psychosomatic Medicine, 50*, 57–63.

Barefoot, J. C., Dahlstrom, W. G., & Williams, R. B. (1983). Hostility, CHD incidence and total mortality: A 25-year follow-up study of 255 physicians. *Psychosomatic Medicine, 45*, 59–63.

Brummett, B. H., Boyle, S. H., Siegler, I. C., Kuhn, C., Ashley-Koch, A., Jonassaint, C. R., et al. (2008a). Effects of environmental stress and gender on associations among symptoms of depression and the serotonin transporter gene linked polymorphic region (5-HTTLPR). *Behavior Genetics, 38*, 34–43.

Brummett, B. H., Muller, C. L., Collins, A. L., Boyle, S. H., Kuhn, C. M., Siegler, I. C., et al. (2008b). 5-HTTLPR and gender moderate changes in negative affect responses to tryptophan infusion. *Behavior Genetics, 38*, 476–483.

Brummett, B. H., Babyak, M. A., Siegler, I. C., Shanahan, M., Harris, K. M., Elder, G. H., et al. (2011). Systolic blood pressure, socioeconomic status, and biobehavioral risk factors in a nationally representative US young adult sample. *Hypertension, 58*, 161–166.

Fukudo, S., Lane, J. D., Anderson, N. B., Kuhn, C. M., Schanberg, S. M., McCown, N., et al. (1992). Accentuated vagal antagonism of beta-adrenergic effects on ventricular repolarization: Differential responses between Type A and Type B men. *Circulation, 85*, 2045–2053.

Kirby, E. D., Williams, V. P., Hocking, M. C., Lane, J. D., & Williams, R. B. (2006). Psychosocial benefits of three formats of a standardized behavioral stress management program. *Psychosomatic Medicine, 68*, 816–823.

Kring, S. I., Brummett, B. H., Barefoot, J., Garrett, M. E., Ashley-Koch, A. E., Boyle, S. H., et al. (2010). Impact of psychological stress on the associations between apolipoprotein E variants and metabolic traits: Findings in an American sample of caregivers and controls. *Psychosomatic Medicine, 72*(5), 427–433.

McKegney, F. P., & Williams, R. B. (1967). Psychological aspects of hypertension: II. The differential influence of interview variables on blood pressure. *The American Journal of Psychiatry, 123*, 1539–1543.

Siegler, I. C., Peterson, B. L., Barefoot, J. C., & Williams, R. B., Jr. (1992). Hostility during late adolescence predicts coronary risk factors at mid-life. *American Journal of Epidemiology, 136*, 146–154.

Stauder, A., Konkolÿ Thege, B., Kovács, M. E., Balog, P., Williams, V. P., & Williams, R. B. (2010). Worldwide stress: Different problems, similar solutions? Cultural adaptation and evaluation of a standardized stress management program in Hungary. *International Journal of Behavioral Medicine, 17*, 25–32.

Williams, R. B. (1994). Neurobiology, cellular and molecular biology, and psychosomatic medicine. *Psychosomatic Medicine, 56*, 308–315.

Williams, R. B., & Chesney, M. A. (1993). Psychosocial factors and prognosis in established coronary artery disease. The need for research on interventions.

Journal of the American Medical Association, 270, 1860–1861.

Williams, R. B., & Eichelman, R. (1971). Social setting: Influence upon physiological responses to electric shock in the rat. *Science, 174*, 613–614.

Williams, R. B., & McKegney, F. P. (1965). Psychological aspects of hypertension: I. The influence of experimental interview variables on blood pressure. *The Yale Journal of Biology and Medicine, 38*, 265–273.

Williams, R. B., & William, V. P. (1993). *Anger kills: Seventeen strategies for controlling the hostility that can harm your health*. New York: Times Books. Trade paperback edition published by Harper-Collins. Spring, 1994.

Williams, V. P., & Williams, R. B. (1998). *LIFESKILLS: 8 simple ways to build stronger relationships, communicate more clearly, improve your health, and even the health of those around you*. New York: Times Books/Random House, Spring. Paperback. April, 1999.

Williams, R. B., Kimball, C. P., & Willard, H. N. (1973). The influence of interpersonal interaction upon diastolic blood pressure. *Psychosomatic Medicine, 34*, 194–198.

Williams, R. B., Bittker, T. E., Buchsbaum, M. S., & Wynne, L. C. (1975). Cardiovascular and neurophysiologic correlates of sensory intake and rejection: I. Effect of cognitive tasks. *Psychophysiology, 12*, 427–433.

Williams, R. B., Haney, T. L., Blumenthal, J. A., & Kong, Y. (1980). Type A behavior, hostility, and coronary atherosclerosis. *Psychosomatic Medicine, 42*, 539–549.

Williams, R. B., Lane, J. D., Kuhn, C. M., Melosh, W., White, A. D., & Schanberg, S. M. (1982). Type A behavior and elevated physiological and neuroendocrine responses to cognitive tasks. *Science, 218*, 483–485.

Williams, R. B., Barefoot, J. C., Califf, R. M., Haney, T. L., Saunders, W. B., Pryor, D. B., et al. (1992). Prognostic importance of social and economic resources among medically treated patients with angiographically documented coronary artery disease. *Journal of the American Medical Association, 267*, 520–524.

Williams, R. B., Barefoot, J. C., Blumenthal, J. A., Helms, M. J., Luecken, L., Pieper, C. F., et al. (1997). Psychosocial correlates of job strain in a sample of working women. *Archives of General Psychiatry, 54*, 543–548.

Williams, R. B., Marchuk, D. A., Gadde, K. M., Barefoot, J. C., Grichnik, K., Helms, M. J., et al. (2003). Serotonin-related gene polymorphisms and central nervous system serotonin function. *Neuropsychopharmacology, 28*, 533–541.

Williams, R. B., Marchuk, D. A., Siegler, I. C., Barefoot, J. C., Helms, M. J., Brummett, B. H., et al. (2008). Childhood socioeconomic status and serotonin transporter gene polymorphism enhance cardiovascular reactivity to mental stress. *Psychosomatic Medicine, 70*, 32–39.

Williams, V. P., Bishop-Fitzpatrick, L., Lane, J. D., Gwyther, L. P., Ballard, E. L., Vendittelli, A. P., et al. (2010a). Video-based coping skills to reduce health risk and improve psychological and physical well-being in Alzheimer's disease family caregivers. *Psychosomatic Medicine, 72*(9), 897–904.

Williams, R. B., Surwit, R. S., Siegler, I. C., Ashley-Koch, A. E., Collins, A. L., Helms, M. J., et al. (2010b). Central nervous system serotonin and clustering of hostility, psychosocial, metabolic and cardiovascular endophenotypes in men. *Psychosomatic Medicine, 72*, 601–607.

Willingness-to-Pay (WTP)

▶ Benefit Evaluation in Health Economic Studies

Wish for a Hastened Death

▶ End-of-Life

Women's Cardiovascular Health

▶ Women's Health

Women's Health

Michael O'Hara
Department of Psychology, University of Iowa, Iowa City, IA, USA

Synonyms

Women's cardiovascular health; Women's mental health; Women's reproductive health; Women's well-being

Definition

A recent Institute of Medicine committee approached women's health as a concept that has expanded beyond the reproductive system and includes "... health conditions that are specific to women, are more common or more serious in women, have distinct causes or manifestations in women, have different outcomes or treatments in women, or have high morbidity or mortality in women (pp. 2–3)" (Institute of Medicine [IOM] 2010). Examples of these conditions include breast cancer, cardiovascular disease, cervical cancer, depression, HIV/AIDS, and osteoporosis, among others.

Description

History

Historically, women's health referred to women's reproductive health – the menstrual cycle, pregnancy, labor, delivery, and menopause. It is only in the past three decades that women's health has been understood to include the full complement of women's health concerns. For example, it was common for women of reproductive potential to be excluded from clinical trials because of the possibility of unknown teratogenic effects of the medication under study. In fact, in 1977, the FDA restricted women of childbearing potential from being in clinical trials. This policy was only reversed in 1993. Moreover, it was assumed that results of clinical trials with men could be extrapolated to women. This was an untested assumption that is now known to be untrue. Additionally, investigators were concerned that the hormonal fluctuations associated with the menstrual cycle would influence study findings in unknown ways. For all of these reasons, the great bulk of health research until recently has either excluded women or included them in small numbers or has not analyzed the data for sex differences. These deficiencies are slowly being remedied.

There have been a number of important milestones in women's health. For example, the publication of *Our Bodies, Ourselves* in 1970 by the Boston Women's Health Book Collective was a landmark event in women advocating for women's health. This organization and its work continue today. It argues that it has brought several key ideas into the public discourse on women's health (Our Bodies Ourselves [OBOS] 2011).

- That women, as informed health consumers, are catalysts for social change
- That women can become their own health experts, particularly through discussing issues of health and sexuality with each other
- That health consumers have a right to know about controversies surrounding medical practices and about where consensus among medical experts may be forming
- That women comprise the largest segment of health workers, health consumers, and health decision-makers for their families and communities, but are underrepresented in positions of influence and policy making
- That a pathology/disease approach to normal life events (birthing, menopause, aging, death) is not an effective way in which to consider health or structure a health system

Change in traditional concepts of women's health did not occur quickly, and it was not until 1980s that clear recognition of the importance of a women's health perspective came into focus. In the forward to a seminal 1985 Public Health Service Task Force report on women's health, Edward Brandt, assistant secretary for health said "This report does not focus strictly on the diseases and problems unique to women in the traditional sense, that is, reproductive problems, but rather is devoted to assessing the problems of women's health, in the context of the lives women in America lead today (p. 74)." Going on the report states: "Good health requires a safe and healthful physical and social environment, an adequate income, safe housing, good nutrition, access to preventive and treatment services appropriate to the persons to be served, and a population that is educated and motivated to maintain healthful behaviors" (p. 77).

In 1990, the Congressional Caucus for Women's Issues (CCWI) pushed through legislation entitled the Women's Health Equity Act. This act created the Office for Women's Health Research at the NIH. It also created a gynecology research program and a Center for Women's Health Research at the NIH. Finally, it required the NIH director to report on progress on women's health and research and that a database be developed of research on women's health and to require the inclusion of women and minorities in NIH trials. The authors of the bill pointed to the then recent Harvard study of 22,000 men (and no women), which demonstrated that daily aspirin could prevent heart attacks as a case of blatant discrimination against women. The CCWI continued to be very active in subsequent congressional sessions in pushing through many additional laws aimed at improving women's health and including women in biomedical research.

Subsequent to the to the Women's Health Equity Act, there has been a great deal of legislation that bears on improving women's health through improved services and research. Most recently, the Patient Protection and Affordable Care Act (Public Law 111–148) formally codified the Office of Women's Health Research at the NIH, and it formally established an Office of Women's Health in the director's office of the Agency for Health Care Research and Quality (AHRQ), Centers for Disease Control and Prevention (CDC), Food and Drug Administration (FDA), Health Resources and Services Administration (HRSA), and Substance Abuse and Mental Health Services Administration (SAMSA). Additionally, it also established a Department of Health and Human Services Coordinating Committee on Women's Health and a National Women's Health Information Center.

Advocacy Matters: The Example of Breast Cancer

Until the 1970s, there was very little public discussion of breast cancer. Often, it was a cause of shame in families. There were several important landmarks in the 1970s that set the stage for the current strong advocacy around breast cancer prevention and treatment. Already mentioned, *Our Body, Ourselves*, helped set the stage for women taking control of their health. In 1974, the first lady, Betty Ford, was diagnosed with breast cancer. She spoke about her experiences in public, and this encouraged others to do the same. At about the time, Rose Kushner, a journalist, was diagnosed with breast cancer. She objected to the then common practice in which a tumor biopsy and radical mastectomy were performed in a single surgical operation while the patient was under anesthesia. Instead she insisted on a two-step procedure in which biopsies and surgery were undertaken as separate procedures, allowing a woman time to consider her options. This was very unpopular with the medical establishment. However, through persistent advocacy, her efforts resulted in a 1977 NIH panel (of which she was a member), concluding that the two-step procedure that she recommended should be adopted, and that in primary breast cancer, the standard treatment should be a total simple mastectomy rather than the more common radical mastectomy.

The first major advocacy organization was the Susan G. Komen Breast Cancer Foundation in 1982. The work of the Foundation has been described as priming the market (step 1), which means drawing attention to breast cancer through personal stories and by communicating the impact of breast cancer in stark and concrete terms (Braun 2003). Important in this effort was portraying that there was hope in the form of prevention and effective treatment. In a related manner, efforts were made to engage consumers (step 2) by sponsoring activities, such as the "Race for the Cure" established in 1983. These activities brought positive media attention and raised money for further advocacy. Political action (step 3) in 1980s and 1990s led to a number of legislative, regulatory, and funding accomplishments, for example, the army took on the task of breast cancer research; the Breast and Cervical Cancer Early Detection Program was established; and federal funding for breast cancer research increased fivefold in the 1990s. Currently, over $700,000,000 dollars in federal funds is allocated to breast cancer research each year. The final step in breast cancer advocacy is that the movement has gone mainstream (step 4). There is little question that breast cancer is firmly entrenched in the American consciousness. The ubiquitous pink ribbons and strong support for breast cancer research in the congress and the strong corporate support and the continuing proliferation of strong national and local advocacy groups speak to the effectiveness of breast cancer advocacy by women over the past 30 years.

Progress in Women's Health Research

In 2010, the Institute of Medicine released a report entitled *Women's Health Research: Progress, Pitfalls, and Priorities*. The committee considered some select diseases of importance to women and characterized the nature of progress that has been made in prevention and treatment. Breast cancer, cervical cancer, and cardiovascular disease are conditions on which research has contributed to major progress. For example, the age-adjusted mortality from invasive breast cancer dropped from 33.1 per 100,000 women in 1990 to 22.8 per 100,000 in 2007 due to increased screening and improved adjuvant therapies. Despite these gains, the incidence of breast cancer is higher today than in 1975. However, there has been a significant decrease in estrogen-positive breast cancers since 2002, probably because of the large decline in hormone replacement therapy for menopause.

HIV/AIDS is an example of a condition in which scientific research has led to some progress in women's health despite the early heavy research emphasis on men. The proportion of AIDS cases represented by women has been increasing steadily since 1985, and women now represent about 27% of cases. Like the case for men, prevention entails decreasing high-risk sexual behavior. However, women suffer from their own high-risk sexual behavior as well as that of their partner, which makes prevention more challenging. Antiretroviral therapy has made a tremendous impact for women (as well as men). However, women seem to be less tolerant of the side effects of these therapies, and treatment toxicity remains a significant problem for women suffering from HIV/AIDs. Treatment and side effects for pregnant women and the offspring can also be problematic.

Autoimmune disorders as a group are common (third only to cardiovascular disease and cancer). Examples of autoimmune disorders include diabetes, thyroid disease, Graves' disease, lupus, rheumatoid arthritis, and multiple sclerosis. They affect 5–8% of population, but over 78% of those affected are women. Advances in knowledge have occurred over the past 20 years, but these advances have not led to treatment advances beyond the treatment of symptoms. These disorders do not have the mortality associated with cardiovascular disease and cancer, but they are associated with significant morbidity and reduced quality of life.

Women's Mental Health

Mental health problems represent a significant burden for women. For example, globally, among women aged 15–44 years, unipolar depressive disorders are the second leading cause of disability (measured in disability-adjusted life years) after HIV/AIDS. Moreover, schizophrenia, bipolar affective disorder, suicide attempts, and panic disorder are in the top 15 conditions causing disability in young women. Depressive and anxiety disorders are much more common in women than men – for depression, the ratio is approximately 2 to 1 around the world. These disorders are found in all societies, not just the societies in the developed nations. In addition to the suffering experienced by women due to mental health problems, there is a large and increasing literature linking maternal mental health problems to behavioral and mental health problems in the offspring. Effective pharmacological and psychotherapeutic interventions exist for depressive and anxiety disorders. Nevertheless, women often go untreated in part because of lack of access but also because the women's depressive and anxiety disorders are often undetected in primary care settings such as prenatal and postnatal health care and routine gynecological care. Major initiatives are underway to develop more effective methods of detecting depression and anxiety among women and primary care and to provide more efficacious and accessible treatment for these women.

Cross-References

▶ Breast Cancer
▶ Cardiovascular Disease
▶ Clinical Trial

- Depression
- Diabetes
- Menopause
- Panic Disorder
- Pregnancy

References and Readings

Boston Women's Health Book Collective. (1973). *Our bodies, ourselves: A book by and for women*. New York: Simon and Schuster.

Braun, S. (2003). The history of breast cancer advocacy. *The Breast Journal, 9*, S101–S103.

Institute of Medicine (IOM). (2010). *Women's health research: Progress, pitfalls, and promise*. Washington, DC: The National Academies Press.

National Cancer Institute. (2011). *Cancer research funding*. From http://www.cancer.gov/cancertopics/factsheet/NCI/research-funding. Accessed 23 Apr 2011.

Our Bodies Ourselves. (2011). From http://www.ourbodiesourselves.org/about/default.asp. Accessed 17 Apr 2011.

US Department of Health and Human Services (HHS). (1985). Women's health. Report of the public health service task force on women's health issues. *Public Health Reports, 100*, 73–106.

World Health Organization (WHO). (1946). *Preamble to the constitution of the World Health Organization as adopted by the International Health conference*, New York, June, 19–22, 1946; Signed on 22 July 1946 by the Representatives of 61 States (Official Records of the World Health Organization, No. 2, p. 100) and Entered into Force on April 7, 1948. From http://www.who.int/about/definition/en/print.html. Accessed 17 Apr 2011.

World Health Organization (WHO). (2001). *The world health report: 2001: Mental health: New understanding, new hope*. Geneva: Author.

Women's Health Initiative (WHI)

Jonathan Newman
Columbia University, New York, NY, USA

Definition

The Women's Health Initiative (WHI) is a long-term, domestic health study that has focused on preventing heart disease, colorectal cancer, and osteoporotic fractures in post-menopausal women, all of which are major causes of death and disability in older women.

Description

The WHI is a multimillion-dollar study sponsored by the National Institutes of Health (NIH) and the National Heart, Lung, and Blood Institute, involving 161,308 women aged 50–79. The study has two major parts: a set of randomized clinical trials and an observational component. The WHI clinical trials (CT) include three overlapping components: the hormone therapy (HT) trials, dietary modification (DM) trials, and the calcium and vitamin D (CaD) trial. Each trial is a randomized comparison among postmenopausal women, age 50–79 at enrollment, who could be randomized into one, two, or three of the CT trials. Women who declined or were unable to participate were invited to participate in the observational study (OS), including 93,976 participants.

The HT trial is one of the most noteworthy within the WHI, and it consists of two separate trials, one for women who were post-hysterectomy at the time randomization (estrogen-alone trial) and one for women with a uterus (estrogen plus progestin trial). Both the hormone therapy trials and the CaD trial had a 1:1 double-blinded, placebo-controlled randomization, while the DM trial randomized 40% of women to a sustained low-fat diet and 60% to self-selected dietary behavior.

After 5.6 years of follow-up, the estrogen plus progestin (E+P) trial was stopped in 2002 because of increased risks of cardiovascular disease and breast cancer among women randomized to active treatment. While at a lower risk for colon cancer and fracture, women on estrogen and progestin had a higher risk of heart disease, stroke, blood clots, and certain types of breast cancer. After stopping the E+P trial, the WHI continued to follow up the women involved. Three years after stopping hormone therapy with estrogen and progestin, the women no longer had an increased risk of cardiovascular disease nor a lower risk of colon cancer compared to women who were randomized to placebo. Further follow-up revealed a nearly twofold increase in the incidence of breast cancer among women who had taken this hormone combination for 5 or more years. However, once estrogen and progestin hormone therapy was stopped, the risk of breast cancer decreased significantly, independent of rates of mammography in the population as a whole during this time.

The estrogen-alone trial was stopped in 2004 after 6.8 years of follow-up. It was found that estrogen alone did not affect the risk of heart disease; however, the risk of stroke was increased by 12 cases per 10,000 women taking estrogen alone and tended to increase the incidence of deep vein thrombosis as well. Similar to the results of the E+P HT trial, estrogen alone decreased the occurrence of both hip and total bone fractures. Colorectal cancer rates were unaffected, and there was a small suggestion of a reduction in breast cancer incidence. In a follow-up study, there was an indication that estrogen alone might decrease the amount of coronary artery calcium, a useful subclinical marker of atherosclerotic risk. Taking into account all the diseases studied during the estrogen-alone trial, the WHI investigators concluded that estrogen should not be used to prevent heart disease specifically, nor chronic diseases overall in postmenopausal women without a uterus.

The DM trials, while largely negative in terms of the effects of fat and caloric restriction on either breast or colorectal cancer in postmenopausal women, did suggest that reductions in saturated and trans fat, along with higher intakes of fruit and vegetables, may have a protective effect on the incidence of cardiovascular disease in these women. The separate CaD trials, while failing to show a protective effect of calcium and vitamin D on the occurrence of hip fracture in all postmenopausal women, did find a protective effect on the occurrence of hip fractures in women over the age of 60. The WHI trialists have recognized that the dose of calcium and vitamin D may have been insufficient to prevent hip fractures and may have contributed to the largely negative findings of this trial. Further, in the CaD trial, there were no beneficial effects of calcium and vitamin D on the occurrence of colon cancer. However, there were small (1%) but significant protective effects on maintenance of bone mineral density seen in women taking calcium plus vitamin D supplements.

References and Readings

Beresford, S., Johnson, K., Ritenbaugh, C., Lasser, N., Snetselaar, L., Black, H., Anderson, G., Assaf, A., Bassford, T., Bowen, D., Brunner, R., Brzyski, R., Caan, B., Chlebowski, R., et al. (2006). Low-fat dietary pattern and risk of colorectal cancer: The women's health initiative randomized controlled dietary modification trial. *Journal of the American Medical Association, 295*, 643–654.

Jackson, R., LaCroix, A., Gass, M., Wallace, R., Robbins, J., Lewis, C., Bassford, T., Beresford, S., Black, H., Blanchette, P., Bonds, D., Brunner, R., Bryzski, R., Caan, B., et al. (2006). Calcium plus vitamin D supplementation and the risk of fractures. *NEJM, 354*(7), 669–683.

The Women's Health Initiative Steering Committee. (2004). Effects of conjugated equine estrogen in postmenopausal women with hysterectomy. The women's health initiative randomized controlled trial. *Journal of the American Medical Association, 291*, 1701–1712.

The Writing Group for the WHI Investigators. (2002). Risks and benefits of estrogen plus progestin in healthy post-menopausal women: Principal results of the Women's health initiative randomized controlled trial. *Journal of the American Medical Association, 288*(3), 321–333.

Women's Mental Health

▶ Women's Health

Women's Reproductive Health

▶ Women's Health

Women's Well-Being

▶ Women's Health

Work

▶ Job Diagnostic Survey

Work Autonomy

▶ Job Satisfaction/Dissatisfaction

Work Engagement

▶ Job Demands

Work Fulfillment/Non-fulfillment

▶ Job Satisfaction/Dissatisfaction

Work Performance Feedback

▶ Job Satisfaction/Dissatisfaction

Work Rehabilitation

▶ Occupational Rehabilitation

Work Satisfaction/Dissatisfaction

▶ Job Satisfaction/Dissatisfaction

Work Tasks

▶ Workload

Work, Lipids, and Fibrinogen (WOLF) Study

William Whang
Division of Cardiology, Columbia University Medical Center, New York, NY, USA

Definition

The WOLF study is a prospective cohort study that was started to analyze the role of adverse occupational conditions in cardiovascular risk and disease development in employed Swedish men and women. Occupational health units carried out baseline screening of employees from approximately 60 companies from 1992 to 1998, including a clinical exam and blood samples. The initial study of 10,382 subjects from WOLF found no associations between job strain and serum total cholesterol and plasma fibrinogen (Alfredsson et al. 2002). Additional studies have examined relationships between cardiac risk and leisure time (Fransson et al. 2003) and managerial leadership behaviors (Nyberg et al. 2009).

References and Further Reading

Alfredsson, L., Hammar, N., Fransson, E., et al. (2002). Job strain and major risk factors for coronary heart disease among employed males and females in a Swedish study on work, lipids and fibrinogen. *Scandinavian Journal of Work, Environment & Health, 28*, 238–248.

Fransson, E. I., Alfredsson, L. S., de Faire, U. H., Knutsson, A., & Westerholm, P. J. (2003). Leisure time, occupational and household physical activity, and risk factors for cardiovascular disease in working men and women: The WOLF study. *Scandinavian Journal of Public Health, 31*, 324–333.

Nyberg, A., Alfredsson, L., Theorell, T., Westerlund, H., Vahtera, J., & Kivimaki, M. (2009). Managerial leadership and ischaemic heart disease among employees: The Swedish WOLF study. *Occupational and Environmental Medicine, 66*, 51–55.

Working Memory

David Pearson
School of Psychology, University of Aberdeen, Aberdeen, UK

Definition

The term "working memory" describes temporary memory systems involved in tasks such as reasoning, learning, and understanding. Examples of everyday tasks that rely on working memory include performing mental arithmetic or remembering a shopping list. While linked to the concept of short-term memory (STM), theories of working memory place greater emphasis on simultaneous storage and processing of information. Memory systems responsible for STM can be regarded as forming part of an overall working memory system. Working memory not only temporarily stores information but also manipulates it during complex cognitive activities. Theories of working memory are highly influential in the fields of cognitive psychology, neuroscience, and behavioral medicine.

Description

An influential model of working memory is the multicomponent approach first proposed by Baddeley and Hitch in Baddeley und Hitch 1974. The original model was tripartite in nature and comprised three separate, limited-capacity components: the phonological loop, the visuospatial sketchpad, and the central executive. The phonological loop and sketchpad are modality-specific "slave systems" that enable individuals to retain verbal speech-based material and visuospatial material, respectively. The phonological loop consists of a passive phonological store containing information that is rehearsed by an active articulatory mechanism closely linked to the production of speech (Baddeley 2007). A similar distinction has been made within the visuospatial component between a passive visual store and an active spatial mechanism involved during the planning and execution of movement (Logie 2003; Pearson 2007). Both the phonological loop and sketchpad are controlled by the central executive, a modality-free system responsible for strategic cognitive control, the coordination of tasks carried out in parallel, and scheduling and planning during multitasking (Law et al. 2006; Logie et al. 2004). The original tripartite model was subsequently modified with the addition of a fourth component, the episodic buffer, which functions to bind together information from working memory and long-term memory into unitary multimodal representations (Baddeley 2000).

An alternative to the multicomponent approach regards working memory as an activated portion of long-term memory rather than as a separate system. According to Cowan (1999), working memory comprises a set of cognitive processes that maintain information in a highly accessible state. Working memory representations are embedded within long-term memory, with the activation of representations controlled by attentional processes. The focus of attention is capacity limited and able to hold up to four activated representations (Cowan 2005). The temporary activation of representations in working memory can be maintained by either continued attention or rehearsal in a verbal subsystem (Cowan 1999).

The interaction between storage and processing in working memory is further explored by the time-based resource sharing model proposed by Barrouillet et al. (2004). In this model, rehearsal in working memory is carried out by an attentional mechanism also implicated during concurrent processing. Rehearsal must therefore take place during small time intervals in which task processing does not place demands upon attention. Forgetting in working memory is predicted by the model to increase with overall cognitive load, in which both the rate of individual processing steps during a task and their duration have a high density.

Theories of working memory have widespread application in behavioral medicine. Evidence suggests that schizophrenia is linked to a reduced ability to maintain information in working memory (Park und Holzman 1992), with deficits also being found in patients' biological relatives (Myles-Worsley und Park 2002). Working memory deficits have also been documented in patients suffering from bipolar affective disorder (Hammar und Ardal 2009), Asperger's syndrome (Cui et al. 2010), multiple sclerosis (McCarthy et al. 2005), Alzheimer's disease (MacPherson et al. 2007), and attention deficit hyperactivity disorder (Holmes et al. 2010). Working memory has also been linked with theories of craving and addiction (Kavangh et al. 2005) and the occurrence of intrusive memories associated with post-traumatic stress disorder (Holmes et al. 2004; Pearson et al. 2012; Pearson und Sawyer 2011).

Cross-References

▶ Executive Function
▶ Post Traumatic Stress Disorder

References and Readings

Baddeley, A. D. (2000). The episodic buffer: A new component of working memory? *Trends in Cognitive Sciences, 4*(11), 417–423.

Baddeley, A. D. (2007). *Working memory, thought, and action.* Oxford: Oxford University Press.

Baddeley, A. D., & Hitch, G. J. (1974). Working memory. In G. Bower (Ed.), *The psychology of learning and motivation* (Vol. VIII, pp. 47–90). New York: Academic Press.

Barrouillet, P., Bernardin, S., & Camos, V. (2004). Time constraints and resource sharing in adults' working memory spans. *Journal of Experimental Psychology: General, 133,* 83–100.

Cowan, N. (1999). An embedded-processes model of working memory. In A. M. P. Shah (Ed.), *Models of working memory* (pp. 62–101). Cambridge: Cambridge University Press.

Cowan, N. (2005). *Working memory capacity.* Hove: Psychology Press.

Cui, J. F., Gao, D. G., Chen, Y. H., Zou, X. B., & Wang, Y. (2010). Working memory in early-school-age children with Asperger's Syndrome. *Journal of Autism and Developmental Disorders, 40*(8), 958–967.

Hammar, A., & Ardal, G. (2009). Cognitive functioning in major depression – a summary. *Frontiers in Human Neuroscience, 3,* 26.

Holmes, E. A., Brewin, C. R., & Hennessy, R. G. (2004). Trauma films, information processing, and intrusive memory development. *Journal of Experimental Psychology: General, 133*(1), 3–22.

Holmes, J., Gathercole, S. E., Place, M., Alloway, T. P., Elliott, J. G., & Hilton, K. A. (2010). The diagnostic utility of executive function assessments in the identification of ADHD in children. *Child and Adolescent Mental Health, 15*(1), 37–43.

Kavangh, D. J., Andrade, J., & May, J. (2005). Imaginary relish and exquisite torture: The elaborated intrusion theory of desire. *Psychological Review, 112*(2), 446–467.

Law, A. S., Logie, R. H., & Pearson, D. G. (2006). The impact of secondary tasks on multitasking in a virtual environment. *Acta Psychologica, 122*(1), 27–44.

Logie, R. H. (2003). Spatial and visual working memory: A mental workspace. In D. Irwin & B. H. Ross (Eds.), *The psychology of learning and motivation* (Vol. 42, pp. 37–38). New York: Academic Press.

Logie, R. H., Cocchini, G., Della Sala, S., & Baddeley, A. D. (2004). Is there a specific executive capacity for dual task coordination? Evidence from Alzheimer's disease. *Neuropsychology, 18*(3), 504–513.

MacPherson, S. E., Della Sala, S., Logie, R. H., & Wilcock, G. K. (2007). Specific AD impairment in concurrent performance of two memory tasks. *Cortex, 43*(7), 858–865.

McCarthy, M., Beaumont, J. G., Thompson, R., & Peacock, S. (2005). Modality-specific aspects of sustained and divided attentional performance in multiple sclerosis. *Archives of Clinical Neuropsychology, 20*(6), 705–718.

Myles-Worsley, M., & Park, S. (2002). Spatial working memory deficits in schizophrenia patients and their first degree relatives from Palau, Micronesia. *American Journal of Medical Genetics, 114*(6), 609–615.

Park, S., & Holzman, P. S. (1992). Schizophrenics show spatial working memory deficits. *Archives of General Psychiatry, 49*(12), 231–246.

Pearson, D. G. (2007). Visuospatial rehearsal processes in working memory. In N. Osaka, R. H. Logie, & M. D'Esposito (Eds.), *The cognitive neuroscience of working memory* (pp. 231–246). Oxford: Oxford University Press.

Pearson, D. G., & Sawyer, T. (2011). Effects of dual task interference on memory intrusions for affective images.

International Journal of Cognitive Therapy, 4(2), 122–133.

Pearson, D. G., Ross, F. D. C., & Webster, V. L. (2012). The importance of context: Evidence that contextual representations increase intrusive memories. *Journal of Behavior Therapy and Experimental Psychiatry, 43*, 573–580.

Workload

Karen Jacobs[1], Miranda Hellman[2], Jacqueline Markowitz[1] and Ellen Wuest[2]
[1]Occupational Therapy, College of Health and Rehabilitation Science, Sargent College, Boston University, Boston, MA, USA
[2]Boston University, Boston, MA, USA

Synonyms

Work tasks

Definition

There is no one widely accepted definition of workload. Hart and Staveland (1988) describe workload as "the perceived relationship between the amount of mental processing capability or resources and the amount required by the task." Another definition is that it represents the relationship between a group or individual human operator and task demands. In simpler terms, it is the volume of work expected of a person. According to Wickens (1984), "the main objective of assessing and predicting workload is to achieve evenly distributed, manageable workload and to avoid overload or underload."

It can be measured in terms of many factors such as the amount of work accomplished over a period of time (number of hours worked or the number of assignments in a course), level of production, or the physical or cognitive demands of the work being performed (working with a person who speaks a different language than your own). There can be constraints to reaching one's workload such as lack of resources, motivation, and sufficient amount of time.

Cross-References

▶ Social Support

References and Readings

Hart, S. G., & Staveland, L. E. (1988). Development of NASA-TLX (Task Load Index): Results of empirical and theoretical research. In P. A. Hancock & N. Meshkati (Eds.), *Human mental workload* (pp. 77–106). New York: Elsevier Science Publishers B.V (North Holland).

Spector, P., & Jex, S. (1998). Development of four self-report measures of job stressors and strain: Interpersonal conflict at work scale, organizational constraints scale, quantitative workload inventory, and physical symptoms inventory. *Journal of Occupational Health Psychology, 3*(4), 4356–4367.

Wickens, C. D. (1984). Processing resources in attention. In R. Parasuraman & D. R. Davies (Eds.), *Varieties of attention* (pp. 63–102). New York: Academic.

Work-Related Health

▶ Occupational Health
▶ Organizational Health Psychology

Work-Related Stress

▶ Job Related to Health

Worksite Health Promotion

Ellinor K. Olander
City, University of London, London, UK

Synonyms

Organizational health promotion

Definition

Worksite health promotion refers to interventions/programs implemented in the workplace that aim to promote health and improve employee well-being.

There are numerous benefits associated with implementing interventions/programs in the worksite setting including a great potential to reach a large number of individuals, provision of existing social support for behavior change, or existing infrastructure making it easy to contact individuals or assess their behavior/health. Examples of worksite health promotion programs include those that target smoking, physical activity, stress management, weight reduction, and nutrition. Most worksite health promotion programs target individual behavior (such as encouraging individuals to stop smoking); others may target the physical environment (e.g., encouraging stair instead of elevator use) or organizational change/policy (such as not selling unhealthy food in the worksite restaurant).

Cross-References

▶ Nutrition
▶ Physical Activity
▶ Smoking Cessation

References and Further Readings

Chenoweth, D. (2006). *Worksite health promotion* (2nd ed.). Champaign: Human Kinetics.
O'Donnell, M. P. (2001). *Health promotion in the workplace* (3rd ed.). Albany: Delmar Cengage Learning.
Pronk, N. P. (Ed.). (2009). *ACSM's worksite health handbook: A guide to building healthy and productive companies (American College of Sports Med)* (2nd ed.). Champaign: Human Kinetics.

World Health Organization (WHO)

Shekhar Saxena and M. Taghi Yasamy
Department of Mental Health and Substance Abuse, World Health Organization, Geneva, Switzerland

Basic Information

The World Health Organization (WHO) was established in 1948 and is the directing and coordinating authority on international health within the United Nation's system (World Health Organization 2006). It is responsible for providing leadership on global health matters, shaping the health research agenda, setting norms and standards, articulating evidence-based policy options, providing technical support to countries, and monitoring and assessing health trends (About WHO n.d.).

WHO's constitution echoes a clear understanding about psychosocial aspects of health. It states that "Health is a state of complete physical, mental and social well-being and not merely the absence of disease or infirmity" (World Health Organization 2007). It also lays emphasis from the beginning on the "happiness, harmonious relations and security to all people..." (World Health Organization 2007).

Major Impact on the Field

WHO has a strong relationship with the Ministries of Health of the member states, and this provides an opportunity for advocating for mental health and integration of mental health into general health-care systems of countries.

For decades, WHO has been generating tools and data on epidemiology of mental disorders, classification of mental disorders, and mapping available resources and services. WHO's ATLAS Mental Health and the WHO Assessment Instrument for Mental Health systems (WHO_AIMS) are well-known resources which are being widely used by mental health planners and policy makers across the globe (http://www.who.int/mental_health/evidence/atlas/en/; Saxena et al. 2006; WHO_AIMS n.d.).

In 2001, when Dr. Gro Harlem Brutland was the Director General, WHO's theme was chosen "mental health, stop exclusion, dare to care." The World Health Report title was selected as "Mental Health: New Understanding, New Hope." The report focused on the fact that mental health is crucial to the overall well-being of individuals, societies, and countries. The report advocated the policies that were required to ensure that stigma and discrimination are broken down and that effective intervention and treatment are put in place (WHO 2001).

WHO promotes the rights of people with mental illness and supports participation of service users at all stages of planning, implementation, and evaluation of mental health interventions (Funk 2005). WHO has also produced intervention guidelines for a wide range of mental, neurological, and substance abuse disorders. In 2008, WHO's Director General launched the Mental Health Gap Action Programme (mhGAP) (World Health Organization 2008) and in 2010 the mhGAP Intervention Guide (World Health Organization 2010). The program and the related guidelines and tools will help poor resource countries in providing basic evidence-based mental health care through nonspecialized health providers.

WHO is also currently developing the International Classification of Diseases (ICD-11) and is collaborating with a wide group of professionals including psychologists to develop the mental and behavioral disorders chapter in ICD-11.

Cross-References

▶ Health Care
▶ Health Care Access
▶ Health Care System
▶ Health Care Utilization
▶ Health Economics
▶ Health Policy/Health-Care Policy
▶ Health Promotion and Disease Prevention
▶ Lifestyle, Healthy
▶ Prevention: Primary, Secondary, Tertiary
▶ Primary Care
▶ Primary Care Providers
▶ Public Health
▶ Quality of Life
▶ Quality-Adjusted Life Years (QALYs)
▶ Reproductive Health
▶ Risk Factors and Their Management
▶ Tobacco Control

References and Further Reading

About WHO. (n.d.). Retrieved March 1, 2011, from http://www.who.int/about/en/

Funk, M. (2005). Advocacy for mental health: Roles for consumer and family organizations and governments. *Health Promotion International, 21*(1), 70–75.

Saxena, S., Sharan, P., Garrido, M., & Saraceno, B. (2006). World Health Organization's Mental Health Atlas 2005: Implications for policy development. *World Psychiatry, 5*(3), 179–184.

WHO. (2001). *The world health report 2001 – Mental health: New understanding, new hope*. Geneva: WHO.

WHO_AIMS. (n.d.). *General information*. Retrieved May 25, 2011, from http://www.who.int/mental_health/evidence/WHO-AIMS/en/

World Health Organization. (2006). *Working for health: An introduction to World Health Organization*. Geneva: World Health Organization.

World Health Organization. (2007). *Basic documents* (46th ed.). Geneva: World Health Organization.

World Health Organization. (2008). *mhGAP: Mental Health GAP Action Programme: Scaling up care for mental, neurological and substance use disorders*. Geneva: World Health Organization.

World Health Organization. (2010). *mhGAP intervention guide for mental, neurological and substance use disorders in non-specialized health settings. Version 1.0.* Geneva: World Health Organization.

World Health Organization. (n.d.). *Project atlas: Resources for mental health.* Retrieved May 25, 2011, from http://www.who.int/mental_health/evidence/atlas/en/

Worldview

▶ Meaning (Purpose)

Worry

J. F. Brosschot and Bart Verkuil
Clinical, Health and Neuro Psychology, Leiden University, Leiden, The Netherlands

Synonyms

Intrusive thoughts; Perseverative cognition; Repetitive thinking; Rumination

Definition

Worry is defined as *"a chain of thoughts and images, negatively affect-laden and relatively uncontrollable. The worry process represents an attempt to engage in mental problem-solving on an issue whose outcome is uncertain but contains the possibility of one or more negative outcomes. Consequently, worry relates closely to fear process"* (Borkovec et al. 1983). Worry can impact health in several ways. First, it is a form of the so-called perseverative cognition (see term), which is defined as "the ongoing cognitive representation of psychological stressors (threat)" (Brosschot et al. 2006). Perseverative cognition is believed to be responsible for a large part of the health impact of psychological stressors, because it prolongs the physiological responses to these stressors. Second, disease-specific worry can lead to maladaptive outcomes in the long or short term, for example, in the aftermath of surgery or other intrusive medical treatments (Verkuil et al. 2010). Third, severe worry about illness can take the form of the anxiety disorder hypochondriasis, or disorders such as somatization or somatoform disorders. In a milder form of illness, worry can increase the number and severity of medically unexplained symptoms, presumably via the excessive activation of illness-related memory networks, that bias perception and behavior in the direction of experiencing and reporting symptoms (Brosschot 2002; Brown 2004). Fourth, a symptom-specific, catastrophizing form, for example "pain catastrophizing," appears to play a role in the maintenance and exacerbation of symptoms. Catastrophizing thoughts about a symptom such as pain may drive the vicious circle that leads from pain to catastrophizing to immobility to more pain, etc. (Vlaeyen and Linton 2000). Last but not least worry and related perseverative thinking styles, such as rumination, play a causal or maintaining role in several forms of psychopathology (Watkins 2008).

Cross-References

▶ Anxiety and Its Measurement
▶ Intrusive Thoughts
▶ Negative Thoughts
▶ Perseverative Cognition

References and Further Readings

Borkovec, T. D., Robinson, E., Pruzinsky, T., & DePree, J. A. (1983). Preliminary exploration of worry: Some characteristics and processes. *Behavior Research and Therapy, 21,* 9–16.

Brosschot, J. F. (2002). Cognitive-emotional sensitization and somatic health complaints. *Scandinavian Journal of Psychology, 43,* 113–121.

Brosschot, J. F., Gerin, W., & Thayer, J. F. (2006). The perseverative cognition hypothesis: A review of worry, prolonged stress-related physiological activation, and health. *Journal of Psychosomatic Research, 60,* 113–124.

Brown, R. J. (2004). Psychological mechanisms of medically unexplained symptoms: An integrative conceptual model. *Psychological Bulletin, 130,* 793–812.

Verkuil, B., Brosschot, J. F., Gebhardt, W., & Thayer, J. F. (2010). When worries make you sick: A review of perseverative cognition, the default stress response and somatic health. *Journal of Experimental Psychopathology, 1*(1), 87–118.

Vlaeyen, J. W., & Linton, S. J. (2000). Fear-avoidance and its consequences in chronic musculoskeletal pain: A state of the art. *Pain, 85*(3), 317–332.

Watkins, E. R. (2008). Constructive and unconstructive repetitive thought. *Psychological Bulletin, 134*(2), 163–206.

Worship

▶ Prayer

Wound Healing

Christopher G. Engeland
Department of Biobehavioral Health,
The Pennsylvania State University, University Park, PA, USA

Synonyms

Tissue repair

Definition

Wound healing pertains to the repair and regeneration of damaged tissue.

Stages of Wound Healing

Tissue repair involves three interdependent and overlapping phases:

1. The inflammatory phase (hours to days) in which blood flow to the injured area is decreased, a blood clot forms, inflammatory cells (e.g., neutrophils, monocytes) are recruited to the site of injury, and bacterial clearance occurs.
2. The proliferative phase (days to weeks) in which fibroblasts, epithelial cells, and endothelial cells are recruited and proliferate for the rebuilding process which involves wound contraction, reepithelialization, and angiogenesis (i.e., formation of new blood vessels).
3. The remodeling phase (weeks to months) in which the connective tissue matrix begun in the previous phase is fully formed and restructured (for review, see Engeland and Marucha 2009). Psychological stress can impair healing through its effects on each of these phases.

Description

Overview

It is generally accepted that a patient's state of mind can modulate immune responses (for reviews, see Christian et al. 2009; Hawkley et al. 2007), affecting factors such as healing rates and surgical outcomes. Numerous psychological factors such as stress, anxiety, depression, hostility, and anger can relate to poor healing, such as slowed wound closure which increases the risk of infection and other complications. Conversely, factors such as positive mood, optimism, conscientiousness, positive social interactions, and emotional stability can improve healing outcomes.

Stress Pathways

The primary effects of stress on wound healing occur through central activation of the hypothalamic pituitary adrenal (HPA) axis and the sympathetic nervous system (SNS). HPA activation promotes the systemic release of glucocorticoids (GCs) (e.g., cortisol in humans) from the adrenal glands. GCs are potently anti-inflammatory and immunosuppressant and act as the body's main brake on inflammation. By dysregulating the release and function of GCs, chronic stress can result in higher inflammatory reactions following immune activation (e.g., response to injury). Activation of the SNS by stress results in vasoconstriction (caused by norepinephrine), which limits blood flow to the site of injury resulting in hypoxia and lowering available nutrient supplies to tissues. Vasoconstriction may also delay the arrival of immune cells, such as neutrophils and monocytes, to the site of injury further impeding the healing process. In addition, norepinephrine (released during stress) reduces the capacity of macrophages to kill bacteria. Through these two pathways, stress can dysregulate immune function and alter early wound repair. The end result is impaired bacterial clearance, prolonged inflammation, higher risk of infection, and greater post-surgical (or post-injury) complications (for reviews, see Marucha and Engeland 2007; Engeland and Marucha 2009).

Stress and Anxiety

Since 1995, numerous studies have demonstrated that stress negatively affects healing, and this notion is now widely accepted. Stressors such as caregiving for a patient with Alzheimer's disease and university examinations, along with preoperative and perceived stress, have each been shown to slow dermal healing (for reviews, see Devries et al. 2007; Engeland and Graham 2011). For instance, stress associated with caregiving slowed the healing of skin wounds by 24%. Such delays are typically accompanied by elevated cortisol levels and reduced inflammation, and similar stress-induced changes have been mirrored in animal research (Engeland and Marucha 2009). Aside from skin, stress affects mucosal inflammation and is a known risk factor for periodontal disease. Stress from university examinations in American dental students slowed the healing of experimental oral mucosal wounds by 40%. It is of note that a stressor as predictable and transient as examinations should delay healing to such a degree in professional students. Interestingly, stress appears to delay healing in mucosal tissues by increasing early inflammation, rather than by inhibiting inflammation as has been shown in skin wounds (Engeland and Graham 2011). Clinically, efforts should be made to reduce both pre- and postsurgical stress and to avoid scheduling elective surgery during or shortly after a period of stress (e.g., university examinations).

Depression and Other Behavioral Constructs

Psychosocial factors other than stress and anxiety also affect immunity. Higher depressive symptoms, marital disagreements, lower levels of anger control, and higher levels of hostility have all been related to slower healing in skin. Similarly, subclinical depression (dysphoria) relates to slower healing of mucosal wounds. Conversely, higher positive mood, optimism, conscientiousness, positive social interactions, and emotional stability relate to faster healing times in skin (for review, see Engeland and Graham 2011), suggesting a positive role for behavioral interventions on wound healing (see below).

Pain

Pain usually accompanies healing and can be viewed as a unique stressor with both physiological and psychological components. Pain can alter immunity directly by promoting cytokine release and indirectly through activation of stress pathways and changes in behavior. Through these different mechanisms, pain exacerbates the negative effects of stress on healing. Greater pain from elective gastric bypass surgery has been related to slower healing of an experimental skin wound placed on the day of surgery. Importantly, pain and stress are not additive but synergistic in their effects. Not only does each negatively affect healing, but each promotes the other through physiological and immune responses and through changes in mood and behavior. For instance, pain can lead to maladaptive health behaviors such as loss of sleep, inactivity, and alcohol use, each of which has been linked with poorer healing. Not only pain, but also its anticipation, can be a tangible source of anxiety for surgical patients, as well as concerns about the healing process. Efforts to minimize not only pain, but also these sources of anxiety, are encouraged (for review, see Engeland and Graham 2011).

Aging

It is known that ageing alters skin morphology. Aged skin undergoes reductions in vascularization, granulation tissue, collagen, elastin, mast cells, fibroblasts, and epidermal turnover, the latter of which is reduced ~50% as one ages from 20 to 70 years. In general, the elderly have slower healing times, increased rates of infection and wound dehiscence, and reduced wound strength. This is primarily caused by reductions in reepithelialization, angiogenesis, macrophage infiltration, and collagen deposition. In women, menopause exacerbates these effects. It is important to note that wound healing is slowed but not impaired in the elderly, and the eventual healing outcome is similar to that of young adults. This appears to hold true for mucosal healing as well. Also, for reasons unknown, wounds in the aged heal better aesthetically with less scarring. However, risk factors for impaired healing occur more commonly in the elderly, such as comorbidity, malnutrition, immobility, and obesity. Psychological stress is also more common in the aged and negatively impacts tissue healing to a greater degree than in young adults. Prior to surgery, when possible, each of these risk factors for impaired healing should be tested for, treated, and monitored to ensure maximal healing outcomes. In the elderly, especially, the presence of any of these risk factors should serve as a red flag to the clinician (for review, see Engeland and Gajendrareddy 2011).

Chronic Wounds

Most wound healing studies have been conducted in a controlled laboratory setting on acute wounds which heal relatively quickly (for a review of wound healing models, see Bosch et al. 2011). Clinical studies, which involve more naturally occurring wounds (e.g., diabetic foot ulcers, surgical wounds, accidents), provide valuable information about how such factors affect larger and more chronic wounds where poor outcomes may have more serious implications. Higher levels of depression and anxiety have been related to slower healing of chronic leg ulcers, with patients who scored in the top 50% of these measures being four times more likely to be categorized as slow healers. Thus, psychological stress has been shown to exert negative effects on the healing of both acute and chronic (nonhealing) wounds.

Skin Barrier Recovery

The skin is an essential barrier for providing resistance to pathogens and limiting water loss. This barrier plays an important factor in numerous skin diseases (e.g., psoriasis, atopic dermatitis) and in dermal healing. Repair to this barrier can be evaluated through tape stripping, in which cellophane tape is repeatedly applied to and removed from a dermal area (e.g., forearm). An evaporimeter is then used to assess transepidermal water loss (TEWL) over time. Stress from public speaking (i.e., Trier social stress test) slows barrier recovery times and is associated with increased levels of cortisol and inflammation. Similar delays in barrier recovery times have been demonstrated with stress stemming from marital dissolution, university examinations, and sleep deprivation. Higher positive mood relates to faster recovery times, indicating the negative effect of stress on skin barrier repair can be buffered by positive emotion. Skin barrier function, which is an important factor in numerous skin diseases (e.g., psoriasis, atopic dermatitis) and in dermal healing, undergoes slower recovery/repair during times of stress (for review, see Engeland and Graham 2011).

Health Behaviors

Stress and pain can affect wound healing indirectly through behavioral alterations such as poor sleep and nutrition, reduced exercise, increased consumption of alcohol or nicotine, and self-neglect (for review, see Guo and DiPietro 2010). For example, sleep deprivation can disrupt macrophage/lymphocyte functions and alter inflammation, thereby hindering immunity. Such changes can themselves promote stress, often in the form of anxiety or depression, which further impact on health creating a downward spiral effect. Smoking, which often increases during times of stress, reduces vitamin C and oxygen levels in blood, impairs collagen deposition and macrophage function, and alters turnover of the extracellular matrix during healing. It has been shown that smoking intervention 6–8 weeks before surgery reduces postoperative morbidity including wound-related complications. In addition, interventions aimed at lowering stress prior to surgeries such as patient education, massage therapy, and relaxation with guided imagery can have positive effects on postsurgical outcomes. Similarly, a 4-week exercise regimen was shown to speed healing rates by 25% in experimental skin wounds, independent of perceived stress. Emotional disclosure interventions, which involve participants writing about traumatic personal events, have been shown to positively affect immunity and speed up the healing of experimental wounds in skin. Such expressive writing appears to accelerate healing times compared to control subjects that write about time management (for reviews, see Engeland and Marucha 2009; Engeland and Graham 2011). Given the impact that such behaviors and interventions have on health, reducing negative behaviors, facilitating positive behaviors, and reducing stress levels around surgery will help to optimize immune responses, tissue repair, and postsurgical outcomes.

Cross-References

▶ Aging
▶ Anxiety
▶ Corticosteroids
▶ Depression
▶ Pain
▶ Stress

References and Further Readings

Bosch, J. A., Engeland, C. G., & Burns, V. E. (2011). Psychoneuroimmunology in vivo: Methods and principles. In J. Decety & J. T. Cacioppo (Eds.), *The Oxford handbook of social neuroscience* (pp. 134–148). New York: Oxford University Press.

Christian, L. M., Deichert, N. T., Gouin, J. P., Graham, J. E., & Kiecolt-Glaser, J. K. (2009). Psychological influences on endocrine and immune function. In G. G. Berntson & J. T. Cacioppo (Eds.), *Handbook of neuroscience for the behavioral sciences* (pp. 1260–1279). Hoboken: Wiley.

Devries, A. C., Craft, T. K., Glasper, E. R., Neigh, G. N., & Alexander, J. K. (2007). 2006 Curt P. Richter award winner social influences on stress responses and health. *Psychoneuroendocrinology, 32*, 587–603.

Engeland, C. G., & Gajendrareddy, P. K. (2011). Wound healing in the elderly. In M. Katlic (Ed.), *Cardiothoracic surgery in the elderly: Evidence based practice* (pp. 259–270). Berlin: Springer.

Engeland, C. G., & Graham, J. E. (2011). Psychoneuroimmunological aspects of wound healing and the role of pain. In D. Upton (Ed.), *Psychological impact of pain in patients with wounds* (pp. 87–114). London: Wounds UK Limited, A Schofield Healthcare Media Company.

Engeland, C. G., & Marucha, P. T. (2009). Wound healing and stress. In R. D. Granstein & T. A. Luger (Eds.), *Neuroimmunology of the skin: Basic science to clinical relevance* (pp. 233–247). Berlin: Springer.

Guo, S., & DiPietro, L. A. (2010). Factors affecting wound healing. *Journal of Dental Research, 89*(3), 219–229.

Hawkley, L. C., Bosch, J. A., Engeland, C. G., Cacioppo, J. T., & Marucha, P. T. (2007). Loneliness, dysphoria, stress, and immunity: A role for cytokines. In N. P. Plotnikoff, R. E. Faith, & A. J. Murgo (Eds.), *Cytokines: Stress and immunity*. Boca Raton: CRC Press.

Marucha, P. T., & Engeland, C. G. (2007). Stress, neuroendocrine hormones, and wound healing: Human models. In R. Ader, D. Felten, & N. Cohen (Eds.), *Psychoneuroimmunology* (pp. 825–835). San Diego: Academic.

Written Disclosure

▶ Expressive Writing and Health

X

X-Ray Computed Tomography

▶ CAT Scan
▶ Computerized Axial Tomography (CAT) Scan

Y

Years of Potential Life Lost (YPLL)

▶ Life Years Lost

Yoga

Melissa M. A. Buttner
Department of Psychology, University of Iowa, Iowa City, IA, USA

Definition

Yoga is an ancient tradition originating in India and is derived from a Sanskrit word meaning "to yoke" or "to unite" (Desikachar 1999). In Western culture, yoga is considered a form of physical activity and, more recently, a mind-body intervention designed to support overall health and well-being. In its full expression, yoga integrates three basic components: breath (*pranayama*), physical poses (*asanas*), and meditation (*dhyana*).

Description

Origins

Yogic philosophy traces back to 3000 BCE, with roots spanning four periods known as the Vedic (2000–600 BC), Preclassical (600–200 BC), Classical (200 BC), and Postclassical periods (Feuerstein 2001). The Preclassical period is associated with the emergence of the *Upanishads* (200 texts influencing Hindu philosophy) and the creation of the *Bhagavad Gita*, considered to be among yoga's oldest written texts. It was during this time that the foundations of meditation and the concept of *samadhi* (a path to enlightenment) surfaced (Feuerstein 2001). Patanjali's *Yoga Sutras* was compiled during the Classical period (Iyengar 1993) and contains 196 sutras describing raja yoga and its underlying eight-limbed path, or *ashtanga* yoga: *yama* (ethical guidelines), *niyama* (spiritual observances), *asana* (physical poses), *pranayama* (breathing exercises), *pratyahara* (control of the senses), *dharana* (concentration), *dhyana* (meditation), and *samadhi* (state of bliss) (Iyengar 2001). During the Postclassical period, *Hatha* yoga emerged, the most common form of yoga practiced in Western culture today (Feuerstein 2001).

Complementary and Alternative Medicine (CAM)

Complementary and alternative medicine (CAM) is a form of medicine consisting of systems, practices, and consumer products that are outside the realm of traditional or conventional forms of medicine (Barnes et al. 2008). Acceptance of this nontraditional form of medicine is growing. Findings from a 2008 survey on Americans' use of CAM published by the National Center for Complementary and Alternative Medicine

© Springer Nature Switzerland AG 2020
M. D. Gellman (ed.), *Encyclopedia of Behavioral Medicine*,
https://doi.org/10.1007/978-3-030-39903-0

(NCCAM) showed that *yoga* was one of the top ten most commonly used CAM therapies among adults, with 6.1% indicating use of yoga in the past year (Barnes et al. 2008). Preference for yoga as a CAM option over that of conventional forms of medicine may be associated with characteristics including decreased stigma, a more gentle form of treatment with minimal side effects, and flexibility in personalizing treatment (Uebelacker et al. 2010).

Yoga's Role in Behavioral Medicine
The past few decades have witnessed a confluence of Western medical science and psychological theories with ideas from Eastern practices such as yoga, which has led to the recent emergence of yoga as a mind-body intervention. In contrast with traditional forms of medicine, yoga offers a holistic approach to treating physical and mental health issues (Hayes and Chase 2010) and is currently being used to address various health conditions (see Table 1 for a detailed list). Recent reviews of the yoga literature suggest that yoga has beneficial effects on pain syndromes, cardiovascular, autoimmune and immune conditions, and on pregnancy (Field 2011). Further, there is evidence to suggest that yoga yields physiological benefits as evidenced in studies showing links between yoga and decreased heart rate and blood pressure, as well as physical effects, such as weight loss and increased muscle tone (Field 2011). More well-established physiological effects of yoga include stress reduction (Ross and Thomas 2010), with psychological effects evidenced by increased mindfulness and reduced symptoms of depression and anxiety (Field 2011; Uebelacker et al. 2010) (see Figs. 1 and 2 for illustrations of yoga poses).

ADHD attention deficit hyperactivity disorder, *OCD* obsessive compulsive disorder, *PTSD* post-traumatic stress disorder, *PNS* parasympathetic nervous system, *SNS* sympathetic nervous system

Stress
Stress has adverse effects as evidenced in many health conditions. Empirical evidence for yoga in combating these adverse effects suggests that controlled breathing helps to focus and relax the mind

Yoga, Table 1 Application of yoga as a therapeutic intervention

Psychological	Physical	Physiological
Anxiety	Arthritis	High blood pressure
ADHD	Cancer	High cortisol levels
Depression	Carpal tunnel syndrome	Increased heart rate
Eating disorders	Diabetes	PNS/SNS activity
OCD	Epilepsy	Poor circulation
Perimenopausal symptoms	Infertility	
Premenstrual syndrome	Insomnia	
PTSD	Irritable bowel syndrome	
Stress	Multiple sclerosis	
	Obesity	
	Pain (chronic)	
	Pregnancy (complications)	
	Sciatica	
	Scoliosis	
	Sinusitis	

through activation of the autonomic nervous system (ANS), which may work to counteract stress (Harinath et al. 2004). To understand the role of stress in disease and the effects of relaxation associated with a yoga practice in prevention and recovery, it is important to understand the function of the ANS. The ANS is responsible for regulating the heart, intestines, and other internal organs through a synergistic relationship between the sympathetic nervous system (SNS) and the parasympathetic nervous system (PNS) (McCall 2007). In general, when activity is high in the SNS, it will be low in the PNS, and vice versa. The SNS, along with the stress hormones cortisol and andrenaline, is responsible for generating a response to stressful situations, leading to physiological changes such as increased heart rate and blood pressure (McCall 2007). Increased mobilization of energy and additional blood and oxygen flowing to the body will enable a person to respond to the stressor, otherwise known as the

Yoga, Fig. 1 *Warrior II Pose* (*Virabhadrasana II*) requires weight bearing and helps to strengthen and stretch the legs and ankles, stimulates abdominal organs, and increases stamina. This pose is recommended for carpal tunnel syndrome, flat feet, osteoporosis, and sciatica (McCall 2007)

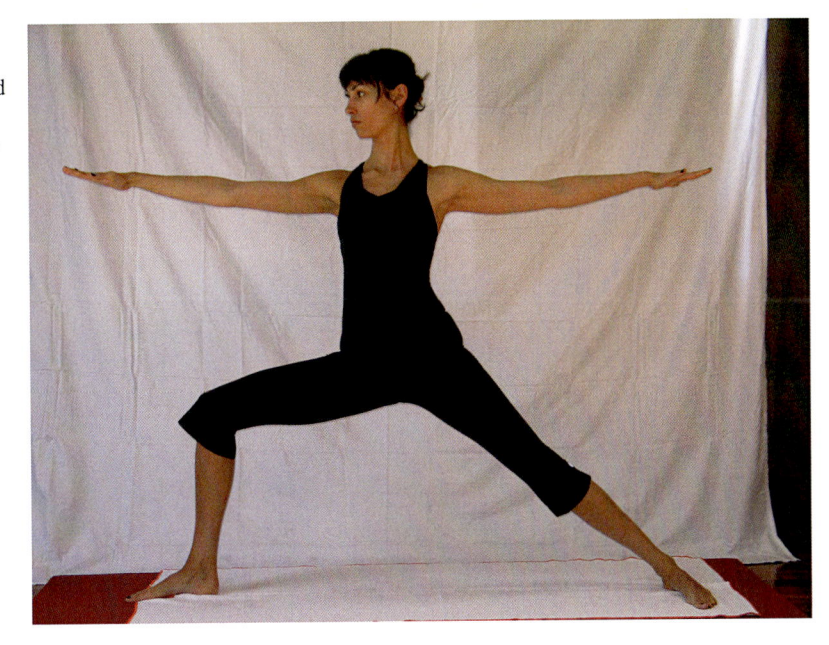

Yoga, Fig. 2 *Cobra Pose* (*Bhujangasana*) helps to strengthen the spine, stretch the chest and lungs, shoulders, and abdomen. It is recommended for stress, fatigue, and sciatica (McCall 2007)

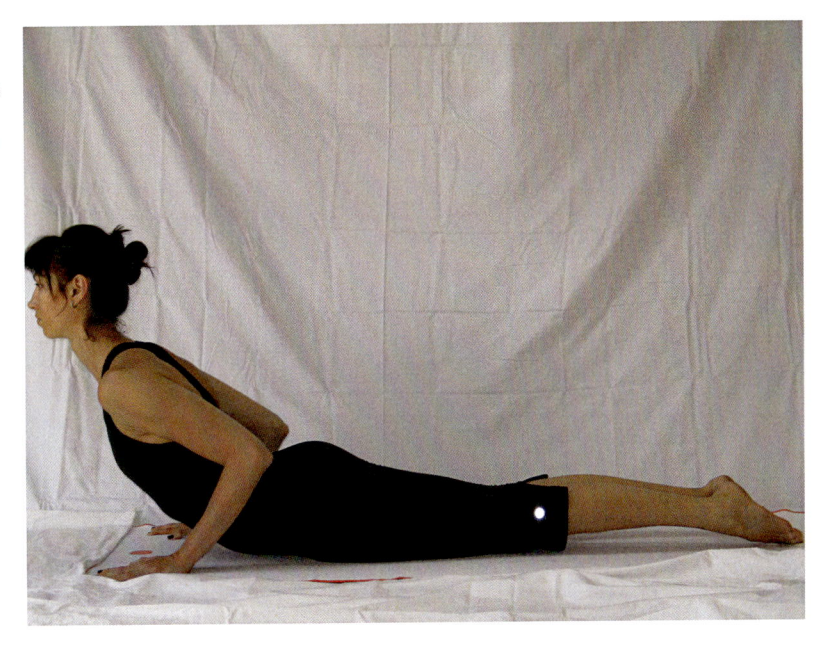

classic "fight or flight" response (McCall 2007). Conversely, the PNS slows the heart rate and lowers blood pressure to support recovery from a stressful situation, thereby functioning as a restorative mechanism that is often referred to as the "relaxation response" (Benson 2000).

The three basic components of yoga – physical postures, breathing, and meditation – interact with the PNS and SNS as potential mechanisms by which yoga has a calming effect on the nervous system, potentially leading to decreased stress reactivity (Ross and Thomas 2010). For example, ujjayi breathing (a form of slow yoga breathing characterized by an oceanic sound) is hypothesized to increase activation of the PNS, leading to a calm but alert state while simultaneously having a restorative effect on the body (McCall 2007). Practicing more rigorous forms of breathing (e.g., *kapalabhati* breathing) and poses (e.g., sun salutations) triggers a sympathetic response similar to that found in traditional forms of aerobic activity. In contrast to a typical aerobic workout, however, a more invigorating yoga practice followed by a sequence of relaxing poses will stimulate the PNS and restore energy (McCall 2007).

Mindfulness

The most commonly used definition of *mindfulness* is that of Jon Kabat-Zinn's, who defined it as "paying attention in a particular way: on purpose, in the present moment and nonjudgmentally" (Kabat-Zinn 1994, p. 4). Support for mindfulness as an agent of change comes by way of its role as an active component of evidence-based psychotherapies (e.g., acceptance and commitment therapy and mindfulness-based cognitive therapy). The practice of mindfulness allows one to experience disengaging from evaluative thinking in the presence of negative stimuli through cultivation of an attitude of curiosity and attention to ongoing reactions to emotions, thoughts, and feelings (Shapiro et al. 2008). In depressed patients, for example, a repetitive focus on negative feelings (rumination) is a typical way of responding and is implicated in the onset and maintenance of depression. *Mindfulness* cultivated in a yoga practice may counteract ruminative thinking by offering participants an alternative focus, such as the breath and physical sensations experienced in the body (Uebelacker et al. 2010). Through a regular yoga practice, yoga practitioners naturally begin to adopt a lifestyle guided by yogic philosophies such as self-acceptance, compassion, and spirituality. In general, the more one commits to the practice, the greater the benefits tend to be, and healthier habits begin to form (McCall 2007).

Yoga Styles

There is a preponderance of *Hatha* yoga styles practiced in the West today, with popular forms including *Anusara, Ashtanga, Bikram, Iyengar, Power, Vinyasa flow*, and *Viniyoga*. Most styles generally incorporate mindfulness with physical activity. Yoga, however, is distinct from traditional forms of physical activity with its focus on breath, and the intentional linking of breath with movement of the body through a sequence of postures (McCall 2007). In addition, there are some forms of *Hatha* yoga that focus on the therapeutic application of poses for various medical conditions, including *Anusara, Iyengar*, and *Viniyoga*.

Anusara yoga was developed by John Friend who integrated his Iyengar background with a "heart-centered" approach to teaching (Friend 2006). The focus in this style of yoga is on the physical poses and precision of alignment; however, chanting, pranayama, and meditation are also woven into many classes (Friend 2006). Although the application of Anusara yoga is not well established in the empirical literature, characteristics such as a focus on alignment may support its use as a therapeutic tool (McCall 2007).

Iyengar yoga, developed by B.K.S. Iyengar, is rooted in Patanjali's *Yoga Sutras* and is known for its therapeutic application based on a large body of literature supporting the benefits of Iyengar yoga and its emphasis on precision and alignment (Iyengar 1995). Iyengar yoga is often employed in research trials examining the effectiveness of yoga for treating mood disorders such as depression and anxiety. This particular style of yoga incorporates the use of props (bolsters, blankets, blocks) to make yoga accessible to beginners, despite limited experience and flexibility, and to help assist in guiding the student into the posture (Iyengar 2001). In this style of yoga, the poses are typically held for a longer duration of time relative to other forms of yoga such as Vinyasa flow. It is thought that holding the poses allows for proper alignment that is the hallmark of Iyengar yoga (Iyengar 2001). Yoga therapy performed according to this lineage of yoga can only be performed by instructors certified at a Junior Intermediate II level or above (see IYNAUS website for instructors and their level of certification). Iyengar yoga is known to have the highest standards in terms of teacher training and certification. Benefits of Iyengar yoga can be seen with many health conditions, ranging from depression to stress-related illnesses (Shapiro et al. 2007).

Viniyoga is a highly therapeutic and gentle style of yoga founded by T.K.V. Desikachar, in which poses and sequences are modified according to the needs of the student (Desikachar 1999). Students practicing this style of yoga will flow from one pose to the next, holding the poses for a brief period of time, minimizing the risk of injury and making this style of yoga suitable for students with chronic diseases (McCall 2007). In addition, pranayama breathing and chanting are integrated into a typical class.

Application of Yoga

Currently, there is no reliable system for identifying the most effective style of yoga for any one individual. Despite the number of studies examining the beneficial effects of yoga, most studies do not compare different styles of yoga or the mechanisms of action by which one particular style of yoga is effective (Uebelacker et al. 2010). In general, it is recommended that the elements of a yoga class (e.g., relaxation, rigorous flow with challenging poses), in addition to the quality of instruction, be considered when starting a yoga practice (McCall 2007). The length of a yoga class may range from 60 to 90 minute, with each posture being held for a few seconds to 1 minute, depending on the style of yoga.

For physically fit individuals with no serious medical conditions contraindicated with yoga, most yoga classes are appropriate. For beginning students, learning yoga in a group environment or through private instruction with a certified instructor is preferable; however, individuals may also learn using audiotapes or DVDs. Individuals presenting with serious medical conditions seeking yoga as a form of therapy should consult with a certified yoga instructor specializing in the medical issue being treated (Shapiro et al. 2008). An increasing number of classes are now being offered that are tailored to the needs of specific populations, such as pregnant and postpartum women. Women practicing yoga during and after pregnancy are advised to attend classes with an instructor knowledgeable in providing modifications specific to the perinatal population. If a woman established a rigorous yoga practice prior to conceiving, it is recommended that she transition to a gentler style of yoga until after childbirth (McCall 2007).

Cross-References

▶ Exercise
▶ Interventions and Strategies to Promote Physical Activity
▶ Meditation
▶ Mindfulness
▶ Physical Activity and Health

References and Readings

Barnes, P. M., Bloom, B., & Nahin, R. (2008). *Complementary and alternative medicine use among adults and children: United States, 2007* (CDC National Health Statistics Report No. 12). Accessed 27 November 2010.
Benson, H. (2000). *The relaxation response.* New York: Harper Paperbacks.
Cope, S. (2006). *The wisdom of yoga: A seeker's guide to extraordinary living.* New York: Bantam Dell.
Desikachar, T. K. V. (1999). *The heart of yoga: Developing a personal practice* (revised ed.). Rochester: Inner Traditions International.
Feuerstein, G. (2001). *The yoga tradition: Its history, literature, philosophy and practice.* Prescott: Hohm Press.
Field, T. (2011). Yoga clinical research review. *Complementary Therapies in Clinical Practice, 17*, 1–8.
Friend, J. (2006). *Anusara yoga teacher training manual* (9th ed.). The Woodlands: Anusara.
Harinath, K., Malhotra, A. S., Pal, K., Prasad, R., Kumar, R., Kain, T. C., Rai, L., & Sawhney, R. C. (2004). Effects of Hatha yoga and Omkar meditation on cardiorespiratory performance, psychologic profile, and melatonin secretion. *Journal of Alternative and Complementary Medicine, 10*, 261–268.
Hayes, S. C. (1999). *Acceptance and commitment therapy: An experiential approach to behavior change.* New York: Guilford Press.
Hayes, M., & Chase, S. (2010). Prescribing yoga. *Primary Care, 37*, 31–47.
International Association of Yoga Therapists. Accessed 29 November 2010.
Iyengar, B. K. S. (1993). *Light on the yoga sutras of Patanjali.* London: Aquarian Press.
Iyengar, B. K. S. (1995). *Light on yoga.* New York: Schocken Books.

Iyengar, B. K. S. (2001). *Yoga: The path to holistic health*. London: Dorling Kindersley.

Iyengar Yoga National Association of the United States (IYNAUS). Retrieved from www.iynaus.org. Accessed 29 November 2010

Kabat-Zinn, J. (1994). *Wherever you go, there you are: Mindfulness meditation in everyday life*. New York: Hyperion.

Kripalu Center for Yoga and Health. Retrieved from www.kripalu.org. Accessed 29 November 2010.

McCall, T. (2007). *Yoga as medicine: The yogic prescription for health and healing*. New York: Bantam Dell.

National Center for Complementary and Alternative Medicine (NCCAM). Retrieved from http://nccam.nih.gov/. Accessed 29 November 2010.

Ross, A., & Thomas, S. (2010). The health benefits of yoga and exercise: A review of comparison studies. *The Journal of Alternative and Complementary Medicine, 16*, 3–12.

Shapiro, D., Cook, I. A., Davydov, D. M., Ottaviani, C., Leuchter, A. F., & Abrams, M. (2007). Yoga as a complementary treatment of depression: Effects of traits and moods on treatment outcome. *Evidence-based Complementary and Alternative Medicine: eCAM, 4*, 493–502. https://doi.org/10.1093/ecam/nel114.

Shapiro, S. L., Oman, D., Thoresen, C. E., Plante, T. G., & Flinders, T. (2008). Cultivating mindfulness: Effects on well-being. *Journal of Clinical Psychology, 64*, 840–862.

Uebelacker, L. A., Epstein-Lubow, G., Gaudiano, B. A., Tremont, G., Battle, C. L., & Miller, I. W. (2010). Hatha yoga for depression: Critical review of the evidence for efficacy, plausible mechanisms of action, and directions for future research. *Journal of Psychiatric Practice, 16*, 22–33.

Yoga Alliance. Retrieved from www.yogaalliance.org. Accessed 29 November 2010.

Yoga Journal. Retrieved from www.yogajournal.com. Accessed 29 November 2010.

Yoga Research and Education Center (YREC). Retrieved from http://www.yrec.org/. Accessed 29 November 2010.

Youth Life Orientation Test (Y-LOT)

▶ Optimism and Pessimism: Measurement

Z

Z Distribution

▶ Standard Normal (Z) Distribution

Zoloft®

▶ Selective Serotonin Reuptake Inhibitors (SSRIs)

Zung Depression Inventory

Maria Kleinstäuber
Department of Clinical Psychology and Psychotherapy, Philipps University, Marburg, Germany

Synonyms

Zung depression rating scale (ZDRS); Zung depression scale; Zung self-assessment depression scale; Zung self-rating depression scale (SDS)

Definition

The Zung Depression Inventory (SDS) is a 20-item self-rating scale which was constructed to simply measure affective, cognitive, behavioral, and somatic symptoms of patients whose primary diagnosis is a depressive disorder (Zung 1965). The SDS was the first self-rating scale which allows to assess depression specifically as a psychiatric disorder. The scale was developed on the basis of the most commonly found diagnostic criteria of depression and patient interviews.

Description

Structure of the SDS

Half of the SDS items are worded positively, and half are phrased negatively. Subjects rate each item according to how they felt during the preceding week. The response categories range from (1) "none or a little of the time" to (4) "most or all of the time." The scale takes on average 5 min to complete. An index for the SDS is derived by summing the item scores. This summary score is then divided by a maximum possible score of 80. The SDS index ranges from 0.25 to 1. The following cutoffs are recommended by the author of the scale: Individuals with an index below 0.62 are considered normal, with an index of 0.62–0.74 are considered to suffer from a mild depression, and with an index of 0.75–0.86 are considered to suffer from a moderate to marked depression. Indices of 0.87 and above indicate severe depression. The SDS is available in about 30 languages (e.g., Brazilian, Arabic, Spanish, etc.).

© Springer Nature Switzerland AG 2020
M. D. Gellman (ed.), *Encyclopedia of Behavioral Medicine*,
https://doi.org/10.1007/978-3-030-39903-0

Psychometric Properties of the SDS

The little available data examining the reliability of the SDS reveals satisfactory *split-half reliability* ($r = 0.73$) and *internal consistency* (Cronbach's alpha $=0.79$). *Concurrent validity* of the scale could be demonstrated by correlating the SDS with other standardized self-rating scales of depression like the Beck Depression Inventory and the Depression Scale of the Minnesota Multiphasic Personality Inventory. Results of correlations between the SDS and clinician-rated instruments like the Hamilton Rating Scale for Depression are less consistent. The authors of the original SDS have not proposed a factorial structure for their scale. However a meta-analysis by Shafer (2006) demonstrated that a substantial number of included studies showed that factors of well-being/positive symptoms (nine items) and depressed affect/negative symptoms (eight items) are the most identifiable factors of SDS. Partly also a third component – somatic symptoms/appetite (three items) – was identified. These results indicate that factorial structure of SDS is not invariant. Sensitivity of the SDS in differentiating between depressed and non-depressed subjects was found to be adequate. The influence of different demographical variables on the SDS index was also examined. There seem to be higher SDS scores for individuals being older than 64 or younger than 20 years in non-patient groups. Associations between SDS score and age in psychiatric populations could not be demonstrated clearly. Women in patient as well as non-patient groups seem to have slightly higher scores than males. Furthermore, SDS scores are slightly negatively correlated with education (range: $r = -0.08$ to -0.28). In summary, evidence of validity supports the use of the SDS as *screening tool* but not as a diagnostic measure of depressive disorder.

Equations for Converting Scores Between SDS and Other Well-Validated Depression Self-Rating Scales

There are several well-validated depression self-rating scales which can be applied in research and clinical settings, including SDS. Although these scales differ in regard to emphasis on individual symptoms, they commonly address the criteria of Major Depression defined in the 4th edition of the Diagnostic and Statistical Manual of Mental Disorders. Accordingly, since they all assess the same construct, they reveal high intercorrelations (between $0.7 \leq r \leq 0.9$). Consequently, Hawley et al. (2013) generated equations in order to translate scores of a specific depression scale into a score of another scale. For example, the equation for predicting a score of SDS from a score of Montgomery-Åsberg Depression Rating Scale (MÅDRS) is SDS = 0.795 * MÅDRS – 16.8. For the Patient Health Questionnaire-9 (PHQ-9), the equivalent equation is as follows: SDS = 1.325 * PHQ-9 + 34.34.

Applications of SDS

The SDS has not only been used in psychiatric settings and in clinical research to monitor for treatment effectiveness or to assess psychopathological profiles but also in behavioral medical settings. In particular, SDS has been administered in a large number of studies to assess depressive symptoms in patients with somatic diseases, e.g., cancer; diabetes; cardiovascular diseases; in patients with functional somatic syndromes, such as irritable bowel syndrome, temporomandibular joint dysfunction, or burning mouth syndrome; and in patients suffering from chronic pain. Specific difficulties have to be considered when the SDS is used for screening depressive symptoms in medically ill patients. For example, somatic symptoms of depression can be confounded with symptoms of the organic illness or side effects of medication. This can lead to an overestimation of depression (e.g., fatigue or insomnia can also be a symptom of cancer or can be a side effect of pain medication). Especially in diseases influencing cognitive functions, the use of reverse coding introduces complexity (e.g., especially in patients suffering from Parkinson's disease who have difficulty in set-shifting).

Cross-References

▶ Beck Depression Inventory (BDI)
▶ Reliability and Validity

References and Further Reading

Hawley, C. J., Gale, T. M., Smith, P. S. J., Jain, S., Farag, A., Kondan, R., Avent, C., & Graham, J. (2013). Equations for converting scores between depression scales (MADRS, SRS, PHQ-9 and BDI-II): Good statistical, but weak idiographic, validity. *Human Psychopharmacology: Clinical and Experimental, 28,* 544–551. https://doi.org/10.1002/hup.2341.

Hedlund, J. L., & Vieweg, B. W. (1979). The Zung self-rating depression scale: A comprehensive review. *Journal of Operational Psychiatry, 10*(1), 51–64.

Shafer, A. B. (2006). Meta-analysis of the factor structures of four depression questionnaires: Beck, CES-D, Hamilton, and Zung. *Journal of Clinical Psychology, 62,* 123–146. https://doi.org/10.1002/jclp.20213.

Zung, W. W. (1965). A self-rating depression scale. *Archives of General Psychiatry, 12*(1), 63–70. https://doi.org/10.1001/archpsyc.1965.01720310065008.

Zung, W. W. (1967). Factors influencing the self-rating depression scale. *Archives of General Psychiatry, 16*(5), 543–547.

Zung, W. W. (1986). Zung self-rating depression scale and depression status inventory. In N. Sartorius & T. A. Ban (Eds.), *Assessment of depression* (pp. 221–231). New York: Springer.

Zung Depression Rating Scale (ZDRS)

▶ Zung Depression Inventory

Zung Depression Scale

▶ Zung Depression Inventory

Zung Self-Assessment Depression Scale

▶ Zung Depression Inventory

Zung Self-Rating Depression Scale (SDS)

▶ Zung Depression Inventory

Zyban®

▶ Bupropion (Wellbutrin, Zyban)